Hyperbaric Medicine Practice

4th Edition

Hyperbaric Medicine Practice

4th Edition

Harry T. Whelan, MD
Eric P. Kindwall, MD
Editors

BEST PUBLISHING COMPANY

Cover Photos: Courtesy of Harry T. Whelan (monoplace hyperbaric chamber); U.S. Navy Public Domain (Harry T. Whelan, diver); Kirill Egorov (back cover, three divers).

Photos, figures, and tables included in this edition without specific recognition were provided by the chapter authors.

This textbook uses the abbreviation HBO_2 for hyperbaric oxygen, which is the official abbreviation used by the Undersea and Hyperbaric Medical Society.

First Edition: 1994
Second Edition: 1999
Second Edition Revised: 2002
Third Edition: 2008

International Standard Book Number: 978-1-947239-00-5
Library of Congress Catalog Number: 2017941450

Best Publishing Company
631 US Highway 1, Suite 307
North Palm Beach, FL 33408

Printed in the United States of America

Foreword

The second edition of *Hyperbaric Medicine Practice* (1999) by Kindwall and Whelan was my first hyperbaric textbook, and I recall studying it extensively during my fellowship (and in the years since) to learn as much as I could about my chosen profession. Back then, the content leaned a little on the anecdotal side with much less concern about evidence-based medicine and systematic meta-analyses. Much has changed in the last quarter century, as our understanding of hyperbaric oxygen physiology has become more sophisticated, and our need for quality, evidence-based practice recommendations has become more urgent.

The field of hyperbaric medicine has changed as well. More facilities focus on the delivery of hyperbaric oxygen therapy for chronic wound patients rather than the treatment of urgent or emergent indications. The modern hyperbaric practitioner is more likely to come from a field with little primary training in hyperbaric physiology and is more likely to spend only a portion of his or her practice treating patients with hyperbaric oxygen. There is great concern amongst veterans of undersea and hyperbaric medicine that the scope of knowledge of the modern hyperbaric practitioner is focused only on a narrow sector of the field rather than appreciating the complexities and nuances of all of the indications for therapy. While some providers may be interested in learning more about the specialty, opportunities for in-depth education are scarce. Fellowship training is preferable for those who wish to devote themselves to the field, but it is often out of reach for established physicians who find themselves practicing hyperbaric medicine as a second career. It is for this reason that we need resources such as *Hyperbaric Medicine Practice* to provide a comprehensive approach for educating practitioners on the full breadth and scope of undersea and hyperbaric medicine.

The Undersea and Hyperbaric Medical Society (UHMS) has devoted itself to promoting the scientific study of hyperbaric oxygen therapy and raising the level of knowledge of hyperbaric practitioners, so it is with great pleasure that we welcome *Hyperbaric Medicine Practice, 4th edition*. This fourth edition includes updates to "classic" chapters, while others have been completely rewritten to address modern-day issues. There are new chapters covering the most recently accepted indications for hyperbaric oxygen therapy while removing some that are less relevant to hyperbaric medicine practice in today's environment. Overall, the fourth edition of *Hyperbaric Medicine Practice* is an impressive work that should serve veterans and newcomers of undersea and hyperbaric medicine alike.

Enoch Huang, MD, MPH&TM, FUHM
President
Undersea and Hyperbaric Medical Society

Contents

Preface xi
Editor xiii
Contributors xv
Acknowledgments xxv

SECTION ONE
Hyperbaric Oxygenation: General Considerations

Chapter 1. ...... Clinical Hyperbaric Facility Accreditation-Process Improvement in Action 29
W.T. Workman

Chapter 2. ...... Physiologic Effects of Hyperbaric Oxygen 39
Gerardo Bosco, Enrico M. Camporesi

Chapter 3. ...... Oxygen Toxicity 49
Heather Annis, Aliyah Keval, Harry T. Whelan

Chapter 4. ...... Management of Critically Ill Patients in the Monoplace Hyperbaric Chamber 67
Lindell K. Weaver

Chapter 5. ...... Multiplace Hyperbaric Chamber 97
Giacomo Garetto, Gerardo Bosco

Chapter 6. ...... Hyperbaric Nursing 111
Valerie Messina

Chapter 7. ...... The Use of Drugs Under Pressure 131
Ryan Feldman

Chapter 8. . . . . . . Myringotomy 159
Michael E. McCormick, Joseph E. Kerschner

Chapter 9. . . . . . . Contraindications and Relative Risks of Hyperbaric Oxygen Treatment 169
Phi-Nga Jeannie Le

Chapter 10. . . . . . Side Effects and Complications: Selected Overview and Brief Guide to Management 199
Phi-Nga Jeannie Le, John B. Slade Jr, Jason A. Kelly, E. George Wolf

Chapter 11. . . . . . Pediatric Considerations for Hyperbaric Medicine 221
Pamela C. Petersen, Michael T. Meyer, Paul A. Thombs

Chapter 12. . . . . . The Role of Oxygen and Hyperbaric Oxygen Mechanisms . . . 237
Michael B. Strauss, Lientra Q. Lu

SECTION TWO
Disorders Approved for Hyperbaric Treatment

Chapter 13. . . . . . Carbon Monoxide 301
Jillian Theobald

Chapter 14. . . . . . Idiopathic Sudden Sensorineural Hearing Loss. 325
Tracy Leigh LeGros, Heather Murphy-Lavoie

Chapter 15. . . . . . Gas Embolism 361
Richard E. Moon

Chapter 16. . . . . . Effects of Hyperbaric Oxygen in Infectious Diseases: Basic Mechanisms. 379
Rodney E. Willoughby Jr., Charles C. Falzon, Aliyah Keval, Harry T. Whelan

Chapter 17. . . . . . Gas Gangrene. 407
Aliyah Keval, Harry T. Whelan

Chapter 18. . . . . . Selected Aerobic and Anaerobic Soft Tissue Infections 433
R.A. van Hulst, D.J. Bakker

Chapter 19. . . . . . Hyperbaric Oxygen in Intracranial Abscess. 465
Lorenz A. Lampl, Guenter Frey, Dietmar Fischer, Enrico Staps

Chapter 20. . . . . . Hyperbaric Oxygen for the Management of Chronic Refractory Osteomyelitis 485
Michael B. Strauss, Stuart S. Miller, Lientra Q. Lu

Chapter 21. . . . . . Strategic Approach to Diabetic Foot and Other Wounds 523
Michael B. Strauss, Anna M. Tan, Lientra Q. Lu

Chapter 22. . . . . . Evaluation and Management of the Diabetic Foot Ulcer 555
Enoch Huang, Marvin Heyboer III

Chapter 23. . . . . . Adjunctive Hyperbaric Oxygen Therapy for Diabetic Foot Ulcers 589
Enoch Huang, Marvin Heyboer III

Chapter 24. . . . . . Fracture Healing and Roles of Hyperbaric Oxygen. 623
Michael B. Strauss, Anna M. Tan, Lientra Q. Lu

Chapter 25. . . . . . The Microcirculation and Ischemia-Reperfusion: Basic Mechanisms of Hyperbaric Oxygen. 641
Richard C. Baynosa, William A. Zamboni, John Brosious

Chapter 26. . . . . . The Roles of Hyperbaric Oxygen in Crush Injury and Other Acute Traumatic Ischemias 659
Michael B. Strauss, Lientra Q. Lu

Chapter 27. . . . . . Hyperbaric Oxygen Use in Exceptional Blood Loss Anemia. . . 691
Keith W. Van Meter

Chapter 28. . . . . . Hyperbaric Oxygen in Skin Grafts and Flaps 707
Jenna Cusic, Chelsea Venditto, Hani S. Matloub

Chapter 29. . . . . . Radiation Injury to Tissue 725
Robert E. Marx

Chapter 30. . . . . . The Use of Hyperbaric Oxygen for Treating Delayed Radiation Injuries in Gynecologic Malignancies 777
Harry T. Whelan, Chris Kilian

Chapter 31. . . . . . Adjunctive Hyperbaric Oxygen Therapy in the Treatment of Thermal Burns. 789
Paul Cianci, Ronald M. Sato, Julia Faulkner

Chapter 32. . . . . . Central Retinal Artery Occlusion 819
Heather Murphy-Lavoie, Tracy Leigh LeGros

SECTION THREE
Hyperbaric Oxygen Used in Off-Label Disorders and Investigational Areas

Chapter 33. . . . . . Off-Label Indications for Hyperbaric Oxygen Therapy 837
Michael H. Bennett, Simon J. Mitchell

Chapter 34. . . . . . Hyperbaric Oxygen Treatment of Avascular Bone Necrosis of the Femoral Head. 861
Giuliano Vezzani, Gerardo Bosco, Enrico M. Camporesi

Chapter 35. . . . . . Use of Adjunctive Hyperbaric Oxygen in the Management of Invasive Fungal Infections. 881
Lisardo Garcia-Covarrubias, Diana M. Barratt

Chapter 36. . . . . . Treatment of the Brown Recluse Spider Bite with Hyperbaric Oxygen Therapy. 895
Matthew Stanton

Chapter 37. . . . . . Hyperbaric Oxygen in Traumatic Brain Injury. 909
Sarah B. Rockswold, Samuel R. Daly, Gaylan L. Rockswold

Chapter 38. . . . . . Neurological Aspects of Hyperbaric Medicine 945
Ann K. Helms, Charles C. Falzon, Aliyah Keval, Harry T. Whelan

Chapter 39. . . . . . Hyperbaric Oxygen in the Treatment of Hansen's Disease 961
David A. Youngblood, Tomaz A.P. Brito

SECTION FOUR
Diving, Submarine Rescue, and Life in the Sea

Chapter 40. . . . . . Emergency Management of Stricken Divers in Remote Areas . 973
Joseph Dituri, Carla Renaldo

Chapter 41. . . . . . Ketogenic Diet and Ketogenic Supplementation for Central Nervous System Oxygen Toxicity. 995
Angela M. Poff, Heather Annis, Harry T. Whelan, Csilla Ari, Joseph Dituri, Dominic P. D'Agostino

Chapter 42. . . . . . Submarine Rescue Diving and Hyperbaric Medicine 1015
Joseph Dituri, Harry T. Whelan

Chapter 43. . . . . . Dive Medicine 1049
Terrance L. Leighton III, Jonathan E. Strain

Chapter 44. . . . . . Closed-Circuit Rebreathers (CCR). 1085
Derek B. Covington, Charlotte Sadler, Richard L. Sadler

Chapter 45. . . . . . Maladies Specific to Technical and Rebreather Divers 1107
Carla Renaldo, Joseph Dituri, Brian P. O'Connell

Chapter 46. . . . . . Ocean Exploration-Living in the Deep Sea. 1133
Harry T. Whelan, Terrance L. Leighton III, Heather Annis, Joseph Dituri

Index 1153

Preface
4th Edition

Eric Kindwall learned to dive while he was in high school and by necessity invented some of his own equipment. He later learned more sophisticated aspects of diving from one of the pioneers in the field, also a Milwaukee physician, Edgar End, MD, who helped develop deep mixed-gas diving with the Diving Equipment and Salvage Company (DESCO.) In his early adult years, he served on the oceans as a merchant seaman and later included an account of that period in his autobiography *Unexpected Odyssey*.

After his residency in psychiatry at Harvard and a brief private practice, Eric was commissioned in the Navy Medical Corps, was a submarine medical officer on the nuclear submarine USS *Robert E. Lee*, then served at the Navy School of Submarine Medicine. When he left the U.S. Navy, he was granted the use of the two large hyperbaric chambers at St. Luke's Hospital in Milwaukee. The catch to that grant was that while the chambers had been donated to the hospital, their plumbing had never been completed, and their intended use had never been considered. Eric saw to the final installations of the plumbing in those chambers, persuaded some experts in chamber use to join him at St. Luke's, and began using the chambers for some of the earliest trials of clinical hyperbaric oxygen as well as treating more familiar dysbaric conditions.

It was my privilege to have known him in his start in clinical hyperbaric medicine as well as his work with dysbaric conditions. Eric became concerned about the caisson workers he was treating for decompression sickness. These men were creating deep tunnels for sewage flow under the city and suburbs of Milwaukee. The tunneling was often through mud and required pressurized tunnel equipment. Eric treated many of these men who had decompression sickness (bends) or one of its delayed complications, dysbaric osteonecrosis, and realized that the decompression schedules they used were inadequate. He gathered data and persuaded state authorities to change the pressure exposure and decompression schedules for caisson workers.

He backed theory with action; I was present when he entered a pressurized tunnel head, deep under Milwaukee streets, to provide first aid to a tunnel worker (sand hog in industrial slang) who had badly injured his hand toward the end of an eight-hour shift. In an unusual application of surface decompression (SUR-D), the worker was rapidly decompressed, hauled by crane through a vertical shaft to the surface, sped through the city by ambulance, and recompressed at the St. Luke's chamber, where a surgeon could attend to his hand.

Eric was one of the founding fathers of the Undersea Medical Society and led the organization as president for a term. The Society later added "hyperbaric" to its name, due in part, to his development of clinical uses of hyperbaric medicine. Among the patients he treated in those early days was a patient with an iatrogenic air embolus, a patient in cardiogenic shock, and several patients unconscious due to carbon monoxide intoxication. Not all of these patients recovered, but those conditions which might benefit from hyperbaric oxygen were not known at that time.

Eric's Hyperbaric Medicine Department at St. Luke's Hospital became a model for other hyperbaric facilities and has remained so. He was an associate professor of the Medical College of Wisconsin. Eric remained in the U.S. Navy Reserve, was consulted frequently by the U.S. Navy, and taught classes to new Undersea Medical Officers at the Navy Diving and Salvage Training Center in Panama City, Florida.

Over the course of his professional career, he led in determining which medical conditions could benefit from hyperbaric oxygen and which did not. These conditions have been accepted by the medical mainstream, and thousands of patients have been helped across the world. Eric was ringside in watching the handful of chambers tentatively used to experiment with clinical hyperbaric oxygen grow to thousands worldwide. Eric also led in setting safety standards for safety and responsibility.

Eric passed his hard-won wisdom into the first editions of this text, as well as many papers and presentations. He remained a strong supporter of professional organizations concerned with diving and clinical hyperbaric medicine.

The current version of this textbook has been created without his assistance since his death in 2012. The authors have tried to meet what they believe was his rigorous attention to first-rate medical care for his special patients—those benefitting from hyperbaric oxygen.

Henry J. C. Schwartz, MD, FACP
Captain, Medical Corps, United States Navy (Retired)
December 18, 2016

Harry T. Whelan, MD

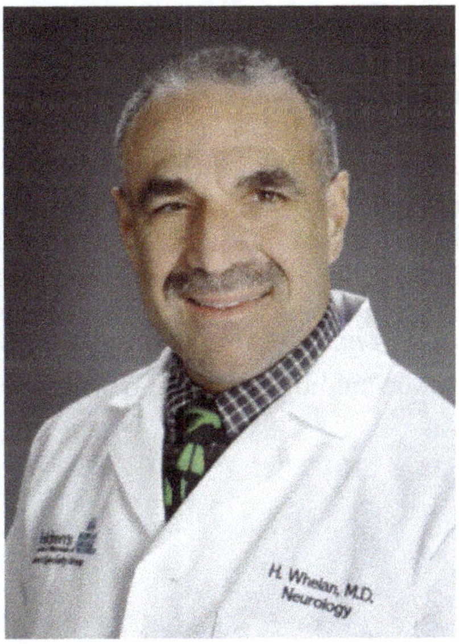

Dr. Whelan, a Milwaukee native, is Professor of Neurology, Pediatrics and Hyperbaric Medicine at the Medical College of Wisconsin. He is also a captain and a diving medical officer (DMO) in the U.S. Navy, a consultant to the Navy Experimental Diving Unit (NEDU), and recently served as Commanding Officer of Marine Air Control Group 48 Medical and Undersea Medical Officer for Deep Submergence Unit, which is the navy's submarine rescue team and its deep sea research component.

He first began scuba diving in 1966 at age thirteen and developed his interest in cellular metabolism during a National Science Foundation Summer Research Program focused on biochemistry at Wesleyan University in Connecticut. After graduating cum laude in chemistry (biochemistry option) from the University of Wisconsin-Milwaukee, he attended the University of Wisconsin Medical School in Madison, where he received his medical degree. He completed his pediatrics internship and residency training at the University of Florida in Gainesville and his neurology fellowship at the University of Minnesota in Minneapolis.

Dr. Whelan then joined the faculty of Vanderbilt University in Nashville, TN, where he developed a laboratory research project involving new types of treatment for brain tumors. For this he received the American Cancer Society's Clinical Oncology Career Development Award.

Dr. Whelan then decided to move back to Milwaukee where he became Professor of Neurology and Pediatrics at the Medical College of Wisconsin as well as accepted a direct commission as lieutenant commander in the U.S. Navy. He developed research ties with the Hyperbaric Medicine Unit at the Medical College of Wisconsin and the U.S. Navy Experimental Diving Unit in Panama City, FL. The navy then trained him at its dive school in Panama City to become a diving medical officer. When he was promoted to full commander, his fellow officers pinned his new rank onto his uniform in an underwater ceremony, 190 feet below sea level. He has since been promoted to captain in the U.S. Navy.

Dr. Whelan has over twenty years' experience conducting research on the use of new light technologies in the treatment of cancer and wounds. His use of NASA space-based light-emitting diode (LED) technology to activate cancer-killing drugs has now extended further into direct effects of near-infrared LED light on human growth stimulation. Potential benefits to Special Operations Forces and space station astronauts include prevention of deep space radiation toxicity and healing wounds, such as traumatic eye and brain injuries. In the year 2000, Dr. Whelan was inducted into the NASA Space Technology Hall of Fame for his photobiology research.

As a renowned expert in the field of hyperbaric medicine, Dr. Whelan made significant contributions to the submarine rescue mission. At the international submarine rescue exercise in Singapore in 2010, he conducted multiple scientific lectures to a multinational media team. His guidance and direction were pivotal in the execution of multiple mass casualty exercises onboard a foreign vessel. His experience and expertise were crucial in planning the medical portions of the exercise, and he received multiple invitations to assist other nations in their submarine rescue medical efforts as a result of his performance.

Dr. Whelan assumed directorship of the Medical College of Wisconsin's Hyperbaric Unit in 1998 and has been awarded the Bleser Foundation Endowed Chair of Neurology. He has over 100 publications including cancer, laser, LED, and diving/hyperbaric studies, and he has served as an advisor to the Director of Net Assessment in the Office of the Secretary of Defense and the Defence Research and Development of Canada (DRDC). In 2015, he was awarded the Legion of Merit medal by the U. S. Marine Corps, which is given for exceptionally meritorious conduct in the performance of outstanding services and achievements.

Contributors

A

Heather Annis, MD
LT MC USN
Risk Manager, Naval Hospital Pensacola

Csilla Ari, PhD
Department of Molecular Pharmacology and Physiology
Hyperbaric Biomedical Research Laboratory
Morsani College of Medicine
University of South Florida
Tampa, FL

B

D. J. (Dirk Jan) Bakker, MD, PhD, FUHM
Professor of Surgery and Medical Director of the Academic Medical Center (Emeritus)
University of Amsterdam

Diana M. Barratt, MD, MPH
Director of Neurology Clerkship and Associate Professor, Florida International University
Herbert Wertheim College of Medicine, Miami, Florida
Neurologist, Camillus Health Concern, Miami, Florida

Richard C. Baynosa, MD, FACS
Associate Professor and Chief, Division of Plastic Surgery
Program Director, Integrated Plastic Surgery Residency
UNLV School of Medicine

Tomaz A.P. Brito, MD
Assistant Instructor, Anesthesiology Medical Resident Program,
Federal University of the State of Rio de Janeiro, School of Medicine,
Gafrée e Guinle Hospital, Rio de Janeiro
Medical Director, Hyperbaric Medicine Centre, OHB-RIO
Silvestre Adventist Hospital, Rio de Janeiro

Gerardo Bosco, MD, PhD
Associate Professor, Environmental Physiology
Dept. of Biomedical Sciences, University of Padova
Padova, Italy

John Brosious, MD
Assistant Professor, Division of Plastic Surgery
University of Nevada School of Medicine
Las Vegas, NV

Michael H. Bennett, MD, MB BS, FANZCA, FFARCSI, MM(Clin Epi), ANZCA Cert DHM, DA, SPUMSDipDHM, FUHMS
Director, Australian Diving and Hyperbaric Medicine Research Group
Prince of Wales Medical School
Faculty of Medicine, University of NSW
Sydney, Australia

C

Enrico M. Camporesi, MD
Emeritus Professor of Surgery/ Anesthesiology
and Molecular Pharmacology/ Physiology
University of South Florida
Attending Anesthesiologist & Director of Research
TEAMHealth Anesthesia
Tampa, FL

Paul Cianci, MD, FACP, FUHM
Emeritus Medical Director, Department of Hyperbaric Medicine
Doctors Medical Center, San Pablo, CA

Derek B. Covington, MD
Assistant Professor
Department of Anesthesiology
University of Florida College of Medicine
Gainesville, FL

Jenna Cusic, MD
Resident Fellow, Department of Plastic Surgery
Medical College of Wisconsin
Milwaukee, WI

D

Dominic P. D'Agostino, PhD
Associate Professor
Department of Molecular Pharmacology and Physiology
Morsani College of Medicine
University of South Florida
Tampa, FL

Samuel R. Daly, B.A.
Division of Neurosurgery
Department of Surgery
Hennepin County Medical Center

Joseph Dituri, MS, CDR, US Navy Saturation Diving Officer (ret)
Director, International Board of Undersea Medicine
Tampa, FL

F

Charles C. Falzon, MD, MBA
Osher Center for Integrative Medicine
Northwestern Medical Group

Julia Faulkner
Research Assistant
Doctors Medical Center, San Pablo, CA

Ryan Feldman, PharmD
Clinical Pharmacy Specialist, Emergency Medicine
Froedtert & The Medical College of Wisconsin
Froedtert Hospital Wisconsin Poison Center
Children's Hospital of Wisconsin

Dietmar Fischer, MD
Deputy Medical Director, Intensive Care Medicine
Federal Armed Forces Hospital
Oberer Eselsberg 40
D-89081 Ulm, Germany

Guenter Frey, MD, LtCol MC (Retired)
Anesthesiology and Intensive Care Medicine
Hyperbaric Medicine Consultant
Tokajerweg 72
D-89075 Ulm, Germany

G

Lisardo Garcia-Covarrubias, MD, FACS
Staff Cardiothoracic Surgeon Baptist Health of South Florida
Associate Professor of Surgery and Chief of Cardiothoracic Surgery
Florida International University Herbert Wertheim College of Medicine
Miami, Florida

Giacomo Garetto, MD
Specialist in Anesthesiology, Intensive Care and Hyperbaric Therapy
Medical Director
ATIP Hyperbaric Medical Center
Padova, Italy

H

Ann K. Helms, MD, MS
Associate Professor
Department of Neurology
Medical College of Wisconsin
Milwaukee, WI

Marvin Heyboer III, MD, FUHM, FACEP, FACCWS
Associate Professor, Emergency Medicine
SUNY Upstate Medical University
Syracuse, NY

Enoch Huang, MD, MPH&TM, FACEP, FUHM, FACCWS
Program Medical Director
Hyperbaric Medicine/ Wound Care Clinic
Legacy Emanuel Medical Center
Affiliate Assistant Professor, Emergency Medicine
Oregon Health and Science University

K

Jason A. Kelly, MD, Lt Col, USAF, MC, SFS
Physician, Hyperbaric Medicine
United States Air Force

Joseph E. Kerschner, MD, FACS, FAAP
Dean of the School of Medicine
Executive Vice President
Professor of Otolaryngology and Communication Sciences,
Microbiology and Immunology
Medical College of Wisconsin
Milwaukee, WI

Aliyah Keval
Undergraduate Student, Chemistry major
University of Wisconsin- Madison

Chris Kilian, MD

Eric P. Kindwall, MD (Deceased)
Associate Professor Emeritus
Medical College of Wisconsin
Executive Director
American College of Hyperbaric Medicine

L

Lorenz A. Lampl, MD, PhD
Professor of Anesthesiology
Medical Director, Anesthesiology and Intensive Care Medicine
Federal Armed Forces Hospital
Oberer Eselsberg 40
D-89081 Ulm, Germany

Phi-Nga Jeannie Le, MD

Tracy Leigh LeGros, MD, PhD, FACEP, FAAEM, FUHM
Associate Clinical Professor
Emergency Medicine Program Director
Undersea and Hyperbaric Medicine
University Medical Center
New Orleans, LA

Terrance L. Leighton III, DO
LT, MC, Undersea/Dive Medical Officer USN
Special Physicals (Team Valor)
USS Tranquillity Branch Medical Clinic
Federal Health Care Center
Chicago, IL

Lientra Q. Lu, BS
Research Coordinator
Tibor Rubin VA Medical Center
Long Beach, CA
Long Beach Memorial Medical Center
Long Beach, CA

M

Robert E. Marx, DDS
Professor of Surgery and Chief
Division of Oral and Maxillofacial Surgery
University of Miami Miller School of Medicine
Chief of Surgery
Jackson South Community Hospital, Miami, FL

Hani S. Matloub, MD, FACS
Professor, Department of Plastic Surgery
Medical College of Wisconsin
Milwaukee, WI

Michael E. McCormick, MD
Assistant Professor
Department of Otolaryngology and Communication Sciences
Medical College of Wisconsin and Children's Hospital of Wisconsin
Milwaukee, WI

Valerie Messina, RN, CWCN
Program Director, Wound Care & Hyperbaric Medicine
Long Beach Memorial Medical Center
Long Beach, CA

Michael T. Meyer, MD, FCCM
Associate Professor and Chief of Pediatrics, Critical Care
Associate Director, Pediatric Intensive Care Unit
Medical College of Wisconsin and Children's Hospital of Wisconsin
Milwaukee, WI

Stuart S. Miller, MD
Medical Director, Hyperbaric Medicine
Long Beach Memorial Medical Center
Long Beach, CA
Associate Clinical Professor, Family Medicine
University of California Irvine School of Medicine
Irvine, CA

Simon J. Mitchell, MB ChB, PhD, FANZCA
Professor, Department of Anaesthesiology
University of Auckland and Auckland City Hospital
Auckland, New Zealand

Richard E. Moon, MD, FACP, FCCP
Professor of Anesthesiology
Professor of Medicine
Medical Director, Center for Hyperbaric Medicine & Environmental Physiology
Duke University Medical Center
Durham, NC

Heather Murphy-Lavoie, MD, FAAEM, FACEP, FUHM
UHMS Education Committee, Chair
Associate Professor
Emergency Medicine Residency
Associate Program Director
Hyperbaric Medicine Fellowship
LSU School of Medicine/ UMC
New Orleans, LA

O

Brian P. O'Connell, Ed.D
International Board of Undersea Medicine, (IBUM)
Training Development

P

Pamela C. Petersen, MD, FAAP
PGY5 Pediatric Critical Care Fellow
Medical College of Wisconsin and Children's Hospital of Wisconsin
Milwaukee, WI

Angela M. Poff, PhD
Research Associate
Department of Molecular Pharmacology and Physiology
Morsani College of Medicine
University of South Florida
Tampa, FL

R

Carla Renaldo, DO
Medical Director, International Board of Undersea Medicine Tampa, FL
Board Certified Internal Medicine & NOAA / UHMS trained Diving Physician

Sarah B. Rockswold, MD
Medical Director, TBI Center
Medical Director, Outpatient TBI Program
Department of Physical Medicine and Rehabilitation, Hennepin County Medical Center
Department of Physical Medicine and Rehabilitation, University of Minnesota
Minneapolis, MN

Gaylan L. Rockswold, MD, PhD
Division of Neurosurgery, Department of Surgery, Hennepin County Medical Center
Department of Neurosurgery, University of Minnesota
Minneapolis, MN

S

Charlotte Sadler, MD
Assistant Clinical Professor of Hyperbaric and Emergency Medicine
University of California-San Diego

Richard L. Sadler, MD, FACS, UHM
Thoracic and Vascular Surgery
Medical Director Dive Rescue International
San Diego, CA

Ronald M. Sato, MD
Plastic Surgeon, former Medical Director
Burn Center, Doctors Medical Center
San Pablo, CA

John B. Slade, Jr., MD
Staff Physician, Hyperbaric Medicine Flight
60th Medical Group, Travis Air Force Base, CA 94535

Matthew Stanton, PharmD, BCPS, DABAT
Emergency Medicine Pharmacist
Froedtert & The Medical College of Wisconsin
Milwaukee, WI

Enrico Staps, MD
Assistant Medical Director, Anesthesiology and Intensive Care Medicine
Federal Armed Forces Hospital
Oberer Eselsberg 40
D-89081 Ulm, Germany

Jonathan E. Strain, MD
LT, MC, Undersea/Dive Medical Officer USN
Special Physicals (Team Valor)
USS Tranquillity Branch Medical Clinic
Federal Health Care Center
Chicago, IL

Michael B. Strauss, MD, FACS, AAOS, AOFAS
Medical Director (Retired) Hyperbaric Medicine
Long Beach Memorial Medical Center
Long Beach, CA
Clinical Professor, Orthopedic Surgery
University of Irvine School of Medicine
Irvine, CA
Consultant Orthopedic Surgeon PAVE (Preservation-Amputation for Veterans Everywhere) Clinic
Tibor Rubin VA Medical Center
Long Beach, CA

T

Anna Maria M. Tan, DPM
Hyperbaric Medicine & Wound Care Program
Long Beach Memorial Medical Center
Long Beach, CA

Jillian Theobald, MD, PhD
Assistant Professor
Department of Emergency Medicine
Section of Medical Toxicology
Medical College of Wisconsin
Milwaukee, WI

Paul A. Thombs, MD
Diplomate, American Board of Pediatrics (ABP) and Hyperbaric and Undersea Medicine (ABPM)
Medical Director Emeritus Hyperbaric Medicine Center
Presbyterian/St. Luke's Medical Center
Denver, CO

V

R.A. (Rob) van Hulst, MD, PhD, FUHM
Professor of Hyperbaric and Diving Medicine
Department of Anesthesiology
Academic Medical Center
Amsterdam, Netherlands
Captain Royal Dutch Navy (retired)
Director of Diving and Submarine Medicine, Royal Netherlands Navy

Keith W. Van Meter, MD
LSU-HSC Emergency Medicine Section Head
Clinical Professor of Medicine, LSU-HSC
Baton Rouge, LA
Clinical Professor of Surgery, Tulane School of Medicine
New Orleans, LA

Chelsea Venditto, MD
Resident Fellow, Department of Plastic Surgery
Medical College of Wisconsin
Milwaukee, WI

Giuliano Vezzani, MD
Professor on contract, II Level Master in Hyperbaric Medicine
Dept. of Biomedical Sciences, University of Padova
Padova, Italy

W

Lindell K. Weaver, MD, FACP, FCCP, FCCM, FUHM
Medical Director and Division Chief, Hyperbaric Medicine
LDS Hospital, Salt Lake City, UT and
Intermountain Medical Center, Murray, UT
Professor of Medicine, University of Utah School of Medicine
Adjunct Professor, Department of Anesthesia, Duke University, Durham, NC

Harry T. Whelan, MD
Bleser Professor, Department of Neurology
Director of Hyperbaric Medicine
Medical College of Wisconsin
Milwaukee, WI

Rodney E. Willoughby, Jr., MD
Professor of Pediatrics
Division of Infectious Diseases
Medical College of Wisconsin
Milwaukee, WI

E George Wolf, MD
59th Medical Wing, Hyperbaric Medicine
JBSA-Lackland, TX

W.T. Workman, MS, CAsP, CHT-A, FAsMA
Director, Quality Assurance & Regulatory Affairs
UHMS San Antonio
San Antonio, TX

Y

David A. Youngblood, MD, MPH&TM

Z

William A. Zamboni, MD (Deceased)
Professor, Division of Plastic Surgery
University of Nevada School of Medicine
Las Vegas, NV

Acknowledgments

This work was supported by the Bleser Endowed Chair in Neurology (to Dr. Whelan) as well as the Baumann Research Endowment (to Dr. Whelan).

The editor would like to thank each one of the authors for contributing their time and expertise to this textbook. It is greatly appreciated.

The editor would also like to acknowledge the valuable contributions of the publishing and design teams and their enthusiastic dedication to the textbook.

The authors and editor wish to greatly acknowledge Lisa Jome for her valuable administrative support in the publication of this textbook.

SECTION 1 SECTION

Hyperbaric Oxygenation: General Considerations

CHAPTER 1 CHAPTER

Clinical Hyperbaric Facility Accreditation-Process Improvement in Action

CHAPTER ONE OVERVIEW

Introduction 31
Background 32
Program Design 33
Status 34
Opportunities for Improvement 35
External Recognition 36
International Expansion 37
Summary 37
References 38

Clinical Hyperbaric Facility Accreditation-Process Improvement in Action

W.T. Workman

INTRODUCTION

In the late 1970s, there were fewer than 30 hyperbaric facilities operational in the United States. Most were military, commercial, or highly specialized research facilities. It is estimated that there are now around 1,350 operating in hospitals and hospital-affiliated facilities.(3) We have seen the primary role of hyperbaric facilities transition from the treatment of diving-related disorders to providing an important primary and adjunct treatment modality for multiple medical conditions as described in this publication. Refined research efforts will no doubt validate continued efficacy and support new indications. The location of facilities is expanding from hospital-based to nonaffiliated outpatient settings, some with appropriate medical supervision, others without. In the past decade, certification in hyperbaric technology and hyperbaric nursing has become a staffing requirement in a growing number of programs. After years of dedicated efforts by many members of the Undersea and Hyperbaric Medical Society (UHMS), the American Board of Preventive Medicine, the American Board of Emergency Physicians, and the American Osteopathic Association have established board certification for physicians in Undersea and Hyperbaric Medicine. Minimum recommended staffing and training standards were first presented in the *UHMS Operations Committee Report* in 2000.(1) Now, they are an important part of a more comprehensive set of guidelines and recommended practices. The *UHMS Guidelines for Hyperbaric Facility Operations, 2nd Edition*, set these foundational standards of practice for hyperbaric medicine.(6)

Each of these milestones reflects a continuing maturation and professional recognition of clinical hyperbaric medicine in the United States. As in any growth process, success has not come easily. There are still many challenges that must be faced. There have been many in the field of hyperbaric medicine who felt an appropriate response to these challenges was to create an external means of quality assurance and performance improvement: a formal clinical hyperbaric facility accreditation program. Programs that evaluate the adequacy of the facility and equipment, the appropriateness of the staff and their training, quality of care, and patient safety have proven useful to professional organizations in ensuring that quality is maintained within their specialty. In 2000, the UHMS accepted this challenge and established a professional, comprehensive clinical hyperbaric facility accreditation program.

The UHMS believes that such a program is the most efficient method to ensure that

- clinical hyperbaric facilities are staffed with the proper specialists who are well trained,
- clinical hyperbaric facilities are using quality equipment that has been properly installed and maintained and is being operated with the highest level of safety possible,
- clinical hyperbaric facilities are providing high quality of patient care, and
- clinical hyperbaric facilities are maintaining the appropriate documentation of informed consent, patient treatment procedures, physician involvement, etc.

BACKGROUND

At the present time, there are approximately 18 different organizations in the United States that have some level of interest in the practice of hyperbaric medicine.[3] They include federal agencies such as the Centers for Medicare and Medicaid Services (CMS/Medicare) and the Food and Drug Administration (FDA); codes and standards organizations like the National Fire Protection Association (NFPA); and professional groups like the UHMS, the American College of Hyperbaric Medicine (ACHM), the Baromedical Nurses Association (BNA), and the National Board of Diving & Hyperbaric Medicine (NBDHMT). With the exception of the professional medical groups, there is little effort to coordinate among these organizations to foster a greater understanding of our community and on matters important to us.

Many advantages can result from accreditation and thus impact the regulatory environment, individual hyperbaric facilities and programs, and the specialty of hyperbaric medicine. Of immediate importance is the community response to the regulatory climate. In October of 2000, the Office of the Inspector General (OIG) of the Department of Health and Human Services released a report on Hyperbaric Oxygen Therapy: Its Usefulness and Appropriateness.[5] Among its findings, the OIG reported that a lack of testing and treatment monitoring raised a variety of quality-of-care concerns and that the Health Care Finance Administration (HCFA, now The Centers for Medicare and Medicaid Services (CMS) guidance to the field of hyperbaric medicine was limited. Specific OIG recommendations were for HCFA to initiate a national coverage decision policy for HBO_2; improve policy guidance (e.g., practice guidelines and physician attendance policy); and improve oversight by requiring contractors to initiate edits and consistent medical review procedures and by exploring the creation of a national registry of facilities and/or physicians. Without a doubt, this report laid the foundation for increased government involvement and intervention. By creating a national clinical hyperbaric facility accreditation program, the UHMS responded proactively to the OIG findings and recommendations. This action was a sign to the various regulatory agencies that the organized hyperbaric medical community was concerned with our current situation and responded to the recognized need to assure quality of care and patient safety across the continuum of clinical hyperbaric facilities are promoted, achieved, and maintained.

Equally important are the advantages that an accredited clinical hyperbaric facility may realize. Though not all-inclusive, some of the more immediate include the following:

- improved quality of care
- enhanced patient safety
- increased efficiency at the facility level
- more effective risk management programs
- outward symbol of code compliance and adherence to recognized standards of practice
- possibly lower liability insurance premiums
- staff motivation and esprit de corps
- maximized public relations and marketing efforts
- ability to recruit and retain quality staff
- alliances developed with other provider groups
- credibility of legitimate nonaffiliated outpatient facilities established among their professional referral base

Achieving the regulatory and facility-level advantages provides the foundation for significant advancements in the acceptance and credibility of hyperbaric medicine as a growing, recognized medical specialty, thus enhancing professional organizations such as the UHMS, the ACHM, the BNA, and the NBDHMT, who are at the forefront of the field. Further, a successful accreditation program will establish nationally recognized Standards of Practice for clinical hyperbaric medicine and brings hyperbaric medicine in line with many other specialties such as radiation oncology and rehabilitative medicine, each of which sponsors specific accreditation programs for their respective specialty.

PROGRAM DESIGN

For the most part, the focus areas of the UHMS accreditation program are a compilation of national codes and standards that relate to hyperbaric medicine and facilities as well as common quality-of-care improvement areas as defined by accrediting organizations such as the Joint Commission (JC), Commission on Accreditation of Rehabilitation Facilities (CARF), and Det Norske Veritas-Germannishcer Lloyd (DNV-GL). Central to the areas that represent compliance to national codes and standards are references from the National Fire Protection Association's (NFPA) Health Care Facilities Code (NFPA 99), the NFPA's Life Safety Code (NFPA 101), the American Society of Mechanical Engineers' Code for Pressure Vessels for Human Occupancy (ASME PVHO-1), the Compressed Gas Association, and others. The focus areas related to staff, training, certification, physician credentialing, supervision, continuing education, and so on are adopted from the *UHMS Guidelines for Hyperbaric Facility Operations, 2nd Edition.*

The above compilation is represented in 24 concentration areas:[4]

- Governance
- Administration
- Operations
- Maintenance
- Facility Construction
- Hyperbaric Chamber Fabrication

- Hyperbaric Chamber Ventilation
- Hyperbaric Chamber Fire Protection
- Hyperbaric Chamber Electrical Systems and Services
- Hyperbaric Gas Handling
- Patient Rights
- Patient Assessment
- Patient Care
- Environment of Care
- Patient Education
- Quality Improvement
- Professional Improvement
- Leadership
- Human Resources
- Information Management
- Infection Control
- Medical Staff
- Teaching and Publication
- Clinical Research

Surveys are conducted by a voluntary team of three highly experienced members: a hyperbaric physician, a board-certified hyperbaric nurse, and a board-certified technologist. Each survey is two full days to allow the team sufficient time to evaluate compliance to all concentration areas noted above. Each facility is provided a written report of the assessment, and recommended improvement areas are identified.

The survey teams do not make the determination for accreditation; that responsibility resides with the UHMS Accreditation Council (AC). Membership of the AC is comprised of a cross section of UHMS members representing physicians, nurses, and technologists. The AC responds to each survey report in the following manner:

- accredit (valid for three years)
- accredit with a written plan of action
- accredit after a written plan of action has been completed
- accredit with distinction (valid for four years)
- do not accredit

STATUS

By the end of 2016, the UHMS had accredited a total of 252 hyperbaric medicine programs, 3 of which were international. Of the remaining 249, 8 were facilities that were not affiliated with a health-care system resulting in approximately 17% of the 1,350 hospital-affiliated hyperbaric medicine programs in the country being accredited.[3]

This figure is impressive when one considers the fact that, with few exceptions, participation is voluntary. There are two notable exceptions. Beginning in 2006, the Utah Medicaid Management Office mandated UHMS-specific accreditation in order for facilities to receive Medicaid funding for hyperbaric oxygen therapy. In 2014, the third-party payor Mohawk Valley Physicians (MVP) began requiring facility accreditation for their beneficiaries in upstate New York, Vermont, and New Hampshire who required hyperbaric oxygen therapy. More specifically, MVP stipulated that physicians, in order to receive payment, must be on staff at an accredited facility.

Hyperbaric facility accreditation has not gone unnoticed by Medicare. A 2013 draft Local Coverage Determination (LCD) for hyperbaric oxygen therapy published by Novitas-Solutions, Inc., a major Medicare Administrative Contractor (MAC) with jurisdiction in 11 states, proposed that UHMS hyperbaric facility accreditation be a mandate for Medicare reimbursement.(2) While this requirement was not retained in what was to be the final LCD, it represented a major acknowledgment of the program and its potential link to Medicare reimbursement on a broad scale. Many believe this is a sign of things to come.

There are those who recognize that there are a variety of issues common to the hyperbaric medicine community regardless of the country of operation. This is especially true when you consider those related to hyperbaric facility safety. This is one common bond that ties the international hyperbaric community together. As a result, the UHMS has been honored to have been asked by international facilities to evaluate their programs for accreditation. Thus, the UHMS has accredited programs in Brazil, Canada, and Thailand. Surveys are pending in 2017 for facilities in Singapore and Saudi Arabia.

OPPORTUNITIES FOR IMPROVEMENT

Preparing for an accreditation survey is a lot of work. There are those who might question if the effort is worth it. If the process does not add value, then why bother? Well, after 15 years of effort, the UHMS can say, without doubt, that the process indeed has merit and has demonstrated that it has succeeded in improving the quality-of-care and patient safety elements in those facilities that have accepted the challenge. Equally important, it has identified a number of areas where opportunities for improvement are most evident. Several of these areas are quite surprising.

The biggest surprise is related to the privileging process for physicians. UHMS accreditation surveyors frequently discover weak or nonexisting policies regarding the granting of physician privileges specifically for hyperbaric medicine. Surveyors have even documented instances in which hyperbaric physicians were not credentialed for hyperbaric medicine at all, yet they were routinely supervising the treatment of hyperbaric patients! An even more egregious omission was one hospital was allowing physicians to practice hyperbaric medicine with no formal training in the specialty! This is not acceptable.

Surveyors rarely find a process to proctor physicians new to the specialty and/or facility for a period of time before they are granted full unsupervised privileges. Credentialing bodies seem to be receptive to allowing a physician who has just completed a recognized 40-hour introductory course in hyperbaric medicine to independently supervise patients. This, too, is not acceptable.

Currency of continuing medical education (CME) related to hyperbaric medicine is also lacking. It is common to survey a facility in which physicians had been practicing for 20 years and have not had a hyperbaric-related CME since their initial course. Can they be considered current in the specialty? I suggest not.

While these opportunities for improvement are prevalent, the UHMS has found that medical staff offices are very receptive to guidance that the UHMS can provide. An excellent source for such guidance is the *UHMS Guidelines for Hyperbaric Facility Operations, 2nd Edition*, which includes a complete section on recommendations for credentialing, etc.

With regard to nurses and allied health-care providers such as respiratory therapists, specialty-specific board certification is not yet the norm. While improvements have been made in recent years in the number of nurses and allied health-care providers who are board certified as a Certified Hyperbaric Registered Nurse (CHRN) or a Certified Hyperbaric Technologist (CHT), there is still much upside potential. Hospitals are strongly encouraged to make board certification a requirement for employment. Proactive hospitals occasionally require certification within two years of employment. This is a reasonable goal.

From an operational safety perspective, one of the biggest concerns is the failure of the designated hyperbaric safety director to assume the responsibilities of the position as outlined in the National Fire Protection Association's NFPA 99, Health Care Facilities Standard, which has now become a national mandate. When the NFPA first established hyperbaric facility safety standards in 1968, they recognized the importance of a hyperbaric facility safety director and stipulated that one be designated at each facility. This requirement went largely ignored until the UHMS implemented their accreditation program in 2000, and surveyors began assessing this requirement. While hyperbaric safety directors are now common in hospital-based or affiliated programs, they are scarce in nonaffiliated, freestanding centers.

Even though safety directors are now being designated in the hospital setting, many are not fulfilling their obligations with regard to creating and managing a comprehensive hyperbaric safety program. An all-too-common finding is the failure to conduct recurring medical and operational emergency drills so that the entire staff is competent in their execution. For many, conducting emergency drills stop at participating in hospital-directed fire drills. The practice of emergency procedures related to loss of chamber pressure, loss of power, communications, contaminated gas, etc. have been absent.

Closely related to the lack of safety director involvement is the availability of additional training to provide the safety director with the added knowledge and tools in order to better fulfill his or her responsibilities as a safety director. It was not until a little more than 15 years ago that there was any additional training that focused on the added skills necessary to be an effective safety director. Today, there are several courses designed to do just that. All hyperbaric facilities, regardless of location or governance, should place this supplemental training on the highest priority for their safety director.

While examples of opportunities for improvement can be provided from each of the 24 hyperbaric facility accreditation concentration areas, those described here are trending as the most obvious.

EXTERNAL RECOGNITION

The value of hyperbaric facility accreditation is not only evident from within the hyperbaric medicine community. The process is also recognized by organizations like The Joint Commission (JC). The JC has a special program called The Cooperative Agreement Program which was established to recognize alternative accrediting bodies representing medical specialties for which the JC surveyors might not have sufficient expertise or experience to allow them to conduct a meaningful assessment. Many of these specialties include a highly specialized technical component. For hyperbaric medicine, that specialized component is the hyperbaric chamber itself. The UHMS is very proud of the fact that their accreditation program is one of four such programs that have been formally endorsed by the JC as a complementary accrediting body.

Equally important to the external awareness of added value for the hyperbaric medicine community is the parallel acknowledgment of compliance to time-honored, internationally recognized management principles of process improvement and the implementation of quality systems control. The UHMS Clinical Hyperbaric Facility Accreditation Program enjoys the singular distinction of being the only ISO 9001:2008–certified hyperbaric facility accrediting program in the world.

INTERNATIONAL EXPANSION

Prior to 2000 and the creation of the UHMS program, there was only one other international effort to implement a meaningful facility accreditation program. This process, which was initially conceived by Dr. John Ross of Aberdeen, Scotland, was developed and managed by the British Hyperbaric Association (BHA). This watershed event, along with the unparalleled success of the UHMS program, has stimulated significant interest within the greater international hyperbaric medicine community. Programs now exist, or are under strategic development, in South Africa, Brazil, Canada, the greater European Community, and Southeast Asia.

In countries where professional hyperbaric medicine societies and hyperbaric specific codes or standards do not exist, program leaders are beginning to seek accreditation through the UHMS. As an international medical society, the UHMS has successfully demonstrated that their process is easily tailored to a specific country's need and that the program standards can be equitably applied to their need. Thus far, the UHMS has accredited programs in Brazil, Canada, and Thailand and are working with programs in Saudi Arabia and Singapore to further expand the program to be truly international.

SUMMARY

A little more than 15 years ago, meaningful hyperbaric facility accreditation did not exist. Today, it is quickly becoming the gold standard throughout the world as an outward symbol of quality of care and patient safety. Facilities that spend the energy to prepare for an accreditation survey, and can demonstrate compliance to high quality and safety standards, are rewarded with the pride that comes along with mastering such a lofty standard. It is clear that staffs of accredited facilities take their responsibilities to their patients seriously and are playing an important role in improving the quality of care and safety one facility at a time. As each new program is added to the growing list of accredited facilities, quality of care and safety of the hyperbaric patient is raised across the entire hyperbaric medicine community. Equally important is that with each newly accredited program, the community is proactively addressing the findings of the infamous OIG report. In spite of accomplishments to date, opportunities for improvement remain numerous. While many believe that facility accreditation will eventually be linked to reimbursement by others beside Utah and Mohawk Valley Physicians, there is still reluctance from many to seek accreditation. There are others who believe that the program has clear value and is simply the right thing to do. I stand with those who believe it is the right thing to do.

REFERENCES

1. Kimbrell PN, editor. Operations Committee report. Kensington (MD): Undersea & Hyperbaric Medical Society; 2000 Jan.
2. Novitas Solutions, Inc. Draft Local Coverage Determination (LCD) for hyperbaric oxygen (HBO_2) therapy (L34794). Novitas Solutions, Inc.; 2014 January.
3. Undersea & Hyperbaric Medical Society (San Antonio), Office of Quality Assurance & Regulatory Affairs, 14607 San Pedro Avenue, Ste 270, San Antonio, TX 28232.
4. Undersea & Hyperbaric Medical Society. Clinical hyperbaric facility accreditation manual. 2005 edition, revision 1. Dunkirk (MD): Undersea & Hyperbaric Medical Society, 2005.
5. U.S. Department of Health and Human Services, Office of the Inspector General. Hyperbaric oxygen therapy: its use and appropriateness. [Washington (DC)]: U.S. Department of Health and Human Services; 2000 Oct. Report No.:OEI 06-99-00090.
6. Workman WT, editor. Guidelines for hyperbaric facility operations. 2nd ed. North Palm Beach (FL): Undersea & Hyperbaric Medical Society; 2015.

CHAPTER 2 CHAPTER

Physiologic Effects of Hyperbaric Oxygen

CHAPTER TWO OVERVIEW

Abstract **41**
Exploring HBO_2: Biologic Effects and Mechanisms of Action **42**
Improved Neovascularization 43
Improved Post-Ischemic Tissue Survivals. 44
Bacteriostatic and Bactericidal Effects 45
Osteogenetic Process Promotion 45
Uncertainty About Oxygen Dosage. 46
Conclusions. **46**
References **47**

Physiologic Effects of Hyperbaric Oxygen

Gerardo Bosco, Enrico M. Camporesi

ABSTRACT

Hyperbaric oxygen therapy exerts its beneficial effects by elevating both the partial pressure of inspired O_2 and the hydrostatic pressure. The latter leads to compression of all gas-filled spaces in the body and is helpful in treating diseases in which gas bubbles are present in the body, such as intravascular embolism and intravascular or intratissue bubbles in decompression sickness. Interestingly, the majority of patients treated with HBO_2 experience clinical improvements from the elevated O_2 partial pressures and do not suffer from bubble-induced injuries. An elevated O_2 partial pressure in certain tissues leads to increased production of reactive O_2 species (ROS) and reactive nitrogen species (RNS) due to hyperoxia. Previously, research studies have demonstrated that the clinical efficacy from HBO_2 comes from the modulation of intracellular transduction cascades, leading to synthesis of growth factors and promoting wound healing and ameliorating post-ischemic and post-inflammatory injuries.

Throughout the first half of the last century, hyperbaric (recompression) chambers were not to be found within the traditional health-care delivery system. Rather, they were located at compressed air tunneling and bridge caisson work sites, within select military facilities, and in support of various underwater operations. In these medically remote settings, chambers were employed to decompress workers from elevated pressures and treat any resulting decompression sickness. It was not until the 1960s that chambers were introduced into hospitals and mainstream medicine. This was the period in which several therapeutic mechanisms associated with exposure to hyperbaric doses of oxygen had been identified and the term "hyperbaric oxygen (HBO_2) therapy" introduced. Previously, chambers were compressed with, and patients breathed, air. Among the newly identified effects there are (a) transport of high levels of oxygen within plasma to acutely ischemic tissues, (b) antimicrobial-like effects on certain anaerobic and aerobic bacteria, (c) enhanced elimination of carbon monoxide, vasoconstriction (without component hypoxia) to augment management of acute peripheral ischemia, and (d) stimulation of repair of hypoxia-mediated deficient wound healing.

The use of oxygen during recompression therapy was first recommended in 1937 by the U.S. Navy physician Albert Behnke to treat the bends. High-pressure oxygen breathing combines the therapeutic mechanisms of elevated pressure and elevated oxygen concentration. Indeed, high pressure increases partial pressure of gases and causes a reduction in the volume of blood's and tissues' gas bubble; moreover, breathed oxygen improves tissues' oxygenation and accelerates nitrogen elimination from affected tissues.

EXPLORING HBO_2: BIOLOGIC EFFECTS AND MECHANISMS OF ACTION

The efficacy of hyperbaric therapy in treating a variety of diseases and syndromes was first reported in 1939, but the most important findings were documented between 1955 and 1962. Churchill-Davidson was the first to suggest that high oxygen pressures may be used to initiate antitumoral radiation therapy in cancer patients. Starting from the knowledge that the sensitivity of cells to X-ray is directly dependent on the level of oxygen dissolved around them, he thought to profit by the increased oxygen tension obtained from HBO_2 to raise radiosensitivity and improve the efficacy of the treatment.

Professor Ite Boerema, chief of surgery at the University of Amsterdam, was the first to publish on the clinical utility of hyperbaric oxygen. He performed a lot of cardiac and surgery experiments, initally on animals, inside a hyperbaric chamber and obtained impressive outcomes before the arrival of effective artificial circulation equipment (1956). Indeed, with his experiments he proved that cardiac arrest induced in hyperbaric condition doubled the time without irreversible damages and supported his idea that "life without blood" under hyperbaric oxygen conditions was possible.(5) The increase in tissue oxygen stores and extension of the respiratory reserves at elevated barometric pressure prior to onset of hypoxic damage were thought to mediate this action.

Though Boerema's research focused on limited application of a biophysical principle, his seminal findings had a lasting impact around the world: hyperbaric chambers were constructed and used to supplement surgical procedures and other treatments at a number of institutions.

Other researchers at the University of Amsterdam also reported that HBO_2 was beneficial for patients affected by clostridial infections or gas gangrene.(7) This finding led to a series of studies to evaluate the antimicrobial activity of HBO_2. Smith and Sharp first described HBO_2's role in hastening cardiac and neurologic recovery following carbon monoxide poisoning. High-pressure oxygen was first proposed from a variety of medical fronts with the assumption that higher oxygen tensions and an elevation of pressure to reduce bubble size in blood and tissues was a natural expansion of commonly accepted physiological principles. This led to an outburst of research, publications, and meetings to understand the potential of this therapy.

Respiratory effects alone cannot explain the beneficial and toxic manifestations of high-pressure oxygen. In order for nonhealing wounds to continue healing over several weeks, the repair mechanisms of multiple tissues must converge.

In other syndromes, repeatedly elevated oxygen pressures induced by HBO_2 cause anti-inflammatory mediators to accumulate over time. This phenomenon was termed the "pharmacological effect" of oxygen, a concept brought forward by Kindwall.(14) With a better understanding of oxygen toxicity and its biologic role on cell signaling and protective antioxidant pathways, this area was explored in more detail.

Oxygen and nitrogen (N_2) radicals were identified as reactive species that are highly toxic for cells because of their ability to induce oxidative stress and propagate cell death pathways. Nevertheless, they also play a protective role by mediating intracellular signaling and impacting immune defenses, inflammatory reactions, and gene expression. Therefore, oxygen and nitrogen reactive species may be harmful or beneficial depending on their intracellular localization and concentration.

Two publications from Thom propose possible mechanisms of action of hyperbaric oxygen therapy via a thorough analysis of O_2 and N_2 radicals produced from breathing O_2 at elevated pressures.[20-21] These publications are significant in this area because they provide both biochemical[21] and clinical[20] explanations for the action of O_2 at higher pressures.

Thom initially noted that the majority of patients who undergo HBO_2 therapy are treated for processes responding slowly over days and weeks to increases in O_2 pressure instead of for bubble-induced injuries. In most instances, O_2 exposure is regulated by the total pressure reached and the length of exposure (e.g., a few minutes or hours each day at 2–3 ATA (202.65–303.98 kPa). These repeated exposures result in time-favorable biological responses while also limiting toxic effects.[21] When O_2 is breathed at pressures greater than 1 ATA, the production of reactive oxygen species and, to a lesser degree, the production of reactive nitrogen species is increased. These newly formed reactive compounds can act as signaling molecules able to modulate transduction cascades and molecular pathways involved in the generation of a variety of growth factors, hormones, and cytokines. Several activation pathways underpinning the therapeutic effect of HBO_2 have been described. Neutrophil beta-actin nitrosylation, lower monocyte chemokine synthesis, and ischemic preconditioning changes in HO-1, SPSs, and HIF-1 are the three mechanisms thought to improve postischemic tissue survival. This critical differentiation may reflect the 2 existing exposure pressures recommended for HBO_2 treatments: the first can be activated at 2 ATA oxygen breathing while the second might require exposure at 2.5 to 2.8 ATA oxygen.

Improved Neovascularization

HBO_2 therapy has been accepted and successfully utilized in nonhealing wound repair. Diabetic wounds and postradiation delayed tissue injuries have been studied at length to understand how HBO_2 therapy affects tissue lesions. Though the pathophysiology of these disorders is distinct, common components include depletion of stromal cells, poor skin surface granulation, chronic inflammation, fibrosis,[10-11,16] and reduced supply of O_2 and mediators.

Even if the exact mechanism explaining the efficacy of hyperbaric oxygen therapy in wound healing is not completely discovered, it seems to imply the combined action of local alterations on wound margins and body-wide systemic events. Two processes lead to neovascularization: (1) the growth of new blood vessels from local endothelial cells, the so-called angiogenesis; and (2) the recruitment and differentiation in the bed of the wound of circulating stem/progenitor cells to form new vessels, or vasculogenesis.

Both angiogenesis and vasculogenesis are affected by HBO_2 treatment, since hyperbaric oxygen can amend the inhibited synthesis of extracellular matrix (collagen) and growth factors of injured tissues. HBO_2 exerts this beneficial effect by distinct mechanisms. One mechanism involves radicals and causes an increased mobilization of bone marrow stem/progenitor cells (SPCs) which, once circulating, can migrate to the open wound bed and expedite the healing. These beneficial effects are produced without increasing the thrombogenic circulating leukocyte count.

In a different mechanism, HBO_2-induced oxidative stress at sites of neovascularization prompt stem and progenitor cells to produce cell growth factors.[13,15] Part of this mechanism has been linked to synthesis and stabilization of hypoxia-inducible factor (HIF). These transcription factors are activated intracellularly by hypoxia and excreted when cells are saturated with O_2. Interestingly, they need the expression of free O_2 radicals, likely as an induced response to thioredoxin (an antioxidant enzyme) and thioredoxin reductase (its regulatory enzyme). Furthermore, the same pathway can be set off by the oxidative stress of the lactate metabolism. HBO_2 also cued synthesis of basic fibroblast growth factors such as growth factor B1 by human dermal fibroblast and basic fibroblast growth factor in ischemic limbs. Thom has proposed a more robust list of putative triggering events and factors[20] for the beneficial effects of HBO_2 in nonhealing wounds. Still, more conclusive studies are needed to more clearly elucidate the timing and optimal doses of HBO_2 administration.

Improved Post-Ischemic Tissue Survivals

Significant recovery with HBO_2 following extremity reimplantation, free-tissue transfer, and crush injury/reperfusion has been noted in clinical studies. Though the evidence is heterogeneous, it applies to visceral tissues and musculoskeletal tissues. For example, HBO_2 can reduce coronary artery restenosis following balloon angioplasty and stenting and can increase myocardial tissue recovery following thrombolytic treatment for acute myocardial infarction.[17-18] HBO_2 can also improve hepatic survival after liver transplantation and reduce the likelihood of encephalopathy seen following cardiopulmonary bypass. Instead of treating patients for weeks for wound healing, they can be effectively treated for reperfusion injuries, a therapy that only includes HBO_2 sessions for a few days at higher pressures of 2.5 to 3 ATA, multiple times in a day. In effect, circulating neutrophils can adhere to vascular endothelium using beta 2 integrins and hinder tissue reperfusion. Exposition to HBO_2 can prevent this adhesion, producing a number of advantages as follows:[23]

- Improved reperfusion following injury in the brain, heart, lung, liver, skeletal muscle, and intestines
- Reduced smoke-induced lung injury and encephalopathy from CO poisoning
- Beneficial effects in decompression sickness
- Reperfusion after gas embolus

The basic mechanism underlying this elective inhibition is regulated by the increase of reactive species from inducible NO synthase and myeloperoxidase, which cause excessive S-nitrosylation of cytoskeletal beta-actin. Though this modification increases the concentration of short, non-cross-linked filamentous actin within the cell,[22] the viability and defense capability of neutrophils is unaffected, as is the phagocytosis or oxidative burst in response to chemoattractants. Secondary inhibition of beta 2 integrins using monoclonal antibodies also ameliorates ischemia reperfusion injuries, but, unlike hyperbaric oxygen, antibody therapy causes the immune system to be profoundly compromised. Further, a separate anti-inflammatory pathway for hyperbaric oxygen does not inhibit neutrophil antibacterial functions because the G-protein-coupled pathway for endoplasmic activation remains functioning. A different anti-inflammatory pathway for hyperbaric oxygen involves impaired production of proinflammatory cytokines due to the action of monocyte-macrophages. This may lead to a reduction in circulating proinflammatory cytokines under stress conditions. A proposed molecular mechanism in this area is the augmentation of heme oxygenase-1 and heat shock protein 20. Lastly, HBO_2 has been shown to increase the ischemic tolerance of multiple organs in a variety of animal models by inducing antioxidant enzymes and anti-inflammatory proteins.[6, 24-25]

Bacteriostatic and Bactericidal Effects

High oxygen concentrations have a notable direct bactericidal effect on obligate anaerobic microorganisms. The absence of scavenger enzymes in anaerobic bacteria makes them sensitive to the elevated concentration in oxygen free radicals. Zanon et al. recently reported on the growth in cultures of a number of bacterial strains directly exposed a single time to HBO_2 or normoxic pressure alone.[27] They investigated possible changes in the minimum inhibitory concentration (MIC) as well as in the minimum bactericidal concentration (MBC) of multiresistant microorganisms following a single hyperbaric exposure. Their findings suggest that HBO_2 is only bactericidal if the total exposure pressure is elevated. This effect does not solely depend on the pO_2 applied.

Almzaiel et al.[3] reported on the interactions between bacteria and neutrophil-like cells and noted that a single 90-minute HBO_2 exposure caused an increase in the respiratory burst activity of neutrophil-like cells following exposure. They also noted an increase in the phagocytosis of *Staphylococcus aureus*. Both the hyperoxia and pressure components of HBO_2 contribute to the increase in antimicrobial activity and apoptosis of the cells. Though enhanced antimicrobial activity is harmful to wound healing because it promotes a proinflammatory environment, enhanced apoptosis addresses inflammation. Together, this encourages wound healing and likely offsets the mentioned detrimental effects.[3]

Osteogenetic Process Promotion

Though the exact cellular and molecular mechanisms through which hyperbaric oxygen therapy exerts its positive effect on chronic osteonecrosis (ON) is elusive, recent data reveal that intermittent supplementation of O_2 to hypoxic bone stimulates osteoblast differentiation and suppresses osteoclast genesis/activation resulting in bone tissue regeneration.[1-2,12] The current reports, performed by Hadi and colleagues, evaluated distinctly the effect of HBO_2, pressure, and hyperoxia on the following:

a) RANKL-induced (receptor activator of nuclear factor–kappa B–induced) osteoclast formation in RAW 264.7 cells and human peripheral blood monocytes (PBMC)
b) osteoblast differentiation and activity in Saos-2 human osteoblast cells cultured in normoxic (21% O_2) or hypoxic (2% O_2) conditions

In detail, researchers found that HBO_2 had a more marked anti-osteoclastic effect than hyperoxia or pressure singularly and also directly stopped osteoclast formation and resorption in hypoxic conditions, an indication for a number of osteolytic skeletal disorders. At least part of the suppressive effect of HBO_2 was mediated *via* reduction in RANK, NFATc1, and Dc-STAMP expression and inhibition of HIF-1alpha, mRNA, and protein expression. Moreover, their in vitro study on Saos-2 cells reveals that HBO_2 enhances the rate of osteoblast differentiation, augments early stages of mineralization, and has a more pronounced effect than treatment with elevated oxygen levels or pressure alone. All these data provide mechanistic evidence to support the use of HBO_2 as an adjuvant therapy in preventing osteoclast formation and bone loss from hypoxic bone lesions. This consideration is supported by the retrospective study conducted by Camporesi et al. that describes the reversal of femoral head necrosis in a 7-year follow-up in a group of patients treated with a series of HBO_2 treatments at 2 ATA (202.65 kPa).[8]

Uncertainty about Oxygen Dosage

The effective use of hyperbaric medicine remains an imprecise science since adequate data are not currently available to support both the ideal dose and the minimally toxic dose necessary to induce the slowly evolving healing mechanisms that provide wound closure, functional restoration, and reperfusion of insured tissues without triggering oxidative stress side effects.

CONCLUSIONS

Hyperbaric oxygen therapy entails intermittent inhalation of 100% oxygen while under a pressure greater than 1 ATA (101.325 kPa). Though this therapy has been used in medical settings for more than a half-century, the use of hyperbaric oxygen is still debated. In the last 20 years, the mechanism of hyperbaric oxygen therapy has been more clearly understood and its benefit more widely accepted. Nevertheless, many health-care providers remain unaware of its therapeutic effect in certain carefully defined disease states.

REFERENCES

1. Al Hadi H, Smerdon GR, Fox SW. Hyperbaric oxygen therapy accelerates osteoblast differentiation and promotes bone formation. J Dent. 2015;43(3):382-8.

2. Al Hadi H, Smerdon G, Fox SW. Osteoclastic resorptive capacity is suppressed in patients receiving hyperbaric oxygen therapy. Acta Orthop. 2015 Apr;86(2):264-9.

3. Almzaiel AJ, Billington R, Smerdon G, Moody AJ. Effects of hyperbaric oxygen treatment on antimicrobial function and apoptosis of differentiated HL-60 (neutrophil-like) cells. Life Sci. 2013 Jul 30;93(2-3):125-31.

4. Boerema I, Kroll JA, Meijne NG, Lokin E, Kroon B, Huiskes JW. High atmospheric pressure as an aid to cardiac surgery. Arch Chir Neerl. 1956;8:193-211.

5. Boerema I, Meyne NG, et al. Life without blood: a study of the influence of high atmospheric pressure on dilution of blood. J Cardiovasc surg 1960;1(2):133-146.

6. Bosco G, Yang ZJ, Nandi J, Wang J, Chen C, Camporesi EM. Effects of hyperbaric oxygen on glucose, lactate, glycerol and anti-oxidant enzymes in the skeletal muscle of rats during ischaemia and reperfusion. Clin Exp Pharmacol Physiol. 2007 Jan-Feb;34(1-2):70-6.

7. Brummelkamp WH, Hogendijk J, Boerema I. Treatment of anaerobic infections (clostridial myositis) by drenching the tissues with oxygen under high atmospheric pressure. Surgery. 1961;49:299-302.

8. Camporesi EM, Vezzani G, Bosco G, Mangar D, Bernasek TL. Hyperbaric oxygen therapy in femoral head necrosis. J Arthroplasty. 2010 Sep;25(6 Suppl):118-23.

9. Churchill-Davidson I, Sanger C, Thomlinson RH. High-pressure oxygen and radiotherapy. Lancet. 1955;1:1091-5.

10. Denham J, Hauer-Jensen M. The radiotherapeutic injury a complex "wound." Radiother Oncol. 2002;63:129-45.

11. Falanga V. Wound healing and its impairment in the diabetic foot. Lancet. 2005;366:1736-43.

12. Hadi HA, Smerdon GR, Fox SW. Hyperbaric oxygen therapy suppresses osteoclast formation and bone resorption. J Orthop Res. Epub 2013 Jul 22.

13. Hunt TK, Aslam RS, Beckert S, et al. Aerobically derived lactate stimulates revascularization and tissue repair via redox mechanisms. Antioxid Redox Signal. 2007;9:1115-24.

14. Kindwall EP. A history of hyperbaric medicine. In: Kindwall EP, editor. Hyperbaric medicine practice. Flagstaff (AZ): Best Publishing Co.; 1994. p. 1-16.

15. Milovanova TN, Bhopale VM, Sorokina EM, Moore JS, Hunt TK, Hauer-Jensen M, Velazquez OC, Thom SR. Lactate stimulates vasculogenic stem cells via the thioredoxin system and engages an autocrine activation loop involving hypoxia-inducible factor 1. Mol Cell Biol. 2008;28:6248-61.

16. Peppa M, Stavroulakis P, Raptis SA. Advanced glucoxidation products and impaired diabetic wound healing. Wound Repair Regen. 2009;17:461-72.

17. Sharifi M, Fares W, Abdel-Karim I, Koch JM, Sopko J, Adler D. Hyperbaric oxygen therapy in percutaneous coronary interventions investigators. Usefulness of hyperbaric oxygen therapy to inhibit restenosis after percutaneous coronary intervention for acute myocardial infarction or unstable angina pectoris. Am J Cardiol. 2004 Jun 15;93(12):1533-5.

18. Sharifi M, Fares W, Abdel-Karim I, Petrea D, et al. Inhibition of restenosis by hyperbaric oxygen: a novel indication for an old modality. Cardiovasc Radiat Med. 2002;3:124-6.

19. Smith G, Sharp GR. Treatment of coal gas poisoning with oxygen at two atmospheres pressure. Lancet. 1962;1:816-9.

20. Thom SR. Hyperbaric oxygen: its mechanisms and efficacy. Plast Reconstr Surg. 2011;127(Suppl 1):131S-141S.

21. Thom SR. Oxidative stress is fundamental to hyperbaric oxygen therapy. J Appl Physiol. 2009;106:988-95.

22. Thom SR, Bhopale VM, Mancini JD, et al. Actin S-nitrosylation inhibits neutrophil beta-2 integrin function. J Biol Chem. 2008;283:10822-34.

23. Weaver LK, Hopkins RO, Chan KJ, Churchill S, Elliott CG, Clemmer TP, et al. Hyperbaric oxygen for acute carbon monoxide poisoning. N Engl J Med. 2002 Oct 3;347(14):1057-67.

24. Yang ZJ, Bosco G, Montante A, Ou XL, Camporesi EM. Hyperbaric O_2 reduces intestinal ischemia-reperfusion-induced TNF-alpha production and lung neutrophil sequestration. Eur J Appl Physiol. 2001 Jul;85(1-2):96-103.

25. Yang Z, Nandi J, Wang G, Bosco G, Gregory M, Chung C, Xie Y, Yang X, Camporesi EM. Hyperbaric oxygenation ameliorates indomethacin-induced enteropathy in rats by modulating TNF-alpha and IL-1beta production. Dig Dis Sci. 2006 Aug;51(8):1426-33.

26. Yarbrough OD, Behnke AR. The treatment of compressed air illness using oxygen. J Ind Hyg Toxicol. 1939;21:213-8.

27. Zanon V, Rossi L, Castellani E, Camporesi EM, Palù G, Bosco G. Oxybiotest project: microorganisms under pressure. Hyperbaric oxygen (HBO) and simple pressure interaction on selected bacteria. Med Gas Res. 2012 Sep 11;2(1):24.

CHAPTER 3 CHAPTER

Oxygen Toxicity

CHAPTER THREE OVERVIEW

Recognition and Prevention of Oxygen Poisoning in Hyperbaric Oxygen Therapy 51
Biochemical Mechanisms of Oxygen Poisoning 51
Manifestations of Oxygen Poisoning 52
Central Nervous System Effects 52
Pulmonary Effects 53
Ocular Effects 55
Modification of Oxygen Tolerance 56
Factors that Decrease Oxygen Tolerance 56
Management of Oxygen-Induced Seizures 57
References 59
Appendix – Measuring Pulmonary Oxygen Toxicity 64
The Unit Pulmonary Toxicity Dose Concept 64
Arithmetic Method 65
Appendix References 66
References Breakdown by Subject Matter 66

Oxygen Toxicity

Heather Annis, Aliyah Keval, Harry T. Whelan

RECOGNITION AND PREVENTION OF OXYGEN POISONING IN HYPERBARIC OXYGEN THERAPY

Although any therapeutic application of hyperbaric oxygen (HBO_2) is intrinsically associated with the potential for producing mild to severe toxic effects,[12,17,36,41,P] the appropriate use of hyperoxia is one of the safest therapeutic procedures available to the modern medical practitioner. A wide margin of safety for oxygen use is provided by potent antioxidant defense mechanisms[31] that slow the development of oxygen poisoning and hasten recovery from its subclinical manifestations. In conditions of prolonged oxygen exposure, however, antioxidant defenses are overwhelmed and toxic manifestations eventually occur. Susceptibility to oxygen toxicity may be influenced by the clinical state of the patient or by the effects of concurrent drug therapy. Both the awareness of such influences and the ability to recognize early manifestations of oxygen poisoning can further enhance the safety and efficacy of HBO_2 therapy.

BIOCHEMICAL MECHANISMS OF OXYGEN POISONING

There is now general agreement that the formation of reactive oxygen species is an intermediate event in the production of oxidant damage to cell membranes and their constituents. The degree of damage appears to be determined by the stoichiometric relationship between the rate of formation of reactive oxygen species and their rate of elimination by antioxidants. Evidence for and against this current concept has recently been the subject of extensive discussion by several authors.[25,39,A,M,Q]

Reduction of molecular oxygen by the sequential addition of electrons results in the formation of superoxide, hydrogen peroxide, hydroxyl radical, and, finally, water. There are indications that superoxide radicals generated in mitochondria are rapidly dismutated to hydrogen peroxide and that these products interact further in the presence of catalytic amounts of iron to potentially generate both highly reactive hydroxyl radicals and singlet oxygen. Initiation of lipid peroxidation by either of these highly reactive radicals could greatly increase oxidant damage by propagating a series of reactions, resulting in possible oxidation of proteins and lipids, inactivation of critical enzymes, and, ultimately, cellular membrane damage. Protein cross-linking, fatty acid oxidation, and oxidation of amino acids are all potential results of free-radical production in hyperoxic environments.[3,4,11,13,25,39]

There are several antioxidant enzymes that oppose the formation of reactive oxygen species, including superoxide dismutase, catalase, glutathione peroxidase, glutathione reductase, and the enzymes of the Hexose Monophosphate (HMP) Shunt. Other compounds that appear to have important antioxidant activity include glutathione, selenium, vitamin E, and vitamin C.

The likelihood of oxygen toxicity manifesting during hyperbaric oxidative therapy is dependent on the intracellular localization and concentration of reactive oxygen species. The nature and degree of oxidant damage during hyperoxia exposure is determined by the net results of the radical-producing and radical-quenching actions. The oxidant damage is determined by the interaction of antioxidant defenses and tissue repair mechanisms.(A,M,P) Antioxidant defenses during the brief exposure to hyperoxia that occurs in clinical hyperbaric oxygen therapy are sufficient to reverse processes associated to upsurges in reactive oxygen species.(50)

Potential insights into mechanisms that cause oxygen convulsions are provided by studies of pharmacologic agents that delay the onset of seizures in animals exposed to toxic oxygen pressures. These agents include diethyldithiocarbamic acid, 1-aminobenzotriazole, 21-aminosteroid compounds (lazeroids),(33,35,49) propranolol,(51,53) and low-dose caffeine.(9,R)

Diethyldithiocarbamic acid and 1-aminobenzotriazole are two examples of antioxidants that effectively inhibit the cytochrome P-450 monooxygenases, a class of enzymes that are known to form reactive oxygen species. These antioxidant compounds are selectively distributed and at their highest concentrations in neuronal tissue, or non-glial cells, where they are most effective.(27) A potential physiological role for cytochrome P-450-dependent enzymes is explained by the fact that neurons contain biochemical machinery for the synthesis of neurotransmitters, neurohormones, and other physiologically active endogenous substances. Inhibiting these enzymes limits the extent of oxidative injury that can occur by decreasing the rate of formation of reactive oxygen species.

Free radical–induced peroxidation of neuronal, glial, vascular cell membranes, and myelin within the central nervous system is catalyzed by release of free iron from injured cells. This suggests a possible role for iron-chelating drugs, such as the 21-amino steroids, in the prevention of lipid peroxidation.(10,A,M,P)

The protective effects of propranolol against neurological manifestations of oxygen toxicity have been attributed to its adrenergic blocking properties.(48,49) However, propranolol also decreases cerebral blood flow and cerebral oxidative metabolism. These additional actions could contribute to the delayed onset of oxygen convulsions by preexposure administration of propranolol.(51,53)

Low-dose caffeine produces cerebral vasoconstriction by acting as an adenosine receptor agonist, and as an antioxidant, which may have antiepileptic properties, delaying the onset of oxygen convulsions.(9,R)

It has been proposed that heat shock protein 27 is an antagonist to the process by which expanded polyglutamine tracts in proteins affected by neurodegenerative disorders induce reactive oxygen species.(55) The protein was expected to achieve this by suppressing the production of reactive oxygen species in cells that express mutant huntingtin through its ability to bind to cytochrome c. This was later found to be unnecessary, and that it is the large oligomeric form of the heat shock protein 27 that is the protective species of the protein. The study extrapolates that the protein protects against oxidative stress, and so, by implication, can be a useful avenue towards apprehending a remedy for oxygen toxicity.(55)

MANIFESTATIONS OF OXYGEN POISONING

Central Nervous System Effects

Grand mal convulsions caused by central nervous system (CNS) oxygen toxicity can occur in patients breathing oxygen at pressures of 2.0 ATA (atmosphere absolute) or greater.[D,G,I,Y] Convulsions may occur abruptly, or may be preceded by other signs of central nervous system irritability (Table 1).

TABLE 1. SIGNS AND SYMPTOMS OF CNS OXYGEN POISONING IN NORMAL MEN (ADAPTED FROM DONALD)

Facial pallor	Inspiratory predominance
Sweating	Diaphragmatic spasms
Bradycardia	Nausea
Palpitations	Spasmodic vomiting
Depression	Fibrillation of lips
Apprehension	Lip twitching
Visual field constriction	Twitching of cheek, nose, eyelids
Tinnitus	Syncope
Auditory hallucinations	Convulsions
Vertigo	

Detection of one or more of the premonitory symptoms of CNS oxygen poisoning should be treated by switching the patient's source of breathing gas from oxygen to chamber air. Reversal of the symptoms while breathing chamber air is consistent with recovery from oxygen poisoning. Once the patient has recovered by showing no evidence of persistent CNS toxicity, treatment with oxygen may be resumed after the patient's treatment protocol is modified to prevent recurrence of toxic symptoms by either inserting additional "chamber air" intervals or by ascending to the depth where the patient was previously asymptomatic.[H] As long as mechanical trauma is avoided while the patient is actively seizing, there should be no residual effects to the oxygen convulsions.

Pulmonary Effects

Prolonged exposure to oxygen pressures greater than 0.5 ATA is associated with the development of intratracheal and bronchial irritation, such as substernal burning, chest tightness, cough, and dyspnea.[13,17,18,52,E,F,S,T,X] With continued oxygen exposure, the patient develops progressive impairment of pulmonary function, and, eventually, acute respiratory distress syndrome (ARDS). Initially, there are indications of capillary endothelial damage, followed by pulmonary edema, protein exudation, and progressive respiratory failure.[52] These changes are seen over the course of days to weeks at lower oxygen pressures and occur more rapidly as the oxygen pressure is increased. The early changes of pulmonary oxygen toxicity generally reverse upon cessation of oxygen therapy. No residual (irreversible) pulmonary effects have been observed after a single administration of any of the therapy protocols listed in Table 2. When oxygen therapy is provided in accordance with the standard HBO_2 treatment protocols outlined in this text, there is little or no danger that patients will experience pulmonary oxygen toxicity.

When patients show signs of pulmonary oxygen toxicity, they must be provided with sufficient time to fully recover before being treated with another course of HBO_2 or receiving supplemental oxygen between treatments. Otherwise, these patients are at risk of developing harmful side effects, as a result of their cumulative

TABLE 2. CUMULATIVE PULMONARY OXYGEN TOXICITY INDICES FOR COMMONLY USED OXYGEN THERAPY TABLES

THERAPY TABLE	UPTD*
Refractory osteomyelitis/radionecrosis	
120 min oxygen at 33 fsw	300
90 min oxygen at 45 fsw	270
Anaerobic infection	401
45 min oxygen/15 min air/45 min oxygen at 60 fsw	
45 min oxygen at 60-0 fsw with 8 min at 20 fsw and 27 min at 10 fsw	
CO intoxication	361
30 min oxygen at 60 fsw	
4 min oxygen at 60-33 fsw	
90 min oxygen at 33 fsw	
10 min oxygen at 33-0 fsw	
USN 5**	66
USN 6	645
USN 6 extended	
20 min oxygen/5 min air at 30 fsw	718
15 min air/60 min oxygen at 30 fsw	787
20 min oxygen/5 min air at 60 fsw and 15 min air/60 min oxygen at 30 fsw	860
USN 6A	690
USN 6A extended	
20 min oxygen/5 min air at 60 fsw	763
15 min air/60 min oxygen at 30 fsw	833
20 min oxygen/5 min air at 60 fsw and 15 min air/60 min oxygen at 30 fsw	906
IFEM 7A (air and oxygen)**	1813
IFEM 7A alternating 50/50 Nitrox with air 30 min on/ 30 min off from 100-70 fsw	2061

*UPTD value indicates duration (minutes) of oxygen breathing at 1.0 ATA that would cause equivalent degree of pulmonary intoxication (measured as decrease in vital capacity). From the Institute for Environmental Medicine. Revision of UPTD concept with addition of new data[16,20] is ongoing.

**USN (United States Navy)

**IFEM (Institute for Environmental Medicine, University of Pennsylvania)

U.S. Navy Diving Manual Rev. 6. Public Domain. [U]

oxygen dose. The progression of intoxication is best monitored by serial pulmonary-function studies; however, direct measurement in this fashion may be difficult or unduly expensive.[11,18,22,49] Consequently, attempts have been made to quantify the degree of pulmonary intoxication from a single hyperoxic exposure,[12,13,17] for two purposes: (1) to compare the degree of toxicity expected from exposure to different oxygen pressures for different lengths of time, and (2) to calculate the cumulative toxicity from repeated hyperoxic exposures. These attempts have led to development of the concept of the unit pulmonary toxic dose (UPTD),[6,54] a standard value that allows physicians to compare the potential pulmonary effects from the various treatment tables. The UPTD is designed to express any pulmonary toxic dose in terms of an equivalent exposure to oxygen at 1.0 ATA. The calculations are based on vital capacity measurements that describe the rate of development of pulmonary intoxication at oxygen pressures above 0.5 ATA.

The UPTD values shown in Table 2 are derived from averaged data obtained during single, continuous-oxygen exposures in healthy male subjects. They should be regarded only as general guidelines for assessing degrees of pulmonary oxygen poisoning in any individual patient. The cumulative effects of pulmonary oxygen toxicity with repeated exposures can be estimated by multiplying the UPTD of the treatment by the number of treatments. In the absence of adequate information about the time course for reversal of pulmonary oxygen poisoning, this value does not provide an estimate of the amount of recovery that can be expected to occur between treatments.

For example, this method would predict that 10 oxygen treatments at 2.4 ATA, or 45 feet of seawater (fsw), for 90 minutes each would give a patient a UPTD of 2700 and should produce significant pulmonary symptoms and a 20% reduction in vital capacity.[54] However, it is common clinical experience that patients are able to tolerate this daily regimen, six days a week, for up to six to eight weeks without reporting any side effects. [24] Pulmonary symptoms, such as inspiratory burning or chest tightness, are occasionally experienced by sensitive individuals during administration of a USN Table 6 or 6A, especially when these tables are extended or repeated for treating severe gas lesion diseases, such as decompression sickness or an arterial gas embolism. In the event that saturation with intermittent hyperoxygenation at increased ambient pressure (Institute for Environmental Medicine, University of Pennsylvania 7A or equivalent) is required for gas lesion diseases that are refractory to standard HBO_2 treatment protocols, the timing and duration of intermittent oxygen periods may be determined partially by the severity of pulmonary symptoms.

Ocular Effects

Progressive myopia has been reported by some patients who receive daily 90- to 120-minute oxygen treatments at 2.0 to 2.4 ATA for various chronic disease states. [3,4,43,47] The overall incidence is approximately 20% to 40%, with some indications of an increased incidence in diabetics and elderly patients. Complete recovery usually occurs within six weeks of terminating of HBO_2 therapy but can also be irreversible in exceptional cases.[43,47] Although the observed myopia appears to be lenticular in origin,[4, C] the exact mechanism remains obscure. Direct exposure of the eye to 100% O_2 in a hood or monoplace chamber is likely, though not yet demonstrated, to produce a higher lens PO_2 than when oxygen is delivered via facemask at depth.

The growth of preexisting nuclear cataracts may be stimulated by prolonged series of hyperbaric oxygen therapies, and new cataracts were found in 7 of 15 patients exposed to 150–850 daily therapies at 2.0–2.5 ATA.[47] The nuclear cataracts were not reversible after cessation of these extremely prolonged therapy series. Published reports,[3,4,43,47] as well as extensive clinical experience in major HBO_2 centers, indicate that new cataracts do not develop within the series of 20–50 therapies that are used to treat most chronic disease states.

Other reversible effects of hyperoxia on visual function in humans include contraction of peripheral visual fields[8,42] and reduction in the electrical response of retinal glial cells to a light flash.[15,21] These effects have been observed only with continuous or intermittent experimental oxygen exposures that greatly exceed the limits of all standard HBO_2 regimens. Visual effects of hyperoxia that have occurred in uniquely susceptible individuals include the development of retrolental fibroplasia in premature infants after exposure to relatively low levels of hyperoxia[48] and a reversible, unilateral loss of vision during a 6-hour oxygen exposure at 2.0 ATA in an individual who had a previous history of retrobulbar neuritis.[45]

MODIFICATION OF OXYGEN TOLERANCE

Susceptibility to developing overt manifestations of pulmonary or CNS oxygen toxicity seems to vary widely among different individuals and animal species.[12,17] Specific chemical manifestations may prove to be less variable. The development rate can also be modified extensively by a variety of conditions, procedures, and drugs.

D'Agostino et al. have found that oxygen toxicity–induced seizures can be avoided by the use of ketone ester to carry out therapeutic ketosis.[23] It involves reference to the metabolic activity of derivation of energy from ketones that occurs in cases of severe carbohydrate deprivation that occur with ketogenic diets. This has the effect of significantly delaying oxygen toxicity in the central nervous system. They hypothesize that oral administration of butanediol acetoacetate diester would mimic the ability of ketosis to inhibit seizures. The use of saturated hydrogen saline is another recent avenue of study. Hydrogen is already known to be an effective antioxidant through the process of rapid diffusion into cells and subsequently tissues. A study involving the use of mice as subjects determined that pulmonary injury induced by hypoxia, which is responsible to some extent for oxidative damage inhibition, is alleviated by saturated hydrogen saline.[56]

Although most of the factors found to modify oxygen tolerance in laboratory animals have not been evaluated in clinical trials, it is assumed that agents with prominent effects on oxygen tolerance in animals should produce similar effects in human subjects.

Factors that Decrease Oxygen Tolerance

Examples of factors that either hasten the onset or increase the severity of overt manifestations of oxygen toxicity are shown on the left side of Table 3. While none of these factors should be considered an absolute contraindication to hyperbaric oxygen therapy for a patient who would benefit from treatment, the presence of one or more of the listed influences should be regarded as an indication for caution. Consideration should be given either to reducing the inspired oxygen pressure or to decreasing the total duration of oxygen exposure.

Other factors, listed on the right side of Table 3, have been found to delay the onset or decrease the severity of overt toxic manifestations. Some factors (indicated by *) are potentially useful as protective agents under appropriate conditions of oxygen exposure. For example, physicians should be cautious when administering Disulfiram (Antabuse) as a neuroprotective agent. While Disulfiram does provide the benefit of delaying the onset of convulsions in animals exposed to oxygen at 4.0

TABLE 3. FACTORS THAT MODIFY RATE OF DEVELOPMENT OF OXYGEN POISONING

HASTEN ONSET OR INCREASE SEVERITY	DELAY ONSET OR DECREASE SEVERITY
Adrenocortical hormones	Acclimatization to hypoxia
CO_2	Adrenergic blocking drugs
Dextroamphetamine	Antioxidants
Epinephrine	Caffeine (low-dose)
Hyperthermia	Chlorpromazine
Insulin	Gamma-aminobutryic acid
Norepinephrine	Ganglionic blocking drugs
Paraquat	Glutathione
Hyperthyroidism	Hypothyroidism
Vitamin E deficiency	Propranolol
	Reserpine
	Starvation
	Succinate
	Trisaminomethane
	Intermittent exposure*
	Disulfiram*
	Hypothermia*
	Vitamin E*

*Potentially useful as protective agents (Adapted from Clark and Lambertsen)[17-19]

ATA,[29,30] it also enhances the progression of pulmonary intoxication in oxygen at 1.0 [26] or 2.0 [32] ATA.

At present, the most rational and practical means for extension of oxygen tolerance in humans is the systematic alternation of oxygen-exposure periods with relatively brief intervals of normoxia. Early studies at the University of Pennsylvania [34,40,H] established the effectiveness of providing these "air breaks" to animal subjects, which led to subsequent validation in humans.[37] Additional studies[14,15,19] extending these observations have been completed, and open literature documentation is in progress. The neuroprotective effect of ketosis is the subject of current human research.

MANAGEMENT OF OXYGEN-INDUCED SEIZURES

Convulsions are hazardous in all patients but particularly so in those with fractures, osseous nonunion, head injury, cardiac abnormality, or recent surgery. In addition to ensuring standard safety measures that prevent the patient from injuring himself or herself or aspirating during a seizure, the attending physician must remember that it is extremely important to avoid decompression during the tonic phase of the convulsion, since expanding pulmonary gas could then rupture the lung and produce a possibly fatal arterial-gas embolism. Once there is evidence of tonic-clonic movements and the patient resumes a normal breathing pattern, the patient may undergo decompression.

One chamber requirement that is critical to preventing CNS toxicity is selecting an oxygen-delivery apparatus which limits the amount of carbon dioxide that patients can rebreathe while at depth. The simultaneous intake of carbon dioxide with oxygen markedly accelerates the onset of oxygen convulsions, even at pressures as low as 2.0 ATA. Elevation of arterial PCO_2 causes cerebral vasodilation with an associated increase in brain oxygen tension. Increased tensions of arterial carbon dioxide partial pressures can also be caused by ventilatory depression following administration of narcotic analgesic drugs such as morphine or meperidine hydrochloride.

Epileptic patients may undergo HBO_2 treatment, but they should be considered much more susceptible to oxygen-induced seizures than patients without a history of seizure disorders. It is prudent to ensure that the patient's anticonvulsant medication regimen has been administered and that he or she is at therapeutic blood levels prior to starting treatment with HBO_2.

Oxygen-induced seizures are usually self-limited and do not require pharmacologic agents to terminate the seizure activity. The occurrence of an oxygen-induced seizure is not a contraindication to further HBO_2 therapy. Additional seizures can be prevented by shortening the duration of oxygen exposure (inserting more air breaks) and/or by decreasing the oxygen pressure. Although administration of diazepam (Valium) before each treatment can also be used to suppress seizures, instituting an anticonvulsant therapy regimen after the completion of an HBO_2 treatment protocol is not indicated for patients without a preexisting seizure history.

REFERENCES

1. Alderman J, Culver BW, Shellenberger MK. An examination of the role of gamma-aminobutyric acid (GABA) in hyperbaric oxygen-induced convulsions in the rat. I. Effects of increased gamma-aminobutyric acid and protective agents. J Pharmacol Exp Ther. 1974;190:334-40.
2. Allen JE, Goodman DB, Besarab A, Rasmussen H. Studies on the biochemical basis of oxygen toxicity. Biochem Biophys Acta. 1973;320:708-28.
3. Anderson B Jr., Farmer JC Jr. Hyperoxic myopia. Trans Am Opthalmol Soc. 1978;76:116-24.
4. Anderson B Jr, Shelton DL. Axial length in hyperoxic myopia. In: Bove AA, Bachrach AJ, Greenbaum LJ, editors. Underwater and hyperbaric physiology IX. Proceedings of the Ninth International Symposium on Underwater and Hyperbaric Physiology. Bethesda (MD): Undersea and Hyperbaric Medical Society; 1987. p. 607-11.
5. Balentine JD. Pathology of oxygen toxicity. New York: Academic Press; 1982.
6. Bardin H, Lambertsen CJ. A quantitative method for calculating pulmonary toxicity. Use of the "Unit Pulmonary Toxicity Dose" (UPTD). In: Institute for Environmental Medicine Report. Philadelphia: University of Pennsylvania; 1970.
7. Becker NH, Galvin JF. Effect of oxygen-rich atmospheres on cerebral lipid peroxides. Aerosp Med. 1962;33:985-7.
8. Behnke AR, Forbes HS, Motley EP. Circulatory and visual effects of oxygen at 3 atmospheres pressure. Am J Physiol. 1936;114:436-42.
9. Bitterman N, Schaal S. Caffeine attenuates CNS oxygen toxicity in rats. Brain Res. 1995;696(1-2):250-3.
10. Braughler JM, Burton PS, Chase RL, et al. Novel membrane localized iron chelators as inhibitors of iron-dependent lipid peroxidation. Biochem Pharmacol. 1988;37:3853-60.
11. Caldwell PRB, Lee WL Jr, Schildkraut HS, Archibald ER. Changes in lung volume, diffusing capacity, and blood gases in men breathing oxygen. J Appl Physiol. 1966;21:1477-83.
12. Clark JM. Oxygen toxicity. In: Bennett PB, Elliott DH, editors. The physiology and medicine of diving. 3rd ed. London: Bailliere, Tindall and Cox; 1982. p. 200-38.
13. Clark JM. Pulmonary limits of oxygen tolerance in man. Exp Lung Res. 1988;14:897-910.
14. Clark JM, Gelfand R, Stevens WC, Lambertsen CJ. Extension of pulmonary oxygen tolerance in man at 2.0 ATA by intermittent exposure on 60:15 oxygen:normoxic pattern in Predictive Studies VI. Undersea Biomed Res. 1990;17(Suppl):25.
15. Clark JM, Gelfand R, Stevens WC, Lambertsen CJ. Comparison of human visual and pulmonary responses to continuous and intermittent oxygen exposure at 2.0 ATA in Predictive Studies V and VI. Undersea Biomed Res. 1991;18(Suppl):86.
16. Clark JM, Jackson RM, Lambertsen CJ, Gelfand R, Hiller WDB, Unger M. Pulmonary function in men after oxygen breathing at 3.0 ATA for 3.5 h. J Appl Physiol. 1991;71:878-85.
17. Clark JM, Lambertsen CJ. Pulmonary oxygen toxicity: A review. Pharmacol Rev. 1971;23:37-133.
18. Clark JM, Lambertsen CJ. Rate of development of pulmonary oxygen toxicity in man during oxygen breathing at 2.0 ATA. J Appl Physiol. 1971;30:739-52.

19. Clark JM, Lambertsen CJ. Principles of oxygen tolerance extension defined in the rat by intermittent oxygen exposure at 2.0 and 4.0 ATA. Undersea Biomed Res. 1989;16(Suppl):99.

20. Clark JM, Lambertsen CJ, Gelfand R, Flores ND, Pisarello JB, Rossman MD, Elias JA. Effects of prolonged oxygen exposure at 1.5, 2.0, or 2.5 ATA on pulmonary function in men (Predictive Studies V). J Appl Physiol. 1999;86(1).

21. Clark JM, Lambertsen CJ, Montabana DJ, Gelfand R, Cobbs WH. Comparison of visual function effects in man during continuous oxygen exposures at 3.0 and 2.0 ATA for 3.4 and 9.0 hours. Undersea Biomed Res. 1988;15(Suppl):32.

22. Comroe JH Jr, Dripps RD, Dumke PR, Deming M. Oxygen toxicity. The effect of inhalation of high concentrations of oxygen for twenty-four hours on normal men at sea level and at a simulated altitude of 18,000 feet. JAMA. 1945;128:710-17.

23. D'Agostino DP et al. Therapeutic ketosis with ketone ester delays central nervous system oxygen toxicity seizures in rats. Am J Physiol Regul Integr Comp Physiol. 2013: 829-39.

24. Davis JC, Dunn JM, Heimbach RD. Hyperbaric medicine: patient selection, treatment procedures, and side effects. In: Davis JC, Hunt TK, editors. Problem wounds: the role of oxygen. New York: Elsevier; 1988. p. 225-35.

25. Dell'Anna AM, Lamanna I, Vincent JL, Taccone FS. How much oxygen in adult cardiac arrest? Crit Care. 2014;18:555.

26. Deneke SM, Bernstein SP, Fanburg BL. Enhancement by disulfiram (Antabuse) of toxic effects of 95 to 97% oxygen on the rat lung. J Pharmocol Exp Ther. 1979;208:377-80.

27. Dhawan A, Parmar P, Seth D, Seth PK. Cytochrome P-450 dependent monooxygenases in neuronal and glial cells: inducibility and specificity. Biochem Biophys Res Commun. 1990;170(2):441-7.

28. Donald KW. Oxygen poisoning in man. I and II. Br Med J. 1947;1:667-72, 712-17.

29. Faiman MD, Mehl RG, Oehme FW. Protection with disulfiram from central and pulmonary oxygen toxicity. Biochem Pharmacol. 1971;20:3059-67.

30. Faiman MD, Nolan RJ, Oehme FW. Effect of disulfiram on oxygen toxicity in beagle dogs. Aerosp Med. 1974;45:29-32.

31. Forman HJ, Fisher AB. Antioxidant defenses. In: Gilbert DL, editor. Oxygen and living processes. New York: Springer-Verlag; 1981. p. 235-49.

32. Forman HJ, York JL, Fisher AB. Mechanism for the potentiation of oxygen toxicity by disulfiram. J Pharmacol Exp Ther. 1980;212:452-5.

33. Frank L, McLaughlin GE. Protection against acute and chronic hyperoxic inhibition of neonatal rat lung development with the 21-aminosteroid U-74389F. Pediatr Res. 1993;33:632-8.

34. Hall DA. The influence of the systematic fluctuation of PO_2 upon the nature and rate of development of oxygen toxicity in guinea-pigs [master's thesis]. University of Pennsylvania; 1967.

35. Haynes J, Seibert A, Bass JB, Taylor AE. U74500A inhibition of oxidant-mediated lung injury. Am J Physiol. 1990;259:H144-8.

36. Helmerhorst HJF, Roos-Blom MJ, van Westerloo DJ, de Jonge E. Association between arterial hyperoxia and outcome in subsets of critical illness: a systematic review, meta-analysis, and meta-regression of cohort studies. Crit Care Med. 2015;43(7):1508-18.

37. Hendricks PL, Hall DA, Hunter WL Jr, Haley PJ. Extension of pulmonary oxygen tolerance in man at 2 ATA by intermittent oxygen exposure. J Appl Physiol. 1977;42:593-9.

38. Hetz SK, Bradley TJ. Insects breathe discontinuously to avoid oxygen toxicity. Letter to: Nature. 2005:516-9.

39. Jamieson D. Oxygen toxicity and reactive oxygen metabolites in mammals. Free Radic Biol Med. 1989;7:87-108.

40. Lambertsen CJ. Respiratory and circulatory actions of high oxygen pressure. In: Goff LG, editor. Proceedings of the Underwater Physiology Symposium. Washington (DC): National Academy of Sciences-National Research Council, Pub 377; 1955. p. 25-38.

41. Lambertsen CJ. Effects of hyperoxia on organs and their tissues. In: Robin E, editor. Extrapulmonary manifestations of respiratory disease. New York: Marcel Dekker; 1978. p. 239-303.

42. Lambertsen CJ, Clark JM, Gelfand R, Pisarello J, Cobbs WH, Bevilacqua JE, Schwartz DM, Montabana DJ, Leach CS, Johnson PC, Fletcher DE. Definition of tolerance to continuous hyperoxia in man. An abstract report of Predictive Studies V. In: Bove AA, Bachrach AJ, Greenbaum LJ, editors. Underwater and hyperbaric physiology IX. Proceedings of the Ninth International Symposium on Underwater and Hyperbaric Physiology. Bethesda (MD): Undersea and Hyperbaric Medical Society; 1987. p. 717-35.

43. Lyne AJ. Ocular effects of hyperbaric oxygen. Trans Opthalmol Soc. 1978;98:66-8.

44. Moore MJ, Hammar T, Arruda J, Cramer S, Dennison S, Montie E, Fahlman A. Hyperbaric computed tomographic measurement of lung compression in seals and dolphins. J Exp Biol. 2011;214: 2390-7. doi:10.1242/jeb.055020.

45. Nichols CW, Lambertsen CJ, Clark JM. Transient unilateral loss of vision associated with oxygen at high pressure. Arch Opthalmol. 1969;81:548-52.

46. Ohlsson WTL. A study on oxygen toxicity at atmospheric pressure. Acta Med Scand. 1947;(Suppl):190.

47. Palmquist BM, Philipson B, Barr PO. Nuclear cataract and myopia during hyperbaric oxygen therapy. Br J Opthalmol. 1984;68:113-7.

48. Patz, A. Effect of oxygen on immature retinal vessels. Invest Opthalmol. 1965;4:988-99.

49. Richards IM, Griffin RL, Fidler SF, Jacobsen EJ. Effect of the 21-aminosteroid U-74389F on hyperoxic lung injury in rats. Agents Actions. 1993;39:C136-8.

50. Thom SR. Hyperbaric oxygen – its mechanisms and efficacy. Plast Reconstr Surg [Internet]. 2011 [cited 26 June 2016];127(Suppl 1):131S–141S. Available from: PubMed Central.

51. Torbati D. Effect of propranolol on brain electrical activity during hyperbaric oxygenation in the rat. Undersea Bio Res. 1985;12:423-9.

52. van Ooij PJAM, Hollmann MW, van Hulst RA, Sterk PJ. Assessment of pulmonary oxygen toxicity: relevance to professional diving; a review. Respir Physiol Neurobiol. 2013;189:117-28.

53. Whelan HT, Bajic DM, Karlovits SM, Houle JM, Kindwall EP. Use of cytochrome-P450 mono-oxygenase 2 E1 isozyme inhibitors to delay seizures caused by central nervous system oxygen toxicity. Aviat Space Environ Med. 1998;69(5):480-5.

54. Wright WB. Use of the University of Pennsylvania Institute for Environmental Medicine procedure for calculation of cumulative pulmonary oxygen toxicity. U.S. Navy Experimental Diving Unit; 1972. Report 2-72.

55. Wyttenbach A, Sauvageot O, Carmichael J, Diaz-Latoud C, Arrigo AP, Rubinsztein DC. Heat shock protein 27 prevents cellular polyglutamine toxicity and suppresses the increase of reactive oxygen species caused by huntingtin. Hum Mol Genet. 2002;11(9):1137-51. doi:10.1093/hmg/11.9.1137.

56. Zheng J et al. Saturated hydrogen saline protects the lung against oxygen toxicity. Undersea Hyperb Med. 2010;185-92.

A. Ahmad S, White CW, Chang LY, Schneider BK, Allen CB. Glutamine protects mitochondrial structure and function in oxygen toxicity. Am J Physiol Lung Cell Mol Physiol. 2001 Apr;280(4):779-91.

B. Balestra C, Germonpre P, Poortmans JR, Marroni A. Serum erythropoietin levels in healthy humans after a short period of normobaric and hyperbaric oxygen breathing: the "normobaric oxygen paradox". J Appl Physiol. 2006 Feb;100(2):512-8.

C. Bantseev V, Oriowo OM, Giblin FJ, Leverenz VR, Trevithick JR, Sivak JG. Effect of hyperbaric oxygen on guinea pig lens optical quality and on the refractive state of the eye. Exp Eye Res. 2004 May;78(5):925-31.

D. Bitterman N. CNS oxygen toxicity. Undersea Hyperb Med. 2004;31(1):63-72.

E. Buhrke T, Lenz O, Krauss N, Friedrich B. Oxygen tolerance of the H2-sensing [NiFe] hydrogenase from ralstonia eutropha H16 is based on limited access of oxygen to the active site. J Biol Chem. 2005 Jun 24;280(25):23791-6.

F. Capellier G, Beuret P, Clement G, Depardieu F, Ract C, Regnard J, Robert D, Barale F. Oxygen tolerance in patients with acute respiratory failure. Intensive Care Med. 1998 May;24(5):422-8.

G. Chavko M, Xing G, Keyser DO. Increased sensitivity to seizures in repeated exposures to hyperbaric oxygen: role of NOS activation. Brain Res. 2001 May 11;900(2):227-33.

H. Clark JM. Extension of oxygen tolerance by interrupted exposure.Undersea Hyperb Med. 2004;31(2):195-8.

I. Hampson N, Atik D. Central nervous system oxygen toxicity during routine hyperbaric oxygen therapy.. Undersea Hyperb Med. 2003;30(2):147-53.

J. Helms AK, Whelan HT, Torbey MT. Hyperbaric oxygen therapy of cerebral ischemia. Cerebrovasc Dis. 2005;20(6):417-26.

K. Huang TY, Tsai PS, Wang TY, Huang CL, Huang CJ. Hyperbaric oxygen attenuation of lipopolysaccharide-induced acute lung injury involves heme oxygenase-1. Acta Anaesthesiol Scand. 2005 Oct;49(9):1293-301.

L. Liang LP, Ho YS, Patel M. Mitochondrial superoxide production in kainate-induced hippocampal damage. Neuroscience. 2000;101(3):563-70.

M. Liang LP, Patel M. Mitochondrial oxidative stress and increased seizure susceptibility in Sod2(-/+) mice. Free Radic Biol Med. 2004 Mar 1;36(5):542-54.

N. Plafki C, Peters P, Almeling M, Welslau W, Busch R. Complications and side effects of hyperbaric oxygen therapy.. Aviat Space Environ Med. 2000 Feb;71(2):119-24.

O. Sheffield PJ. How the Davis 2.36 ATA wound healing enhancement treatment table was established. Undersea Hyperb Med. 2004;31(2):193-4.

P. Shinkai M, Shinomiya N, Kanoh S, Motoyoshi K, Kobayashi H. Oxygen stress effects on proliferation rates and heat shock proteins in lymphocytes. Aviat Space Environ Med. 2004 Feb;75(2):109-13.

Q. Smerz RW. Incidence of oxygen toxicity during the treatment of dysbarism. Undersea Hyperb Med. 2004;31(2):199-202.

R. Stephens M, Frey M, Mohler S, Khamis H, Penne R, Bishop J, Bowden A. Effect of caffeine consumption on tissue oxygen levels during hyperbaric oxygen treatment. Undersea Hyperb Med. 1999;26(2):93-7.

S. Suttner DM, Sridhar K, Lee CS, Tomura T, Hansen TN, Dennery PA. Protective effects of transient HO-1 overexpression on susceptibility to oxygen toxicity in lung cells. Am J Physiol. 1999 Mar;276(3 Pt 1):443-51.

T. Topal T, Oter S, Korkmaz A, Sadir S, Metinyurt G, Korkmazhan ET, Serdar MA, Bilgic H, Reiter RJ. Exogenously administered and endogenously produced melatonin reduce hyperbaric oxygen-induced oxidative stress in rat lung. Life Sci. 2004 Jun 11;75(4):461-7.

U. U.S. Navy Diving Manual Rev. 6. Washington, DC: Supervisor of Diving, U.S. Navy, U.S. Government Print Office; 2008.

V. van Hulst RA, Haitsma JJ, Lameris TW, Klein J, Lachmann B. Hyperventilation impairs brain function in acute cerebral air embolism in pigs.. Intensive Care Med. 2004 May;30(5):944-50.

W. Vann RD. Lambertsen and O_2: Beginnings of operational physiology. Undersea Hyperb Med. 2004;31(1):21-31.

X. Weaver LK, Churchill S. Pulmonary edema associated with hyperbaric oxygen therapy. Chest. 2001 Oct;120(4):1407-9.

Y. Yildiz S, Aktas S, Cimsit M, Ay H, Togrol E. Seizure incidence in 80,000 patient treatments with hyperbaric oxygen.. Aviat Space Environ Med. 2004 Nov;75(11):992-4.

APPENDIX – MEASURING PULMONARY OXYGEN TOXICITY

The Unit Pulmonary Toxicity Dose Concept (Original Definition)*

Using the standard treatment protocols as outlined in this manual, there is little or no danger that patients will experience pulmonary oxygen toxicity. If, however, patients must be carried on supplemental O_2 between treatments, pulmonary oxygen toxicity can become a real problem. The UPTD method allows one to predict how soon someone will become toxic when continuously exposed to high partial pressures of oxygen.

The following section is adapted from Rutkowski and Wells outline of this method for "bookkeeping" the pulmonary effects of oxygen exposure as presented in the UHMS/NOAA diving medicine course for physicians. This method was originally developed at the University of Pennsylvania.[1,4]

The "Unit Pulmonary Toxicity Dose" (UPTD) concept of Wright [54] allows one to estimate the degree of pulmonary toxicity incurred by breathing oxygen at partial pressures in excess of 0.5 ATA. Oxygen exposures should be planned so as not to exceed the following limits. During decompression and for treatment of mild decompression sickness, the total oxygen exposure should be limited to that which yields a UPTD of 615 or less. In the use of oxygen for medical therapy or treatment of serious decompression sickness which is responding poorly, an extreme limit of oxygen exposure which yields a UPTD of 1425 or less should be planned. A dose of 1425 will produce a predicted 10% decrease in vital capacity. U. S. Navy Table 6 gives a UPTD of 645. Occasionally these limits are knowingly exceeded when medically required (a Table 6 with multiple extensions, for example).

Having derived a formula for calculating a UPTD, Wright developed a simplified arithmetic method and constructed a table which may be used to calculate oxygen exposure from 0.6 to 5.0 atmospheres. The following arithmetic method enables the calculation of the total UPTD for a given oxygen exposure or sequences of exposures. This method, however, makes no provision for interrupted exposures to elevated oxygen partial pressures. Such interruptions are known to increase oxygen tolerance, but the expected improvement in tolerance has not yet been fully quantitated for humans. Doses of 600 UPTD given in 2 treatment sessions have been administered on a daily basis with no evidence of cumulative toxicity.

*UPTD concept is under revision with addition of new data.

ARITHMETIC METHOD

1. Convert the partial pressure of oxygen breathed at each depth to pO_2 in atmospheres (pO_2 = fraction of inspired O_2 x total pressure in atmospheres).
2. Select the corresponding Kp from Table 1 (above).
3. Multiply the time of exposure (in minutes) at that pO_2 by the corresponding Kp to get the UPTD for that depth.
4. Add the UPTDs for each pO_2 in the complete exposure together to get the total UPTD for the exposure.

APPENDIX REFERENCES

1. Bardin H, Lambertsen CJ. A quantitative method for calculating pulmonary toxicity. Use of the "Unit Pulmonary Toxicity Dose" (UPTD). In: Institute for Environmental Medicine Report. Philadelphia: University of Pennsylvania; 1970.
2. NOAA Diving Manual. Best Publishing Company. GPO #003-017-00468-6.
3. U.S. Navy Diving Manual. Best Publishing Company. NAVSEA 0994-LP-001-9010.
4. Wright WB. Use of the University of Pennsylvania Institute for Environmental Medicine procedure for calculation of cumulative pulmonary oxygen toxicity. U. S. Navy Experimental Diving Unit; 1972. Report 2-72.

REFERENCES BREAKDOWN BY SUBJECT MATTER

Biochemical Mechanisms of Oxygen Poisoning
(1-10)
Manifestations of Oxygen Poisoning: Central Nervous System Effects
(9, 11-15) (16)
Pulmonary Effects
(7, 16-19)
Ocular effects
(20)
Modifications of Oxygen Tolerance
(7, 21, 22, 24)
Management of Oxygen-Induced Seizures
(11, 13, 15, 26)

CHAPTER 4 CHAPTER

Management of Critically Ill Patients in the Monoplace Hyperbaric Chamber

CHAPTER FOUR OVERVIEW

Preface....69
Introduction....69
Approach to the Critically Ill Patient....70
The Hyperbaric Unit....71
Defibrillation....71
Intrahospital Transport of Critically Ill Patients....72
Preparing the Critically Ill Patient for Monoplace HBO_2....73
Patient Monitoring in the Monoplace Chamber....77
Patient Management During HBO_2....82
Intravenous Therapy....82
Ventilation....87
Conclusion....91
Acknowledgments....91
References....92

Management of Critically Ill Patients in the Monoplace Hyperbaric Chamber

Lindell K. Weaver

PREFACE

The most important element of treating critically ill patients with hyperbaric oxygen in the monoplace chamber is the experience of the staff. At our facility, the monoplace chamber is an extension of the critical care environment: in proximity, in equipment, and in personnel. In fact, at one of our two hospitals, the monoplace chamber is moved into the ICU for the treatment of a critically ill patient. Having extensive experience in critical care is vital to managing critically ill patients. This is especially true when performing interventions that effect significant cardiovascular changes, such as hyperbaric oxygen therapy. This chapter is an overview of the manner in which we treat critically ill patients with hyperbaric oxygen at our institutions. To apply some of the techniques that are presented in this chapter to any monoplace unit would be inappropriate. For example, I state that we often intubate, sedate, and paralyze critically ill or comatose patients to carry out hyperbaric treatment. These are skills that are performed on a daily basis in the critical care units. We feel competent with the procedures, drugs, and expected patient responses. However, hyperbaric staff without this background may not feel as comfortable with these aspects of care. Certainly, a brief book chapter cannot train people in critical care. This requires specialized training and years of experience. It is the goal of this chapter to focus on the treatment of critically ill patients in the monoplace hyperbaric chamber. What I hope to do is demonstrate the hyperbaric department as part of a critical care system, which may be of value to others caring for patients in monoplace hyperbaric chambers.

INTRODUCTION

In the past several years, there has been rapid growth in the number of clinical hyperbaric facilities, due in part to the availability of the monoplace, or single-person, hyperbaric chamber and the proliferation of outpatient wound care centers. Monoplace chambers are relatively inexpensive, require fewer personnel, and require less space to operate and maintain than multiplace (walk-in) chambers. Another advantage of the monoplace over the multiplace chamber is that attendants need not enter the hyperbaric chamber with the patient. However, some hyperbaric physicians express concerns about treating unstable or critically ill patients in the monoplace chamber, because of the lack of "hands-on" care during hyperbaric exposure, the lack of suitable equipment for optimal patient care, and the limitations of treatment pressures to 3 atmospheres absolute pressure (ATA). We have found that with a well-trained staff and the availability of appropriate equipment, critically ill patients can be treated safely in the monoplace chamber. We, and others, have presented monoplace chamber use in critically ill patients.[8,20-21,24-25,45-46,48,51,53-56,60-61,63] Anyone who anticipates treating critically ill patients in a monoplace chamber should be familiar with this work.

Also, ground and air transport move critically ill patients frequently. The treatment of critically ill patients in the monoplace chamber, in many ways, is much easier and safer than the care of patients during transport, particularly air transport, with limited access to the patient, cramped spaces, high ambient noise conditions, and no access to personnel or equipment other than the transport team.

APPROACH TO THE CRITICALLY ILL PATIENT

The team concept is an important element of the optimal management of patients in the intensive care unit (ICU). Successful patient management depends upon the integration of physicians, advanced practice clinicians (nurse practitioners and physician assistants), nurses, respiratory therapists, social workers, case managers, ethicists, and others. For the ICU patient requiring hyperbaric oxygen (HBO_2) therapy, it is imperative that the hyperbaric unit be staffed and configured as an extension of the ICU; otherwise, there is risk that the level of care may be lower than in the ICU, which is potentially dangerous to the patient. Therefore, the HBO_2 unit should be staffed with nurses, therapists, and physicians knowledgeable in the management of the critically ill patient, as well as possessing a thorough understanding of hyperbaric physiology and the medical techniques unique to HBO_2.

Furthermore, since the patient generally must be transported to and from the ICU to the chamber, perhaps several times per day, the patient may be exposed to additional risks.[7,30,35] Alternatively, the monoplace chamber either resides in the ICU or is moved to the ICU for the treatment of critically ill patients.[62] The risk/benefit ratio of HBO_2 and the risk of transport must be carefully evaluated in critically ill patients. A hypothetical example would be a patient with respiratory distress syndrome with multiple chest tubes requiring intravenous pressors, high partial pressures of oxygen (O_2), and high airway pressures, who develops clostridial gas gangrene. Most hyperbaric physicians would agree that gas gangrene should be treated with HBO_2, but to move such a patient to the chamber, much less to treat him or her in the chamber (monoplace or multiplace), may present more risk than withholding HBO_2. Experience and careful weighing of the risk versus the benefit in these situations is important.

There are many details of the ICU patient that require attention prior to the transport of the patient to the chamber for hyperbaric treatment. These include informed consent, recording of the ventilator settings and blood gases, filling the endotracheal tube cuff with sterile saline, capping off unnecessary intravenous catheters and drains, placing chest tubes to Heimlich one-way valves, changing arterial pressure and electrocardiograph (ECG) monitors to the appropriate portable units, and adequately sedating the patient if clinically indicated. Also, it is very important to conduct a safety time-out[3] and ensure no prohibited items enter the chamber prior to compression. In addition, the patient will need to be able to equalize middle-ear pressure during compression and decompression. These items will be discussed in more detail below.

In addition, it is critically important that mistakes are not made regarding any lines that are disconnected and reconnected. Treating critically patients in monoplace chambers requires multiple lines and monitoring devices and catheters to be disconnected and reconnected multiple times per HBO_2 treatment. This Food and Drug Administration (FDA) website discusses such mishaps: https://www.fda.gov/MedicalDevices/Safety/AlertsandNotices/TubingandLuerMisconnections/ucm313275.htm. In addition to verifying that no prohibited items enter the chamber, a safety time-out is also critically important to verify all intravenous (IV), connections, proper drugs, correct IV drip rates, security of mechanical ventilation tubing, adequacy of mechanical ventilation, and no disallowed items in the chamber.[3]

THE HYPERBARIC UNIT

If the hyperbaric unit anticipates treating critically ill patients, appropriate emergency medical equipment and supplies need to be readily available, and the staff need to be trained and familiar with the equipment function. This includes equipment for maintenance of an artificial airway, ventilators, hemodynamic monitors, a defibrillator, suction apparatus, oximeters, IV catheters, IV tubing sets, extension tubing, infusion pumps, chest tube insertion trays, and the drugs employed in the management of critically ill patients.

Ample space in the chamber area is requisite. There may be several medical personnel attending to the critically ill patient prior to the HBO_2 treatment, so it is important to have enough room for access to both sides of the patient (Figure 1).

Special equipment is necessary to deal with the ICU patient in the monoplace chamber. This includes electrical pass-throughs for monitoring of the ECG and pressures from invasive catheters, IV pass-throughs, and a gas pass-through for the ventilator. We have designed or modified other equipment that permits

1. suctioning of tubes and drains,[41]
2. use of air-breaks with mechanical ventilation during HBO_2,[42]
3. noninvasive blood pressure (BP) monitoring,[47,64]
4. monitoring of pulmonary artery hemodynamics, measurement of thermodilution of cardiac output, and mixed venous blood oximetry,[48] and
5. simultaneous use of up to four IV lines through a single monoplace chamber hatch penetrator.

Subsequent sections will discuss these modifications and techniques.

DEFIBRILLATION

I have defibrillated one patient and cardioverted another patient after their rapid removal from the monoplace chamber for dysrhythmias. Some hyperbaric practitioners have recommended that patients exiting the oxygen-filled chamber be moved some distance away from the chamber prior to defibrillation, because of concerns about the risk of combustion. The patient's tissues (including the brain and heart) presumably will have high concentrations of O_2, so taking a few extra seconds to move the patient to an area with a lower ambient concentration of O_2 should be acceptable. In the two cases commented upon above, a few seconds elapsed following extraction of the patients from the chamber before defibrillation. Both patients were defibrillated/cardioverted while on the gurney attached to the monoplace chamber. There was no evidence of sparks or fire. Provision for cardiac monitoring, defibrillation, bag-valve-mask ventilation, and

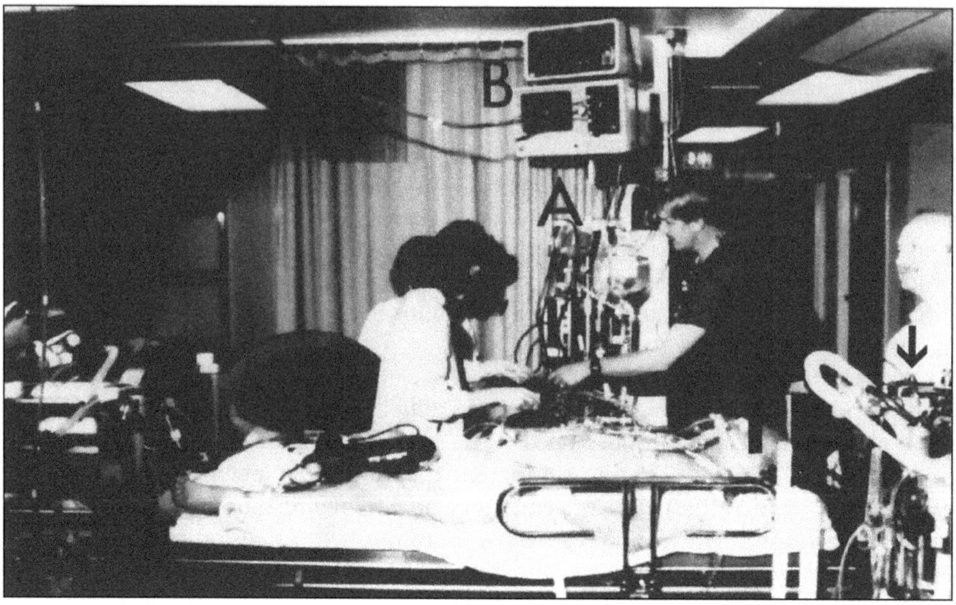

Figure 1. Preparing to place a critically ill patient with necrotizing fasciitis and septic shock in the monoplace chamber. A liquid oxygen–powered transport ventilator (arrow) ventilated the patient during transport. The patient received intravenous total parenteral nutrition, blood transfusion, and continuous infusions of levophed, fentanyl, and propofol (A). The physiologic monitor and end-tidal CO_2 monitor (B) is located in a position that is easily observed by the chamber operator. Ample room is important.

intubation must be readily available if the hyperbaric unit anticipates treating critically ill patients. [Former editor's note (Dr. Eric Kindwall): We have measured oxygen levels in the room after emergency decompressing and opening a monoplace chamber. The cold oxygen falls to the floor and dissipates in about 30 seconds. It does not measurably remain elevated at the level of the patient or rise in other parts of the room.]

INTRAHOSPITAL TRANSPORT OF CRITICALLY ILL PATIENTS

Paramount in the safe transport of critically ill patients is a knowledgeable and experienced staff. Critically ill patients can be safely transported to the HBO_2 chamber, but it is important to recognize that ICU care must continue without disruption during the transport to minimize adverse consequences to the patient. If the patient requires mechanical ventilation and positive-end expiratory pressure (PEEP), ventilation with a portable transport ventilator or a manually operated bag-valve incorporating a PEEP attachment are suggested. If PEEP is removed for patient transport, the patient's pulmonary gas-exchange efficiency may decrease, which may reduce the ability of the patient to oxygenate into the hyperbaric range during HBO_2. If there is concern about the adequacy of ventilation, arterial blood gases (ABG) may be necessary to inspect the pH and arterial carbon dioxide tension ($PaCO_2$). Monitoring of the end-tidal CO_2 ($EtCO_2$) and pulse oximetry during transport can serve as aids in determining the adequacy of pulmonary gas exchange and alert the transport team to potential ventilation and/or oxygenation problems.

The ECG rhythm and BP should be monitored if the patient is at risk for hemodynamic instability or if the patient is receiving continuous infusions of cardiovascular-active drugs such as levophed or nitroprusside. Several portable transport monitors are available that are compact and battery operated. A transport defibrillator may be necessary if the patient has dysrhythmias or if the critical staff are concerned in this regard.

Critically ill patients commonly have continuous IV infusions of maintenance fluids, cardiovascular drugs, total parenteral nutrition (TPN), insulin, antibiotics, analgesics, and sedatives. Some of these can be withheld for the transport, but some must be continued. Utilizing volumetric infusion pumps facilitates the administration of IV agents during transport. The team needs to take emergency drugs (e.g., lidocaine, epinephrine, etc.) along with the patient.

A transport cart that attaches to the patient's gurney is useful to carry multiple IV pumps, monitors, O_2 cylinders, a portable suction device, and containers with clearly labeled emergency drugs.

PREPARING THE CRITICALLY ILL PATIENT FOR MONOPLACE HBO_2

The cardiac rhythm and BP (if an arterial catheter is present) should be monitored during the time that preparations are underway for placing the patient in the chamber. The patient's endotracheal tube can be connected to the hyperbaric ventilator circuit, and appropriate adjustments can be made in the minute ventilation (VE). The Sechrist 500A hyperbaric ventilator (Sechrist Industries, Inc., Anaheim, CA) entrains ambient gas (air if the chamber hatch is open) to deliver an appropriate tidal volume (VT). If the patient requires high fractional inspired concentrations of O_2 (FiO_2), the patient may develop arterial hypoxemia, unless supplemental O_2 is provided to the entraining valve area. Pulse oximetry can be useful to monitor for hypoxemia. The patient needs to be clothed in a gown endorsed by the chamber manufacturer such as 100% cotton or an appropriate blend.[29] According to the National Fire Protection Association Section 14.3.1.5.4.1:

> *"Except where permitted in 14.3.1.5.4.3 silk, wool, or synthetic textile or synthetic textile materials, or any combination thereof, shall be prohibited in Class A or Class B chambers."* [29]

Section 14.3.1.5.4.2 states:

> *"Garments permitted inside of chambers shall be as follows: (1) Garments fabricated of 100 percent cotton or a blend of cotton and polyester fabric shall be permitted in Class A chambers. (2) Garments fabricated of 100 percent cotton, or a blend of cotton and polyester fabric containing no more than 50 percent polyester, shall be permitted in Class B chambers."* [29]

Comatose patients, or patients pharmacologically sedated, should be physically restrained to prevent them from inappropriately pulling on lines and tubes and to position their extremities in safe positions. We restrain a patient by placing soft restraints on the wrists, pulling one of the restraints under the ipsilateral buttock and up through the groin, then tying the restraint from the contralateral wrist to the other. If the elbows splay out too far (now that monoplace chambers are larger, this is less of a need), or if the IV catheters are kinked by binding of the arms at the elbow, we wrap

Kerlex gauze around the elbows and tie the ends together, pulling the elbows inward. Care must be taken to ensure that the gauze does not cause excessive local pressure. Combative or anxious patients should be pharmacologically sedated and, if intubated, possibly pharmacologically paralyzed as well. The staff that sedates patients must have the requisite training, experience, and credentialing by the institution. Surgical drains may be capped off. If the drain requires suction during HBO_2, or if a wound is covered by a vacuum closure device, suction can be performed in the monoplace chamber.(41) Chest tubes need to have the drainage system removed and a Heimlich valve inserted. The drainage tubing can then be placed to suction or left open to ambient pressure. In my experience, commercially available pleural drainage systems generally break when compressed in the chamber, so chest tubes need to be connected to Heimlich valves.

Some monoplace chambers are limited in the number of IV pass-through ports. This aspect of the chamber requires careful consideration of which drugs and IV solutions are necessary during HBO_2. For example, if the patient is receiving separate infusions of TPN and insulin, those two infusions could be joined together before infusing the solution through the chamber. If the patient is receiving drugs such as levophed, nitroprusside, midazolam, or potent analgesics by continuous infusion, then do not anticipate using that particular IV line for anything else during the course of HBO_2, since "pushing" another drug in that IV line would result in a bolus of a potent cardiovascular agent to the patient, with concomitant potential adverse consequences. A knowledge of which drugs are compatible with one another is important when combining IV agents in the same IV line.

Some critically ill patients require more IV lines than are available in some monoplace chambers. Our solution to this limitation was to develop special pass-through penetrators that allow up to four IV lines to pass through 1 chamber hatch orifice (Figure 2, Figure 3, Figure 4). Details of this solution are available (the appendix of reference 46). Similarly, another special chamber hatch penetrator permits passage of the Sechrist 500A ventilator gas supply and provides pass-through ports for the suction device(41) and for monitoring $EtCO_2$ during HBO_2 (Figure 5).(13) A port for supplying either O_2 or air to an anesthesia bag fixed about the Sechrist 500A ventilator entraining venturi is a modification that permits intermittent air breathing to mechanically ventilated patients undergoing HBO_2.(42) This specially manufactured pass-through conserves the other chamber hatch orifices, permitting them to be available for IV use, an important factor in treating critically ill patients in the monoplace chamber. Some monoplace chambers have sufficient pass-throughs for critical care, and some chambers have metal plates that can be machined to accommodate more than one IV port.

Preferably, intubated patients should have an endotracheal (ET) tube that is a low-pressure, high-volume design (to reduce the risk of tracheal necrosis). Prior to HBO_2, air is evacuated from the ET tube cuff, and the cuff is gently filled with sterile saline to achieve an appropriate seal with as minimal pressure as possible. After HBO_2, the saline is removed, and the cuff is filled with air, with documentation of an acceptable cuff pressure. The ET tube needs to be securely tied in the appropriate position. Restraining the patient, to prevent the patient from self-extubation or from pulling IV catheters, should be considered.

Some hyperbaric physicians recommend that myringotomies be performed on all intubated patients to prevent middle- and inner-ear barotrauma.(15) However, other hyperbaric practitioners, including myself, do not routinely perform prophylactic myringotomies in intubated patients. If myringotomies are not performed, our

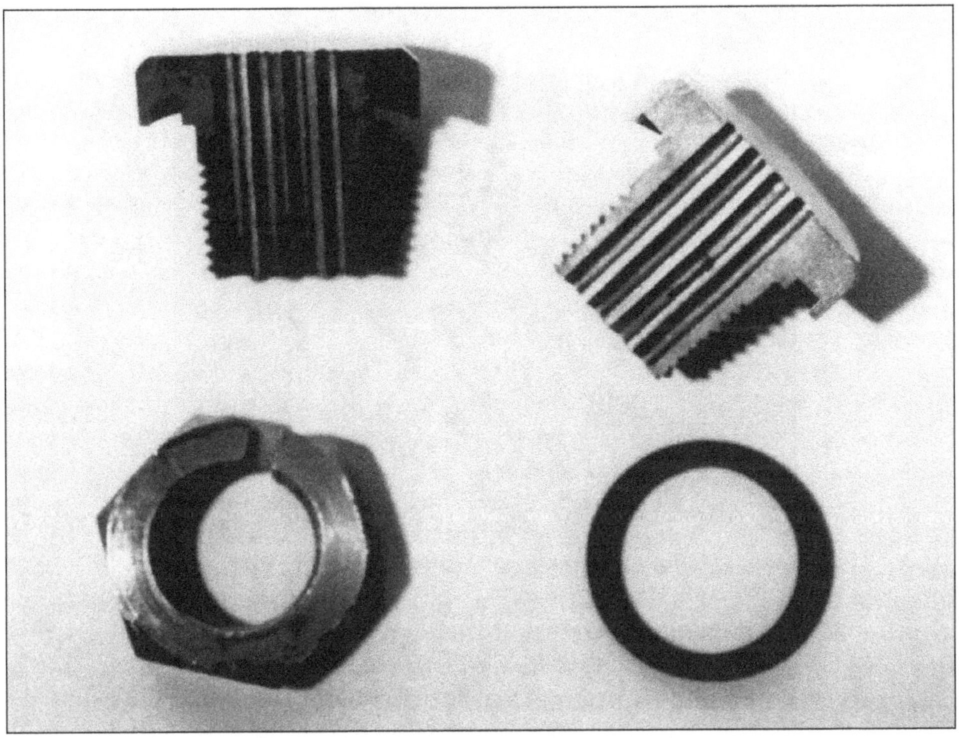

Figure 2. Split bolt pass-through, nut, and O-ring that permits up to four intravenous (IV) pressure lines to pass through a single Sechrist chamber hatch pass-through orifice.

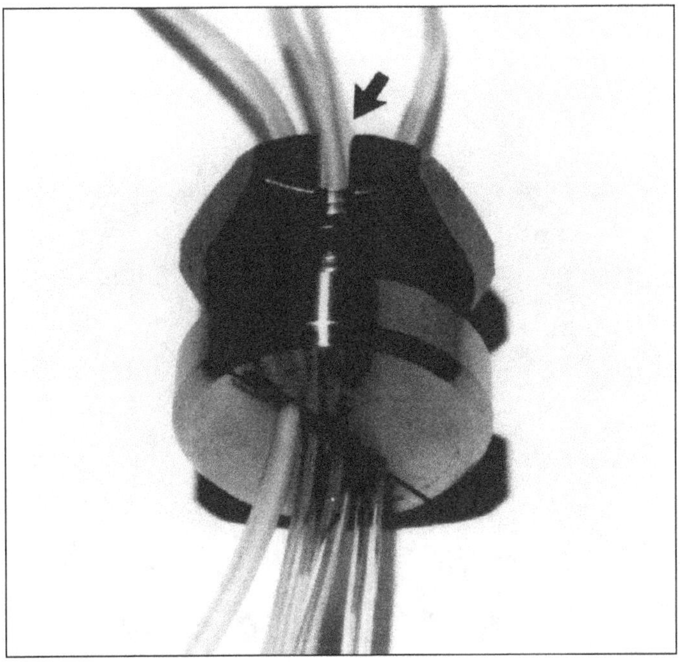

Figure 3. Ratchet and special socket (arrow) to tighten the nut onto the split bolt. The bolt is slightly tapered so as the nut is tightened, the bolt halves are drawn tightly together.

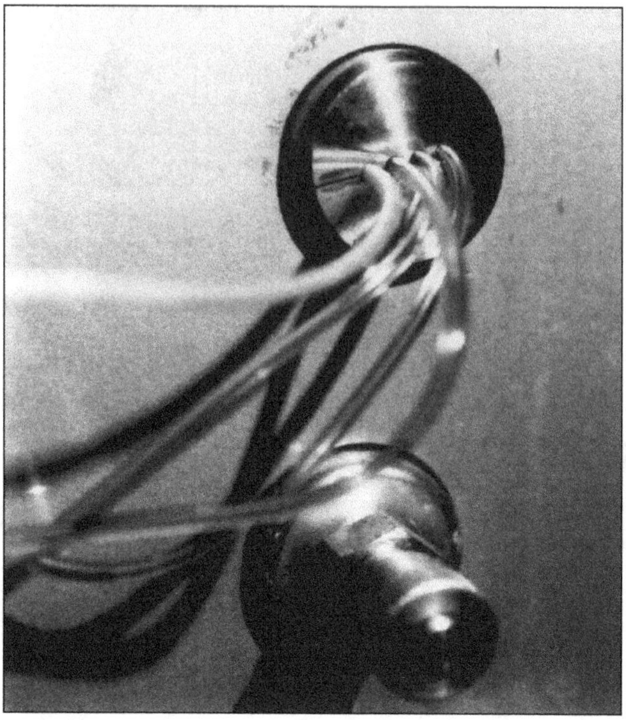

Figure 4. Split bolt pass-through and four IV lines installed in the door of the Sechrist chamber. One-way back-check valves are located between the IV tubing connections and the catheters inside the chamber (not shown).

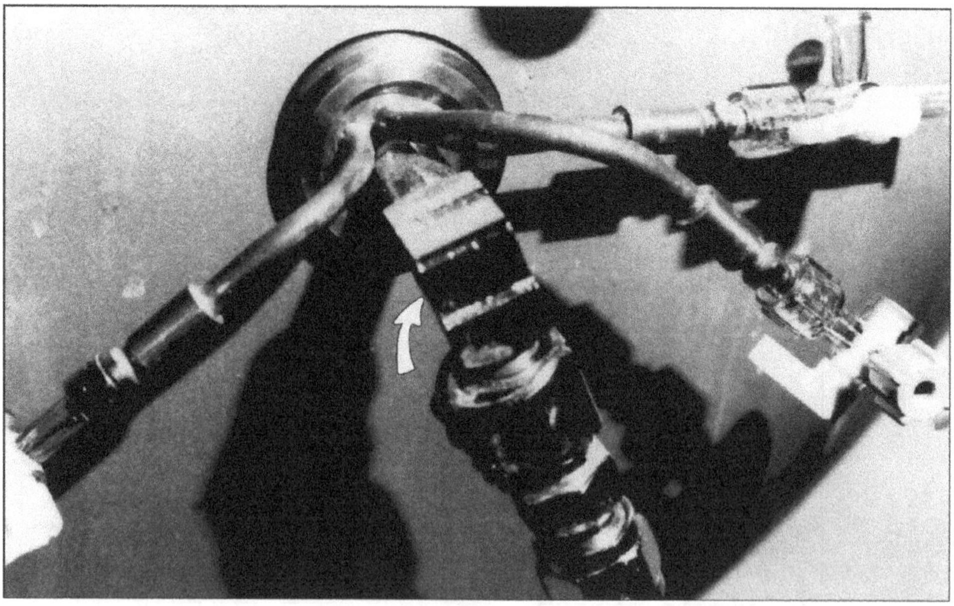

Figure 5. Four-in-one modified pass-through. This pass-through permits passage of a 1/8-inch NPT for the ventilator gas supply (arrow) and three additional ports (e.g., suction $EtCO_2$ monitoring and operation of the Doppler noninvasive blood pressure device).

practice style has been to sedate the intubated patient to facilitate passive inflation of the middle-ear space during hyperbaric compression. Presently, there is no controlled clinical information indicating that myringotomies are absolutely required in intubated patients treated with HBO_2.

If the individual hyperbaric physician deems that the patient requires myringotomies, I recommend specific training in this procedure, ideally from otolaryngologists.

PATIENT MONITORING IN THE MONOPLACE CHAMBER

The majority of patients (non-critically ill) treated in monoplace chambers can be safely monitored by direct observation alone. The respiratory rate is evident, as well as manifestations of anxiety which can be a warning sign of central nervous system (CNS) O_2 toxicity.[12] Critically ill patients require additional monitoring, which is determined clinically.

The cardiac rhythm is easily monitored during HBO_2 by placing electrocardiographic leads on the patient which pass out of the chamber via an electrical pass-through (the Sechrist monoplace chambers incorporate a 19-pin electrical pass-through) (Figure 6) allowing electrical leads to pass from the chamber to a physiologic monitor. The hospital bioengineering personnel can make the appropriate cables in this regard. The monitoring system should permit graphing and the delayed inspection of adverse or suspected dysrhythmic events.

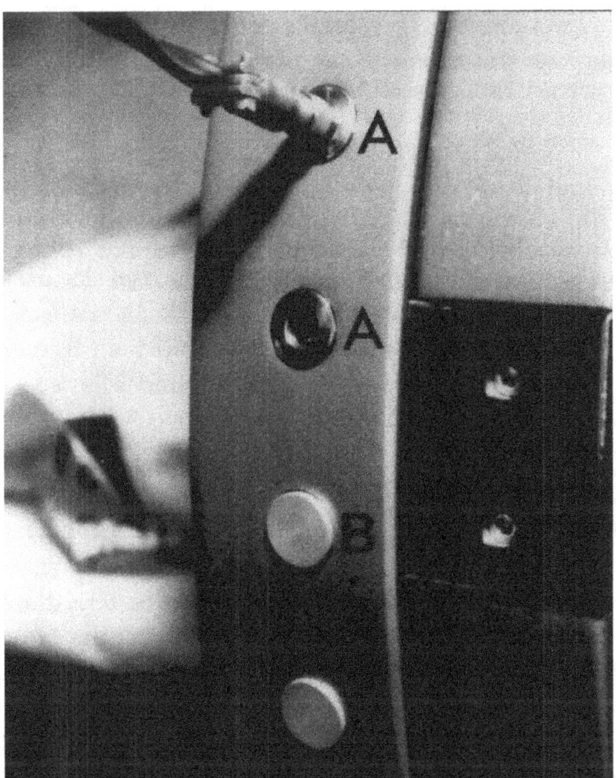

Figure 6. Sechrist monoplace 19-pin electrical pass-throughs (A) and blank plugs (B).

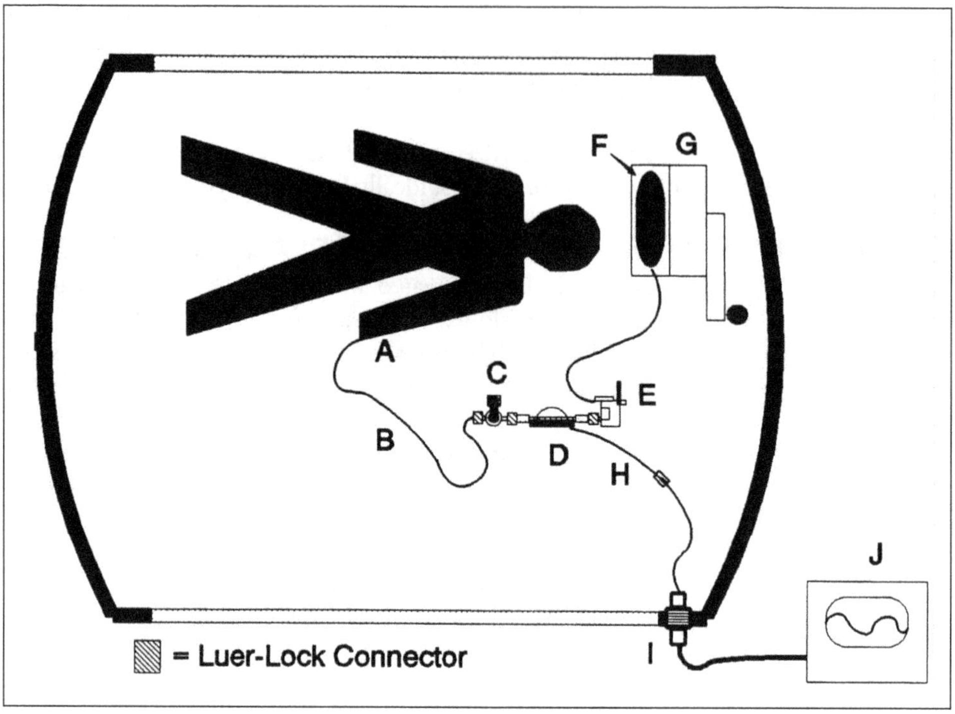

Figure 7. Schematic representation of invasive blood pressure monitoring system in the monoplace chamber. The arterial catheter (A) is connected to 4-foot neonatal Argon pressure tubing (B). A stopcock (C) is placed proximal to the pressure transducer (D). An intraflow (E) flushes the transducer and catheter continuously at 3 ml/hr. Saline (F) is pressurized (300 mmHg) by a Ethox Infuser (G) to provide the intraflow with adequate pressure to maintain system patency. The transduce signal is passed out of the chamber by its electrical leads (H) connected to the Sechrist 19-pin electrical pass-through (I) and displayed by a physiologic monitor (J).

In critically ill patients, the BP is generally measured by an indwelling arterial catheter connected to a pressure transducer through which an electrical signal is passed out of the chamber to a physiologic monitor (Figure 7). The catheter and transducer are continually flushed with sterile saline at three ml per hour by a continuous flush device, which is standard in intensive care.[18] The continuous flush device is connected to a bag of saline maintained at 300 mmHg pressure by a Surgi-press pressure infuser made for HBO_2 applications (Ethox Corp., 251 Seneca St., Buffalo, NY 14204). A formerly available pressure infuser (Tycos) had a petroleum-based grease as a bearing lubricant which should not be used in the hyperbaric O_2 environment because of the risk of fire,[40] so cannot be placed inside an oxygen-filled monoplace chamber. Prior to chamber compression, the pressure transducer should be zeroed to the appropriate reference level. Also, the arterial pressure waveform should be inspected to ensure that adequate dynamic response is present in the system for interpretation.[16-17] If the BP monitoring system has inadequate dynamic response, the pressure and waveform will not be an accurate representation of the patient's true BP; this is a significant implication considering the potent drugs often infused in patients to raise or lower the BP. Gardner's review and recommendations are strongly encouraged for anyone practicing invasive monitoring.[17]

Noninvasive BP monitoring can be accomplished in the monoplace chamber. We developed a system for noninvasive BP monitoring, incorporating a Doppler flow detector to determine the systolic BP.[47,64]

An automated BP system (Oscillomate 1630, CAS Medical Systems, Inc., Branford, CT) once existed.[28] This BP monitoring device inflates the cuff automatically from outside the chamber, at a preset interval. The instrument also displays the mean arterial pressure and the heart rate and has adjustable alarms. Unfortunately, this system is no longer available.

Mechanically ventilated patients should have several respiratory variables monitored during HBO_2. These include ventilatory rate (VR), expired VT, PEEP, airway pressure with an analog monitor, ventilator O_2 supply pressure, and presence of spontaneous breathing by the patient.

The $EtCO_2$ can be followed during HBO_2 and may provide useful information regarding the adequacy of alveolar ventilation.[13] Sidestream $EtCO_2$ measurements may be performed by placing the sampling port at the proximal airway adjacent to the ET tube and passing this sampling line out of the chamber. Gas is analyzed by a CO_2 detector. The expected $EtCO_2$ would be the predicted value x atmospheric pressure/chamber pressure (in absolute units). For example, assume the $EtCO_2$ is 40 Torr at our altitude (0.85 ATA). At a chamber pressure of 3.0 ATA, the displayed $EtCO_2$ ideally would be 11.3 Torr (40 x 0.85/3.0). Measuring $EtCO_2$ is helpful in adjusting the mechanical ventilator and provides a continuous display for respiratory rate. $EtCO_2$ can also be monitored in nonintubated, spontaneously breathing patients who are wearing a low-volume nasal cannula as a sampling catheter that is passed out of the chamber and analyzed by the $EtCO_2$ monitor. As expected, there is more variability in the measurement, but it can be useful to follow trends in the individual patient, particularly if the patient is given sedatives or analgesics.

Arterial blood gases of patients treated with HBO_2 can be monitored. This technique requires a setup permitting aspiration of arterial blood out of the pressurized chamber (Figure 8). It is important to use Luer-Lock connections and hard-pressure tubing. The continuous flush device can be used by placing a four-way stopcock between the arterial pressure transducer and the continuous flush device. The handle of the four-way stopcock should be positioned so that the continuous flush device, the sampling line, and the transducer are all in direct communication. Incorporating the continuous flush device in this system prevents the arterial catheter from clotting. We have demonstrated that the ABL 330 blood gas instrument (Radiometer, Copenhagen, Denmark) can accurately measure O_2 tension of saline and blood in tonometry experiments.[44] Further studies have verified that the ABL 330 can also measure accurately the arterial O_2 tension (PaO_2), pH, and arterial carbon dioxide tension ($PaCO_2$) of subjects[49] and patients exposed to HBO_2.[52] Unfortunately, the ABL 330 is no longer available or supported by Radiometer, including service and parts. More recent versions of Radiometer blood gas instruments appear capable of measuring hyperbaric oxygen tensions too,[50,59] although in my experience they are not as accurate as the ABL 330, especially with O_2 tensions above 1,500 Torr.

We often measure ABGs to determine the adequacy of mechanical ventilation (pH and $PaCO_2$) during HBO_2. Personnel who perform ABG measurements of patients in the monoplace chamber need to be aware of several potential risks. Retrograde arterial gas embolism can occur if any gas is introduced into the arterial catheter.[9] Inadvertent rapid loss of blood could ensue if a catheter or connector becomes accidentally disconnected. Embolic phenomena may occur if clots or thrombi are infused into the

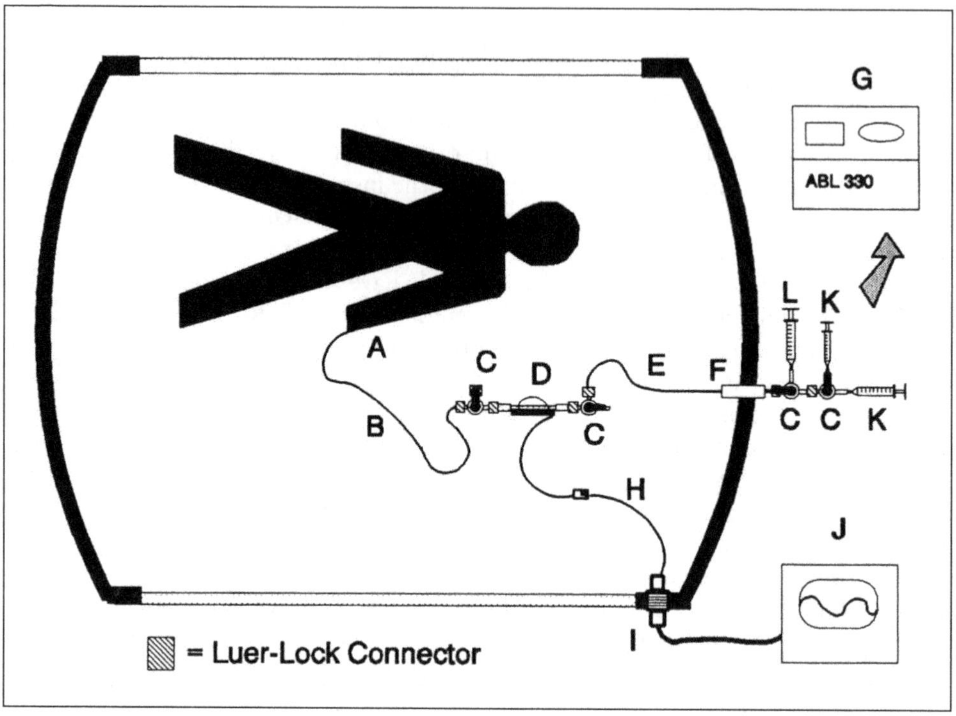

Figure 8. Schematic representation of the system we use to aspirate arterial blood out of the compressed monoplace chamber. The pressure monitoring system is analogous to Figure 8. Arterial blood can be withdrawn by connecting a stopcock (C) to the distal side of the pressure transducer (D). A 4- or 6-foot neonatal Argon pressure line (E) connects to a Argon hyperbaric sterile, disposable pass-through (F) (See blow-up of pass-through in Figure 10). A 10 ml Luer-Lock syringe (L) collects the dead-space volume during sampling, and a 3 ml blood gas syringe (K) is used to collect the arterial sample in a midstream fashion. The sample is analyzed immediately in the Radiometer ABL 330, ABL 500, or ABL 800 blood gas machines (G).

arterial catheter. Iatrogenic blood loss is possible, since one should ideally withdraw three times the system dead space prior to obtaining the arterial blood sample to reduce preanalytical errors. For an ABG sample, typically this volume is approximately 10cc. If no contraindications, and if obtained using strict aseptic technique, and with physician order, the dead-space blood can be heparinized and given back to the patient in a venous line.

Patients who have pulmonary dysfunction, requiring supplemental O_2 at atmospheric pressure to have adequate arterial O_2 content, may require higher chamber pressures to have similar hyperbaric PaO_2 as patients with normal lungs at lower chamber pressures [52] (Table 1). Therefore, it may be reasonable to treat patients with abnormal lungs (i.e., an increased right-to-left intrapulmonary shunt fraction) with chamber treatment pressures higher than for patients with normal lungs, but there is no evidence doing so alters outcome favorably.

Accurate measurement of PaO_2 during treatment may be important to titrate the treatment pressure. This observation also has implications for patients who are mechanically ventilated with the Sechrist 500A ventilator, because its performance is marginal at chamber pressures > 2.0 ATA.[43] The optimal PaO_2 of patients requiring HBO_2 is unknown. Tissue PO_2 is the measurement that is likely to aid in titrating the dose of HBO_2. Unfortunately, invasive tissue O_2 tension measurements are not easily

TABLE 1. ARTERIAL OXYGEN TENSION OF PATIENTS WITH ABNORMAL PULMONARY FUNCTION[52]

PCH (ATM)	N	PaO_2*	PaO_2 MEAS	PaO_2 CORR	PaO_2 (a/A2 ratio)	PaO_2 (from pre HBO_2 a/A)
0.85**	22	564±10	269±81	269±81	0.487±0.14	0
2	6	1433±10	1083±232	1162±232	0.76±0.16	278±138
2.4	15	1740±8	1168±293	1272±293	0.67±0.17	394±242
2.9	32	2113±11	1282±230	1416±230	0.61±11	396±266
3	19	2195±7	1420±185	1561±185	0.61±0.17	531±306
0.85***	9	562±7	254±144	254±144	0.45±0.25	0
0.85****	18	219±75	95±49	95±49	0.48±0.25	0

*Alveolar PO_2-O_2 values expressed as mean ± 1 S.D. **a/A ratio from 0.85 ATA pre HBO_2 data
100% O_2 *<100% O_2

performed and are certainly not yet practical as a useful tool to titrate HBO_2 dosing. Also, even the process of measuring tissue O_2 tensions may alter the local tissue O_2 tension.

We generally do not offer HBO_2 to patients requiring > 50% FiO_2 for adequate arterial saturation at atmospheric pressure unless the risk/benefit ratio clearly favors treating with HBO_2. If we do treat such patients with HBO_2, ABG measurements are performed during HBO_2. Even at 3 ATA, some of these patients have such severe pulmonary dysfunction that they are unable to achieve PaO_2 values > 1000 Torr, and frequently considerably lower. Furthermore, these patients generally require PEEP and high VE so adequate ventilation becomes a significant limitation with the Sechrist 500A ventilator. The PaO_2 during HBO_2 cannot be predicted in patients with abnormal pulmonary function (arterial/alveolar ratio < 0.75) from measurements made at atmospheric pressure.[52] In patients with considerable pulmonary dysfunction who require high FiO_2s, we generally withhold HBO_2 until the patient's pulmonary function improves.

It is possible to monitor the intracranial pressure (ICP) during HBO_2 in the monoplace chamber with a transducer system analogous to the invasive BP monitoring system.[20,36] Similarly, the electroencephalogram (EEG) signal can be passed out of the chamber via 19-pin electrical pass-throughs.

Transcutaneous oxygen ($PtcO_2$) measurements are commonly employed by both multiplace and monoplace chambers.[22,27,58] Radiometer (Copenhagen, Denmark) has developed a transcutaneous O_2 monitor that is intrinsically, electrically safe, meeting Underwriter's Laboratories' criteria for use in a 100% O_2 environment.[33] Other transcutaneous manufacturers offer monitors that can measure $PtcO_2$. Special cables to pass the transcutaneous probes into chambers are usually available from the chamber manufacturers. The $PtcO_2$ data may be useful in predicting the response to HBO_2 in problem wounds.[14,20,27,39]

To summarize, with innovation and modifications to existing equipment, patients can be monitored in the monoplace hyperbaric chamber similarly as in the ICU. The degree of monitoring required for the individual patient depends upon the clinical scenario and the physician's and hyperbaric staff's experience with critical care in the monoplace chamber. Most patients can be sufficiently monitored with the ECG and BP, whether noninvasive or invasive. If clinically indicated, other monitoring modalities such as EEG, ICP, and $PtcO_2$ measurements are relatively straightforward to accomplish.

PATIENT MANAGEMENT DURING HBO_2

A staff that has experience treating critically ill patients is the most important element of delivering HBO_2 to critically ill patients. The hyperbaric staff needs to be familiar with hyperbaric medicine and physiology, but it is also mandatory that they are skilled in dealing with critical care. If the HBO_2 unit only sees critically ill patients rarely (e.g., a septic patient with gas gangrene or necrotizing fasciitis once per year), that level of experience may be inadequate to maintain proper skills. Training evolutions can be can be useful to maintain practice skills of treating critically ill patients. Also, rotating the HBO_2 staff through the ICU is a method of maintaining their critical care medicine skills. The HBO_2 unit must have physicians trained in critical care and hyperbaric medicine immediately available if the unit is treating critically ill patients.

If the patient is not alert, prior to HBO_2, it may be prudent to intubate the patient for airway protection. Assuming the staff has adequate expertise, it may be safer to pharmacologically control combative or semicomatose patients who require HBO_2. Patients who are at risk of vomiting and aspiration, or of awakening abruptly inside the chamber in an anxious or combative state, may pull out lines and possibly harm themselves before sedatives can be provided. It is mandatory that paralytic agents not be used unless the patient is adequately sedated. Anesthesiology can offer guidance for sedation. Typically, our center uses continuous infusions of fentanyl and propofol to achieve adequate sedation of mechanically ventilated adult patients treated with HBO_2. These patients need arterial pressure monitoring, preferably with an arterial catheter, and often need levophed delivered via a central venous catheter and titrated to maintain adequate blood pressure.

Neuromuscular blocking agents are used to pharmacologically paralyze patients. The patient must be adequately sedated prior to use of paralytic agents, since these drugs have no sedative or amnestic properties. Obviously, if patients are paralyzed, or even sedated, they will not demonstrate with compression the typical expected clinical responses from a pneumothorax, seizure, or auditory or sinus pain. It is critical that chamber personnel pay close attention to the patients' exhaled VTs, airway pressures, and evidence of auto-PEEP. Air breaks[42] may be provided to intubated patients to reduce the risk of CNS O_2 toxicity, especially in patients who are paralyzed and who cannot demonstrate the typical manifestations of O_2 toxicity. It is mandatory that the staff administering sedation, analgesia, and paralysis have credentials to do so and the necessary training and experience to essentially render general IV anesthesia during HBO_2.

INTRAVENOUS THERAPY

Intravenous infusions are provided to compressed patients in the monoplace chamber by passing the IV tubing through the chamber bulkhead via a special sterile IV pass-through (Figure 9, Figure 10).

The IV line passes from inside the chamber hatch to outside. It is unnecessary to completely disassemble the IV pass-through device. By loosening the knurled pass-through fitting, the sterile, disposable pass-through can be inserted. Once inserted, the knurled fitting is tightened down to achieve a seal. The hyperbaric IV pass-through and

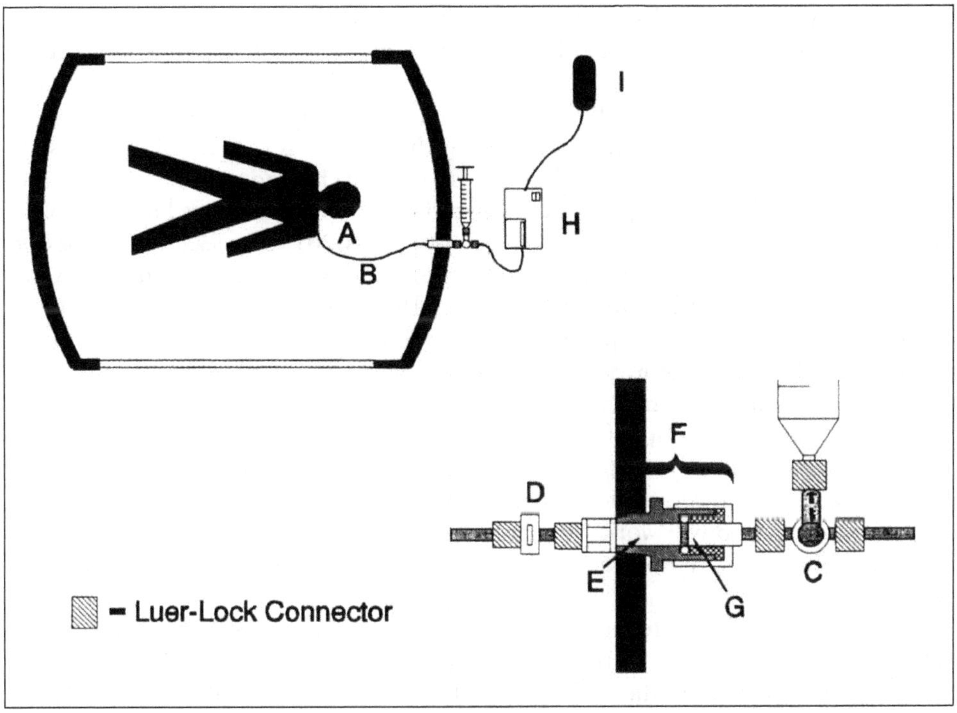

Figure 9. Schematic representation of method of delivering intravenous (IV) solutions to patients compressed in the monoplace chamber. The IV catheter (A) is Luer-Lock connected to pressure tubing (B). The pressure tubing is connected to a one-way back-check valve (D) located inside the chamber. This valve permits unidirectional flow of fluids towards the patient. Shown is a Argon hyperbaric pass-through (E). The pass-through is passed out of the chamber by a Swagelok metal fitting (F). A pressure seal is accomplished by an O-ring (G). A stopcock (C) is located just outside the chamber. Medications are pushed at this point. IV solutions (I) are pumped into the patient by a high pressure pump (H).

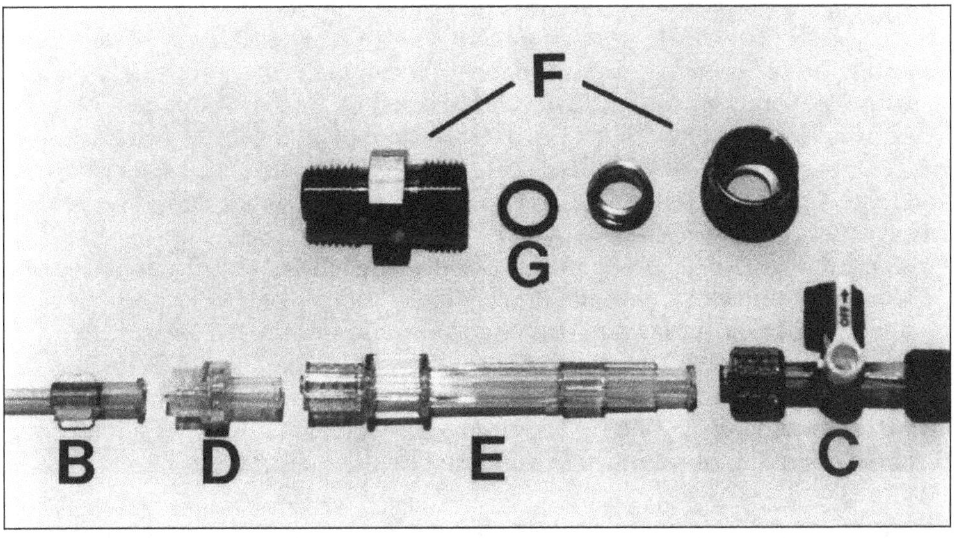

Figure 10. Argon sterile disposable hyperbaric IV pass-through (E). Use the legend and schematic in Figure 9. The Swagelok fitting (F) is shown disassembled.

back-check valve (Argon Medical Devices, Athens, TX) (Figure 10) allows removal of the back-check valve (e.g., for blood gas measures) and has a relatively low dead-space volume of approximately 6 ml. The IV line must be flushed with IV solution. For continuous infusions of drugs, the line is flushed with the appropriate solution.

High-pressure IV infusion pumps permit the controlled delivery of IV fluids. At this time there is no FDA-approved IV infusion pump for monoplace chamber use. However, several IV infusion pumps can infuse fluids to patients treated in monoplace hyperbaric chambers. One such pump is the Flo-Gard® #6201 volumetric pump (Baxter, Deerfield, IL) (Figure 11). This pump is no longer available from the manufacturer but may be available by chamber supply companies. This pump can deliver up to 1,999 ml per hour of IV crystalloid to a patient compressed to 19 psig (2.1 ATA at our altitude of 1,430 m). During compression the occlusion alarm is activated, but once 2 ATA pressure is reached, the alarm can be reset and the pump operates satisfactorily. The FlowGuard® pump will not infuse IV fluids above approximately 2 ATA unless the occlusion alarm sensitivity is altered or defeated, an alteration that is not endorsed by the manufacturer. However, the hospital bioengineering department can adjust this alarm, and this pump will work satisfactorily to 3 ATA chamber pressures.[5,31,57] For accurate IV infusions, the Baxter pump requires a specially designed IV infusion set, available from Baxter.

Other IV pumps that can infuse crystalloid fluids up to 3 ATA are the Zyno-800F (Zyno Medical LLC, Natick, MA) (Figure 12) and the CME 323 Bodyguard Color Vision (Caesarea Medical Electronics, Caesarea, Israel.[5] At this time the CME 323 is not available in the United States.

It is important to have a one-way or back-check valve in-line in the IV tubing (Figure 9, Figure 10). The back-check valve prevents retrograde blood return in case of an IV-line disconnect outside the pressurized hyperbaric chamber. The back-check valve can be located inside the chamber anywhere along the IV line. Luer-lock pressure tubing should be used inside the chamber to prevent inadvertent IV-tubing

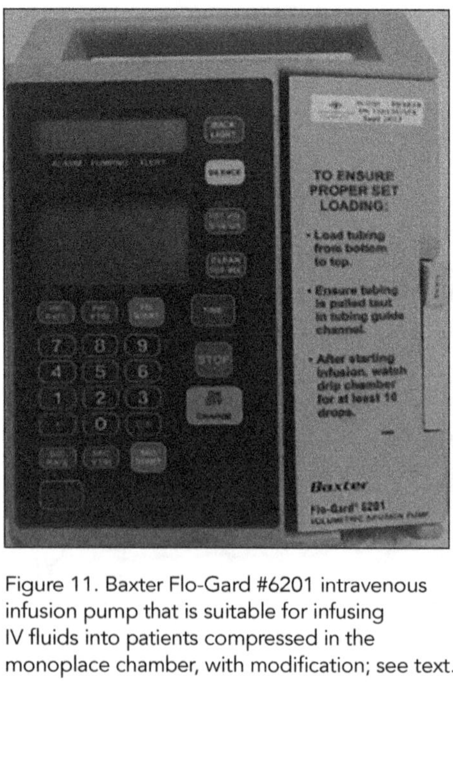

Figure 11. Baxter Flo-Gard #6201 intravenous infusion pump that is suitable for infusing IV fluids into patients compressed in the monoplace chamber, with modification; see text.

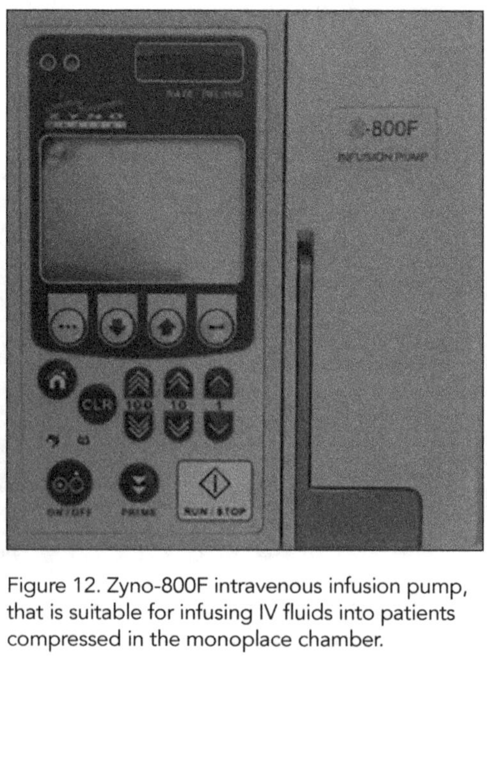

Figure 12. Zyno-800F intravenous infusion pump, that is suitable for infusing IV fluids into patients compressed in the monoplace chamber.

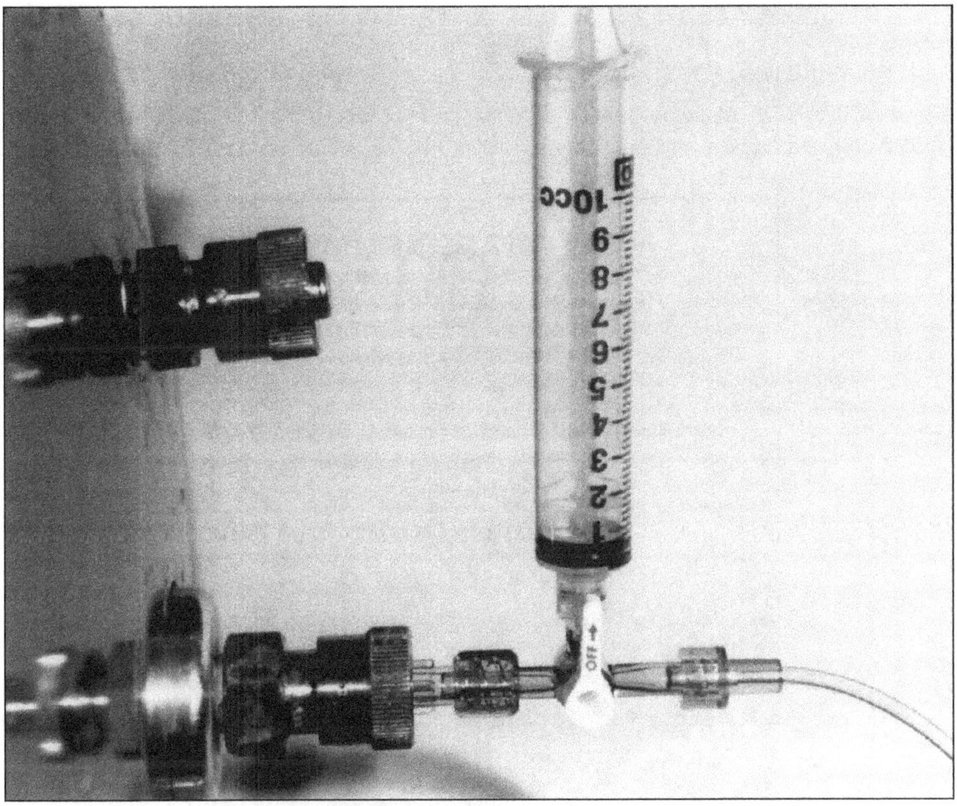

Figure 13. Medications are pushed into the IV line by a syringe Luer-Lock connected to a 3-way stopcock located at the chamber pass-through. Adequate volumes of IV fluid must be pushed behind the medication to push it through the tubing dead-space (generally 6–15 ml) in order for the medication to reach the patient.

disconnections or kinking of the IV tubing. At the present time, there is only 1 manufacturer for IV tubing, back-check valves, and pass-throughs (Argon Medical Devices, Athens, TX).

Intravenous medications are given as controlled infusions or as bolus injections. To give a bolus injection, the drug is drawn up in a 3 ml luer-lock syringe. The needle is removed, and the syringe tightly luer-lock connected to a three-way stopcock located just outside the chamber bulkhead hatch (Figure 9, Figure 10, Figure 13). The drug is injected into the IV line. The drug must be flushed through the IV tubing dead space to arrive at the patient. This is accomplished by drawing up approximately 10 ml of compatible IV solution and injecting it behind the medication. The smaller the syringe plunger diameter, the easier it is to push the fluid into the IV line (e.g., force = pressure x area). The amount of flush solution is determined by the volume of tubing dead space. With adult six-foot Argon tubing the system dead space is 6 ml. With six-foot Argon neonatal tubing the dead space is approximately 2.5 ml. To initiate a potent pressor such as levophed in a hypotensive patient inside the chamber requires either that levophed has been primed in a dedicated IV line in anticipation or that it must be started once the patient has been compressed. To begin levophed in the latter circumstance requires the clinical team to know precisely when the levophed has been flushed through the tubing dead space and when it reaches the patient, to avoid administering the patient a levophed bolus which could be harmful.

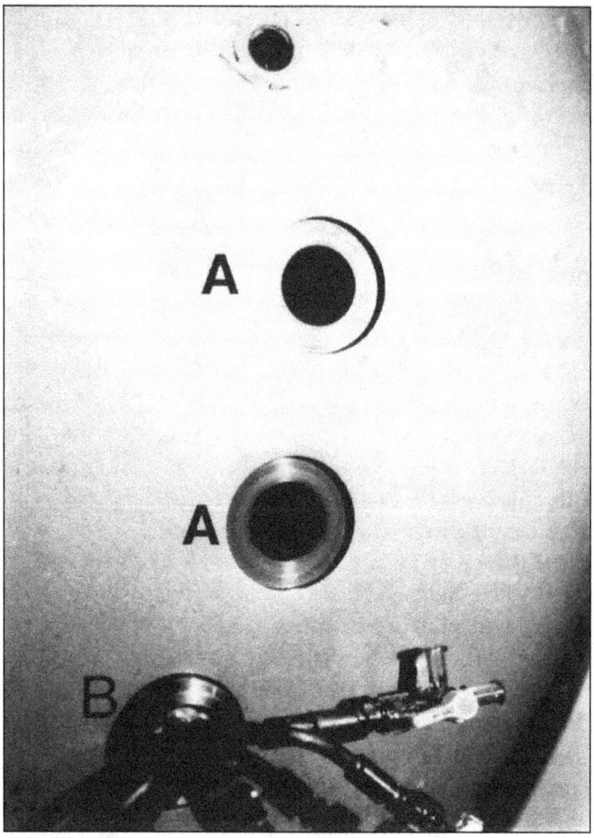

Figure 14. Sechrist 2500B monoplace chamber hatch. Depicted are 2 open orifices which measure 13/16-inch diameter (A). it is possible to pass more than 1 line or tube through these orifices (See Figures 2-4). Notice the 4-in-1 pass-through (B) (See Figure 5).

Total parenteral nutrition and insulin infusions are sometimes discontinued during HBO_2.[32] We generally do not discontinue TPN or insulin during HBO_2. Generally, we favor continuing TPN during HBO_2 because discontinuing the TPN predisposes to hypoglycemia, reduces the net caloric balance per day, and potentiates swings in the patient's nutritional balance. Total parenteral nutrition requires a dedicated IV line. Also, enteral feeding can be continued during HBO_2. By passing the enteral feeding tube into the chamber via an Argon disposable IV pass-through, continuous enteral feeds can be continued during HBO_2 by infusing the feeding solution with the IV infusion pump. Strict adherence to insuring the enteral feeding tube is not mistakenly connected to a vascular catheter is mandatory.

The patient's response should be monitored after infusing medications. Sedatives may contribute to hypercarbia, a risk factor for CNS O_2 toxicity.[12] Analgesics can cause hypotension, so BP monitoring of patients who are receiving these agents may be necessary. A flow sheet can be helpful in documenting physiologic responses to medications. Also, communication and documentation in the patient's inpatient record of the type, dose, route, and time of medications is important.

Some monoplace hyperbaric chambers have limited numbers of IV pass-through ports. Although not commonly in use, the Sechrist 2500B monoplace chamber only has five pass-through orifices in the chamber hatch, each of 13/16-inch diameter (Figure 14). The hatch may not be altered, according to American Society of Mechanical Engineers - Pressure Vessel for Human Occupancy (ASME-PVHO) guidelines. However, the newer, larger-diameter chambers have more pass-through capability than the 2500B. It is difficult, and potentially dangerous for the physician, to treat critically ill patients with HBO_2 if there are inadequate numbers of IV pass-throughs. For the HBO_2 session, certain IV infusions can be discontinued or run piggyback. However, some critically ill patients may still require more than five IV lines (fewer than five are available if mechanically ventilating the patient or if inspecting ABGs during HBO_2). Our solution to the limited number of pass-throughs in the 2500B chamber was to design a pass-through permitting several IV lines to pass through a single chamber hatch orifice.[(48)]

Septic patients requiring pressors frequently drop their BP during chamber compression and decompression. Intravascular volume expansion and/or increasing the dose of their pressor is often required to treat the hypotension. The BP reduction during chamber compression is likely due to a reduction in the dose of pressor delivered to the patient by the IV infusion pump[(5,31)]. This hypotension is managed by transiently increasing the infusion rate of the pressor while monitoring blood pressure continuously.

VENTILATION

Patients with gas gangrene, necrotizing fasciitis, carbon monoxide poisoning, or arterial gas embolism may be intubated and require mechanical ventilation. Mechanical ventilation can be performed in the monoplace chamber. Some aspects of mechanical ventilation that are particularly important are described here.

The endotracheal tube (ET) needs to have an adequate internal diameter. Gas density is greater in the compressed chamber, so the minute ventilation (VE) and the ability of the patient to exhale will be limited if the ET tube lumen is too small. This is a problem if the VE is high (> 10 liters/minute) and if the lungs are stiff, requiring high airway pressures and positive end-expiratory pressure (PEEP) > 5 cm H_2O.

If the maintenance of an adequate airway is questionable, the patient should be intubated prior to HBO_2. Likewise, if the patient is combative and requiring IV sedation, it may be prudent to intubate such a patient to prevent possible aspiration and hypercarbia, a risk factor for CNS O_2 toxicity during HBO_2.[(12)]

There are several ventilators commercially available for use in the monoplace chamber in the United States. The 500A hyperbaric ventilator (Sechrist Inc., Anaheim, CA) dates back to the 1970s and is one that is commonly used in the United States. The 500A ventilator circuit is located inside the chamber hatch (Figure 15), and the ventilator controls are located outside the chamber (Figure 16). The 500A is a pneumatic, time-cycled ventilator that permits adjustments for flow, inspiratory time, and expiratory time (Figure 16). When the ventilator cycles, O_2 moves through the ventilator control unit into the ventilator block supply hose and into the ventilator block, simultaneously closing the exhalation valve to augment VT. Some O_2 is routed through a water-filled nebulizer to provide humidity to the inspiratory circuit. VT is measured with a spirometer located inside the chamber connected to the expiratory limb of the ventilator circuit. Airway pressure is measured in the ventilator block, not at the proximal airway (Figure 15). PEEP is provided by placing PEEP valves in the expiratory circuit (Figure 17).

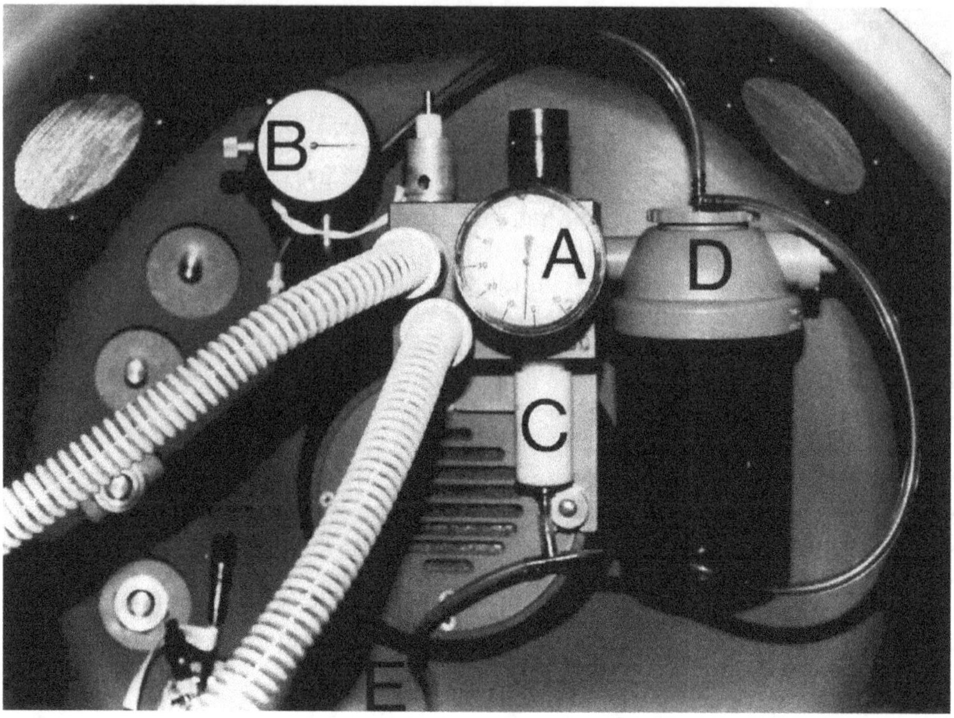

Figure 15. Sechrist 500A hyperbaric ventilator block and circuit are positioned inside the chamber hatch. Airway pressure is measured by a manometer (A). A spirometer (B) located on the exhalation side of the circuit measures exhaled tidal volumes. The entraining venture (C) augments tidal volume. The nebulizer (D) is also powered from the control module (Figure 16) located outside the chamber.

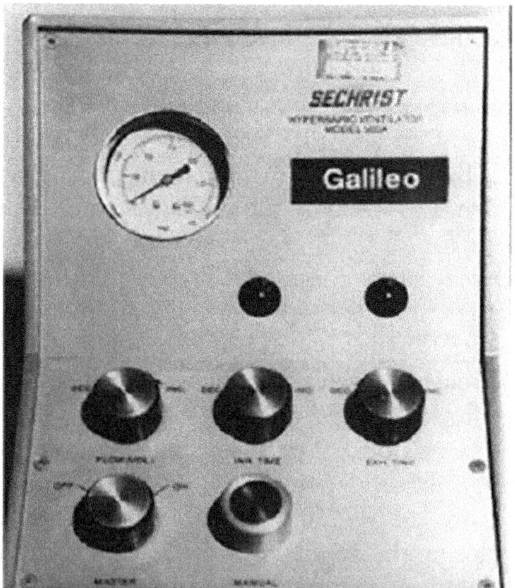

Figure 16. Control unit of the Sechrist 500 hyperbaric ventilator. Flow, inhalation time, and exhalation time are adjusted by turning the appropriate knobs.

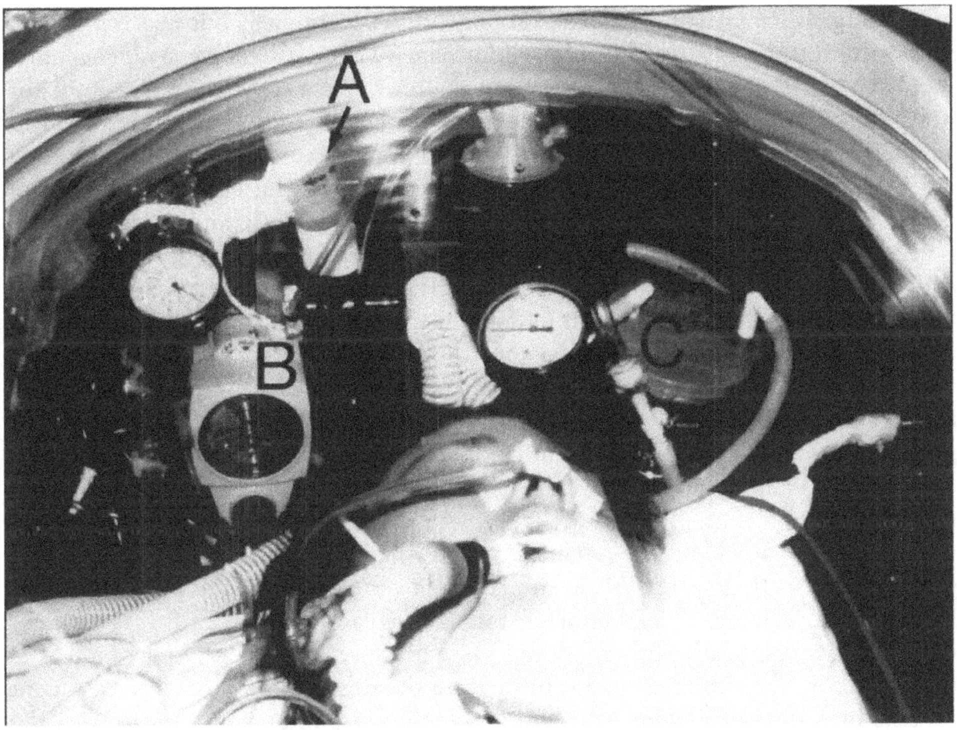

Figure 17. Positive and expiratory pressure (PEEP) is provided to patients in the monoplace chamber by placing PEEP valves (A) at the exhalation port of the 500A ventilator circuit. A vacuum regulator (B) and suction canister (C) are also being used in this patient with necrotizing fasciitis and myonecrosis.

Ventilator controls allow changes in inspiratory time, expiratory time, and inspiratory gas flow. The tidal volume is delivered by adjusting the inspiratory time and flow, whereas the ventilation rate is primarily determined by adjustments in expiratory time.

A single O_2 hose leads from the controls through a ventilator pass-through in the chamber hatch and connects to the inlet hose of the ventilator block (Figure 5, Figure 14, Figure 15).

A peak pressure pop-off valve is located on the 500A ventilator block and should be adjusted prior to use for each particular patient. A 1-way valve permits the patient to inspire (nonmechanical breath). As originally designed, the 500A provides only a fractional inspired concentration of 1.00 O_2. With modifications, the 500A ventilator can deliver air as well as O_2,[42] which may be important to prevent CNS and pulmonary O_2 toxicity.[6,12,23]

Because the 500A operates in the control mode only, generally the patient will need to be sedated and, rarely, may need neuromuscular blocking agents. Also, sedation is often important to minimize patient-ventilator asynchrony which could result in gas-trapping or auto-PEEP; or, the patient could resist a breath during a controlled mechanical breath which could result in pulmonary barotrauma, a serious complication in a compressed patient.

The 500A performance is particularly limited with a VE > 15 liters/minute, especially at chamber pressures > 2.0 ATA.[43] For optimal ventilator performance, the ventilator driving pressure must be at least 65 psig and preferably up to 85 psig.

Most hospitals have wall O_2 pressures of only 50 to 55 psig, which is unacceptable to supply the 500A ventilator. The 500A performance was evaluated over a range of inlet supply pressures, test lung compliances, and chamber pressures.[43] The 500A ventilator performance is inadequate to ventilate patients with a compliance < 60 ml/cm H_2O who require > 5 cm H_2O PEEP, with a VE > 15 liters/minute at chamber pressures > 2.0 ATA. Furthermore, the VT and VR change significantly during pressurization and depressurization of the chamber.[40] Careful monitoring of VT, VR, and airway pressures is necessary, as the chamber pressure is altered with titration of flow, inspiratory time, and expiratory time to achieve the desired VE. There are no alarms incorporated in the 500A ventilator, so astute attention to detail is mandatory when using it. One needs to weigh carefully the risk/benefit ratio of treating mechanically ventilated patients in the monoplace chamber, especially if the patient has pulmonary dysfunction requiring higher airway pressures and high VE. The measurement of pH and $PaCO_2$ can help guide the adequacy of mechanical ventilation. Inspecting ABG measurements prior to compression, while the patient is ventilated with the 500A, and during HBO_2, should be considered.

In order to provide a VE > 10 liters/minute, the 500A ventilator uses an inverted/ expiratory ratio (I-time exceeds E-time). An inverted I/E ratio is not necessarily harmful, but operators of this ventilator must be vigilant of auto-PEEP. If the patient is hypotensive, especially with a reduced pulse pressure, it very likely may be due to the ventilator. The treatment is not to increase the dose of levophed. The treatment consists of adding expiratory time and shortening inspiratory time. Even with the 500A flows set to maximum, small VTs are the rule. Some mechanically ventilated patients must be hypoventilated (increased $PaCO_2$) to prevent auto-PEEP. Presumably, hypoventilation increases the risk of CNS O_2 toxicity.[12] Use of the 500A ventilator in critically ill patients treated in the monoplace chamber is one of the skills requiring the highest level of expertise and attention.

Other ventilators are available for monoplace chamber use. The Omni-vent (Allied Healthcare Products, St. Louis, MO), $MaxO_2$ (Medical Support Products, Lancaster, PA), and Magellan (Oceanic Medical Products, Atchison, KS) are all very similar to each other and in some regard to the 500A. These ventilators are all pneumatic and allow adjustments of the inspiratory and expiratory times and inspiratory flow. The performance of the Omni-Vent can exceed that of the 500A,[10-11] but this ventilator requires considerable experience and attention to detail. The FDA has approved one ventilator for monoplace chamber use, the Atlantis (Atlantis BaroVent, Providence Global Medical, Holladay, UT; and the PGM Atlantis, AHV-1, Perry Baromedical, Riviera Beach, FL). This ventilator is similar to the Omni-Vent, but I cannot comment about its performance. I have not comprehensively evaluated this ventilator although brief information about bench testing is available[19]. The "Sieretron 1000 IPER lung ventilator for hyperbaric chamber" (Siare Engineering International Group, s.r.l., Valsamoggia, Italy, distributed by West Care Medical, Ltd., Chilliwack, BC, Canada) is electronic and similar to ventilators used in the ICUs. It does not have FDA approval for use with monoplace chambers, and there are no publications about its performance available with monoplace chamber use, but this ventilator potentially offers several advantages, such as alarms, adjustable PEEP, different ventilator modes, etc. Of note, for this ventilator to be used in the monoplace chamber, the chamber must be filled with air, rather than oxygen, and the exhaled gas must be "dumped" overboard from the chamber to minimize fire risk.

CONCLUSION

Critically ill patients can be treated with HBO_2 in the monoplace chamber. Just as with treating critically ill patients in general, treating them with HBO_2 requires attention to detail. The critically ill patient needs to have an adequate airway, adequate numbers of IV lines, and caregivers who possess a thorough understanding of the limitations of IV infusion pumps, monitoring, and mechanical ventilation in the monoplace chamber. Suction, $EtCO_2$ monitoring, measurement of hyperbaric PaO_2, and increased numbers of IV lines increase the ability of monoplace units to offer HBO_2 to critically ill patients safely.

A thoroughly knowledgeable staff, skilled in the management of critically ill patients, is the most important element in delivering HBO_2 to these patients. Next, this staff must do critical care to maintain high-level competency. Also important is a hyperbaric medicine department that has the required additional equipment readily available to treat critically ill patients. The close proximity of the HBO_2 chambers to the ICU area facilitates the delivery of HBO_2 to critically ill patients. Obviously a sound foundation in HBO_2 physiology, risks, and benefits is central to applying HBO_2 to patients, especially if they are critically ill.

ACKNOWLEDGMENTS

I wish to thank Steve Howe, MA, for drawing the schematic figures. Appreciation is extended to George Hart, MD, Eric Kindwall, MD, Robert Goldmann, MD, and Gaylan Rockswold MD for building the foundation for treating critically ill patients in the monoplace chamber.

REFERENCES

1. American Society of Mechanical Engineers. Safety Standard for Pressure Vessels for Human Occupancy. American Society of Mechanical Engineers, United Engineering Center, New York, NY. 2016.
2. Bell JE, Weaver LK, Churchill SC, Holm JR. Survey of UHMS members regarding the use of 100% cotton or a blend in Class A and B chambers. Undersea Hyperb Med. 2008;35(4):267.
3. Bell JE, Christoffersen PB, Holm JR, Churchill SK, Weaver LK. Implementing a safety "time out" in the hyperbaric setting. Undersea Hyperb Med. 2008;35(4):268.
4. Bell J, Weaver LK, Deru K. Performance of the Hospira Plum A+ (HB) hyperbaric infusion pump. Undersea Hyperb Med. 2014;41(3):235-43.
5. Bell J, Weaver LK, Deru K. Performance of the Z-800F, Body Guard 323 Color Vision™ & Flo-Gard® 6201 infusion pumps for monoplace chamber use. Undersea Hyperb Med. 2016;43(1):9-19.
6. Bleiberg B, Kerem D. Central nervous system oxygen toxicity in the resting rat: postponement by intermittent oxygen exposure. Undersea Biomed Res. 1988;15(5):337-52.
7. Braman SS, Dunn SM, Amico CA, et al. Complications of intra-hospital transport in critically ill patients. Ann Int Med. 1987;107:469-73.
8. Camporesi EM, Moon RE. Management of critically ill patients in the hyperbaric environment [editorial]. J Hyperbaric Med. 1987;2(4)195-8.
9. Chang C, Dughi J, Shitabata P, et al. Air embolism and the radial arterial line. Crit Care Med. 1988;16:141.
10. Churchill S, Weaver LK, Haberstock D. Omni-vent: another option for mechanical ventilation in the monoplace hyperbaric chamber. Undersea Hyperbaric Med. 1998;25(Suppl):24.
11. Churchill S, Weaver LK, Haberstock D. Performance of the Omni-vent mechanical ventilator for use with the monoplace hyperbaric chamber. Undersea Hyper Med. 1999;26(Suppl):70-1.
12. Clark JM, Thom SR. Oxygen under pressure. In: Brubakk AO, Neuman TS, editors. Bennett and Elliot's physiology and medicine of diving. 5th ed. London: WB Saunders Company, Ltd.; 2003. p. 358-418.
13. Eskelson MI, Weaver LK, Greenway LG. End-tidal CO2 monitoring within the monoplace hyperbaric chamber [abstract]. Undersea Biomed Res. 1989;16(Suppl): 18-19.
14. Faglia E, Favales F, Aldeghi A, et al. Change in major amputation rate in a center dedicated to diabetic foot care during the 1980s: prognostic determinants for major amputation. J Diabetes Complications. 1998;12(2):96-102.
15. Farmer JC Jr. Ask the expert. Pressure. 1998;27(5):12-3.
16. Gardner RM. Direct blood pressure measurement – dynamic response requirements. Anesthesiology. 1981;54:227-36.
17. Gardner RM. Hemodynamic monitoring: from catheter to display. In: Weil MH, editor. Acute care. Basel, Switzerland: S. Karger AG; 1986; p. 3-33.
18. Gardner RM, Bond EL, Clark JS. Safety and efficacy of continuous flush systems for arterial and pulmonary artery catheters. Ann Thorac Surg. 1977;23:534-8.
19. Gates W, Redd A. The Atlantis mechanical ventilator, specifically developed for hyperbaric chamber utilization. Undersea Hyperb Med. 2011;38(5):439-40.

20. Gossett WA, Rockswold GL, Rockswold SB, Adkinson CD, Bergman TA, Quickel RR. The safe treatment, monitoring and management of severe traumatic brain injury patients in a monoplace chamber. Undersea Hyperb Med. 2010 Jan-Feb;37(1):35-48.
21. Hart G. Equipment and procedures – monoplace chambers. In: Shilling CW, Carlson CB, Mathias RA, editors. The physician's guide to diving medicine. New York: Plenum Press; 1984. p. 621-5.
22. Hart GB, Meyer GW, Strauss MB, et al. Transcutaneous partial pressure of oxygen measured in a monoplace hyperbaric chamber at 1, 1.5, and 2 ATA oxygen. J Hyperbaric Med. 1990;5(4):223-9.
23. Hendricks PL, Hall DA, Hunter WH Jr, Haley PJ. Extension of pulmonary oxygen tolerance in man at 2 ATA by intermittent oxygen exposure. J Appl Physiol: Resp Environ Exercise Physiol. 1977;42:593-9.
24. Holcomb JR, Matos-Navarro AY, et al. Critical care in the hyperbaric chamber. In: Davis JC, Hunt TK, editors. Problem wounds. New York: Elsevier; 1988. p. 200-9.
25. Kindwall EP, Goldmann RW. Hyperbaric medicine procedures. 7th ed. Milwaukee (WI): St. Luke's Medical Center; 1995.
26. Layton W, Weaver L, Haberstock D. Modifications to the Omni-Vent ventilator for use within the monoplace hyperbaric chamber. Undersea Hyperbaric Med. 1998;25(Suppl):56.
27. Mathieu D, Wattel F, Bouachour G, et al. Post-traumatic limb ischemia: prediction of final outcome by transcutaneous oxygen measurement in hyperbaric oxygen. J Trauma. 1990;30(3):307-14.
28. Meyer GW, Hart GB, Strauss MB. Noninvasive blood pressure monitoring in the hyperbaric monoplace chamber. J Hyperbaric Med. 1990;4(4):211-6.
29. National Fire Protection Association (Quincy, MA), NFPA 99, 2015 Edition, Chapter 14 Section 14.3.1.5.4.1 & 14.3.1.5.4.2. http://www.nfpa.org/
30. Nuckols TK. Reducing the risks of intrahospital transport among critically ill patients. Crit Care Med. 2013;41(8):2044-5.
31. Ray D, Weaver LK, Churchill S, Haberstock D. Baxter Flo-Gard 6201 volumetric infusion pump for monoplace chamber applications. Undersea Hyperb Med. 2000;27(2):107-11.
32. Riseman JA, Zamboni WA, Curtis A, et al. Hyperbaric oxygen therapy for necrotizing fascitis reduces mortality and the need for debridements. Surgery. 1990;108:847-50.
33. Salomon A. Safety of the Radiometer transcutaneous monitors when measuring in hyperbaric chambers. TC109 Bulletin, Radiometer. Copenhagen, Denmark: A/S; 1990. p. 1-10.
34. Sheffield PJ. Tissue oxygen measurements. In: Davis JC, Hunt TK, editors. Problem wounds. New York: Elsevier; 1988. p. 17-51.
35. Stevenson VW, Haas CF, Wahl WL. Intrahospital transport of the adult mechanically ventilated patient. Respir Care Clin N Am. 2002;8(1):1-35.
36. Sukoff MH, Ragatz RE. Hyperbaric oxygenation for the treatment of acute cerebral edema. Neurosurgery. 1982;10:29-38.
37. Voigt LP, Pastores SM, Raoof ND, Thaler HT, Halpern NA. Review of a large clinical series: intrahospital transport of critically ill patients: outcomes, timing, and patterns. J Intensive Care Med. 2009;24(2):108-15.
38. Wattel FE, Mathieu DM, Fossati P, et al. Hyperbaric oxygen in the treatment of diabetic foot lesions. J Hyper Med. 1991;6(4):263-8.

39. Wattel F, Pellerin P, Mathieu D, et al. Hyperbaric oxygen therapy in the treatment of wounds, in plastic and reconstructive surgery. Ann Chir Plast Esthet. 1990;35(2):141-6.

40. Weaver LK. Tycos Pressure Infuser: some precautions before using in the chamber. Pressure. 1987;16(6):15.

41. Weaver LK. A functional suction apparatus within the monoplace hyperbaric chamber. J Hyperbaric Med. 1988;3(3):165-71.

42. Weaver LK. Air breaks with the Sechrist 500A monoplace hyperbaric ventilator. J Hyperbaric Med. 1988;3(3):179-86.

43. Weaver LK, Greenway L, Elliott CG. Performance characteristics of the Sechrist 500A hyperbaric ventilator in a monoplace hyperbaric chamber. J Hyperbaric Med. 1988;3(4):215-25.

44. Weaver LK, Howe S, Berlin SL. Normobaric measurement of O2 tension of blood and saline tonometered under hyperbaric O2 conditions. J Hyperbaric Med. 1990;5(1):29-38.

45. Weaver LK. Monitoring and life support. In: Weaver LK, Strauss MB, editors. Monoplace hyperbaric chamber safety guidelines. Bethesda (MD): Undersea and Hyperbaric Medical Society; 1991 Sep. p. 31-48.

46. Weaver LK. Clinical applications of hyperbaric oxygen-monoplace chamber use. In: Moon RE, Camporesi EM, editors. Problems in respiratory care – clinical application of hyperbaric oxygen. Philadelphia: JB Lippincott; 1991. : p. 189-214.

47. Weaver LK, Howe S. Noninvasive Doppler blood pressure monitoring in the monoplace hyperbaric chamber. J Clin Monit. 1991;7:304-8.

48. Weaver LK. Technique of Swan-Ganz catheter monitoring in patients treated in the monoplace hyperbaric chamber. J Hyperbaric Med. 1992;7(1):1-18.

49. Weaver LK, Howe S. Normobaric measurement of arterial oxygen tension of normal human subjects exposed to hyperbaric oxygen. Chest. 1992;102:1175-81.

50. Weaver LK, Ershler L, Howe S. Accuracy of the Radiometer ABL 500 measuring hyperbaric blood gases at atmospheric pressure. Undersea Biomed Res. 1992;19(Suppl):105.

51. Weaver LK. Management of critically ill patients in the monoplace hyperbaric chamber. In: Kindwall EP, editor. Hyperbaric medicine practice. Flagstaff (AZ): Best Publishing Company; 1994. p. 173-246.

52. Weaver LK, Howe S. Arterial oxygen tension of patients with abnormal lungs treated with hyperbaric oxygen is greater than predicted. Chest. 1994;106:1134-9.

53. Weaver LK, Strauss MB, editors. Monoplace hyperbaric chamber safety guidelines. Bethesda (MD): Undersea & Hyperbaric Medical Society; 1997.

54. Weaver LK. Operational use and patient care in the monoplace chamber. In: Moon R, McIntyre N, editors. Resp care clinics of N Am – hyperbaric medicine, part I. Philadelphia: W.B. Saunders Company; 1999 March. p. 51-92.

55. Weaver LK. Hyperbaric treatment of respiratory emergencies. Resp Care. 1992;37(7):720-38.

56. Weaver LK. The treatment of critically ill patients with hyperbaric oxygen therapy. In: Brent J, Wallace KL, Burkhart KK, Phillips SD, Donovan JW, editors. Critical care toxicology: diagnosis and management of the critically poisoned patient. Philadelphia: Elsevier Mosby; 2005. p. 181-7.

57. Weaver LK, Ray D, Haberstock D. Comparison of three monoplace hyperbaric chamber intravenous infusion pumps. Undersea Hyperb Med. 2005;32(6):451-6.

58. Weaver LK. Transcutaneous oxygen and carbon dioxide tensions compared to arterial blood gases in normals. Respir Care. 2007;52(11):1490-6.

59. Weaver LK, Christoffersen PB, Churchill SK, Deru K. Accuracy of the Radiometer ABL 800 measuring hyperbaric blood gases at atmospheric pressure. Undersea Hyperb Med. 2008;35(4):283.

60. Weaver, LK. Monoplace hyperbaric chambers. In: Thom SR, Neuman T, editors. The physiology and medicine of hyperbaric oxygen therapy. Philadelphia: Saunders/Elsevier; 2008. p. 27-35.

61. Weaver, LK. Critical care of patients needing hyperbaric oxygen. In: Thom SR, Neuman T, editors. The physiology and medicine of hyperbaric oxygen therapy. Philadelphia: Saunders/Elsevier; 2008. p. 117-29.

62. Weaver LK, Churchill SC, Bell JE. Taking the chamber to the critically ill patient. Undersea Hyperb Med. 2010;37(5):347.

63. Weaver LK. Hyperbaric oxygen in the critically ill. Crit Care Med. 2011;39(7):1784-91.

64. Weaver LK, Bell JE, Medina T, Laveder T. Non-invasive Doppler blood pressure monitoring in the monoplace hyperbaric chamber. Undersea Hyperb Med. 2011;38(5):445.

CHAPTER 5 CHAPTER

Multiplace Hyperbaric Chamber

CHAPTER FIVE OVERVIEW

Introduction 99
Construction Requirements 99
Multiplace Hyberbaric Chamber 100
Pressurization 102
What You Can and What You Should *Not* Introduce in the Room 104
Hyperbaric Chamber Attendant 105
Medical Devices 106
Continuous Infusion Pumps 107
Hyperbaric Ventilators 107
References 109

Multiplace Hyperbaric Chamber

Giacomo Garetto, Gerardo Bosco

INTRODUCTION

The multiplace hyperbaric oxygen therapy chamber has reached safety and comfort levels for occupants that were unthinkable a few years ago. Advancements in this apparatus have significantly challenged builders who had to comply with a myriad of rules and regulations to certify their product as a potent medical therapy and not just a space under pressure. They consist normally of a cylindrical structure with diameter sufficient to allow access to the standing occupants. However, more recently, there are several hyperbaric facilities built with square dimensions simulating standard therapeutic room space (see Karolinska Hospital-Stockholm), ideal to make the most of the internal space available.

To minimize the risk of fire, pressurization occurs with compressed air rather than with oxygen. This key feature of multiplace chambers makes them preferable to monoplace chambers, which are usually compressed with 100% O_2. Within the walls of a hyperbaric multiplace chamber, it is possible to treat patients from intensive care units (ICUs), while they are still attached to electronic medical equipment to ensure continuity of care and maintain ventilator support if necessary. Some monoplace chambers can also be configured to provide most specialized implements, but personnel need to remain outside the compressed space.

The initial cost for multiplace chambers is very high because of the space construction and the equipment necessary for the operation of the hyperbaric chamber (i.e., pressurized air production and storage, dryers, humidity control equipment, sprinklers and water deluge systems to extinguish fires, and filters for air quality according to strict standards of control). Maintaining these complex pieces of equipment also requires specially trained personnel who are kept abreast of advancements.

The following table summarizes these key points (Table 1).

CONSTRUCTION REQUIREMENTS

The hyperbaric chamber is not simply a pressurized vessel but rather an officially recognized medical device named Device Class IIB (Rule 11, Subset IX, Directive 93/42/EEC; also named in guidelines MEDDEV 2.4/1 2010) (European Standards).[1,3] The European Community marking is affixed outside the chamber, and the manufacturer must submit a technical file with notification of the equipment's compliance with required directives. Below is a list of European standards to which the manufacturer must comply in the construction of the product. To those there are

TABLE 1. ADVANTAGES AND DISADVANTAGES OF MULTIPLACE HYPERBARIC CHAMBERS VERSUS MONOPLACE HYPERBARIC CHAMBERS

ADVANTAGES	DISADVANTAGES
Greater fire safety	High costs of purchase and management
Enhanced comfort for patients	Risk for service staff (physician, nursing, and technical personnel)
Possibility of treating patients from ICU with suitable support and monitoring equipment	
Higher working pressures	
Abililty to deal with emergencies without having to decompress the chamber	

additional regulations for individual components of the hyperbaric chamber which are added to the facility. [(1)]

The U.S. regulations can be traced to a single important document: the National Fire Protection Association NFPA-99-2015, Chapter 14, which defined Class A hyperbaric chambers as chambers which could accommodate two or more people simultaneously.[(5)]

MULTIPLACE HYBERBARIC CHAMBER

These multiplace clinical hyperbaric chambers consist of large rooms designed to accommodate more occupants inside simultaneously, with a maximum limit imposed by the European standard of 14 patients (Figure 1). They are usually constructed from two adjoining structures to simultaneously allow treatment of several people in a so-called "master pressurized chamber" with individual workstations dedicated to each patient for treatment and a pressurization compartment, usually smaller (Figure 2).

Hyperbaric chambers are normally made up of two adjoining sections separated by an airtight door: a main compartment used for therapy and a secondary compartment called a pressure lock, which can be pressurized when it is necessary to enter or exit the main compartment, while the main compartment remains under pressure (Figure 2).

The main treatment room usually consists of a cylindrical body enclosed by a rounded ceiling on the top and a flat bottom below, fitted with a flat door with a pressurized closure, usually with a rubber O-ring but without locking devices or additional mechanical closures, for safety (Figure 3).

A rectangular door facilitates the entry of patients with walking difficulties and is large enough to allow passage of wheelchairs and stretchers. The pressure inside the chamber is ensured by an airtight simple seal. The main body of the chamber is made of carbon steel, suitable for pressure equipment and hyperbaric chambers, painted with enamel epoxy 2-component polyacrylic, subject to corrosion. In particular, the interior finish will be inorganic zinc epoxy fire retardant, without exhalation of toxic vapors or combustible mixtures production in case of fire, as provided by law.

The main treatment chamber can be accessed directly from outside through the appropriate door when the chamber is not pressurized, or through the airlock if it is

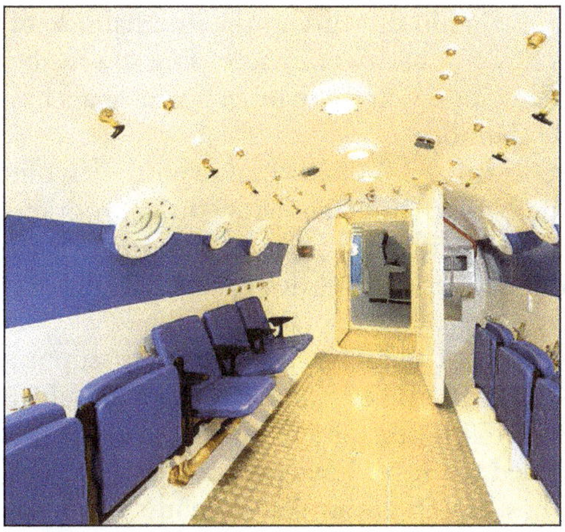

Figure 1. In the hyperbaric chamber with HCV-12d Vecom SRL (Padova, Italy).

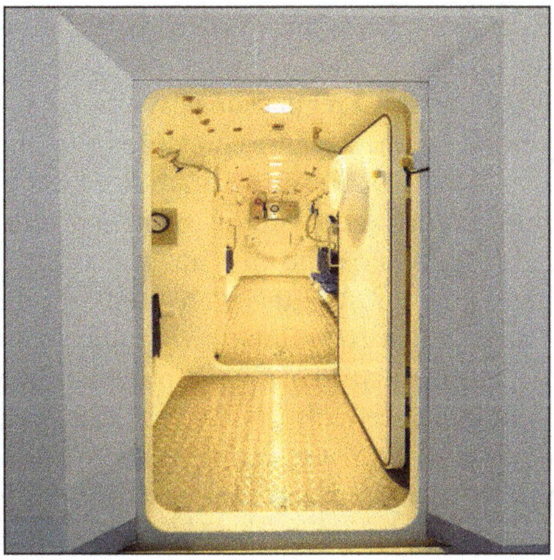

Figure 3. Main entry through the airlock which is made up of a rectangular door with an O-ring.

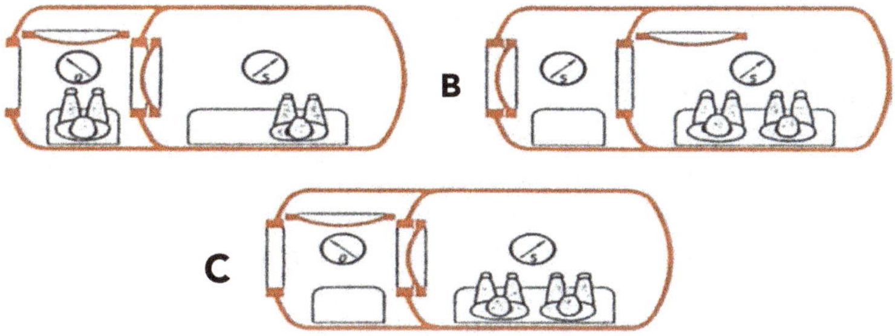

Figure 2. Pressurization schematic between the main treatment room and airlock. In A, we have a patient inside the treatment chamber at high pressure while a second individual is in the room with air entering the lock of the compression chamber. In B, the compression compartment is compressed at the same pressure as the treatment chamber, and the individual can enter the treatment chamber. In C, the compression lock is decompressed to be available at the surface again. Both subjects are inside the multiplace chamber.

necessary to access a pressurized chamber. In this case, the airlock is closed, and the pressure inside the airlock is increased to reach the same pressure as the treatment chamber (Figure 2). When the two compartment pressures are equal, then open access will be involved between the airlock and the treatment chamber. As illustrated in Figures 2 and 3, the doors of the main treatment chamber and the access to the airlock are O-ring–lined without lock mechanism, and they will passively open when pressures are equal in the two compartments, in agreement with the regulation.

The main treatment chamber is also equipped with a special device called an object pass-through lock, normally located on the farther side of the chamber and open to the outside with interposition of dual doors. Pressure seals are built in to allow passage, in and out, of small objects to use or small medical devices for medical personnel, while the chamber is under pressure. There are doors on both sides of the pass-through lock to enable the pressure equalization while the treatment chamber is at pressure.

There are transparent portholes on the side walls of the main room to ensure the vision from the outside and inside of the treatment chamber and of the airlock (Figure 4). The window material is made of a clear Perspex cover which is also scratch resistant. This is annealed with "O" rings to maintain pressure in the internal side of the chamber. The portholes are made of thick acrylic safety glass according to specific ASME PVHO regulations: two layers for each window, and the inner acrylic glass has a small hole to equalize pressure to the inside chamber.

Smaller observatories are also planned, constructed similarly to side portholes, but smaller and placed on the top area of the hyperbaric chamber, to allow the appropriate lighting fixtures and provide at least 300 lux level with the option of dimming to 10 lux. Similar observatories are used for internal observation via video cameras (Figure 4). The chamber is equipped with video cameras which allow digital recording.

Emergency lighting is provided independent of the main lighting power supply, in compliance with EN 14931 (paragraph 4.2.13) in case of failure or blackout. When designing and constructing the body of the room, it is necessary to grant access to some pipe penetrations and cable connections intended for instrumentation control, excess in number compared to the penetration used. Those not in use are sealed tightly.[4]

These multiplace chambers are pressurized with air; patients are exposed to oxygen or other breathing-gas mixtures through various devices (mask, helmet, endotracheal tube) via a demand valve connected to a gas circuit separate from the inside of the room, which emits exhausted gas to the outside.

PRESSURIZATION

Pressurization systems and control for the treatment chamber and airlock are completely independent and autonomous, as specified in the standard (Figure 6). There is a line of compressed air supply, with dual power supply upstream as required by standard, which can power the room either from the control system or manually. This is achieved by valve bypasses for maneuvers in the event of an emergency or breakdown.

Power lines, both automatic (control system) and manual (for emergency maneuvers), are automatically stopped in case of maximum chamber pressure. These lines are designed for a minimum inlet pressure of at least 30–40 m3/min. These

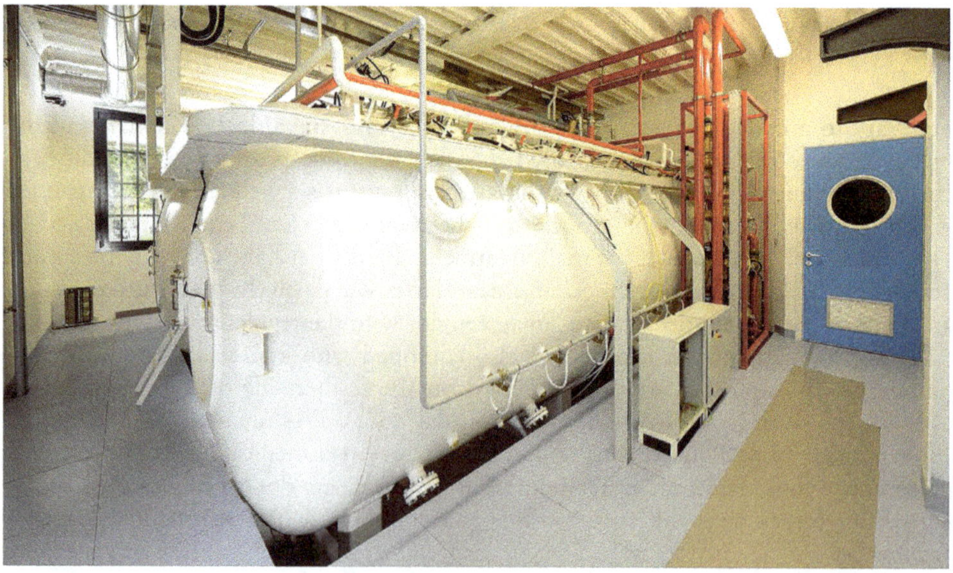

Figure 4. Rear view of the hyperbaric chamber. Sprinkler lines can be identified (red) and the portholes (on both walls) of larger size for direct vision inside the room and to admit light from outside. Smaller portholes are used to house video cameras to record activities inside the chamber.

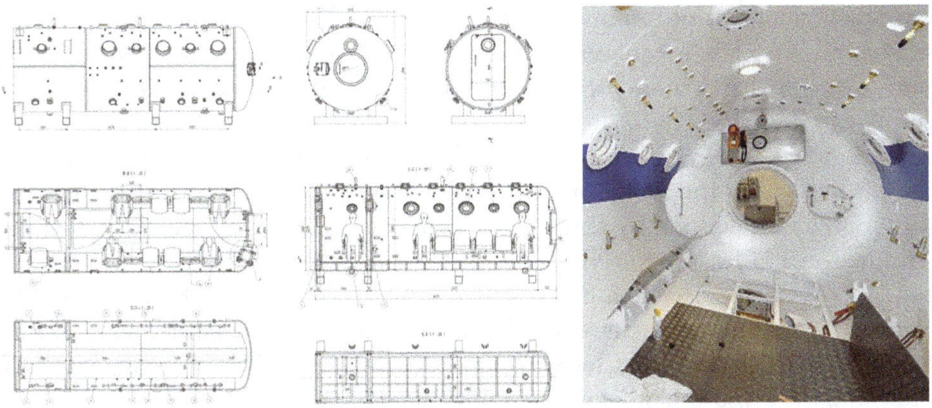

Figure 5. Outline design of a hyperbaric chamber. You can see the numerous necessary hull penetrators (Vecom, SRL). Pictured beside the schematic is a photo demonstrating penetrations.

courses are those expected to reach the maximum speed limit pressure within the range established by EN 14931. The loads are fitted with a silencer.

The power system and distribution of oxygen is made with external systems to the hyperbaric chamber. The oxygen supply to the main room is via external manifolds, with inside-the-room shut-off valves prior to the attack on the regulator. Similarly, there are two outside collectors, for connecting the exhalations of patients being treated (gas vented). The supervision of pressurization and control and the administration of oxygen or other breathable mixtures is managed by specially trained technicians, via a control panel.

Breathing systems, which are used in the administration of pure oxygen to patients, consist of a normal oxygen tap which is opened and closed by the operator every time therapy is needed, a "demand valve," similar to an underwater breathing valve, which will provide gas-derived oxygen through a flexible hose connected to an oronasal mask applied to the patient's face snugly to prevent the entry of air into the mask; that would lower the percentage of oxygen breathed, making it a less effective therapy. Expiration is allowed through a corrugated tube similar to the expiration circuit.

The other possibility is a "dispensing controller," which measures the amount of gas in liters per minute to be transferred to the patient through a helmet. This case requires continuous flow to keep the helmet inflated. However, any increase in percentage of oxygen in the room, which could be caused by leakage of oxygen from the helmet, makes this potentially dangerous, and possibility of fire hazard exists. European legislation is rigid and requires no more than a single helmet used during the therapy session.

Fuel system and distribution of medical air is operated from control system (console) and bypass with solenoid valves and manual valves in case of emergency. Medical air supply and distribution is controlled with solenoid valves and manual valves in case of emergency. Medical air supply and distribution can be intentionally sent to supply mask if the sensor encounters oxygen concentration exceeding 23% (23.5% max limit allowed by this from EN14931). The breathing system includes valves that prevent oxygen flushing into the chamber accidentally.

The water sprinkler can be located in the main treatment chamber or in the airlock chamber as required by 14931. It must provide compressed water deluge, pressurized water to flood, with pressures and flow rates of no less than guaranteed minimum standards or minimum pressure > 8.5 bar and capacity of at least 50 L/m2 per minute. This is equivalent to approximately 1000 L/min altogether (640 L/min for main chamber and 360 L/min for airlock), which must be distributed by sprinklers throughout both chambers.

A great deal of emphasis has been placed on fire alarms, fire suppression, and active surveillance. The activation of the fire-extinguishing system is by two opposing, distinct fire extinguishing systems, both in the Penal Code, and are C.E. identified, (required in EU legislation, NFPA standards optional) that are activated only with simultaneous flame detection by both within a maximum time of one second. The alarm can be manually deactivated within three seconds. In this short interval of time, it is still possible to exclude deluge fire protection with the appropriate action manual present in the console in order to avoid flooding in case of false alarms.

Two water spray extinguishing systems can still be activated manually by the operator in the console or intentionally by staff inside the room, using manual valves identified. Within airlock and treatment chambers a special hose for manual intervention will also be installed, as specified in the standard. In the case of automatic activation of sprinklers, gas flow blocks the administration of oxygen or breathing gas, and the bottom valve of the interested area is decompressed. The tanks are always loaded with water pressure maintained at the chamber pressure; their pressurization occurs through the high-pressure cylinders pack, 200–220 bar stored on specially crafted storage tanks and led to low working pressure via a pressure reducer.

WHAT YOU CAN AND WHAT YOU SHOULD NOT INTRODUCE IN THE ROOM

Hyperbaric chambers are pressurized with compressed air environments and oxygen is supplied by an independent circuit, thus keeping the oxygen percentage values between 20.9%–22%. The fire risk is controlled, not completely cancelled. To increase security, it is forbidden to introduce a series of potentially dangerous elements inside the room. Here is a list of these materials or equipment that are absolutely prohibited:

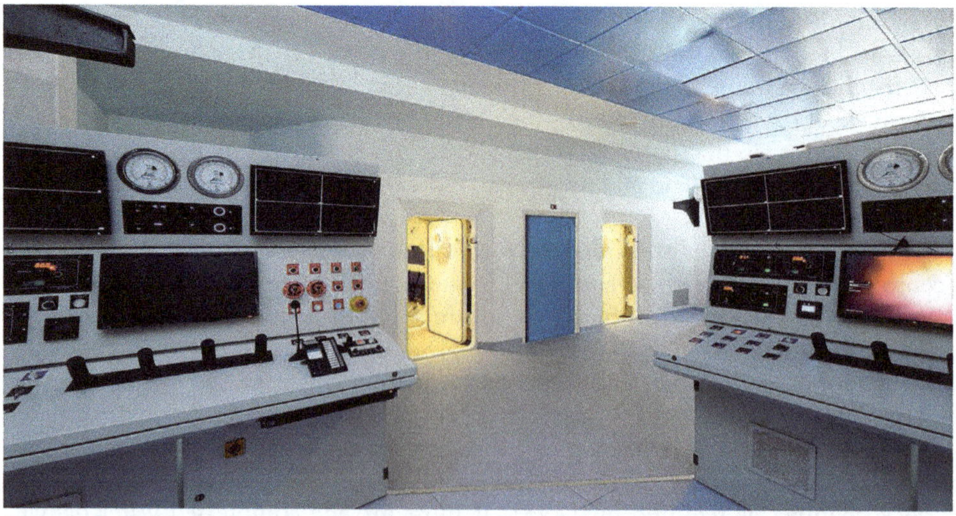

Figure 6. Control panel of a modern hyperbaric chamber (hyperbaric chamber at ATIP, Padova, Italy).

- lighters and matches (for possibility of open flames)
- gas hand warmers (for possibility of open flames)
- battery-powered equipment, e.g., phones, remote controls, music players (for possibility of sparks)
- fully synthetic clothing (for possibility of electrostatic discharge sparks)
- uncertified equipment and medical equipment not tested by the physician in charge of the hyperbaric chamber
- furnishings (pillows, blankets, mattresses) not certified for hyperbaric environments (flame retardant and antistatic) to minimize the danger of fire
- cosmetics on the patient's face, directly in contact with 100% oxygen mask used in the environment
- newspapers (usually these papers are impregnated with oil products in the ink to write)

Inside the room one can take the following items:

- magazine or book
- eyeshades of any material
- pencil to write (pens are not dangerous but may stain for excessive leakage of ink due to pressure changes)
- implanted medical devices (pacemakers or cardiac defibrillators) if they are hyperbaric eligible; if they were not tested, these could have serious consequences for the patient due to malfunctions
- soft contact lenses

HYPERBARIC CHAMBER ATTENDANT

Personnel providing assistance – technical assistance, nursing staff, or a physician – depending on the needs of the patient are permitted inside the multiplace chamber during therapeutic activities. When the chamber is under pressure, these assistants breathe compressed air at the pressure of treatment. The therapies vary depending on the pathology of the disease being treated from 2.0 to 2.8 ATA, for a total time varying from 95 to 115 minutes. In case of therapy for a decompression sickness accident, depth and time of exposure increase substantially (see Table 6 U.S. Navy, and Table 6A U.S. Navy). It is important to adopt procedures to protect the hyperbaric chamber attendant to avoid incurring a decompression accident.

The most straightforward method is to adopt no-decompression limits shown in the U.S. Navy tables for the depths reached in the chambers during therapy. After that time limit, the assistant will not breathe compressed air but will don a mask breathing oxygen (Figure 7).

This procedure, in addition to limiting the further accumulation of nitrogen in the tissues, accelerates nitrogen washout while breathing oxygen at pressure.

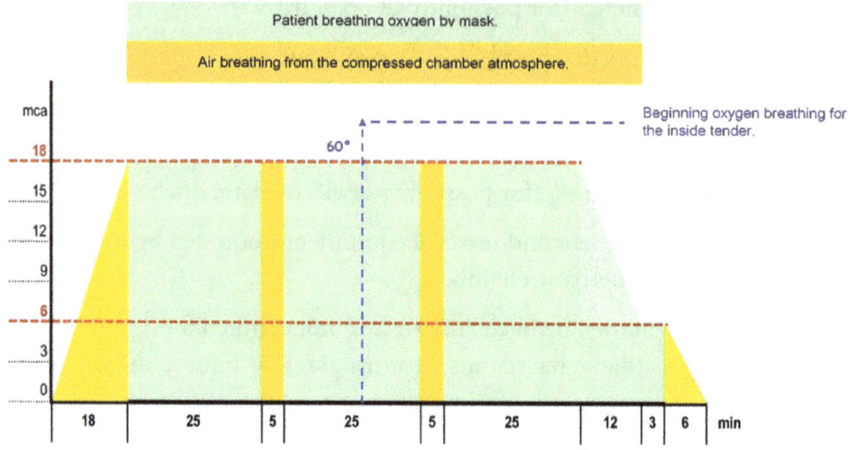

Figure 7. Example of therapy to 2.8 ATA (60 feet). The chamber attendant starts breathing oxygen after 60 minutes. No decompression limits at a given altitude exist according to the U.S. Navy tables.

MEDICAL DEVICES

Medical electrical equipment involves intensive patient care within the hyperbaric chamber during the session and should have the same characteristics as those that are used for monitoring in the intensive care unit.

The hyperbaric environment is a particular environment, both for the increase in air pressure inside the chamber (a factor that can alter the parameters set at atmospheric pressure) and for environmental safety regulations (power supply and fire risk), factors that severely limit the usability of the equipment normally and make it difficult to find suitable material.[6]

In the selection of medical equipment for use within hyperbaric chambers, one must first seek material the use of which is certified in a hyperbaric oxygen–enriched environment. Clinical parameters to be monitored will be corrected at various pressures of therapy because technicians at designated time will have taken into account the possible environmental variations by affixing corrections.

If certified material is not available, the doctor of the hyperbaric chamber is directly responsible for what is used for monitoring.

- Must be certain that the clinical parameters measured, fluids injected, and ventilation mode set are kept constant, even by changing to the ambient pressure, with the basal setting
- Should ensure that even under pressure, equipment does not lose its functions but retains the ability to change parameters at any time during the therapy
- Should ensure that the exercise is far superior to the duration of the therapy session
- Lower alert thresholds and in response to the increase of oxygen in the room, check the relative humidity in the room by increasing the percentage over the values normally used, thus reducing the possibility of electrostatic current and increasing environmental safety

- Must reduce the number of people in the chamber to just the physician and single patient
- Monitor vital signs
    - ECG/HR: 3-5 leads are sufficient.
    - IBP/NIBP: IBP, always present in patients from ICU. More widespread use of NIBP, even in situations of unstable pressure supported by pharmacologic means. The small compressor for inflating the cuff is running on battery power, and its repeated use significantly reduces the duration of battery power. Must be taken into account in the choice of monitor. The newer models and compatibles use compressed air to inflate the cuff. Does not affect the battery life and is safer as there are no moving parts in compression.
    - SpO_2: this parameter is not required in treating a normal patient but becomes very important in a critical patient. The sensor shows the saturation of the hemoglobin in the blood that normally takes values close to 100% in room air, and therefore does not detect the significant increase of oxygen dissolved plasma by hyperbarism. In critical patients, assisted breathing can be a sensitive index of ineffective ventilation and therefore poor oxygenation of the blood.

CONTINUOUS INFUSION PUMPS

Continuous infusion pumps are necessary for the continuity of drug therapy in the ICU.

To ensure safety of the subject, equipment must be designed in a manner that allows for the changing of parameters at any time during the session. Furthermore, working autonomy of at least 1.5 the duration of therapy must be maintained (practicing 50% more safety than required).

HYPERBARIC VENTILATORS

We analyze the following characteristics that a ventilator must have when used inside a hyperbaric chamber:

- Maintain a steady gas flow despite different pressures inside the chamber
- Maintenance of a constant ventilator rate at different pressures
- The ability to provide different types of ventilation (volume-controlled, SIMV, pressure-controlled, pressure-assisted ventilation)
- Ability to set PEEP (positive end-expiratory pressure)
- If battery operated, there should be sufficient electrical power for the length of the given treatment

The environment at higher pressure than the atmospheric alters volumes, due to the increase of the ambient pressure and increasing resistance to increased density of gases. This is reflected with hypoventilation and increasing work of breathing.

There can be both types of ventilators in use: constant volume ventilators and constant pressure ventilators. In constant volume ventilators (VCV), the density of the gas increases with increasing pressure, causing a decreased flow which results in a decrease of tidal breathing volume at different pressures. These ventilators require continuous adjustments to tidal volume at different pressures.

In pressure-controlled ventilation (PCV), the pressure values to be reached are constant over time, and the ratio of inspiration to expiration (I-E ratio) is kept constant. In this case, the tidal volume may vary in different breaths. Every reduction of flow induced by an increase in ambient pressure is recorded by transducers of the volume expired by the patients and is compensated and offset by a stability control algorithm of pressure, and thus the tidal volume remains almost constant.

REFERENCES

1. BS EN 14931:2006 Pressure vessels for human occupancy (PVHO). Multi-place pressure chambers for hyperbaric therapy – performance, safety requirements and testing. British Standards Institution; 2008 Jul.
2. Citti P, Delogu M. Studio di un approccio operativo integrato al progetto e sviluppo delle attrezzature a pressione a fronte dell'entrata in vigore della direttiva 97/23/CE: "PED." In: Convegno, A.T.T.I. SAFAP 2016. 2016. Italian.
3. Direttiva ONDR. 93/42/CEE e successiva modifica 2007/47/CE. Dispositivo medico classe II a. (2005). Italian.
4. European Commission. Classification of medical devices (MEDDEV 2.4/1 Rev. 9) [Internet]. 2010 Jun. Available from: http://ec.europa.eu/consumers/sectors/medicaldevices/files/meddev/2_4_1_rev_9_classification_en.pdf
5. National Fire Protection Association. NFPA 14 Standard for Installation of Standpipe and Hose Systems. 2010.
6. Workman WT. Hyperbaric facility safety: a practical guide. Best Publishing Co.; 1999.

CHAPTER 6 CHAPTER

Hyperbaric Nursing

CHAPTER SIX OVERVIEW

Introduction 113
Historical Perspectives 113
Hyperbaric Nursing as a Specialty 115
Qualifications for Hyperbaric Nurses 116
Hyperbaric Oxygen Therapy Training 117
The Role of the Hyperbaric Nurse 118
The Hyperbaric Nurse Clinician 119
The Nurse as Educator 123
The Nurse as Researcher 124
The Nurse as Manager 124
Advanced Practice Nursing in Hyperbaric Medicine 125
Pediatrics 125
Trends 125
Acknowledgments 126
References 127

Hyperbaric Nursing

Valerie Messina

INTRODUCTION

The specialty of hyperbaric nursing has evolved since the 1950s along with the practice of hyperbaric medicine. Nurses, qualified by education, experience, and professional licensure, provide care for patients in the altered environment of the hyperbaric chamber. The art and science of nursing are uniquely combined in this setting as nurses not only deal with the technology of the hyperbaric chamber, the physiological monitoring and life-support equipment, but also with the art of psychologically adapting the patient and providing emotional support and patient and family education.

The administrative aspects of setting up a hyperbaric medicine department and training and developing staff also fall into the realm of nursing. This chapter discusses these aspects as well as the practical aspects of hyperbaric nursing.

HISTORICAL PERSPECTIVES

Clinical hyperbaric oxygen (HBO_2) therapy evolved from research and experience of physicians primarily in Europe, with Dr. Boerema from Amsterdam being the most recognized. His experimental work in hyperbaric chambers of the Dutch Royal Navy was conducted with a team of divers/technicians from the Dutch Navy as well as one male nurse.

In 1959, a large multiplace hyperbaric chamber facility at the Wilhelmina Gasthuis in Amsterdam was used primarily for open-heart surgery. The first hyperbaric nurses were qualified operating-room nurses who volunteered to participate in this unique work environment.[5, 16] When patients with carbon monoxide poisoning, gas gangrene, and other anaerobic necrotizing infections began being treated with hyperbaric oxygen at the Wilhelmina Gasthuis, patient care inside the chambers began to be provided by nurses. These pioneer hyperbaric nurses received on-the-job training. Later, formal training in hyperbaric therapy was provided by the Dutch Royal Navy in Den Helder, and by the hyperbaric medicine department at the Wilhelmina Gasthuis. When specialization in intensive care and coronary care nursing evolved in the 1960s, this training and experience also became a prerequisite for becoming a hyperbaric nurse.[5]

The multiplace clinical hyperbaric facility at Western Infirmary in Glasgow, Scotland, began treatment of various nonhealing wounds, as well as acute carbon monoxide poisoning and anaerobic infections. Specially trained nursing staff were integrated as members of the team taking primary charge of patients in the chamber.[24]

With the introduction of the Vickers monoplace pressure chamber in England, nurses were trained to operate these chambers and to provide care prior to, during, and after hyperbaric treatment. Later nursing auxiliaries were trained as hyperbaric nurse technicians to assist with these treatments.[31] In 1964, a hyperbaric program in Stockholm, Sweden obtained a Vickers chamber[9] and use of these monoplace chambers spread throughout the world in the later 1960s. A variety of personnel, including nurses,technicians, and respiratory therapists were trained to operate these chambers.

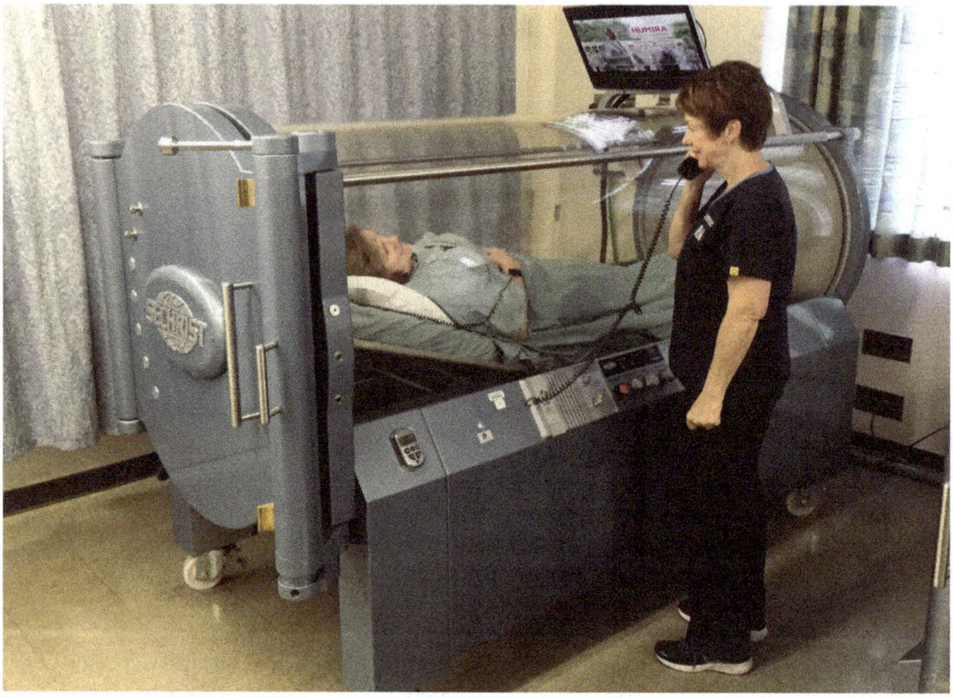

Figure 1. A monoplace chamber. Photo courtesy of Long Beach Memorial.

Clinical hyperbaric research was being done by surgeons from Harvard using an old U.S. Navy decompression chamber to evaluate surgical procedures for correcting heart abnormalities under pressure. This led to the installation of a multiplace hyperbaric facility in the 1960s at Children's Hospital Medical Center in Boston which was used primarily for cardiovascular surgery.[2] Other multiplace facilities at Lutheran General Hospital in Park Ridge, Illinois, Duke University in North Carolina, Mount Sinai in New York, St. Barnabas Medical Center in New Jersey, Millard Fillmore Hospital in Buffalo, New York and the University of Maryland Hospital, soon followed. [1, 44] The Royal Victoria Hospital in Montreal established the first Canadian medical hyperbaric facility in 1963. Toronto General Hospital opened its unit in 1964, and Vancouver General Hospital opened its facility in 1965.[54] Vickers monoplace chambers were also being installed in some hospitals including the unit at the United States Naval Hospital in Long Beach, California.[19]

As in Europe, some of the first American hyperbaric nurses were operating-room nurses. HBO_2 was being used to treat many other conditions, so nurses with experience primarily in critical care, as well as emergency room nursing and medical-surgical nursing, were being trained in the specialty of hyperbaric oxygen therapy. An interest in research was also a prerequisite. Some hyperbaric units like the one at Lutheran General used registered nurses exclusively for patient care during hyperbaric treatment.[22, 43]

Nursing had the opportunity to be involved in the planning and development of some of these early hyperbaric programs. The most publicized of these was at Mount Sinai Hospital in New York. Venger and Jacobson described this program's development as an ideal project for showing the value of cooperation between the nurse, the clinician, and the administrator.[50] Nursing needs were identified and divided into two areas: selection of personnel and staffing; training and staff development. Patient care needs focused around emotional support, patient teaching, medical therapy, surgical procedures, and experimental research. Venger described the potential of hyperbaric nursing as being founded on the medical program and on the findings relative to research.[51] Further, she challenged that nurses had an innate responsibility to keep pace as their role broadened and expanded.[49] It is noteworthy that the hyperbaric department at Mount Sinai was organizationally under the department of nursing.

During the 1960s and early 1970s, the subject of hyperbaric oxygen therapy received considerable attention in nursing journals around the world. Although physicians contributed some of these articles, the majority of these were published by nurses working in hyperbaric therapy.[13,17,20,23,25,34,36,37,38,46,48] While these articles addressed nurses in general, one publication in a nursing textbook provided an in-depth analysis of the nurse's role in hyperbaric therapy.[32]

At the Fifth International Hyperbaric Congress in Vancouver, B.C., Canada, in 1973, a small group of nurses and respiratory therapists met for half a day and presented papers, as well as shared experiences. In 1982 in Norfolk, Virginia, the Undersea Medical Society (UMS) Associates sponsored a half-day program of presentations by technicians, nurses, and respiratory therapists. This was the first time that the UMS Associates had conducted their own program in conjunction with the UMS Annual Scientific Meeting. Since that time, the Associates continued to grow into an active organization with a rapid increase in membership, including nurses, and representation on the UMS Executive Committee.

The annual conferences on the clinical application of HBO_2 therapy sponsored by the Baromedical (Hyperbaric Medicine) Department at Memorial Medical Center in Long Beach, California, attracted many hyperbaric nurses as well as physicians, respiratory therapists and technicians. In 1978, this conference began including workshops specifically for nurses.

HYPERBARIC NURSING AS A SPECIALTY

The specialty of hyperbaric nursing was formally recognized with the founding and incorporation of the Baromedical Nurses Association (BNA) in 1985. The BNA was established with 35 founding RN members at the joint meeting of the UMS Annual Scientific Meeting and the Long Beach Clinical Hyperbaric Conference. The BNA, which is international in scope, maintains a membership of 250 registered nurses from approximately five countries. Functions of the BNA include promoting professional activities that enhance the effectiveness of hyperbaric nursing in the health-care system and promoting educational opportunities and networking for nurses practicing in the specialty. Educational activities of the BNA can now be accessed online and focus on chamber and patient safety, patient compliance, evidence-based best practices, and quality improvement programs. The BNA develops and maintains standards-of-care guidelines in hyperbaric nursing and supports nursing research efforts.[6,8] Hyperbaric nurses may now achieve specialty certification as a certified or advanced-certified hyperbaric nurse or as a hyperbaric nurse clinician. Since its inception, the face of the BNA has aged, but its mission to serve nurses practicing in the field of clinical hyperbaric nursing is essentially unchanged. Information and an application for membership can be obtained from the Baromedical Nurses Association through Internet access at www.hyperbaricnurses.org.

In hyperbaric medicine, a collegial role between the nurse and the physician exists – roles both independent and interdependent.[21] This collegial role has been described throughout the evolution of hyperbaric nursing, and it continues as the BNA joins the Undersea and Hyperbaric Medical Society (UHMS) for their annual scientific meetings, providing a forum for sharing scientific knowledge between the members of the hyperbaric health-care team. The BNA is also represented on the UHMS Committees by the UHMS Associate Liaison.

QUALIFICATIONS FOR HYPERBARIC NURSES

The patient population treated at hospital-based hyperbaric departments is quite diverse in age, diagnosis, and degree of acuteness. Because of this diversity, the hyperbaric nurse should be experienced and competent in medical-surgical nursing of ill adults and children. One year of critical care experience is highly recommended and is required at most hyperbaric facilities as well as Advanced Cardiac Life Support (ACLS) and Pediatric Advanced Life Support (PALS) certifications. Good communication skills are essential both for patient care and for working with other departments and other hospitals involved in the care of the patient receiving HBO_2 therapy. Good leadership skills are needed to coordinate and provide continuity of care to patients and to direct patient care provided by nonnursing staff. A high degree of technical skill and expertise is also beneficial in the hyperbaric setting, as the hyperbaric chambers and ancillary equipment are technologically state-of-the-art. Hyperbaric staff may also be required for on-call coverage in departments that provide care for emergencies such as carbon monoxide poisoning or decompression sickness.[53] Nursing staff must be licensed in the state in which they practice and must function within the guidelines of the Nurse Practice Act of that state.

Nurses who are applying for work inside a multiplace hyperbaric chamber must also meet specific physical requirements.[30,47] These nurses are subject to an evaluation including medical history, physical examination, and relevant radiological and laboratory tests as indicated. In case of a disease affecting the ears, sinuses, upper respiratory tract, or lungs, the hyperbaric nurse is evaluated by a relevant physician for fitness to be pressurized in the multiplace chamber. Disqualifications for work inside the chamber include history of seizure disorder, insulin-dependent diabetes, or claustrophobia which could render the inside attendant unconscious or incapacitated. Preexisting conditions, such as certain orthopedic injuries, may increase the risk of developing decompression sickness and would be a disqualifying factor, as would conditions involving chronic pain, even if intermittent, that could be confused with symptoms of decompression sickness.

Pregnancy is an absolute contraindication to working in a high-pressure environment, and all female inside-chamber attendants must be warned of potential danger to the fetus. Any female attendant trying to become pregnant must avoid hyperbaric exposure. While these physical requirements are very specific, hyperbaric inside-attendant staff do not need to meet the physical requirements of recreational divers, such as stamina and the ability to swim. Applicants for hyperbaric inside-attendant positions need to be evaluated by a physician knowledgeable in diving and hyperbaric medicine.[14,45]

Staffing for a hyperbaric department is dictated by the state and country laws in which the facility operates. The Joint Commission (TJC) and Joint Commission International guidelines influence the staffing and the practice of nursing in hyperbaric units.[26-27] Accountability to these legislative and organizational guidelines is paramount to a department's success.

HYPERBARIC OXYGEN THERAPY TRAINING

All hyperbaric personnel involved in patient care and chamber operations are trained in hyperbaric medicine theory and clinical practice, including technical procedures and patient safety. Effective patient management and safety procedures cannot be learned in the classroom alone. Hands-on training and precepted on-the-job experience are essential to develop a level of expertise necessary for providing safe, comprehensive, quality patient care. The level of training and experience required is relative to the patient's condition, clinical indications, and whether hyperbaric is provided in the ambulatory care setting or in the acute care hospital setting. Treatment of the critical care patient necessitates additional training for the hyperbaric nurse, including critical care monitoring and life-support equipment used with the hyperbaric chamber.[29]

Hyperbaric departments utilizing multiplace chambers usually have a facilities manager with knowledge and expertise in chamber systems operation and maintenance, as well as expertise in the use of treatment protocols. Personnel for these positions usually come from the military or from a commercial diving setting. Patient care planning and delivery of patient care, however, is in the domain of nursing. It is important that an RN be in charge of this activity for both multiplace and monoplace chamber facilities. The Joint Commission guidelines require that the delivery of nursing care, treatment, and services be directed by a nurse executive who is a licensed professional registered nurse and qualified by advanced education and management experience.[26]

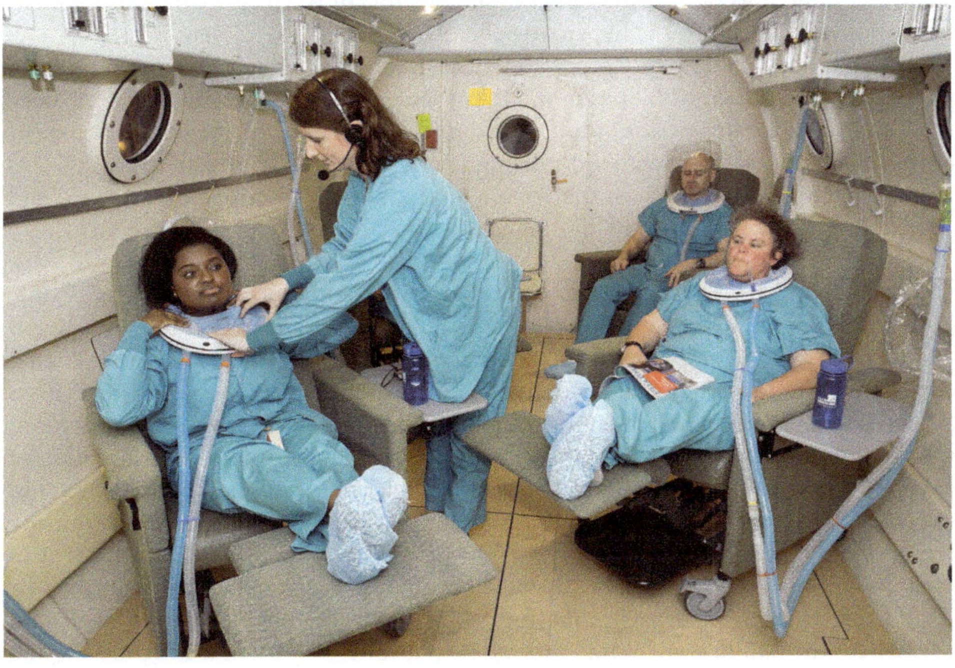

Figure 2. A multiplace chamber. Photo courtesy of Virginia Mason Medical Center.

The most efficient use of staff in a multiplace hyperbaric facility is obtained through cross-training. Registered nurses should be trained to operate the chamber, and technical staff should have Emergency Medical Technician or Diver Medical Technician training and certification to work inside the chamber during patient treatments. The use of on-call or resource staff in addition to full-time staff provides for better treatment coverage and reduces the risk of staff burnout and the risk of developing decompression sickness. The use of resource and on-call staff has a favorable impact on the budget; it decreases overtime pay, nonproductive paid time, and the indirect costs from benefits.

There are several medical centers and educational companies that sponsor hyperbaric training programs for physicians, nurses, and technicians in either monoplace or multiplace chamber settings. These training programs are ideal for staff starting out in a newly established hyperbaric program. The Undersea and Hyperbaric Medical Society provides a directory of UHMS-approved hyperbaric medicine training courses that meet the educational criteria for nurses seeking specialty certification. Information from the UHMS can be obtained through Internet access at www.uhms.org. Some hyperbaric chamber manufacturers also provide training in the operation of their equipment. Established hyperbaric departments often provide their own training program for new staff. Businesses that start up hyperbaric medicine departments in clinics and hospitals also provide training for the hyperbaric staff.

Course content for nurses includes didactic sessions and clinical practicum on the following topics: introduction and history of hyperbaric medicine; mechanisms of HBO_2; gas laws and HBO_2 physiology; standards for the clinical use of HBO_2; complications of HBO_2 and contraindications; adaptation of the patient to the hyperbaric chamber; chamber safety requirements and precautions; pharmacology of HBO_2; application of HBO_2 in medicine; diving; orthopedics; neurology compromised wound healing; infectious disease conditions; the role of the hyperbaric nurse; care of the critically ill patient in the hyperbaric chamber; and reimbursement issues.

Nurses also participate in relevant continuing-education programs to remain prepared for their responsibilities in the hyperbaric specialty unit. In order to practice in this setting, the hyperbaric nurse must be knowledgeable of the complex patient environment found in hyperbaric nursing. Basic and critical care nursing skills, as well as hyperbaric skills such as transcutaneous oxygen monitoring, are reviewed and validated annually per state and TJC standards.(26)

THE ROLE OF THE HYPERBARIC NURSE

Hyperbaric nursing was defined in the BNA position statement as the diagnosis and treatment of human responses to actual or potential health problems in the altered environment of the hyperbaric chamber.(7) This further expands the American Nurses Association social policy statement which defines nursing as the protection, promotion, and optimization of health and abilities, prevention of illness and injury, alleviation of suffering through the diagnosis and treatment of human response, and advocacy in the care of individuals, families, communities and populations.(3) Hyperbaric nursing was further defined in the publication *Hyperbaric Nursing and Wound Care,* a text of essential and practical information devoted to the specialty of hyperbaric nursing.(30)

The hyperbaric nurse has a multifunctional role – that of clinician, educator, and researcher. The administrative role may also be an integral function in managing the department and supervising patient care. The nurse may also function as the safety director of the department and be responsible for developing, directing, and enforcing safety guidelines and standards.[35] The goal of hyperbaric nursing is to provide safe, cost-effective, quality patient care, according to established standards.[15]

The Hyperbaric Nurse Clinician

Hyperbaric nurse clinicians utilize the nursing process to provide direct patient care. Hyperbaric patients are first assessed using the nursing theoretical framework of the institution in which the hyperbaric facility is located. Nurses assess for risks related to hyperbaric medicine and the psychological and physiological status of the patient. The assessment is then used as a database to develop a care plan for the hyperbaric patient. HBO_2 treatment is administered according to hyperbaric protocol, physician orders, and clinical practice guidelines. Patients are continually assessed during treatment, and nursing actions are provided as necessary to prevent or manage any complications and to continue medical and nursing interventions. After treatment, evaluation is done to assess the response to treatment and the presence of complications. The nursing process is documented in the health team record. Electronic medical records implemented in hyperbaric units for documenting the treatment, nursing process, and outcomes may include the information demonstrated in Table 1.

TABLE 1. HYPERBARIC OXYGEN TREATMENT RECORD

Date/Time
Treatment Number/Series Number
Time In/Time Out of Chamber
Pressure (ATA)/Total Time (minutes)
HBO Chamber FiO_2 (monoplace) or Hood/Mask FiO_2 (multiplace)
Oxygen/Air Breaks (minutes)
Pre-HBO_2 Assessment
Safety/Fire Hazard Checks
Post-HBO_2 Evaluation
HBO_2 Treatment Administered/Standards Met
Physiological Monitor/Life Support Equipment/Transcutaneous Monitor
Nursing Diagnosis: Potential for Injury RT HBO_2 Treatment
Protocol Implemented (Barotrauma, Anxiety)
+Outcome Evaluation Note
+Multidisciplinary Team Rounds Note
+Vital Signs and Medications Documented in Patient Record

Part of nursing practice involves activities within the medical domain. Administering medications, performing treatments, and monitoring physiological changes are delegated medical functions. The domain of nursing practice, however, deals with activities that address human responses to actual or potential problems related to an altered health status (physiological, psychological, sociological, and cognitive). It is the nurse who helps patients and their families manage illness and medical treatment as it impacts their ability to cope and their activities of daily living.[11]

The hyperbaric nurse provides emotional support for the patient and family, and a therapeutic relationship develops that involves mutual trust and respect. Patient satisfaction is an important quality indicator, as patients are asked to rate their experience with the treatments, the nursing staff, and the teamwork of the physicians and staff. Hyperbaric departments are responsible for improving patient satisfaction ratings and for meeting the patients' perceived needs. Patient compliance and adherence to treatment regimen are often reflective of the patients' satisfaction with the delivery of treatments and nursing care. Reimbursement and health-care systems ranking may also be linked to patient satisfaction scores.

Patient care standards reflect the application of the nursing process for specific patient care situations. They establish nursing diagnoses of patient and family problems associated with illness and medical treatment, they identify patient and family-focused desired outcomes of nursing care, and they develop nursing interventions that will assist the patient and family in preventing, relieving, or coping with identified problems in daily living.[42]

Standards help to operationalize the nursing process and to provide baseline criteria for evaluating the quality of nursing care delivered to patients. They provide the basis for continuity of care delivered to one patient by many caregivers or for continuity within groups of patients with common problems and needs.[42]

Within the following patient care standards, there are nursing diagnostic statements related to common human responses, either actual or potential, associated with a medical condition or treatment. The desired outcomes are derived from the nursing diagnosis, and the interventions are specific statements of nursing actions that address the nursing diagnosis. While these interventions are specific in nature, they still allow for flexibility to include the unique variability of individuals. The patient care standards in Table 2 represent examples that apply to patients receiving HBO_2.[39] The Baromedical Nurses Association Standards of Care[8] are available online and revised as indicated. Clinical practice guidelines for hyperbaric oxygen therapy which are integrated with the electronic medical record are utilized by some health-care systems. These address the standardized approach to support consistent patient care and identify potential problems for which the patient is at risk and can be individualized by adding patient-specific information to the plan of care.[10]

TABLE 2. CARE OF THE PATIENT RECEIVING HYPERBARIC OXYGEN THERAPY[8,10,39,40]

I. A. NURSING DIAGNOSIS/PROBLEMS

Potential complications: barotrauma to ears, sinuses, and lungs related to changes in atmospheric pressure inside the HBO_2 chamber; cerebral gas embolism associated with gas expansion during decompression.

B. DESIRED OUTCOMES

1. Barotrauma and gas embolism will be prevented.
2. Signs and symptoms of barotrauma or gas embolism will be recognized and promptly treated if present.

TABLE 2 (CONTINUED)

C. NURSING INTERVENTIONS

1. Prior to HBO_2 treatment, instruct patient in ear equalization techniques such as swallowing, chewing, yawning, and modified Valsalva maneuver.
2. Prior to HBO_2 treatment, administer decongestants as indicated, and assist patient, if necessary, with decongestant nasal spray per physician orders.
3. Monitor patients during HBO_2 therapy for signs and symptoms of barotrauma including the following:

   a. signs and symptoms of middle-ear or sinus barotraumas

   b. increased rate or decrease in depth of respirations

   c. signs and symptoms of pneumothorax

   d. observed swallowing of gas
4. Stop chamber pressurization or slightly decrease chamber pressure to allow additional time for pressure equalization if patient is not successful in doing so. Notify physician if patient is unable to clear his/her ears and discontinue the HBO_2 treatment.
5. Remind patient to breathe normally during pressure changes.
6. Document instruction, observations, and patient's ability to follow instructions.

II. A. NURSING DIAGNOSIS/PROBLEMS

Potential anxiety and fear related to feelings of claustrophobia associated with confinement in HBO_2 chamber.

B. DESIRED OUTCOMES

Patient will be able to tolerate being in the HBO_2 chamber for duration of treatment.

C. NURSING INTERVENTIONS

1. Monitor and document patient's behavior for symptoms of confinement anxiety including the following:

   a. restlessness

   b. inability to tolerate face mask or head hood

   c. statements of feeling confined or trapped
2. Talk to patient with a calm voice.
3. Assure patient of nurse presence throughout treatment.
4. Reassure patient that he/she is safe.
5. Engage patient in problem-solving his/her feelings of confinement anxiety such as visualization, distraction, listening to music, etc.
6. Notify physician if patient is having problems with confinement anxiety.
7. Administer antianxiety medications per physician's orders.
8. Monitor and document patient response to antianxiety medication and other interventions.

TABLE 2 (CONTINUED)

III. A. NURSING DIAGNOSIS/PROBLEMS

Potential complication: oxygen toxicity related to administration of 100% oxygen at increased atmospheric pressure.

B. DESIRED OUTCOMES

1. Signs and symptoms of oxygen toxicity will be promptly recognized, reported, and treated.
2. Oxygen toxicity seizure will be avoided.

C. NURSING INTERVENTIONS

1. Instruct patient how to recognize signs and symptoms of oxygen toxicity.
   a. Central nervous system (CNS) oxygen toxicity: numbness and tingling, ringing in ears, vertigo, blurred vision, nausea, restlessness, difficulty breathing, and/or palpitations.
   b. Pulmonary oxygen toxicity: tightness in chest, dry hacking cough, and/or difficulty inhaling a full breath.
2. Monitor for oxygen toxicity risk factors.
3. Monitor for signs and symptoms of CNS and pulmonary oxygen toxicity. Notify physician. Document.
4. Immediately switch breathing gas from oxygen to air if patient has symptoms of CNS oxygen toxicity.
5. Initiate emergency protocol if patient has a CNS oxygen toxicity seizure. Notify physician. Document.

IV. A. NURSING DIAGNOSIS/PROBLEMS

Potential complication: HBO_2 treatment-aggravated hypoglycemic event in diabetic patients.

B. DESIRED OUTCOMES

1. Signs and symptoms of hypoglycemia will be promptly recognized, reported, and treated.
2. Hypoglycemic events and hypoglycemia induced seizure will be avoided.

C. NURSING INTERVENTIONS

1. Pre- and post-HBO_2 treatment monitoring of blood sugars with administration of nutritional correction and adjustment of diabetes medications per physician orders.
2. Monitor for signs and symptoms of hypoglycemia, including shakiness, decreased concentration, tremors, diaphoresis, changes in body temperature, palpitations, headache, dry mouth, hunger, tingling in extremities, irritability, anxiety, altered speech and coordination, marked change in mental status, seizures, coma, hypertension, tachycardia, decreased blood glucose level.
3. Instruct patient how to recognize signs and symptoms of hypoglycemia.
4. Initiate emergency protocol for hypoglycemic events. Notify physician. Document.

The Nurse as Educator

Facilitating the educational process of patients and families is an accountability of the hyperbaric nurse. Patient education helps maximize the benefit of hyperbaric therapy's integration into the total health-care delivery system and helps improve cost effectiveness and maintain patient safety and facilitate care. The principles of teaching/learning are utilized as the nurse assesses for readiness to learn and adapts the teaching process to the individual patient and family. A thorough orientation to HBO_2, including the concepts and patient objectives in Table 3, is facilitated with the use of audiovisual aids such as videos and brochures.

TABLE 3. PATIENT ORIENTATION TO HYPERBARIC OXYGEN THERAPY

CONCEPT:	Effects of hyperbaric oxygen therapy.
OBJECTIVES:	Verbalizes purpose, indication, and expected outcomes of treatment.
CONCEPT:	Psychological adaptation to the hyperbaric chamber.
OBJECTIVES:	Verbalizes self-control for exiting chamber prn.
	Identifies/refines own relaxation techniques.
	Demonstrates technique for calling for nurse.
	Discusses when/how to request sedative for relaxation prn.
CONCEPT:	Signs & symptoms (S & S) of possible complications.
OBJECTIVES:	Verbalizes/recognizes S & S of middle-ear and sinus barotrauma.
	Identifies/verbalizes S & S of visual acuity changes.
	Identifies/verbalizes S & S of oxygen toxicity.
	Identifies/verbalizes S & S of hypoglycemia (diabetic patients).
CONCEPT:	Safety protocols for hyperbaric oxygen treatments.
OBJECTIVES:	Demonstrates knowledge of safety protocols – 100% cotton patient gown on, toiletries removed, jewelry off, battery-operated devices off, no electronics in chamber.
	Verbalizes/recognizes need to empty bladder before treatment.
CONCEPT:	Middle-ear equalization.
OBJECTIVES:	Demonstrates technique for "clearing ears."
	Discusses ability to request decongestants for congestion.
CONCEPT:	Smoking cessation.
OBJECTIVES:	Verbalizes importance of cessation: effect on tissue oxygenation.
	Verbalizes resources/mechanisms to assist with cessation.

Participation in educational programs for the community and for the health-care team enhances the advancement of the specialty and the effectiveness of hyperbaric medicine in the health-care system. As examples of the educator role, nurses facilitate patient care conferences, inservices, and other formal classes on hyperbaric medicine for their medical centers and participate in interdisciplinary rounds on hyperbaric patients. Nurses also contribute to websites for health-care institutions and professional organizations that provide hyperbaric medicine education.

The Nurse as Researcher

Nurses are frequently involved in the arena of medical research, in cooperation with the hyperbaric physician, administering HBO_2 treatments according to investigational protocols, developing research protocols and their implementation, and reporting and publishing the results. The testing of new technology in the hyperbaric field is often delegated to nurses who will be utilizing the equipment.

Nurses working in hyperbaric departments centered at academic institutions will find opportunities to be involved in research projects at the basic laboratory stage. Working in these types of settings requires the professional nurses to draw upon their scientific background and training. These nurses perform experiments, collect and analyze data, and document results. The nurse becomes integral to the research team when the project advances from the laboratory stage to human studies. Nurses involved in research being conducted in the area of wound healing are helping to define and document the benefit of new technology.[52] The unique perspective that nursing provides aids in the design of functional, effective, and patient-friendly equipment that will be used as an adjunct to hyperbaric oxygen treatments to serve the population of patients with problem wounds.

As health-care resources diminish, hyperbaric nurses are also challenged to conduct nursing research to define and validate their role and to describe the client's response to actual or potential health problems in the altered environment.[21] Nurses also support the development and trials of evidence-based practices related to hyperbaric treatments. An example is the evaluation of methods for monitoring and controlling blood glucose levels during hyperbaric treatments.[40] Nursing research has been presented at recent BNA and UHMS meetings, but wider publication of these results should be encouraged in order to better disseminate the acquired knowledge.

The Nurse as Manager

Responsibility for management of resources in the hyperbaric department often is in the realm of the hyperbaric nurse who functions in a management position. Accountabilities may include management of resources – staffing, supplies and services, and supervision of patient care. Responsibilities may include coordination of clinical and educational activities and research within the department. In the multiplace setting, this may be a shared responsibility with a facilities manager. The nurse manager is accountable for directing and monitoring the department's adherence to state laws, Joint Commission standards, and NFPA codes and standards. These monitors include fire drills, disaster preparedness, and environment-of-care reviews.[26,27,35] The nurse manager may function in the role of safety director of the department.[35]

ADVANCED PRACTICE NURSING IN HYPERBARIC MEDICINE

Advanced practice nurses (APN), nurse practitioners (NP), and/or clinical nurse specialists (CNS) are nurses with a master's or doctoral degree in nursing and advanced clinical education. Many states have granted APNs independent prescriptive authority, and insurance companies, Medicare, and Medicaid reimburse for care provided by APNs, including supervising outpatient hyperbaric treatment under the direction of a physician.

Proper utilization of the APN in the hyperbaric medicine unit will increase the opportunity for research and coverage of increased patient populations in the units. The APN may be responsible for pretreatment history and physicals, as well as care and intervention needed during HBO_2 therapy. APNs maintain quality health care, and add to the research potential of HBO_2 therapy.

PEDIATRICS

Use of HBO_2 in the pediatric population requires skill and knowledge in the care and treatment of children's physical as well as emotional conditions. Children present a particular challenge based on age and cognition. Fears of confinement anxiety and separation need to be addressed. Hyperbaric nurses need to show evidence of age-specific training and skills which are reviewed and validated annually. Some facilities require Pediatric Advanced Life Support (PALS) certification for hyperbaric nurses treating children in the hyperbaric chamber.

Parents can and should be present to talk and interact with their child. Reading stories or watching a favorite movie are helpful distractions. In cases in which a child becomes fearful or anxious before entering the chamber, the use of guided imagery is beneficial. Asking the child to name his/her special place, such as a castle, rocket ship, etc., and helping to make up a story about it can keep him/her occupied. Writing the story down or recording it can be used for future treatments. Age-appropriate guided imagery and movies can be used for distraction in the chambers. Multiplace hyperbaric facilities allow closer contact with children and can alleviate anxiety due to separation. NFPA guidelines for hyperbaric facilities define Class B chambers for single occupancy, thus prohibiting facilities from placing a family member inside the chamber with the child.[(35)]

TRENDS

Demand for hyperbaric nurses has grown as the number of hyperbaric facilities and the number of patients receiving hyperbaric treatment has increased.[(18,41)] The focus of most hyperbaric facilities currently centers on the management of problem wounds.[(28,33)] Some hyperbaric departments have changed their names to reflect the emphasis on wound management. Many hyperbaric nurses have become experts in wound care; some also serve as wound-care consultants to nonhyperbaric patients within their medical centers. Just as the practice of hyperbaric medicine is dynamic, so is the process of defining and advancing the role of nurses practicing within this unique specialty. Hyperbaric nursing continues to be responsive to the changing health-care needs of our patients and the health-care environment.[(4,12)] Maintaining patient safety and quality of care while ensuring adequate reimbursement challenges the hyperbaric nurse providing health care in the twenty-first century.

ACKNOWLEDGMENTS

The author wishes to thank Diane Norkool, deceased, for her work in previous editions of this chapter, which greatly contributed to this edition's chapter.

REFERENCES

1. Abbott C. The use of the hyperbaric chamber as an auxiliary curing aid. AORN J. 1969;9(5):80-4.
2. Adams J. Hyperbaric oxygen therapy. Am J Nurs. 1964;64(6):76-9.
3. American Nurses Association. Nursing's Social Policy Statement: The Essence of the Profession. Silver Spring, Maryland, 2010, American Nurses Association, p.10.
4. Baines C, Sykes P. Professional capability within the Australian hyperbaric nursing workforce. Aust J Adv Nurs. 2014 Dec-2015 Feb;32(2):6-13.
5. Bakker D. Letter of personal communication. 1991 Apr 8.
6. Baromedical Nurses Association. Rules, Article 1, Section 1. 1985.
7. Baromedical Nurses Association. BNA Update. 1987 Jul. Position statement of the BNA.
8. Baromedical Nurses Association [Internet]. Baromedical Nurses Association. Guidelines for: standards of care for the patient receiving hyperbaric oxygen therapy; 2007 [cited 2017 Mar 27]. Available from: http://hyperbaricnurses.org/about-us/standards-of-care/.
9. Barr P. Personal communication. 1991 May 2.
10. CPM Resource Center. Clinical practice guideline: hyperbaric oxygen therapy (HBO2T). Elsevier Clinical Solutions, Inc.; 2015.
11. Carnevali D, Mitchell P, Woods N, Tanner C. Diagnostic reasoning in nursing. Philadelphia: J.B. Lippincott Co.; 1984.
12. Carney AY. Hyperbaric oxygen therapy: an introduction. Crit Care Nurs Q. 2013;36(3):274-9.
13. Cockerill G, O'Conner R. Hyperbaric oxygenation – a new field opened for nurses. Nurs Times. 1967;63:216-8.
14. Davis J. Medical examination of sport scuba divers. San Antonio (TX): Medical Seminars, Inc.; 1986.
15. De Jesus-Greenberg D, Messina V, Mones C, Chase P. Hyperbaric oxygen therapy in critical care. In: Zschoche D, editor. Comprehensive review of critical care. 3rd ed. St. Louis (MO): The C.V. Mosby Co.; 1986. p. 301-10.
16. Fegan F. Hyperbaric oxygen therapy centers. Nurs Forum. 1964;III(2):90-101.
17. Fegan F. What is hyperbaric oxygen therapy? Am Assoc Ind Nurses J. 1964;12(2):11-3.
18. Gaskill M. Deep impact. NurseWeek. 2003;8(1-3).
19. Gaul A, Thompson R, Hart G. Hyperbaric oxygen therapy. Am J Nurs. 1972;72(5):892-6.
20. Gaul A, Hart G. Baromedical nursing combines critical, acute, chronic care. AORN J. 1975;21(6):1038-47.
21. Gaul A. Keynote address to: 1st Annual Baromedical Nurses Association Meeting; 1986 Apr; Key Biscayne, FL.
22. Gaynor M. Nursing under pressure [editorial]. Nurs Outlook. 1964;12 (5):29.
23. Greenberg D, Messina V, Reichow W, MacLean C. Hyperbaric oxygen: exciting new clinical results. RN. 1979;42(9):52-7.
24. Griffiths J. Oxygen therapy in a high pressure environment: recent advance in treatment. Nurs Mirror. 1962;115:171-3.

25. Hanson G. Hyperbaric oxygenation. Nurs Times. 1967;63:213-6.
26. Joint Commission. 2015 comprehensive accreditation and certification manual. Oak Brook(IL): Joint Commission E-dition; 2017.
27. Joint Commission International. 2014 accreditation standards for hospitals. 5th ed. Oakbrook (IL): Joint Commission International; 2013.
28. Kob DG, Gesell LB, Spadafora MP, Liu T. Utilization and staffing of monoplace hyperbaric facilities in the United States. Undersea Hyperb Med. 1998;25(Suppl):25.
29. Kot J. Staffing and training issues in critical care hyperbaric medicine. Diving Hyperb Med. 2015;44(1):47-50.
30. Larson-Lohr V, Norvell H, Josefsen L, Wilcox J, editors.

    Hyperbaric nursing and wound care. Flagstaff (AZ): Best Publishing Co.; 2011.
31. Maudsley R, Mandow G, Lustig E, Daly B. Experience with a hyperbaric oxygen unit. Nurs Mirror. 1966;9:x-xii.
32. Molbo D. The nurse's role in hyperbaric therapy. In: Bergersen BS et al, editors. Current concepts in clinical nursing. St. Louis (MO): The C.V. Mosby Co.; 1967. p. 57-75.
33. Moon RE. Use of hyperbaric oxygen in the management of selected wounds. Adv Wound Care. 1998;11(7):332-4.
34. Nash M. Hyperbaric medicine. Aust Nurses J. 1974;3(8):24-6.
35. National Fire Protection Association. NFPA-99: health care facilities code handbook. Quincy (MA): National Fire Protection Association; 2015.
36. Neelon V, McIntosh H. Hyperbaric oxygenation. Part I: therapeutic benefits. Cardiovasc Nurs. 1971;7(3):69-72.
37. Neelon V, McIntosh H. Hyperbaric oxygenation. Part II: hazards and implications. Cardiovasc Nurs. 1971;7(4):73-6.
38. Norkool D. Current concepts of hyperbaric oxygenation and its application in critical care. Heart Lung. 1979;8(4):728-35.
39. Norkool D. Care of the patient receiving hyperbaric oxygen therapy (HBO2). In: Reiner A, editor. Manual of patient care standards. Gaithersburg (MD): Aspen Publications; 1992.
40. Nwafor TS, Collins N. Managing low blood glucose levels in patients undergoing hyperbaric oxygen therapy. Ostomy Wound Manage. 2014;60(4):12-5.
41. Paez N, Wilcox JR. Hyperbaric nursing. Crit Care Nurs Q. 2013;36(3):316-20.
42. Reiner A, editor. Manual of patient care standards. Gaithersburg (MD): Aspen Publications; 1991.
43. Robinson A. Hyperbaric oxygen unit. Nurs Outlook. 1964;12:40-1.
44. Shaw B. Whatever happened to hyperbaric medicine? RN. 1969;32(11):50-5.
45. Sheffield P, Davis J, Bell G, Gallagher T. Hyperbaric chamber clinical support multiplace. In: Davis J, Hunt T, editors. Hyperbaric oxygen therapy. Bethesda (MD): Undersea Medical Society; 1977. p. 25-39.
46. Thompson M. Treating a patient in the pressure chamber. Nurs Times. 1964;60:174.
47. Uzun G, Mutluoglu M, Ay H, Yildiz S. Decompression sickness in hyperbaric nurses: retrospective analysis of 4500 treatments. J Clin Nurs. 2011;20:1784-7.
48. Vaughan P. Success of hyperbarics in modern medicine. Nurs J India. 1966;57(9):264.

49. Venger M, Jacobson J. Nursing plans for a hyperbaric unit. Am J Nurs. 1964;64(10):79-81.

50. Venger M, Jacobson J. Hyperbaric oxygenation: a nursing challenge. Int Nurs Rev. 1965;12(1):17-9.

51. Venger M. Hyperbaric oxygenation: nursing responsibility in planning for a new clinical service. Nurs Clin North Am. 1966;1(1):131-42.

52. Whelan HT, Houle JM, Donohoe DL, Bajie DM, Schmidt MH, Reichert KW, Weyenberg GT, Lasron DL, Meyer GA, Caviness JA. Medical applications of space light-emitting diode technology – space station and beyond. Space Technol Appl Int Forum. 1999;458(1):3-15

53. Wills-Long S, Long C, Laybourne M. Hyperbaric oxygen therapy – nursing opportunity. Dimens Crit Care Nurs. 1989;8(3):176-82.

54. Zilm G. Hyperbaric oxygen units – high pressure nursing. Can Nurse. 1969;65(2):37-40.

CHAPTER 7 CHAPTER

The Use of Drugs Under Pressure

CHAPTER SEVEN OVERVIEW

The Hyperbaric Oxygen Environment and Oxygen as a Drug **133**
Practical Considerations **133**
Vials 133
Intravenous Infusions 134
Infusion Pumps 134
Routes of Administration 134
Pharmacokinetic Considerations **134**
Absorption 135
Intramuscular and Subcutaneous Routes 135
Oral Routes 135
Transmucousal Routes 135
Pulmonary Route 135
Distribution 136
Metabolism 136
Elimination 137
Practical Kinetic Application **139**
Pharmacodynamic Considerations **139**
Drugs Decreasing Tolerance to Oxygen Toxicity 139
Agents Increasing or Decreasing Metabolic Rate *139*
Thyroid Replacement *139*
Glucocorticoids *140*
Sympathetic Stimulation *140*
Central Vasodilators (Mafenide Acetate and Acetazolamide) *140*
Drugs Increasing Tolerance to Oxygen Toxicity 141
Vitamin E (Alpha Tocopherol) *141*
Propranolol *141*
Tromethamine (THAM) *141*
Chlorpromazine and Promethazine *141*

Considerations for Commonly Used Drugs in the Chamber . . . 141
Anticonvulsants . . . *141*
Barbiturates . . . *142*
Phenytoin . . . *142*
Benzodiazepines . . . *142*
Opioid Analgesics . . . *143*
Analgesics, Non-opioid . . . *143*
Drugs Incompatible with Hyperbaric Oxygen Due to Enhanced Drug Toxicity . . . 143
Cisplatin . . . *143*
Doxorubicin . . . *144*
Drugs Commonly Used with Hyperbaric Oxygen or That May Have Special Consideration . . . 144
Insulin and Antihyperglycemics . . . *144*
Sympathomimetics, Vasoactive Compounds, and Antihypertensives . . . *145*
Bleomycin Sulfate . . . *146*
Disulfiram . . . *146*
Ethanol . . . *147*
Anesthetics . . . *147*
Lidocaine . . . *148*
Digitalis/Digoxin . . . *148*
Heparin . . . 148
Phenothiazines, Antipsychotics, and Antidepressants . . . *149*
Antimicrobials . . . *149*
Conclusion . . . 150
References . . . 151

The Use of Drugs Under Pressure

Ryan Feldman

THE HYPERBARIC OXYGEN ENVIRONMENT AND OXYGEN AS A DRUG

A hyperbaric and hyperoxic environment creates numerous considerations for the use of drug therapies within it. First, the physical stress of hyperbaria impacts drug storage and has implications on which containers are most appropriate for use. Second, physiologic changes to the body from hyperbaria and hyperoxia may lead to pharmacokinetic changes in drug disposition. Lastly, hyperbaric oxygen acting as a drug can interact and enhance or ameliorate the physiologic effect of a drug.

Most drugs will not interact unfavorably with oxygen, and to study each and every drug in its interaction with hyperbaric oxygen would be not feasible. Unless specific contraindications or precautions have been addressed, it is generally safe to assume a medication can be used. Significant known exceptions and their evidence will be discussed in this chapter, along with the implications of hyperbaric oxygen use on drug disposition.

PRACTICAL CONSIDERATIONS

The mechanical effects of pressure on the drug container are our first concern. Medications stocked are subjected to continual compressions and decompressions and must retain their absolute seal at the maximum pressure anticipated.

Vials

Glass vials appear to resist pressures ranging up to 6 atmospheres (ATM). Caution should be exercised when opening glass vials of 10 ml or larger at pressures greater than 3 atmospheres. To avoid operator harm from vial implosion, the vial should be wrapped in gauze when accessed. Alternatively, the contents of the vial could be withdrawn outside of the chamber and brought into the chamber in a syringe. Small vials of 3 milliliters or less appear stable to opening at pressures of 3 ATM or greater.

If a multidose vial is accessed, it should not undergo pressurization again. Introduction of a needle through the rubber stopper allows air to be forced in during subsequent compression cycles, and the contents can be expelled during decompression. Accessing multidose vials also risks contamination of the sterile environment within. The vial should be discarded at the end of decompression regardless of the amount used.

Intravenous Infusions

The preferred storage for intravenous solutions in the chamber is flexible plastic bags which can adapt to changing pressures. Glass vials can be used only in conjunction with vented tubing with a needle that reaches to the bottom of the vial or far enough into the vial to pass the liquid phase and enter the compartment of air within the bottle.

During compression, vented tubing is not required; increasing pressure causes air to bubble freely through the contents of the intravenous (IV) bottles and gather at the top. During decompression, however, an air vent tube is mandatory; the expanding air in the IV bottle above the liquid will forcefully drive the entire contents of the bottle into the patient's circulation. This will be followed by a bolus of air, which may vary in amount from a few milliliters to over a liter depending on the size of the vial. If a glass bottle is used with no vent tubing extending through the contents to the bottom, during decompression the infusion may be stopped and the bottle may be turned over so that the vent needle is on top. This will allow any air in the bottle to escape during decompression without emptying the bottle of its contents.

Sealed glass vials that have not been accessed may also be vulnerable to air entry. Prior editions of this text report a case of a sealed 500 ml saline vial exploding after decompression from 6 ATM. The vial had been exposed to many compression cycles, and the cause was thought to be related to air being forced in.

Infusion Pumps

Infusion pumps may be used in the multiplace chamber if battery powered. If supplied from line voltage, the plug must be of the explosion-proof type, which positively locks, and the current must be supplied through an isolation transformer. It should be noted the National Fire Protection Agency NFPA code has been revised, and the chamber atmosphere is no longer classified as explosive, but is now classified as hazardous. This will mean that some electrical equipment that was banned in the past is now permitted.

Routes of Administration

The intravenous route is the most reliable choice for delivering drugs in the chamber. Hyperbaric oxygen causes a vasoconstriction in normal tissues resulting in up to a 20% reduction in blood flow.[50,90] It was thought that this same vasoconstriction would also severely impede the normal absorption of drugs injected intramuscularly and subcutaneously. This theoretical interaction is not supported by the literature. (See the next section on pharmokinetic considerations.) Oral absorption also does not seem to be affected despite theoretical interactions. Transdermal absorption is highly variable and dependent on solvents used to help diffuse the drug across the membrane. It is recommended that all patches and creams be removed from patients prior to entrance into a chamber; this route of administration should not be considered.

PHARMACOKINETIC CONSIDERATIONS

Oxygen under pressure induces numerous physiologic changes which may have an impact on the pharmacokinetic disposition of a drug. Generally, the pharmacokinetic properties of a drug are described as a function of four separate phases: absorption into the body, distribution to tissue, metabolism into a new chemical moiety, and elimination from the body. A change to any of the above four factors would change serum concentration and may alter therapeutic efficacy or toxicity. In this section, theoretical changes to pharmacokinetic parameters will be discussed. It should be noted that while theoretical interaction exists, the majority of available evidence supports that single-dose pharmacokinetics are unchanged with acute exposure to hyperbaric oxygen.

Absorption

Absorption into the body is a function of route of administration and bioavailability (the total amount of drug available for systemic use from a given dose). The most reliable method of delivering a drug is via the intravenous route where absorption and bioavailability are 100%.

Intramuscular and Subcutaneous Routes

Intramuscular and subcutaneous injections retain high bioavailability, but absorption is dependent on drug diffusion from the tissue depot into systemic circulation. This diffusion is dependent on intrinsic drug properties such as size and lipophilicity as well as the rate of tissue perfusion. As hyperbaric oxygen has been shown to decrease cardiac output by 10%–20%, and hyperoxia leads to vasoconstriction, both delayed and decreased peak absorption from subcutaneous or intramuscular injections would be expected. However, when 20 normal volunteers were injected with midazolam intramuscularly and placed in a chamber, there was not a delay or decrease in peak level as compared to those in normobaria.[(30)] In 65% of the subjects, peak levels occurred earlier while at 2.8 atmosphere absolute (ATA). Peak levels occurred significantly later at 2.8 ATA in only 15%. The mean time to peak level at 2.8 ATA was 33 minutes, and 41 minutes at 1 ATA. Midazolam is a highly lipophilic drug, which would aid in diffusion across biologic membranes but limits its dissolution into the serum. Studies with more hydrophilic drugs that are more rapidly dissolved in serum are not available for analysis.

Oral Routes

Oral absorption is dependent on drug bioavailability and splanchnic perfusion. Oral bioavailability is reduced by the amount of drug not absorbed into the gastrointestinal tract, the amount metabolized by the gastrointestinal tract cells, and the amount metabolized by the liver before reaching systemic circulation. Any alteration to the metabolic rates of the gastrointestinal and hepatic enzymes will alter the amount of drug available for systemic use. Hyperoxic conditions can alter metabolic systems responsible for drug metabolism. [(4)] (See the following section on metabolism.) Decreased splanchnic blood flow that can be seen with HBO_2 would also theoretically delay or decrease peak oral absorption.[(50,90)] Interactions with oral absorption are, however, largely theoretical, and no studies to date have evaluated the effect of HBO_2 on this route of administration.

Transmucousal Routes

Intranasal and buccal-delivered medications bypass gut and liver metabolism and would be less likely to be affected by changes in drug metabolism from hyerpoxia. Intranasal absorption, however, is sporadic and less reliable than intramuscular (IM) or subcutaneous injection.

Pulmonary Route

Pulmonary medicines that are aerosolized should not exhibit a change in absorption as these medications are contained in aerosolized droplets and do not behave in the gaseous phase. Any drug delivered as a gas via the pulmonary route will have an increased partial pressure and thus an increased diffusion gradient across the alveoli which would lead to an increase in absorption.

Distribution

Distribution of drug into tissue is dependent on its inherent chemical properties that influence biologic membrane permeability. Molecular weight, degree of ionization at physiologic pH, affinity for drug transport proteins, and protein binding all affect total drug distribution. When drug distribution is increased (through greater tissue penetration), serum concentrations may appear lower for the same given dose. Protein binding may be affected in hyperoxic conditions due to excess free radicals.(92,100) This may affect drugs that are highly protein bound such as phenytoin or valproic acid. No current literature has evaluated the impact of this theoretical interaction however.

Some reviews have suggested that increased negatively charged free radicals generated from increased oxygen partial pressures may increase the permeability of biologic membranes.(92,100) This postulate is not supported in animal trials assessing the permeability of the blood-brain barrier. Rabbits injected with the antimicrobial tobramycin did not have significantly changed ratios of blood to cerebrospinal fluid concentration when measured at baseline and at 90 minutes of 3 ATA hyperbaric oxygen.(59) Similar studies with gentamicin in rabbits also showed no difference.(94) Few interactions between HBO_2 and drug distribution are likely to exist.

Metabolism

Drug metabolism is a biological process for structurally modifying a pharmaceutical to enhance its elimination. While each individual drug has its own specific metabolic pathway, it can generally be considered to occur in two phases. Phase I metabolism is carried out primarily by a set of monooxygenase enzymes known as cytochrome oxidase P-450 (CYP450), and its reactions are characterized by oxidation or reduction such as hydroxylation, acetylation, or hydrolysis. Just three families of this enzyme, CYP 1, 2, and 3, account for 79% of phase I metabolism of some of the most commonly prescribed drugs.(120)

Phase II reactions are conjugation reactions and involve the attachments of a large hydrophilic group to the chemical moiety to increase its solubility and enhance renal excretion. Generally, phase II reactions occur at the site previously modified by the phase I reaction. Some examples of phase II reactions include sulfation, methylation, and glucuronidation. These metabolic steps are carried out by a variety of transferase enzymes such as methyltransferase, sulfotransferase, and UDP-glucuronyltransferase.(54,28)

Conditions that increase or decrease the metabolizing capacity of an enzyme utilized in a drug's metabolism can alter the clearance of the drug. Enzyme activity can be altered in three ways. The first is to up- or downregulate gene expression and increase or decrease enzyme transcription and translation (transcriptional induction or inhibition). The next is allosteric binding of a substance which induces a structural change to enzyme and increases or decreases reaction rate (allosteric induction or inhibition). The final interaction is through competitive inhibition from shared drug metabolism. When two substrates share a metabolic pathway that is maximally saturated, the elimination of both substances is decreased due to competition for enzyme binding site (competitive inhibition).

Hyperoxia alone has shown increases in cytochrome oxidase p-450 transcription and translation in animals.(72) When mice were exposed to oxygen at 1–3 ATA for 15 minutes to 4 hours there was an increase in CYP450 production. This increase was proportional with the total amount of oxygen exposure. The effects were not seen when nitrogen or air were used under pressure, leading to the conclusion that hyperoxia was the stimulus for increased transcription and translation. In vitro hepatocyte suspensions also show increased CYP450 production when exposed to hyperoxia. Hyperbaric oxygen also induces the production of superoxide dismutase RNA in rats after only 1 hour of 100% oxygen at 1 ATA.(39) Superoxide dismutase, however, is not an enzyme involved in metabolism of most drugs, and this clinical effect is unknown. The results of these studies would suggest the possibility of transcriptional induction of metabolic enzymes from hyperbaric oxygen.

To evaluate the effects of HBO_2 on drug-metabolizing enzyme systems, rat microsomes were subjected to oxygen at 2.96 ATM, 4.93 ATM, and 6.9 ATM, and their catabolic activity was measured.(4) Aniline hydroxylation, a CYP450 reaction, was reduced by 34%, 57%, and 64% respectively. Amidopyrine demethylation, another CYP450 isoenzyme reaction, was unaffected, suggesting variability with specific isoenzymes in inhibitory effect. Conversely, when rat liver and lung microsomes are first exposed to hypoxia (0.286 ATM O2 x 1 h) and subsequent hyperoxia (1.97 ATM x 1 h), increases in both aninline and amidopyrine metabolism are seen.(98) Hypoxia increased the reaction rate for amidopyridine by 57%. Subsequent hyperoxia led to a 114% increase in aniline hydroxylation and a 148% increase in amidopyridine metabolism.(97)

The interactions described above occurred during in vitro experiments; however, similiar results are seen in-vivo. Liver microsomes were prepared and analyzed from rats that underwent 12 days of continuous exposure to either normoxic air, 1.2 ATA He-O_2, or 21 ATA He-O_2. Specimens continuously exposed to HBO_2 environments had increased rates of morphine n-dealkylatytion and p-nitroanisole O-dealkylation. Cocaine n-dealkylation was not affected, however, highlighting the variability in effect with specific isoenzymes. Another study utilizing the same conditions looked at chronic exposure for 23–84 days. Once again, p-nitroanisole O-dealkylation was increased; however, both morphine and cocaine n-dealkylation were not affected during this more prolonged exposure.(41-42)

In vivo drug metabolism pathways differ substantially between agents. Given the complex interaction of in vivo metabolism, these in vitro animal results are not directly interpretable in human models. They do suggest that changes in phase I monooxygenase enzyme systems may occur in hyperbaric oxygen. When considering drug-metabolizing enzymes, transcription interactions typically occur on a time course of days to weeks after consistent substrate exposure. However, as cited above, more acute increases in CYP450 production may occur in hyperoxia.

Enzymatic reactions rates also appear to have been decreased in some systems suggesting possible inhibitory effects of HBO_2 on enzyme metabolism, but the effects were highly variable. Data analyzing human enzymatic rates or metabolic product analysis after exposure to HBO_2 are lacking. It has been shown that drugs such as caffeine do not appear to have increased metabolic rates in humans under hyperbaric oxygen.(91) It should be considered, however, that metabolic changes for drugs are possible when patients are exposed to hyperbaric oxygen.

Elimination

Elimination is the process of drug removal from systemic circulation, and in clinical practice is most often measured via serum concentration decay. For first-order elimination drugs, the serum concentration decay can be expressed as an elimination rate constant known as Ke, which represents the slope of a log-linear transformed serum concentration versus time graph. In a multicompartment model, the drug is administered to the vascular compartment, and the initial serum decay occurs by distribution to other compartments (i.e., adipose) as well as elimination by normal routes. This results in a very large elimination rate known as αKe, which correlates with a very short drug half-life known as $\alpha T_{1/2}$. As this elimination rate represents primarily distribution as well as clearance and not clearance alone, it is not clinically as useful. After initial distribution is complete, a smaller elimination rate remains known as βKe, which is reliant only on drug clearance from the serum compartment. This is representative of drug elimination from the body. **The more relevant value to clinicians, the terminal elimination half-life ($\beta T_{1/2}$), can be expressed as $\beta T_{1/2}$ = Ln(2)/βKe.**[28]

The βKe is determined by the rate of drug removal from serum (known as clearance, CL) and the volume of tissue needing to be cleared of drug (Vd). The elimination rate constant βKe can be expressed as βKe = CL/Vd. Clearance (CL), the amount of serum that is cleared of drug by the eliminating organ per unit time, is expressed in volume/time (i.e., ml/min). Clearance is additive, where the total clearance of drug for the body is the sum of the clearance value of all eliminating organs. It can usually be thought of as CL = renal CL + nonrenal CL. As the primary eliminating organs in the body are the kidneys and liver, it can be thought of as CL= CL renal + CL hepatic.

For primarily renal-excreted drugs that do not undergo metabolic transformation, their clearance can be defined as CL = renal CL. Renal clearance is dependent on renal perfusion. Hyperoxia and hyperbaria induce a decrease in cardiac output and vasoconstriction and cause decreased renal perfusion.[50, 90] Decreased renal perfusion should decrease renal clearance and thus reduce the βKe (prolonging half-life) of primarily renal-cleared medications. This observation was not reflected when healthy adult males were given 1.5 mg/kg of the renal-cleared drug gentamicin.[81] Pharmacokinetic assessments during normobaric oxygen were compared with the same dose given under hyperbaric oxygen after a two-week wash-out period. In their study, no difference was observed in the HBO_2 group in $\beta T_{1/2}$ (112 versus 115 min), volume of distribution (0.201 versus 0.184 L/kg), or total clearance (0.0754 versus 0.0676 L/kg).

For drugs that undergo primarily hepatic clearance, their total clearance can be expressed as CL = hepatic CL. Hepatic clearance varies depending on the hepatic extraction ratio of the drug. For drugs with a high hepatic extraction ratio, 70%–100% of the drug is cleared upon reaching the liver; thus, clearance is limited by the rate of drug delivery to the liver and is perfusion dependent. As increased hepatic perfusion has been demonstrated in rat models, the clearance of high–hepatic extraction ratio drugs would be expected to increase with HBO.[50,90]

When the high–hepatic extraction drug meperidine was given to dogs during normobaria, 2.8 ATA with 100% O_2, and 6.9 ATA, no change was seen in drug clearance.[64] Rump et al., 1999, describe human data that echo this finding. Healthy human males were given the high-extraction drug lidocaine at both 1 and 2.5 bar and demonstrated no change in lidocaine disposition.[92] These findings suggest that high–hepatic extraction drugs are unaffected by increases in hepatic perfusion or that the hepatic perfusion in humans is not significantly altered. Lastly, highly protein-bound drugs that have a high hepatic extraction ratio would have increased clearance if HBO decreased protein binding and made more free drug available for metabolism. (See the previous section on distribution.) No studies currently exist to evaluate this theoretical interaction.

Clearance of low–hepatic extraction drugs is dependent on intrinsic enzymatic reaction rate and is independent of hepatic perfusion. These drugs exhibit maximal, or saturated, enzymatic metabolism, and thus delivery of more drug to the liver does not increase clearance; only a change in metabolic reaction rate or enzyme quantity would alter clearance. As it has been previously demonstrated that HBO_2 may increase or decrease the rate of metabolite production by CYP450 enzymes, it is reasonable to assume that low extraction drugs may be affected by changes in intrinsic enzyme activity.

This conclusion was refuted when dogs were exposed to the low-extraction drugs theophylline and pentobarbital at normobaric, hyperbaric, and hyperbaric hyperoxic conditions.(63,65) No change was seen in the total clearance or disposition in these drugs. The effects on low–hepatic extraction drugs were also evaluated in humans utilizing caffeine. Two healthy adult males were administered caffeine at normobaria, and the βKe was evaluated at 0.25 MPa, alternating 100% O_2 breathing for 20 min and air breathing for 5 min. While there was no comparator in this evaluation, the kinetic parameters derived from serum sampling did not differ significantly from prior reported literature at normobaric kinetics.(91) Caffeine and theophylline both undergo CYP1A2 metabolism; theophylline also is targeted by CYP2E1 and CYP3A4. Results for drugs that are metabolized via other enzyme systems may vary.

PRACTICAL KINETIC APPLICATION

As discussed above, while many theoretical interactions exist, the available limited medical literature has not supported significant changes in drug disposition with acute exposure to hyperbaric oxygen. Clinicians should be aware interactions may occur through changes in perfusion, and it is possible enzymatic processes may be affected, but currently no significant kinetic effects have been noted. While no data exists to support change in oral, IM, or subcutaneous injection, the most reliable route of administration for acute therapies is intravenous injection to avoid possible interactions in the chamber.

PHARMACODYNAMIC CONSIDERATIONS

Pharmacodynamic interactions result in modification of the pharmacologic effect of a drug after administration. These interactions will increase or decrease the effects of oxygen or the drug. The remainder of the chapter will discuss known evidence behind pharmacodynamic interactions between HBO_2 and prescribed therapies.

Drugs Decreasing Tolerance to Oxygen Toxicity

Agents Increasing or Decreasing Metabolic Rate

Elevation in temperature and metabolism leads to an increased susceptibility to oxygen toxicity. Hypothermia also has a protective effect upon oxygen toxicity.(10) Agents that alter metabolic rate or temperature may alter oxygen toxicity thresholds.

Thyroid Replacement

Iatrogenic production of hyperthyroidism with the administration of synthetic thyroid in experimental animals results in very pronounced enhancement of O_2 toxicity at atmospheric pressure and at increased ambient pressure. A thyroidectomy has the opposite effect. This has been demonstrated in animal studies, and one may reasonably assume that these factors would also be operative in human subjects selected for clinical exposure to hyperbaric oxygen. Presumably, this is due to the increased metabolic rate.

Hypophysectomy also counters oxygen seizures.[10] Active Graves's disease predisposes to seizures as the patient is hyperthyroid. There is no danger of oxygen toxicity in a patient taking thyroid supplement to maintain a euthyroid state.

Glucocorticoids

Steroids and adrenaline have a sensitizing effect on oxygen toxicity, while adrenalectomy in rats has protective effects.[10] In clinical practice, hyperbaricists are often called upon to treat people who are receiving steroids. Careful monitoring of the patient who is receiving large doses of steroids is warranted, and prophylactic anticonvulsants may be necessary. Frequent air breaks are often used. It has been reported in prior editions that patients on steroids may develop premonitory signs of oxygen toxicity more quickly than normal. Steroid-mediated seizures have not been seen in patients exposed to U.S. Navy Tables 5 and 6, probably because of the short exposures to oxygen between air breaks.

Sympathetic Stimulation

Drugs that increase sympathetic stimulation may increase the susceptibility to oxygen toxicity by similar means to enhanced metabolic rate. The mechanisms of pulmonary and neurologic oxygen toxicity have not been fully elucidated. Evidence in humans on the risks associated with central nervous system (CNS) stimulants and sympathomimetics is lacking. The clinician should be mindful of the possibility of increased risk for oxygen toxicity in humans with excessive sympathetic stimulation.

Animal research using histochemical staining shows that norepinephrine-containing cells are activated during HBO_2 seizure in larger quantities than control.[5] Pulmonary oxygen toxicity is also increased in rats by exposure to isoproterenol.[24] Animal data is conflicting; however, some animal studies have shown low doses of caffeine and amphetamine to have protective effects.[22,15]

Central Vasodilators (Mafenide Acetate and Acetazolamide)

Carbonic anhydrase catalyzes the metabolism of carbon dioxide to a bicarbonate and hydrogen ion. Pharmacologic inhibition of this process leads to an increase in carbon dioxide retention. Hyperbaric oxygen causes decreased response to carbon dioxide in the respiratory centers of the brain, leading to an even further retention of carbon dioxide. Carbon dioxide retention promotes vasodilation and leads to an increase in cerebral blood flow, enhancing oxygen delivery and decreasing the time to oxygen toxicity.

Mafenide acetate is a sulfonamide antimicrobial cream that inhibits the growth of a variety of microbial organism. While its antimicrobial effect stems from targeting the folate production pathway, it also has carbonic anhydrase–inhibiting effects in humans. It is recommended in practice that this cream be removed from any patient entering the chamber. No evidence currently exists evaluating the depth or severity of this interaction but it is thought risk outweighs benefit.

Numerous studies in rats with the carbonic anhydrous inhibitor acetazolamide demonstrate that the latency period to oxygen-induced seizures is decreased.[51-52,116] However, a study has also demonstrated a protective effect when a lower dose is utilized.[52] While no human data is available to evaluate the depth of this interaction, it may be wise to consider prophylactic antiepileptics, if the drug must be used at higher pressures. If a patient is already taking acetazolamide when referred for treatment, or requires emergent treatment, there may be a higher risk of oxygen seizure at pressures greater than 2 ATA. It should be avoided at pressures greater than 2 ATA whenever possible.

Drugs Increasing Tolerance to Oxygen Toxicity

Vitamin E (Alpha Tocopherol)

Vitamin E acts as an antioxidant and scavenges free radicals formed by oxygen. Vitamin E–deficient mice have a higher mortality in HBO_2.[57,84] Vitamin E also appears to protect against pulmonary oxygen toxicity and prolong life in mice an average of 1.6 days compared to vitamin E–deficient mice when exposed to 100% oxygen.[87] The seizure threshold also appears to be raised by supplemental vitamin E.[70] Some hyperbaric clinicians recommend a dosage of 400 units p.o. per 90-minute treatment, given at any time preceding treatment, allowing time for absorption.

Propranolol

Propranolol is a beta-adrenergic blocker that has good penetration into the central nervous system. Whelan and colleagues administered propranolol to mice and found a significant increase in time to oxygen-induced seizure as compared to other substances (dilsufiram, diethyldithiocarbamate, and 21-aminosteroid).[113] When rats were pretreated with a stimulator of cyclic adenosine monophate (cAMP) (glucagon or isoproterenol) or an inhibitor (propranolol, practolol), the propranolol-treated rats had an increase in time to seizure by 70%.[24] Necropsy of propranolol-treated rats suggests that the mechanism may be related to prevention of glycogen depletion in the central nervous system. While propranolol is not recommended as a seizure-preventing medication, those who are on it may be more resilient to demonstrating signs of toxicity. (See the sections on sympathomimetics, vasoactive compounds and antihypertensives.)

Tromethamine (THAM)

Tromethamine is a buffering agent that will generate bicarbonate from carbonic acid. It appears to protect against pulmonary oxygen toxicity as well as neurologic toxicity when administered to rats. It is thought this is mediated via a reduction of HBO_2-induced hypercapnia as THAM will drive the production of bicarbonate from carbonic acid instead of CO_2. While the interplay of CO_2 in oxygen toxicity is complex, it is known that 5% CO_2 environments appear to potentiate oxygen toxicity.[10] Increases in CO_2 are seen in HBO via decreased ventilatory rates and CO_2 displacement from hemoglobin in hyperoxia, which increase tissues and plasma CO_2 levels.

Chlorpromazine and Promethazine

Chlorpromazine and promethazine have been shown to reduce pulmonary and neurologic oxygen toxicity in rats.[10] The mechanism is thought to be related to sympatholytic properties of the drugs. (See the following section on phenothiazines, antipsychotics, and antidepressants.)

Considerations for Commonly Used Drugs in the Chamber

Anticonvulsants

The use of anticonvulsants in connection with hyperbaric therapy may be either prophylactic or for the treatment of seizures which do not stop when oxygen inhalation is terminated. If anticonvulsants are used prophylactically to suppress convulsions, it is critically important that the usual oxygen pressure/time limits be observed. Suppression of convulsions, if exposure is carried beyond the normal latent period for oxygen toxicity, can allow permanent oxygen-induced damage to the CNS. This has been well demonstrated by Gutsche, et al.[44] In dogs exposed to 5 ATA of oxygen for 4 hours, convulsive seizures were suppressed by anesthetics. Post decompression, the surviving animals had permanent paralysis and severe neurologic damage.

In clinical exposures of no more than 90 minutes limited to 3 ATA, permanent damage has not been reported in humans. Even though there is still disagreement among some hyperbaricists regarding seizure prophylaxis, it is safe in selected cases, so long as these limits are not exceeded. In the patient who is febrile, toxic from gas gangrene, taking steroids, or has an idiopathic-low seizure threshold, prophylactic administration of a suitable anticonvulsant may be indicated.

Barbiturates

Barbiturates function via allosteric modulation of central nervous system gama-amino-butryic acid (GABA) receptors to depress CNS function and may depress respiratory function, leading to increased CO_2 retention in a similar mechanism to opioids. Rodent studies of thiopental and pentobarbital also demonstrate the duration and potency of action may be reduced by certain hyperbaric environments or increased by hyperbaric nitrogen.[78,99]

Phenobarbital has been used as an agent in preventing oxygen convulsions. Prior editions of this text report lengthy experience utilizing phenobarbital as a prophylactic drug for those at high risk for seizure and noted no adverse effects. Patients receiving this medication should have respiratory status monitored and capnography measured. If increased CO_2 retention in noted, the patient should be instructed to take multiple deep breaths to reduce systemic CO_2.

Phenytoin

Phenytoin has been widely used in epilepsy, but its efficacy in preventing oxygen convulsions is not as well established. Marks, in early animal experiments, did not find phenytoin to be effective in delaying or preventing oxygen convulsions.[76] This was corroborated by data from Bitterman and colleagues that demonstrated no change in the latency time to seizure for rats undergoing 100% O_2 at 6 ATA compared to saline-injected controls.[14] It is probable that, in animals with a normal seizure threshold, no effect could be observed.

Human data is not well documented. One case describes a 27-year-old male patient being treated for cerebral air embolism who developed seizures after 11 minutes of 100% $O_{2.}$[111] Oxygen was removed, but the patient was not able to tolerate any further HBO until 15 mg/kg of phenytoin was administered, at which point the patient and attendants completed all prescribed therapies. Clinical experience dictates that its effect in stopping oxygen seizures can be substantial in the acute situation.

Benzodiazepines

Benzodiazepines work in a similar fashion to barbiturates; they bind via allosteric interaction to GABA receptors and induce a decrease in the resting threshold of the neuron from increased chloride permeability, inhibiting depolarization. Many different benzodiazepines exist, all with slightly different duration of action due to biologic half-life and presence of active metabolites. Diazepam has been used prophylactically during HBO_2 in patients who are thought to be at high risk for oxygen convulsions.

Prior editions of this text report no adverse effects utilizing diazepam in their facility to premedicate against oxygen-induced seizures.

Clonazepam has been shown to be effective in reducing latency to seizure occurrence in cats; however, it is only available as an oral option and would not be sufficient during acute seizure activity.[12] Diazepam, midazolam, and lorazepam are recommended for terminating seizures in convulsive disorders of non-hyperbaric origin and are useful for terminating seizures in the chamber.[17] Frequently, patients under hyperbaric therapy will require larger doses than would be expected. The reason for this is unclear. Studies in mice suggest a possible decrease in diazepam allosteric modulation of GABA-A receptors.[25] Courtiere et al. has shown a 29% decrease in cortical benzodiazepine receptors under hyperbaric hyperoxia.[21] Clinical experience demonstrates that there does not seem to be any evidence of rebound sedation following cessation of therapy when larger than usual dosages of diazepam (15 to 50 mg) have been used. Monitoring of respiratory and mental status is recommended for patients who receive benzodiazepines prophylactically or emergently.

Opioid Analgesics

The clinician should be especially vigilant for oxygen toxicity in patients receiving opioid analgesics, which will enhance risk of oxygen toxicity via CO_2 retention, leading to central vasodilation similar to carbonic anhydrase inhibitors. Opioid analgesics depress respiration by reducing the reactivity of the medulla to CO_2.[66-68] When respiration is decreased by opioid analgesics, a rise occurs in the alveolar and arterial PCO_2. In addition, oxygen can have a depressant effect on respiration. This exaggerated depression of ventilation leads to a still-greater rise in arterial PCO_2 above normal. The blood vessels of the brain dilate as a result of this increased PCO_2, and, because of the increased blood flow, the amount of dissolved oxygen rises in brain tissue. The increased amount of oxygen in brain tissue speeds the development of oxygen convulsions. One should be particularly watchful if the patient has received one of these agents. If the patient's respirations are noted to be slowed, he or she should be instructed or stimulated to take a number of deep breaths to ventilate and reduce the CO_2 levels.

It has also been demonstrated that an HBO_2 environment can exhibit antinocioceptive effects at μ and κ opioid receptors in rats.[121] This effect is less pronounced in rats that are opioid tolerant, likely due to receptor downregulation. The action of opioid drugs does not appear to be affected by this shared interaction, and their pharmacodynamics properties are retained under HBO_2.[2]

Analgesics, Non-opioid

Non-narcotic pain medicationsand nonsteroidal anti-inflammatory drugs such as aspirin, acetaminophen, and ibuprofen, when given in the usual therapeutic dosage, are not known to have any potentiating effects on oxygen toxicity. Their efficiency under increased partial pressure of oxygen appears to be unimpaired. Although some feel that aspirin may potentiate oxygen toxicity, there is little clinical evidence to support this.

Drugs Incompatible with Hyperbaric Oxygen Due to Enhanced Drug Toxicity

Cisplatin

Cisplatin is a chemotherapeutic that interferes with DNA synthesis, affecting fibroblast production and collagen synthesis. When mice were exposed to cisplatin, wound breaking strength was found to be adversely affected by HBO_2 when compared to controls.[82] In other rodent models, HBO_2 has had variable effects on ameliorating cisplatin nephrotoxic and ototoxic effects.[6-7,117] As HBO_2 may impede wound healing in combination with cisplatin, any patient who has a wound healing problem (such as radionecrosis) should not be treated concomitantly. However, in a life-threatening situation such as CO poisoning, gas gangrene, or necrotizing fasciitis, wound healing concerns are overridden by the emergency indication.

Doxorubicin

Doxorubicin is an antineoplastic agent that exerts its effect through generation of free radicals and has a dose-limiting cardiac toxicity as a consequence of therapy. It has been considered contraindicated in HBO_2 therapy based on the work of Upton and colleagues. They attempted to determine if tissue damage caused by extravasation of doxorubicin could be counteracted by four weeks of hyperbaric oxygen therapy.[108] By the fourth week, animals exposed to HBO_2 experienced 87% mortality when concomitantly receiving doxorubicin. Further studies carried out on rats involving IM injection of doxorubicin and subsequent HBO did not find an increased rate of rat mortality and found statistically significant increases in wound healing compared to control at three to four weeks of HBO_2.[1] Given the conflicting evidence, a further study was conducted evaluating the cardiac effects of doxorubicin and HBO_2 in rats using cardiac ultrasound and histopathologic evaluation of cell damage.[58] It was found that the use of doxorubicin and HBO_2 together did depress cardiac output compared to control but faired better than doxorubicin alone. The cardiac depression and cardiac cellular damage were less than that of doxorubicin alone suggesting that HBO_2 may have ameliorated the damaging effects.

In a long-term follow-up of humans pretreated with HBO_2 prior to doxorubicin versus those receiving doxorubicin alone, 5-year survival in the HBO_2 group was 73%. The mortality rate was not different between groups, and all mortality was cancer related.[47] Given the lack of strong evidence and possibility of harm, HBO_2 and doxorubicin should be avoided in combination. Some recommend at least three days to elapse between the last doxorubicin dose and the initiation of a course of HBO_2. The conflicting evidence, and possibility of myocardial protectant effects in rats, suggests further research is warranted, however.

Drugs Commonly Used with Hyperbaric Oxygen or That May Have Special Consideration

Insulin and Antihyperglycemics

The effects of HBO_2 on insulin activity are not completely understood but are clearly potentiated by HBO_2. Blood glucose levels have consistently been shown to fall in diabetic patients who are undergoing HBO_2 therapy.[56,73,101,104] Average drops in blood glucose levels during a single hyperbaric oxygen treatment range between 31 and 51 milligrams per deciliter. In a prospective observational study of the effects of 15–40 sessions of HBO_2 on blood pressure and glycemic levels of hypertensive diabetics, blood glucose levels were lowered by 23% post session.[3] If the pretreatment glucose was between 120–170 mg/dl, a treatment reduction to < 100 mg/dl occurred 52% of the time. If the glucose was < 120 mg/dl before treatment, a reduction to < 70 mg/dl occurred 23.5% of the time.

Oral glucose tolerance tests and fasting glycemic levels are improved significantly by 20 sessions of HBO_2 therapy in diabetic patients.[109] While the effect is most pronounced in diabetic patients, there may be a moderate effect in nondiabetic patients as well.[115] Obese or overweight males with (n = 7) and without (n = 10) diabetes were subjected to HBO_2 therapy for 3 sessions. Insulin sensitivity was measured via maximal glucose uptake into cells using a hyperinsulinaemic euglycaemic clamp (80 $mU{\cdot}m^{-2}{\cdot}min^{-1}$) at baseline and during the third session as well as 30 minutes after the session. Maximal glucose infusion rate was increased by 29% +/- 32(p = 0.01) in nondiabetics and by 57% +/- 66 in diabetics (p = 0.04) at the third session. Similar effects were seen in nonobese nondiabetics when subjected to 100% oxygen at 2 ATA 6 times a week for 5 weeks.[114] Insulin sensitivity was tested by the same method described above; all participants had an increase in glucose infusion rate requirements by the third treatment, and it was maintained throughout the study.

The reason for increases in insulin sensitivity is unknown and may differ between diabetics and nondiabetics. Plasma glucagon levels have been shown to decrease in diabetics receiving HBO_2, but insulin level does not appear to increase.[104] Others have postulated a variety of mechanisms including inhibition of carotid body chemoreceptors, increases in interleukin-6, and increased muscle oxidative capacity as possible factors in this phenomenon.[77,109,115,118]

The pharmacodynamic increase in effect may be multifactorial, but it should be accounted for. The highest-risk population for hypoglycemia is the diabetic patient. One large retrospective cohort identified 3136 diabetic patients undergoing HBO_2 over a 77-month period.[102] The incidence of blood glucose reading < 70 mg/dl was 1.5%, and symptomatic hypoglycemia was rare. A pretreatment blood glucose value of 150 mg/dl and type 1 diabetes were independently associated with hypoglycemia, but insulin use was not.

Insulin requirements in diabetics may change rapidly, precipitating unexpected hypoglycemia. HBO_2 patients should be constantly monitored for glucose levels; empiric reductions may be needed. Additionally, while no data exists, insulin sensitizer and oral hypoglycemic may also have a pronounced effect under HBO_2. It is a good idea to have on hand in the hyperbaric unit orange juice and 50% glucose for injection to manage hypoglycemia. All diabetic patients must have their blood glucose levels recorded immediately prior to treatment and supplemental glucose given if needed. A pretreatment threshold for glucose supplementation of 110 mg/dl has been suggested by some clinicians.

Sympathomimetics, Vasoactive Compounds, and Antihypertensives

Hyperbaric oxygen appears to potentiate the vasoconstrive and negative chronotropic effects of vasoactive drugs and reduce the effectiveness of vasodilatory and sympathetic inhibitory drugs. In vitro rat aortas appear to constrict in response to HBO_2, but the response to both nitric oxide and norepinephrine is blunted.[49] Further rat studies show the antihypertensive effects mediated by central α2 agonism, β2 receptor agonism, and α1 or β1 antagonism were blunted while vasoconstrictive α1 stimulation and β1 effects were potentiated.[37]

The same effects are demonstrated in vitro with human participants. In a prospective trial of hypertensive diabetics undergoing multiple HBO_2 treatments, the use of beta blockers was associated with an increased blood pressure, and further studies have shown its negative chronotropy to be potentiated.[3,95] A prospective trial of nine healthy adults measured the effect of phentolamine (α-1 blockade) and tyramine on forearm blood flow.[19] Participants performed forearm exercises, and forearm blood flow was measured in normoxia and hyperoxia via arterial catheterization. The subjects were then given the α1 adrenergic blocker phentolamine; the sympatholytic response was more pronounced in the normoxic group, showing some decreased efficacy of the hypotensive effect under hyperoxia. The participants were also exposed to tyramine to release norepinephrine at both normoxic and hyperoxic conditions; the amount of vasoconstriction that occurred did not differ between normoxia and hyerpxoia. Data is limited for other antihypertensives, but dihydropyridine calcium channel blockers appear safe, and their reflex tachycardia effect from lowering systemic vascular resistance is blunted via HBO_2.[95]

As the negative chronotropic effects of drugs appear to be potentiated, it may be best to give drugs such as beta blockers (and possibly nondihydropyridine calcium channel blockers) after HBO_2. Patients on cardiovascular medications should have monitoring of heart rate and blood pressure while under pressure.

Bleomycin Sulfate

Bleomycin is an antineoplastic that causes DNA chain scission by utilizing ferrous irons and oxygen free radicals, disrupting the G2 phase of the cell cycle. The primary dose-limiting toxicity of bleomycin is the development of pulmonary toxicity ranging from radiographic changes to pneumonitis and fatal pulmonary fibrosis. The pulmonary toxicity appears to be enhanced in the presence of free radicals and reduced by antioxidants.[55] Experience with this toxicity is most well described in patients receiving therapy for germ cell tumors, and incidence of fatal toxicity has been estimated to be between 1%–3% in those receiving courses of bleomycin.[26] Risk factors include renal function and age, but exposure to supplemental oxygen therapy is also thought to predispose to toxicity.[85] For these reasons, bleomycin was thought to be a strong contraindication to use within a supplemental oxygen chamber. These theoretical risks are substantiated by animal studies in rats that demonstrate a synergism in pulmonary toxicity when rats were exposed to 100% oxygen and bleomycin compared to control or bleomycin alone.[13,55]

Despite the theoretical risk, no documented cases of bleomycin pulmonary toxicity from hyperbaric oxygen exist. The only published work is a case series that demonstrates HBO_2 is safe to administer to patients who have a remote history of bleomycin use.[107] These patients received a treatment protocol that involved pretreatment evaluation with chest radiograph and pulmonary function testing; a 2-atmospheres absolute (atm abs), 120-minute HBO_2 treatment; and slow increase in frequency of HBO_2 over 1 week depending on clinical findings. Median bleomycin-to-HBO_2 time was 34 months (range 1–279). There were no adverse findings to the patients throughout the study and no persistent post-HBO_2 pulmonary complications on follow-up. It is felt that as long as the patient has no signs of pulmonary compromise from fibrosis, and it has been over three months since he or she was treated with bleomycin, his or her exposure to bleomycin should not be a health factor.

Disulfiram

Disulfiram inhibits ethanol oxidation to acetic acid and halts metabolism in the acetaldehyde stage. This metabolite causes flushing, nausea, and vomiting and is intended to deter the user from ingesting alcohol. Conflicting evidence exists regarding its ability to enhance or ameliorate oxygen toxicity.

A theoretical risk with using disulfiram in the chamber is that it, or its reduced metabolite diethyldithiocarbamate, blocks the production of superoxide dismutase (SOD), a major protective enzyme against oxygen toxicity.[46] Disulfiram was shown to increase pulmonary oxygen toxicity in rats as well as increase the incidence of mortality in rats that have been continually exposed to oxygen.[27,38] Based on the animal data, it was thought that disulfiram might pose a risk if taken in concert with HBO_2 therapy. The doses given to animals in these studies were much higher (200 mg/kg) than the typical dose administered to humans (250–500 mg daily) and may not reflect effects during clinical conditions. There have been no reports of humans developing oxygen toxicity while taking disulfiram.

The effect of disulfiram in ameliorating oxygen toxicity was tested by Faiman. He showed that mice could be exposed to 6 atmospheres of oxygen, exercising for 1 hour, without convulsing, when pretreated with intraperitoneal disulfiram.[33] Subsequent necropsy failed to demonstrate any CNS or pulmonary oxygen damage. This work was also repeated in beagle dogs at pressures of 4 atmospheres with little or no evidence of oxygen toxicity.[34] Disulfiram may act in competition with enzymes containing sulfhydryl (SH) bonds for the free radical oxygen and thereby exerts a protective effect by reducing circulating free radicals. This medication's efficacy in blocking seizures has not been demonstrated in a controlled trial with humans. Given the lack of clinical data for harm and possible protective effect, it is no longer considered a contraindication. See disulfiram information in Chapter 9: Contraindications and Relative Risks of Hyperbaric Oxygen Treatment.

Ethanol

Alcohol intoxication is a common comorbidity of carbon monoxide, trauma, or decompression sickness. In rat studies, hyperbaria appears to have an antagonizing effect on motor impairment and intoxication, despite increased brain serum concentration.[40,75,103] This was, however, only seen with pressures > 12 ATA. In humans, hyperbaric oxygen does not lower blood alcohol levels significantly faster or induce a sobering effect, as measured by performance testing.[53] The postalcoholic state appears to predispose to decompression sickness in divers, probably secondary to dehydration. Fortunately, acute alcoholic intoxication does not seem to seriously predispose to oxygen toxicity or seizures.

Anesthetics

The basics concerning the administration of anesthetic drugs have been well covered elsewhere by Severinghaus.[96] When volatile or gaseous anesthetics are used, the concentration or percentage must be reduced in proportion to the number of atmospheres of pressure at which it is used. That is to say, the effective percentage is the actual percentage multiplied by the number of atmospheres of pressure at which it is administered. Strict attention must be paid to containing the gas so that it does not contaminate the chamber atmosphere, and adequate chamber ventilation must be assured. Needless to say, flammable anesthetics cannot be used.

Nongaseous anesthetics have many potential advantages for use under hyperbaric conditions, in that one does not have to be concerned about the changing effective percentages of anesthetic gas. Ketamine is administered intravenously. Its use involves risks similar to all general anesthetics and must be administered by physicians specifically trained in its use. Local anesthetics and regional blocks work well under hyperbaric conditions and require no modification in technique.

Generally, the employment of a general anesthetic in a hyperbaric chamber, regardless of the route of administration, requires all of the safeguards and equipment of a modern operating room. The special conditions imposed by increased barometric pressure are additive to the routine considerations of general anesthesia. Today, surgery requiring general anesthesia in the chamber is rare.

Lidocaine

Lidocaine is both a local anesthetic and Class Ib anti-arrhythmic sodium channel blocker. Experimentally it has been used with conflicting results in antiarrhythmic doses to evaluate whether it protects the brain after air embolism.(31,79) It was shown to significantly enhance neural recovery in the cat after embolism, but a separate study demonstrated no difference compared to HBO_2 alone. A retrospective analysis was conducted of divers who received lidocaine for neurologic decompression sickness compared to those who did not.(112) There was no difference in neurologic outcomes or adverse effects; however, the study was underpowered. The benefit of lidocaine in this disease requires further investigation. It is, however, safe for administration, and its kinetics appear unchanged by HBO_2.

Digitalis/Digoxin

Digoxin is a cardiac glycosyide that enhances inotropy and chronotropy through sodium and potassium ATP pump inhibition, increasing resting membrane potential leading to easier depolarization. Very limited evidence exists evaluating the effect of hyperbaric oxygenation on digoxin effect. The limited available animal evidence shows that HBO_2 but not hyperbaria alone increases the required digitalis dose to induce ventricular fibrillation in guinea pigs.(8) The effectiveness of hyperbaric oxygen in the treatment of digitalis toxicity has not been studied in humans, and it is not a routinely recommended antidote. Nor have the effects at normal dosages been studied. Given that HBO_2 decreased cardiac output via a reduction in heart rate, there may be additive effects with HBO. Patients taking digitalis should have heart rate and ECG monitored closely.

Heparin

Heparin induces anticoagulation via allosteric modulation of antithrombin III to increase deactivation of factors II and X. It is unknown if hyperbaric oxygen alters the effects of heparin, but it may predispose to bleeding from hyperoxic toxicity. Some clinicians discourage use of heparins during decompression sickness due to risk of tympanic membrane hemorrhage. Data describing this risk is sparse. A prospective cohort study evaluated incidence of middle-ear barotrauma during HBO in patients taking anticoagulants and patients not taking them.(36) No patients in the anticoagulant group (0/34) experienced tympanic membrane bleeding, while 2 of 39 patients in the control group did (defined as TEED score > 3). The anticoagulant group did, however, have two patients who reported epistaxis, compared to zero in the control group. In dog studies utilizing heparin for air embolism conducted by Waite, one of the dogs developed an intracranial bleed following embolization which was documented photographically.(110) Rat studies have also demonstrated a possible effect of increased bleeding from hyperoxic pulmonary lesions when rats were heparinized during HBO_2.(106)

Heparin has been used in a variety of experimental conditions treated with hyperbaric oxygen. Cockett et al. pretreated dogs with heparin prior to rapid decompression from depth, which produced severe decompression sickness. The unheparinized control dogs all died, whereas the heparinized animals survived.(20) Philp has shown that it ameliorates decompression sickness (DCS) in congenitally obese rats.(88) On the other hand, Reeves and Workman found it to have no effect in dogs suffering mild to moderate decompression sickness.(89) There are no human studies to determine its effect in the bends, but some clinicians may administer heparin empirically in severe cases. The use of heparin has also been considered in air embolism, as it would appear that the no-reflow phenomenon is mitigated in situations where heparinization is in effect before embolization (cardiovascular pump bypass patients and animal studies). There are no controlled studies in humans where it has been given post embolization. Nevertheless, Hart routinely used heparin in the treatment of 30 air embolism cases and 14 decompression sickness patients with no apparent deleterious effect.[45]

Phenothiazines, Antipsychotics, and Antidepressants

Antipsychotics exhibit a variety of effects on serotonin, dopamine, and acetylcholine receptors in the brain. Of the phenothiazines, chlorpromazine and prochlorperazine have been shown to reduce incidence of oxygen-induced pulmonary edema and seizure in mice.[11,18] Bean et al. have demonstrated that chlorpromazine has a considerable protective action in the CNS against the seizure-producing propensity of oxygen under high pressure.[11] In mice, lithium salts, haloperidol, and apomorphine also appear to have a seizure reducing effect.[18,23] Bean felt that the protective action of the phenothiazines is due in large measure to a suppressant action on sympathetics at the hypothalamic and medullary levels. Others suggest a decrease in central nervous system loss of gamma-aminobutyrate plays a role.[18]

Few studies have been conducted to elucidate the true mechanism; these medications, however, appear safe to be used in conjunction with HBO_2. Again, it must be borne in mind that the absence of seizures does not necessarily mean absence of toxicity or absence of the possibility of permanent damage if pressure/time limits are exceeded. Very little data exist on the use of antidepressants in conjunction with hyperbaric oxygen. One study of fluoxetine on decompression sickness in rats infers there may be a slight benefit due to anti-inflammatory effects.[16]

Antimicrobials

Hyperbaric oxygen itself has antimicrobial properties and is used to aid in the treatment of many different infections including necrotizing fasciitis, Fournier's gangrene, diabetic foot infections, and brain abscesses. It may enhance killing of bacteria through generation of oxygen free radicals or direct hyperoxic toxicity on anaerobic bacteria. Briefly data regarding hyperbaric oxygen interactions with antimicrobials will be discussed.

Penicillin: *Staphylococcus aureus* resistance to penicillin was increased by 23% in vivo when exposed to greater than 36 bar heliox.[48] Murine models of *Streptococcus pyogenes* myositis in combination with penicillin and HBO reduced bacterial colony forming unit (CFU) at necroscopy and increased survival more than either alone.[86]

Cephalosporins: Murine osteomyelitis models with *S. aureus* demonstrate that HBO in combination with cefazolin was more effective than either alone at reducing four-week bacterial CFU.[80]

Vancomycin: Nephrotoxicity of vancomycin was enhanced compared to controls in rats exposed to 60-minute sessions of HBO at 2 ATM for 7 days. Histopathological and laboratory value determined nephrotoxicity was increased; however, the dose of 500 mg/kg vancomycin that the rats received is extremely high compared to human dosing.[93]

Ciprofloxacin: Penetration of *Pseudomonas aeruginosa* biofilms was enhanced by hyperbaric oxygen.[60]

Imipenem: 100% oxygen at 3 ATA for 5 h enhanced imipenem killing of *P. aeruginosa* bacterial counts in vitro.[71]

Amphotericin B: After a single dose of amphotericin B 75 mg/kg, daily hyperbaric oxygen x 3 days reduced rat nephrotoxicity determined by serum creatinine and blood urea nitrogen.[83] The killing effect of amphotericin B on *Candida albicans* was increased at 1800 mmHg in vivo.[43] Amphotericin B inhibition of zygomycetes growth was enhanced by hyperbaric oxygen in vitro compared to amphotericin B alone.[35] However in vivo murine models of zygomycosis do not show any difference in cure between amphotericin B alone and amphotericin B + HBO_2.[9]

Aminoglycosides: Hyperbaric oxygen did not increase blood-brain barrier penetration of gentamicin or tobramycin in rabbits (see the section on distribution in pharmokinetic considerations); it also did not reduce the ototoxicity of amikacin in rodent studies.[29,59,94] The combination of HBO_2 and amikacin increased survival in *P. aeruginosa*–infected mice compared to HBO_2 alone.[74] *Escherichia coli* and *Salmonella typhimurium* resistance to gentamicin was increased as measured by MIC when exposed to heliox at 36 and 71 bar in vivo.[48]

Linezolid: Linezolid wound tissue penetration was enhanced in two diabetic patients undergoing hyperbaric oxygen for foot ulcers. Tissues penetration was measured via concentration of linezolid in wound effluent compared to serum concentration. The 12-hour AUC ratio of tissue effluent to blood was collected before and after HBO_2 sessions. The tissue penetration was 0.474 and 0.479 at the beginning of HBO_2. After completing HBO_2, penetration improved in both patients to 0.757 (after 5 weeks) and 0.950 (after 8 weeks).[62]

Ketoconazole: In vivo experiments exposing *C. albicans* to ketoconazole at pressures of 900 mmHg oxygen showed protective effects of HBO_2 for the MIC of ketoconazole to candida albicans.[43]

CONCLUSION

The theoretical implications and known literature regarding interactions amongst drugs and hyperbaric oxygen has been summarized. While many drugs appear to retain their effects, there are specific considerations. The scarcity of data in humans and improbability of assessing interactions between hyperbaric oxygen and all possible drugs leaves much unknown. Whenever the physician uses a new drug, he or she should consider the pharmacology of the drug and the possible kinetic or dynamic changes that may occur under the effects of hyperbaric oxygen. This may allow him or her to anticipate any theoretical adverse effects that would arise before employing it.

REFERENCES

1. Aktaş S, Toklu AS, Olgaç V. Hyperbaric oxygen therapy in Adriamycin extravasation: an experimental animal study. Ann Plast Surg. 2000 Aug;45(2):167-71. PubMed PMID: 10949345.
2. Alkana RL, Davies DL, Mørland J, Parker ES, Bejanian M. Low-level hyperbaric exposure antagonizes locomotor effects of ethanol and n-propanol but not morphine in C57BL mice. Alcohol Clin Exp Res. 1995 Jun;19(3):693-700. PubMed PMID: 7573795.
3. Al-Waili NS, Butler GJ, Beale J, Abdullah MS, Finkelstein M, Merrow M, Rivera R, Petrillo R, Carrey Z, Lee B, Allen M. Influences of hyperbaric oxygen on blood pressure, heart rate and blood glucose levels in patients with diabetes mellitus and hypertension. Arch Med Res. 2006 Nov;37(8):991-7. PubMed PMID: 17045116.
4. Ananian AA, Miliutina WP, Shugalei VS, Sherstner KB, Kostkin VB. The cytochrome P-450 content and catalytic activity in rat liver microsomes during hyperbaric oxygenation. Biol Nauki. 1991;12:28-33.
5. Arai M, Takata K, Takeda Y, Mizobuchi S, Morita K. The excitement of multiple noradrenergic cell groups in the rat brain related to hyperbaric oxygen seizure. Acta Med Okayama. 2011 Jun;65(3):163-8. PubMed PMID: 21709713.
6. Atasoyu EM, Yildiz S, Bilgi O, Cermik H, Evrenkaya R, Aktas S, Gültepe M, Kandemir EG. Investigation of the role of hyperbaric oxygen therapy in cisplatin-induced nephrotoxicity in rats. Arch Toxicol. 2005 May;79(5):289-93.
7. Aydinoz S, Uzun G, Cermik H, Atasoyu EM, Yildiz S, Karagoz B, Evrenkaya R. Effects of different doses of hyperbaric oxygen on cisplatin-induced nephrotoxicity. Ren Fail. 2007;29(3):257-63.
8. Bachand RT Jr, Somani P. Digitalis intoxication: protection with hyperbaric oxygen. Life Sci. 1967;6:739-42.
9. Barratt DM, Van Meter K, Asmar P, Nolan T, Trahan C, Garcia-Covarrubias L, Metzinger SE. Hyperbaric oxygen as an adjunct in zygomycosis: randomized controlled trial in a murine model. Antimicrob Agents Chemother. 2001 Dec;45(12):3601-2. PubMed PMID: 11709348; PubMed Central PMCID: PMC90877.
10. Bean JW. Factors influencing clinical oxygen toxicity. Ann NY Acad Sci. 1965;117:645-755.
11. Bean JW, Wagemacker H. Brain blood flow, chlorpromazine (thorazine) and protective action against the toxicity of O2 at high pressure. Am J Physiol. 1960;198:(2)341-5.
12. Beckman DL, Crittenden DJ. Protection from oxygen-induced seizures by clonazepam and propylene glycol. Proc Soc Exp Biol Med. 1981 Oct;168(1):45-8. PubMed PMID: 6798572.
13. Berend N. The effect of bleomycin and oxygen on rat lung. Pathology. 1984 Apr;16(2):136-9. PubMed PMID: 6205354.
14. Bitterman N, Katz A. The effect of sodium phenytoin on central nervous system oxygen toxicity. Aviat Space Environ Med. 1987 Mar;58(3):224-6. Erratum in: Aviat Space Environ Med. 1987 Jun;58(6):616. PubMed PMID: 3579804.
15. Bitterman N, Schaal S. Caffeine attenuates CNS oxygen toxicity in rats. Brain Res. 1995 Oct 23;696(1-2):250-3. PubMed PMID: 8574677.
16. Blatteau JE, de Maistre S, Lambrechts K, Abraini J, Risso JJ, Vallée N. Fluoxetine stimulates anti-inflammatory IL-10 cytokine production and attenuates sensory deficits in a rat model of decompression sickness. J Appl Physiol (1985). 2015 Dec 15;119(12):1393-9. doi: 10.1152/japplphysiol.00602.2015. PubMed PMID: 26494447.

17. Brophy GM, Bell R, Claassen J, Alldredge B, Bleck TP, Glauser T, Laroche SM, Riviello JJ Jr, Shutter L, Sperling MR, Treiman DM, Vespa PM; Neurocritical Care Society Status Epilepticus Guideline Writing Committee. Guidelines for the evaluation and management of status epilepticus. Neurocrit Care. 2012 Aug;17(1):3-23. doi: 10.1007/s12028-012-9695-z. PubMed PMID: 22528274.

18. Calcet J, Joanny P, Corriol J, Dimov S. The protection against the cerebral and pulmonary effects of hyperbaric oxygen by pharmacological agents and lithium salts in mice. Resuscitation. 1973 Apr;2(1):37-50. PubMed PMID: 4146241.

19. Casey DP, Joyner MJ, Claus PL, Curry TB. Vasoconstrictor responsiveness during hyperbaric hyperoxia in contracting human muscle. J Appl Physiol (1985). 2013 Jan 15;114(2):217-24. doi: 10.1152/japplphysiol.01197.2012. PubMed PMID: 23154993; PubMed Central PMCID: PMC3774558.

20. Cockett ATK. Presentation at: Journees Int d'Hyperbarie et Physiol Subaquat; 1970 Jun; Marseille, France.

21. Courtiere A, Reybaud J, Camilla C, Lobert P, Drouet J, Jadot G. Oxygen-induced modifications of benzodiazepine receptors and D2 dopamine receptors in the rat under hyperoxia. Free Rad Res Comms. 1991;15(1):29-34.

22. Criborn CO, Clemedson CJ, Henriksson C. Amphetamine as a protective agent against oxygen-induced convulsions in mice. Aviat Space Environ Med. 1986 Aug;57(8):777-81. PubMed PMID: 3753361.

23. Criborn CO, Henriksson C, Ahlenius S, Hillegaart V. Partial protection against hyperbaric oxygen induced convulsions by dopaminergic agents in mice: possible involvement of autoreceptors? J Neural Transm. 1987;69(3-4):277-85. PubMed PMID: 3625196.

24. Crittenden DJ, Beckman DL. Beta adrenergic receptors and glucagon in seizures from exposure to oxygen at high pressure (OHP). Life Sci. 1983 Nov 14;33(20):1959-64. PubMed PMID: 6316053.

25. Davies DL, Bejanian M, Parker ES, Mørland J, Bolger MB, Brinton RD, Alkana RL. Low level hyperbaric antagonism of diazepam's locomotor depressant and anticonvulsant properties in mice. J Pharmacol Exp Ther. 1996 Feb;276(2):667-75. PubMed PMID: 8632335.

26. Delanoy N, Pécuchet N, Fabre E, Combe P, Juvin K, Pujade-Lauraine E, Oudard S. Bleomycin-induced pneumonitis in the treatment of ovarian sex cord-stromal tumors: a systematic review and meta-analysis [review]. Int J Gynecol Cancer. 2015 Nov;25(9):1593-8. doi: 10.1097/IGC.0000000000000530. PubMed PMID: 26308607.

27. Deneke SM, Bernstein SP, Fanburg BL. Enhancement by disulfiram (Antabuse) of toxic effects of 95 to 97% O2 on the rat lung. J Pharmacol Exp Ther. 1979 Mar;208(3):377-80. PubMed PMID: 219176.

28. DiPiro JT, Sprull WJ, Wade WE, Blouin RA, Preumer Jane M. Concepts in clinical pharmacokinetics. In: DiPiro JT, Talbert RL, Yee GC, Matzke GR, Wells BG, Posey LM, editors. Pharmacotherapy: a pathophysiologic approach. 8th ed. New York City: McGraw-Hill; 2011. p. 943-5.

29. DJ. The effects of hyperbaric oxygen therapy upon ototoxic injuries produced by amikacin in guinea pigs. Braz J Otorhinolaryngol. 2013 May-Jun;79(3):342-8. English, Portuguese. doi: 10.5935/1808-8694.20130060. PubMed PMID: 23743750.

30. Emerson G, Hackett P. Hyperbaric oxygen does not delay the absorption of intramuscular midazolam. SPUMS J. 1998;28(3):122-5.

31. Evans DB, McDermott JJ, Kobrine AI, Flynn ET. Effects of intravenous lidocaine in experimental cerebral air embolism [abstract]. Undersea Biom Res. 1988;15(Suppl):17.

32. Faiman MD, Mehl RG. Effect of high oxygen pressure on brain norepinephrine and serotonin turnover. Eur J Pharmacol. 1973 Nov;24(2):123-30. PubMed PMID: 4765737.

33. Faiman MD, Mehl RG, Oehme FW. Protection with disulfiram from central and pulmonary oxygen toxicity. Biochem Pharmacol. 1971;20:3059-67. Great Britain: Pergamon Press.

34. Faiman MD, Nolan RJ, Oehme FW. Effect of disulfiram on oxygen toxicity in beagle dogs. Aerosp Med. 1974 Jan;45(1):29-32. PubMed PMID: 4811136.

35. Farina C, Marchesi G, Passera M, Diliberto C, Russello G, Favalli A. In vitro activity of amphotericin b against zygomycetes isolated from deep mycoses: a comparative study between incubation in aerobic and hyperbaric atmosphere. Med Mycol. 2012 May;50(4):427-32. doi: 10.3109/13693786.2011.614964. PubMed PMID: 21954953.

36. Fijen VA, Westerweel PE, van Ooij PJ, van Hulst RA. Tympanic membrane bleeding complications during hyperbaric oxygen treatment in patients with or without antiplatelet and anticoagulant drug treatment. Diving Hyperb Med. 2016 Mar;46(1):22-5. PubMed PMID: 27044458.

37. Filatov AF, Reznikov KM. [Effect of adrenomimetic, adreno- and ganglionic-blocking agents during hyperbaric oxygenation]. Farmakol Toksikol. 1982 Mar-Apr;45(2):35-9. Russian. PubMed PMID: 6122598.

38. Forman HJ, York JL, Fisher AB. Mechanism for the potentiation of oxygen toxicity by disulfiram. J Pharmacol Exp Ther. 1980 Mar;212(3):452-5. PubMed PMID:6244385.

39. Freiberger J, Coulombe KA, Suliman HB, Piantadosi CA. The time course of changes in superoxide dismutase isoforms induced by HBO [abstract]. Undersea and Hyperbaric Medical Society Annual Meeting; 2002.

40. Garcia-Cabrera I, Berge OG. Pressure reversal of the depressant effect of ethanol on spontaneous behavior in rats. Pharmacol Biochem Behav. 1988 Jan;29(1):133-41. PubMed PMID: 3353418.

41. Geiger JD, Akers TK, Parmar SS. Effects of helium-oxygen and hyperbaric helium-oxygen environment on drug-metabolizing enzyme activity in rat liver. Undersea Biomed Res. 1983 Dec;10(4):321-9. PubMed PMID: 6675228.

42. Geiger JD, Brumleve SJ, Boelkins JN, Parmar SS. Selective induction of liver drug-metabolizing enzymes in rats exposed to a 21 ATA He-O2 environment. Aviat Space Environ Med. 1977 Aug;48(8):737-40. PubMed PMID: 889548.

43. Gudewicz TM, Mader JT, Davis CP. Combined effects of hyperbaric oxygen and antifungal agents on the growth of Candida albicans. Aviat Space Environ Med. 1987 Jul;58(7):673-8. PubMed PMID: 3304267.

44. Gutsche BB, Harp JR, Stephen CR. Influence of anesthetic drugs on dogs subjected to oxygen at 5 atmospheres. In: Proc of 3rd Intl Conf on Hyperbaric Med. Natl Acad Sciences, Natl Research Council; 1966. p. 300-6.

45. Hart GB. Treatment of decompression illness and air embolism with hyperbaric oxygen. Aerospace Med. 1974;45(10):1190-3.

46. Heikkila RE, Cabbat FS, Cohen G. In vivo inhibition of superoxide dismutase in mice by diethyldithiocarbamate. J Biol Chem. 1976;251:2182.

47. Heys SD, Smith IC, Ross JA, Gilbert FJ, Brooks J, Semple S, Miller ID, Hutcheon A, Sarkar T, Eremin O. A pilot study with long term follow up of hyperbaric oxygen pretreatment in patients with locally advanced breast cancer undergoing neo-adjuvant chemotherapy. Undersea Hyperb Med. 2006 Jan-Feb;33(1):33-43. PubMed PMID: 16602255.

48. Hind J, Attwell RW. The effect of antibiotics on bacteria under hyperbaric conditions. J Antimicrob Chemother. 1996 Feb;37(2):253-63. PubMed PMID: 8707735.

49. Hink J, Thom SR, Simonsen U, Rubin I, Jansen E. Vascular reactivity and endothelial NOS activity in rat thoracic aorta during and after hyperbaric oxygen exposure. Am J Physiol Heart Circ Physiol. 2006 Oct;291(4):H1988-98. PubMed PMID: 16648176.

50. Hordnes C, Tyssebotn I. Effect of high ambient pressure and oxygen tension on organ blood flow in conscious trained rats. Undersea Biomed Res. 1985;12:115-28.

51. Huang JL, Ma YW, Lian QL, Xu JP, Jiang CL, Guo MZ, Sun XJ. [Effect of acetazolamide on the latency of hyperbaric oxygen-induced convulsion]. Sheng Li Xue Bao. 2004 Apr 25;56(2):158-62. Chinese. PubMed PMID: 15127124.

52. Huang JL, Zhang YL, Xiao X, Zhang JH, Lian QL, Liu Y, Sun XJ. Bidirectional influences of acetazolamide on central nervous system oxygen toxicity of rats. Undersea Hyperb Med. 2010 Sep-Oct;37(5):271-80. PubMed PMID: 20929184.

53. Jacobson GR, Kindwall EP. Effects of hyperbaric oxygenation on acute alcohol intoxication. J Hyperbaric Med. 1991;6(2):119-31.

54. Jakoby WB, Ziegler DM. The enzymes of detoxication [review]. J Biol Chem. 1990 Dec 5;265(34):20715-8. PubMed PMID: 2249981.

55. Jamieson DD, Kerr DR, Unsworth I. Interaction of N-acetylcysteine and bleomycin on hyperbaric oxygen-induced lung damage in mice. Lung. 1987;165(4):239-47. PubMed PMID: 2442568.

56. Kakhnovskii IM, Efuni SN, Khodas MY, Bolshakova TD, Gitel EP. The mechanism of hypoglycemic effect of hyperbaric oxygenation in diabetes mellitus patients. Klin Med (Mosk). 1981 Sep;59(9):83-8. HBO Rev. 1983 July;4(3):143.

57. Kann HE Jr et al. Oxygen toxicity and vitamin E. J Aerosp Med. 1964;35:840-4.

58. Karagoz B, Suleymanoglu S, Uzun G, Bilgi O, Aydinoz S, Haholu A, Turken O, Onem Y, Kandemir EG. Hyperbaric oxygen therapy does not potentiate doxorubicin-induced cardiotoxicity in rats. Basic Clin Pharmacol Toxicol. 2008 Mar;102(3):287-92. doi: 10.1111/j.1742-7843.2007.00196.x. PubMed PMID: 18248515.

59. Kent TA, Sheftel TG, Sutton TE, Morrison LT, Mader JT. Effect of hyperbaric oxygen on the blood cerebrospinal fluid transfer of tobramycin. Aviat Space Environ Med. 1986;57:664-6.

60. Kolpen M, Mousavi N, Sams T, Bjarnsholt T, Ciofu O, Moser C, Kühl M, Høiby N, Jensen PØ. Reinforcement of the bactericidal effect of ciprofloxacin on Pseudomonas aeruginosa biofilm by hyperbaric oxygen treatment. Int J Antimicrob Agents. 2016 Feb;47(2):163-7. doi: 10.1016/j.ijantimicag.2015.12.005. PubMed PMID: 26774522.

61. Kong Y, Lunzer S, Heyman A, et al. Effects of acetazolamide on cerebral blood flow of dogs during hyperbaric oxygenation. Am Heart J. 1969;78:229-37.

62. Koomanachai P, Keel RA, Johnson-Arbor KK, Suecof LA, Nicolau DP, Kuti JL. Linezolid penetration into wound tissue of two diabetic patients before and after hyperbaric oxygen therapy. Undersea Hyperb Med. 2011 Jan-Feb;38(1):11-6. PubMed PMID: 21384759.

63. Kramer WG, Gross DR, Fife WP, Chaikin BN. Theophylline pharmacokinetics during hyperbaria and hyperbaric hyperoxia in the dog. Res Commun Chem Pathol Pharmac. 1981;34:381-8.

64. Kramer WG, Gross DR, Moreau PM, Fife WP. Drug disposition under hyperbaric and hyperbaric hyperoxic conditions: meperidine in the dog. Aviat Space Environ Med. 1983;54:410-2 .

65. Kramer WG, Welch DW, Fife WP, Chaikin BN, Medlock C, Gross DR. Pharmacokinetics of pentobarbital under hyperbaric and hyperbaric hyperoxic conditions in the dog. Aviat Space Environ Med. 1983;54:1005-8.

66. Lambertsen CJ. Drugs and respiration. Ann Rev Pharmacol. 1966;6:327-78.

67. Lambertsen CJ, Hall P, Wollman H, Goodman MW. Quantitative interactions of increased PO2 and PCO2 upon respiration in man. Ann NY Acad Sci. 1963;109:731-41.

68. Lambertsen CJ, Kough RH, Cooper DY, Emmel GL, Loeschske HH. Oxygen toxicity. Effects in man of oxygen inhalation at 1 and 3.5 atmospheres upon blood gas transport, cerebral circulation and cerebral metabolism. J Appl Physiol. 1953;5:471-86.

69. Lembeck F, Beubler E. Convulsions induced by hyperbaric oxygen: inhibition by phenobarbital, diazepam and baclofen. Naunyn Schmiedebergs Arch Pharmacol. 1977 Mar;297(1):47-51. PubMed PMID: 870832.

70. Levy SL, Burnham WM, Bishai A, Hwang PA. The anticonvulsant effects of vitamin E: a further evaluation. Can J Neurol Sci. 1992 May;19(2):201-3. PubMed PMID: 1623446.

71. Lima FL, Joazeiro PP, Lancellotti M, de Hollanda LM, de Araújo Lima B, Linares E, Augusto O, Brocchi M, Giorgio S. Effects of hyperbaric oxygen on Pseudomonas aeruginosa susceptibility to imipenem and macrophages. Future Microbiol. 2015;10(2):179-89. doi: 10.2217/fmb.14.111. PubMed PMID: 25689530.

72. Longmuir IS, Gottlieb SF, Pashko LL, Martin P. In vivo and in vitro induction of cytochrome P-450 synthesis in hyperoxia. Undersea Biomed Res. 1980 Sep;7(3):161-70. PubMed PMID: 7423654.

73. Longoni C, Camporesi EM, Buizza M, et al. Reduction in insulin requirements during HBO therapy. UBR. 1988;15(Suppl):16-7.

74. Luongo C, Imperatore F, Matera MG, Mangoni G, Marmo M, Baroni A, Catalanotti P, Rossi F, Filippelli A. Effect of hyperbaric oxygen therapy in experimental subcutaneous and pulmonary infections due to Pseudomonas aeruginosa. Undersea Hyperb Med. 1999 Spring;26(1):21-5. PubMed PMID: 10353181.

75. Malcolm RD, Alkana RL. Hyperbaric ethanol antagonism: role of temperature, blood and brain ethanol concentrations. Pharmacol Biochem Behav. 1982 Feb;16(2):341-6. PubMed PMID: 7071084.

76. Marks HP. Interim report on oxygen intoxication in animals and the effect of drugs on sensitivity to oxygen intoxication. Med Res Counc, R.N. Personnel Res Comm Report; 1944. 44/001.

77. Martindale VE, Dixon PA. Fresh dissected mouse diaphragms take up glucose more rapidly during hyperbaric oxygenation. Undersea Hyperb Med. 1993 Jul;20(Suppl):33.

78. McCracken LE, Nicodemus HF, Tobey RE, Bailey RC. Ketamine and thiopental sleep responses in guinea pigs in hyperbaric helium-oxygen. Undersea Biomed Res. 1979 Dec;6(4):329-38. PubMed PMID: 538861.

79. McDermott JJ, Dutka AJ, Evans DE, Flynn ET. Treatment of experimental cerebral air embolism with lidocaine and hyperbaric oxygen. Undersea Biomed Res. 1990 Nov;17(6):525-34. PubMed PMID: 2288043.

80. Mendel V, Reichert B, Simanowski HJ, Scholz HC. Therapy with hyperbaric oxygen and cefazolin for experimental osteomyelitis due to Staphylococcus aureus in rats. Undersea Hyperb Med. 1999 Fall;26(3):169-74. PubMed PMID: 10485518.

81. Merritt GJ, Slade JB. Influence of hyperbaric oxygen on the pharmacokinetics of single-dose gentamicin in healthy volunteers. Pharmacotherapy. 1993 Jul-Aug;13(4):382-5. PubMed PMID: 8361865.

82. Nemiroff PM. Effects of cis-platinum and hyperbaric oxygen on wound healing in mice [abstract]. Undersea Biomed Res. 1988;15:(Suppl):40.

83. Nir H, Berkovitch M, Youngster I, Kozer E, Goldman M, Abu-Kishk I. Effect of hyperbaric oxygen therapy on amphotericin-B induced acute renal failure in rats. Minerva Urol Nefrol. 2015 Jun;67(2):97-102. PubMed PMID: 25847867.

84. Okamoto H, Isa P. Protective effects of alpha-tocopherol nicotinate against oxygen effects in mouse and rat [abstract]. Jap J Anesth. 1975;24:468-471. English abstract.

85. O'Sullivan JM, Huddart RA, Norman AR, Nicholls J, Dearnaley DP, Horwich A. Predicting the risk of bleomycin lung toxicity in patients with germ-cell tumours. Ann Oncol. 2003 Jan;14(1):91-6. PubMed PMID: 12488299.

86. Oztas E, Kiliç A, Ozyurt M, Korkmaz A, Başustaoğlu A. Effect of hyperbaric oxygen and penicillin in a murine model of streptococcal myositis. Undersea Hyperb Med. 2001 Fall;28(4):181-6. PubMed PMID: 12153145.

87. Pauland RL, Bollinger RO, Bozynski ME, Karna P, Perrin EVD. Effect of vitamin E deficiency on pulmonary oxygen toxicity. Pediatr Res. 1977;11(4):577.

88. Philp RB. The ameliorative effects of heparin and depolymerized hyaluronate on decompression sickness in rats. Can J Physiol Pharmacol. 1964;42:819-29.

89. Reeves E, Workman RD. Use of heparin for the therapeutic/prophylactic treatment of decompression sickness. Aerosp Med. 1971;42(1):20-3.

90. Risberg J, Bergo GW, Hordnes C, Tyssebotn I. Distribution of cardiac output in awake rats during exposure to 5 bar. Undersea Biomed Res. 1990;17:503-14.

91. Rump AFE, Siekmann U, Dreja M, Kalff G. Caffeine pharmacokinetics during hyperbaric hyperoxia in humans. Aviat Space Environ Med. 1997;68:142-6.

92. Rump AF, Siekmann U, Kalff G. Effects of hyperbaric and hyperoxic conditions on the disposition of drugs: theoretical considerations and a review of the literature. Gen Pharmacol. 1999;32(1):127-33.

93. Sabler IM, Berkovitch M, Sandbank J, Kozer E, Dagan Z, Goldman M, Bahat H, Stav K, Zisman A, Klin B, Abu-Kishk I. Exposure to hyperbaric oxygen intensified vancomycin-induced nephrotoxicity in rats. PLoS One. 2016 Apr 19;11(4):e0152554. doi: 10.1371/journal.pone.0152554. PubMed PMID: 27092557; PubMed Central PMCID: PMC4836689.

94. Schaeffer DO, Caprile KA, Strain GM, Bivin WS, Cohn GH. Effect of hyperbaric oxygen on cerebrospinal fluid gentamicin concentrations J Vet Pharmac Ther. 1992;15:104-6.

95. Seriakov VV, Sidorenko BA, Efuni SN. [Interaction of hyperbaric oxygenation with nifedipine and propranolol at the level of autonomic regulation of the heart in patients with angina pectoris]. Kardiologiia. 1992 Jan;32(1):50-3. Russian. PubMed PMID: 1614022.

96. Severinghaus JW. Anesthesia and related drug effects. In: Fundamentals of hyperbaric medicine. Washington (DC): Natl Acad of Sci. 1966;9:115-27.

97. Shchugale� VS, Ananian AA, Miliutina NP, Sadekova SI. [The effect of hypoxia and of subsequent baro-oxygenation on the function of the microsomal oxidation system in the rat liver]. Nauchnye Doki Vyss Shkoly Biol Nauki. 1992;(7):86-94.

98. Shugale� VS, Ananian AA, Sadekova SI, Miliutina NP. [Cytochrome P-450 activity and lipid peroxidation in rat liver and lung microsomes during hypoxia and followed by pressure oxygenation]. Vopr Med Khim. 1991 Sep-Oct;37(5):19-21.

99. Sledkov AIu, Troshikhin GV. [Duration of the narcotic action of nembutal under hyperbarism]. Farmakol Toksikol. 1986 May-Jun;49(3):32-5. Russian. PubMed PMID: 3720931.

100. Smith RG. An appraisal of potential drug interactions regarding hyperbaric oxygen therapy and frequently prescribed medications. Wounds. 2011;23(6):147-59.

101. Springer R. The importance of glucometer testing of diabetic patients pre and post-dive [abstract]. UBR. 1991;18(Suppl):20.

102. Stevens SL, Narr AJ, Claus PL, Millman MP, Steinkraus LW, Shields RC, Buchta WG, Haddon R, Wang Z, Murad MH. The incidence of hypoglycemia during HBO_2 therapy: a retrospective review. Undersea Hyperb Med. 2015 May-Jun;42(3):191-6. PubMed PMID: 26152103.

103. Syapin PJ, Chen J, Finn DA, Alkana RL. Antagonism of ethanol-induced depression of mouse locomotor activity by hyperbaric exposure. Life Sci. 1988;43(26):2221-9. PubMed PMID: 3210903.

104. Takahashi H, Kobayshi S, Sakakibara K. Effect of HBO on the endocrine system and metabolism of diabetic patients [abstract]. Undersea Biomed Res. 1990;17(Suppl):52.

105. Torbati D. Effect of propranolol on brain electrical activity during hyperbaric oxygenation in the rat. Undersea Biomed Res. 1985 Dec;12(4):423-9. PubMed PMID: 4082345.

106. Torbati D. Heparin effects during hyperbaric oxygenation in rats. Life Sci. 1985 Jan 14;36(2):147-51. PubMed PMID: 3965847.

107. Torp KD, Carraway MS, Ott MC, Stolp BW, Moon RE, Piantadosi CA, Freiberger JJ. Safe administration of hyperbaric oxygen after bleomycin: a case series of 15 patients. Undersea Hyperb Med. 2012 Sep-Oct;39(5):873-9. PubMed PMID: 23045915.

108. Upton PG, Yamaguchi KT, Myers S, Kidwell TD, Anderson RJ. Effects of antioxidants and hyperbaric oxygen in ameliorating experimental doxorubicin skin toxicity in the rat. Cancer Treat Rep. 1986;70(4):503-7.

109. Vera-Cruz P, Guerreiro F, Ribeiro MJ, Guarino MP, Conde SV. Hyperbaric oxygen therapy improves glucose homeostasis in type 2 diabetes patients: a likely involvement of the carotid bodies. Adv Exp Med Biol. 2015;860:221-5. doi: 10.1007/978-3-319-18440-1_24. PubMed PMID: 26303484.

110. Waite CL, Mazzone WF, Greenwood ME. Cerebral air embolism 1. Basic studies. Washington (DC): Navy Department, Bureau Med and Surg.; 1967. U.S. Naval Submarine Med Ctr Report No.: 493.

111. Weaver, LK. Phenytoin sodium in oxygen toxicity-induced seizures. Ann Emerg Med. 1983;12(1):81-4.

112. Weenink RP, Hollmann MW, Zomervrucht A, van Ooij PJ, van Hulst RA. A retrospective cohort study of lidocaine in divers with neurological decompression illness. Undersea Hyperb Med. 2014 Mar-Apr;41(2):119-26. PubMed PMID: 24851549.

113. Whelan HT, Bajic DM, Karlovits SM, Houle JM, Kindwall EP. Use of cytochrome-P450 mono-oxygenase 2 E1 isozyme inhibitors to delay seizures caused by central nervous system oxygen toxicity. Aviat Space Environ Med. 1998 May;69(5):480-5. PubMed PMID: 9591618.

114. Wilkinson D, Chapman IM, Heilbronn LK. Hyperbaric oxygen therapy improves peripheral insulin sensitivity in humans. Diabet Med. 2012 Aug;29(8):986-9. doi: 10.1111/j.1464-5491.2012.03587.x. PubMed PMID: 22269009.

115. Wilkinson D, Nolting M, Mahadi MK, Chapman I, Heilbronn L. Hyperbaric oxygen therapy increases insulin sensitivity in overweight men with and without type 2 diabetes. Diving Hyperb Med. 2015 Mar;45(1):30-6. PubMed PMID: 25964036.

116. Wood CD. Acetazolamide and CO2 in hyperbaric oxygen toxicity. Undersea Biomed Res. 1982 Mar;9(1):15-20. PubMed PMID: 6806959.

117. Yassuda CC, Righetti AE, Cury MC, Hyppolito MA, Oliveira JA, Féres O. The role of hyperbaric oxygen therapy (hot) as an otoprotection agent against cisplatin ototoxicity. Acta Cir Bras. 2008;23(Suppl 1):72-6; discussion 76.

118. Yasuda K, Adachi T, Gu N, Matsumoto A, Matsunaga T, Tsujimoto G, Tsuda K, Ishihara A. Effects of hyperbaric exposure with high oxygen concentration on glucose and insulin levels and skeletal muscle-fiber properties in diabetic rats. Muscle Nerve. 2007 Mar;35(3):337-43. PubMed PMID: 17094100.

119. Yilmaz MI, Korkmaz A, Kaya A, Sonmez A, Caglar K, Topal T, Eyileten T, Yenicesu M, Acikel C, Oter S, Yaman H, Aktug H, Oguz Y, Vural A, Ikizler TA. Hyperbaric oxygen treatment augments the efficacy of a losartan regime in an experimental nephrotic syndrome model. Nephron Exp Nephrol. 2006;104(1):e15-22. PubMed PMID: 16699289.

120. Zanger Ulrich M, Turpeinen Miia, Klein Kathrin, Schwab Matthias. Functional pharmacogenetics/genomics of human cytochromes P450 involved in drug biotransformation. Analytical and bioanalytical chemistry. 2008;392:1093-108. Cited in: PubMed.

121. Zhang Y, Stolz PA, Shirachi DY, Quock RM. Reduced antinociceptive responsiveness to hyperbaric oxygen in opioid-tolerant mice. Eur J Pain. 2014 Aug;18(7):1032-9. doi: 10.1002/j.1532-2149.2013.00448.x. PubMed PMID: 24390852.

CHAPTER 8 CHAPTER

Myringotomy

CHAPTER EIGHT OVERVIEW

Introduction 161
Pathophysiology of Barotitis 161
Decongestants and Ear Plugs 163
Myringotomy: Indications 163
Myringotomy: Technique 163
Pressure Equalization Tubes 167
Acknowledgment 167
References 168

Myringotomy

Michael E. McCormick, Joseph E. Kerschner

INTRODUCTION

Air-containing spaces within the skull and facial skeleton include the middle-ear cleft (tympanum) and the paranasal sinuses. Air pressure within these spaces must equilibrate with ambient pressure in order for a person undergoing pressurization or depressurization to remain asymptomatic. The most common problem encountered in patients undergoing hyperbaric treatment is "ear squeeze," which is an inability to equalize pressure in the middle-ear clefts during compression. Less commonly, the air pressure in one or more of the paranasal sinuses may not equalize, resulting in facial or head pain. Acute barotitis (ear) or barosinusitis (paranasal sinuses) are terms used to describe pain, transudation of fluid, and/or hemorrhage resulting from failure of this equilibration process.[2-5,7] This chapter will deal primarily with acute barotitis and its management.

PATHOPHYSIOLOGY OF BAROTITIS

A diagnosis of barotitis can be inferred if the patient complains of deep ear pain, either unilateral or bilateral, during hyperbaric pressurization. Examination of the ear using an otoscope may show retraction, engorgement, or hypervascularity of the tympanic membrane, blood within the middle-ear cleft (hemotympanum), or even perforation of the tympanic membrane with or without hemorrhagic otorrhea. Because the eustachian tube is unable to equilibrate the air pressure in the middle-ear space with that of the ambient environment, a relative vacuum develops within the middle-ear cleft. Depending on how rapidly this negative pressure develops and how great the pressure differential is, the patient may experience one or more of the signs or symptoms mentioned above. Sometimes patients may be able to equilibrate if the pressurization is done very gradually, but they are unable to do so if the compression is rapid. Although the eustachian tube serves other important functions (e.g., protection of the middle ear from pharyngeal secretions), the focus in this chapter is on the eustachian tube as a conduit for pressure equalization.

The eustachian tube (Figure 1) is the only natural communication between the middle-ear cleft and the ambient air, and it is normally closed in its resting state. It opens briefly with swallowing or yawning or during a modified Valsalva maneuver. Air can passively exit the middle-ear cleft through the eustachian tube, since the lateral tympanic portion of the tube is bony and rigid. However, entrance of air into the middle-ear cleft depends on active contraction of the palatine and pharyngeal musculature (in particular, the tensor veli palatini) to open the collapsible cartilaginous medial portion of the eustachian tube. Functional integrity of the eustachian tube may be impaired by a number of pathologies: edema or hypersecretion of the tubal

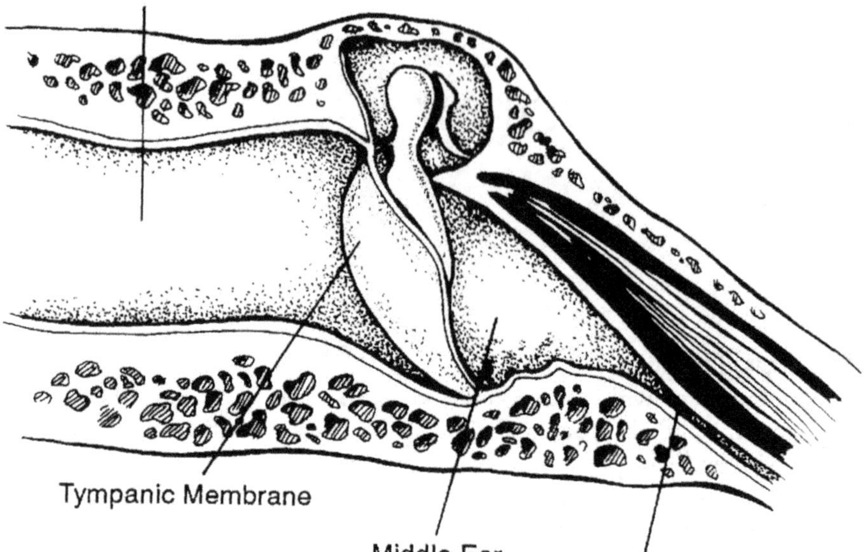

Figure 1. Cutaway coronal view of external canal, middle-ear, auditory tube, and tympanic membrane.

mucosa; failure of the mucociliary blanket within the tube; adenoid hypertrophy or other nasopharyngeal mass obstruction; altered function of the muscles which open the eustachian tube, as in patients with cleft palate; or obstruction of the tube by inspissated mucus or exudates. Mucosal edema and dysfunction of the mucociliary blanket may be due to factors such as infection, allergy, tobacco smoking, dry air, and exposure to noxious chemicals.

The distinction between a Valsalva maneuver and a modified Valsalva maneuver should be understood. A Valsalva maneuver, which has no effect on opening the eustachian tube, is performed by closing the glottis and increasing intrathoracic pressure. Examples of the Valsalva maneuver include straining during heavy lifting, defecation, or childbirth. The modified Valsalva maneuver is performed by maintaining an open glottis, closing the mouth, occluding the nose (e.g., pinching the nostrils closed), and then increasing intrathoracic pressure). In effect, this latter maneuver should force air up through the eustachian tube into the middle ear. The modified Valsalva maneuver is not recommended as a way to equalize middle-ear pressure because it can also raise intracranial pressure to dangerously high levels and, in susceptible individuals, result in retrograde flow of cerebrospinal fluid through the cochlear aqueduct into the inner ear. A much safer and equally effective method of inflating the middle ear is the Toynbee maneuver – the patient simply pinches the nostrils closed and swallows. This facilitates opening the eustachian tube without raising intracranial pressure.

"Locking" of the eustachian tube – a situation where no amount of swallowing, yawning, or modified Valsalva maneuver is able to open the medial pharyngeal end of the tube and equalize pressure – occurs when the pressure differential between the ambient air and the middle-ear cleft reaches or exceeds about 125 torr. This differential is about one atmosphere of pressure change. When this occurs, the patient must be carefully returned to sea-level pressure and compression restarted and progressed very slowly.

DECONGESTANTS AND EAR PLUGS

Spraying the nose liberally with a topical sympathomimetic like oxymetazoline (Afrin®), xylometazoline (Otrivin®), or phenylephrine (Neo-Synephrine®) may help to decongest the eustachian tube and facilitate tubal opening and pressure equilibration. The use of oral decongestants or decongestant/antihistamine preparations is less predictable. In general, oral decongestants have no preferential effect on the vascularity of the eustachian tube, so in order to obtain meaningful vasoconstriction in these target tissues, a patient would require doses high enough to also potentially cause cardiac dysrhythmias and hypertension. Consequently, oral decongestants are not generally recommended for these situations.

There are a few commercially available earplugs that help to regulate the pressure changes experienced by the patient during hyperbaric therapy and other environments that modify the atmospheric pressure. Examples of these products include Ear Planes™, Aqua Ears™, and hep/O2™ ear plugs.[6] These have been demonstrated to be effective aids for adults who chronically have difficulty clearing their ears. Caution is advised with children who require hyperbaric therapy, since it may be difficult to obtain an appropriate seal with these earplugs so that they function properly. These products work by permitting a slow and gradual pressurization within the external auditory canal. They can be purchased at nominal cost in most pharmacies or ordered online without a prescription.[6] The authors are not aware of any controlled trials of these devices for hyperbaric therapy, but they might be worth considering in patients who may otherwise require myringotomy.

MYRINGOTOMY: INDICATIONS

Myringotomy (a small incision or perforation of the tympanic membrane) is indicated when acute otalgia, secondary to middle-ear barotraumas, develops during pressurization and cannot be relieved by previously described nonsurgical measures. A prospective study of a group of hyperbaric patients identified several risk factors for middle-ear barotrauma and need for tympanostomy tubes: older age, history of ENT radiation, anticoagulant use, history of cardiovascular disease, treatment for an infective condition, history of difficulty equalizing pressure, and female gender. However, they were unable to recommend prophylactic tympanostomy tube insertion for any specific group of patients.[1]

Performing a myringotomy in an unconscious patient where there is potential for middle-ear barotrauma (e.g., carbon monoxide poisoning) who is not experiencing pain is not advisable or necessary. If the tympanic membrane does rupture spontaneously or if the middle ear fills with blood or transudate, these occurrences will almost always heal or resolve spontaneously. The risk of inner-ear damage resulting from middle-ear barotrauma in an unconscious patient is extremely unlikely and does not justify routine performance of myringotomy.

MYRINGOTOMY: TECHNIQUE

As with any surgical procedure, exposure of the operative site is paramount. In the ear, this means a nonobstructed external auditory canal, coaxial bright light, and the largest speculum which the ear canal will comfortably accommodate. The light source may be an electric otoscope (Figure 2) with an operating head that allows instrumentation of the ear canal and eardrum, a head mirror, an electric headlight, or a binocular operating microscope. Retracting the pinna upward and backward straightens the cartilaginous

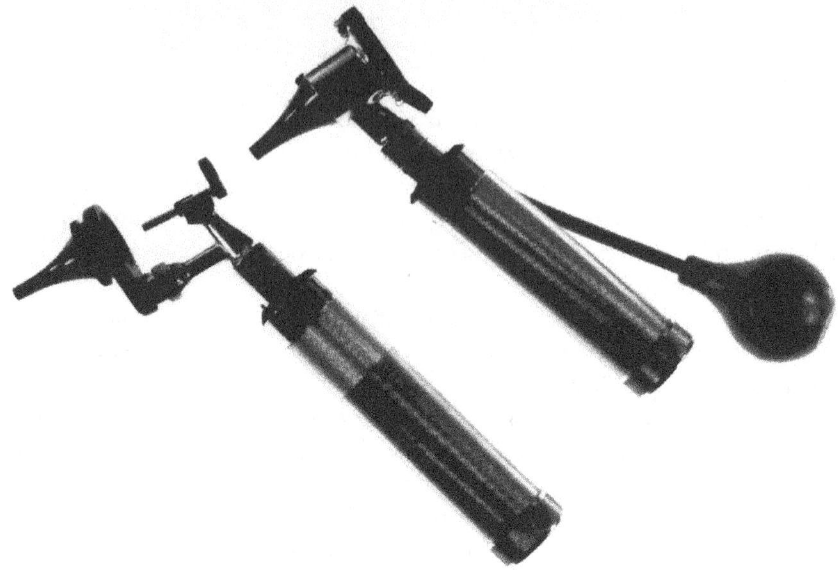

Figure 2. Two electric otoscopes. Left, open "operating" head. Right, closed "diagnostic" head; pneumatic oloscopy bulb attached.

ear canal and provides an optimal view of the tympanic membrane, assuming an obstructed view.[2,5]

When obstructive, cerumen and desquamated skin debris should be removed from the external auditory canal to allow complete visualization of the tympanic membrane landmarks. Removal of debris must be done gently and carefully, since the skin of the external ear canal, and especially the medial bony portion of the canal, is delicate and easily traumatized. While cerumen removal may be safely performed by an experienced clinician using a wax removal loop, a safer method for removing wax under less than ideal conditions is to irrigate the wax using warm water close to or at body temperature. At body temperature, the irrigation will be comfortable and should not elicit vertigo or nausea. While many cerumen irrigation devices are commercially obtainable, an easy method using readily available supplies is the following: a large plastic syringe (preferably 30 to 50 ml) with Luer-Lock tip attached to a 14- or 16-gauge, 3 to 5 cm long, flexible plastic intravenous catheter (e.g., Angiocath®) (Figure 3). It is important to use a Luer-Lock syringe and to be certain the catheter is securely attached so that it does not become a missile and perforate the tympanic membrane during irrigation. This apparatus produces a fine, hard stream of water which will dislodge and flush out most ear canal debris with little chance of abrading the delicate skin of the external auditory canal or traumatizing the tympanic membrane.[2,5]

The question of whether it is safe to irrigate an ear canal filled with cerumen before one has determined that there is no perforation is not really a problem. If, during pressurization in the chamber, the patient experiences otalgia, it is virtually certain that the tympanic membrane is intact, since a perforation allows automatic equalization of pressure through the perforation, and the patient would experience relief of any ear pain that may have developed during pressurization.

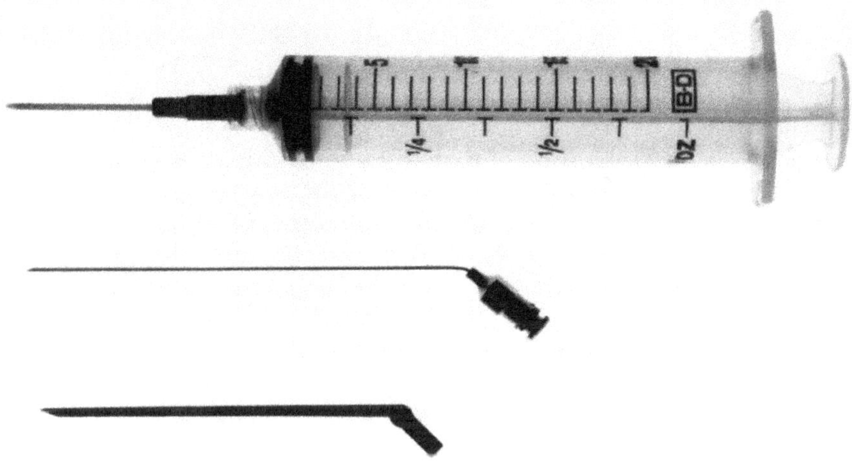

Figure 3. Top, large plastic syringe with flexible short catheter attached; note Luer-Lock tip. Middle, 22 gauge spinal needle, angled near hub. Bottom, disposable Beaver® myringotomy knife blade.

It is best to position the patient supine with the head at an angle away with the contralateral side of the head resting firmly on the mattress or pillow to minimize movement. Children and anxious or less cooperative adult patients may need to be restrained and immobilized using a papoose board or similar method to minimize movement and make the procedure safer.[3-4]

The basic instruments (Figure 2, Figure 3) needed for a myringotomy are an otoscope with an operating head (i.e., one which permits visualization of the tympanic membrane and simultaneous instrumentation); an ear speculum of adequate size; and a myringotomy knife, preferably a sharp disposable knife whose blade can be angled to permit an accurately placed incision. Lacking a myringotomy knife, a simple, inexpensive, readily available substitute is a 25- or 22-gauge, disposable spinal needle which may be angled as needed. Alternative ways of visualizing the tympanic membrane are with a head mirror or headlight which provides illumination coaxial to the line of vision or with a binocular operating microscope.[3-4]

Anesthetizing the tympanic membrane is usually not necessary for a myringotomy done as an emergency procedure to relieve acute barotitis. The momentary pain of the myringotomy is usually overshadowed by the discomfort the patient is already experiencing and is followed by immediate relief. Often the application of an anesthetic, either topical or infiltration, is likely to produce as much or more discomfort than the myringotomy itself, assuming the procedure is performed carefully and skillfully.

Otolaryngologists divide the tympanic membrane into four quadrants (Figure 4). A vertical line through the umbo divides the eardrum into anterior and posterior halves; a horizontal line through the umbo divides it into superior and inferior halves. The intersection of these two imaginary lines produces four quadrants.

Because of the location of structures contained within the middle ear (Figure 5) and their susceptibility to penetrating injuries, it is imperative that a blind or random puncture of the eardrum be avoided. With few exceptions, the myringotomy should be made in either of the inferior quadrants, preferably in the anterior-inferior

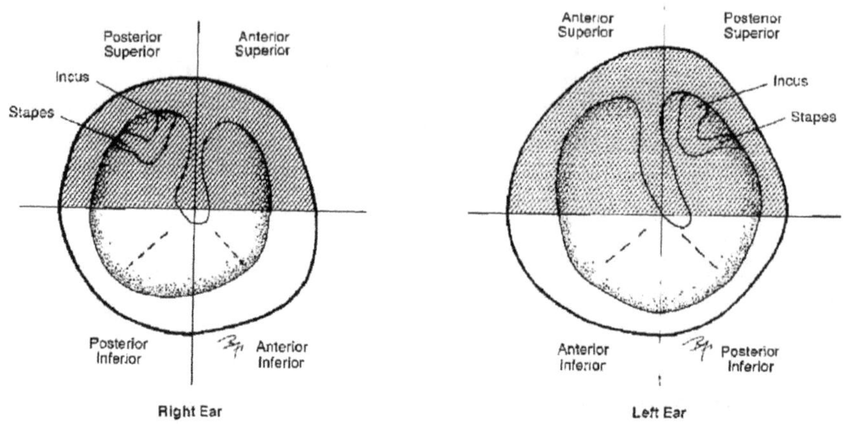

Figure 4. View of tympanic membrane, showing division into quadrants. Incise inferior quadrants. Avoid incising posterior-superio quadrant.

quadrant. However, that option is sometimes precluded by an obstructing bulge in the anterior bony external ear canal. In such cases, the myringotomy is made either directly inferiorly or in the posterior-inferior quadrant.[2-5,7]

The superior quadrants (Figure 4, Figure 5) should be avoided because several middle-ear structures lie just medial to the tympanic membrane superiority. These include the handle of the malleus, the long process of the incus, the stapes, the oval window, and the horizontal portion of the facial nerve. If the myringotomy is made too cephalad, even in the posterior-inferior quadrant, the aforementioned structures could potentially be injured with complications such as hearing loss, bleeding, and facial weakness. It is therefore safest to incise either inferiorly or anterior-inferiorly to avoid these complications.

The myringotomy need not be a long incision if a ventilation tube is not to be inserted. A simple full-thickness puncture of the tympanic membrane will suffice. Admittedly, the perforation usually heals in a day or two, but such an opening will provide immediate pain relief from acute barotitis. The clinician must remember that the tympanic membrane is usually retracted medially and is often, at least in its central portion, in contact with the bony bulge (promontory) of the medial wall of the tympanum. Furthermore, the tympanic membrane is typically extremely thin (0.1 mm). Therefore, it is advisable to keep the myringotomy entrance site peripheral, a few millimeters from the tympanic membrane annulus, to minimize the chance of impinging the tip of the knife or needle on the medial bony wall of the middle-ear cleft.[2-5,7]

As a result of previous middle-ear inflammatory disease, some tympanic membranes may contain hard plaques of myringosclerosis, a hyalinization of the subepithelial connective tissue layer of the eardrum. These usually appear as white, chalky patches within the tympanic membrane. It is best to avoid incising one of these plaques, since they are often difficult to penetrate.

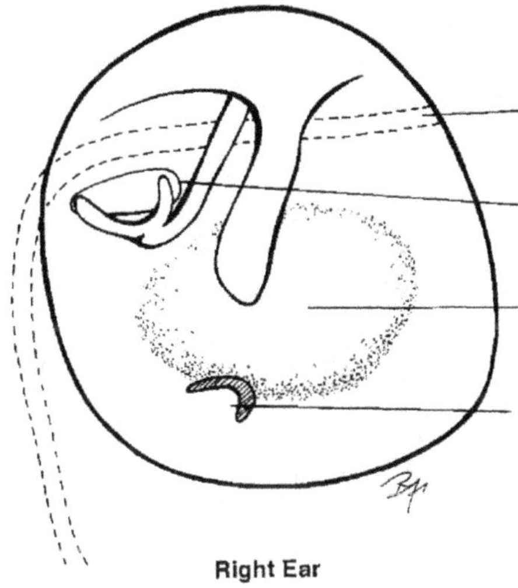

Figure 5. Drawing of medial wall of tympanum with tympanic membrane removed to show middle-ear structures.

PRESSURE EQUALIZATION TUBES

For the patient who is unable to equalize middle-ear pressure readily and will require a series of hyperbaric treatments (e.g., for osteomyelitis, flap survival, or radionecrosis), otolaryngologic consultation for placement of middle-ear vent tubes is recommended. For patients in whom generalized edema is expected to occur as a result of the injury or disease (e.g., burn victims), it is advisable to consider myringotomy and insertion of vent tubes at the time of the first hyperbaric treatment. This can be done, usually at the bedside, using topical or infiltration local anesthesia. Hyperbaric treatments can be commenced immediately after placement of the vent tubes, and the tubes will migrate out of the tympanic membrane spontaneously after several months leaving a healed, intact tympanic membrane in the majority of patients. Patients with middle-ear vent tubes are generally advised to keep water out of the ear canals until the tubes have extruded from the eardrums, and the perforations have healed. While studies show that bath water and most chlorinated pool water does not risk infection, unlike most natural water, especially lakes, rivers, and ponds, it still may be uncomfortable to get water in the middle-ear space.[2-5,7] "Dry ear protection" is easily accomplished by using small, soft earplugs that can be purchased at most pharmacies for exposures to water.

ACKNOWLEDGMENT

The authors wish to acknowledge Dr. Thomas Kidder for his contributions to the original version of this chapter which has formed the basis for this ongoing work.

REFERENCES

1. Commons KH, et al. A prospective analysis of independent patient risk factors for middle ear barotrauma in a multiplayer hyperbaric chamber. Diving Hyperbaric Med. 2013 Sep;43(3):143-7.
2. English G, ed. New York City: Lippincott Williams and Wilkins; 1991. Otolaryngology.
3. Flint PW et al, editors. Cummings otolaryngology – head and neck surgery. 5th ed. Philadelphia: Mosby Elsevier; 2010.
4. Naumann HH, ed. Head and neck surgery. 2nd ed. Vol. 2: Ear. Philadelphia: Thieme; 1996.
5. Paparella M et al. Otolaryngology. 3rd ed. Vol. II, The Ear. Philadelphia: Saunders; 1991.
6. Sea-Long Medical Systems, Inc [Internet]. Louisville (KY): Sea-Long Medical Systems, Inc. Sea-Long Medical Systems Product Information Page. Available from: http://www.sea-long.com/products/index.php
7. Shambaugh GE. Surgery of the ear. 2nd ed. Philadelphia: Saunders; 1967.

CHAPTER 9 CHAPTER

Contraindications and Relative Risks of Hyperbaric Oxygen Treatment

CHAPTER NINE OVERVIEW

Introduction 171
Logistical Contraindications 172
Contraindications 172
Relative Risks 173
Specific Patient Conditions *Not* Contraindicated 174
Conflicting Data of Benefit Versus Contraindication Versus Complication 177
Contraindications – Management 177
Relative Risks – Management 178
Conflicting Data of Benefit Versus Contraindication Versus Complication – Management 188
Actual Case Samples 190
Answers and Explanations 192
References 193

Contraindications and Relative Risks of Hyperbaric Oxygen Treatment

Phi-Nga Jeannie Le

INTRODUCTION

In selecting appropriate patients, it is as important to screen patients for conditions that can pose relative risks for treatment with hyperbaric oxygen (HBO_2). The importance of obtaining a thorough history during the initial consultation cannot be emphasized enough. All medical treatments and procedures inherently entail a benefit-risk analysis. The more complete and accurate are the data from a patient's medical history, the more reliable the benefit-risk analysis can be. It is not possible to account for every situation about which a physician must determine if the risks of hyperbaric oxygen therapy (HBO_2 therapy) would outweigh the benefits; however, if fundamental principles are kept in mind, then one can try to extrapolate and make a reasonable decision.

Key concepts:

* 100% oxygen is a metabolic gas that has both therapeutic effect and toxicity correlative to the elevated O_2 partial pressure.(14,104)
* Increasing and decreasing pressure will always enforce the gas laws on any gas-filled space.(101)

When confronted with a condition that is not explicitly addressed here, ask the fundamental question: how could this condition, drug, or device be complicated by high O_2 tension, and how could it be complicated by increased or decreased ambient pressure? In general, the literature is sparse for evidence to contraindicate a condition, drug, or device for HBO_2. There is only one true contraindication for which there is scientific certainty, based upon Boyle's law: trapped gas that expands in volume under decreasing pressure that can then cause barotrauma, the most described and exemplified being an unvented pneumothorax that can evolve into a tension pneumothorax. Virtually all other risks are theoretical, experiential, circumstantial, or anecdotal. Other than gas trappings of various types, the overwhelming majority of risks are relative – if not simply being conditions with potential for complication rather than being actual risks themselves.

In this chapter, risk factors have been categorized according to the mechanism of action, e.g., mechanism by trapped gas, by oxygen toxicity, or by pressurization/ depressurization. Following this, management considerations are provided for each risk factor. Where relevant, a notation will be made if there is expert disagreement regarding a relative risk or the management thereof.

It is important to keep in mind that the management considerations described herein are based on clinical application by various academic institutions and by various practicing authorities – who have differing practice iterations themselves – founded on decades of expert diving and hyperbaric medicine practice, outcomes data, manufacturer product information, and culled published studies. While providing clinical management recommendations, the content of this review does not constitute a formal, statistically validated clinical practice guideline and should not be utilized as a dichotomous "go" or "no go" algorithm template. The information and recommendations are presented to assist clinicians in their calculation of the benefit versus risk of a patient's specific conditions affecting the outcomes of HBO_2 treatment. Each patient's condition comes with a multitude of variables that must be factored into the benefit-risk analysis, but it is not known how much any of the factors listed in this review increase a patient's chance of a particular HBO_2 side effect. As with any drug, which 100% oxygen is, HBO_2 has side effects, of which no physician can predict or control the occurrence. By applying one's knowledge and understanding of the physiology and mechanism of hyperbaric oxygen therapy to a particular medical situation, a physician can make a reasonable judgment of whether the benefit of a specific outcome is worth sustaining certain side effects – whether, for example, salvaging a limb at risk of amputation is worth sustaining otic barotrauma.

LOGISTICAL CONTRAINDICATIONS

- **Safety:** Technical competence of staff, functioning adequate equipment
- **Hazards:** Stability for transport, inclement weather, safe mode of transport
- **Coercion:** Parent who insists on being inside chamber with child

CONTRAINDICATIONS

Due to trapped gas

- Pneumothorax (unvented)
- Intraocular gas (except from bubble manifestation in decompression sickness, or DCS)
- Hollow orbital prosthesis
- Acute severe bronchospasm (unresolved)
- Other rare, gas-filled structures that might develop gas trapping: pneumatoceles, laryngocele, esophageal diverticulum[71]

Due to oxygen toxicity

- Considerable question regarding two particular drugs as being contraindicated or a relative risk: bleomycin and doxorubicin, with bleomycin being the most under question. The current literature does not support the supposition that bleomycin and doxorubicin are contraindicated in HBO_2.

- HBO_2 candidates who are on active, current therapy with either bleomycin or doxorubicin ought to be considered on a case-by-case basis as to the urgent need for HBO_2. However, prior exposure to either bleomycin or doxorubicin does not preclude patients from HBO.
- For the purpose of this textbook resource, the current use of bleomycin or doxorubicin is considered a relative risk.

RELATIVE RISKS

Due to trapped gas

- Chronic obstructive pulmonary disease (COPD), particularly emphysema
- Recent pneumothorax
- History of spontaneous pneumothorax
- Chest surgery/trauma
- Dental problems: cavities, incomplete or cracked root fillings, periapical cysts, devitalized pulp

Due to oxygen toxicity

- Optic neuritis – if acute (not just history of optic neuritis without exacerbation as seen in multiple sclerosis)
- Retrobulbar optic neuritis
- Retinopathy of prematurity (a.k.a. retrolental fibroplasia) – premature infants
- Current bleomycin
- Current doxorubicin

Due to pressure change

- Acute upper respiratory infection (URI) – inability to equalize middle-ear pressure
- Otitis media – inability to equalize middle-ear pressure
- Mastoidectomy – inability to equalize middle-ear pressure; damage to inner ear with increased pressure
- Stapedectomy – dislodgment of stapes prosthesis, damage to labyrinthine membranes; inner-ear barotrauma if perilymph fistula present
- Tympanoplasty – risk of recurrent rupture
- Cochlear implant – malfunction of internal components rather than removable external hardware
- Total ossicular prostheses – inner-ear damage due to penetration of stapes plate by prosthesis
- Implanted devices (pacemakers, defibrillators, shunts) – malfunction above pressure threshold of device
- Untested devices

Various other systemic effects

- Unstable congestive heart failure (CHF)

- Uncontrolled seizure disorder – organic seizure disorder is a different mechanism than hyperoxia-induced seizure activity
- Uncontrolled hypertension
- Chronic respiratory failure and hypercapnia
- Claustrophobia
- Brittle diabetes with hypoglycemia

Various other drugs – relative risks due to weak published evidence

- Cis-Platin
- Disulfiram (Antabuse)
- Mafenide acetate (Sulfamylon)
- Anti-angiogenic cancer drugs
- Amiodarone

SPECIFIC PATIENT CONDITIONS *NOT* CONTRAINDICATED

Pregnancy

- Physiologic effect of premature but reversible closure of fetal ductus arteriosum by hyperoxia.
    a. Based on animal studies using O_2 partial pressures at higher than the doses used for clinical treatment in humans.
- Multiple reports of pregnant women, including one prospective trial of 44, treated with HBO_2 for carbon monoxide poisoning demonstrated no increased risk of spontaneous abortion or other adverse effects related to HBO_2 in the fetus and mother.[11,30,74,97,111]
- Evidence not demonstrated for deleterious effects or teratogenicity occurring in humans based on considerable Russian experience of treating a prodigious number (> 700) of pregnant women in all trimesters for a multitude of conditions; with report of HBO_2 improving condition of and reducing perinatal complication and mortality of both mother and fetus.[11,74]
- Recent nonrandomized cohort study conducted in Russia for the purpose of assessing effectiveness of HBO_2 in the treatment of chronic anemia and prevention of perinatal complications (both nonindications in the United States) in 65 pregnant women (unequal distribution of 40 patients in HBO_2 group and 25 in control group), reported no adverse or deleterious effects related to HBO_2. Improved conditions in the mother and neonate were observed in HBO_2 group: threat of spontaneous abortion less frequent in HBO_2 group (9 women, 22.5%) compared to control group (15 women, 60%); preeclampsia less frequent in HBO_2 group (4, 10%) versus control group (14, 56%); Apgar scores at 1 and 5 mins higher in HBO_2 group (7.6, 8.4) versus control group (7.2, 7.8).[52]
- HBO_2 ought to be provided to pregnant women as with any other patient, particularly for urgent or emergent indications for HBO_2 treatment.
- The same criteria to meet indication for treatment should be applied to pregnant women as to any other patient, with some academic physicians

applying a lower threshold in criteria to treat pregnant women for certain emergent indications, such as for carbon monoxide poisoning,[29] though there are no prospective studies of efficacy or effectiveness of accepted HBO_2 indications in pregnancy.[43]

Malignancy

- A 1950s study demonstrated that oxygen concentration influences the effect of radiation therapy.[42,72] A modern meta-analysis elucidated that, of all the tumor hypoxia modification techniques, HBO_2 has the most marked effect on tumor sensitization to radiation.[82]
- Among early research conducted in 1960s and 1970s using HBO_2 as chemo- and radiosensitizer, one particular study made the first report of malignancy progression among some of 25 cervical cancer patients undergoing radiation therapy enhanced by HBO_2 radiosensitization. Concern that HBO_2 enhances tumor growth when these adjunctive HBO_2-treated patients were found to have higher incidences of metastases and earlier than expected deaths with distal metastases.[56]
    a. Same researchers demonstrated in their sequential controlled trial in 1974 of 25 cervical cancer (CA) patients treated under adjunctive HBO_2 and 25 cervical CA patients in air group that 5-year survival rate was higher for HBO_2 group at 44% compared to 16% for air group; but serious bowel complication rate was higher in HBO_2 group.[57]
- Additional human clinical studies followed that suggested possible HBO_2 enhancement of cancer progression.
    a. 1967: Controlled trial including 40 patients with bladder CA showed increased metastases; but control and HBO_2 group were not well matched for tumor grade, with HBO_2 group comprised of increased number of patients with advanced stage and more aggressive histology.[9,33]
    b. 1987: Three anecdotal cases of patients with urothelial tumors from indwelling catheters had existing cancer that seemed to progress rapidly after HBO_2 therapy.[31]
    c. 1996: Four patients with advanced head and neck CA treated with HBO_2 for delayed radiation injury displayed recurrence and rapidly progressing tumors after HBO_2. However, two of the four patients already had recurrence before starting HBO_2 therapy. One of the four had a six-month delay of radiation therapy following surgical resection due to pneumonia.[4,33]
- In contradiction, many more human clinical studies evinced neutral or beneficial effects. Highlighted studies follow:
    a. 1978: Controlled trial of 238 bladder CA patients randomized to HBO_2 or air showed no difference in local tumor control or morbidity between the two groups.[8]
    b. 1978: Randomized controlled trial of 320 patients with cervical CA demonstrated metastatic rate was the same in HBO_2 and control groups.[114]
    c. 1979: Clinical trial of 1500 patients to compare treatment with HBO_2-enhanced radiation therapy versus air showed improved local

cure and survival in patients with head/neck and cervical cancers, benefit in bronchial CA, but no beneficial effect in bladder cancer in the HBO_2-treated group compared to control.[25]
d. 1987: 201 patients with squamous cell CA of head and neck treated with HBO_2 radiosensitized radiation therapy between 1960 and 1980 had "perceptibly" better, though not statistically different, 5-year survival rate than contemporary cohorts treated in air from 1970 to 1980.[22]
e. 1999: Case series of 405 head and neck CA patients, with 245 patients receiving HBO; 19.6% of patients in HBO_2 group developed tumor recurrence versus 28% in control group; decreased recurrence rate of head and neck CA in HBO_2-treated patients.[69]
f. 2004: Transplanted human prostate cancer cells were injected into severe combined-immunodeficient mice that were then treated with HBO; tumor microvessel density, proliferative index, and differentiation and apoptosis markers were similar in HBO_2 and control groups. Conclusion: HBO_2 does not accelerate growth of prostate CA cells.[13]
g. 2005: HBO_2 increased tumor O_2 but no growth of irradiated or unirradiated tumors; no increase in vascularity or vascular endothelial growth factor (VEGF) seen. Conclusion: No promotion of tumor growth with HBO_2 exposure.[95]

- In 2003, a group of international radiation oncology specialists conducted a comprehensive review of experimental and clinical data and evidence, concluding that HBO_2 does not promote primary or metastatic cancer progression and that the application of HBO_2 treatment is safe in patients with prior history of malignancy.[33]
  a. Contended that though 72 patients in 3 published clinical trials displayed possible promotion of cancer growth by HBO_2, over 3000 patients treated with HBO_2 in 12 clinical trials exhibited either neutral or cancer-suppressive effect.
  b. Affirmed that the pathophysiology of angiogenesis occurring in malignant tumor growth differs from the physiology of HBO_2-induced angiogenesis occurring in nonhealing hypoxic wounds.
- In 2006, another comprehensive review of experimental and clinical data was conducted demonstrating the same conclusions.[18]
- HBO_2 should not be withheld from cancer patients when needed.
- HBO_2 ought not to be pursued when it may interfere with treatment for malignancy, which must take priority over HBO_2 therapy.

Glaucoma

- Open-angle glaucoma: Not fully understood; intraocular pressure (IOP) related to retinal ganglion cell death; characterized by increased resistance to aqueous humor outflow drainage through trabecular meshwork.[115]
- Closed-angle glaucoma: Obstruction of the aqueous outflow occurs at the angle (the location of aqueous outflow in eye) by apposition of the iris, causing physically closed angle; aqueous humor amasses behind iris.[115]

- The increase in intraocular pressure in glaucoma is due to aqueous humor liquid accumulation, which is a different IOP mechanism than gas accumulation in the eye that can cause ophthalmic barotrauma.
- IOP decreases with increasing ambient pressure by either HBO_2 or diving.[32,37,80,110]
- Conflicting results of high altitude or hypobaric environments on IOP.[52]

CONFLICTING DATA OF BENEFIT VERSUS CONTRAINDICATION VERSUS COMPLICATION

Theoretical mechanism due to trapped gas

- Pneumocephalus
  a. Also identified as pneumocephaly, intracranial aerocele, or intracranial pneumatocele.

CONTRAINDICATIONS – MANAGEMENT

Due to trapped gas – leading to barotrauma

- Pneumothorax (unvented)
  a. Untreated pneumothorax (PTX) can convert to tension pneumothorax during decompression stage of HBO_2 treatment when gas expands faster than it can escape, causing respiratory and hemodynamic collapse.
  b. Types: spontaneous, traumatic, postsurgical, secondary to pulmonary disorders, iatrogenic.
  c. Screening chest X-ray (CXR) as part of initial consultation to rule out presence. CXR is inaccurate in assessing the volume of the PTX.[15]
  d. When PTX present, chest tube placement with Heimlich valve or water seal to equalize pulmonary pressure with ambient chamber pressure, with mandatory CXR after chest tube placement to confirm resolved PTX.
  e. Treatment can proceed after chest tube placement, particularly if emergent HBO_2 is necessary.
  f. Asymptomatic small PTX of < two cm from lung edge to chest wall may be treated with normobaric O_2 and inpatient observation,[10,45] but this does not ensure the patient will be safe for HBO_2 at later time, as intervention with pressure equalization procedure, e.g., chest tube thoracostomy, has not been conducted to ensure gas egress during the decompression stage of HBO_2 treatment.
  g. Of the different types of pneumothorax, the most concerning is the spontaneous PTX for which no antecedent cause can be identified. History of spontaneous PTX does not contraindicate a patient to HBO_2, but, if a recent PTX occurred, consider delay of non-emergent HBO_2 until about 6 weeks from time of occurrence.
  h. Watchful surveillance of patient with history of spontaneous PTX during and throughout HBO_2 therapy course is warranted for symptoms of respiratory distress.

- Intraocular gas (except from bubble manifestation in DCS)
  a. Used as a tamponade in ophthalmologic surgeries and procedures.
  b. Gases commonly used: air, sulfur hexafluoride (SF_6), perfluoroethane (C_2F_6), and perfluoropropane (C_3F_8).[55,73]
  c. Resorbs eventually into circulation; about 2–9 weeks relative to particular gas used.[48]
  d. Computerized tomography scan (CT) of head to confirm complete resorption when medical history indicates possible presence.
  e. May already be resorbed if placed in distant past from vitreoretinal surgery.
  f. Decompression during HBO_2 treatment causes gas expansion, resulting in marked elevation in intraocular pressure (IOP).[53]
  g. Increased IOP can lead to barotrauma, reduced ocular blood flow, or compression and occlusion of the central retinal artery, resulting in ischemia and possibly blindness.[6,34,48,55]
  h. HBO_2 should not proceed in the presence of an existing intraocular gas.

- Hollow orbital prosthesis
  a. Hollow orbital prosthesis collapsible under hyperbaric condition.
  b. Silicone-based hollow prosthesis reported collapsing during diving at shallow 10-feet depth.[52]
  c. Double-walled glass hollow prosthesis reported imploding during diving at 18-meters depth.[59]
  d. If removable, then remove for each treatment; otherwise HBO_2 therapy ought not to be undertaken.
  e. Solid prosthesis does not have collapsible tissue under increased pressure.[7]

- Acute severe bronchospasm
  a. Must be resolved or controlled with inhaled bronchodilators or steroids or ventilated.
  b. Be prepared with in-chamber nebulizer for patients at risk of exacerbation.
  c. Frequent auscultation during HBO_2 treatment to assess for developing acute bronchospasm, especially during change of depth.
  d. Frequent nebulized bronchodilators as needed.

- Other rare, gas-filled structures that might develop gas trapping: pneumatoceles, laryngocele, esophageal diverticulum.
  a. CT scan to assess for presence when history indicates possible formation secondary to prior medical condition or surgical procedure.

RELATIVE RISKS – MANAGEMENT

Due to trapped gas

- COPD, particularly emphysema
  a. Screening CXR during initial consultation.

b. High-resolution chest CT to look for blebs, bullae, cysts, or other trapped gas in lung.
c. Evaluate for symptomatic or unstable condition.
d. Consider pulmonary risk assessment.
   - ◊ Pulmonary function tests (PFT): spirometry, diffusing capacity of lung for carbon monoxide (DL_{CO}), plethysmography, inert gas ventilation scan/washout study, or arterial blood gas (ABG) to determine level of lung function or for when blebs, bullae, or other air trappings exist. The University of Pennsylvania Undersea and Hyperbaric Medicine program utilizes the xenon (inert gas) ventilation scan/washout study.[108]
   - ◊ Optional approach of maximizing corticosteroid and bronchodilator therapy for a time period to assess bronchodilator response followed by PFT.
   - ◊ Optional approach of counseling patient regarding higher risk of pulmonary barotrauma than those patients without air trapping and proceed with HBO_2 therapy without risk assessment workup if risk acceptable to patient.[51]

e. Once risk determined, and HBO_2 proceeds, slow the decompression time. University of Pennsylvania method: Slow decompression time to 5–6 times the gas half-life previously determined on the inert gas (xenon) ventilation scan.[108]
f. Pretreat with inhaled bronchodilators prior to each HBO_2 treatment; maximize corticosteroid therapy.
g. Relative to severity, periodic auscultation during HBO_2 treatment to assess for developing acute bronchospasm, especially during change of depth (multiplace chamber).
h. Consider periodic in-chamber nebulizer for patients at risk of exacerbation (multiplace).
i. In emergency HBO_2 treatment, if patient appears to be developing acute bronchospasm, treat with fast-acting bronchodilator as needed.

- Asthma and other pulmonary conditions affecting lung function
  a. Screening CXR during initial consultation.
  b. Evaluate for symptomatic or unstable condition.
  c. For pulmonary risk assessment, consider approaches as discussed above for COPD.
  d. Pretreat with inhaled bronchodilators prior to each HBO_2 treatment.
  e. Relative to severity, periodic auscultation during HBO_2 treatment to assess for developing acute bronchospasm, especially during change of depth (multiplace).
  f. Consider periodic in-chamber nebulizer for patients at risk of exacerbation (multiplace).
  g. In emergency HBO_2 treatment, if patient appears to be developing acute bronchospasm, treat with fast-acting bronchodilators as needed.

- Recent pneumothorax
  a. Consider type, e.g., spontaneous, traumatic, tension, iatrogenic.
  b. Wait about six weeks from time of event.[108]
  c. Recognize risk of recurrence of spontaneous PTX and problem of turning into tension PTX during HBO_2 treatment.

- History of spontaneous pneumothorax
  a. Consider possible cause of spontaneous PTX.
  b. Wait about six weeks from time of event.[108]
  c. Recognize risk of recurrence of spontaneous PTX and problem of turning into tension PTX during HBO_2 treatment, particularly if patient has bullous emphysema.

- Chest surgery/trauma
  a. Consider air-trapping secondary to surgery or scarring.
  b. Chest CT
  c. If air trapping present, consider inert gas ventilation/washout study (see COPD section above).
  d. Ajust rate of decompression (see COPD section above).

- Dental problems
  a. Resulting in barodontalgia and odontocrexis
  b. Air-trapping from prosthesis or dental surgeries
  c. X-rays

Due to oxygen toxicity

- Optic neuritis
  a. A type of optic neuropathy of unknown etiology demonstrating demyelinating inflammation and swelling of the optic nerve, causing acute decreased visual acuity or complete blindness, with painful ocular movements.[27,36]
  b. Often confused with the term "optic neuropathy," which is the general disease state of optic nerve disorders inclusive of optic neuritis.
  c. Occurs in many disease states, including infections and diabetes mellitus, but mostly and highly associated with multiple sclerosis (MS).[27,36,89]
  d. History of optic neuritis in MS does not preclude HBO.
  e. *Active* optic neuritis precludes HBO_2 treatment.
  f. Over 14,000 cases of MS patients treated with HBO_2 reported in literature as having been treated without report of complications from HBO_2 in patients who had *no active* optic neuritis.[61,92]
  g. One published case report of vision loss in patient treated with HBO_2, whose vision gradually returned to pretreatment baseline visual acuity upon cessation of HBO.[62]
  h. Anecdotal personal report by an editor of the previous edition of this textbook noting knowledge of a case in which a woman with history of optic neuritis was being treated for multiple sclerosis and became completely blind during the course of HBO.[60]

i. Unpublished direct clinical experience of this author who treated an MS patient for chronic refractory osteomyelitis who had exacerbation of optic neuritis during course of HBO_2 and subsequently developed precipitous marked decline in bilateral visual acuity. Due to the temporal occurrence of the acute visual deterioration, HBO_2 could not be excluded as the cause. HBO_2 therapy was suspended and then completely discontinued due to risk of complete blindness.[108]
j. Occurrence or exacerbation of optic neuritis resulting in worsened visual acuity or vision loss during course of HBO_2 necessitates a pause in, if not the complete cessation of, treatment.
k. Resumption of HBO_2 is dependent on case and assessed risk.
l. Surveil patient frequently for visual decline during course of HBO_2. A decline in visual acuity during treatment of a patient with a history of optic neuritis must be assumed to be recurrent optic neuritis exacerbated by HBO_2 until proven otherwise.
m. Communication and consultation with patient's ophthalmologist.
n. May be extremely difficult to distinguish HBO_2-induced acute visual decline of exacerbated optic neuritis versus hyperoxia-induced myopia versus hyperoxia worsening of cataracts.

- Retrobulbar optic neuritis
  a. An optic neuritis occurring in the segment of the optic nerve posterior to globe.
  b. A specific case report in 1969 of a 21-year-old male who was participating in an experimental study of human pulmonary oxygen tolerance who developed unilateral vision loss after 6 hours of inspired O_2 at 2 ATA.[78,108]
     ◊ subject already had history of unilateral retrobulbar optic neuritis with recurrent bouts of pain, transient scotomas in his right eye, and intermittent reduced visual acuity, which were not reported to physician researchers at time of experiment.
     ◊ Pre-HBO_2 screening exam had demonstrated no scotoma but presence of "slight" right optic disc pallor.
     ◊ During HBO_2 experimental study, subject had progressively worsened vision that he did not report until developing vision loss to degree of only light perception.
     ◊ Visual loss began to minimally improve 15 minutes after cessation of HBO_2, with continued improvement in visual acuity over following 2 months.
     ◊ Normal visual acuity returned, but the "slight" right optic disc pallor was now larger area of temporal pallor.
     ◊ Subject was diagnosed with recurrence of retrobulbar optic neuritis with transient unilateral vision loss secondary to HBO_2 exposure.
  c. Very rare case of extreme exposure to HBO_2 in experimental environment that would not normally be experienced by patients in clinical treatment.
  d. Case has been source of citation contraindicating optic neuritis for HBO.

e. In clinical practice, discuss with affected patient the risk of vision loss versus risk of not conducting HBO_2 treatment.
f. Surveil patient daily for visual decline if risk of treatment acceptable.
g. Cease HBO_2 with any visual change or decline.
h. Communication and consultation with patient's ophthalmologist.

- Retinopathy of prematurity (aka retrolental fibroplasia)
  a. Condition of abnormal retinal development of premature (< 35 weeks) or young infants exposed to hyperoxia, causing permanent blindness.
  b. High inspiratory supplemental oxygen provided to treat respiratory distress syndrome in premature infants with immature retinas was described to cause vasoconstriction of the developing retinal vessels, suppression of angiogenic mediators of normal retinal vascularization in hyperoxic environment, followed by hypoxic retina on return to normobaric environment, and then subsequent abnormal uncontrolled neovascularization resulting in retinal detachment and ultimately blindness.(14,44,83,85,93,103)
  c. Varying degree of severity
  d. Weigh necessity of HBO_2 for chronic versus acute indication.
  e. Consider adjusting PaO_2 by lowering ATA without compromising effective HBO_2 treatment.
  f. Communication and consultation with infant's neonatologist and ophthalmologist.
  g. No report of retrolental fibroplasia developing in babies born from pregnant women treated with HBO.

- Current doxorubicin (Adriamycin)
  a. Antineoplastic chemotherapy drug with serious side effects including cardiotoxicity.
  b. Experimental animal studies investigating various use of HBO_2 as enhancement effect with doxorubicin on tumor cells or as protective mechanism against doxorubicin adverse effects instead showed increased cytotoxicity, particularly lethal cardiotoxicity, in animals treated with combination of doxorubicin and HBO; with very high doses of HBO_2 used.(75,109)
  c. Theoretical risk to humans based on these animal studies, but no human clinical studies.
  d. Contradictory experimental animal studies showed either no cardiotoxicity or actual cardioprotective effect.(58,102)
  e. Doxorubicin is cleared from body in 24 hours, but there appears to be a dose-response curve with higher dose having higher cardiotoxicity.
  f. Due to half-life of doxorubicin, suggest waiting two to three days from last dose before proceeding and holding doxorubicin during treatment if not detrimental to patient.

- Current or recent bleomycin
  a. Antineoplastic chemotherapy drug with serious side effects including pulmonary toxicity (pulmonary fibrosis, pneumonitis, acute respiratory distress syndrome (ARDS).
  b. Experimental animal studies, human case series, and case reports described normobaric oxygen induced/exacerbated pulmonary toxicity occurring with the application of increased inspiratory oxygen for different purposes (anesthesia, intraoperative, mechanical ventilation) at broad-ranging various times following bleomycin treatment.[3,39,50,66]
  c. Evidence and many more case series reports indicate that pulmonary toxicity (fibrosis, pneumonitis, ARDS) occurring in bleomycin treatment is due to the direct cellular and tissue damage caused by bleomycin itself, rather than a deleterious synergistic effect with normobaric increased FiO_2 or hyperbaric oxygen exposure.[26,28,40,79,98,105,112,116]
  d. Patients at highest risk of lung dysfunction or death due to bleomycin toxic drug effect are those who are age > 70, are within 2 months of last bleomycin dose, received total dose > 450 units, and decreased renal function of CrCl < 35 mL/min.[70,105]
  e. Withholding HBO_2 from patients with history of previous bleomycin treatment is not warranted.
  f. A safe interval of time to administer HBO_2 following bleomycin treatment has not been established, but a range of three months to one year has been applied to patients on a case-by-case basis.[29,105,108]
  g. Prior to initiating HBO_2 therapy, evaluate for existing or degree of lung damage with CT scan and PFT or combination of PFTs (spirometry, DL_{CO}, plethysmography, inert gas ventilation scan, ABG).
  h. Surveil for developing pulmonary dysfunction or worsening clinical condition during course of HBO_2 therapy.
     ◊ DL_{CO} is the most predictive PFT of potential problems arising.
     ◊ Baseline DL_{CO} with periodic DL_{CO} as surveillance.
  i. If emergent HBO_2 required, consider N-acetylcysteine administration, but evidence for this is weak and found only in animal studies.[54,94]

Due to pressure change

- Acute upper respiratory infection (URI)
  a. Evaluate for ability to equalize middle-ear pressure.
  b. Treat symptomatically with appropriate medication.

- Otitis media
  a. Evaluate for ability to equalize middle-ear pressure.
  b. Consider tympanostomy tube placement in non-emergent HBO_2 for chronic indication or myringotomy in emergent situation.

- Mastoidectomy
    a. Evaluate for ability to equalize middle-ear pressure.
    b. Discuss potential damage to inner ear.
    c. Communication and consultation with patient's ear, nose, and throat specialist (ENT).

- Stapedectomy
    a. Evaluate for presence of perilymph fistula.[96]
    b. Evaluate for ability to equalize middle-ear pressure.
    c. Discuss risk of dislodgment, damages to inner structures.[96]
    d. Communication and consultation with ENT.

- Tympanoplasty
    a. Evaluate for ability to equalize middle-ear pressure.
    b. Risk of rerupture higher.[96]

- Cochlear implant
    a. Determine pressure threshold of implant from manufacturer.

- Total ossicular prostheses
    a. Evaluate for ability to equalize middle-ear pressure.
    b. Discuss risk of dislodgment.[96]
    c. Communication and consultation with ENT.

- Implanted devices (pacemakers, defibrillators, shunts, pumps)
    a. Determine pressure threshold of implant from manufacturer.

- Untested devices
    a. Weigh risk of malfunction with benefit of HBO_2 treatment.
    b. Prudent to avoid HBO_2 with untested devices for chronic indications.
    c. Weigh risks/benefits for emergent condition.

Various other systemic effects

- Unstable congestive heart failure (CHF)
    a. Clinical status of patient is important: if frequent CHF exacerbations or easily exacerbated, risk of HBO_2 treatment outweighs benefit.
    b. Baseline left ventricular ejection fraction (EJF) is *not* a predictor of CHF outcomes.[76]
    c. The EJF percentage ought not to be used as a criterion for inclusion or exclusion from HBO.
    d. If echocardiogram already done, repeat echo not likely to offer additional information, as EJF is not indicative of current clinical status.
    e. Ensure medical compliance and maximize medical management.
    f. Communication and consultation with patient's cardiologist for accurate clinical status.

- Uncontrolled seizure disorder
    a. History of a seizure disorder is not a contraindication to HBO.

  b. Epileptic and nonepileptic seizure disorders involve mechanisms different from hyperoxia-induced seizure activity.(5,14,38,99,113)
  c. The concern is the manageability of the seizure during HBO_2 treatment and being able to discern from hyperoxic seizure in order to intervene appropriately, as elevated PaO_2 lowers the seizure threshold.
  d. Hypercapnia from comorbidities is added risk.
  e. Determine degree of stability and medical compliance.
  f. Screen for therapeutic level of anticonvulsants.
  g. Use of benzodiazepine is beneficial for existing organic seizure disorder, not for preventing or managing oxygen toxicity seizure activity.
  h. Multiplace chamber preferable over monoplace for possible medical intervention in event of seizure occurrence.
  i. If seizure occurs, switch gas to air, and do not decompress during tonic phase of seizure. Upon cessation of tonic-clonic movements along with return of regular respiration, decide whether to resume treatment or to begin decompression.

- Uncontrolled hypertension (HTN)
  a. Screening vital signs before, during, and after HBO.
  b. Screen for symptomatic uncontrolled HTN.
  c. Ensure medical compliance.
  d. Monitor for symptoms of hypertensive urgency/emergency during treatment.

- Congenital spherocytosis
  a. Theoretical risk of hemolysis due to high PaO_2.
  b. Should not preclude HBO_2 for emergency indication, as long as patient is not significantly anemic.
  c. Prepare to treat complications of hemolysis and acute anemia.

- Chronic respiratory failure and hypercapnia
  a. Hyperoxia could reduce respiratory drive.
  b. Monitor patient with SaO_2, $TcPO_2$, $TcPCO_2$.
  c. Risk is low, but prepare for hypoventilation.

- Claustrophobia
  a. Consider trial run of HBO_2 treatment.
  b. Consider anxiolytic.

- Brittle diabetes with hypoglycemia (not all diabetics who are already well-controlled on oral medication).
  a. Correction of hypoglycemia to prevent hypoglycemic seizure and other symptoms is necessary prior to HBO.
  b. Have the patient consume steady nutrition (protein with carbohydrate) prior to each HBO.
  c. Monitor blood sugar prior and during HBO_2 therapy as necessary. Note that the status of being diabetic does not mandate nor require the routine checking of random blood sugar before every HBO_2 treatment.
  d. Prepare for hypoglycemic episode during treatment.

e. Diabetic patients most at risk of hypoglycemia are the ones who require insulin and had insulin adjusted higher during active infection but did not have insulin adjusted back down after infection resolved.
f. If patient is exceptionally brittle with constant hypoglycemic episodes that are not managed well, then cessation of HBO_2 therapy is warranted.
g. The checking of blood sugar pre- and post-HBO_2 on every diabetic – whether T1DM, T2DM, or T2DM on insulin – is a wholly facility-centric practice decision rather than a scientific rigor. There is much variation in opinion on the necessity of daily routine finger-stick blood sugar on every diabetic prior to and post-HBO_2, regardless of insulin-requiring or only oral medication-requiring.

Various other drugs

- Cis-Platin
    a. More an issue of wound care than HBO.
    b. Some evidence of delayed wound healing.[86]
    c. HBO_2 can be given to non-wound-care patients.

- Disulfiram (Antabus)
    a. Theoretical risk of increased seizures due to reduction in superoxide dismutase antioxidant production leading to oxygen toxicity.[21,35]
    b. Multiple HBO_2 treatments appear to be the highest risk; single treatment for emergent condition possible.

- Mafenide acetate (Sulfamylon)
    a. Used as topical antimicrobial on burn patients.[20,77,107]
    b. Inhibits carbonic anhydrase, causing vasodilation,[20,77,107] and thus counteracts vasoconstriction in HBO_2 leading to impaired wound healing.
    c. Theoretical risk of increased seizures if absorbed.
    d. Remove from burn patient receiving HBO.
    e. Use alternate antimicrobial for burn wounds during HBO_2 therapy (e.g., silver sulfadiazine).

- Anti-angiogenic cancer drugs
    a. Check all of patient's anticancer drugs for mechanism of action.
    b. HBO_2 not likely effective in presence of antiangiogenic drug if goal is to induce angiogenesis to treat indication.

- Amiodarone
    a. Known potential fatal adverse effects, including pulmonary toxicity (hypersensitivity pneumonitis or interstitial/alveolar pneumonitis) in 10%–17% of patients with existing ventricular arrhythmias when given at doses of about 400 mg/day. Some pulmonary effects appear as abnormal diffusing capacity without symptoms in a much higher percentage of patients, with pulmonary toxicity being fatal 10% of the time. The mechanism of action of toxicity *may* result from the release of oxygen radicals and/or phospholipidosis (foamy

macrophages). This is an inherent component of amiodarone use and can occur any time from a few days to a few weeks.[87]

b. Amiodarone pulmonary toxicity risks highest for age > 60 and duration of treatment 6–12 months[31A]
   - ◊ dose 400 mg/day > 2 months or 200 mg/day for 2 years being highest duration risk.[115A]

c. A small number of amiodarone patients subjected to increased FiO_2 were reported to have developed ARDS, but a causal association has not been established.[87]

d. There is no evidence or reports in the literature that suggest hyperbaric oxygen and amiodarone are synergistic in inducing or increasing the risk of pulmonary toxicity.

e. Pulmonary oxygen radicals formation occurs with normobaric oxygen, and evidence is lacking to demonstrate that hyperbaric oxygen increases pulmonary oxygen radicals formation.

f. In a patient undergoing amiodarone treatment, any new respiratory symptoms should suggest the possibility of pulmonary toxicity due to the medication itself, and patient should receive pulmonary specialist evaluation and intervention, rather than pursue HBO_2 therapy at that time, as HBO_2 therapy should not interfere with treatment for amiodarone-induced pulmonary toxicity.

g. If there is pulmonary toxicity in a patient taking amiodarone and receiving HBO_2 therapy concurrently, it is likely due to the amiodarone rather than to HBO_2.

h. Pre-HBO_2-therapy screening to establish baseline pulmonary status and function with CXR, high-resolution CT (HRCT), PFT (e.g., spirometry), and lung diffusing capacity (DL_{CO} – refer to COPD section for pulmonary risk assessment).
   - ◊ Recommend at least HRCT and DL_{CO} as baseline screening in patient with already existing risk factors for amiodarone-induced pulmonary toxicity.

i. Possible findings in patient with existing amiodarone pulmonary toxicity:[115A]
   - ◊ PFT – low lung volumes and a restrictive pattern.
   - ◊ DL_{CO} – diminished diffusing capacity.
   - ◊ HRCT – possible bilateral interstitial, alveolar, or mixed interstitial/alveolar infiltrates; better than CXR for detection of extent of disease.
   - ◊ CXR – nonspecific ground glass, patchy, or diffuse infiltrates.

j. Surveil patient for developing pulmonary dysfunction or worsening clinical condition during course of HBO_2 therapy.
   - ◊ DL_{CO} is the most predictive PFT of potential problems arising.
   - ◊ Baseline DL_{CO} with periodic DL_{CO} as surveillance.

k. Discussion with the patient and his or her referring physician on existing factors and possible risks, with decision to continue or discontinue HBO_2 therapy based upon change in clinical condition.

CONFLICTING DATA OF BENEFIT VERSUS CONTRAINDICATION VERSUS COMPLICATION – MANAGEMENT

Pneumocephalus/pneumocephaly/intracranial aerocele/ intracranial pneumatocele

- Intracranial air
- Not uncommon or rare occurrence
- Detectable by skull X-ray, but CT scan is preferred diagnostic choice as very small volume (0.5 cm^3) of air can be detected with sensitivity 10 times greater than plain film.[(1,119)]
- Tension pneumocephalus is a rare adverse evolution of simple pneumocephalus of cranial air trapped under pressure and considered a neurosurgical emergency.[(24,88,90)]
- Possible sequela from trauma, surgical procedures (especially craniotomy), intracranial tumors, intracranial infections, diving, iatrogenic intravenous retrograde injection of air, cerebral air embolism, neural tube defects, nontraumatic CSF fluid leak, air travel.[(2,12,19,23,49,65,68,91,106,118,120)]
- Can be asymptomatic or symptomatic, leading to adverse effects.[(68,88,106)]
  1. Severe: CSF leakage, rhinorrhea, meningitis, syncope, aphasia, confusion, lethargy, seizure, hemiparesis, ataxia, lack of pupillary response.
  2. Less severe: Fever, nausea, vomiting, headache, agitation.
  3. Adverse effects: Tension pneumocephalus (mass effect), meningitis.
- A conundrum condition characterized by three possible situations.
  a. A condition that benefits from HBO_2
  b. A complication of HBO_2
  c. A contraindication to HBO_2
- Pneumocephalus as a condition *benefitting* from HBO_2
  a. Standard noninvasive treatment: Normobaric supplemental O_2 through non-rebreather mask to increase rate of air absorption.[(16,23,41,46)]
  b. A 2014 prospective, nonrandomized cohort study in Brazil of 24 patients (22 traumatic brain injury patients and 2 post-surgical cerebellar tumor patients, all hospital inpatients) with symptomatic or persistent pneumocephalus assigned 13 patients to the HBO_2 treatment arm at 2.5 ATA and 11 patients to the control arm receiving continuous normobaric O_2 at 5 L for 5 days. The study demonstrated 1) sooner radiological resolution of the pneumocephalus in the HBO_2-treated group, 2) no incidence of meningitis in the HBO_2 group versus four in control group, 3) significantly longer hospital stay in the control group, 4) clinical improvement in all patients, and 5) no acute complications related to HBO_2.[(84)]

- Pneumocephalus as a *complication* of HBO_2
  a. Rare incidence of tension pneumocephalus development in a head trauma patient given adjunctive HBO_2 while still with unrepaired basilar skull fracture and persistent CSF leakage, resulting in a vegetative state.[63]
  b. Rare incidence of tension pneumocephalus development in a head trauma patient treated with HBO_2 for recovery of function 15 months after an unrepaired basilar skull fracture and a CSF diversion using a ventriculoperitoneal shunt, resulting in protracted loss of consciousness.[64]
  c. Report of development of tension pneumocephalus during air travel in patient who had rare complication of ethmoid sinus osteoma eroding through the dura mater.[67]
  d. While HBO_2 would rapidly resorb pneumocephalus during compression, question remains of potential residual air possibly expanding during depressurization due to obstructed gas egress.
  e. Life-threatening complications appear to be highest in patients presenting with CSF leakage (presenting as rhinorrhea).

- Pneumocephalus as a *contraindication* to HBO_2
  a. Several case reports of pneumocephalus developing upon air travel in patients with past medical history of cranial surgical or invasive spinal procedures.[49,67,100]
  b. Tension pneumocephalus resulting during flight due to existing known pneumocephalus.[67,100]
  c. Extrapolating from air travel cases and from HBO_2 treatment cases of simple pneumocephalus developing tension pneumocephalus complication, HBO_2 can also be contraindicated in pneumocephalus patients.

- Appears that the mechanism of the originating structural insult, the subsequent malformed intracranial defect creating a one-way valve tract, and the resultant decrease in intracranial pressure are likely combined complex factors determining whether the pneumocephalus will be characterized as benefitting from or pose as a complication of or contraindication to HBO_2.

- Two possible mechanisms
  1. "Inverted soda bottle effect" theory – negative intracranial pressure created by CSF leak draws air into intracranial cavity with the air replacing the lost fluid volume due to a pressure gradient.[47]
  2. "Ball-valve" theory – extracranial air enters cranium through defect in dura, acting as one-direction valve by permitting air to enter but preventing air exit.[17]

- Due to conflicting reported experiences and sparse mechanism data in the available literature, no recommendation can be made either in support of or against the use of HBO_2 in the case of pneumocephalus.

ACTUAL CASE SAMPLES

1. A 70-year-old man with history of prostate cancer treated with radiation therapy now has hemorrhagic radiation cystitis and presents for evaluation for HBO_2 therapy. Being thorough with your history taking, you discover that he has COPD, which he says is under control with inhalers, but you see that he seems slightly short of breath when talking. Lung exam is equal, with equal expansion, clear auscultation, and good air movement. The medical records you requested for this initial consultation include a previous chest CT from one year ago with a report of minimal air trapping at the base of the right lung. The spirometry report from one year ago notes mild obstruction with responsiveness to bronchodilator. What would be an appropriate next step in your evaluation?

    a. Start the patient that day with HBO_2 therapy because he has gross hematuria and is at risk of severe anemia, as evidenced by his being short of breath when talking.
    b. Since he has a normal lung exam and had a PFT that showed only mild obstruction with responsiveness to bronchodilator, inform the patient he is not contraindicated for HBO_2 therapy and can be placed on the schedule starting next week.
    c. Order an inert gas ventilation scan and a new high-resolution chest CT.
    d. Inform the patient he is contraindicated for HBO_2 therapy because of the air trapping found on the chest CT from one year ago.

2. A 54-year-old woman with type 2 diabetes mellitus on insulin was admitted into the hospital to receive parenteral antibiotics for cellulitis. An inpatient consultation request was made for a Wagner Grade 3 ulcer on her right plantar foot for which treatment was begun during this current admission and for which the primary physician wants HBO_2 therapy started immediately while inpatient. During evaluation, the patient reports past medical history including childhood asthma, hypertension, and hypercholesterolemia and past surgical history including appendectomy, cholecystectomy, and squamous cell carcinoma (SCCA) removal. At the end of the exam, you discuss the risks and benefits with the patient and explain to her the mechanism of action of HBO_2 therapy and how it may affect people with asthma or any condition where there might be gas trapping. The patient now remembers to tell you that she had eye surgery two months ago and that a gas bubble was put into her eye for the procedure. You delve more into this, but she can tell you only that the surgery involved her retina and cannot remember what kind of gas was used. What would be the appropriate next step?

    a. Proceed with HBO_2 therapy as soon as possible since the patient is currently inpatient, has a Grade 3 Wagner wound, and the consulting surgeon is pushing for HBO_2 therapy.
    b. Inform the patient and the surgeon that the patient is contraindicated for HBO_2 therapy until the intraocular gas bubble has been proven to no longer be present.

c. Inform the patient and surgeon that the patient currently does not meet criteria for HBO_2 therapy since the ulcer has not been shown to be nonhealing and since conventional wound treatment has not been maximized. Recommend reevaluation in one month for HBO_2 therapy.
d. Consult the ophthalmologist who conducted the eye surgery and obtain a head CT with focus on the eyes.
e. B, C, and D are correct.

3. A 39-year-old woman with multiple sclerosis has been consulted for chronic refractory osteomyelitis that has been resistant to parenteral antibiotic treatment for 6 weeks. She has OD 20/200 and OS 20/100 visual acuity. She was diagnosed with optic neuritis at the same time that she was diagnosed with MS and has had three optic neuritis flares since then, but none in the last seven months. She meets criteria for and wants to proceed with HBO_2 therapy, with the understanding and acceptance of the risks involved. Which of the following is the best indicator for discontinuing HBO_2 therapy completely?

   a. The patient experiences a seizure during her first HBO_2 treatment.
   b. She is found to have TEED 4 otic barotrauma after her first HBO_2 treatment.
   c. She feels claustrophobic and requires an anxiolytic during her first HBO_2 treatment.
   d. She develops blurry vision after the 7th HBO_2 treatment with OD visual acuity change to 20/300 and OS to 20/200.
   e. She develops OU cataracts after the tenth treatment.

4. A 71-year-old man with osteoradionecrosis of the mandible has type 1 diabetes mellitus, CHF, 3-vessel coronary artery bypass graft (CABG), and glaucoma. Which of the following conditions would be a reason not to proceed forward with HBO_2 therapy?

   a. An ejection fraction of 25% with no history of decompensation
   b. An ejection fraction of 55% with multiple episodes of decompensation with the last one being 1 month ago
   c. Prior thoracic surgery with chest CT one year ago showing no acute lesions or abnormality
   d. Worsening glaucoma
   e. Diabetes with history of multiple hypoglycemic episodes

5. A 42-year-old woman with history of breast cancer treated with radiation therapy (XRT) has a nonhealing wound at the Port-a-Cath site that was placed in the subcutaneous tissue that was exposed to XRT. She is currently inpatient and has metastases. She has been consulted to hyperbaric medicine for the refractory wound on her chest wall. Initial consultation reveals the following past and current medications: doxorubicin stopped one week ago, disulfiram stopped three years ago, current tamoxifen, current Avastin, current Zosyn, current vancomycin, and current

paroxetine. Which of the following medications would contraindicate the patient for HBO_2 therapy?

a. Avastin
b. Tamoxifen
c. Doxorubicin
d. Disulfiram
e. None of the above

ANSWERS AND EXPLANATIONS

1. **C** This patient poses high risk of pulmonary barotrauma. The presence of the gas trapping one year ago does not necessarily mean it is currently present, but it could also have expanded in the interval. A high-resolution chest CT is warranted to evaluate for expansion and/or presence of other lesions that might require intervention. While a spirometry was done one year ago, pulmonary function may have worsened in the last year, and a ventilation scan would provide better information on how to adjust HBO_2 protocol to manage the pulmonary risk. However, the patient has not yet proven himself to have a current absolute contraindication.
2. **E** An intraocular gas bubble placed for vitreoretinal surgery is an absolute contraindication to HBO_2 therapy. It must be proven first that the gas bubble is no longer present before HBO_2 therapy can proceed. Though the patient does have a Wagner Grade 3 diabetic foot ulcer, she currently does not meet criteria, though she might have cause to worsen with the cellulitis. A case could be argued that HBO_2 therapy ought to be conducted rather than waiting for conventional wound care to be ineffective after one month first before starting HBO_2 therapy, but neither her inpatient status nor the pressure from another physician constitutes valid reason to begin HBO_2 therapy immediately.
3. **D** The other listed complications do not preclude further HBO_2 therapy, but with the obvious decline in vision that could progress towards blindness – even if the decline is actually a natural course of optic neuritis flare rather than HBO_2 exacerbation of flare – the risk is too high to continue.
4. **B** Clinical instability of CHF is a better predictor of decompensation by HBO_2 than the numerical value of the EJF.
5. **A** Avastin is antiangiogenic and would counter the mechanism of HBO_2 in inducing angiogenesis for soft-tissue radionecrosis.

REFERENCES

1. Ani CC, Ismaila BO. Tension pneumoventricle: a report of two cases. Nigerian J Clin Pract. 2016;19(4):559-62.
2. Baba M, Tarar O, Syed A. A rare case of spontaneous pneumocephalus associated with nontraumatic cerebrospinal fluid leak. Case Rep Neurol Med. 2016;ID1828461:3pp.
3. Berend N. The effect of bleomycin and oxygen on rat lung. Pathology. 1984;16:136-9.
4. Bradfield JJ, Kinsella JB, Mader JT, et al. Rapid progression of head and neck squamous carcinoma after hyperbaric oxygen. Otolaryngol Head Neck Surg. 1996;114:793.
5. Bromfield EB, Cavazos JE, Sirven JI, editors. An introduction to epilepsy [Internet]. West Hartford (CT): American Epilepsy Society; 2006. Available from: https://www.ncbi.nlm.nih.gov/books/NBK2510/pdf/Bookshelf_NBK2510.pdf
6. Brosh K, Strassman I, Seelenfreund M. High intraocular pressure in four vitrectomized eyes with intravitreal C3F8 without high altitude travel. Eye. 2014;28(7):892-4.
7. Butler FK, Hagan C, Murphy-Lavoie H. Hyperbaric oxygen and the eye. Undersea Hyperbar Med. 2008;35(5):327-81.
8. Cade IS, Dische S, Watson ER, et al. Hyperbaric oxygen and radiotherapy: a Medical Research Council trial in carcinoma of the bladder. Br J Radiol. 1978;51:876-8.
9. Cade IS, McEwen JB. Megavoltage radiotherapy in hyperbaric oxygen. Cancer. 1967;20:817-21.
10. Chadha TS, Cohn M. Noninvasive treatment of pneumothorax with oxygen inhalation. Respiration. 1983;44(2):147-52.
11. Chaika V. The immediate and long term results to development of children born by mother with hyperbaric oxygenation. In: Yefuni SN, editor. Proceeding of the 7th International Congress on Hyperbaric Medicine; 1981; Moscow. Moscow: Nauka; 1983. p. 364-7.
12. Choi Y-Y, Dong D-K, et al. Pneumocephalus in the absence of craniofacial skull base fracture. J Kor Neurotraumatol Soc. 2006;2(2):128-31.
13. Chong KT, Hampson NB, Bostwick DG, et al. Hyperbaric oxygen does not accelerate latent in vivo prostate cancer: implications for the treatment of radiation-induced haemorrhagic cystitis. BJU Internat, 2004;94:1275–8.
14. Clark J. Oxygen toxicity. In: Neumann T, Thom S, editors. Physiology and medicine of hyperbaric oxygen therapy. Philadelphia: Saunders; 2008. p. 527-63.
15. Currie GP, Alluri Ratna, et al. Pneumothorax: an update. Postgrad Med J. 2007 Jul;83(981):461-5.
16. Dabdoub CB, Salas G, et al. Review of the management of pneumocephalus. Surg Neurol Int. 2015;6:155.
17. Dandy WE. Pneumocephalus (intracranial pneumatocele or aerocele). Arch Surg. 1926;12(5):949-82.
18. Daruwalla J, Christophi C. Hyperbaric oxygen therapy for malignancy: a review. World J Surg. 2006;30:2112–31.
19. DelGaudio JM, Avani IP. Treatment of pneumocephalus after endoscopic sinus and microscopic skull base surgery. Am J Otolaryn. 2010;31(4):226-30.
20. Demling RH, DeSanti L. The use of moist wound healing with infection control in the burn wound [Internet]. Eplasty. Available from: http://www.eplasty.com/images/PDF/MoistWoundHealing.pdf

21. Deneke SM, Bernsetein SP, Fanburg BL. Enhancement by disulfiram (antabuse) of toxic effects of 95% to 97% O2 on rat lung. J Pharmacol Exp Ther. 1979;208(3):377-80.

22. Denham JW, Yeoh, Wittwer G, et al. Radiation therapy in hyperbaric oxygen for head and neck cancer at Royal Adelaide Hospital – 1964 to 1980. Internat J Radiat Onc Biol Phys. 1987;13(2):201-8.

23. Dexter F, Reasoner D. Theoretical assessment of normobaric oxygen therapy to treat pneumocephalus: recommendations for dose and duration of treatment. J Am Soc Anesthesiologists. 1996;84:442-7.

24. Di Lorenzo N, Caruso R, Floris R, et al. Pneumocephalus and tension pneumocephalus after posterior fossa surgery in the sitting position: a prospective study. Acta Neurochirurgica. 1986;83(3):112-5.

25. Dische S. Hyperbaric oxygen: the medical research council trials and their clinical significance. Br J Radiol. 1979;51(611):888-94.

26. Donat SM, Levy DA. Bleomycin associated pulmonary toxicity: is perioperative oxygen restriction necessary? J Urology. 1998;160(4):1347-52.

27. Dooley MC, Foroozan R. Optic neuritis. J Ophthalmic Vis Res. 2010;5(3):182-7.

28. Douglas MJ, Coppin CM. Bleomycin and subsequent anaesthesia: a retrospective study at Vancouver General Hospital. Canad Anaesth Soc J. 1980;27(5):449-52.

29. Duke University, Duke Center for Hyperbaric Medicine and Environmental Physiology. Durham, NC.

30. Elkharrat D, Raphael JC, Korach JM, et al. Acute carbon monoxide intoxication and hyperbaric oxygen in pregnancy. Intensive Care Med. 1991;17(5):289-92

31. Eltorai I, Hart GB, Strauss MB, et al. Does hyperbaric oxygen provoke an occult carcinoma in man? In: Kindwall EP, editor. Proceedings of the 8th International Congress on Hyperbaric Medicine. San Pedro (CA): Best Publishing Co.; 1987. p. 18-29.

31A. Ernawati DK, Stafford L, Hughes JD. Amiodarone-induced pulmonary toxicity. Br J Clin Pharmacol. 2008;66(1):82-7.

32. Ersanli D, Akin T, Yildiz S, et al. The effect of hyperaric oxygen on intraocular pressure. Undersea Hyperbar Med. 2006;33(1):1-4.

33. Feldmeier J, Carl U, et al. Hyperbaric oxygen: does it promote growth or recurrence of malignancy? Undersea Hyperbar Med. 2003;30(1):1-18.

34. Ferrini W, Pournaras JA, Wolfensberger TJ. Expansion of intraocular gas bubbles due to altitude: do meteorological factors play a role? Klin Monbl Augenheilkd. 2010;227(4):312–4.

35. Forman HJ, JLYork. Mechanism for the potentiation of oxygen toxicity by disulfiram. Pharmacol Exp Ther. 1980;212(3):452-5.

36. Foroozan R, Buono LM, Savino PJ, Sergott RC. Acute demyelinating optic neuritis. Curr Opin Ophthalmol. 2002;13:375.

37. Gallin-Cohen PF, Podos SM, Yablonski ME. Oxygen lowers intraocular pressure. Investig Ophthal Vis Sci. 1980;19:43-8.

38. Garcia Cabrera I, Milgram NS, Berge OG. Electroencephalographic and behavioral correlates of seizure development in rats in response to hyperbaric exposure. Epilepsy Res. 1990;7(1):65-71.

39. Goldiner PL, Carlon GC, Cvitkovic E, et al. Factors influencing postoperative morbidity and mortality in patients treated with bleomycin. BMJ. 1978;1(6128):1664-7.

40. Goldiner PL, Schweizer O. The hazards of anesthesia and surgery in bleomycin-treated patients. Semin Onc. 1979;6(1):121-4.

41. Gore PA, Maan H, Chang S. Normobaric oxygen therapy strategies in the treatment of postcraniotomy pneumocephalus. J Neurosurg. 2008 May;108(5):926-9.

42. Gray LH, Conger AD, Ebert M, Hornsey S, Scott OC. The concentration of oxygen dissolved in tissues at the time of irradiation as a factor in radiotherapy. Br J Radiol. 1953;26:638–48.

43. Hampson NB, Piantadosis CA, Thom SR, Weaver LK. Practice recommendations in the diagnosis, management, and prevention of carbon monoxide poisoning. Am J Resp Crit Care Med. 2012;186:1095-101.

44. Hartnett ME, Hane RH. Effects of oxygen on the development and severity of retinopathy of prematurity. J Am Assoc Pedi Ophthalmol Strabismus. 2013;17(3):229-34.

45. Henry M, Arnold T, Harvey J. BTS guidelines for the management of spontaneous pneumothorax. Thorax. 2003;58(Suppl II):ii39–52.

46. Hong B, Biertz F, Raab P, Scheinichen D, et al. Normobaric hyperoxia for treatment of pneumocephalus after posterior fossa surgery in the semisitting position: a prospective randomized controlled trial. PLoS ONE. 2015;10(5):e0125710. doi: 10.1371/journal.pone.0125710.

47. Horowitz M. Intracranial pneumocoele. An unusual complication following mastoid surgery. J Laryngol Otol. 1964;78:128-34.

48. Houston S, Graf J, Sharkey J. Commercial air travel after intra-ocular gas injection. Aviat Space Environ Med. 2012;83:809-10.

49. Huh J. Barotrauma-induced pneumocephalus experienced by a high risk patient after commercial air travel. J Korean Neurosurg Soc. 2013;54:142-4.

50. Ingrassia TS, Ryu JH, et al. Oxygen-exacerbated bleomycin pulmonary toxicity. Mayo Clinic Proc. 1991;66(2):173-8.

51. Intermountain Medical Center, Hyperbaric Medicine. Salt Lake City, UT.

52. Isenberg SJ, Diamant A. SCUBA diving after encucleation [letter]. Am J Ophthalmol. 1985;100:616-7.

53. Jackman SV, Thompsom JT. Effects of hyperbaric exposure on eyes with intraocular gas bubbles. Retina. 1995;15(2):160-6.

54. Jamieson DD, Kerr DR, Unsworth I. Interaction of N-acetylcysteine and bleomycin on hyperbaric oxygen-induced lung damage in mice. Lung. 1987;165:239–47.

55. Jamil A. Managing patients after retinal surgery. Rev Ophtho [Internet]. 2009. Available from: https://www.reviewofophthalmology.com/article/managing-patients-after-retinal-surgery

56. Johnson RJ, Lauchlan SC. Epidermoid carcinoma of the cervix treated by 60Co therapy and hyperbaric oxygen. In: Brown IW, Cox BG, editors. Proceedings of the 3rd International Congress on Hyperbaric Medicine. Washington (DC): National Academy of Sciences; 1966. p. 648-52.

57. Johnson RJ, Walton RJ. Sequential study on the effect of the addition of hyperbaric oxygen on the 5 year survival rates of carcinoma of the cervix treated with conventional fractional irradiations. Am J Roentgen. 174;120(1):111-7.

58. Karagoz B, Suleymanoglu S, Uzun G, et al. Hyperbaric oxygen therapy does not potentiate doxorubicin-induced cardiotoxicity in rats. Basic Clin Pharmacol Toxicol. 2008 Mar;102(3):287-92.

59. Khan K, Wegewitz D, Drone D. Implosion of an artificial eye during a scuba dive at 18 metres depth. Dtsche Z Sportmed. 2011;62(10):334-6.

60. Kindwall EP. Personal report. In: Kindwall EP, Whelan HT, editors. Hyperbaric medicine practice. 3rd ed. Flagstaff (AZ): Best Publishing Co.; 2008. p. 278.

61. Kindwall EP et al. Treatment of multiple sclerosis with hyperbaric oxygen: results of a national registry. Arch Neurol. 1991:195-9.

62. Lambrou GN, Kopferschmitt J, Jaeger A, Brini A. Slowly reversible central scotoma: iatrogenic effect of hyperbaric oxygenation in the treatment of multiple sclerosis. J Fr Ophtalmol. 1987;10(1):51-9.

63. Lee C-H, Chen W-C, et al. Tension pneumocephalus: a rare complication after hyperbaric oxygen therapy. Am J Emerg Med. 27(2):257.e1-e3

64. Lee LC, Lieu FK, Chen YH, et al. Tension pneumocephalus as a complication of hyperbaric oxygen therapy in a patient with chronic traumatic brain injury. Am J Phys Med Rehabil. 2012 Jun;91(6):528-32

65. Leong KM, Vijayananthan A, et al. Pneumocephalus: an uncommon finding in trauma. Med J Malaysia. 2008;63(3):256-8.

66. Luis M, Ayuso A, Martinez, et al. Intraoperative respiratory failure in a patient after treatment with bleomycin: previous and current intraoperative exposure to 50% oxygen. Eur J Anaesth. 1999;16(1):66-8.

67. Mahabir RC, Szymczak A, Sutherland GR. Intracerebral pneumatocele presenting after air travel. J Neurosurg. 2004;101(2):340-2.

68. Markham JW. The clinical features of pneumocephalus based upon a survey of 284 cases with report of 11 additional cases. Acta Neurochir (Wien). 1967;16:1–78.

69. Marx RE. Radiation injury to tissue. In: Kindwall EP, Whelan HT, editors. Hyperbaric medicine practice. 2nd ed. Flagstaff (AZ): Best Publishing Co.; 1999. p. 720.

70. Mathes DD. Bleomycin and hyperoxia exposure in the operating room. Int Anesth Research Soc. 1995;81(3):624-9

71. Mathieu D. Contraindications to hyperbaric oxygen therapy. In: Neumann T, Thom S, editors. Physiology and medicine of hyperbaric oxygen therapy. Philadelphia; Saunders: 2008. p. 587-98.

72. Moen I, Stuhr LE. Hyperbaric oxygen therapy and cancer – a review. Targ Oncol. 2012;7:233-42.

73. Mohamed S, Lai TY. Intraocular gas in vitreoretinal sugery. HKJOphthalmol. 14(1):8-13.

74. Molzhaninov E, Chaika V, Domanova A. Experience and prospects of using hyperbaric oxygenation in obstetrics. In: Yefuni SN, editor. Proceeding of the 7th International Congress on Hyperbaric Medicine; 1981; Moscow. Moscow: Nauka; 1983. p. 139-41.

75. Monstrey SJ, Mullick P, et al. Hyperbaric oxygen therapy and free radical production: an experimental study in doxorubicin (Adriamycin) extravasation injuries. Ann Plast Surg. 1997;38(2):163-8.

76. Moreo A, de Chiara B, Cataldo G, et al. Prognostic value of serial measurements of left ventricular function and exercise performance in chronic heart failure. Revista Espanola Cardiol. 2006;59(9):905-10.

77. Mylan Institutional. Sulfamylon – mafenide acetate cream drug information. Rockford(IL); 2013.

78. Nichols CW, Lambertsen CJ, Clark JM. Transient unilateral loss of vision associated with oxygen at high pressure. Arch Ophthal. 1969;81:548-52.

79. O'Sullivan JM, Huddart RA, Norman AR, et al. Predicting the risk of bleomycin lung toxicity in patients with germ-cell tumours. Anns of Onc. 2003;14:91–6.

80. Oguz MD, Sobaci G. The use of hypebaric oxygen therapy in ophthalmology. Survey Ophthal. 2008;53(2):112-20.

81. Orasmuradov AA, Paendi OL, Paendi FA. Modern possibilities of hyperbaric oxygen therapy in pregnant women with anemia. Internat J BioMed. 2014;4(2):82-4.

82. Overgaard J. Hypoxic modification of radiotherapy in squamous cell carcinoma of the head and neck – a systematic review and meta-analysis. Radiother Oncol. 2011;100:22–32.

83. Ozgurtas T, Tekin S, Yesildal F, et al. A novel model of retinopathy of prematurity in normobaric hyperoxic conditions. Int J Ophthalmol. 2016;9(0):1265-70.

84. Paiva WS, Andrade AF, Fegueiredo EG, et al. Effects of hyperbaric oxygenation therapy on symptomatic pneumocephalus. Ther Clin Risk Manag. 2014;10:769-73.

85. Patz A. The effect of oxygen on immature retinal vessels. Invest Ophthalmol. 1965;4:988-99.

86. Payne WG, Naidu DK, Wheeler CK, et al. Wound healing in patients with cancer. Eplasty. 2008;8:68-90.

87. Pfizer Canada Inc. Cordarone (amiodarone HCl) product monograph. Quebec; 2016. p. 1-75.

88. Pillai P, Sharma R, MacKenzie L, et al. Traumatic tension pneumocephalus – two cases and comprehensive review of literature. Internat J Critical Illness Injury Sci. 2017;7(1)58-64.

89. Plant GT. Optic neuritis and multiple sclerosis. Curr Opin Neurol. 2008;21(1):16-21.

90. Rao V, Fredriksli O, Gulati S. Post-traumatic epidural tension pneumocephalus: a case report. J Med Case Reports. 2015;9:151.

91. Reasoner DK, Todd MM, Scumman FL, Warner DS. The incidence of pneumocephalus after supratentorial craniotomy: observations on the disappearance of intracranial air. Anesthesiology. 1994;80:1008-12.

92. Register SD, Aaron ME, Gelly HB. Hyperbaric oxygen therapy and optic neuritis: case report and literature review. Undersea Hyperb Med. 2011 Nov-Dec;38(6):557-9.

93. Reynolds JD. The management of retinopathy of prematurity. Paediatr Drugs. 2001;3:263–72

94. Serrano-Mollar A, Closa D, Prats N. In vivo antioxidant treatment protects against bleomycin-induced lung damage in rats. Br J Pharmacol. 2003;138,1037-48.

95. Shi Y, Lee CS, Wu J, et al. Effects of hyperbaric oxygen exposure on experimental head and neck tumor growth oxygenation, and vasculature. Head Neck. 2005;27(5):362-9.

96. Shupak A, Gilbey P. Effects of pressure. In: Neumann T, Thom S, editors. Physiology and medicine of hyperbaric oxygen therapy. Philadelphia: Saunders; 2008. p. 513-26.

97. Silverman RK, Montano J. Hyperbaric oxygen treatment during pregnancy in acute carbon monoxide poisoning. A case report. J Reprod Med. 1997;42(5):309-11.

98. Simpson AB, Paul J, et al. Fatal bleomycin pulmonary toxicity in the west of Scotland 1991-95: a review of patients with germ cell tumours. Br J Cancer. 1998;78(8):1061-6.

99. Staley K. Molecular mechanisms of epilepsy. Nat Neurosci. 2015;18(3):367-72.

100. Sweni S, Senthilkumaran S, et al. Tension pneumocephalus: a case report with review of literature. Emerg Radiol. 2013;20(6):573-8.

101. Taylor LH. Diving physics. In: Bove A, editor. Bove and Davis' diving medicine. Philadelphia: Saunders; 2004. p. 11-35.

102. Teczan O, Karahan O, Alan M, et al. Hyperbaric oxygen preconditioning provides preliminary protection against doxorubicin cardiotoxicity. Acta Cardiol Sin. 2017;33:150-5.

103. Terry TL. Extreme prematurity and fibroblastic overgrowth of persistent vascular sheath behind each crystalline lens: a preliminary report. Am J Ophthalmol. 1942;25:203.

104. Thom SR. Oxidative stress is fundamental to hyperbaric oxygen therapy. J Appl Physiol. 2009;106:988-95.

105. Torp KD, Carraway MS, Ott MC, et al. Safe administration of hyperbaric oxygen after bleomycin: a case series of 15 patients. Undersea Hyperb Med. 2012 Sep-Oct;39(5):873-9.

106. Tran P, Reed E, Hahn F, et al. Incidence, radiographical features, and proposed mechanism for pneumocephalus from intravenous injection of air. West J Emerg Med. 2010 May;11(2):180-5.

107. UDL Laboratories. Sulfamylon (mafenide aetate) drug information.

108. University of Pennsylvania, Undersea and Hyperbaric Medicine. Philadelphia, PA.

109. Upton PG, Yamaguchi KT, Myers S, et al. Effects of antioxidants and hyperbaric oxygen in ameliorating experimental doxorubicin skin toxicity in the rat. Cancer Treat Rep. 1986;70:503-7.

110. Van de Veire S, Germonpre P, Renier C, et al. Influences of atmospheric pressure and temperature in intraocular pressure. Investig Ophthal Vis Sci. 2008;49(12):5392-6.

111. Van Hoesen K, Camporesi E, Moon R, et al. Should hyperbaric oxygen be used to treat the pregnant patient for acute carbon monoxide poisoning? A case report and literature review. JAMA. 1989;261:1039-43.

112. van Hulst RA, Rietbroek RC, et al. To dive or not to dive with bleomycin: a practical algorithm. Aviat Space Environ Med. 2011 Aug;82(8):814-8.

113. Vion-Dury J, LeGal La Salle G, et al. Effects of hyperbaric and hyperoxic conditions on amygdala-kindled seizures in rat. Exp Neurol. 1986:92(3):513-2.

114. Watson ER, Halnan KE, Dische S, et al. Hyperbaric oxygen and radiotherapy: a Medical Research Council trial in carcinoma of the cervix. Br J Radiol. 1978;51:879-87.

115. Weinreb RN, Aung T, Medeiros FA. The pathophysiology and treatment of glaucoma: a review. JAMA. 2014;311(18):1901–11.

115A. Wolkove N, Baltzan M. Amiodarone pulmonary toxicity. Can Respir J. 2009;16(2):43-8.

116. Wuethrich PY, Burkhard PY. No perioperative pulmonary complications after restricted oxygen exposition in bleomycin-treated patients: a short report. ISRN Anesthesology. 2011;2011(art ID 143189):1-3.

117. Yates H, Hamill M, Borel CO, Toung TJ. Incidence and perioperative management of tension pneumocephalus following craniofacial resection. J Neurosurg Anesthesiol. 1994;6(1):15–20.

118. Yin J-H, Chuang Y-J, Hu H-H. Pneumocephalus associated with massive cerebral air embolism. Acta Neurol Taiwan. 2013;22:93-4.

119. Zasler ND. Posttraumatic tension pneumocephalus. J Head Trauma Rehabil. 1999;14:81-4.

120. Zeba I, Barkovic I, Knezevic S, et al. Pneumocephalus after an uneventful scuba dive. Aviat Space Environ Med. 2010;81:511-3.

CHAPTER 10 CHAPTER

Side Effects and Complications: Selected Overview and Brief Guide to Management

CHAPTER TEN OVERVIEW

Introduction **201**
Otic Barotrauma **201**
Middle-Ear Barotrauma **202**
Anatomy 202
Pathophysiology 203
Clinical Presentation 204
Management 205
Inner-Ear Barotrauma **207**
External-Ear Barotrauma **207**
Paranasal Sinus Barotrauma (Barosinusitis) **207**
Anatomy 207
Clinical Presentation 208
Management 209
Barodontalgia **209**
Anatomy 209
Clinical Presentation 210
Pathophysiology 210
Management 211
Visual Changes **211**
Myopia/Cataracts 211
Seizures **212**
Pulmonary Barotrauma **213**
Pneumothorax 213
References **217**

Side Effects and Complications: Selected Overview and Brief Guide to Management

Phi-Nga Jeannie Le, John B. Slade Jr., Jason A. Kelly, E. George Wolf

INTRODUCTION

One hundred percent oxygen, whether normobaric or hyperbaric, is a drug and, as with any drug, there are known side effects. What is unique to this drug is that it is delivered to a patient inside a sealed chamber under increasing pressure for the purpose of amplifying the drug concentration in order to achieve certain physiological responses that could not otherwise be attained at regular surface atmosphere. The addition of pressurization by a chamber introduces other known effects to the treatment, which adds complexity to the benefit-risk analysis that a physician must do for every patient, every treatment, every day. This does not make the hyperbaric oxygen (HBO_2) therapy any less acceptable or less valuable than, for instance, a chemotherapy drug with known side effects and known complications. When an oncologist has made the benefit-risk analysis that the adjunctive use of temozolomide to treat brainstem glioma is worth the known common side effect of nausea/vomiting and the known uncommon reactions of seizures and hepatotoxicity, the actual appearance of these side effects and complications are not surprising and would not be considered adverse events since they are expected to possibly take place. Similarly, hyperbaric oxygen therapy has known effects from the common otic barotrauma to the very rare pulmonary barotrauma. Common side effects and uncommon complications are anticipated to potentially occur during the course of hyperbaric oxygen therapy, for which awareness, surveillance, preparation, and intervention should be maintained and provided in response.

OTIC BAROTRAUMA

Otic barotrauma, in varying degrees of presentation, is the most common side effect of HBO_2 treatment. It can manifest in any part of the otic structures, from the external to the middle to the inner ear, with side effects ranging from the most minor otalgia to the more serious but very rare loss of hearing.

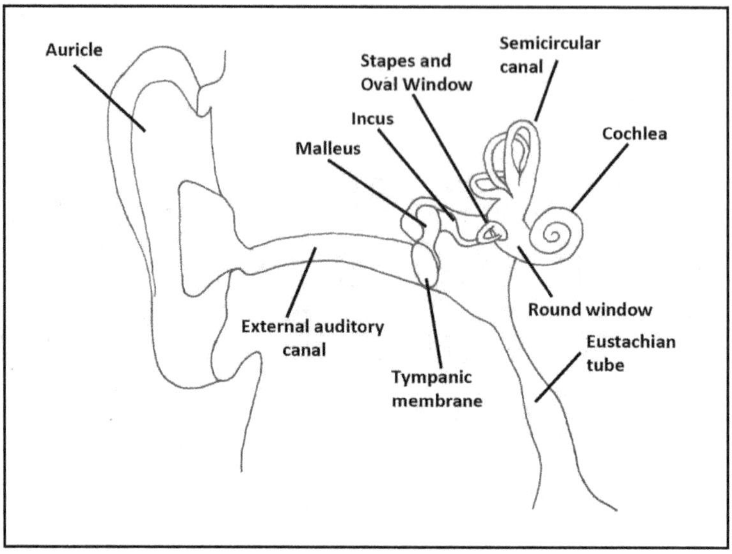

Figure 1.

MIDDLE-EAR BAROTRAUMA

Middle-ear barotrauma, often referred to historically as barotitis media, is frequently cited as the most common medical side effect of both hyperbaric oxygen therapy and underwater diving. In 1999, Fitzpatrick et al. performed a retrospective analysis showing 35 of 111 patients (32%) at the U.S. Army Lyster Army Community Hospital hyperbaric facility reported symptoms of barotrauma in the ear or sinuses throughout their treatment course.[23] Fifty-one percent of these experienced symptoms only during their first treatment session. In the same year, Zwart reported a lower incidence of 2%–6% in patients treated at the U.S. Air Force Davis Hyperbaric Laboratory.[58] In older reports, middle-ear symptoms have been reported in as high as 82% of patients.[13,18] In 2007, Beard et al. presented data showing a 0.75%–0.89% rate of ear barotrauma per patient treatment in a review of over 90,000 hyperbaric treatments.[4] Recent unpublished data from the David Grant U.S. Air Force Medical Center show an overall rate of 1.3% out of 2995 patient treatments with only 0.2% of treatments being aborted for ear pain.

Anatomy

The human ear is a fascinating organ that collects external sound waves and then conducts and converts them into electrochemical signals that allow interpretation within the central nervous system. This complex sensory organ consists of three distinct areas: the external, middle, and inner portions.

The external ear is comprised of the auricle and the external auditory canal. Their function is to capture sound so that it may be carried to the middle ear. The external auditory canal is a space formed by bone and cartilage and covered by epithelium that is continuous with the tympanic membrane. Cerumen is a waxy, slightly acidic substance produced by sebaceous and apocrine sweat glands within the outer cartilaginous canal that serves to clean and lubricate the canal and restrict microbial growth.

The middle ear is an air-filled cavity that begins with the tympanic membrane laterally and ends at the round and oval windows medially. It contains three bony structures: the malleus, incus, and stapes. The tympanic membrane is a semitransparent membrane that transmits sound waves to the bony structures of the middle ear. As the middle ear is typically air-filled, it is particularly vulnerable to changes in pressure, and its only direct communication with ambient pressure is through the eustachian tube.

The inner ear conducts sound to the central nervous system and provides input regarding balance and spatial orientation. The inner ear consists of membranous structures – the cochlea, the vestibule, and the semicircular canals – which contain endolymph and are surrounded by perilymph. Acoustic energy conducted through the oval window enters the cochlea, resulting in an electrical charge which is transmitted to the central nervous system via the cochlear nerve. The three semicircular canals are positioned to detect angular acceleration and transmit this information by the vestibular nerve.

As mentioned, the eustachian tube serves as the direct connection between the middle-ear space and the nasopharynx, allowing equalization of pressure and drainage of middle-ear secretions. This tube is approximately 36 mm long in adults and consists of a lateral bony portion and a medial cartilaginous portion which opens near the inferior turbinate in the fossa of Rosenmueller. The eustachian tube has a slit-like opening which is positioned in a manner best suited to allow escape of secretions and air into the nasopharynx. Four muscles aid in voluntary opening of the tube and are typically activated during swallowing.

Pathophysiology

Barotrauma, or "squeeze" of a body tissue such as the middle ear, is a result of a pressure difference between the particular body cavity and the surrounding space. The pressure of that surrounding space can vary significantly from low ambient air pressure at high altitudes to increased hydrostatic pressure at depth. The U.S. Navy Diving Manual Revision 7[(49)] references four criteria that must be met for a body cavity to be susceptible to barotrauma: A gas-filled space must be present. That space must have rigid walls so that collapse of the space cannot occur. The space must be enclosed so that gas or liquid cannot freely enter the space to allow pressure equalization. The space must have a membrane with arterial supply and venous drainage. A fifth factor necessary for barotrauma to occur in a space meeting these criteria is that there must be a change in ambient pressure.

During pressurization of the hyperbaric chamber, pressure within the middle-ear cavity remains constant, becoming relatively negative as compared to ambient pressure. For example, during a compression that begins at a surface pressure of 760 mmHg, the middle-ear pressure begins in equilibrium with ambient pressure at 760 mmHg. Upon compression to 3 fsw, the ambient pressure increases to 829 mmHg. The external auditory canal and nasopharynx, as open spaces, are at ambient pressure, and a pressure difference of 69 mmHg exists between the middle ear and its surroundings. This results in deflection of the tympanic membrane and the round and oval windows into the middle ear. At a differential of around 60 mmHg, a pressure sensation and pain can be detected by the patient. As the differential increases to around 90 mmHg, it becomes impossible to equalize pressure within the middle ear through techniques that will be discussed later. This situation has often been referred to as a "locked ear." These pressure differences represent a depth of only 2–4 fsw. As the pressure differential continues to increase, stress is placed on the tympanic membrane and the vascular lining of the middle ear, resulting in leakage from and rupture of the blood vessels. With continued pressurization, the tympanic membrane may tear, which allows equalization of pressure with the surrounding environment. Alternatively, the middle ear may fill with blood, also allowing equalization of pressure. Rupture of the tympanic membrane has been demonstrated to occur anywhere between 100 and 500 mmHg (4–21 fsw).[2,33,35]

Middle-ear barotrauma can also occur during depressurization, on ascent of the chamber. This is often referred to as a "reverse squeeze." As ambient pressure increases, the pressure within the middle ear is relatively positive. This creates a force deflecting the tympanic membrane outwards and creates pressure against the opening of the eustachian tube. During normal function, the eustachian tube opens passively as a result of the pressure differential, allowing equalization and a "popping" sensation in the ear before a painful sensation can develop. However, edema and secretions may obstruct the eustachian tube, preventing this passive opening. This is often seen in the case of a patient who has difficulty with equalization during initial pressurization that results in damage to the middle-ear lining and tympanic membrane, allowing buildup of fluid and edema during the course of the hyperbaric treatment. This can produce a unique challenge as attempts at necessary depressurization may continue to worsen the problem.

Clinical Presentation

Symptoms of middle-ear barotrauma are readily recognizable. A sensation of pressure and pain initially develops. This is often accompanied by a mild decrease in hearing in the affected ear that is conductive in nature. As the pressure differential increases, the severity of symptoms increases as well. In some cases, vertigo or tinnitus may occur. This vertigo has been demonstrated to occur specifically in the situation where one ear equalizes and the other does not, resulting in unequal pressures within the vestibular system. This condition is known as "alternobaric vertigo" and can be quite distressing for a patient who is already trying to manage worsening ear pain. The pain peaks at the point of rupture of the tympanic membrane. Otoscopic findings can be seen fairly quickly after the onset of injury and may progress over the following minutes to hours. In 1944, Wallace Teed developed a scale for describing the clinical appearance and severity of injury from otic barotrauma.

TEED 0 is a normal tympanic membrane without evidence of injury despite the presence of symptoms.

TEED 1 is defined by erythema over part of the tympanic membrane as a result of inflammation. This may be particularly noted around the handle of the malleus.

TEED 2 involves erythema of the entire tympanic membrane.

TEED 3 involves hemorrhage into the membrane that appears as darker red patches.

TEED 4 is represented by frank hemorrhage into the middle-ear space. This may include drainage of blood through the eustachian tube into the nasopharynx.

TEED 5 includes any of the previous findings along with perforation of the tympanic membrane and may involve hemorrhage into the external auditory canal.

Other staging systems have been developed and are in use as well. As these staging methods may involve some variability in interpretation among health-care providers, the most appropriate method for communicating the level of tympanic membrane trauma is to simply describe the otoscopic findings.

Management

Prevention of middle-ear barotrauma is clearly the best management technique. Prevention involves appropriate patient instruction, evaluation of risk factors, and rapid recognition of patients who experience difficulty with middle-ear pressure equalization. The most common risk factors for middle-ear barotrauma include conditions which adversely impact proper function of the eustachian tube. This may include acute or chronic rhinitis from an upper respiratory infection or from allergic rhinitis. Trauma to the area may negatively affect pressure equalization and fluid drainage, whether it be from surgical procedures or radiation. Fiesseler et al. compiled retrospective data showing that 15% of all patients in 1 facility required tympanostomy tubes prior to or after the start of hyperbaric oxygen therapy, while 29% of patients with a history of head/neck radiation required such treatment.(22) A history of difficulty with equalization during prior activities such as flying or SCUBA diving may indicate subsequent difficulty during hyperbaric treatments. During the previously mentioned retrospective analysis, Fitzpatrick noted that higher rates of symptomatic barotrauma were reported in females and in patients under age 40.(23) Conversely, a 1-year survey of 2,690 hyperbaric patients by Corigliano uncovered no trends in patient histories correlating with an increased risk for otic barotrauma.(15) Multiple evaluations have indicated that greater speed of compression increases the likelihood of middle-ear barotrauma.(23,40)

It is likely that many patients experience middle-ear barotrauma during their initial hyperbaric treatment, not due to underlying dysfunction, but due to lack of experience in techniques for pressure equalization. Prior to initiation of treatment, it is essential that the patient be instructed on pressure equalization. Patients should be advised to actively equalize middle-ear pressure every 1–2 fsw, prior to the development of pressure or pain. Once pain has developed, staff must be notified, and chamber pressurization should cease to avoid further damage to the middle ear. There are many techniques that patients may use for equalization, and there appears to be no strong consensus regarding which techniques are most effective. Many patients may demonstrate pressure equalization simply by opening the jaw widely (yawning) or swallowing. The yawning maneuver may be modified by moving the jaw forward as well as down. Patients should be provided with liquids to aid in swallowing. Others may be able to contract the muscles of the soft palate and nasopharynx without swallowing or moving the jaw. The Toynbee maneuver is quite simple and easy for all patients to understand and demonstrate but may have limited effectiveness. With this technique, the patient simply closes the mouth and nose and swallows, resulting in a brief initial increase in nasopharyngeal pressure. The Valsalva maneuver is performed by forcefully blowing (or increasing intrathoracic pressure) against a closed nose and mouth with the modification of maintaining an open glottis. While frequently taught and used, the Valsalva maneuver is less favorable due to the risk of increased intracranial pressure that is transmitted through the inner ear, resulting in round-window rupture. Finally, the Frenzel maneuver is performed by elevating the floor of the mouth and tongue while the nose, mouth, and glottis are closed thereby increasing nasopharyngeal pressure. This maneuver is both effective and safe. Tilting the head to place the affected ear in an up position may provide added benefit by stretching the involved muscles and eustachian tube opening. Patients should be advised to perform these maneuvers only during compression or when the chamber is not moving. Maneuvers should not be performed during decompression due to the risk of overpressurization of the inner- and middle-ear spaces.

During both compression and decompression, hyperbaric staff must be attentive to difficulties that patients may have with equalization. In the event that a patient is unable to equalize middle-ear pressure, chamber movement should immediately cease. Care must be taken to ensure the chamber pressure remains constant during equalization attempts. If a "locked ear" occurs, chamber pressure may be decreased by 2–3 fsw to allow equalization. If barotrauma occurs during depressurization, then pressure may be increased by the same magnitude to alleviate symptoms. If a patient demonstrates repetitive difficulty with equalization of pressure, then compression or decompression rate may be slowed. Caution should be taken in aggressively attempting to reach full pressurization for a patient who is experiencing difficulty. Damage to the middle-ear and eustachian-tube vasculature during pressurization may result in edema and fluid buildup that results in further difficulty with equalization on subsequent ascent. In emergency situations where timely continuation of the hyperbaric treatment is essential, bedside or in-chamber myringotomy may be performed.

For patients who are unsuccessful or who have repetitive difficulty in equalizing middle-ear pressure, or in those where significant difficulty is anticipated, pressure equalization tubes may be placed prophylactically. Alternatively, pharmacological therapy may be initiated prior to hyperbaric treatment. Patients with acute conditions affecting pressure equalization may simply have elective hyperbaric treatments delayed until symptom resolution. Those patients with subacute or chronic conditions such as allergic rhinitis should have maximal symptom reduction through standard therapies prior to initiation of hyperbaric treatment. Topical decongestants such as oxymetazoline hydrochloride are used frequently for prophylaxis and treatment of acute middle-ear barotrauma with good anecdotal results. However, in 1992, Carlson evaluated 60 hyperbaric patients who were randomized to oxymetazoline or sterile water spray prophylaxis and found no difference in ear pain, TEED scores, hearing loss, or tinnitus and concluded that topical decongestants may not be effective in preventing barotrauma.[(13)] In the same year, Brown randomized 120 SCUBA divers to an oral decongestant (pseudoephedrine) or placebo 30 minutes prior to diving. Symptomatic ear discomfort or blockage was noted in 8% of the pseudoephedrine group as compared to 32% of the placebo group. A TEED score of greater than 1 was observed in 22% of the pseudoephedrine group and 46% of the placebo group.[(8)] This data would indicate that prophylactic pseudoephedrine may be more effective than oxymetazoline for prophylactic therapy although no direct comparison studies have been performed. Caution must be used with these medications in patients where contraindications may exist. Prophylactic treatment with an intranasal corticosteroid spray may also be considered. These medications have an onset of action of a few hours but may take several days for maximal effect.

Once middle-ear barotrauma has occurred in non-emergent cases, continuation of hyperbaric therapy is determined by the severity of tympanic-membrane and middle-ear trauma and the subsequent therapy initiated. In patients who receive pressure equalization tubes, treatment may commence immediately. In patients with tympanic membrane perforation, treatment should not resume until complete healing of the tympanic membrane occurs, or pressure equalization tubes are placed. For all other patients, there is no clear timeframe for resumption of treatment. The patient should be able to demonstrate the ability to successfully perform pressure equalization techniques at surface level. The presence of blood or edema within the middle ear or eustachian tube may predispose the patient to further difficulty with equalization, so it would be prudent to allow any visible hemorrhage to resolve prior to resuming treatment.

INNER-EAR BAROTRAUMA

Inner-ear barotrauma is an infrequent, but more serious, result of differential pressures within the ear. The round and oval windows represent areas of susceptibility to pressure within the fluid-filled inner ear. The footplate of the stapes displaces the oval window as sound energy is conducted to the cochlea. Flexibility of the round window allows movement of endolymph within the cochlea as the oval window is displaced. Rupture of the round or oval window occurs at greater pressures than that required for tympanic membrane rupture. Research done in cats by Harker et al. has shown round window rupture occurring when cerebrospinal fluid (CSF) pressure reached 120 to 300 mmHg.[29] Kringlebotn demonstrated in cadaver cattle that the round window ruptured at 1,520 mmHg, with tympanic membrane rupture at approximately 300 mmHg, roughly the same as in humans.[35]

Inner-ear barotrauma may occur from increased hydrostatic pressure within the inner ear relative to middle-ear pressure or from increased middle-ear pressure relative to the inner-ear hydrostatic pressure. Unsuccessful, vigorous Valsalva attempts can increase intracranial and CSF pressure which displaces the round window outwards and may result in rupture. Alternatively, increased middle-ear pressure from forceful Valsalva or overpressurization on ascent may displace the round or oval window inward, resulting in rupture. Due to the relative weakness of the tympanic membrane as compared to the round and oval windows, this mechanism would appear to be unlikely to occur.

Rupture of the round or oval window typically results in sudden onset of vertigo, tinnitus, and loss of hearing. These symptoms are generally more profound than those noted with middle-ear barotrauma. Suspicion of inner-ear barotrauma should result in prompt consultation with an otolaryngologist. Treatment consists of avoidance of any maneuvers that increase intracranial pressure such as straining, coughing, or Valsalva. Bed rest with elevation of the head is recommended. Surgical intervention may be required. Eventual return to hyperbaric therapy should be considered only following close coordination with the otolaryngologist. Placement of pressure equalization tubes may be used to avoid the need for future pressure equalization maneuvers.

EXTERNAL-EAR BAROTRAUMA

The external auditory canal is readily exposed to ambient pressure and is subject to barotrauma only if obstructed, thereby creating an enclosed space. This is quite uncommon in the hyperbaric environment. Potential causes of obstruction include cerumen impaction, use of earplugs, and severe edema from otitis externa. This can result in edema of or hemorrhage into the external auditory canal or trauma to the tympanic membrane. As with other forms of otic barotrauma, prevention is paramount. The use of nonvented earplugs should be forbidden, particularly during compression or decompression. In patients known to produce large amounts of cerumen, the ears should be periodically examined, and patients should be screened frequently for any otic symptoms.

PARANASAL SINUS BAROTRAUMA (BAROSINUSITIS)

Anatomy

The paranasal sinuses consist of four sets of air-filled spaces located within the skull and facial bones. These include the frontal, maxillary, sphenoid, and ethmoid sinuses. They function in air humidification, speech resonation, protection of underlying structures,

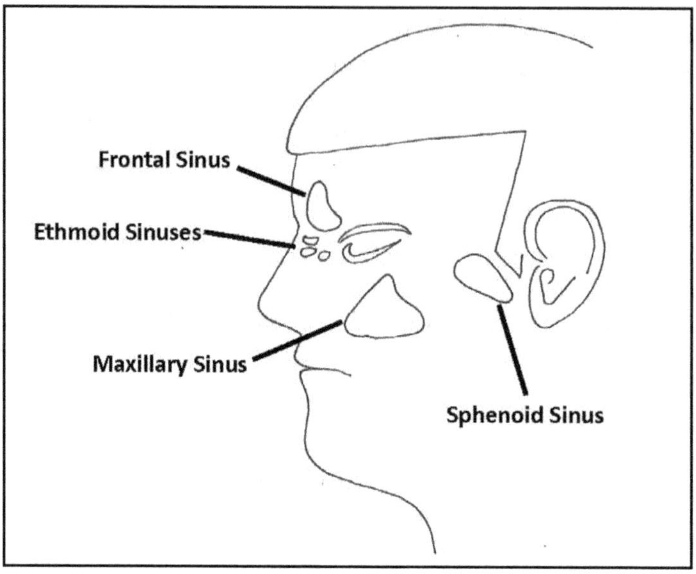

Figure 2.

and decreasing the weight of the anterior skull. The sinuses open to the nasal cavity through small ostia. The frontal sinus is located superior to the eyes, and it has the longest and narrowest duct. The large maxillary sinus sits inferior to the eyes and above the maxillary molar teeth. It contains the infraorbital nerve superiorly, which provides sensory innervation to the soft tissues of the cheek. The sphenoid sinus is variable in size and originates from the sphenoid bone, centrally in the skull. The ethmoid sinuses consist of several pyramid-shaped cells between the eyes.

Clinical Presentation

In their normal state, the ostia of the sinuses are open, allowing continuous equalization with ambient pressure. In a diseased state, these ostia may become closed or obstructed. During acute or chronic nasal inflammatory conditions, the sinus lining is edematous, and the cavities may fill with mucous. Nasal or sinus polyps can develop with chronic inflammatory conditions such as allergic rhinitis or recurrent infections.

During hyperbaric compression, if the ostia is obstructed due to an external polyp or edema, the sinus cavity will experience a negative pressure relative to the nasal cavity. This is often referred to as a "sinus squeeze." This creates a vacuum effect on the mucosal lining and results in pain, edema, fluid secretion, and bleeding. During decompression, the ostia may become obstructed by edema, mucous, or an internal sinus polyp, resulting in a relative overpressurization of the sinus and similar symptoms.

Although not always reliable, the location of pain can provide an indication of the diagnosis and specific sinus cavity involved. Frontal sinus pain is the most common and is typically quite severe, located in the area of this sinus above the eyes. In 1975, Fagan et al. reported that 68% of cases of sinus barotrauma in 50 Royal Australian Navy divers occurred in the frontal sinuses.[21] Maxillary sinus pain may be located over the face in the region of the sinus but may also be felt in the maxillary teeth. Sphenoid sinus pain may be felt in the occiput or vertex of the skull, and ethmoid sinus pain occurs between the eyes and may be accompanied by ocular symptoms.

Because of the important neurovascular structures housed around the paranasal sinuses, other symptoms and deficits may develop as a result of sinus barotrauma. Multiple reported cases exist of facial numbness following maxillary sinus barotrauma. Butler and Bove reported on a case of maxillary sinus barotrauma in a SCUBA diver that resulted in decreased sensation over the cutaneous distribution of the infraorbital nerve.[9] Neuman et al. also reported on a case of maxillary sinus barotrauma in a SCUBA diver resulting in numbness of the upper lip, teeth, and side of the face as a result of cranial nerve involvement.[42] Reports of sinus barotrauma during hyperbaric treatments are scarce in the medical literature.

Management

The management of sinus barotrauma is similar to that of otic barotrauma. Primary management involves prevention through patient evaluation and education. Although not specifically researched in this setting, topical and systemic decongestants and nasal corticosteroids may provide some benefit in prevention. In known nasal and sinus disease, to include the presence of polyps, maximal therapy by an otolaryngologist or allergist is warranted prior to initiation of hyperbaric treatments if able. As no invasive procedure is available to relieve sinus barotrauma pain while in the hyperbaric chamber, the use of nasal decongestants and slow decompression are the only emergency treatment options. If symptoms of sinus barotrauma develop during compression, then the treatment session should be aborted to avoid the potential of more problematic barotrauma upon subsequent decompression. A return to hyperbaric treatment should not be attempted until symptoms have resolved, and the underlying disease process has been appropriately treated.

BARODONTALGIA

Anatomy

Barodontalgia, previously referred to as aerodontalgia, is an oral pain condition resulting from changes in barometric pressure. In order to understand the potential causes of barodontalgia, a basic comprehension of tooth structure and disease is necessary. The tooth consists of three distinct regions: the crown, neck, and root. The visible crown consists of mineralized enamel, the hard, white outer layer of the tooth. Once the tooth is fully developed, there is no process for enamel regeneration. Beneath the enamel and surrounding the pulp is the dentin, which has thousands of fluid-filled tubules per square millimeter. Dentinal tubules communicate directly with pulpal nociceptors. Flow of fluid within these tubules, as occurs with thermal assault and other stimuli, may result in depolarization of nociceptors in the pulp. The dentin and the pulp are located within the crown as well as in root regions where the tooth is surrounded by alveolar bone and gingival tissue. The neurovascular structures exit the pulp at the root end and extend into the underlying maxilla or mandible. Dental caries occurs when bacterial metabolism of sugar results in acid production which demineralizes enamel and dentin. When the rate of demineralization is greater than the rate of remineralization, cavitation of tooth structure and further bacterial colonization occurs. Repair or restoration of dental caries involves the removal of carious tooth structure and replacement with various restorative products. Pulpitis is inflammation that occurs when trauma, tooth fracture, or dental caries approach the pulp, leading initially to inflammation and eventual pulp necrosis and infection. In more extensive disease involving the pulp, endodontic therapy such as root canal therapy is indicated.

This involves removal of all carious tooth structure along with the diseased pulp and its neurovascular structures, followed by root filling and coronal restoration.

Clinical Presentation

Barodontalgia, as its name implies, involves pain in the teeth with a change in barometric pressure. The pain may be sharp and localized or dull and generalized. The majority of cases described in the literature involve changes in pressure experienced during aviation and have occurred during ascent. In a study involving French Armed Forces diving personnel, 7.3% of divers experienced at least 1 episode of barodontalgia. A number of cases (62.2%) were noted to be in the maxillary teeth, and 77.3% of episodes were experienced upon descent.(26) Clinical findings by hyperbaric personnel may be limited and nonspecific but may include sensitivity of specific teeth to air flow, liquids of various temperatures, and percussion. Careful evaluation to differentiate maxillary sinus barotrauma from barodontalgia is warranted.

Pathophysiology

Historically, the hyperbaric, diving, and aerospace medicine literature has focused on trapped gas as the cause of barodontalgia. It has been hypothesized that, following dental restoration procedures, a small amount of air may become trapped between the filling material and the underlying tooth structure. During compression, this air reduces in volume, creating an implosive force on the surrounding structures. On subsequent decompression, the air increases in volume, creating an expansive force on the tooth and filling material. In the aviation environment, the air expansion occurs initially and has been attributed to numerous anecdotal reports of tooth fracture or lost fillings. Unfortunately, this method of barodontalgia remains yet unproven. Data published in 1945 by Devoe and Motley and unpublished data by Kollman revealed no occurrences of barodontalgia upon ascent to altitude when air was intentionally introduced beneath restorative fillings.(20,34)

Dental literature includes several other explanations for barodontalgia. While much of the focus has been on hypobaric exposure at altitude in the aviation environment, the pathophysiology remains applicable in the hyperbaric environment. All proposed mechanisms of action involve pulp inflammation, or pulpitis. In his excellent summary of prior research, Zadik cites six suggestions that explain the pathogenesis of barodontalgia:(57)

1. Direct ischemia resulting from pulp inflammation
2. Indirect ischemia resulting from intrapulpal increased pressure as a result of the vasodilatation and fluid diffusion
3. The result of intrapulpal gas expansion
4. The result of gas leakage through the vessels because of barometric-related reduced gas solubility
5. Hyperemia in the pulp canal system caused by decompression
6. Changes in barometric pressure in the case of a defective restoration may cause dentinal tubule fluid flow which leads to depolarization of communicating pulpal nociceptors

Assault to the pulp through carious processes and subsequent restorative treatment may result in reversible or irreversible pulpitis. From 1986–1990, Kollman reviewed 11,617 simulated altitude flights in a hypobaric chamber.(34) Twenty-eight simulated flights (0.26%) resulted in the subject having dental pain. Each subject was evaluated, and those with prior dental restorations (23/28) had fillings removed. Twenty-two subjects (78.6%) were noted to have irreversible pulpitis, 2 (7.1%) were diagnosed with maxillary sinus barotrauma, and 4 (14.3%) had an unknown cause of their symptoms. Those who received subsequent endodontic treatment to remove the affected pulp had no recurrence of symptoms on subsequent hypobaric exposure. Kollman concluded that his data supported the hypothesis that barodontalgia is due to either an infected maxillary sinus or stimulation of nerve endings in irreversibly inflamed pulp. The presence of existing pulpitis in cases of barodontalgia is supported by other reports in the literature.(47) While pulpitis has been shown to be present in a large percentage of cases of barodontalgia, there is no clear explanation regarding the mechanism of pain induction in the affected pulp during pressure change.

In 1983, Carlson et al. published research examining the penetration of methylene blue in a tooth under hyperbaric conditions.(12) The researchers demonstrated that the dye did penetrate the dentin when placed in an artificially created cavity and penetrated along the pulp chamber wall in some cases. Carlson postulated that sharp, localized pain may occur in a carious or previously restored tooth under hyperbaric conditions due to displacement of dentinal fluid towards the pulp, regardless of the presence or absence of pulp inflammation. Dull, prolonged, generalized pain is likely due to diseased pulp and warrants endodontic intervention.

Management

As with other forms of barotrauma, prevention is essential. Hyperbaric staff with frequent exposures in a multiplace chamber should be screened for good oral health to include periodic dental examinations with special attention to defective restorations, restorations with poor retention, and secondary caries. Periodic panoramic radiographs for those at risk of barodontalgia may be considered.(57) If barodontalgia develops during the course of nonurgent hyperbaric oxygen therapy, subsequent treatments should be halted until further evaluation by a dentist. Exposure to changes in barometric pressure should be avoided for 24–72 hours following any dental restoration or endodontic therapy.(31,57)

VISUAL CHANGES

Myopia/Cataracts

Vision changes as a side effect of HBO_2 therapy have been well documented since first described by Anderson and Farmer in 1978.(1) The etiology for the advancing myopia and accelerated cataracts under hyperoxic influence remains unknown but is likely related to lenticular changes. Advancing myopia usually reverses completely within weeks to months after the last HBO_2 treatment. In contrast, cataract progression is not as reversible, as it is thought to be a more severe form of hyperoxia-induced toxic effect on the lens.(43) Common risk factors for cataract formation include diabetes, corticosteroid use, radiation therapy to the head and neck, and excessive exposure to ultraviolet light.(11) In mice, methionine sulfoxide reductase A (MsrA) is important for the maintenance of lens transparency, and MsrA repair of mitochondrial cytochrome C may defend against oxidative stress-induced cataract formation of the lens.(6)

Lyne showed that 18 of 26 patients (including all 4 diabetics) treated for 60 minutes at 2.5 ATA and oxygen breathing for a 30-minute compression and a 30-minute decompression for 4–52 weeks developed myopia ranging from 0.5–5.5 diopters. Post-HBO_2, vision recovery was initially rapid, then slowed, lasting up to one year. No new lens opacities formed, and, in patients with preexisting opacities, none progressed.(37) In a Swedish study, all but 1 of 25 patients treated with 150–850 exposures at 2–2.5 ATA 7 days/week showed myopic refractive changes; 7 of 15 developed new, well-defined nuclear cataracts, earliest at 150 sessions. The nuclear cataracts were not reversible after cessation.(43) In a study of 96 HBO_2 patients treated an average of 26 times (range 6–59) at 2.0 or 2.5 ATA for 90 minutes, 5 times/week, visual acuity decreased an average of 2.13 lines on the Snellen chart. There was a greater-than-average change in 31%, no change in 10%, and change ≥ 3 lines in 46% of 50–60 year-olds. Four percent more diabetics had a greater-than-average change, and 8% more nondiabetics had no change. A plateau in myopic shift was noted around treatment 25.(39) In a retrospective review of 52 patients treated with ≥ 20 HBO_2 sessions, 81% experienced vision change at the 20th treatment (compared to pretreatment). Myopic change was most common, but 25% experienced hyperopia.(48)

A case report describes a 49-year-old female who developed bilateral cataracts and associated progressive myopic shift after only 48 HBO_2 treatments at 2.5 ATA for 90 minutes with 2 five-minute air breaks. Prior to HBO_2 therapy, formal ophthalmic exams revealed baseline myopia but no evidence of cataract formation. The cataracts and myopic changes remained progressive and persisted until the last follow-up at 11 months post therapy.(25) With this one possible exception to date, new cataracts are not reported during the 20–50 treatments commonly used in U.S. centers. Even when progressive myopia occurs during HBO_2, the visual changes almost always reverse completely. However, extension of a series beyond 100 sessions is associated with an increased risk of irreversible refractive changes or development of new cataracts.(11)

Clinical Recommendations

Information about vision change should be a part of the informed consent for each HBO_2 patient. Consider a baseline ophthalmology exam in patients with risk factors. Patients who develop vision change during HBO_2 should avoid the expense of obtaining new glasses (or use a less-expensive alternative in the interim) until enough time has elapsed for the changes to reverse. In those patients who have persistent change, consider ophthalmology referral to assess for other causes.

SEIZURES

The link between hyperbaric oxygen and seizures was recognized as early as 1878 by Paul Bert.(5) A hyperoxia-induced seizure represents the central nervous system (CNS) effect of oxygen toxicity. Early estimates of seizure incidence at 2.4 ATA with air breaks was 1 in 10,000 to 12,000 patient treatments.(17-18) More recently, seizure incidences at 2.4/2.5 ATA for 90 minutes of oxygen in three 30-minute periods with 2 air breaks are reported as 1 in 3,725 treatments (overall seizure rate of 1 in 6,704),(53) 1 in 2,844,(45) and 1 in 3,388.(27) A 2014 report of an incidence of 1 in 231 treatments using the same protocol is far greater and out of line with the prior reports.(30) The same group reported that air breaks were a risk factor for having a seizure ($p < .001$), and there were 0 per 10,000 seizures at 2 ATA (0/16, 430 treatments). The incidence of seizures at 2 ATA has been reported to be 4–5 times lower than at 2.4–2.5 ATA (with varying air break schedules).(3) One study reported a statistically significant difference ($p = 0.032$) among 300 consecutive patients treated at different pressures for carbon monoxide (CO) poisoning. There was 1 seizure at 2.45 ATA (0.3%), 9 seizures at 2.8 ATA (2.0%), and 6 seizures at 3 ATA. The authors conclude that this potential difference in seizure risk should be considered when selecting the HBO_2 treatment pressure for CO poisoning.(28)

Seizure risk is higher with certain diagnoses, including carbon monoxide poisoning[28] and acute traumatic peripheral arterial insufficiency,[3] and may be higher for patients with a history of febrile seizures. Other risk factors may include hypercapnia due to chronic obstructive pulmonary disease (COPD), narcotic use and withdrawal, alcohol dependence, and antidepressant, tramadol, or cephalosporin/ceftriaxone use. There may be other factors not yet identified.[46] The use of a mask for oxygen delivery may be associated with a lower seizure incidence.[56] This has been suggested to be due to the approximately 80% O_2 actually delivered by mask compared to the 100% O_2 delivered by hood,[56] and thus a lower partial pressure of O_2 received by patients during hyperbaric oxygen treatment.

Central nervous system oxygen toxicity can be manifested by a spectrum of effects including vertigo, twitching, syncope, sleepiness, apprehension, behavioral changes, and seizures.[14] Premonitory signs and symptoms may provide the clinician with an opportunity to avert an impending seizure.[36] Seizures are generally tonic-clonic convulsions that usually resolve without residual effects when the patient resumes room air breathing.[14] In one study, patients that had HBO_2-induced seizures did not require anticonvulsant medications, and there were no untoward neurologic sequelae post seizure.[27] Four of the six patients continued HBO_2 sessions and had no recurrent seizure.

Clinical Recommendations

In the event of an oxygen toxicity seizure during a hyperbaric oxygen treatment, oxygen should be discontinued, the gas switched to air to reduce the FiO_2, and the patient allowed to breath air in the chamber while the treatment pressure is maintained at a constant level until the seizure terminates, usually within two minutes. Do not decompress the chamber or accelerate the rate of decompression during active seizure activity. There is a case report of an air embolism occurring in a patient who developed a seizure during HBO_2 due to mismanagement by an inexperienced staff member who decompressed the chamber while the patient was still seizing. As with any other types of seizures, there will be a postictal phase, and the patient should be given clinical support as per usual following any seizure activity. Neurology consultation should be requested for prolonged seizure activity or recurrent seizures and treated appropriately. The appearance of a hyperoxic seizure does not necessitate the cessation of HBO_2 therapy, nor does it contraindicate the patient for future HBO_2 treatments, nor is it predictive of any future occurrence of seizure activity. The resumption of HBO_2 therapy is appropriate and normal at any time as determined by the physician and patient.

PULMONARY BAROTRAUMA

Pneumothorax

Pneumothorax is a very uncommon presentation of pulmonary barotrauma and, when seen, usually occurs in diving-related incidences.[50] The presence of a pneumothorax is usually detected before HBO_2 initiates since it is contraindicated in the therapy. If it presents during HBO_2 therapy, it is likely due to existing pulmonary trauma that causes gas expansion to the point of creating a tension pneumothorax. In this setting, it is also likely to appear in 5% to 10% of arterial gas embolism (AGE) cases.[44] (Please refer to the relevant chapter on AGE.)

Pneumothorax, or in the layman's term "collapsed lung," by definition is a collection of air or gas in the chest or pleural space that causes part or all of a lung to collapse. Causes are chest injury from blunt or penetrating trauma including medical procedures, underlying lung disease, or conditions such as chronic pulmonary disease, cystic fibrosis or pneumonia, or blebs where adhesions can cause tissue trauma.(38) From a diving and hyperbaric medicine perspective, the concern is for any condition or event that causes airway obstruction, resulting in alveoli expansion beyond their elastic limit and resultant rupture.(51) The most common situation is inadequate expiration upon ascent (usually emergent) in which the alveoli expand due to Boyle's law and eventually rupture. The rate in diving is about 1/50,000. Controlled ascent conditions in hyperbaric chambers will logically be much less. Forced alveolar rupture can also occur with ventilators. Spontaneous pneumothorax is identified as such when there is no apparent provoking factor such as trauma or stress. Seventy-two percent of spontaneous pneumothoraces have no known underlying lung disease.(32) The incidence of spontaneous pneumothorax is 7/100,000 for men and 1/100,000 for women.(52) It usually occurs at rest.

Clinical Presentation

Diagnosis is mainly by history and physical. Classic physical findings in noncomplicated pneumothorax include diminished or absent breath sounds upon auscultation, tympani upon percussion of the affected chest (watch out for bilateral pneumothorax), and voice impairment. Tests to confirm the diagnosis are usually X-rays or computed tomography scan. Tension pneumothorax is the condition in which the pneumothorax air cannot escape the chest cavity, continues to collapse the lung, and pushes against the mediastinum and heart resulting in hemodynamic instability. Common symptoms of tension pneumothorax include acute chest pain, shortness of breath, and tachycardia, and may worsen to hypotension and hypoxia. Physical signs of tension pneumothorax include absent breath sounds or voice, jugular venous distention, rales, and tracheal deviation away from the affected side.(19) This is an emergent condition, and immediate intervention should never be delayed for X-ray confirmation.

Management in Multiplace Chambers

Standard treatment of a pneumothorax may be just observation and allowing the air to be absorbed from the chest cavity. Invasive treatment is usually done when symptoms become severe. Needle thoracotomy (second intercostal space along midclavicular line) is generally a temporary solution, with chest tube thoracotomy the definitive treatment. Needle aspiration, however, can be considered a definitive treatment (three-way stopcock with syringe to draw out the air) and has shown decreased pain and length of hospital stay versus chest tube placement.(52) Surgery is used in persistent or complicated pneumothorax.

One case series discussed three pneumothorax cases during hyperbaric oxygen therapy in which all the patients sustained carbon monoxide poisoning and required cardiopulmonary resuscitation (CPR).(41) All three individuals developed tension pneumothorax in the multiplace chamber at depth (3 ATA). They completed the CO profile and were decompressed to surface. Two of the three received chest tubes that stabilized the hemodynamic compromise but were declared brain dead the following day. Though the tension pneumothorax may have resulted in enough pulmonary trauma to cause fatal cardiopulmonary decompensation, it could just as likely be that the severe carbon monoxide poisoning caused the lethal cardiopulmonary and central nervous system collapse. In emergent situations such as CO poisoning or tension pneumothorax, ultrasound should be considered. Ultrasound has been utilized increasingly and has a pneumothorax detection sensitivity ranging from 86 to

98% with minimal training and can be performed in 2–3 minutes.[54-55] Gawthrope described the use of ultrasound equipment in chamber following biomedical services modification and testing.[24]

Management in Monoplace Chambers

Invasive treatments can be done on patients in a multiplace chamber by trained individuals. As monoplace chambers have no patient accessibility for invasive treatments, alternative interventions must be employed. Daugherty[16] described two cases using inherent unsaturation in treating pneumothorax. Both took place in multiplace chambers for DCI treatment when the tension pneumothorax occurred. One developed pneumothorax at 50 msw and was decompressed on a slow linear rate 1.2 m/hour, with oxygen initiated when 18 msw was achieved. The rate was continued until 15 msw was reached, at which time the rate was decreased to 0.9 m/hr. To avoid oxygen toxicity, Daugherty recommends cycles of 20–25 minutes on oxygen with a 5-minute air breathing period. After six cycles, the patient is allowed to breathe air for two to four hours, and then the oxygen/air cycles are repeated.

Broome and Smith[7] reported the cases of the successful treatment of two Royal Naval Submarine Escape Training Tank (SETT) trainees who had developed neurological and respiratory decompensation following pulmonary barotrauma during the escape tank training. The condition of both students was complicated by bilateral pneumothoraces due to the pulmonary barotrauma. Once the diagnosis was made, the trainees' treatment tables were modified according to ability to decompress. One student trainee was treated on an air treatment table and the other on an oxygen treatment table. The trainee treated on the air treatment table required in-chamber chest tube thoracentesis, but the one treated on an oxygen treatment table averted the need for in-chamber thoracentesis despite the presence of the large bilateral pneumothoraces. While the trainee treated with an oxygen treatment table did eventually require thoracentesis and lung aspiration after reaching surface, he was able to tolerate decompression and reach surface in stable, nondistressed respiratory condition without requiring immediate in-chamber chest tube thoracentesis for the tension pneumothorax. Broom and Smith then reviewed the records of the Royal Naval and the U.S. Naval SETT accident cases. They found 126 Royal Naval cases and 113 U.S. Naval cases of recompression for suspected cerebral arterial gas embolism (CAGE), of which 15 had an associated pneumothorax, with six having bilateral pneumothoraces. Of the 15 cases, 12 were treated using air-only treatment tables and three on oxygen treatment tables. Out of the 15, three needed in-chamber thoracentesis. All three of the thoracentesis cases came from the air-only therapeutic tables, which were the routine intervention at a time before the advent of oxygen-based therapeutic tables. From these incidents, Broom and Smith proposed that oxygen-based therapeutic recompression tables should be the primary treatment option in the event of a pneumothorax diagnosed while under pressure, rather than resorting to formal chest tube thoracentesis, which would otherwise be appropriate under controlled conditions at surface.

They further asserted that the threat from pneumothorax during therapeutic recompression for CAGE has been overstated and had plausibly stemmed from the legacy of routinely applied air-based therapeutic recompression tables. Broom and Smith created a decision algorithm for chamber management of pneumothorax that follows TT6 or TT6A without modification unless symptoms of tension pneumothorax occur, at which time recompression is done to depth of relief. At that point, a prolonged decompression is suggested based on Dougherty's ascent rates.

It should be noted that thoracentesis, repeated as necessary, is one of the steps undertaken if a tension pneumothorax recurs. In a monoplace chamber, this is not possible. As the cases described by Dougherty and Broome/Smith demonstrate, it is possible to decompress a patient with a pneumothorax if an oxygen treatment table or algorithm is employed. The treatment steps without the thoracentesis option would be as follows when a tension pneumothorax occurs in a monoplace chamber: 1) Stop ascent. Descend to depth of relief if severe symptoms are present. 2) Apply an oxygen treatment table, rather than air, if possible, and conduct a slow ascent on oxygen. If the pressure is greater than 3 ATA, then a slow air (or oxygen-enriched nitrox) ascent is done until 100% oxygen can be breathed. Here, the decision algorithm stops with no thoracentesis option. Hence, the slow ascent rate of 0.9 m/hr (3 fsw/hour) would be used along with air breaks as above. As the monoplace chamber has the patient on 100% oxygen during the indication treatment, there is no air to be absorbed.

One case report(10) described a blunt trauma from an earthquake that resulted in subsequent wounds for which HBO_2 treatment was provided. The patient developed cardiopulmonary arrest during the seventh treatment and subsequent tension pneumothorax. Due to the cardiac event, a decompression to surface from 45 fsw at a rate of 2 fsw/min was initiated. Upon removal from the chamber, chest tube insertion and cardiac resuscitation were executed with success. This case is mentioned only as an emergent intervention when there is a team ready to treat the patient immediately upon surfacing.

Although rare, preventive measures and risk assessment should always be considered when each patient is initially reviewed and examined. If any pulmonary trauma has occurred emergently or recently, or the patient has had CPR recently, pneumothorax may be a possibility. If time allows, CT or ultrasound examination should be done. Technicians and staff should review actions needed to be taken if a patient develops a pneumothorax.

REFERENCES

1. Anderson B, Farmer JC. Hyperoxic myopia. Trans Am Opthalmol Soc. 1978;76:116-24.
2. Armstrong HG, Heim JW. Effect of flight on middle ear. JAMA. 1937;109:417-21.
3. Beard T, Warriner RA, Pascer P, et al. Adverse events during hyperbaric oxygen therapy (HBO2T), a retrospective analysis from 25 centers [abstract]. UHMS Annual Scientific Meeting; 2005; Las Vegas, NV.
4. Beard T, Warriner RA 3rd, Pasceri P, Otto GH, Smith M, Hayes C, Fife CE. Hyperbaric oxygen therapy (HBO2T) related adverse events in relation to treatment depth and blood glucose level, an on-going study from 48 centers. Abstract presented at: Undersea and Hyperbaric Medical Society, Inc. Annual Scientific Meeting; 2007 Jun 14-16; Maui, Hawaii.
5. Bert P. La pression barométrique. Paris: Masson Dt Cie; 1878.
6. Brennan LA, Lee W, Cowell T, Giblin F, Kantorow M. Deletion of mouse MsrA results in HBO2-induced cataract: MsrA repairs mitochondrial cytochrome c. Mol Vis. 2009;15:985-99.
7. Broome JR, Smith DJ. Pneumothorax as a complication of recompression therapy for cerebral arterial gas embolism. Undersea Biomed Res. 1992;19(6):447-55.
8. Brown M, Jones J, Krohmer J. Pseudoephedrine for the prevention of barotitis media: a controlled trial in underwater divers. Ann Emerg Med. 1992;21(7):849-52.
9. Butler FK, Bove AA. Infraorbital hypesthesia after maxillary sinus barotrauma. Undersea Hyperb Med. 1999;26(4):257-9.
10. Cakmak T et al. A case of tension pneumothorax during hyperbaric oxygen therapy in an earthquake survivor with crush injury complicated by ARDS (adult respiratory distress syndrome). Undersea Hyperb Med. 2015;42(1):9-13.
11. Camporesi EM. Side effects. In: Weaver LK, editor. Hyperbaric oxygen therapy indications. 13th ed. North Palm Beach (FL): Best Publishing Co.; 2014. p. 247-8.
12. Carlson OG, Halverson BA, Triplett RG. Dentin permeability under hyperbaric conditions as a possible cause of barodontalgia. Undersea Biomed Res. 1983;10(1):23-8.
13. Carlson S, Jones J, Brown M, Hess C. Prevention of hyperbaric-associated middle ear barotrauma. Ann Emerg Med. 1992;21(12):1468-71.
14. Clark J. Oxygen toxicity. In: Neuman T, Thom S, editors. Physiology and medicine of hyperbaric oxygen therapy. Philadelphia: Saunders Elsevier; 527-63.
15. Corigliano J, Josefsen L, Warriner RA. A comprehensive review of outcomes using uniform barotrauma prevention protocols during hyperbaric exposure. Undersea Hyperb Med. 2001. Abstract available from: http://archive.rubicon-foundation.org/250.
16. Daugherty CG. Inherent unsaturation in the treatment of pneumothorax at depth. Undersea Biomed Res. 1990;17(2):171-7.
17. Davis JC. Hyperbaric oxygen therapy. J Intensive Care Med. 1989;4:55-7.
18. Davis JC, Dunn JM, Heimbach RD. Hyperbaric medicine: patient selection, treatment procedures, and side-effects. In: Davis JC, Hunt TK, editors. Problem wounds. The role of oxygen. New York: Elsevier Science Publishing; 1988. p. 225-35.
19. DeGowin EL, DeGowin RL. DeGowin and DeGowin bedside diagnostic examination. MacMillan Publishing Co.; 1976. p. 314-8.
20. Devoe K, Motley HL. Aerodontalgia. Dent Dig. 1945;51:16-8.

21. Fagan P, McKenzie B, Edmonds C. Sinus barotrauma in divers [Internet]. Royal Australian Navy; 1975. Available from: http://archive.rubicon-foundation.org/4966.

22. Fiesseler FW, Silverman ME, Riggs RL, Szucs PA. Indication for hyperbaric oxygen treatment as a predictor of tympanostomy tube placement. Undersea Hyperb Med. 2006;33(4):231-5.

23. Fitzpatrick DT, Franck BA, Mason KT, Shannon SG. Risk factors for symptomatic otic and sinus barotrauma in a multiplace hyperbaric chamber. Undersea Hyperb Med. 1999;26(4):243-7.

24. Gawthrope IC. Ultrasound in diving and hyperbaric medicine. Diving Hyperb Med. 2012;42(1):36-9.

25. Gesell LB, Trott A. De novo cataract development following a standard course of hyperbaric oxygen therapy. Undersea Hyperb Med. 2007;34(6):389-92.

26. Gunepin M, Derache F, Blatteau JE, Zadik Y. Incidence and features of barodontalgia among military divers. Aviat Space Environ Med. 2016;87(2):137-40.

27. Hampson NB, Atik DA. Central nervous system oxygen toxicity during routine hyperbaric oxygen therapy. Undersea Hyperb Med. 2003;30:147-53.

28. Hampson NB, Simonson SG, Kramer CC, Piantadosi CA. Central nervous system oxygen toxicity during hyperbaric treatment of patients with carbon monoxide poisoning. Undersea Hyperb Med. 1996;23:215-9.

29. Harker L, Norante J, Rzu J. Experimental rupture of the round window membrane. Trans Am Acad Ophthalmol Otol. 1974;78:448-52.

30. Heyboer M, Jennings S, Grant WD, Ojevwe C, Byrne J, Wojcik SM. Seizure incidence by treatment pressure in patients undergoing hyperbaric oxygen therapy. Undersea Hyperb Med. 2014;41(5):379-85.

31. Hodges FR. Barodontalgia at 12,000 feet. J Am Dent Assoc. 1978;97:66-8.

32. Inouye WY, Berggren RB, Johnson J. Spontaneous pneumothorax: treatment and mortality. Chest. 1967;51(1):67-73.

33. Keller AP. A study of the relationship of air pressure to myringopuncture. Laryngoscope. 1958;68:2015-29.

34. Kollman W. Incidence and possible causes of dental pain during simulated high altitude flights. J Endod. 1993;19(3):154-9.

35. Kringlebotn M. Rupture pressure of membranes in the ear. Ann Otol Rhinol Laryngol. 2000;109(10 Pt 1):940-4.

36. Kruckeberg S. Airbreaks during monoplace operations: why it matters, what works best. UHMS Annual Scientific Meeting; 2005; Las Vegas, NV. p. 310.

37. Lyne AJ. Ocular effects of hyperbaric oxygen. Trans Ophthalmol Soc UK. 1978;98:66-8.

38. Mayo Clinic [Internet]. Mayo Foundation for Medical Education and Research (MFMER). Pneumothorax [cited 2017 Apr 13]. Available from: http://www.mayoclinic.org/diseases-conditions/pneumothorax/symptoms-causes/dxc-20179900

39. McEwan S. Myopic changes during HBO2 therapy measured with the Snellen eye chart. Abstract presented at the 2009 Undersea and Hyperbaric Medical Society Annual Scientific Meeting. Undersea Hyperb Med. 2009;36(4):278.

40. Minkiewitz K. The effects of compression rates on middle ear barotrauma. Abstract presented at: Undersea and Hyperbaric Medical Society, Inc. Annual Scientific Meeting; 1985 Jun 11-14; Long Beach, CA.

41. Murphy DG, Sloan EP, Hart RG, et al. Tension pneumothorax associated with hyperbaric oxygen therapy. Am J Emerg Med. 1991;9(2):176-9.

42. Neuman T, Settle H, Beaver G, Linaweaver PG Jr. Maxillary sinus barotrauma with cranial nerve involvement: case report. Aviat Space Environ Med. 1975;46(3):314-5.

43. Palmquist BM, Philipson B, Barr PO. Nuclear cataract and myopia during hyperbaric oxygen therapy. Br J Ophthalmol. 1984;68:113-7.

44. Pearson RR. Diagnosis and treatment of gas embolism. In: Shilling CW, Carlston CB, Mathias RA, editors. The physician's guide to diving medicine. New York: Plenum Press; 1984. p. 333-67.

45. Pflaki C, Peters P, Almeling M, Welslau W, Busch R. Complications and side effects of hyperbaric oxygen therapy. Aviat Space Environ Med. 2000;71:119-24.

46. Seidel R, Carroll C, Thompson D, Diem RG, Yeboah K, Hayes AJ, Hall B, Whelan HT. Risk factors for oxygen toxicity seizures in hyperbaric oxygen therapy: case reports from multiple institutions. Undersea Hyperb Med. 2013 Nov-Dec;40(6):515-9.

47. Senia ES, Cunningham KW, Marx RE. The diagnostic dilemma of barodontalgia. Oral Surg Oral Med Oral Pathol. 1985;60:218-23.

48. Smerz RW, Sanders RW. Visual changes in patients undergoing HBO2T. Abstract presented at the 2009 Undersea and Hyperbaric Medical Society Annual Scientific Meeting. Undersea Hyperbar Med. 2010;36(4):297.

49. U.S. Navy Diving Manual. Revision 7. Vol. 1. U.S. Naval Sea Systems Command; 2016. Chapter 3-6, Mechanical effects of pressure on the human body – barotrauma during descent.

50. Van Hoesen K, Neuman TS. Gas embolism. In: Neumann T, Thom S, editors. Physiology and medicine of hyperbaric oxygen therapy. Philadelphia: Saunders; 2008. p. 257-81.

51. Veale A. Tension pneumothorax in divers. SPUMS J [Internet]. 1998 [cited 2017 Apr 13];28(3). Available from: http://archive.rubicon-foundation.org/xmlui/bitstream/handle/123456789/5969/SPUMS_V28N3Supl_4.pdf?sequence=1 Supplement

52. Wakai AP. Spontaneous pneumothorax. BMJ Clin Evid [Internet]. 2008 Mar 10 [cited 2017 Apr 13];2008:1505. Available from: https://www.ncbi.nlm.nih.gov/pmc/articles/PMC2907964/.

53. Welslau W, Almeling M. Toxicity of hyperbaric oxygen (HBO2) – incidence of major CNS-intoxications. Strahlenther Onkol. 1996;172(S2):10-2.

54. Wernecke K, Galanski M, Peters PE, Hansen J. Pneumothorax: evaluation by ultrasound. J Thoracic Imaging. 1987;2:76-8.

55. Wilkerson R, Stone M. Sensitivity of bedside ultrasound and supine anteroposterior chest radiographs for the identification of pneumothorax after blunt trauma. Acad Emerg Med. 2010;17:11-7.

56. Yildiz S, Aktas S, Cimsit M, Ay H, Togrol E. Seizure incidence in 80,000 patient treatments with hyperbaric oxygen. Aviat Space Environ Med. 2004 Nov;75(11):992-4.

57. Zadik Y. Barodontalgia. J Endod. 2009;35(4):481-5.

58. Zwart BP. The smooth ride profile: development, implementation and evaluation of a hyperbaric chamber descent and ascent based on a constant rate of volume change with time – a retrospective comparative analysis. Undersea Hyperb Med. 1999;26(Suppl):70.

CHAPTER 11 CHAPTER

Pediatric Considerations for Hyperbaric Medicine

CHAPTER ELEVEN OVERVIEW

Introduction **223**

Risks and Benefits **223**

Retinopathy of Prematurity 225

Bronchopulmonary Dysplasia 225

Ductus Arteriosus Closure 225

Risks in Older Pediatric Patients 226

Benefits of HBO_2 in Pediatric Patients 226

Practical Considerations in the Treatment of Children **226**

Logistics and Collaboration in the Care of Children 226

Thermal Protection 227

Psychological Preparation and Sedation 228

Middle-Ear Equalization 229

Equipment Challenges 230

Pediatric Disease Indications and Controversies **230**

Indications 230

Contraindications 230

Acute, Critical Illness 231

Wound Healing 231

Autism 231

Cerebral Palsy 232

Traumatic Brain Injury 232

Oxygen Administration Schedules **232**

Conclusion **232**

References **234**

Pediatric Considerations for Hyperbaric Medicine

Pamela C. Petersen, Michael T. Meyer, Paul A. Thombs

INTRODUCTION

Children are treated with hyperbaric therapy (HBO_2) for various acute and chronic indications worldwide, predominantly in adult-based hyperbaric practices and facilities. In this chapter we will review the practical considerations required for the care of children in adult-based facilities, review the indications for HBO_2 in children, and address controversies in the literature. Unfortunately, there is not an abundance of evidence-based literature available for many of the pediatric indications where HBO_2 has been described. The care of children in any adult care setting requires close communication between pediatric and hyperbaric specialty teams to understand the unique logistical and care needs of children required to meet the standards of pediatric care.

This chapter will address two major goals. The first is to provide both the pediatric care teams and emergency teams the basic knowledge of the indications for pediatric HBO_2 therapy and/or referral. This goal is complicated since there are numerous reports available in the literature regarding pediatric HBO_2; unfortunately, many are observational in nature or extrapolations from adult experiences, and evidence-based pediatric studies are lacking. The relatively small number of pediatric patients with acute life-threatening diseases where HBO_2 has been utilized (carbon monoxide intoxication, necrotizing soft-tissue infections) eliminates the feasibility of a randomized, controlled trial, adding to the complexity. Finally, HBO_2 has been reported in multiple uncontrolled settings for a myriad of pediatric conditions where patient families have wanted to proceed with therapy based on preliminary results where the reported positive results may actually be the result of random chance, placebo effect, or other unidentified variables. The second major goal is to describe the special care needs of children; this is especially important since the vast majority of hyperbaric chambers are located in adult-based care organizations where the routine or critical care needs of children are outside of regular workflow.

RISKS AND BENEFITS

Prior to any therapy initiation, the potential risks must be weighed against the potential benefits. Oxygen is one such therapy and is used ubiquitously in health-care settings and considered relatively harmless in most clinical settings. Unfortunately, oxygen toxicity occurs, with symptoms most evident in the pulmonary, neurological, and ocular systems. Oxygen toxicity results from oxygen free-radical formation following prolonged exposure to high concentrations of oxygen at atmospheric pressure or with short exposures to oxygen at hyperbaric pressures. At atmospheric pressure, pulmonary oxygen toxicity does not usually occur below 50% FiO_2 and usually requires anywhere from 4–22 hours to develop. During exposure to hyperbaric oxygen therapy with 100% oxygen at 2–3 atmosphere absolute (ATA), pulmonary oxygen toxicity symptoms can develop within as few as 3 hours. In order to standardize the amount of oxygen being given, ATA is the product of the concentration of oxygen (100% in HBO_2) multiplied by the pressure experienced if one descends in seawater to that depth. This can be expressed in multiple ways, one of which is that a 33-foot depth of seawater equals 1 ATA if breathing 100% oxygen. The symptoms of pulmonary oxygen toxicity include tracheobronchial irritation from decreased ciliary activity which presents as prominent substernal or pleuritic pain. This may progress to decreased vital capacity, progressive abnormalities in carbon monoxide diffusing capacity, and eventual atelectasis. Introduction of inert gases such as nitrogen can prevent the atelectasis from occurring. Prolonged exposure to oxygen can lead to chronic pulmonary fibrosis and emphysema which is worsened by medications which increase cell metabolism such as dexamethasone, epinephrine, estrogen, amphetamines, and thyroid hormones. Bleomycin further exacerbates oxygen-induced lung injury via its metabolism which produces free-radical intermediates.[(36)]

Central nervous system (CNS) oxygen toxicity symptoms consist of visual changes, tinnitus, nausea, facial twitching, dizziness, and confusion and may progress to seizures. Seizures related to oxygen toxicity are reversible without residual neurologic damage if inspired oxygen partial pressure is reduced. Seizure is a commonly feared complication of HBO_2; however, the evidence does not support this fear given a reported incidence of 1:62,614 treatment sessions in 1 large retrospective review. The study was predominantly based on adult patient findings, but did include 240 patients < 16 years of age and included patients with known neurological disorders. In all patients, the minimum effective hyperbaric oxygen exposure dose was used, with the majority of treatments at no more than 2 ATA.[(11)] Neurological toxicity is most commonly associated with short exposure to high concentrations of oxygen at hyperbaric pressures; exposure to oxygen at 4–5 ATA may result in CNS toxicity in as little as 10 minutes. Finally, hyperoxic myopia is a self-resolving ocular toxicity symptom specific to HBO_2 in older patients. It is associated with an increased refractive power of the lens that resolves with time.[(36)]

There are unique pediatric age-associated complications with HBO_2 that are roughly based on patient age groups, most commonly seen in premature and young infants. In general, the complications seen in older children and adolescents are similar to those in the adult population. In the youngest of pediatric patients, term and preterm infants at birth, it is well established that normobaric, 100% oxygen has significant physiologic effects which include a reduction in cerebral blood flow, altered tidal volume, and changes in the ratio of reduced to oxidized glutathione. In this population, most complications focus around the development of retinopathy of prematurity (ROP), the development of bronchopulmonary dysplasia (BPD) or chronic lung disease (CLD), and premature closure of the ductus arteriosus. It has been suggested that HBO_2 eligibility be based on predicted maturity of the antioxidant defense system, therefore not being recommended for neonates younger than 34.5 weeks postmenstrual age and weighing less than 1.2 kg.[31]

Retinopathy of Prematurity

The development of ROP is associated with exposure to elevated partial pressures of oxygen; however, several studies have shown that ROP is multifactorial and has occurred without exposure to elevated partial pressures of oxygen.[22,27,12] Data has been inconclusive on whether oxygen minimization actually reduces the rate of ROP; however, this practice may increase the risk of hypoxic-related complications.[36] The combination of neonatal sepsis, oxygen exposure, and low gestational age has been shown to significantly increase the risk of ROP.[3] Also, the risk of ROP related to oxygen therapy within the first 28 days of life was greatest in infants 23–25 weeks gestational age. Interestingly, randomized clinical trials and cohort studies have shown that high oxygen supplementation may have protective effects by minimizing the hypoxia-induced retinal neovascularization characterizing the second phase of ROP which begins around 32–34 weeks postmenstrual age, but this risk reduction should not be expected until approximately 33 weeks postmenstrual age.[3] Two small case series utilizing HBO_2 for necrotizing enterocolitis (NEC) reassuringly described resolution of the NEC without retinal abnormality or CNS toxicity.[32-33] A careful examination of the retina to ascertain the degree of vascular maturity may be helpful in assessing the risk of hyperbaric oxygen therapy in premature patients.

Bronchopulmonary Dysplasia

Bronchopulmonary dysplasia (BPD) is serious sequelae of barotrauma associated with mechanical ventilation and the elevated inspired partial pressures of oxygen used in the treatment of respiratory distress syndrome in premature infants. The mechanism for BPD development is not clear, but likely includes some, if not all, of the mechanisms of pulmonary oxygen toxicity described above. Animal studies have shown that oxygen is a direct toxin to the bronchial and alveolar epithelium, and the rising partial pressure of blood oxygen causes CNS and retinal toxicity. Similarly, several animal experiments have demonstrated that excess oxygen damages lung growth in the first few weeks after birth. Unfortunately, there are no studies on human infants that reflect these findings.[37]

Ductus Arteriosus Closure

Finally, when considering use of HBO_2 in infants, one must recall that oxygen is a potent stimulus for closure of the ductus arteriosus. Studies on pregnant ewes have shown that the ductal flow was significantly reduced during HBO_2 even though total aortic flow was preserved due to increased transpulmonic flow, which disappeared promptly post HBO_2.[1] This does not represent a problem for HBO_2 in pregnancy, but it does represent a potential problem for patients with ductal-dependent congenital heart disorders. In the setting of severe congenital pulmonic outflow obstruction, systemic blood flow may depend on persistent ductal patency. The increase in blood oxygen tension with hyperbaric oxygen could result in a sudden and catastrophic decrease in cardiac output due to ductal constriction. This is a rare constellation of events; however, the possibility should be kept in mind if treating an infant with complex congenital heart disease. This risk may be excluded by an adequate physical examination, chest radiograph, and, if indicated, echocardiography.

Risks in Older Pediatric Patients

The risks of HBO_2 in older pediatric patients differ from those in premature infants. One published report has systematically explored the occurrence of side effects in children treated with oxygen greater than 1.0 ATA: in 153 patients reviewed over a 20-year period, a 1.7% incidence of side effects and complications occurred which is similar to that in adults. Middle-ear barotrauma was the most frequently seen problem (6.0%) and showed a higher frequency in 11- to 16-year-olds than in younger patients. Central nervous system oxygen toxicity (0.7%) occurred only in critically ill, unconscious, and ventilator-dependent patients. There was no evidence that the dose-response curve for hyperbaric oxygen versus neurologic or pulmonary toxicity is different for term infants versus older children. As seen in adults, reducing the incidence of otic barotrauma depends on both patient education and screening for eustachian tube dysfunction. Undiagnosed congenital malformations of the lung can lead to air trapping and pulmonary overinflation with the sequelae of alveolar rupture, pneumothorax, and potential air embolism.[32] A chest radiograph should be obtained in infants and children prior to HBO_2 since the clinical presentation of the underlying malformation may be delayed.

Benefits of HBO_2 in Pediatric Patients

Although there are several differences in the risks of HBO_2 in pediatric patients, the benefits are similar to those seen in adults. Hyperbaric oxygen at 3.0 ATA increases the dissolved oxygen in the plasma enough to meet the average requirements of resting tissue with dissolved oxygen alone, without contribution of the oxygen bound to hemoglobin. These high oxygen concentrations may indirectly reduce the inflammatory response by reducing levels of hypoxic inducible factor-1a (HIF-1a).[36] Theoretically, the major benefit of HBO_2 seen in children rather than adults is that the benefits obtained in children by preventing permanent neurological disability (carbon monoxide poisoning) or preventing the need for ablative surgery (necrotizing infections) can often be measured in decades of preserved function, not just in months or years.

PRACTICAL CONSIDERATIONS IN THE TREATMENT OF CHILDREN

Successful treatment of children must take into account the physiological and psychological changes of maturation as well as the logistical challenges of transferring a critically ill child from a pediatric intensive care unit (PICU) to the HBO_2 center. In administering hyperbaric oxygen, these axioms apply to the physical environment of the chamber, middle-ear physiology, psychological preparation and support, managing with parent-child interactions, and medical support. Problem prevention and solutions may be quite different depending upon whether one uses a monoplace or multiplace chamber. Including pediatricians on the hyperbaric medicine treatment team, pretreatment planning, and ongoing communication makes the task easier.

Logistics and Collaboration in the Care of Children

HBO_2 therapy is usually provided at predominantly adult institutions, necessitating the transfer of pediatric patients from pediatric hospitals to adult hyperbaric chambers for therapy. One study of HBO_2 in pediatric patients younger than 16 years old found that 54 pediatric patients were treated in the 12-year study period,

9 of which were hospitalized in the PICU. From a resource-utilization standpoint, there were 40 required transfers facilitated by a specialized pediatric emergency transport service between the PICU and the hyperbaric unit. The transfer also required the patient to be accompanied by PICU nurses and intensivists. In an example of logistical ingenuity, to facilitate twice-daily treatments in 3 patients with acute necrotizing fasciitis, the children were admitted to an adult ICU cubicle during the day which was staffed by a PICU nurse and physician; the pediatric patients and staff were transported back to the pediatric hospital every evening. Only two equipment-related complications were noted throughout these processes, both with infusion/syringe pumps failing. The authors noted that children were most likely to receive HBO_2 at the right time and for the correct duration if interfacility transfers were not required, and daily admission to an adult ICU location that was staffed with a PICU nurse and intensivist may assist in facilitating multiple hyperbaric treatments per day as indicated for specific disease states. Overall, children from a PICU can be safely and effectively treated in adult hyperbaric facilities with a low incidence of complications during transfer and treatment. Therefore, the need to transport children for HBO_2 should not prevent its use in children.[(9)]

Thermal Protection

Hypothermia is a genuine concern when utilizing HBO_2 on infants. This hypothermia occurs for multiple reasons including that the body surface-to-mass ratio increases with decreasing age, resulting in a greater relative heat loss for infants; core temperature maintenance is a biological priority, and calories will be diverted to preserve it; and the body's ability to generate heat is finite. Adiabatic cooling on chamber decompression further increases convective and conductive losses. Ventilation of the chamber imposes an added stress by increasing evaporative heat loss. Special attention must be directed to detecting and preventing heat loss, especially in the pre-verbal infant, since by the time a child has developed the language skills sufficient to express the concept of being cold, the body surface-to-mass ratio has changed, and the potential for rapid, dangerous heat loss has diminished. Likewise, the physical assessment of skin looking for piloerection ("goosebumps"), shivering, cool skin, or mottling identifies the presence of hypothermia once it has already occurred and caused potential harm.

Regular monitoring of core temperature is the most sensitive method for early detection of significant losses and affords the opportunity for prevention. It should be utilized for all infants to establish, at a minimum, that heat loss is not a significant problem. If supplementary warming is needed, continued assessment of temperature must be carried out to ensure that the plan for thermal regulation is working. Use of continuous thermal monitoring in the form of cutaneous, rectal, vascular, or urinary bladder probes is likely to be needed during monoplace operations where patient access is limited once the hatch is sealed. Intermittent rectal, cutaneous, or otic monitoring, using a hyperbaric-environment-compatible thermometer, may be sufficient during multiplace operations. Once the temperature is being maintained, further monitoring may not be necessary if the treatment environment is reproducible and major changes in caloric intake or heat loss do not occur.

The requirement for preventing excessive heat loss and reduction of evaporative, conductive, and convective losses is the same in monoplace and multiplace chambers.

In both chamber types, blanket usage decreases evaporative losses by preventing skin exposure to air currents, as well as limiting convective and conductive losses through insulating effects. In small infants (<2500 gm), the ability to generate metabolic heat is extremely limited, and in the face of a relatively large radiating surface, or where mild hypothermia is already present, heat must be added to the environment through the use of external warmers such as hot water bottles or prewarmed blankets. Radiant heaters or devices heated by an electrical resistor are not safe in either the monoplace or multiplace environment.[26] In the monoplace chamber, devices that act as heat reservoirs must provide a sufficient heat gradient during the entire treatment without inflicting a thermal injury early in the course of the exposure. Additionally, the heat must be sufficient to offset increased heat losses during decompression due to adiabatic cooling. In multiplace chambers equipped with a medical transfer lock, heat sources may be replaced as needed.

Psychological Preparation and Sedation

For both medical and ethical reasons, patients should not be subjected to excessive anxiety; yet anxiety is a classical human response to the unknown. For young children with limited life experience, nearly every situation is likely to hold some degree of the unknown. The combination of illness, a novel environment such as a hyperbaric chamber, and parental separation can produce profound anxiety or fear. There are several techniques available for nonpediatric caregivers to manage the anxiety and fear that a child may demonstrate, and addressing these issues beforehand will make treatment much less stressful for the patient and staff. We must remember, for techniques to be effective in children, one must consider the developmental age of the child and that illness in a child usually causes behavior regression and the ability to reason is likely to be a casualty of the illness. Appealing to a child's logic is unlikely to be a useful tactic, but it is appropriate to explain to children beyond the age of three to four years, in simple terms, that the treatment is to make them better. The next task is to make the treatment as stress-free as possible.

When the initial treatment is elective, pretreatment teaching, like preoperative teaching, using pictures, dolls, models, and child-oriented stories provides facts and dispels fears. Child Life Education specialists can help by making the format and content of the presentation age appropriate. In non-emergent situations with children preschool age and older, examining the facility and equipment prior to treatment, with a parent present, also makes the environment less anxiety provoking. If possible, the staff member carrying out the orientation should also carry out the first treatments, either as the internal caregiver in multiplace operations or as the operator in monoplace chamber. Consistency of procedure is also important in reducing novelty. In emergent or semi-emergent situations, this orientation will need to be truncated or omitted.

In elective as well as emergent situations, distraction during treatment is a valuable tool for mitigation of anxiety. Controlled breathing, virtual reality, guided imagery/relaxation, interactive toys, and electronic games in addition to passive distractions including music and television have all been shown to be effective for pain and anxiety reduction in patients of all ages. Additionally, allowing patients to choose their distraction activity provides the additional benefit of giving patients a sense of control, partially compensating for the lack of control involved in their treatment.[18] In HBO_2, items used for distraction cannot represent a safety hazard in the chamber (i.e., toys should not produce sparks, or fabrics incorporated in the toy cannot produce static electricity) and the items must be age appropriate to be effective. The 100%-oxygen atmosphere of a monoplace chamber significantly limits the type of items that can be placed in the chamber with the child, whereas a multiplace chamber allows a range of items that can be safely introduced. The child's parent and Child Life Educators are invaluable resources for age-appropriate distractions, and the chamber operators can assist with assessment of object safety.

Procedures that are painful or frightening should be performed under carefully controlled sedation, allowing the procedures to be done in the shortest time possible and facilitating repetition of the therapy as needed. When psychological preparation and distraction alone are insufficient in preventing significant anxiety, sedation is indicated to successfully complete HBO_2. The American Academy of Pediatrics (AAP) has published extensive guidelines for sedating a pediatric patient, especially when completed by nonpediatric providers. Sedation is a common procedure but is not benign, and pediatric patients can easily slip into deeper levels of sedation than were intended, resulting in complications such as respiratory depression, laryngospasm, impaired airway patency, apnea, loss of protective airway reflexes, and cardiovascular instability. At a minimum, practitioners providing sedation must have the skills to rescue a patient from a deeper-than-intended level of sedation which includes familiarity with management of airway obstruction, laryngospasm, and apnea. Certification in Pediatric Advanced Life Support (PALS) is strongly recommended. Practitioners must have immediate access to an emergency cart or kit containing the necessary age-appropriate equipment needed to resuscitate a child.(5) In the case of HBO_2 where pediatric patients may be transported to an adult facility for treatment, the necessary equipment could be provided by the specialized medical team accompanying the patient. Proper monitoring and documentation pre-, during, and postsedation must be completed. Providers must have adequate familiarity with the pharmacologic properties of the medications being administered and have access to reversal agents if indicated. In all cases, the minimal amount of sedation required to complete the procedure safely should be used, and polypharmacy is discouraged.(5)

Middle-Ear Equalization

Middle-ear and paranasal sinus pressure equalization is no different in children than in adults, and freedom from ear discomfort is perhaps even more important for children. An adult may be able to rationalize some discomfort if, in the long term, he or she will benefit. Children find this much more difficult, and one painful experience may make further treatment impossible. The process of pressure equalization is complicated by two factors: first, a certain level of cognitive function is required to understand the need to equalize pressure, to follow instructions, and to carry out the procedure, and second, eustachian tube dysfunction is common in children which may prohibit even cooperative children from successfully equalizing.

At approximately four to six years, a child may be able to focus his or her attention sufficiently to be taught to clear via Valsalva or Frenzel maneuver or via other eustachian tube–stretching exercises such as yawning, swallowing, or gum chewing. Phenylephrine nasal drops (0.125% for ages 2–6 years and 0.25–0.5% beyond 6 years), may be helpful. Sucking, as from a baby bottle nipple, may lead to eustachian tube opening, presumably from a Frenzel-type maneuver. Screaming or crying at times also produces eustachian tube opening but is difficult for those involved in the child's care to tolerate and could just as well be a sign of excruciating pain. Extremely slow compression rates may be effective in the monoplace setting to manage the pain associated with eustachian tube dysfunction, but in multiplace operations, prolonged descents increase inert gas accumulation for inside attendants, and decompression schedules may need to be altered accordingly.

The sequelae of barotrauma are the same for children as in adults; however, middle-ear effusions may take longer to resolve in children and may be associated with bacterial otitis media. Myringotomy must be considered for every toddler or infant, as preverbal status may slow provider recognition of otic pain. Hemotympanum may also occur and is most likely related to difficulty equalizing the pressure between the middle ear and eustachian tubes in small children. This problem may be exacerbated by the additional obstruction from endotracheal intubation. As a result, some surgeons routinely place prophylactic myringotomy tubes in children less than one year old prior to hyperbaric oxygen therapy.[16] The myringotomy, for hyperbaric treatments over a one to three day period, may not require insertion of a ventilating tube; however, the procedure will likely require sedation for pain control and to ensure that movement of the child's head does not occur and cause middle-ear ossicular injury. When treatment is expected to continue for more than three days, myringotomy and tube insertion are indicated and should be performed by an otolaryngologist.

Equipment Challenges

All equipment utilized in a hyperbaric chamber must be adapted because of the pressurized environment and the fire risks. This includes the equipment needed for mechanical ventilation in addition to intravenous infusion pumps and monitoring equipment such as telemetry.[16,21] Since the majority of hyperbaric chamber utilization is in adult patients, finding pediatric-sized equipment poses an additional challenge.

PEDIATRIC DISEASE INDICATIONS AND CONTROVERSIES

Indications

Approved indications for hyperbaric oxygen therapy by the Undersea and Hyperbaric Medical Society (UHMS) do not vary for adults versus pediatric patients. Indications include air or gas embolism, carbon monoxide poisoning, clostridial myositis and myonecrosis (gas gangrene), crush injury, compartment syndrome, acute traumatic ischemias, decompression sickness, arterial insufficiencies, severe anemia, intracranial abscess, necrotizing soft-tissue infections, refractory osteomyelitis, delayed radiation injury (soft tissue and bony necrosis), compromised grafts and flaps, acute thermal burn injury, and idiopathic sudden sensorineural hearing loss.[38] Several uses of hyperbaric oxygen therapy have been documented in the literature for pediatric patients, and this section will address some of the approved and experimental indications.

Contraindications

Absolute contraindications to hyperbaric oxygen therapy include untreated pneumothorax and the use of some chemotherapeutic agents, including but not limited to disulfiram, cisplatin, adriamycin, doxorubicin, sulfamylon, and bleomycin.[16,20] Relative contraindications include asthma, claustrophobia, congenital spherocytosis,

Eustachian tube dysfunction, high fever, pacemakers or epidural pain pump, pregnancy, seizures, and active upper respiratory infection.[20] Other proposed contraindications include active cancer and active viral infection.[6]

Acute, Critical Illness

The UHMS recommends HBO_2 for patients with carbon monoxide poisoning and for patients with combined carbon monoxide and cyanide poisoning, a combination that often occurs in smoke inhalation, and pediatric patients have been shown to benefit from this therapy.[7] Approximately 18% of the patients receiving HBO_2 for carbon monoxide exposure in the United States over an 18-month period were under the age of 18 years.[4] Pediatric patients are often also treated for acute bubble injury defined as decompression sickness and arterial gas embolism, acute arterial ischemia, and acute severe infection[7] In 2011, the treatment of idiopathic sudden sensorineural hearing loss was added as an indication for HBO_2.[38] There have been several reports demonstrating the effectiveness of HBO_2 in pediatric patients with this condition, including a report showing improvement in a patient with sudden sensorineural hearing loss with preexisting large vestibular aqueduct syndrome.[34]

Wound Healing

The mechanisms of action of HBO_2 in severe infections include restoration of normoxia or achievement of hyperoxia in previously hypoxic tissues, inhibition of exotoxin production, enhancement of neutrophil function, and synergistic enhancement of antibiotic activity in addition to decreased edema and promotion of capillary angiogenesis. There have been several case reports of HBO_2's effectiveness as an adjunct in treating clostridial infections, gas gangrene, and necrotizing fasciitis. Although the majority of the reports are in adults, pediatric literature on this topic is established and continues to emerge.[35,9,7] A retrospective chart review in 2001 showed a synergistic effect of surgical debridement, HBO_2, and granulocyte colony-stimulating factor in seven cases of necrotizing fasciitis with myonecrosis in neutropenic pediatric oncology patients,[15] and a more recent case report reiterated the importance of early surgery and antibiotics with use of hyperbaric oxygen as an adjunct in a previously healthy patient.[17] There are also unclear but potential benefits of HBO_2 therapy in purpura fulminans during the phase of acute arterial ischemia, during resolution of the ischemia perfusion injury, and during the healing phase.[9,7] HBO_2 also shows promise in the treatment of pediatric hemorrhagic cystitis; however, the vast majority of case reports continue to be in the adult population.[6] The success of HBO_2 in wound healing has led to investigation of the benefits of prophylactic HBO_2 to prevent wound infections. In one such study of pediatric patients undergoing neuromuscular scoliosis surgery, the use of HBO_2 was found to significantly decrease the incidence of postoperative infections.[14]

Autism

The use of HBO_2 for autism spectrum disorder was first proposed in 2006 by Rossignol, who hypothesized that HBO_2 may help with cerebral hypoperfusion and neuroinflammation which sometimes characterize autism.[2] In 2009, Rossignol conducted a multicenter, randomized, and double-blind controlled trial of hyperbaric oxygen exposure for the treatment of autism spectrum disorder. This study concluded that children exposed to the hyperbaric treatment at 1.3 ATA and 24% oxygen for 40 hourly sessions had significant improvements compared to the control group of 21% oxygen at 1.03 absolute atmosphere.[28] This study has subsequently come under great scrutiny for several reasons including the fact that, according to the definition of HBO_2 set forth by the UHMS, this study did not use HBO_2 at all. Additionally, the assessment tools used have no widely accepted levels of improvement that would be considered clinically significant.[2] A subsequent randomized, blinded, controlled trial of HBO_2 as a treatment for autism spectrum disorder using levels of therapy consistent with the UHMS definition of HBO_2 concluded that there was no clinically significant benefit of HBO_2.[30] Thorough literature reviews of this topic have independently concluded that there is insufficient evidence to recommend HBO_2 for autism spectrum disorder, and the existing evidence showing treatment benefit is extremely weak including only the one, likely flawed, randomized controlled study showing some benefit.[23,10] The UHMS currently agrees with these reviews and currently does not recommend routine treatment of autism spectrum disorder with HBO_2.[2]

Cerebral Palsy

In 2014, a controlled longitudinal study showed improvements in gross motor function in children with cerebral palsy with intensive rehabilitation combined with HBO_2 beyond those observed with intensive rehabilitation alone.[25] These results opposed the findings of a previous study by Lacey et al. which compared HBO_2 to a control group without any other interventions and found no significant improvements in the HBO_2 group.[19] The official position of the UHMS regarding this matter was last updated in November 2003, and at that time use of HBO_2 for cerebral palsy was not supported.[13] The UHMS has continued to evaluate this use and has taken into account these and other more recent studies, and the use of HBO_2 for treatment of cerebral palsy continues to lack sufficient evidence to be supported.[24]

Traumatic Brain Injury

The use of HBO_2 for the treatment of traumatic brain injury has been occurring sporadically since 1965. Although several adult studies have been published, there currently has been no clear correlation between HBO_2 and improved neurologic outcomes, and as such, the treatment of traumatic brain injury with HBO_2 is not currently recommended by the UHMS.[29,13,24]

OXYGEN ADMINISTRATION SCHEDULES

Detailed studies have clearly defined the safe limits of exposure to hyperbaric oxygen for adults. As yet, no such study has been carried out to delineate these limits for pediatric age groups. Based on the literature describing the hyperbaric treatment of children, as well as practical experience, they do not in general appear to be at increased risk for developing pulmonary or neurological oxygen toxicity. Currently, adult treatment tables are used in the treatment of pediatric patients, and there is no evidence to support that oxygen administration tables need to be routinely altered for the treatment of pediatric patients.[7]

CONCLUSION

As the use of hyperbaric oxygen increases in clinical practice, the likelihood of being asked to treat children grows. The chance of a facility needing to treat children with carbon monoxide poisoning emergently is virtually 100%. Being prepared for this eventuality will improve patient safety and reduce stress on the staff. All units should have skilled, experienced personnel and suitable equipment available for advanced life support, in-chamber oxygen administration, and ventilation. Additionally, establishment of a working relationship with a pediatrician or pediatric facility is beneficial.

REFERENCES

1. Assali NS, Kirschbaum TH, Dilts PV Jr. Effects of hyperbaric oxygen on uteroplacental and fetal circulation. Circ Res. 1968;22:573-88.
2. Bennett M, Hart B. UHMS position paper: the treatment of autism spectrum disorder with hyperbaric oxygen therapy. Undersea Hyperb Med. 2009.
3. Chen M et al. Infection, oxygen, and immaturity: interacting risk factors for retinopathy of prematurity. Neonatology. 2011;99(2):125-32.
4. Clower JH et al. Recipients of hyperbaric oxygen treatment for carbon monoxide poisoning and exposure circumstances. Am J Emerg Med. 2012;30:846-51.
5. Cote CJ, Wilson S. Guidelines for monitoring and management of pediatric patients before, during, and after sedation for diagnostic and therapeutic procedures: update 2016. Pediatr Dent. 2016;38(4):13-39..
6. Decker DB, Karam JA, Wilcox DT. Pediatric hemorrhagic cystitis [review]. J Pediatr Urol. 2009;5:254-64.
7. Frawley G et al. Australian paediatric hyperbaric oxygen therapy. Anaesth Intensive Care. 2013;41(1):74-81.
8. Frawley G et al. Australian paediatric hyperbaric oxygen therapy. Anaesth Intensive Care. 2015;41(1):74-81.
9. Frawley GP, Fock A. Pediatric hyperbaric oxygen therapy in Victoria, 1998-2010. Pediatr Crit Care Med. 2012;13(4).
10. Ghanizadeh A. Hyperbaric oxygen therapy for treatment of children with autism: a systematic review of randomized trials. Med Gas Res. 2012;2(13).
11. Hadanny A et al. Seizures during hyperbaric oxygen therapy: retrospective analysis of 62,614 treatment sessions. Undersea Hyperb Med. 2016;43(1):21-8.
12. Higgins RD. 50 years ago in the Journal of Pediatrics: incidence of retrolental fibroplasias: past and present. J Pediatr. 2006;148(6).
13. Hyperbaric oxygen therapy for chronic brain injury. Undersea Hyperb Med. 2003.
14. Inanmaz ME et al. Can hyperbaric oxygen be used to prevent deep infections in neuro-muscular scoliosis surgery? BMC Surg. 2014;14(85).
15. Johnston DL, Waldhausen JHT, Park JR. Deep soft tissue infections in the neutropenic pediatric oncology patient. J Pediatr Hematol Oncol. 2001;23(7): 443-7.
16. Keenan HT et al. Delivery of hyperbaric oxygen therapy to critically ill, mechanically ventilated children. J Crit Care. 1998;13(1):7-12.
17. King E, Chun R, Sulman C. Pediatric cervicofacial necrotizing fasciitis a case report and review of a 10-year national pediatric database. Arch Otolaryngol Head Neck Surg. 2012;138(4):372-5.
18. Koller D, Goldman R. Distraction techniques for children undergoing procedures: a critical review of pediatric research. J Pediatr Nurs. 2012;27:652-81.
19. Lacey DJ, Stolfi A, Pilati LE. Effects of hyperbaric oxygen on motor function in children with cerebral palsy. Ann Neurol. 2012;72(5):695-703.
20. Latham E. Medscape [Internet]. Hyperbaric oxygen therapy; 2016 July 22 [cited 2016 August 5]. http://emedicine.medscape.com/article/1464149-overview
21. Lefebvre JC et al. Bench testing of a new hyperbaric chamber ventilator at different atmospheric pressures. Intensive Care Med. 2012;38:1400-4.
22. Lucey JF, Dangman B. A reexamination of the role of oxygen in retrolental fibroplasia. Pediatrics. 1984;76:339-44.

23. Martin R et al. Using hyperbaric oxygen for autism treatment: a review and discussion of the literature. Undersea Hyperb Med. 2015;42(4):353-9.

24. Mitchell SJ, Bennett MH. Unestablished indications for hyperbaric oxygen therapy. Diving Hyperb Med. 2014;44(4):228-34.

25. Mukherjee A et al. Intesive rehabilitation combined with HBO_2 therapy in children with cerebral palsy: a controlled longitudinal study. Undersea Hyperb Med. 2014;41(2):77-85.

26. PRESSURE. Newsletter of the Undersea and Hyperbaric Medical Society, Inc. 1989 May/June.

27. Ricci B, Calogero G. Oxygen-induced retinopathy in newborn rats: effects of prolonged normobaric and hyperbaric oxygen supplementation. Pediatrics. 1988;82:193-8.

28. Rossignol DA et al. Hyperbaric treatment for children with autism: a multicenter, randomized, double-blind, controlled trial. BMC Pediatr. 2009;9(21).

29. Sahni T et al. Use of hyperbaric oxygen in traumatic brain injury: retrospective analysis of data of 20 patients treated at a tertiary care centre. Br J Neurosurg. 2012;26(2):202-7.

30. Sampanthavivat M et al. Hyperbaric oxygen in the treatment of childhood autism: a randomised controlled trial. Diving Hyperb Med. 2012;42(3):128-33.

31. Sanchez EC. Use of hyperbaric oxygenation in neonatal patients. Crit Care Nurs Q. 2012;36(3):280-9.

32. Sanchez EC, Myers RAM. Hyperbaric oxygen therapy in the pediatric patient, a 20 year experience. Undersea Biomed Res. 1992;19(Suppl):109.

33. Sanchez EC. Case presentations. National Meeting of Pediatric Critical Care; 1988 Sept 12-15; Veracruz.

34. Shilton H, Hodgson M, Burgess G. Hyperbaric oxygen therapy for sudden sensorineural hearing loss in large vestibular aqueduct syndrome. J Laryngol Otol. 2014;128(Suppl S1):S50-4.

35. Smith-Slatas CL, Borque M, Salazar JC. Clostridium septicum infections in children: a case report and review of the ilterature. Pediatrics. 2006;117(4).

36. Thomson L, Paton J. Mini-symposium: oxygen and infancy: oxygen toxicity. Paediatr Respir Rev. 2014;15(2):120-3.

37. Tin W, Hey E. The medical use of oxygen: a century of research in animals and humans. NeoReviews. 2003;4(12):E349-55.

38. UHMS Indications for Hyperbaric Oxygen Therapy [Internet]. North Palm Beach (FL): Undersea and Hyperbaric Medical Society; 2016 [cited 2016 August 03]. Available from: https://www.uhms.org/resources/hbo-indications.html

CHAPTER 12 CHAPTER

The Role of Oxygen and Hyperbaric Oxygen Mechanisms

CHAPTER TWELVE OVERVIEW

PART 1: Wound Oxygenation and an Introduction to Hyperbaric Oxygen Therapy; Interventions for the Hypoxic/Ischemic Wound

Introduction **239**

Oxygen Requirements for Wound Healing and Infection Control **239**

Interventions to Increase Blood Flow and Oxygen Delivery to Wounds **243**

Evaluation of Wound Perfusion and Oxygenation 243

Improving Perfusion-Oxygenation through Revascularization Techniques 244

Improving Perfusion-Oxygenation through Edema Reduction 246

Improving Perfusion-Oxygenation through Medical Interventions 249

Improving Perfusion-Oxygenation through Rheological Interventions 249

Improving Perfusion-Oxygenation through Hyperbaric Oxygen **251**

Summary **253**

PART 2: Primary Mechanisms of Hyperbaric Oxygen; Hyperoxygenation and Pressurization

Introduction **255**

Hyperoxygenation **256**

Blood Oxygen Content and Henry's Law **256**

Arterial-Venous Oxygen Extraction **258**

Hyperoxygenation Physiology **259**

Clinical Applications of Hyperoxygenation **260**

Oxygen Transfer through Relative Barriers 260

Gas Washout 261

Compensation for Decreased Oxygen-Carrying Capacity in the Blood 261

Mass Effect of Hyperoxygenation **262**

Mitigation of Sluggish Perfusion in the Microcirculation with Hyperbaric Oxygen **264**

Clinical Aspects of Hyperoxygenation **266**

Topical Oxygen 268
Pressurization Effects 270
Summary 271

PART 3: Secondary Mechanisms of HBO_2 – Tissue Consequences of Hyperoxygenation and Pressurization

Introduction 272
Secondary Effects of Hyperbaric Oxygen 273
Vasoconstriction 273
Host Cellular Functions 276
Microbiological Applications of Hyperbaric Oxygen 282
Mitigation of the Reperfusion Injury 285
Gas Washout (and Isobaric Counter Diffusion) 286
Other Theoretical Secondary Mechanisms of Hyperbaric Oxygen 289
Red Blood Cell Deformability 289
Alteration of the Blood-Brain Barrier 290
Conclusions 292
Acknowledgments 293
References 294

The Role of Oxygen and Hyperbaric Oxygen Mechanisms

Michael B. Strauss, Lientra Q. Lu

PART 1

WOUND OXYGENATION AND AN INTRODUCTION TO HYPERBARIC OXYGEN THERAPY; INTERVENTIONS FOR THE HYPOXIC/ISCHEMIC WOUND

INTRODUCTION

Wound oxygenation is an essential strategy for the management of wounds regardless of their severity. Fortunately, in most wound healing situations, autoregulatory mechanisms ensure that oxygen is adequate to meet metabolic requirements. When not adequate, wound healing may be impeded or even totally interrupted, infection may not be controlled, and tissues may die, leading to limb amputations. Wound oxygenation is a function of perfusion. This part of the three-part series discusses oxygen requirements for wound healing and control of infection and methods (and their rationale) for augmenting wound perfusion-oxygenation and introduces the subject of hyperbaric oxygen (HBO_2) as a tactic for mitigating hypoxia in wounds in particular and in other conditions where HBO_2 is useful in general.

OXYGEN REQUIREMENTS FOR WOUND HEALING AND INFECTION CONTROL

Two sources of information demonstrate the critical role oxygen has for wound healing and infection control. This first arises from T.K. Hunt and his associates, who showed that for these processes to occur, juxta-wound tissue fluid oxygenation tensions in the 30 to 40 mmHg range are required (Figure 1).[7-11,14] Others have used this information for making decisions at what levels lower limb amputations are likely to heal.[27] If the juxta-wound oxygen tension is less than 30 mmHg, healing is unlikely. In these situations, methods to improve wound oxygenation and perfusion need to be employed for wound healing to occur. If the juxta-wound oxygen tensions are between 30 and 40 mmHg, wound healing may occur depending on the characteristics of the wound and the wound management. Wound management is optimized by employing five strategies which include 1) debridements and other surgical care for the wound base,

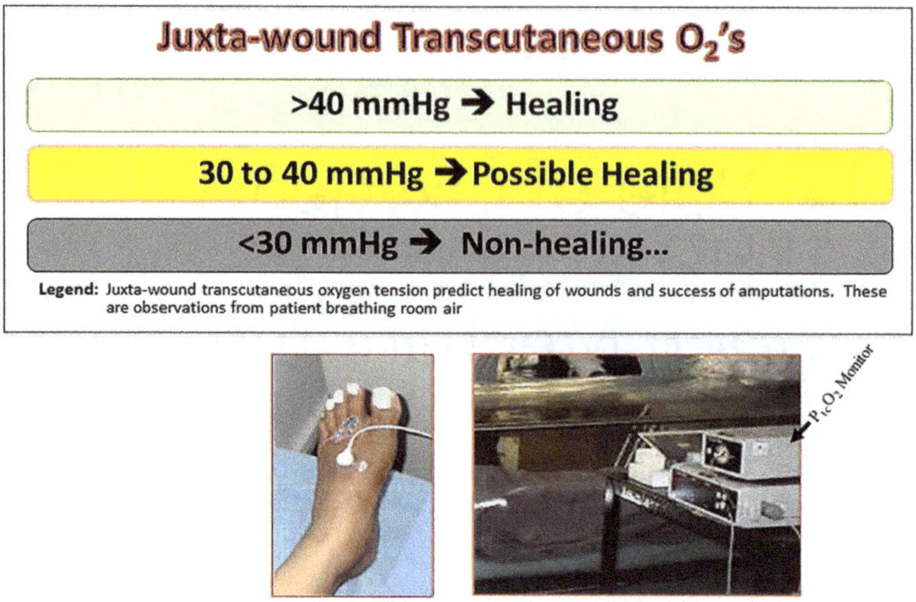

Figure 1. Use of transcutaneous O_2 measurements to predict wound healing.

TABLE 1. THE FIVE STRATEGIES FOR MANAGEMENT OF THE PROBLEM WOUND

Strategy	Providers	Goals	Comments
Medical Management	Primary care physicians (PCP's), medical specialists, nutritionists	Make the host (i.e. the patient) as healthy as possible	PCP's for impairments; specialists for decompensating conditions
Preparation of the Wound Base	Surgeons, wound care providers, physical therapists	Make the wound environment as healthy as possible	Achieved through debridements and precise surgical procedures
Protection & Stabilization of the Wound	Orthopaedists, podiatrists, cast technicians, orthotists	Rest & protect the wound environment	Often neglected; most likely strategy to lead to complications
Selection of Wound Dressing Agents	Wound care providers	Optimize dressing agent choice for the particular healing stage of the wound	Over 3,000 options! As wounds improve dressing choices--preferred agents change
Wound Oxygenation	Medicine specialists, vascular surgeons, interventional radiologists, hyperbaric medicine physicians, pharmacists	Improve perfusion and oxygenation to the wound site	Tactics include improving cardiac function, reducing edema, angioplasty/ revascularization, hyperbaric O_2 and pharmacological interventions

2) protection and stabilization of the wound, 3) appropriate medical management, 4) selection of the most appropriate wound dressing agents, and 5) augmentation of wound oxygenation (Table 1). The latter strategy is the focus of this three-part chapter.

The second source of information regarding perfusion-oxygen needs for wound healing arises from indirect information. It is obvious that markedly increased blood flow and oxygen availability are required to heal a wound and control infection.[19] Perfusion and oxygen requirements are minimal for noncritical tissues that do not have wounds or infections because they are in a steady-state, resting status. An example of this would be the feet of the patient with advanced peripheral artery disease. If a relatively minor wound occurs in one foot, healing may not occur, and a lower limb amputation becomes necessary. In contrast, in the opposite limb that does not have a wound, but perfusion is equally poor, the foot is not immediately at risk for an amputation.

Observations such as this have led us to conclude that perfusion-oxygen and metabolic requirements for wound healing and resolution of infection need to increase 20-fold or more. This is based on several anatomic and physiologic explanations. The first is the reserve capacity of the vascular tree that is highly regulated by activity of the sympathetic nervous system coupled with metabolic demands. An average-sized human has a blood volume of approximately five liters. The calculated potential capacity of the vascular system is over 20 liters when every vascular component such as arteries, veins, sinusoids, arterial-venous shunts, and bone marrow are maximally filled with blood.[(4,12)] From this information, we reason that there is the potential to increase blood flow to a noncritical tissue with increased metabolic demands (for example, for wound healing and/or managing infection) that approaches a factor of 20. This is further supported by the classical findings of hyperemia, increased temperature, and swelling/engorgement (i.e., rubor, calor, and tumor) observed in healing wounds. Another observation of how much blood flow can increase is observed in skeletal muscle. Greater than 20-fold increases in muscle blood flow have been observed between resting states and maximal exercise.[(4)]

With respect to infections, during the oxygen bust to kill bacteria in the phagocyctic vesicle, oxygen uptake increases more than a hundredfold.[(1,5,17-18)] This increased oxygen requirement, of necessity, arises through the mechanism of increased blood flow. During healing of fractures, blood flow increases six- to eightfold. Cardiac outputs have the ability to increase fivefold through filling and rate changes. From the pathology lab, we have observed blood vessels whose lumens were reduced more than 80% from atherosclerosis, yet amputations did not become necessary until wound problems developed (Figure 1). Many revascularizations occlude with time after wound healing has occurred. Usually, the limb is not in jeopardy because of the decreased metabolic demands tissues have after healing and infection control. The growth of collateral vessels, even though perfusion may be a fraction of what the normal perfusion was, is sufficient to meet steady-state metabolic demands. Finally, even with tenfold increases in tissue fluid oxygenation that HBO_2 provides, some wounds do not heal (Figure 2). This suggests that a factor over tenfold is necessary to achieve wound healing and infection control. When observations such as these are

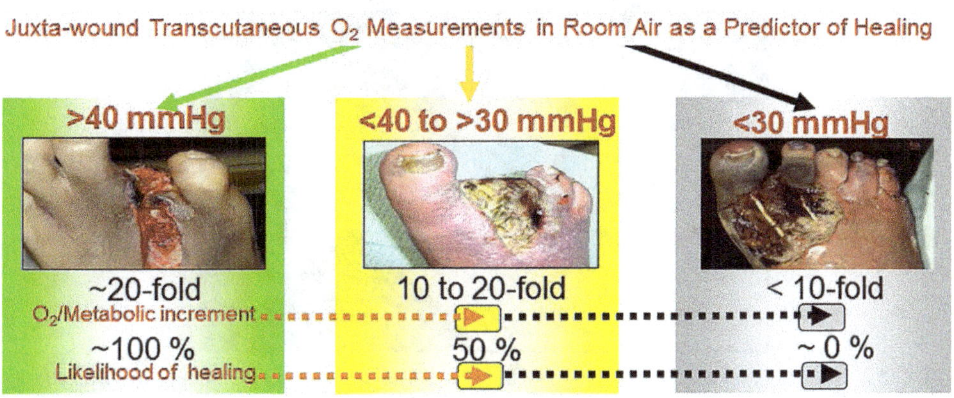

LEGEND: Juxta-wound transcutaneous oxygen ($P_{tc}O_2$'s) measurements predict which wounds will heal. The ability to increase O_2 and metabolic activity in the wound is reflected by the juxta-wound $P_{tc}O_2$'s.

Figure 2. Increments in oxygen and metabolic activity for wound healing to occur.

considered, increased blood flow and oxygen deliver to heal the wound approaches the 20-fold number stated above.

There are eight potential reasons why perfusion and oxygen delivery are not able to increase to levels sufficient for healing in "problem wounds," especially those in diabetics (Table 2). Many of these are remedial, as will be discussed later in this chapter. The most prevalent reason for the inability to increase blood flow and oxygen delivery is atherosclerosis with narrowing of lumen of the blood vessel either with plaques, localized obstructions, or diffuse calcification along the blood vessel, i.e., "arteriogram effect" seen on plain X-rays (Figure 3). Although flow in such vessels may be adequate for steady-state, non-wound-healing situations, it does not have the potential to increase enough to meet the demands for wound healing and infection control. Revascularizations including angioplasty, stenting, and bypass surgery are used to improve perfusion. Hyperbaric oxygen improves oxygen delivery to the wound site through its hyperoxygenation mechanism. Medical interventions also have the ability to increase perfusion and oxygen delivery to tissues as will be described next.

TABLE 2. ETIOLOGIES OF IMPAIRED PERFUSION

Condition	Effects, Comments, Causes
Peripheral artery disease	Decreased flow; inability to increase flow for the demands of wound healing, infection control or activity
Trauma	Physical disruption and/or injury to the vessel
Outflow obstruction	Venous stasis disease, external compression (casts/tourniquets), fluid retention and compartment syndromes
Vasculitis, Raynaud's	Associated with collagen vascular diseases; sympathetic (vasoconstriction) over activity may be a component
Thromboembolism	Associated with hyper coagulation conditions
Hypotension	Cardiac, hypovolemia, anemia & septic causes
Vasospasm	Associated with trauma, hypothermia & surgery
Medication induced	Ergotamine, alpha adrenergic agents, medication infiltrations and nicotine (smoking)

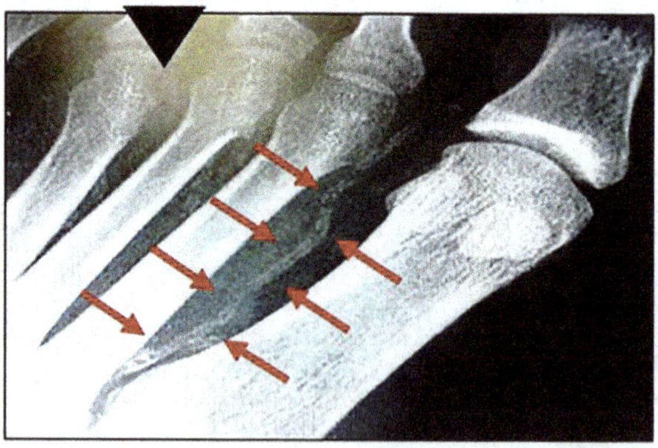

LEGEND: The calcified vessel is no longer able to dilate in response to increased metabolic demands. The atherosclerotic narrowed lumen is able to carry enough blood to meet the low demands of steady-state needs. If infection and/or a wound develops in the foot, perfusion may not be able to increase enough to meet the new demands.

Figure 3. Arteriogram effect from atherosclerosis arteriogram effect from atherosclerosis.

INTERVENTIONS TO INCREASE BLOOD FLOW AND OXYGEN DELIVERY TO WOUNDS

Adequate wound perfusion and its delivery of oxygen to the healing tissues is fundamental to wound healing as just explained. Revascularization invariably is the first intervention considered to achieve this goal. Hyperbaric oxygen all too often is not considered in the management. In addition, other interventions can improve perfusion-oxygenation (Table 3). These include edema reduction, improvement in cardiac function through medical management, and enhanced blood rheology using pharmacological methods. In contrast to the other four treatment strategies where typically a single technique is utilized, the methods to improve the perfusion-oxygenation strategy are complimentary, and typically two or more techniques are employed simultaneously.

TABLE 3. MEASURES TO INCREASE PERFUSION AND OXYGENATION

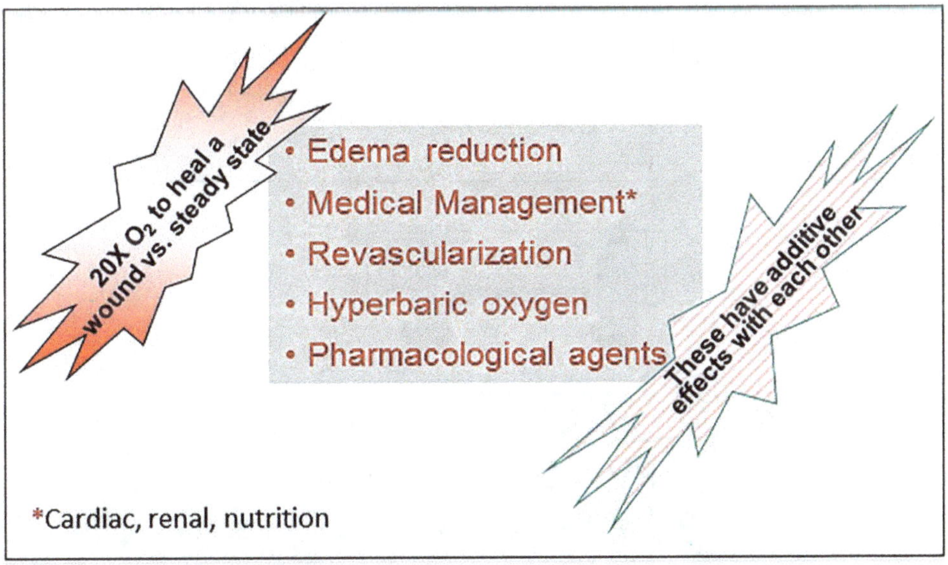

Evaluation of Wound Perfusion and Oxygenation

Determination of blood flow is always a crucial component of the wound evaluation. Important considerations in the history that suggest wound perfusion-oxygenation is not adequate include failure of the wound to improve or infection to be controlled, claudication and/or rest pain, need to keep knee in the hyper-flexed position when lying in bed, and need to hang the leg over the end of the bed to mitigate pain. Examination findings include nonpalpable or barely palpable pulses, rubor (i.e., red but cold skin), dusky or pale appearance of the periwound integument, cool to cold temperature of the skin, and delayed capillary refill. The Doppler is a useful technique to determine perfusion especially when edema, obesity, scar tissue, and/or previous surgeries obscure the palpation of pulses. The latter three findings are the secondary (to pulses) techniques to assess wound perfusion-oxygenation (Table 4). Tertiary techniques to evaluate perfusion-oxygenation include angiography with or without computerized tomography or contrast agents. Juxta-wound transcutaneous oxygen (TCOMs) and carbon dioxide

TABLE 4. PRIMARY, SECONDARY, AND TERTIARY METHODS TO ASSESS PERFUSION

Technique	2 Points	1 Point	0 Points
	Point grading in conjunction with the Wound Score		
Primary Assessment			
Pulses	Palpable	Doppler	Non-detectable or monophasic Doppler
Secondary Assessments			
Temperature	Warm	Cool	Cold
Coloration	Pink, rosy	Dusky, pale	Cyanotic, purplish, black
Capillary Refill	< 2 Seconds	2-5 Seconds	> 5 Seconds
Tertiary Assessments			
Juxta-wound Transcutaneous O_2's	< 40 mmHg	30-40 mmHg	< 30 mmHg
Imaging studies	Descriptions of findings		

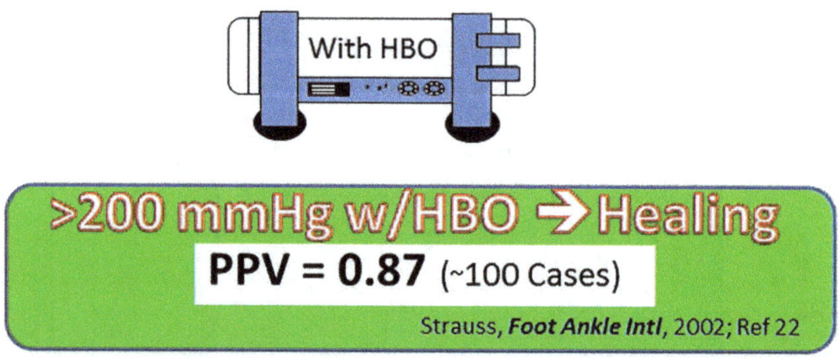

LEGEND: If the juxta-wound transcutaneous oxygen measurement exceeds 200 mmHg with HBO_2, we observed that nearly 90% of the hypoxic wounds healed regardless of the room air readings. In this sense, HBO_2 is both a diagnostic tool and a therapeutic agent.

Figure 4. Using a hyperbaric oxygen challenge to predict healing of the ischemic/ hypoxic wound.

measurements are another tertiary technique to assess wound oxygenation directly and wound perfusion indirectly. Wound healing is likely to occur if TCOMs are over 40 mmHg in room air and, if not, if over 200 mmHg with a hyperbaric oxygen (HBO_2) challenge and continuation of HBO_2 treatments (Figure 4).[22]

Improving Perfusion-Oxygenation through Revascularization Techniques

The value of arterial revascularization for the ischemic wound is without question. Techniques include angioplasty, stenting, and bypass surgery. Great advancements have been made in angioplasty equipment, and now this minimally invasive procedure, when feasible, is especially useful even in medium-sized and small-sized arteries. The vascular surgeon with experience in distal bypass surgeries can be an invaluable asset to the wound team and can often make the difference whether healing is successful or not. Obviously, without adequate perfusion, wound healing is impossible. Lower limb amputation then becomes the option for the nonhealing wound. We label the severely ischemic-hypoxic wound the "end-stage" wound. So-called "last resort" revascularizations may be attempted. Last-resort bypass surgeries are undertaken with the patient and/or family informed that if revascularization is not feasible (e.g., inadequate outflow at the distal end of the revascularization), a lower limb amputation will be done at the time of surgery. The patient's function and goals are critical determinants in the decision to attempt salvage of the end-stage wound. They can be quantified with our user-friendly Wellness Host and Goal Scores (see descriptions of these scoring in tools in our diabetic foot wound chapter 21).[25]

The challenge is the situations where the perfusion is marginal, but revascularization is not feasible or will only be of limited value. Predictors of failure in lower extremity revascularizations include 1) impaired ambulation before surgery (an assessment in the patient's Wellness Score), 2) serious medical problems such as end-stage kidney disease and/or decompensated heart disease (another Host Score assessment), 3) hyperlipidemia, 4) gangrene, and 5) bypass surgery distal to the trifurcation area.[6] Likewise, success of the revascularization should not only be measured by patency of the graft, but also by wound healing, not any need for additional bypass surgery, independent living status, and continued ability to ambulate.[6]

Revascularization for the patient with peripheral artery disease is not always an option, and, if it is an option, does not always provide sufficient blood flow to ensure healing. About ⅓ of the patients in our experiences who have ischemia-hypoxia severe enough that wound healing is not occurring are either not candidates for revascularization, or, if it has been done, the improved blood flow is insufficient to meet the metabolic demands for wound healing. This is related to diffuse vessel disease, microangiopathy, or both. The result is the inability to meet the estimated 20-fold increment in perfusion-oxygenation required for wound healing.

While some may dispute that microangiopathy is a factor in wound perfusion-oxygenation problems, it cannot be discounted in those patients whose wounds do not improve after revascularization. Microangiopathy occurs distal to the distal extent of any possible vascular repair. That is, the vessel disease is occurring in vessels that qualify as microvasculature since loupes or surgical microscopes are needed to visualize blood

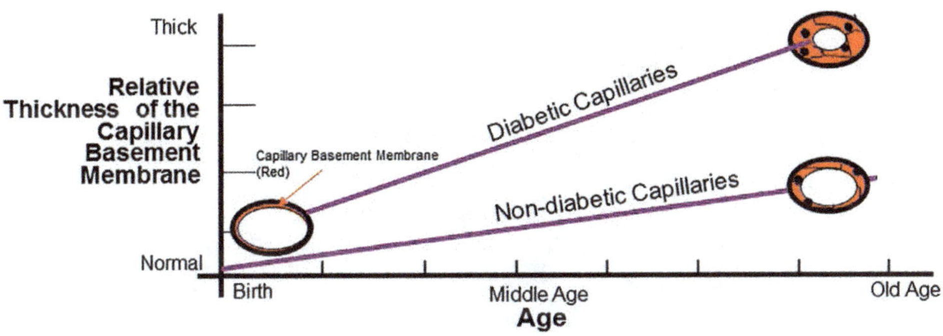

LEGEND: The capillary basement membrane (depicted in red) thickens as a person ages. This processes accelerates in diabetic patients. The thickened basement membrane becomes a diffusion barrier to oxygen and other substances that must move from the capillary to the cell and vice verse. The thickened capillary basement membrane meets the definition of microangiopathy.

Figure 5. Thickening of the capillary basement membrane with aging and in diabetics.

vessels at these levels. In addition, thickening of the capillary basement membrane, a phenomenon of aging and accelerated in diabetics, is an undisputable example of microangiopathy (Figure 5).[2,20]

The consequence of not being able to perform revascularization, or, if done, its benefits not being immediately apparent does not always make a lower limb amputation necessary. This is because optimal wound management, including the concomitant use of the other tactics to supplement wound perfusion-oxygenation, often leads to slow, sustained improvement of the wound.[24] In these situations, the wound is observed to pass through four definable stages. Each stage may take days to months to occur. In other situations, the patient may opt to live with a chronic, stable wound that only requires minimal wound care in deference to an amputation.[24] Finally, minimally invasive, often percutaneous (as an outpatient or bedside), procedures can be done to promote healing without appreciably increasing metabolic demands for wound healing. Examples include percutaneous tenotomies, debridements of fibrous and/or biofilm coverings of the wound base, use of sutures to partially approximate the wound edges, ostectomies to eliminate bone extending beyond the soft-tissue margins, narrowing of forefoot with external fixation for obliterating cavitary defects, and percutaneous drilling of metatarsal necks with controlled fracture through the drill holes to off-load malperforans ulcers under metatarsal heads.[21]

Improving Perfusion-Oxygenation through Edema Reduction

Edema can lead to three causes of wound ischemia and hypoxia. First, edema increases the diffusion distance of oxygen and nutrients from the capillary to the target cell (Figure 6). Oxygen diffuses relatively poorly through tissue fluids, especially as compared to carbon dioxide, which has 20 times the diffusing capacity in tissue fluids as oxygen does.[3] Oxygen tensions in tissue fluids decrease rapidly as the diffusion distance increases. The falloff is calculated to be proportional to the square root of the oxygen concentration in the tissue fluids adjacent to the capillary.[16] Consequently, edema

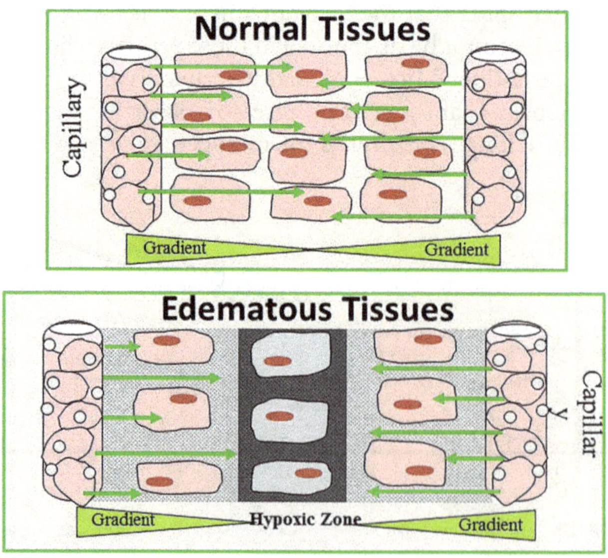

LEGEND: Edema increases the diffusion distance O_2 needs to travel from capillaries to target cells. With increased diffusion distance, the distance O_2 must diffuse exceeds the gradient of O_2 fall-off from the capillary. Cells then reside in a hypoxic environment.

Figure 6. Oxygen diffusion from capillary to cell through normal and edematous tissues.

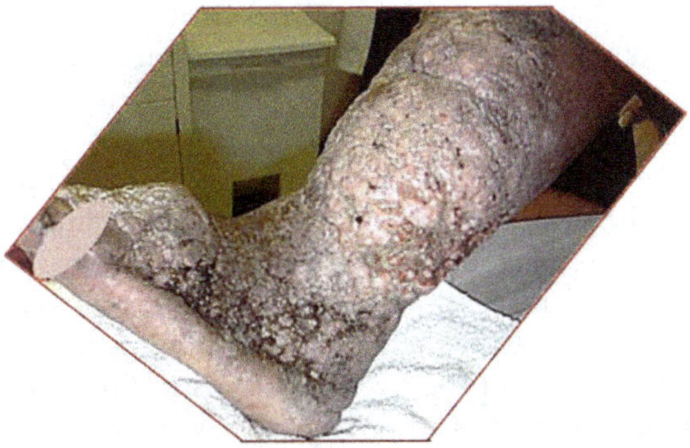

LEGEND: Limb edema has undergone metaplasia from soft pitting, to brawny, to dense, almost avascular nodular cicatrix. Wraps are almost futile in mitigating the edema. If a wound develops, the patient is at risk of a leg amputation. Debridement to healthy fascia with delayed split thickness skin grafting is a consideration if other comorbidities are not contraindications for this surgery.

Figure 7. Limb edema that has evolved into dense, nodular cicatrix.

can severely interfere with oxygenation of cells and tissues and be very detrimental to wound healing and infection control.

Second, edema accumulation in closed, unyielding spaces such as myofascial compartments, within joint capsules (especially metatarsals), casts, tight bandages, and/or wounds encased with cicatrix can lead to collapse of the capillary circulation. When the microcirculation is collapsed from external pressure, flow ceases and all off-loading of oxygen and nutrients to tissues and exchange of waste products of metabolism is obliterated. This defines a compartment syndrome. While this problem is not typically observed in nonhealing wounds, it is associated with trauma to the extremities and prolonged ischemia times associated with delayed revascularizations from traumatic disruption of the blood vessel, thrombosis, or embolization. In the intermediate situation between no edema and an established compartment syndrome, edema interferes with wound oxygenation by increasing the distance-limited diffusion distance of oxygen.

Third, another harmful effect of edema is metaplasia from soft pitting, to brawny, to dense cicatrix especially with chronicity and associated hypoxia (Figure 7). Fibroblasts generate a dense cicatrix induced by transforming growth factor beta 1 (TGF-β1). This growth factor is expressed in hypoxic wounds and is postulated to be the reason fibroblasts form cicatrix (hard scar) rather than the more desirable soft, pliable scar generated by fibroblasts in normoxyic environments.[(15)]

Sclerosis is often found in radiation-associated wounds and is explained by fibrosis initiated by radiation damage to blood vessels. Cicatrix is a greater barrier to oxygen diffusion than edema. More importantly, in conjunction with wound healing, cicatrix becomes a barrier to angiogenesis and keratinization. Cicatrix obviously thwarts wound healing and provides justification for surgical removal of this "pathological" tissue to obtain wound healing. This is especially apparent in large, chronic venous stasis ulcers where skin grafting has been successful after optimizing edema, removing plate-like cicatrix to the myofascial level, and then skin grafting over a vascular bed free of cicatrix. We have observed this in patients who have had failed skin grafts over poorly vascularized cicatrix and/or failed to get ulcer healing with biologic wound-covering agents.

Edema reduction is accomplished by a variety of interventions, many of which can be done simultaneously and complement each other. The first is leg elevation. Patients with edema should be advised to avoid sitting with their feet in the dependent position or standing for sustained periods in one spot. Walking is encouraged, if feasible, because of the desirable effect of the "pumping action" of muscle activity on fluid mobilization plus the benefit of movement on cardiac and musculoskeletal function. This advice becomes a challenge when the patient sleeps in a chair because of spine or breathing problems. Often, the only out-of-bed activity that can be tolerated is sitting in a wheelchair because of the infirmities. The use of reclining chairs or motorized chairs with lower extremity lifts may mitigate these challenges. When the above impediments to lower extremity edema control exist, then other methods to control edema must be utilized.

The use of wraps or compression stockings is the next intervention to control edema. Elastic wraps require diligence. If put on too loosely, they are ineffective. If applied too tightly, they can impede circulation. With activity, they tend to slip and may require reapplication several times a day. If the patient is active, we advise rewrapping several times a day. Many times, the patient is too obese or lacks sufficient joint mobility to apply wraps himself or herself. In these situations, multilayer short-stretch wraps (e.g., Profore or Dynaflex) can be used and left in place for weekly or semiweekly changes, or the patient's caregivers can be taught how to apply and remove elastic wraps daily. If fluid accumulation from the wound is excessive, absorptive dressings are placed over the wound and moisture barrier agents such as zinc oxide applied around the wound edges to prevent maceration of adjacent skin.

Elastic support stockings should always be considered when lower extremity edema reduction is the goal, and wounds are not present. For many patients, their infirmities make it impossible to apply or remove the tightly fitting support hose, so other devices need to be employed. For legs that are not uniform in contour, custom-measured and -fitted stockings (e.g., Jobst) are advised. More user-friendly compression devices are those of two- to four-inch-wide elastic straps attached to a posterior spine of semi stiff material. Simple Velcro or interlocking buttonhole strapping make application and removal easy as well as accommodate almost any leg shape (Figure 8). The ultimate in compression devices, in our opinion, are the custom-fitted intermittent pneumatic devices. These are costly and not authorized for out-of-hospital use by many payers. They require precise application to be effective. Care for edema can be optimized

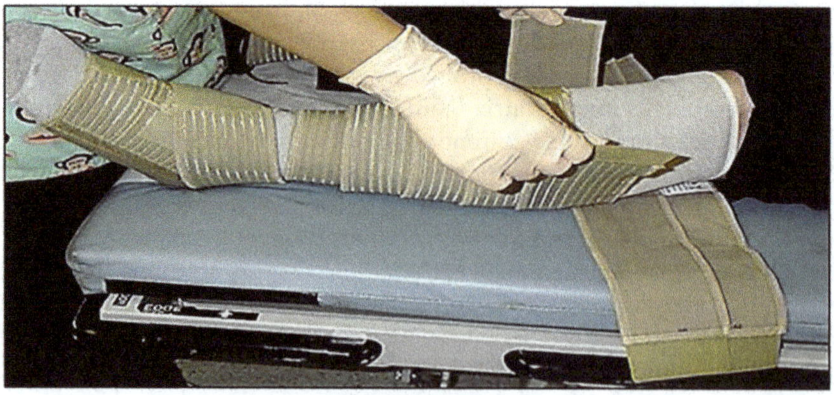

Hook and Loop Fastener (Velcro®)

LEGEND: The segmental straps make this leg compression easy to apply and remove. More importantly, the straps make it possible to apply effective compression to almost any shaped leg.

Figure 8. User-friendly segmental compression stocking.

at lymphedema clinics where all the above interventions may be used plus manual massage and brief applications of very constrictive bandaging to mobilize edema fluid.

Unfortunately, when edema has evolved to brawny and scarified enlargement of the legs and feet, interventions other than surgery are ineffective. Endovascular varicose and superficial to deep feeder vein occlusion with laser techniques may be effective in situations where edema is not massive, or the edema has not undergone metaplasia to scar tissue. In particular, this technique is useful when the varicosities or venous insufficiency sites are immediately proximal to a nonhealing venous stasis ulcer.

Improving Perfusion-Oxygenation through Medical Interventions

The third technique to reduce edema is through medical interventions. These include use of diuretics, medicines to manage congestive heart failure, antibiotics with reduction of inflammation from the infection, optimization of nutrition, and correction of hypoxia. In many patients with diabetic foot and leg wounds, heart failure and chronic kidney disease are comorbidities. Consequently, fluid mobilization may be a major-medical challenge. With those on dialysis, body water can be removed during dialysis sessions. Many patients with leg wounds have borderline heart failure. This can be verified with the brain natriuretic peptide (BNP) blood test and medical management assessed by serial measurements of this peptide. Infection, whether in soft tissues or bone, can also be a cause for edema associated with wounds. Obviously, appropriately selected antibiotics should be considered an edema reduction technique by reducing inflammation associated with the infection.

Optimizing nutrition must not be overlooked as an edema reduction technique. When visceral proteins, namely albumin and pre-albumin, are low, fluids shift from the intravascular compartments to the extravascular spaces. This contributes to edema; with improvements in nutrition, edema decreases. Nutrition can always be improved with increasingly more aggressive techniques ranging from food supplements, to feeding tubes, to percutaneous endoscopic gastrostomy, and finally to hyperalimentation. Salt reduction is another nutrition measure that needs to be managed in patients with edema. Hypoxia at the cell level initiates a chain of reactions starting with interference of metabolic responses, shifts in electrolytes (i.e., the sodium pump), loss of intracellular water to the extravascular spaces, and edema formation. The most apparent presentation of these events is in the patient with severe shock. All the techniques to improve wound oxygenation and edema reduction help to manage this cause of edema. Like the primary care physician and the medical specialists, the clinical nutrition specialist is an integral part of the wound team with respect to edema reduction.

Improving Perfusion-Oxygenation through Rheological Interventions

The term "rheological" applies to "flow of materials." For our purposes, we use this term to elaborate how pharmacological agents can be used to alter blood flow favorably. Five mechanisms, including red blood cell deformability, anti-adhesive/anti-sludging platelet effects, systemic vasodilatation, local vasodilatation, and anticoagulation, have the potential to favorably affect perfusion and oxygen delivery to tissues (Table 5). Whereas the beneficial effects of revascularization, edema reduction, and medical interventions can be readily appreciated and the effects of hyperbaric oxygen quantified with juxta-wound transcutaneous oxygen measurements, the effects of rheological agents on improving wound perfusion and oxygenation are more subtle. Their effects are largely at the microcirculation level, are slow to occur, and many times can only be surmised that they were beneficial in the healing of the ischemic-hypoxic wound.

TABLE 5. PHARMACOLOGICAL AGENTS TO IMPROVE PERFUSION AND OXYGENATION

- **RBC Deformability** Pentoxifylline (Trental®)
- **Anti-adhesive/platelet**
  - Acetylsalicylic acid (Bayers® Aspirin)
  - Clopidogrel (Plavix®)
- **Systemic vasodilators**
  - Nifedipine (Procardia®)
  - Xylocaine (Lidocaine®)
- **Local vasodilators**
  - Nitroglycerin paste/patch (Nitro-Bid®, Nitro-Dur®)
  - Cilostazol (Pletal®)
- **Anticoagulants**
  - Heparin
  - Enoxaparin (Lovenox®)
  - Warfarin (Coumadin®)

These agents often used in combination with each other and even more frequently in combination with other methods to improve perfusion such as revascularization

Generally, the agents are prescribed for reasons other than specifically to improve perfusion and oxygenation to the wound. For example, warfarin (Coumadin) may be ordered by the vascular surgeon after bypass surgery, clopidrogrel (Plavix) and aspirin by the cardiologist after coronary artery stenting, and enoxaparin (Lovenox) by the primary care physician to prevent deep vein thrombosis. If a coexistent ischemic-hypoxic wound is present, these agents may serendipitously improve perfusion and oxygenation to the wound. Two or more agents may be prescribed concurrently, such as clopidrogrel and aspirin for their additive effects on platelet antiaggregation or warfarin and pentoxifyline (Trental®) for different mechanisms that complement each other. For example, warfarin is used to maintain vessel patency (i.e., anticoagulation) after revascularization, while pentoxifyline promotes red blood cell deformity to improve flow through the microcirculation. Without deformation, the 7.5μ in diameter red blood cell will not be able to pass through the 5μ in diameter capillary and off-load its oxygen to cells.

After surgery, when skin flaps appear pale or dusky, nitroglycerin (Nitro-Dur®, Nitro-Bid®) patches may be useful for their local vasodilation effects. The patches are placed over the principal arteries supplying the ischemic portion of the flap and just proximal to the area of discoloration. They should be reapplied daily until the ischemic flap conditions stabilize. Our initial observations using juxta-wound transcutaneous oxygen measurements before and after applying nitroglycerin patches demonstrated that the transcutaneous oxygen measurements of the flaps improved after applying them.[23] Based on the mechanism of action of the nitroglycerin patch and these observations, this technique is used in conjunction with hyperbaric oxygen treatments when a flap appears threatened after surgery.

The pharmacological agents used to compliment blood flow may increase bleeding risks during surgeries, wound debridements at the bedside, or clinic visits. In the non-operating-room setting, short periods of direct pressure over the bleeding site, application of a compression dressing,and/or cauterization of the bleeding sites with silver nitrate applicators are usually sufficient to control bleeding. If the wound is cavitary, a wadded-up piece of Xeroform® tightly packed into the cavity has been an effective hemostatic technique for the wounds that continue to bleed after the simpler techniques were not effective. If these measures are not sufficient, then hemostatic agents such as Gelfoam and thrombin or Surgicel can be obtained from the operating room and placed on the bleeding sites and held in place with a compression dressing. If bleeding continues, placement of "hemostatic" (i.e., continued passes of the suture through the bleeding site, with simple ties/half hitches with each pass until bleeding controlled) or seton-like sutures proximal to the bleeding site and/or identifying, clamping and ligation of the pumping vessel are effective to control bleeding. Finally, tranexamic acid (Cyklokapron®, Lysteda®) given orally, intravenously, or locally applied aids in bleeding control. In the operating room, in addition to the previously mentioned measures, electrocautery and tourniquet application are available.

IMPROVING PERFUSION-OXYGENATION THROUGH HYPERBARIC OXYGEN

After revascularization, hyperbaric oxygen (HBO_2) therapy should be the next option considered in managing the ischemic-hypoxic wound and/or threatened flap. Hyperbaric oxygen has special merits when used as an adjunct for managing wound hypoxia. The merits are that it is both a therapeutic intervention as well as it can be a diagnostic tool for justifying HBO_2 treatments and predicting outcomes when used with transcutaneous oxygen measurements. These two considerations will be elaborated on in this part, while that of the physiology of hyperoxygenation and the secondary mechanisms of HBO_2 will appear in succeeding parts of this chapter.

Hyperbaric oxygen therapy is an inhalation therapy where the partial pressure is increased to levels that exceed what can be achieved by breathing pure oxygen in room air. This is achieved by having the patient breathe pure oxygen in a chamber

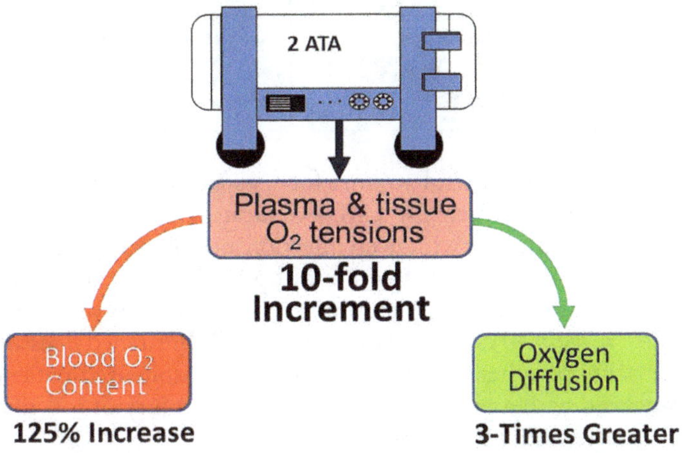

LEGEND: These clinical effects of hyperoxygenation are substantiated by physics and physiology. They provide the basis for understanding how it works and why it is beneficial for a multitude of medical problems.

Figure 9. Physiological benefits of hyperbaric oxygen.

pressurized to two to three atmospheres greater than sea level pressure. Most treatments are done at 2 or slightly greater atmospheres absolute pressure, which is equivalent to breathing pure oxygen at a 33-foot depth in sea water. The immediate effects are a tenfold increase in plasma oxygen content which, in turn, increases tissue fluid oxygen content tenfold and oxygen diffusion distance threefold (Figure 9).

The measurement of juxta-wound transcutaneous oxygen (TCOM) and carbon dioxide (CO_2) tensions in room air and with a hyperbaric oxygen challenge can predict outcomes in ischemic-hypoxic wounds and guide decision-making. The oxygen tensions reflect wound oxygenation, while the CO_2 tensions reflect perfusion. If juxta-wound TCOMs in room air are less than 40 mmHg, measurements should be repeated while the patient is undergoing a HBO_2 exposure. If the TCOMs exceed 200 mmHg, the positive predictive value for healing a wound is nearly 90%.[13,22] A simple, four-cell matrix simplifies decision-making for oxygen supplementation interventions (Table 6). If the TCOMs are in the normal range in room air, HBO_2 is not needed for its ability to improve tissue oxygenation. If the TCOMs are low in room air, but exceed 200 mmHg with the HBO_2 exposure, and the CO_2 tensions are in the normal range, healing is predicted with the adjunctive use of HBO_2. If oxygen tensions are normal in room air, but the CO_2 tensions are elevated, flow and/or oxygen extraction problems probably exist. Considerations to explain this observation include venous stasis disease, arterial-venous malformations, compartment syndromes, and/or anaerobic metabolism is occurring in the tissues. If the oxygen tensions are low with the HBO_2 challenge and the CO_2 tensions elevated, perfusion is inadequate to delivery oxygen as well as remove CO_2. In this permutation, healing is probably not possible without a successful revascularization.

TABLE 6. TRANSCUTANEOUS O_2 AND CO_2 TENSIONS FOR DECISION-MAKING IN USING HBO_2

Transcutaneous O_2 Measurements

CO_2 Measurements	Normal >40 mmHg	Low (<30 mmHg)
Normal 40 +/- 5 mmHg	**Healing with Room Air** Wound healing expected without the need for hyperbaric oxygen	**Healing with HBO** Hypoxic wound with enough perfusion to carry off CO_2, but inadequate O_2 for healing without HBO
High > 45 mmHg	**Special Situations** Outflow and/or O_2 utilization problems such as venous stasis, A-V shunts, compartment syndrome or anaerobic metabolism	**Revascularization or Limb Amputation** Hypoxic wound without enough perfusion to carry off CO_2 or provide enough O_2 for healing

Hyperbaric oxygen is a useful adjunct for six specific wound types, all of which are authorized for reimbursement by CMS/Medicare and most other payers. These include 1) diabetic foot wounds with deep infection and/or osteomyelitis (not showing signs of improvement after a 30-day period of optimal management), 2) progressive necrotizing soft-tissue infections, 3) chronic refractory osteomyelitis persisting after antibiotics and/or surgery, 4) clostridial myonecrosis, 5) threatened flaps and grafts after surgery, and 6) acute peripheral artery ischemia (in a hospitalized patient). Although not always associated with a problem wound, radiation injury of soft tissue and bone is an additional authorized use of HBO_2.

Hyperbaric oxygen has primary effects that are immediate, dose-duration related, and transient.[26] These include hyperoxygenation and the direct effects of pressure. Whereas the direct effects of pressure are usually associated with bubble reduction for decompression sickness and arterial gas embolism, this effect "drives" oxygen into the plasma and provides enhanced gradients for oxygen to diffuse from tissue fluids to the metabolizing target cells. Secondary effects of HBO_2 arise from the effects hyperoxygenation has on tissues. These effects are accumulative rather than dose-duration related, much like radiation therapy, and result in the healing and durable responses seen when the secondary effects of HBO_2 manifest themselves.

Hyperbaric oxygen has remarkably few side effects and contraindications. The most serious side effect is an oxygen induced seizure which occurs once in about every 10,000 treatments,. Middle-ear barotrauma from pressurization occurs in about ⅓ of the patients. Only a small percentage of patients who experience ear barotrauma with pressurization require placement of ventilation tubes through the tympanic membrane to continue HBO_2 treatments. Anxiety in the confines of the hyperbaric oxygen chamber is also observed. In the motivated, well-informed, and fully comprehending patient, the use of sedatives and counseling usually make it possible to continue treatments regardless of the patient's claustrophobia history. A fourth side effect is the transient decrease in distance visual acuity noted after 30 to 40 HBO_2 treatments with the concomitant improvement in near vision. These effects are usually transient, with vision returning to the pre-HBO_2 acuity levels six weeks to six months after completion of the HBO_2 treatments.

Contraindications to HBO_2 treatments may be absolute such as "do not resuscitate" code status, intra-aortic balloon pumps, an untreated major pneumothorax and severe shock requiring high doses of vasopressors, morbid obesity where repeated transfers to gurneys for HBO_2 treatments risk injury to the patient and/or the attendants transferring the patient, and uninterrupted breathing of oxygen percentages greater than 50%. This latter contraindication is due to the increased risk of pulmonary oxygen toxicity that might be precipitated by the added oxygen exposure to the lung tissue with HBO_2. Relative contraindications for HBO_2 treatments include smoking in between HBO_2 treatments, pregnancy (although not a contraindication for carbon monoxide poisoning), active cancer, and juxta-wound transcutaneous oxygen tensions that do not improve with a hyperbaric oxygen exposure. With relative contraindications, the decision to use HBO_2 depends on the seriousness of the problem, the wellness of the patient, and the patient's goals. Temporary contraindications are those conditions such as hyper- and hypoglycemia, hypovolemic shock, severe pain, or ear barotrauma, where established interventions are likely to mitigate the contraindication for HBO_2.

SUMMARY

Adequate wound oxygenation is essential for wound healing. It is one of the three confounders invariably associated with nonhealing wounds and probably the most critical of the three. Metabolism and blood flow must increase markedly (estimated to be about 20-fold) for wound healing and control of infection to occur. If less than this, the tissues may remain alive, but healing does not proceed. If drastically low, tissues die and amputations become necessary.

Much can be done to assess wound oxygen and perfusion with information from the history, examination (Table 3), and specialized testing including angiography and juxta-wound transcutaneous oxygen measurements. Likewise, there are five interventions that can improve perfusion-oxygenation to the wound, including revascularizations (angioplasty, stenting, and/or bypass surgery), edema reduction, optimization of medical management, use of pharmacological agents to affect blood rheology, and hyperbaric oxygen therapy.

The recognition and utilization of HBO_2 for management of problem wounds is gaining increasing recognition. Hyperbaric oxygen treatments are authorized by CMS/Medicare and most other insurance payers for the treatment of six specific, wound-related conditions. There are more than 1,400 wound treatment centers in the United States where HBO_2 therapy is available. Hyperbaric oxygen has double benefits in wound management. With the use of juxta-wound transcutaneous oxygen measurements, it can provide objective indications for when it should be used as well as predict outcomes. As a treatment modality, it increases tissue oxygen tensions tenfold. This increment, coupled with the other perfusion-oxygenation improving tactics, can make the difference whether or not the ischemic-hypoxic wounds heal.

PART 2

PRIMARY MECHANISMS OF HYPERBARIC OXYGEN; HYPEROXYGENATION AND PRESSURIZATION

INTRODUCTION

The effects of hyperbaric oxygen are achieved through its primary and secondary mechanisms (Table 7).[37] The primary mechanisms (hyperoxygenation and pressurization) begin exhibiting their effects as soon as pressurization begins in the hyperbaric chamber. The greater the pressure and the longer the duration of exposure, the more the effects will be manifested. In this sense, hyperbaric oxygen acts like a drug with a dose-duration effect (Figure 10).[26]

The primary mechanisms are the direct effects increased oxygen partial pressures, increased ambient pressures, or combinations of these have on tissue hypoxia and consequences of bubble-related phenomena (for example, arterial gas embolism and decompression sickness). The primary effects are transient. Once the hyperbaric exposure is completed, the effects decrease almost immediately. In contrast, the secondary mechanisms tend to be accumulative and long lasting. Secondary mechanisms occur due to the effects hyperoxia has on cellular functions as well as the effects increased ambient pressures have in producing gradients between gases in

> Is hyperbaric oxygen a drug? This is a debatable question. In terms of its hyperoxygenation effect, it could be considered such with its dose-duration effects. However, like radiation therapy, many of its secondary mechanisms are additive. For classification purposes, hyperbaric oxygen is labeled a respiratory gas rather than a drug. This has important ramifications for the hyperbaric medicine community. If it were considered a drug, any use of HBO_2 would need to go through phased trials before it could be used for other than off-label, nonformulary purposes.

TABLE 7. MECHANISMS OF HYPERBARIC OXYGEN

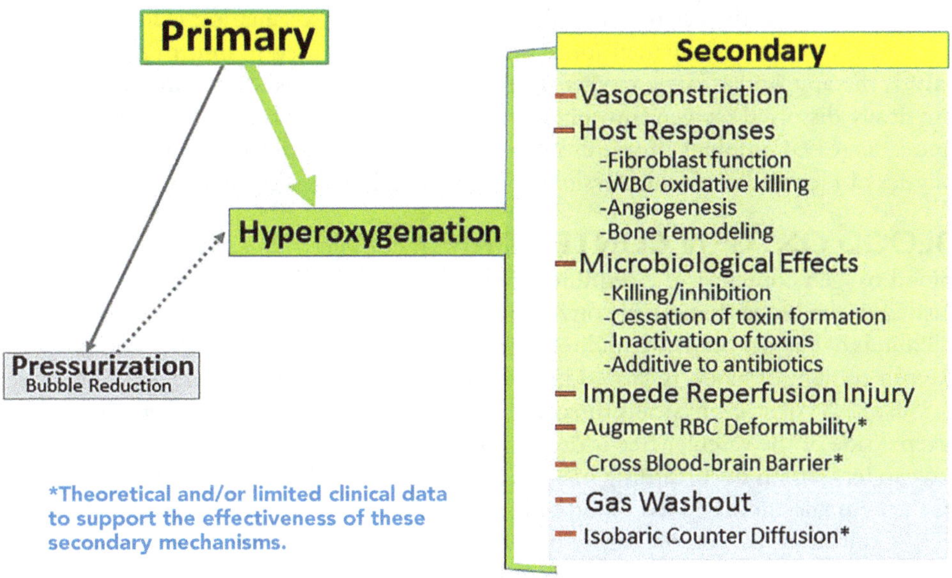

*Theoretical and/or limited clinical data to support the effectiveness of these secondary mechanisms.

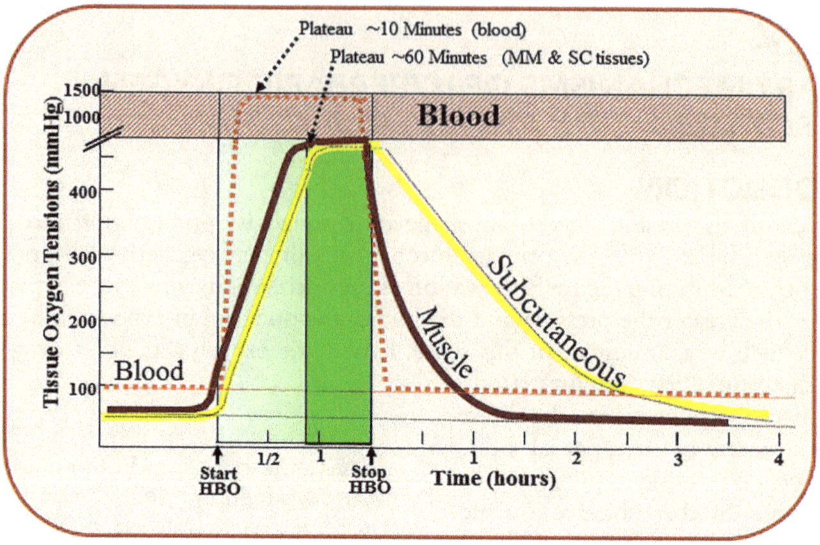

LEGEND: In many respects the hyperoxygenation effect of HBO_2 acts like a drug with its dose-duration effects. Oxygen tensions remain elevated in subcutaneous tissues for four hours after a hyperbaric O_2 exposure. It takes about an hour exposure to HBO_2 before the O_2 tensions in muscles (MM) and subcutaneous tissues (SC) plateau.

Figure 10. Dose-duration effects of hyperoxygenation.

body tissues. This chapter portion (Part 2) describes the physics and physiology of the primary mechanisms of hyperoxygenation and pressurization, both of which are direct effects of increased ambient pressure.

HYPEROXYGENATION

Increased oxygenation of hypoxic tissues is the fundamental and most important mechanism of HBO_2 therapy. Physics confirms how hyperoxygenation works. Physiology explains why it works. When the physics and physiology of hyperoxygenation are combined, there is sound justification for using HBO_2 in hypoxia-related conditions. When the use of HBO_2 is considered, hyperoxygenation is invariably the mechanism that is initially mentioned and the one that is used to inform patients how HBO_2 therapy works. Hyperoxygenation, in simplified terms, is the augmentation of physically dissolved oxygen into plasma and tissue fluids by breathing 100% oxygen under increased ambient pressure. Hyperoxygenation is appreciated by applying the physics of Henry's law to the physiology of the blood oxygen content.

BLOOD OXYGEN CONTENT AND HENRY'S LAW

Blood oxygen content is the terminology used for designating the amount of oxygen carried in the bloodstream. By convention, it is expressed in volumes percent, that is, milliliters of oxygen per 100 milliliters of blood. Normally 97.5%, or 19.5 vol%, of the oxygen content of blood is carried in the hemoglobin of the red blood cell. The other 2.5%, or 0.5 vol%, is physically dissolved in the plasma. Ordinarily, hemoglobin on the arterial side of the vascular tree is nearly fully saturated with oxygen, that is, increased oxygen tensions in the breathing medium do not increase the oxygen-carrying capacity of the hemoglobin in the red blood cell.

Conversely, oxygen physically dissolved in the plasma increases proportionally to increasing oxygen tensions in the breathing medium. Henry's law explains this effect,

In a liquid-gas system, the amount of gas that dissolves in the liquid is a function of the partial pressure of the gas in the system.

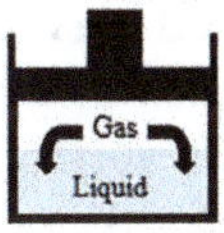

A piston with a liquid and gas phase is a good analogy to explain Henry's law. With compression of the gas phase by lowering the piston, more gas is forced into the liquid phase. Hyperoxygenation with HBO works in an analogous fashion.

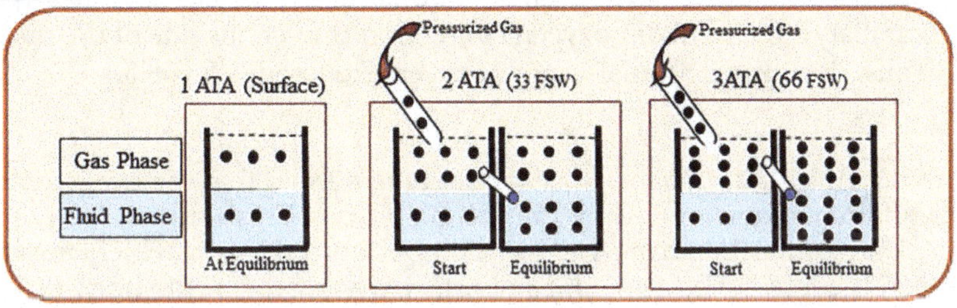

LEGEND: With pressurization of the gas phase of a liquid-gas system, gas is proportionally forced into the liquid phase. It takes time for the gas to come to equilibrium in the two phases. Other factors influence the amount and time that gas is forced into the liquid phase such as solubility coefficients and temperature. In the human the amount of blood flow to the region is a critical consideration for how quickly the breathing of HBO_2 comes into equilibrium with the extracellular tissue fluids. This explains the physics of hyperoxygenation with HBO_2 therapy and as illustrated in Figure 10, how HBO_2 acts like a drug with a dose-duration effect.

Figure 11. Henry's Law.

stating the amount of gas physically dissolved in a gas-liquid system is proportional to the pressure of the gas in the system (Figure 11). When breathing pure oxygen at room air pressure, the oxygen percentages increase approximately fivefold from 20.9% to almost 100%. This is reflected in the partial pressure of oxygen increasing from 160 mmHg to almost 760 mmHg and the blood oxygen content from 0.5 vol% to 2.5 vol%. With doubling the ambient pressure with HBO_2, the blood oxygen content in the plasma doubles so that 5 vol% of oxygen becomes physically dissolved in the plasma.

The physiology just described explains how methods to increase the oxygen-carrying capacity of blood are different between the red blood cell and the physically dissolved oxygen in the plasma. Transfusions increase the oxygen-carrying capacity of blood by adding more hemoglobin to carry oxygen. This is quantified by the formula 1.39 vol/gm X Hbgm%. This means that for each one point rise in blood hemoglobin, 1.39 volumes percent (100 cc of pure hemoglobin) via red blood cells must be transfused.

In contrast, physically dissolved oxygen in the plasma occurs in direct proportion to the partial pressure of oxygen in the breathing medium according to the formula 0.003 vol%/mmHg x ppO_2 (mmHg). When breathing pure oxygen at two atmospheres absolute (ATA) pressure, 4.6 vol% (1520 mmHg x 0.003 vol%/mmHg) of oxygen is physically dissolved in the plasma, and, at 3 ATA, the vol% is 6.8. Thus, with each mmHg increase in oxygen pressure in the breathing medium, 0.003 vol% of oxygen is added to the plasma.

In summary, transfusions increase the oxygen-carrying capacity of the blood by adding to the red blood cell mass; the breathing of increased pressures of oxygen do such by adding oxygen to the plasma. Hyperbaric oxygen therapy achieves this latter effect.

ARTERIAL-VENOUS OXYGEN EXTRACTION

All oxygen extraction from the bloodstream occurs at the capillary level. The difference in the oxygen tensions from the time the blood enters the arterial end of the capillary to the time it exits the venous end is expressed as the arterial-venous (A-V) oxygen extraction or A-V O_2 difference (Figure 12). From the Henderson-Hasselblad curves, it is known that the normal blood oxygen content (of which 97.5% is carried in the hemoglobin) is 20 volumes percent on the arterial side of the capillary. After 5 vol% of oxygen is extracted (the O_2 extraction under normal conditions as the blood passes through the capillary), the resultant oxygen content on the venous side of the capillary is 15 vol%. Thus, the normal arterial-venous oxygen extracton is 5 vol%.

In the early 1900s, J.B.S. Haldane of diving table fame said that the body tissues could only utilize oxygen carried by the red blood cell. This was labeled by Dr. George B. Hart as the "Haldane Hex" and impeded the use of HBO_2 therapy worldwide. In the late 1950s, Dr. C.J. Lambertsen declared that the body tissues did not discriminate from where they got their oxygen (that is, from the hemoglobin or the plasma) as long as 5 vol% of oxygen was able to diffuse from the capillary to the tissue fluids where it could move into the cell and be utilized for tissue metabolism. Dr. Lambertsen informed Dr. Boerema, a Dutch thoracic surgeon who was very interested in the effects of HBO_2.

Dr. Boerema, as a result, did a study where he extracted the red blood cells from piglets and kept them alive by maintaining their fluid volume with low molecular weight dextran and their tissue oxygenation with physically dissolved oxygen in the plasma achieved through HBO_2 exposures. This study resulted in Boerema and his associates' quintessential paper entitled "Life without Blood" and dispelled the Haldane Hex.[28] The publication of this paper gave HBO_2 a solid physiological basis and ushered in the modern era of HBO_2 therapy.

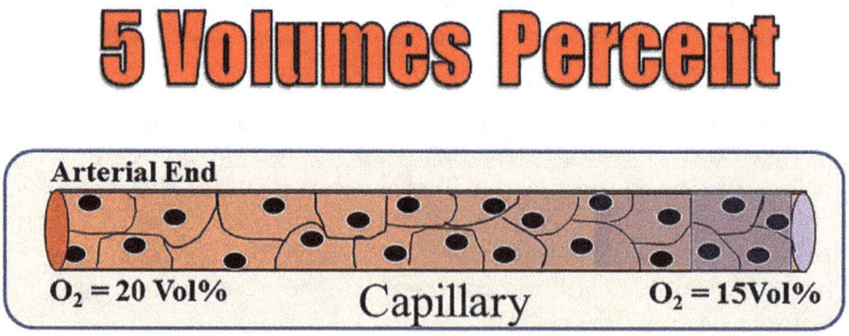

LEGEND: As blood flows through the capillary, 5 vol% of oxygen is offloaded to the tissue fluids. This is the arterial-venous (A-V) O_2 difference between the arterial and venous ends of the capillary.

Ordinarily 97.5% of the oxygen in the blood is carried by the red blood cell. With HBO_2 enough O_2 can be carried in the plasma to meet the A-V O_2 extraction that occurs at the capillary level.

Figure 12. Arterial-venous oxygen extraction.

HYPEROXYGENATION PHYSIOLOGY

Information from the preceding paragraphs helps explain the physiology of hyperoxygenation resulting from a HBO_2 exposure (Figure 13). Once hemoglobin becomes fully saturated, no additional blood oxygen-carrying capacity occurs in the hemoglobin even if the partial pressure of the inspired oxygen increases. The dissolved oxygen in the plasma, as just explained, increases in a linear fashion as the oxygen partial pressure of inspired gas is increased. In room air, this is only a small fraction (2.5%) of the total blood oxygen content. However, with hyperbaric oxygen this increases enough to meet the arterial-venous oxygen difference. The body apparently does not differentiate the source of the 5 volumes percent, that is, whether it is from oxygen extracted from hemoglobin or physically dissolved in the plasma. Remember, only about 25% of the oxygen carried in the hemoglobin is off-loaded as the blood passes from the arterial to the venous side of the capillary (that is, from 20 vol% to 15 vol%). Boerema confirmed that the 5 volume percent of oxygen physically dissolved in plasma through the hyperoxygenation effect of HBO_2 was sufficient to transiently meet oxygenation requirements of the piglet.

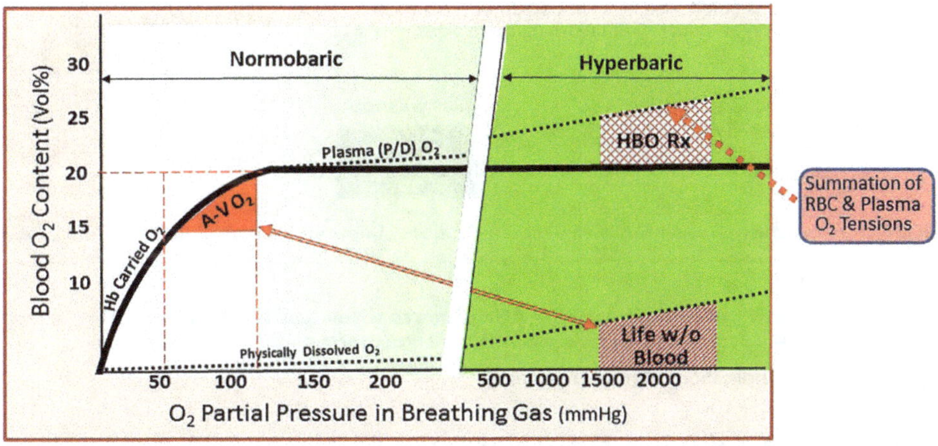

LEGEND: Physically dissolved oxygen in the plasma adds to the blood O_2 content. In room air 97.% of the O_2 is carried in the RBC. HBO_2 adds O_2 to the plasma. Eventually with HBO, enough O_2 becomes physically dissolved in the plasma to meet the normal A-V O_2 extraction and amounts to 5 vol%. When this occurred in Boerema's study, he was able to sustain life in piglets without RBC's.

KEY: A-V = Arterial-venous, HBO = Hyperbaric oxygen, RBC = Red blood cell, P/D = Physically dissolved, Rx = Treatment, w/o = Without

Figure 13. The physiological basis of hyperoxygenation and how "life without blood" is possible.

CLINICAL APPLICATIONS OF HYPEROXYGENATION

Each drop of plasma in the hyperbaric oxygen environment at 2 ATA carries 10 times the amount of oxygen as in room air. This effect has four clinical applications (Figure 14). The first of these is for **Impaired Perfusion**. This problem is especially associated with problem wounds that occur in the presence of peripheral artery disease. Other related conditions include acute skeletal muscle-compartment syndromes, acute arterial insufficiency, threatened tissue loss with Raynaud's disease, purpura fulminans, reperfusion injury, ergot poisoning, frostbite, and septic shock.

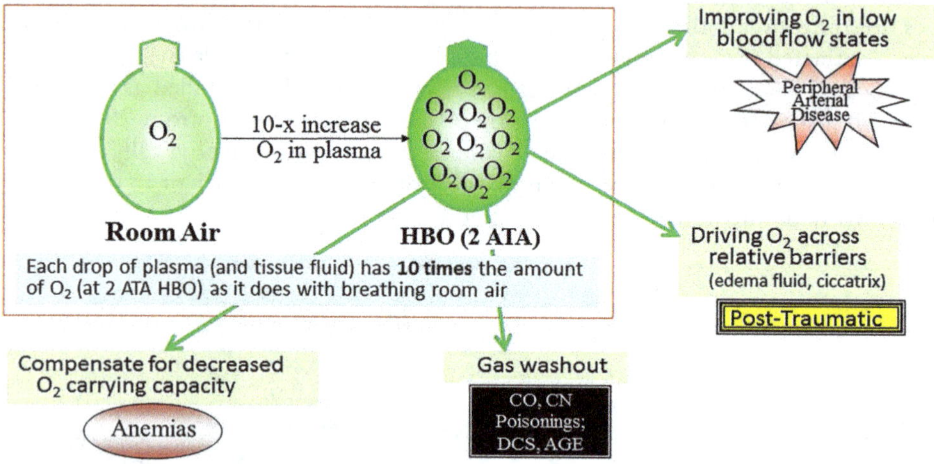

LEGEND: Hyperoxygenation has 4 clinical applications. Improving O_2 availability in low blood flow states is the most frequent clinical application of HBO_2 and is most frequently used as adjunct to managing problem wounds.

KEY: AGE = Arterial gas embolism, ATA = Atmospheres absolute, CN = Cyanide, CO = Carbon monoxide, DCS = Decompression sickness, HBO = Hyperbaric oxygen, O_2 = Oxygen

Figure 14. Clinical applications of hyperoxygenation.

Oxygen Transfer through Relative Barriers

Oxygen Transfer through Relative Barriers is a second clinical application of the hyperoxygenation effect (Table 8). This effect is especially desirable where barriers impede the movement of oxygen through tissue fluids from the capillary to the cell. The most frequent cause is that of edema. Oxygen diffuses through tissue fluids poorly, and at about only 1⁄20 of carbon dioxide's diffusion ability. Hyperoxygenation, through its mass effect, predictably increases the diffusion distance of oxygen through tissue fluids. This concept will be further explained shortly. Oxygen transfer through relative barriers is particularly applicable to traumatic ischemias where edema becomes a significant consideration in crush injuries, compartment syndromes, burns, and threatened flaps and grafts/reimplantations. Other conditions where HBO_2 has the potential to improve clinical outcomes are traumatic brain injuries, acute strokes, encephalopathy associated with near drowning, and acute spinal cord injuries. The common findings in these conditions include traumatic-induced edema and tissue hypoxia secondary to tissue disruption and/or edema.

There are other relative barriers to oxygenation. The most common ones are cicatrix that forms in hypoxic environments and hypertrophic bursas that develop over deformities. Both are associated with chronic wounds. The biochemistry of the cicatrix formation is explained by a signaling factor that is activated by hypoxic environments around a wound. Other relative barriers to oxygenations include pus, biofilms, cartilage (which also forms in hypoxic environments), thickening of the capillary basement membrane (which is accelerated in diabetics), dead bone, implants, and foreign objects. Most of these need to be addressed surgically, but the hyperoxygenation effect of HBO_2 is often a useful adjunct in their management.

Gas Washout

Gas Washout is the third clinical application of hyperoxygenaton. When the body tissues are poisoned with toxic gases or overloaded with inert gas (as observed with decompression sickness), these gases are carried away (that is, "washed out") with blood flow. This occurs as a stepwise process. The first step is movement of the undesirable gas from the tissues into the tissue fluids. Next, the undesirable gas moves into the blood stream by diffusion through the capillary. In the third step, blood flow carries the adverse gas to the lungs. In step four, the gas from the bloodstream moves into the air in the alveoli, and, finally is exhaled to the outside air. While HBO_2 does not ordinarily increase blood flow (exceptions may be with the reperfusion injury and vasospasm), all the steps in gas offloading are responses to gradients. With hyperoxygenation, the gradients are increased in favor of removing the noxious elements which, in turn, speeds the off-loading. This effect is appreciated with off-loading of carbon monoxide from the hemoglobin molecule and inert gas in decompression sickness.

Compensation for Decreased Oxygen-Carrying Capacity in the Blood

As predicted from Dr. Boerema's "Life without Blood" study, hyperoxygenation of the blood can compensate for anemia conditions and is the fourth clinical application of the hyperoxygenation effect.[28] Whereas a patient cannot survive for sustained periods in the HBO_2 environment due to oxygen toxicity, and red blood cells are needed to help carry off the carbon dioxide metabolic waste product, transient exposures to HBO_2 can be life sustaining. This benefit is appreciated for patients who are profoundly hypoxic from anemia as occurs with sickle cell crises and in patients who refuse blood transfusions as those of the Jehovah Witness faith do. Although the body can gradually accommodate to chronic anemia states, in acute blood loss situations, such as after surgeries and trauma, the acute anemia conditions may be life threatening. Infection often complicates these problems and interferes with body's abilities to generate red blood cells.

Although carbon dioxide retention is generally not a problem in anemia conditions, it appears to be a problem when there are almost no red blood cells (RBC) to help carry away this metabolic waste gas. Carbon dioxide retention was apparently the reason the exposure times for HBO_2 in the piglets who were devoid of red blood cells were not longer than 15 minutes in Boerema's study.

Ordinarily, about ⅓ of the carbon dioxide transported in the blood is done via hemoglobin.[32] Carbon dioxide combines with amine radicals in the hemoglobin molecule. Carbaminohemoglobin forms a loose bond in the RBC that is easily reversible in response to the hundredfold gradient of carbon dioxide between inspired air (0.5% carbon dioxide) and expired air (5% carbon dioxide).

Another consideration is the fact that the diffusion capacity of carbon dioxide in tissue fluids is 20 times greater than that of oxygen. Consequently, carbon dioxide retention is not the problem in the acute anemia situations, but rather hypoxia is.

Blood transfusions are the standard of practice for handling sickle cell crises. Unfortunately, as often occurs because of so many previous transfusions, typing and cross-matching may be delayed while a suitable donor is located (through a nationwide network). The sickle cell crisis patient in shock typically responds dramatically to HBO_2 exposures due to the hyperoxygenation of plasma effect. We have observed about a 25% decrease in heart rates with the initial HBO_2 exposure. The benefit lasts four to six hours, at which time the increasing heart rate justifies a repeat treatment. Usually after a day or two, a suitable blood donor is located, and the HBO_2 treatments are then discontinued.

It is noteworthy that the Bible addresses the importance of blood flow. In Deuteronomy, it is stated that the "Life of all tissue is the blood thereof." (New World Translation of the Holy Scriptures). Jehovah Witnesses cite this quotation as their reason for refusing blood transfusions. From a physiology perspective, nothing could be truer with wound healing, control of infection, and ischemia conditions.

Again, the hyperoxygenation effect of HBO_2 can compensate for these problems. As in the sickle cell crisis, the frequency of HBO_2 treatments is based on clinical signs such as pulse rates, cognitive function, appetite, and/or healing responses.

MASS EFFECT OF HYPEROXYGENATION

The mass effect of increased physically dissolved oxygen in plasma and tissue fluids helps to move oxygen through relative barriers. The initial relative barrier (after oxygen diffuses from the lungs to the blood) is the capillary basement membrane at the microcirculation level. Once oxygen moves into the tissue fluids, edema and the other relative barriers previously summarized are mitigated by the increased tension in the plasma (Table 8). In 1918, Krogh studied the diffusion distance of oxygen from the arterial and venous ends of the capillary through muscle tissue fluid.[34] At 4 ATA, the distance was 4 times greater than at the surface level just as predicted by Henry's law (Figure 16). This is consistent with the hypothesis that oxygen diffusion distance through tissue fluids increases in a linear fashion as the oxygen tension in the capillary blood increases.

The concept of mass effect as a benefit of hyperoxygenation is analogous to the pressure head or gradient in fluid flow (Figure 15). The greater the pressure or gradient, the greater the flow of the fluid, and the further it will travel. This has two analogies to the mass effect of hyperoxygenation: First, the higher the concentration (or oxygen tension) of oxygen on one side of a semipermeable barrier, the more oxygen movement through the barrier per unit of time. The second is that the diffusion distance of oxygen through the relative barrier increases proportionally to the oxygen tension of the plasma. This second corollary is of particular benefit in the presence of edema. It also supports the "dose" effect concept of hyperoxygenation; that is, the higher the ambient oxygen partial pressure, the greater the diffusion of oxygen through tissue fluids.

Pierce used a different approach to calculate oxygen diffusion distance. He reported that the oxygen diffusion distance from the capillary through the

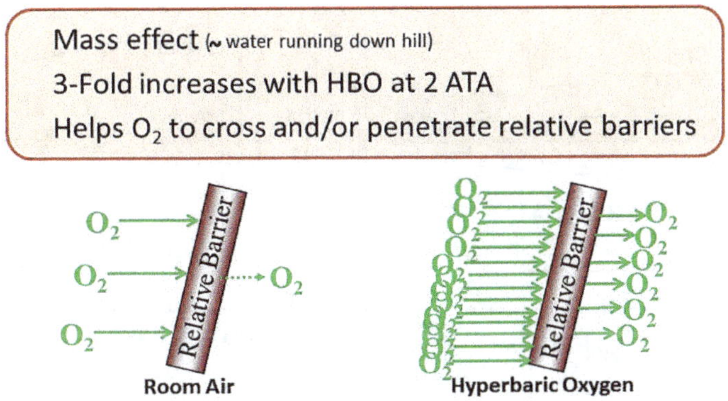

LEGEND: The increased concentration of O_2 molecules in the tissue fluids achieved with HBO_2 provides a "driving force" for oxygen to move through and/or penetrate relative barriers such as edema fluid, cicatrix, thickened capillary basement membranes, suppuration, avascular bone, etc.

KEY: ATA = Atmospheres absolute, HBO = Hyperbaric oxygen, O_2 = Oxygen, ~ = Similar to/ as for example

Figure 15. The "driving force" for moving oxygen across relative barriers.

TABLE 8. RELATIVE BARRIERS FOR OXYGEN TO MOVE FROM THE CAPILLARY INTO TISSUE FLUIDS AND THE INTO THE CELL

Barrier	Causes	Comments
Capillary Basement Membrane	Thickens with age; accelerated thickening in diabetics	Deserves to be labeled a microangiopathy
Edema Fluid	Trauma, inflammation, venous stasis disease, dependent positioning of feet	O_2 diffuses through tissue fluids poorly; CO_2 has 20 times the diffusing ability through tissue fluids as O_2; HBO at 2 ATA increases diffusing distance 3-fold
Cicatrix	Forms in hypoxic tissues by growth factors elaborated in low O_2 tensions	Usually needs to be managed by debridement
Hypertrophic Bursa	A "protective" response generated by the body as an attempt to mitigate the effects of underlying deformities	Debridement and off-loading is the indicated initial management; if not effective then deformity correction and bursa excision necessary
Suppuration	The body's WBC response to pyogenic infections	Many analogies to edema in increasing diffusion distance of O_2 from the capillary to the cell; Neutrophils are unable to perform oxidative killing functions in hypoxic environments
Miscellaneous	Sequestra, foreign objects, implants, bone cement, etc.	Surgical management usually required to resolve the problem

KEY: ATA= Atmospheres absolute, CO_2 = carbon dioxide, HBO = Hyperbaric oxygen, O_2 = Oxygen

tissue fluid increased by the square root of the oxygen partial pressure in the plasma.[16] Consequently, if the oxygen tension in the plasma increases tenfold with HBO_2 at 2 ATA, the diffusion distance through tissue fluids spreads about threefold, which is approximately the square root (3.16) of ten.

Regardless, both Krogh's and Pierce's computations generate results that are quite similar for appreciating the increments in diffusion distance/mass effect from HBO_2 through tissue fluids. The physiological effect is that, with HBO_2, the diffusion distance of oxygen on the venous side (efferent) end of the capillary becomes equivalent to the diffusion distance at the arterial (afferent) end of the capillary when breathing room air.

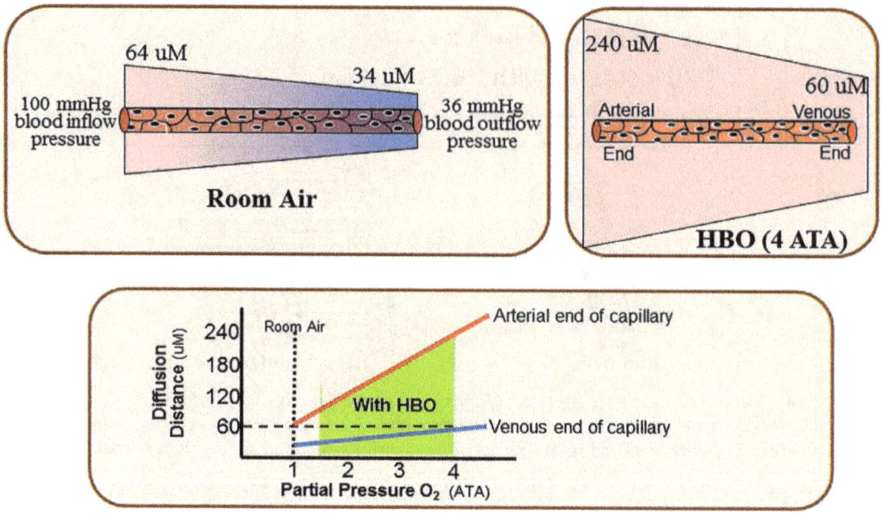

LEGEND: Krogh reported on oxygen diffusion distance from the arterial and venous ends of the capillary. With increased O_2 tensions, the distances increase in a linear fashion. Note that at 4 ATA as large a diffusion distance on the venous end of the capillary occurs as on the arterial end of the capillary in room air. This phenomenon is termed "arterialization" of the venous blood.

KEY: ATA = Atmospheres absolute, HBO = Hyperbaric oxygen, uM = Micrometers

Figure 16. Krogh's capillary oxygen diffusion distance observations.

The clinical term for this state is "arterialization of the venous blood," and the finding is that, with HBO_2, the mixed venous blood has the same oxygen tension as the arterial blood does when breathing room air.

From the clinical perspective, the mass effect of HBO_2 is particularly useful for improving survival of threatened flaps and grafts where tissue oxygenation is compromised by edema. When edema is coupled with ischemia concerns, HBO_2 should be used as an adjunct to improve salvage and/or survival of tissues such as in crush injuries, compartment syndromes, and burns in addition to threatened flaps and grafts.

MITIGATION OF SLUGGISH PERFUSION IN THE MICROCIRCULATION WITH HYPERBARIC OXYGEN

Hemoglobin oxygen transport is the most flow limited of all the substances carried in the blood. This is because of the mass of the red blood cell. All the other substances (except leucocytes and platelets) are physically dissolved in the plasma, and their mass is inconsequential compared to the mass of the red blood cell. Consequently, in sluggish flow states due to partial clotting of blood vessels, sludging, vasospasm, Rouleaux formation from abnormal proteins in the blood (associated with multiple myeloma, inflammatory and connective tissue disorders, and cancers), atherosclerosis with plaques, rewarming after frostbite injury, and reperfusion injury, red blood cell flow through the microcirculation may be severely impaired. Before total occlusion (that is, thrombosis), a fibrin clot network forms. The fibrin network precludes the passage of red blood cells while still allowing plasma to flow through the relative obstruction (Figure 17).

With oxygen physically dissolved in the plasma under HBO_2 conditions, oxygen delivery through the plasma becomes no more flow dependent than the other substances physically dissolved in the plasma. The important corollary to this is that if there is impaired blood flow, but plasma continues to flow through the microcirculation, the physically dissolved oxygen carried in the plasma under HBO_2 conditions will help maintain tissue viability. Obviously if there is no blood flow, HBO_2 will not prevent tissue death. However, in situations where demarcation between viable and nonviable tissue is not clear, it can assist in the demarcation process.

When amputations become necessary because of ischemia (other causes of amputation include pain, nonunion, uncontrolled infection, deformities that severely interfere with function, cancers, or combinations of these), the reason is attributed to lack of adequate blood supply with inadequate oxygen availability to maintain tissue viability. The reason for amputation in the ischemic limb is never given as due to the inability to deliver growth factors, wound healing mediators, and precursors . This is because these substances are carried physically dissolved in the plasma.

Thus, in acute low-flow states such as occurring with sludging, fibrin bridging (as a precursor to thrombosis), Rouleaux formation, and reperfusion injury, the "lack of mass" of the physically dissolved oxygen in the plasma with intermittent HBO_2 treatments can help to maintain viability until perfusion improves. Perfusion is improved physiologically with autologous clot lysis and vasorelaxation, pharmacologically with anticoagulants, thrombolytics, and antiadherent agents, or interventionally with angioplasty, bypass surgery, and/or stenting. Hyperbaric oxygen can be the important "bridging" therapy that maintains tissue viability until the circulation is improved with one or more of the above techniques. In these situations, in accordance with the dose-duration effects of HBO_2, hyperbaric oxygen, treatments need be done frequently. We recommend three to four HBO_2 treatments in the first 24 hours. Then treatments can be tapered and eventually discontinued when it is ascertained that circulation has been reestablished or demarcation becomes defined.

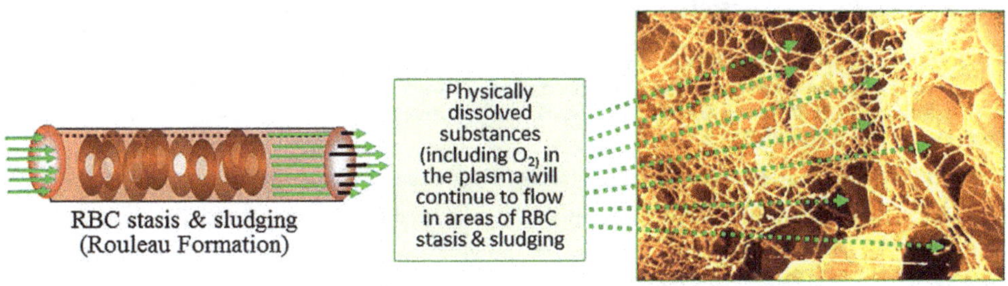

LEGEND: Hemoglobin O_2 transport is the most flow limited of the substances carried in the blood due to the mass of the RBC. HBO_2 results in the physically dissolved O_2 in the plasma being no more flow limited than any of the other substances dissolved in the plasma

KEY: HBO_2 = Hyperbaric oxygen, RBC = Red blood cell

Figure 17. Plasma flow with hyperbaric oxygen through partially occluded microcirculation.

Observations from both laboratory and clinical studies back the value of plasma delivery of oxygen with HBO_2 in sluggish or short-term no-blood-flow states.[39] Thomas, in a well-designed study in canines, compared the infarct size after occlusion of the anterior descending coronary artery for two hours with a copper coil and the benefits of reducing infarct size with recombinant tissue plasma activator (rt-PA), HBO_2, and combinations of the two.[38] Measurements of metabolic enzyme restoration revealed a 35.9% improvement with HBO_2 alone, a 48.9% improvement with rt-PA alone, and a 96.9% improvement with a combination of HBO_2 and rt-PA ($p = 0.001$). Equally striking was the reduction in infarct size (Figure 18).

Two clinical studies have demonstrated the benefits of HBO_2 in reducing cardiac injury via enzyme studies and earlier appearance of the transient arrhythmia verifying restoration of flow in the occluded coronary artery and restoration of function in the cardiac muscle.[35-36]

Zamboni, a plastic surgeon, embraced the role of HBO_2 for reducing tissue damage after threatened microvascular free flaps.[40] These observations were supported by his intravital microscopy studies demonstrating the value of HBO_2 in reducing neutrophil adherence to the microvasculature endothelium.[41] Neutrophil adherence to the microvascular endothelium is the precursor to the cascade of events causing tissue damage from the reperfusion injury.

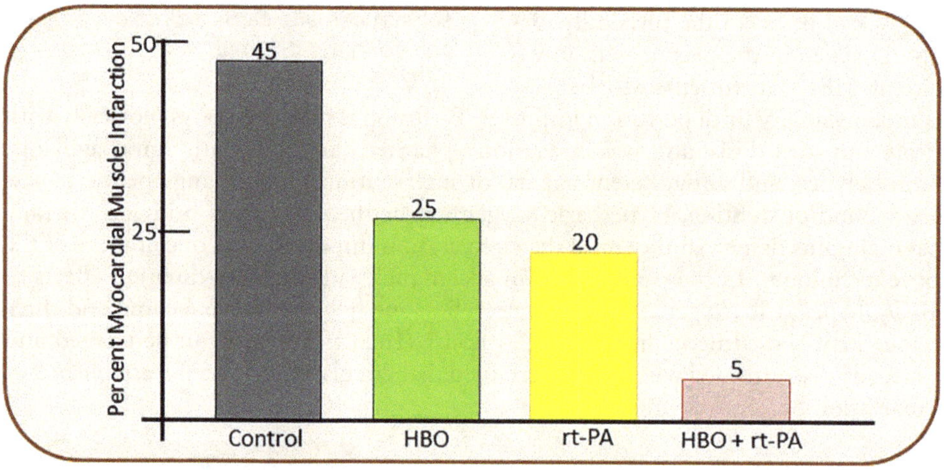

LEGEND: Although both HBO and rt-PA markedly reduced myocardial injury as compared to the controls, the best results were observed where the combinations of the two interventions were utilized. This information lead to two clinical myocardial infarction studies in humans (Shandlin[35] & Stavitsky[36]).

KEY: HBO = Hyperbaric oxygen, rt-PA = Recombinant tissue plasma activator

Figure 18. Muscle infarction after coronary artery occlusion in the canine heart (aka Thomas).

CLINICAL ASPECTS OF HYPEROXYGENATION

The above information on the mechanisms and benefits of HBO_2 support four clinical observations. First, the **effects of hyperoxygenation occur rapidly** (Figure 19). Within ten minutes of starting the HBO_2 exposure, plasma is fully saturated with oxygen at the new ambient pressure (Figure 10). In muscle and subcutaneous tissue, the plateau is reached after about one hour of HBO_2 exposure.[26] This effect is especially important in threatened flaps and graphs. When this benefit is observed with the initial HBO_2 treatment, repeat HBO_2 treatments every six to eight hours may be needed to sustain the ischemic flaps and grafts. The six-to-eight-hour interval equates to over 50 percent of the time elevated oxygen tensions remain in the threatened tissues i.e. 90 minutes for the HBO_2 exposure plus 4 ½ hours post treatment elevations in the subcutaneous tissues. Usually, after 24 to 48 hours, the tissues of concern stabilize enough with

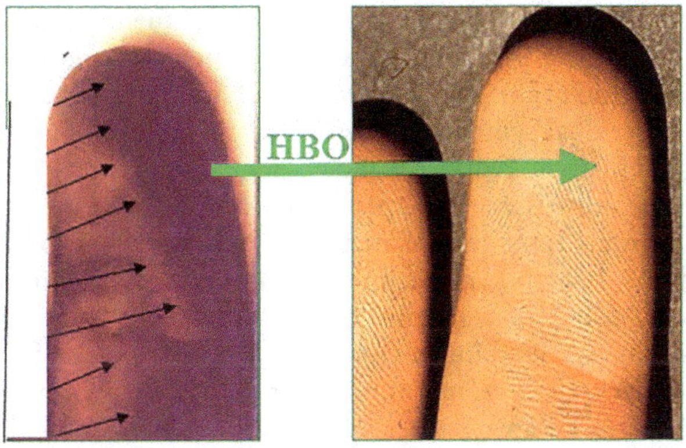

LEGEND: This patient lacerated his long finger when he was a youngster. The radial side of the distal half of the finger became cyanotic after re-traumatizing the finger. The coloration immediately improved with the first HBO treatment. Twelve hours later the injured part of the finger became dusky again. A second HBO treatment restored normal coloration to the finger and the result persisted.

This clinical observation demonstrated the rapid response observed with HBO. The resolution of the problem was attributed to HBO maintaining oxygenation through a vasospastic digital artery. The need for the repeat treatment was consistent with the dose-duration effect of hyperoxygenation.

Figure 19. Immediate improvement of severely ischemic finger with hyperbaric oxygen (HBO_2).

edema reduction and/or mitigation of the reperfusion injury that HBO_2 treatments can be reduced to once a day.

Second, **the hyperoxygenation effects of HBO_2 are transient**, as just described. However, the transient effects appear to be sufficient to activate factors instrumental for wound healing and infection control. The "pulses" of HBO_2 given once or twice a day for these indications appear to be sufficient to maintain the healing process in contrast to the need for more frequent treatments to preserve ischemic tissues. The mechanisms of HBO_2 secondary to hyperoxygenation are the ones benefited by its transient effects and will be described in the secondary mechanisms part of this chapter.

Third, **the hyperoxygenation effects are proportional to the partial pressures of the inspired oxygen**. That is, the higher the treatment pressure, the greater the plasma and tissue tensions of oxygen. This corresponds to the dose response of the dose-duration effects of HBO_2 and supports the decision for initial treatments of carbon monoxide poisoning, gas gangrene, decompression sickness, and arterial gas embolism and possibly sickle cell disease crisis at the highest possible pressures safe for breathing oxygen. In decompression sickness and arterial gas embolism, pressure (the second primary effect of HBO_2, i.e., bubble reduction) also contributes to resolution of the problem and will be discussed shortly. Usually, after the first exposure for the above-mentioned conditions, repeat HBO_2 treatment pressures are reduced to 2 to 2.4 ATA. The justification for the first treatment being at the higher pressure is for the establishment of maximum gradients (the mass effect) to wash out the undesired gases in the tissues and/or maximally oxygenate the involved tissues as well as reduce the bubble volume.

Finally, **hyperoxygenation effects are dependent on plasma transport of oxygen**. If there is no perfusion, attempts to oxygenate tissues with HBO_2 will obviously be futile. The question arises, should HBO_2 be used when the cessation of blood flow is transient? This is often the situation after revascularizations, thrombectomies, and bubble reductions in gas embolisms. Clinical judgment is required whether to use

HBO_2 after the primary pathology appears remediated. If there is a concern that tissue damage occurred during the period of ischemia, elements of the reperfusion injury exist, or latent effects could occur, an additional HBO_2 treatment is recommended after recovery. If there are residual symptoms, then HBO_2 treatments should be continued for 10 to 14 days for its edema reduction and angiogenesis effects.

For muscle and soft-tissue ischemia that occurs in connection with crush injuries, revascularizations, and reimplantations, HBO_2 is an approved indication. Acute peripheral artery ischemia and acute skeletal muscle-compartment syndromes are other indications for HBO_2 in this category of generic indications. Central retinal artery occlusion is a new indication (by *Undersea Medical Society Hyperbaric Oxygen Therapy Committee Guidelines*) for similar reasoning. Acute brain and spinal cord injuries continue to be an off-label use even though substantial benefits could be realized with the immediate use of HBO_2. Unfortunately, there is reluctance by the physicians managing these problems to use HBO_2. Nonetheless, its mechanism of hyperoxygenation, edema reduction, and reperfusion injury mitigation are logical interventions for the pathophysiology of these conditions. HBO_2 may be the "wave of the future" for acute brain and spinal cord injuries.

TOPICAL OXYGEN

It is essential, when discussing the hyperoxygenation effect of HBO_2, to differentiate it from topical oxygen. Topical oxygen is an intervention where a bag or cylinder is placed around an extremity wound and the device inflated with a very low pressure of oxygen (Figure 20). In order to maintain inflation, the proximal edge of the bag must be sealed with a tie or a gasket.

There are published reports that topical oxygen improves healing of diabetic foot wounds.[31,33] However, we are perplexed by its mechanisms of action. That is because the amount of oxygen delivered to the surface of the wound with topical oxygen is only about 1/33 as much as is achieved with HBO_2 (Table 9). In many reports, the mechanisms attributed to HBO_2 are mentioned as justification for the use of topical oxygen.

> Since the definition of HBO_2 was established by a Medicare committee in Dr. Hart was a member in the 1970s, topical oxygen has not been a reimbursable service by the government. According to Dr. Hart, the committee was convened for the purposes of defining HBO_2 and adjudicating whether or not topical oxygen was a variant of HBO_2 therapy.

Topical oxygen (in the reports that show it to be beneficial) appears to work by a mechanism other than hyperoxygenation. In addition, topical oxygen is delivered through the open wound in contrast to HBO_2 where oxygen diffuses into the deeper portions of the wound from the hyper oxygenated tissue fluids. While epithelialization of the superficial portion of the wound might be benefited by low increments in oxygen tensions, the deeper portions where repair and remodeling are occurring are not likely to be affected.

Fischer found that topical oxygen penetrated a fingertip wound to a depth of only one mm.[30] In another study, topical oxygen was found to reduce the juxta-wound oxygen tensions when measurements were made with transcutaneous oxygen monitoring.[29] The decrements in oxygen tensions were attributed to the seals that are used to maintain the minimally increased oxygen pressures in the device. Even though the topical oxygen treatment pressures are very low, the seals are apparently tight enough to impede venous return (Table 9).

In summary, topical oxygen therapy should not be considered a variant of HBO_2. Although reports indicate topical oxygen may be beneficial for improving superficial wounds, it cannot be compared to HBO_2 with its well-documented mechanisms and its multitude of uses.

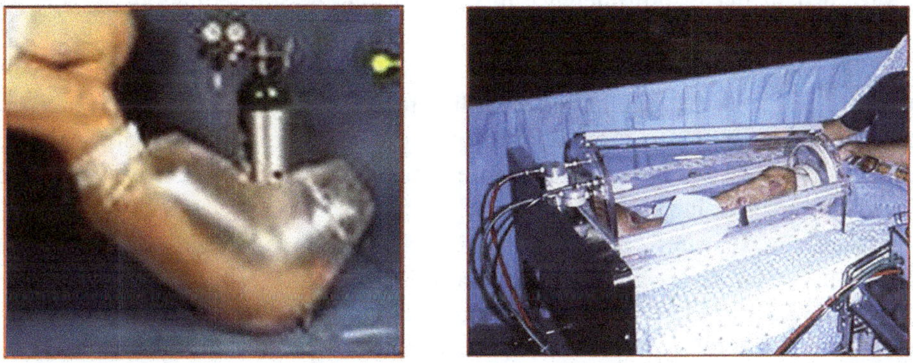

LEGEND: Topical oxygen should not be considered a variant of HBO therapy. Although it appears to enrich the oxygen environment of the superficial portions of a wound, it does not penetrate more than a millimeter or two into deeper tissues.

Note the constricting bands (elastic type on the left and rubber gasket on the right) used to maintain a positive pressure in the devices. These appear to interfere with venous return and lower the juxta-wound transcutaneous oxygen tensions.

Figure 20. Methods of implementing topical oxygen.

TABLE 9. COMPARISONS OF OXYGEN PRESSURES; HBO_2 versus TOPOX

Situation In usual terminology	**fsw* Conversions** For comparison purposes
HBO_2 (2 ATA)	33 Feet of seawater*
Systolic (120 mmHg)	5 fsw
Topox (1.03 ATA)	0.99 fsw
Venous (10 cm H_2O)	0.33 fsw

COMMENT: In terms of oxygen tension increments to the wound, topical oxygen only provides 1/33rd as much as hyperbaric oxygen.

Because of the constricting band or seal to maintain pressure in the topical oxygen system, the inflation pressure exceeds that of the venous return pressure. This may explain why the lowered transcutaneous oxygen tension measurements were observed with topical oxygen (Cotto-Cumba[29]).

PRESSURIZATION EFFECTS

This is the second primary mechanism of HBO_2 therapy. Its primary effect is bubble reduction for managing decompression sickness and arterial gas embolism. Its effects occur instantaneously and are proportional to the magnitude (i.e., depth) of pressurization. The pressurization effect of hyperbaric therapy is independent of the gas breathed. It makes no difference in terms of bubble size reduction whether the pressurization is done with air or oxygen.

Like hyperoxygenation, the physics of pressurization effects on bubbles is fully established. Bubbles decrease in size according to Boyle's law. The decrease is inversely proportional to the pressure; that is, as the pressure increases, the bubble size decreases (Table 10). As this table shows, the volume of bubble reduction successively decreases with each increment in pressure.

Greater and greater pressures are not the answer for managing decompression sickness in sports divers and iatrogenic arterial embolisms. When breathing pure oxygen, the risks of oxygen toxicity seizures become unacceptably high at pressures greater than 3 ATA (66 feet of sea water). Contemporary practice is to utilize maximum pressures of 60 to 66 feet of sea water (2.8–3.0 ATA) for 30 minutes (or longer with air breaks) to achieve the most bubble reduction for the maximal allowable pressure to breathe pure oxygen. The combined effect of this regimen is optimal bubble reduction

TABLE 10. BUBBLE REDUCTION WITH INCREASING PRESSURES/DEPTHS

Pressure/Depth	Volume Ratio	Reductions in Volume (%)	
		Vs. initial volume	From prior volume
Surface 1 ATA/33FSW	1	100	
			50
2 ATA/33 FSW	1/2	50	
			17
3 ATA/66 FSW	1/3	33	
			8
4 ATA/99 FSW	1/4	25	
			5
5 ATA/132 FSW	1/5	20	
			3 1/3
6 ATA/165 FSW	1/6	16 2/3	

COMMENT: With each atmosphere (ATA) of increased pressure, the percentage of bubble reduction volume decreases.

At 3 ATA/33 fsw (feet of sea water) the bubble volume is reduced by 67 =%. Pressurizing from 3 to 6 ATA only decreases the bubble size an additional 16 2/3%.

3 ATA is the maximum depth to breathe pure O_2. Consequently, the "best possible" combination to achieve bubble reduction but still maximize the benefits of breathing pure oxygen for gradient and washout effects would be a depth of 66 fsw.

plus accelerated nitrogen (or other inert gas) washout from the gradient achieved by breathing pure oxygen.

When breathing gases at greater than 3 ATA, air (79% nitrogen and 20.9% oxygen) gas mixtures with lowered oxygen percentages are desirable in order to avoid oxygen toxicity. This adds more inert gases to the body tissues and requires the victim as well as the tender to undergo decompression stops. In addition, to pressurize patients greater than 3 atmospheres absolute pressure, multiplace chambers and technicians who are familiar with using gas mixtures are required.

Bubble reduction is not the only desirable effect of pressurization. Pressurization is the force that "drives" oxygen through relative barriers (Figure 9). Also, it augments gas washout by increasing the gradients between the undesirable gases in the tissues (e.g., nitrogen in the case of decompression sickness and carbon monoxide in poisonings) and the oxygen physically dissolved in the plasma. These desirable effects will be more fully elaborated when secondary mechanisms of HBO_2 are discussed in the next part.

SUMMARY

Many superlatives can be used when considering the primary mechanisms of HBO_2 therapy. For hyperoxygenation, it is the most important mechanism of HBO_2 therapy. Almost all effects of HBO_2 are directly or indirectly attributable to hyperoxygenation. Finally, hyperoxygenation is fraught with the most serious side effects of HBO_2, namely oxygen-induced seizures and pulmonary edema. For pressurization, the main superlative is that it is the easiest mechanism to understand. This is true for bubble reduction, but is not so evident when considering how pressurization provides the driving force for oxygen to move into the plasma and the tissues as well as providing the gradients for gas washouts.

Hyperoxygenation has four major effects, namely 1) augmentation of oxygen delivery to ischemic tissues in low-flow states, 2) increased oxygen diffusion distance through relative barriers, 3) gas washout, and 4) compensation for decreased oxygen-carrying capacity in the blood secondary to anemia. In many of the clinical situations, the major effects complement each other. For example, in peripheral artery disease, the benefit of the augmented oxygen delivery will be enhanced by the improved oxygen diffusion through relative barriers such as cicatrix and edema fluid. With hyperoxygenation making oxygen delivery to tissues no more flow dependent in situations where the circulation is impaired by sludging, fibrin bridging, or plaques, the improved oxygen delivery can make the difference between limb salvage and amputation.

Three cardinal effects occur from hyperoxygenation at 2 atmospheres absolute (Figure 9). Plasma oxygen content increases tenfold. This, in turn, increases the blood oxygen-carrying capacity by 125% and is reflected in a tenfold increase in tissue oxygen tensions. Finally, the combinations of these effects increase oxygen diffusion through relative barriers by a threefold factor. For bubble reduction in diving and gas embolism problems, pressurization effects of bubble size conform to Boyle's law. With doubling the pressure (i.e., from sea level to 33 fsw = 2 ATA), the volume of the bubble decreases by 50%; with tripling the pressure to 3 ATA (66 fsw), the bubble volume is decreased to ⅓.

PART 3

SECONDARY MECHANISMS OF HBO_2 – TISSUE CONSEQUENCES OF HYPEROXYGENATION AND PRESSURIZATION

INTRODUCTION

While hyperoxygenation and pressurization are the primary mechanisms of hyperbaric oxygen (HBO_2) with immediate, transient, and dose-duration effects, the secondary mechanisms of HBO_2 are almost always additive, require repetitive treatments, and give the durable benefits realized from HBO_2 treatments. Part 3 of this chapter explains how HBO_2 has physiological justification for such widespread disease processes as crush injury, compartment syndromes, carbon monoxide poisoning, diabetic foot ulcers, gas gangrene, nonhealing wounds, radiation injury, and other conditions through its seven secondary mechanisms (Table 11).[55,84] Boerema's "Life without Blood" study gave science to the use of HBO_2.[28] It ushered in the modern era of HBO_2 therapy and provided the basis for understanding the physiology of the secondary mechanisms of this modality.

The classification of HBO_2 mechanisms as primary and secondary appears to be unique to our classification system.[70] We feel it has merits because it reconciles the dichotomy between immediate and delayed benefits of HBO_2. It also provides plausible explanations for not fully understood effects of HBO_2 on the blood-brain barrier, the role in red blood cell deformability, and the significance of isobaric counter diffusion. Each decade adds additional information to support the secondary mechanisms of HBO_2. The expectation is that expanded applications of the secondary mechanisms and perhaps the discovery of additional new mechanisms will justify the use of HBO_2 for new and so-called "off-label" applications of this modality.

Most of the more frequently mentioned off-label applications of HBO_2 are supported by mechanisms of HBO_2. Examples include acute traumatic brain and spinal cord injuries/central nervous system hypoxic insults, enhanced recovery for sports-

TABLE 11. SECONDARY MECHANISMS OF HYPERBARIC OXYGEN

• **Vasoconstriction**	• **Inert gas washout** (& isobaric counterdiffusion)
• **Host Responses**	• RBC Deformability
• **Microbiological Effects**	• Blood Brain Barrier Permeability
• **Reperfusion injury**	

Viability	**Primary mechanisms keep tissues alive**
Repair & Function	**Secondary mechanisms resolve the problem**—the long term, durable effects

NOTE: Several of the 2° mechanisms (in smaller font) have theoretical justification at this time. As more information becomes available, we anticipate these will receive further attention & help to justify HBO_2 for "off-label" uses.

related injuries, arrest of early-stage femoral head necrosis, amelioration of sickle cell crises, management of systemic sepsis, and mitigation of acute myocardial infarctions. Advocates of these off-label uses of HBO_2 usually cite mechanisms of HBO_2 in one form or another, the observed outcomes/benefits, or both for justification for using HBO_2 in these conditions.

Other possible off-label applications of HBO_2 include "neuroprotection" for high-risk surgeries such as done on the heart and brain; lessening/arrest of established or worsening disabilities from multiple sclerosis, cerebral palsy, autism, residuals of traumatic brain injury, strokes, spinal cord injuries, and age-related dementia; and enhancement of tumor killing and palliative therapy for cancers. The justification for using HBO_2 for these conditions is less apparent and largely based on anecdotal reports.

SECONDARY EFFECTS OF HYPERBARIC OXYGEN

Vasoconstriction

Hyperbaric oxygen initiates a generalized vasoconstriction of healthy blood vessels mediated through the sympathetic nervous system. This is a consequence of the primary mechanism of hyperoxygenation. Bird and Telfer reported a 20% reduction in blood flow and corresponding edema reduction under HBO_2 conditions (Figure 21).[43] Analogous reports of edema reduction were observed in our canine compartment syndrome studies, as well as brain, burn, and smoke inhalation studies by other investigators (Figure 22).[52,67-68,71-72,74] Reduction of blood flow reduces vasogenic edema formation in posttraumatic conditions such as crush injuries, compartment syndromes, burns, and reimplantations. It also reduces cytotoxic edema in brain, spinal cord, and radiation-induced ischemia by helping to reestablish more normal redox potentials. The consequence is improved intracellular oxygen tensions. This, in turn, maintains cell metabolic functions to keep water in the cell. The result is decreased leakage of water from the ischemic cell to the extracellular spaces.

Edema can be detrimental to cell function. It increases the diffusion distance of oxygen from the extracellular fluid to the cell (Figure 23). Oxygen diffuses poorly through tissue fluids and only a few microns from the capillary (where all oxygen exchange in the vascular system occurs) to the cell in a gradient fashion from high adjacent to the capillary to low as the distance from the capillary to the cell increases. As edema increases, diffusion distances increase, and the result is decreased oxygen availability to the cell.

Another harmful effect of edema is that it can cause collapse of the microcirculation. This occurs with edema fluid accumulation in closed spaces such as myofascial compartments as well as the analogous situation in the brain cavity, spinal canal, and abdominal cavity. As fluid accumulates in a closed compartment, the tissue fluid pressure in the compartment increases. The thin-walled capillary collapses when the tissue fluid pressure exceeds the capillary perfusion pressure. The result is

> Carbon dioxide diffusion is 20 times greater through tissue fluids than is oxygen diffusion.[3] In situations where tissues die or wounds fail to heal because of peripheral artery disease, failure to offload carbon dioxide from tissues is never attributed as the cause. Rather, the cause is attributable to hypoxia. This reflects the markedly improved diffusion ability of carbon dioxide through tissue fluids as compared to oxygen. Once carbon dioxide is in the plasma, it is transported by the bloodstream to the lungs, where it is offloaded with exhalation.

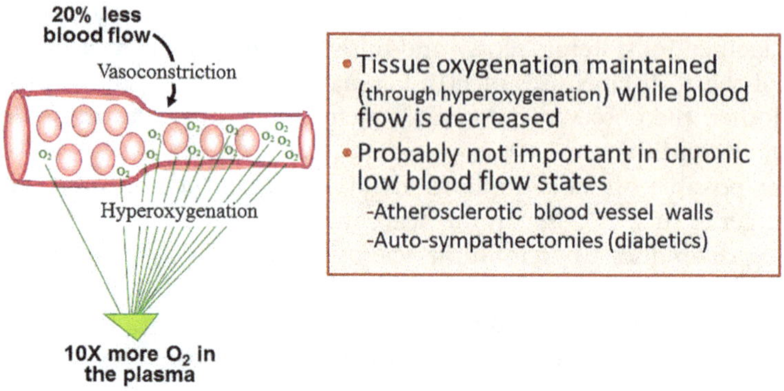

LEGEND: HBO_2 reduces blood flow in healthy blood vessels regulated by the sympathetic nervous system. With hyperoxygenation, oxygen tensions are maintained due to increased physically dissolved oxygen in the plasma.

KEY: HBO = Hyperbaric oxygen, O_2 = Oxygen

Figure 21. Vasoconstriction as secondary mechanism to hyperoxygenation.

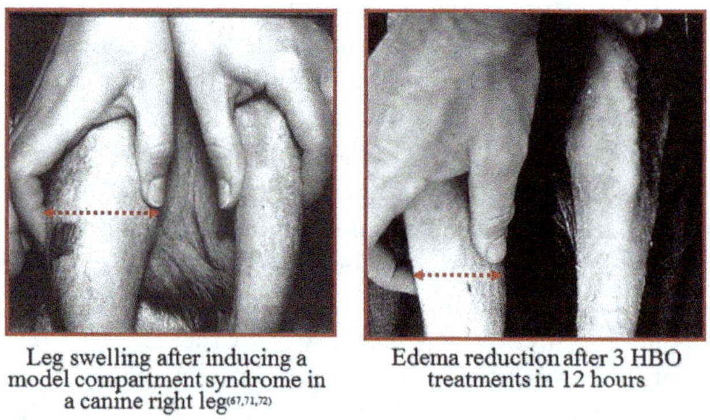

LEGEND: Swelling reduction is clinically obvious after the HBO_2 (hyperbaric oxygen) treatments. This was further substantiated with microscopic examinations and volume-weight measurements.

Figure 22. Edema reduction in a canine compartment syndrome model with HBO_2.

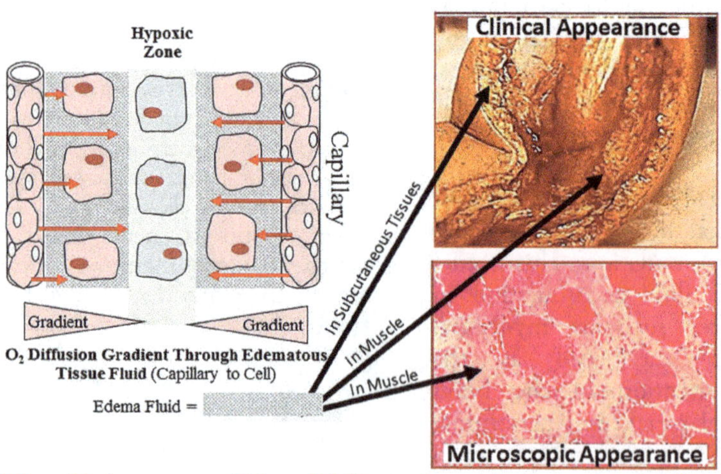

LEGEND: Edema hinders oxygen (O_2) availability to tissues by increasing the distance O_2 must diffuse through tissue fluids. Oxygen diffusion from the capillary to the cell decreases in a gradient fashion. Oxygen diffusion through tissue fluids is only 1/20th that of carbon dioxide.

Figure 23. Edema's harmful effects on tissue oxygenation.

interruption of blood flow through the capillary bed and cessation of oxygen delivery from the capillary to the cell. This defines the pathophysiology of the skeletal muscle-compartment syndrome.

The mechanisms that explain how vasoconstriction reduces edema become clear when the fluid filtration and reabsorption physiology of the capillary are examined (Figure 24). Normally fluid in the capillary and in the surrounding tissue fluids is in balance. What is important to appreciate is that as blood flows through the capillary, there are dynamic fluid exchanges. Due to the perfusion pressure at the arterial end of the capillary, fluid filters through the capillary to the tissue fluid space. Almost all the fluid is reabsorbed on the venous (lower perfusion pressure) side of the capillary due to the oncotic pressure of the blood in the capillary. The lymph system carries off the small remaining fluid excess in the tissue fluids. With trauma, there is increased blood flow to the injury site, so the capillary perfusion pressure increases. The result is increased filtration of fluid from the capillary to the tissue fluids. Since the oncotic pressure in the capillary does not change, fluid reabsorption on the venous side of the capillary remains the same, and the net effect is fluid accumulation, that is, edema in the tissues. With HBO_2's 20% reduction in flow, filtration decreases proportionately while reabsorption remains the same (due to the oncotic pressure in the capillary). The result is a reduction in edema.

At first inspection, the reduction in blood flow to traumatized tissues would seem to be counterproductive. However, Bird and Telfer observed that tissue oxygenation was maintained in the presence of HBO_2-induced vasoconstriction.[43] This is because the oxygen-carrying capacity of blood is increased by 125% under HBO_2 conditions.[73] Skeptics might also argue that vasoconstriction is undesirable when ischemia is associated with peripheral artery disease. In the diabetic, vasoconstriction is probably inconsequential in the peripheral vasculature because atherosclerosis and auto-sympathectomy prevent blood vessels from responding to sympathetic nervous system and metabolic stimuli input.

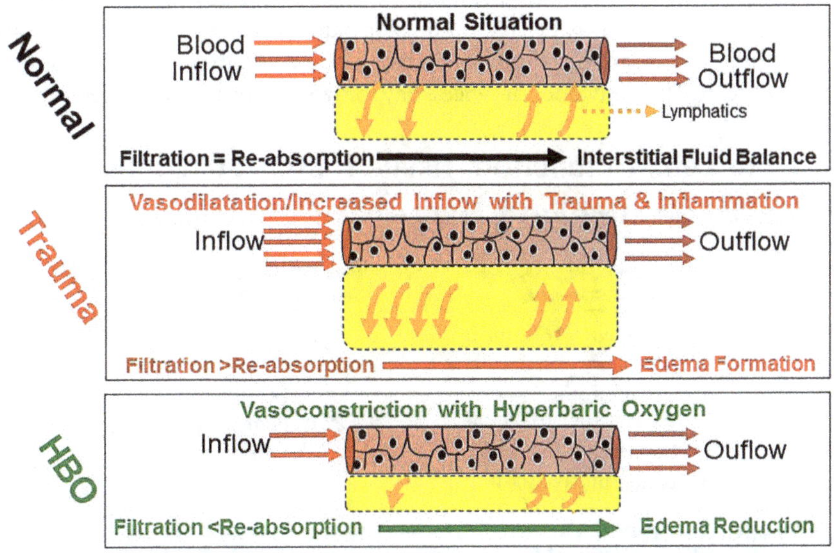

LEGEND: Normally fluid is filtered from the capillary to the tissue fluid spaces on the arterial side of the capillary due to perfusion pressure and reabsorbed on the venous side due to oncotic pressure. Trauma/inflammation increase inflow; HBO_2 decreases inflow 2° to vasoconstriction.

Figure 24. Mechanism of edema reduction with HBO_2.

Approved uses of HBO_2 where vasoconstriction improves outcomes: Crush injuries, compartment syndromes, threatened flaps, grafts, and re-implantations, and burns are approved by the Undersea and Hyperbaric Society, while all but burns are approved by CMS/Medicare.

Off-label considerations for HBO_2 where vasoconstruction may improve outcomes: Sports injuries, femoral head necrosis, cosmetic surgeries especially on exposed portions of the body, acute brain and spinal cord trauma, acute hypoxic brain insults including near-drowning, and multiple sclerosis (in edema stage before plaques form on nerves).

Host Cellular Functions

In the 1970s, Hunt and co-investigators confirmed that 30 to 40 mmHg tissue oxygen tensions are necessary for wound healing.(7-11,14) Although their studies dealt primarily with fibroblasts and neutrophils, ancillary information has shown that angiogenesis as well as bone formation and remodeling are equally dependent on these oxygen tensions to accomplish their functions. Oxygen tensions decrease along a gradient from room air to the mitochondria where all energy production for cell activities occur (Figure 25). The tissue fluid oxygen tension is the transitional zone between oxygen carried in the blood and oxygen within the cell. Any decreases in the oxygen tension along the oxygen gradient will cause proportional decreases along the gradient and will be detrimental to cellular function.

Although the mitochondria oxygen tension is less than 1⁄100 of the inspired oxygen tension, if it does not receive this amount of oxygen, cell metabolic functions will be impeded. If oxygen delivery is reduced anywhere along the gradient (e.g., with peripheral artery disease, edema with decreased oxygen diffusion through tissue fluids, etc.), the falloff will continue to the mitochondria and interfere with their function. Conversely, if oxygen tensions are low in the tissue fluids, HBO_2 can improve them. The effect will be transmitted along the gradient to the mitochondria, which, in turn, will continue to generate energy for all the cell's metabolic processes. "Pulses" of HBO_2 rather than sustained hyper oxygenated tissue oxygen tensions are all that seem to be necessary for these metabolic processes to continue. This justifies (and is substantiated by outcomes) giving HBO_2 treatments only once or twice a day for wound healing and infection control

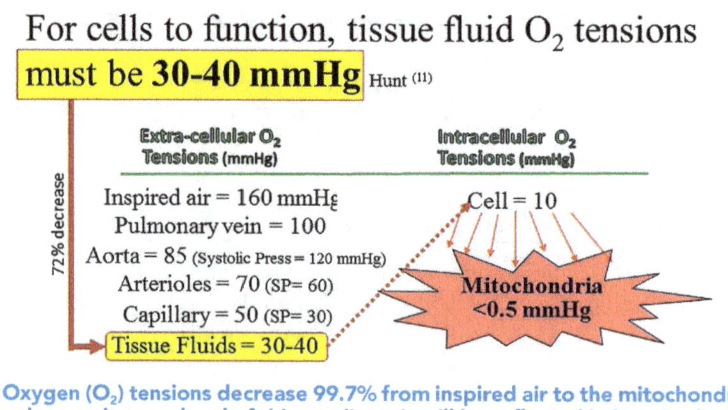

LEGEND: Oxygen (O_2) tensions decrease 99.7% from inspired air to the mitochondria. If the O_2 tensions are lowered at any level of this gradient, it will be reflected in impaired mitochondrial function and will inhibit their ability to carry out energy generation. Mitochondrial hypoxia is compensated by breathing pure O_2 and even more so with HBO_2.

Figure 25. The oxygen gradient from inspired air to the mitochondria.

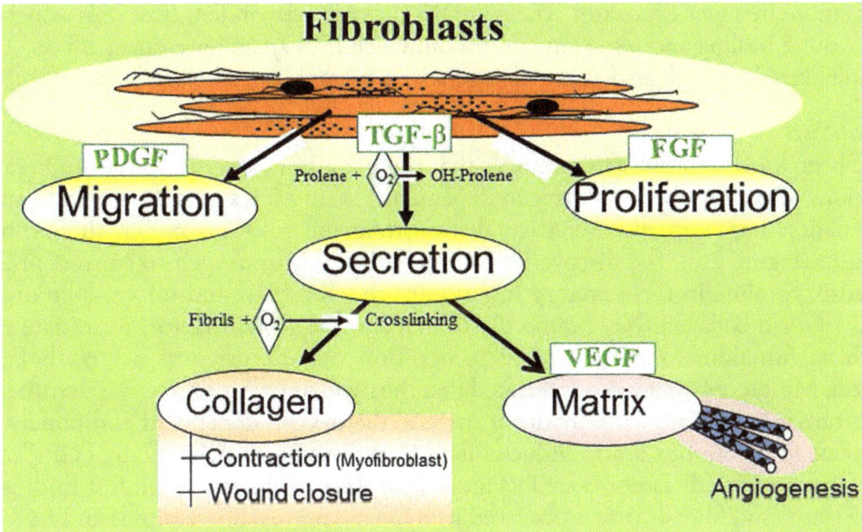

LEGEND: Oxygen has multiple roles in fibroblast function that include growth factor inductions of its three primary functions (migration, secretion and proliferation) to biochemical reactions needed for collagen formation.

KEY: FGF = Fibroblast growth factor, HBO_2 = Hyperbaric oxygen, O_2 = Oxygen, PDGF = Platelet derived growth factor, TGF-β = Transforming growth factor beta, VEGF = Vascular endothelial growth factor

Figure 26. Oxygen roles in fibroblast functions.

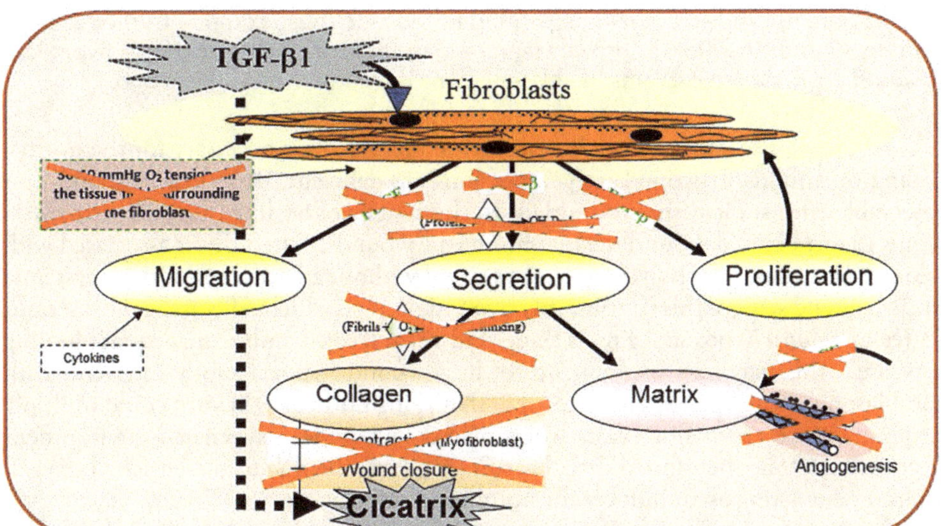

LEGEND: In hypoxic environments , TGF-β1 is induced to form cicatrix, a dense, hypovascular type of scar tissue. The ✕'s indicate where hypoxia could interfere with the normal fibroblast oxygen dependent mechanisms. TGF-β1 appears to bypass these mechanisms (thick, dotted black arrow) to form cicatrix and is induced by a hypoxic environment.

Figure 27. The effects of hypoxia on fibroblast function and as an induction of transforming growth factor-beta1 (TGF-β1).

versus more frequent exposures. There are three oxygen-dependent host cells associated with wound healing and infection control on which HBO_2 can have direct effects. They include fibroblasts with associated angiogenesis, neutrophils, and osteoclasts.

Fibroblasts

It has been known for over five decades that the migration, secretion, and proliferative functions of the fibroblast are oxygen dependent. With each succeeding decade, more information has been discovered to demonstrate the roles of oxygen in fibroblast function (Figure 26). The discoveries started with need for oxygen to convert proline to hydroxyproline in the secretory function of the fibroblast and for cross-linking of fibrils to form collagen. Next came the role of specific growth factors to initiate each fibroblast function, followed by the recognition that oxygen was a growth factor inducer. Most recently, it was appreciated that the hypoxic environment was detrimental to fibroblast function. Not only did it impede the oxygen dependent components of fibroblast function, but it also induced it to form a dense cicatrix due to TGF-β_1, i.e. transforming growth factor-beta 1 (Figure 27). This explains the clinical finding of dense scar tissue/fibrosis that is observed in hypoxic, nonhealing wounds and its rapid reappearance after repeated debridements.

Dr. George B. Hart made some astute clinical observations in the late 1970s about the differences between wound healing in well-oxygenated wounds and those that healed in a hypoxic environment. He noted that "soft scar" formed in the well-oxygenated healing wound. This is the desirable, pliable, thin, cosmetically-desired scar that forms in healthy wounds and is always the goal of plastic surgery procedures. Conversely, Dr. Hart said "hard scar," the type characterized by dense cicatrix and/or fibrosis, formed in the hypoxic wound. Although the biochemical mechanisms were not known at the time Dr. Hart formulated these comments, the recent recognition of the TGF-β_1 growth factor as an inducer of cicatrix in the hypoxic wound environment explains the observations he made over 40 years ago.

As mentioned previously, adequate oxygen tensions are necessary for the normal healing of wounds. If wound oxygen tensions are deficient, there is a continuum of observable effects. First, the wound fails to show signs of healing; next, dense cicatrix begins to form in and around the margins of the wounds. Often this is associated with colonization, usually by polyflora, of the wound without adjacent cellulitis or systemic sepsis. The end stage of this continuum is wound necrosis which reflects the most serious degree of wound hypoxia. Aging is associated with delayed and/or inadequate healing responses. This may be a consequence of how wound hypoxia subtly interferes with fibroblast function. Reenstra reported that that aging fibroblasts in vitro could multiply as rapidly as newborn fibroblasts when placed in a hyper oxygenated environment (Figure 28.)[(66)] She mentioned that these findings may be due to the enriched oxygen environment acting as an inducer for fibroblast proliferation.

Angiogenesis Dependence on Fibroblast Secretory Activity

Angiogenesis is an essential component of wound healing and is of paramount importance in the ischemic wound where perfusion already is marginal. Angiogenesis is dependent on the secretory function of the fibroblast lying down a matrix that can be invaded by capillary budding into it. The other essential component of angiogenesis is a gradient of well-oxygenated to near-anoxic tissues (Figure 29). Adequately oxygenated tissues (30–40 mmHg tissue fluid O_2 tensions) at the margin of the wound, fibroblast

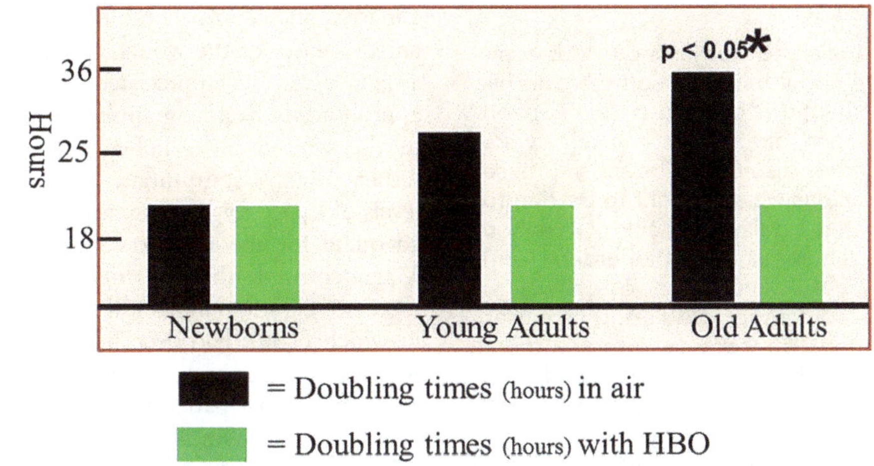

LEGEND: Renstra et al.[21] demonstrated in an in vitro study that HBO_2 significantly reduced the doubling times of fibroblasts from older aged subjects. They speculated that HBO_2 may have acted as a signaling mechanism, inducer of the proliferative function of the fibroblast.

Figure 28. Different aged group fibroblasts doubling times in room air and with hyperbaric oxygen (HBO_2).

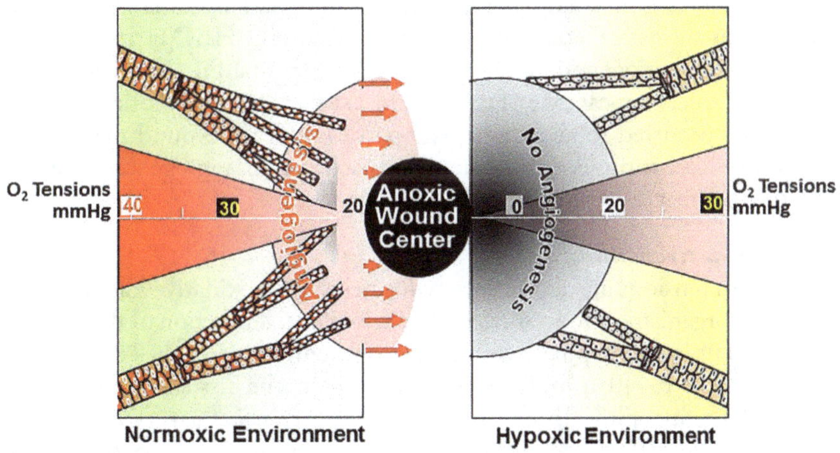

LEGEND: Angiogenesis is dependent on the fibroblast laying down a matrix for capillary budding to invade. This advances the oxygenated environment of the wound (red arrows) so angiogenesis can eventually reach the anoxic wound center. Matrix generation is an oxygen (O_2) dependent secretary function of the fibroblast. Without adequate O_2 tensions at the wound margins angiogenesis will not occur.

Figure 29. Angiogenesis in the normoxic environment versus interruption of angiogenesis in the hypoxic environment.

production of the matrix, and secondary capillary budding into it will be thwarted. The vascular endothelial growth factor (VEGF) is the initiator of these processes and appears, like the fibroblast growth factors, induced by oxygen. Hunt and others have demonstrated that VEGF is increased with increased oxygen tensions.[53,64]

Hyperbaric oxygen appears to be especially important for angiogenesis to proceed in the hypoxic wound and for healing to progress. Hyperbaric oxygen increases tissue oxygen tensions tenfold at the ischemic wound margin (as described in Part 2 of this chapter) and oxygen diffusion distances threefold. These increments can help achieve a wound margin that is adequately oxygenated for inducing VEGF, fibroblast secretion of

> A corollary to Dr. Hart's previous comment about hard and soft scar was his comment that delayed-onset radiation injury and refractory osteomyelitis were ischemic disorders. Previously, these conditions were thought to be due to direct, but delayed, effects of radiation killing tissue and the bioburden being the cause of refractory osteomyelitis. Now contemporary thinking espouses Dr. Hart's concepts, with delayed-onset radiation injury being attributed to a progressive sclerosing arteritis and refractory osteomyelitis being due to ischemic and/or avascular bone at the focus of infection. This insightful thinking supported the approval process of HBO_2 for these two diseases.

a matrix, and capillary budding into the anoxic center of the wound. Clinically, angiogenesis is appreciated by the appearance of healthy granulation tissue in the wound base. Pulses of HBO_2 rather than continuous, sustained levels of hyperoxygenation appear to be adequate for these processes to occur. Marx showed that vascular density increased eightfold in mandibular tissues in which HBO_2 had been used to help manage infection and osteoradionecrosis as compared to patients not receiving HBO_2 for these conditions.[(61)]

Clinical observations indicate that angiogenesis is a delayed effect of HBO_2. Appearance of granulation tissue in a hypoxic wound base is usually not apparent until 10 days to 2 weeks of HBO_2 treatments have been completed. Once granulation tissue is well established, it indicates adequate oxygenation of the wound base, and HBO_2 treatments are no longer needed for angiogenesis to continue. This termination point for HBO_2 is justified by the clinical appearance of the wound as well as the assumption that enough angiogenesis has occurred to allow adequate perfusion at the wound margins for the healing processes to continue. Consequently, to achieve an angiogenesis effect, 14 to 21 HBO_2 treatments are recommended.

Neutrophil Oxidative Killing

Adequate oxygen tensions are also necessary for neutrophil oxidative killing of bacteria and other microorganisms. Hohn showed that this essential function of the white blood cell does not occur in the hypoxic wound environment.[(7)] Again, the "magic number" appears to be a 30 to 40 mmHg oxygen tension in the tissue fluid environment surrounding the neutrophil. These oxygen tensions are necessary for neutrophils to kill bacteria by generating peroxides and superoxides in their phagocytic vesicles. During the actual killing of bacteria, the oxygen consumption in the phagocytic vesicle increases a hundredfold or more (Figure 30).[(49)] When angiogenesis improves perfusion and oxygen tensions in the wound sufficiently, HBO_2 is probably no longer needed for this cellular function to occur. Thus, as in angiogenesis, 14 to 21 treatments are

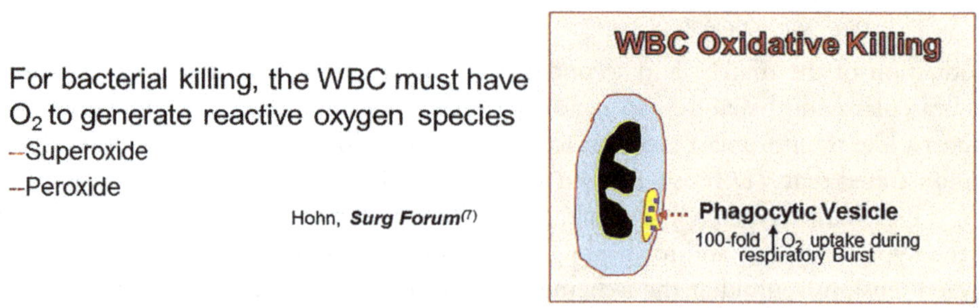
For bacterial killing, the WBC must have O2 to generate reactive oxygen species
--Superoxide
--Peroxide
Hohn, Surg Forum(7)
WBC Oxidative Killing
Phagocytic Vesicle
100-fold ↑ O2 uptake during respiratory Burst

LEGEND: The oxidative burst in the phagocytic vesicle is oxygen dependent.

Figure 30. White blood cell (neutrophil) killing.

probably needed to optimize the effects of HBO_2 for neutrophil oxidative killing of bacteria in the hypoxic wound.

Bone Cell Responses

The cells responsible for bone formation and bone remodeling, the osteoblast and the osteoclast, respectively, like the other cellular elements previously discussed, require adequate oxygen tensions to function. They respond to oxygen gradients in a fashion similar to angiogenesis. Without adequate oxygenation at the margins of the healing/remodeling bone, these cellular functions will not occur. The osteoclast, in particular, exhibits great metabolic activity and consequently has high oxygen demands. The osteoclast is a multinucleated giant cell derived from macrophage linage that has 100 times the metabolic activity of the osteoblast and consequently has very high oxygen demands.[56] The osteoclast is induced (in the environment of bone) to remove calcified tissues by generating acid and alkaline phosphatases.

Although HBO_2 augments osteoclast function to speed removal of necrotic and infected bone, it also increases bone formation, since the osteoblast, like the other cells described in this section, is dependent on oxygen for its metabolic activity (Figure 31).[57] In osteomyelitis, the effects of HBO_2 on the osteoclast can be very beneficial. Hyperbaric oxygen, by improving tissue

The pathophysiology of stress fractures is readily appreciated when the rate of osteoblastic (bone building) activity is compared with the rate of osteoclastic (bone removal) activity. Bone normally undergoes constant remodeling in response to stresses. This remodeling process maintains the structural integrity (i.e., soundness, ability to tolerate stresses and strains, avoidance of pathological fractures, etc.) of bone.

However, osteoclastic ability to remove bone is 100 times greater than osteoblastic ability to form bone. When new stresses arise (e.g., beginning a running program), both cell types are activated. Since bone removal in response to stresses is 100 times faster than new bone formation, these initial responses temporarily make the bone weaker and vulnerable to stress fractures.

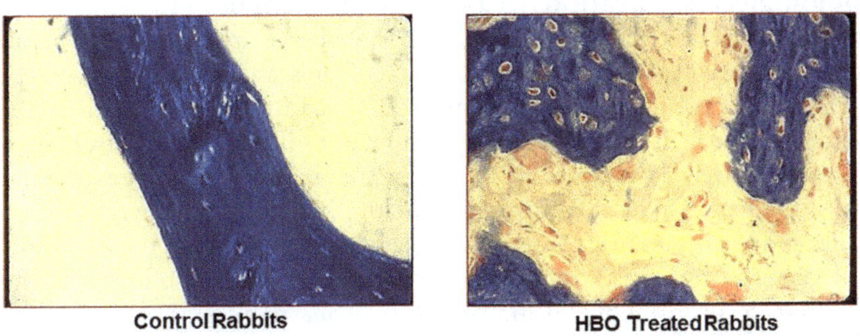

LEGEND: In these microscopic sections, Jones et al. showed the effects of HBO_2 on bone remodeling in the osteotomized femoral necks of rabbits. In the control animals the bone cell activity was quiescent. In the HBO_2 treated group very active cellular activity was present with plump osteocytes within the purple bone spicules, osteoclasts remodeling of the margins of the bone spicules, osteoblasts lining up along the periphery of the bone spicules and markedly increased presence of cells in the bone marrow space.

Even with the significantly increased, osteoclast function, the bone volume (documented with histomorphometric analysis) was maintained in the HBO_2 treated group.

Figure 31. Effects of hyperbaric oxygen on bone activity in osteotomized femoral necks of rabbits (Jones [16]).

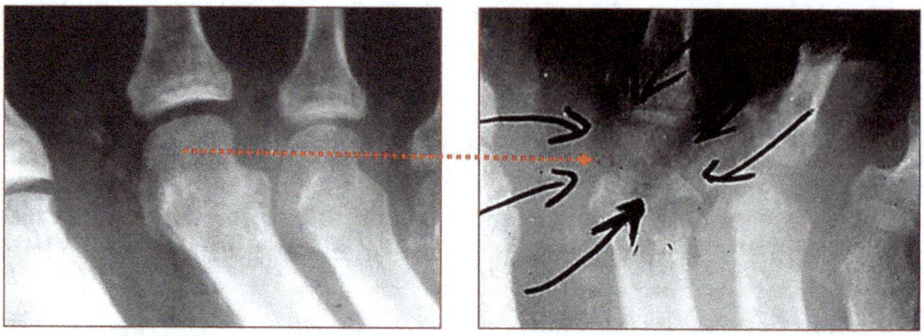

Appearance of Metatarsal Head after 4 weeks of antibiotics, debridements and wound care

Marked Resorption of Metatarsal Head Bone after 2 Weeks of HBO Treatments

LEGEND: A malperforans ulcer in a dysvascular diabetic foot was limb threatening after failing to improve over a month's time. HBO_2 treatments were then initiated in an attempt to avoid a lower limb amputation.

Marked resorption of the infected metatarsal head (encircled by black arrows) became apparent on x-rays. With this information, the metatarsal head was removed and the wound healed. The resorption of dead, infected bone was attributed to HBO_2's stimulation of the osteoclast.

Figure 32. Bone Resorption after initiating HBO_2 treatments in an infected metatarsal head.

oxygen tensions in the hypoxic environment, makes it possible for the osteoclast to function and remove necrotic, infected bone from the wound site (Figure 32).

> **Approved uses of HBO_2 enhance host cellular functions and improve outcomes:** Diabetic foot infections, refractory osteomyelitis, progressive necrotizing infections, radiation injury to tissues, and threatened flaps and grafts.
>
> **Off-label considerations for using HBO_2 for host cellular functions thought to improve outcomes:** Osteonecrosis, systemic sepsis syndrome, fracture healing, autism (pathogenic bowel flora).

Microbiological Applications of Hyperbaric Oxygen

At one time the major effect of HBO_2 on infections, whether in soft tissues or in calcified tissues, was thought to be direct killing of microorganisms. However, this was proven incorrect with aerobic organisms which were observed to thrive in hyper oxygenated environments. Often the bioburden seems to worsen during initial HBO_2 exposures and then progressively decreases as HBO_2 treatments are continued. The explanation for this is that the host responses (neutrophil oxidative killing and angiogenesis to deliver antibiotics and leucocytes to the infection site) are much slower than the rapid doubling times of bacteria. Today, we recognize four beneficial microbial effects of HBO_2 in the management of infections including bactericidal/static effects, cessation of toxin production, inactivation of toxins, and augmentation of the effects of antibiotics.

Bacteriostatic and Bactericidal Effects

There is a continuum of responses of bacteria to HBO_2 exposures. As just mentioned and as would be expected, facultative aerobes such as *Staphylococcus*, *Pseudomonas*, and coliforms appear to thrive in HBO_2 environments. Surprisingly, next in the oxygen continuum responses are the clostridial organisms.[51] Although these organisms are known to thrive and multiply in anaerobic environments, they are not killed by hyperoxic environments – rather, they stop multiplying. Anaerobic *Streptococcus*, *Peptostreptococcus*, and other related species are killed by enriched oxygen environments, while *Bacteroides* species seem to be the bacteria most readily killed by hyperoxia.[44,48] Growth of fungus infections, especially *Actinomyces* species, are also inhibited by HBO_2.[44]

Cessation of Toxin Production

A second microbiological effect of hyperbaric oxygen is that of cessation of endotoxin formation produced by clostridial organisms.[60] *Clostridium perfringens* and other pathogenic clostridial organisms elaborate deadly endotoxins such as the alpha toxin, a C-lecithinase, and theta toxins. These endotoxins cause the life- and limb-endangering effects of cardiovascular collapse and myonecrosis. Hyperbaric oxygen stops these organisms from generating their deadly endotoxins but, as just stated, is not bactericidal. Consequently, cessation of toxin formation is the primary indication for using HBO_2 in clostridial myonecrosis infections. Demello convincingly demonstrated the role of HBO_2 in a canine study (Figure 33).[47] When clostridial infections were introduced into the abdominal cavities, all animals died if only surgery or only HBO_2 was the treatment. Fifty percent of the animals survived with antibiotics alone. Seventy percent survived with surgery plus antibiotics, while a combination of antibiotics, surgery, and HBO_2 improved the survival rate to 95%.

Gas Gangrene

Antibiotics vs. HBO_2*

***Clostridium perfringens* infection in dogs treated with antibiotics, surgery and hyperbaric oxygen**

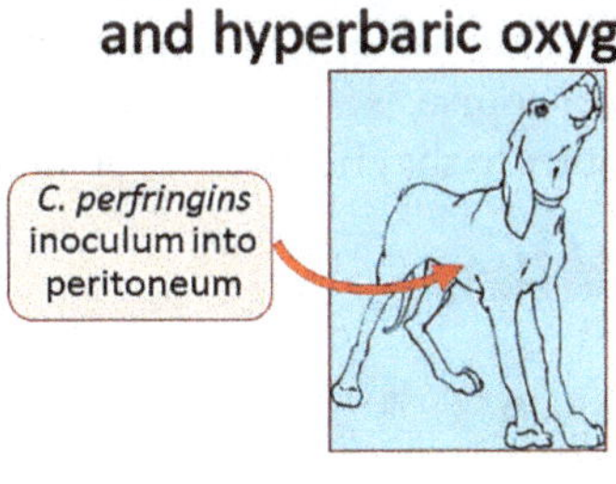

Permutation	% Survival
Surgery	0
HBO_2	0
Antibiotic	50
Surgery + Antibiotics + HBO_2	**95**

*Demello, ***Surgery*** [47]

Figure 33. Effect of different treatment modalities in a canine gas gangrene model.

Although the incidence of clostridial myonecrosis infections has dropped precipitously in recent decades, it always remains a threat in injuries where contamination and severe tissue disruption have occurred. The decreased incidence of clostridial myonecrosis is attributed to the increased diligence of clinicians in preventing clostridial organisms from proliferating. This has been realized through the immediate initiation of antibiotics in open injuries, the use of prophylactic antibiotics in surgeries, and the appreciation of the value of meticulous debridements in injuries where massive contamination (e.g., farm-related), severe trauma to tissues (e.g., combat-related), and tissue death from hypoxia have occurred.

Questions related to clostridial infections had been frequently asked on examinations, especially with respect to HBO_2. Typical questions included, what is *(continued)*

(continued) the most important role of HBO_2 in clostridial infections? The answer is that it prevents the clostridial organisms from generating their deadly endotoxins. Another group of questions relate to management with HBO_2. The answer is that HBO_2 is third in the line of interventions after appropriate antibiotics and debridement surgeries. A third line of questions deal with *C. septicum* infections and their high associations with bowel tumors. Finally, *C. oedematiens* infections are tissue toxic and do not produce gas, but cause massive edema in conjunction with systemic sepsis.

Toxin Inactivation

Toxin inactivation is a third microbiological effect of HBO_2. This has been best appreciated with the theta toxin produced by clostridial organisms.[51,60] It appears that HBO_2 also inactivates the toxin of the brown recluse spider. Tissue necrosis and typical worsening of the wounds after debridements has been observed from these spider bites. Although some of the laboratory studies are contradictory with respect to the benefit of HBO_2 for brown recluse spider bites, clinical observations strongly support its effectiveness.[58,63,76]

Additive to Antibiotics

The fourth microbiological effect of HBO_2 is its additive, possibly synergistic, effect with certain antibiotics. Verklin reported that the effectiveness of aminoglycosides and amphotericin are markedly reduced when these antibiotics are administered in hypoxic environments.[81] The explanation for these observations is that the above-mentioned antibiotics, to be effective, must be actively transported across the cell wall in order to enter the bacteria. The active transport mechanism is oxygen dependent and requires an adequately oxygenated environment (e.g., tissue fluids in the in vivo situation) for the transport to occur. This may also be true for vancomycin. Verklin reported that these antibiotics' effectiveness was reduced by 80% in susceptible organisms when administered in hypoxic environments. Hyperbaric oxygen, of course, is an intervention that effectively improves tissue oxygenation and hence contributes to the effectiveness of these antibiotics.

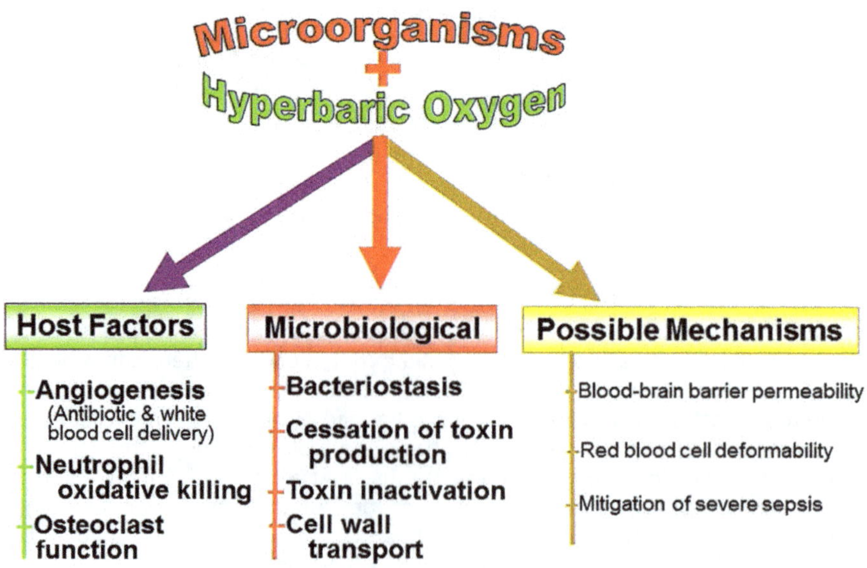

LEGEND: Hyperbaric oxygen has many roles, both well documented as well as potentially beneficial in mitigating the harmful effects of microorganisms.

Figure 34. Hyperbaric oxygen as an antibiotic with multiple mechanisms.

In summary, as described in this section, four microbiological effects, namely (1) direct effects on microorganisms, (2) cessation of toxin formation, (3) toxin inactivation, and (4) additive effect to antibiotics are attributed to HBO_2. When these are combined with host factors and postulated effects of HBO_2 to mitigate sepsis (to be described later), HBO_2 deserves to be labeled "an antibiotic" (Figure 34).

Approved uses of HBO_2 where microbiological effects improve outcomes: Diabetic foot infections, clostridial myonecrosis, necrotizing soft-tissue infections including Fournier's gangrene.

Off-label considerations for HBO_2 where microbiological effects may improve outcomes: Anaerobic infections, mixed aerobic-anaerobic synergistic infections (Meleney's ulcer), brown recluse spider bites, meningitis, systemic sepsis, infections not responding to aminoglycosides in hypoxic wounds.

Mitigation of the Reperfusion Injury

When body tissues are temporarily deprived of a blood supply and oxygen availability, reperfusion injury can occur when perfusion is reestablished. All tissues can survive and resume function after transient periods of ischemia that range from 3 to 4 minutes in the brain, to 4 to 6 hours in muscles, to 12 to 24 hours in bone and even longer for connective tissues and skin. However, during the period of ischemia, the endothelium appears to become "sensitized" due to the hypoxic insult. This activation leads to attachment of neutrophils to the sensitized endothelium. Critical tissues such as brain, heart, and skeletal muscle seem to be most susceptible to these effects.

Once attached, the neutrophil becomes activated and releases the superoxides and peroxides that this cell ordinarily uses for killing bacteria. These reactive oxygen species then attack the surrounding tissues (in a manner analogous to bacteria killing in the phagocytic vesicle). However, intrinsic substances in the tissues such as nitric oxide also combine with the reactive oxygen species to form even more toxic substances such as peroxynitrite (⁻00N), the most toxic oxygen species radical formed in the human body. The consequences are an intense vasoconstriction, the so called "no-reflow phenomenon" of the reperfusion injury, and irreversible tissue damage. The latter occurs because of hypoxia from the vasoconstriction coupled with the destructive effects of the oxygen radicals.

Hyperbaric oxygen interferes with these cascades of events. Thom reported that HBO_2 exposures interrupt the neutrophil adherence to the endothelium through inactivating the beta integrin attachment mechanism in benchwork biochemical studies.[79]

In our "Hot Myocardial Infarction" study, HBO_2 was started within one hour after initiating thrombolysis.[35] Did this prevent the reperfusion injury? Although this question was not specifically addressed, transient arrhythmias signaling reperfusion appeared earlier and lower cardiac enzyme levels were reported in the HBO_2-treated patients. The best explanation for this is that HBO_2 mitigated the effects of the reperfusion injury.

Another potential benefit of HBO_2 mentioned in the citation is that it helps generate oxygen radical scavengers such as superoxide dismutase and peroxidase to inactivate the reactive oxygen species. Scavenger generation is an oxygen-dependent process. Consequently, in the hypoxic environment, a primary consideration of the reperfusion injury, this autoregulating mechanism may be hindered.

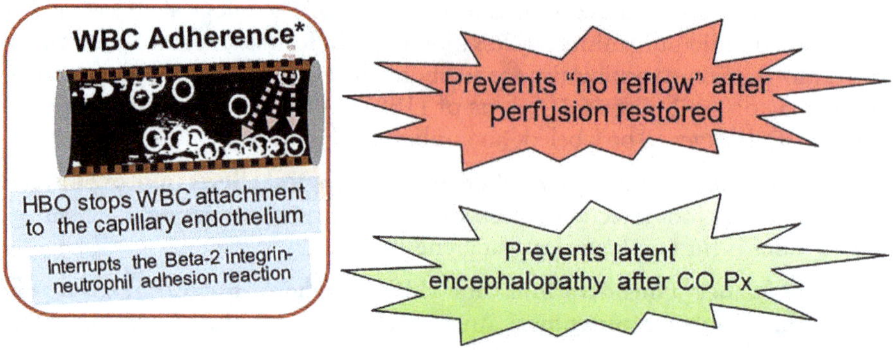

LEGEND: Mitigation of neutrophil adherence to the capillary endothelium sensitized by hypoxia reduces/eliminates the release of toxic O_2 radicals (peroxides and superoxides) that cause the harmful effects of the reperfusion injury.

In addition, this prevents the cascade of reactive oxygen species with nitric oxide (NO)--in hypoxic environments--from forming highly toxic degradation products such as peroxynitrite (-OON).

NOTES & KEY: *Neutrophils adhering to the sensitized capillary endothelium are so indicated by white circles around them (Zamboni[10]); CO Px = Carbon monoxide poisoning, HBO_2 = Hyperbaric oxygen, WBC = White blood cell

Figure 35. Morphology of the reperfusion injury and roles of HBO_2 in mitigating its effects.

Subsequently, Zamboni demonstrated with intravital microscopy that HBO_2 impeded the attachment of the neutrophil to the sensitized endothelium in a reperfusion injury animal model (Figure 35).[85] The clinical benefits of HBO_2 for mitigating the reperfusion injury have not been fully appreciated. A major challenge is starting HBO_2 at the time reperfusion commences, which undoubtedly varies with tissue type and the extent of the ischemia. Obviously, if the ischemia time is lengthy, the hibernating tissues (i.e., the tissues not being perfused) will eventually die. We recommend starting HBO_2 as soon as possible after an extended period of ischemia in critical tissues such as the brain and heart as well as skeletal muscles and perhaps in other organs such as the liver, kidney, pancreas, etc. Finally, HBO_2 should be considered after revascularization surgeries associated with long ischemia times, viability concerns associated with reimplantations, threatened flaps, and other situations where there is a possibility that reperfusion injury will contribute to more morbidity.

> **Approved uses of HBO_2 where reperfusion injury mitigation improves outcomes:** Crush injuries, compartment syndromes.
>
> **Off-label considerations for HBO_2 where reperfusion injury mitigation may improve outcomes:** Acute strokes, acute spinal cord injuries, acute myocardial infarctions, prolonged ischemia times associated with revascularization surgeries, reimplantations, and frostbite.

Gas Washout (and Isobaric Counter Diffusion)

Gas diffusion responds to gradients whether in liquid, gas, or combined phases. This is the principal for understanding decompression science in diving medicine. [69] Gases in high concentrations in liquid and gas mediums will move to mediums with the lower concentrations until equilibrium is reached. This mechanism of HBO_2 is useful for washing out carbon monoxide (and cyanide) in the blood and tissues after poisoning from these agents. By hyper oxygenating blood, there is a steep gradient for carbon monoxide to move from the body tissues to the bloodstream and then be carried to the

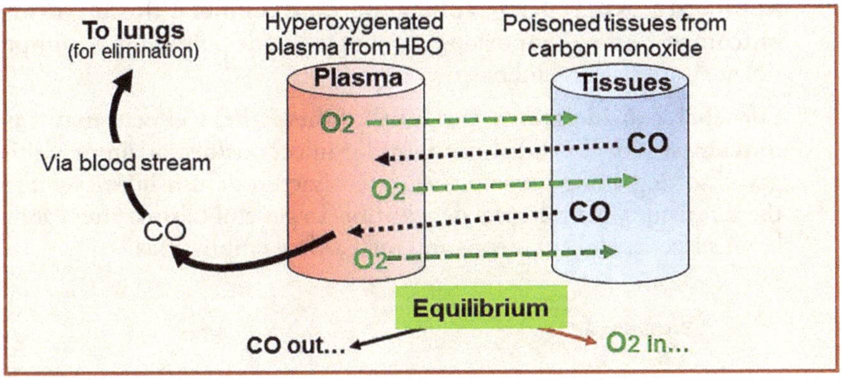

LEGEND: Gases in tissues equilibrate with gases in the plasma.

With high plasma O_2 partial pressures, inert gases & carbon monoxide move from tissues → plasma →lungs → expired air.

KEY: CO = Carbon monoxide, HBO = Hyperbaric Oxygen, O_2 = Oxygen, Via = By way of

Figure 36. Carbon monoxide (and inert gas) "washout" in response to gradients from HBO_2.

lungs and offloaded by exhalation(Figure 36). This effect is appreciated clinically when comparing times to decrease carboxyhemoglobin levels by 50% in the bloodstream.[80] In the carbon monoxide-poisoned victim, carboxyhemoglobin decreases by 50% in 4 hours when breathing room air. With breathing 100% oxygen, the half time is reduced to 1 hour, and with HBO_2 at 2.8 to 3.0 atmospheres absolute, it is reduced to 23 minutes.

In treating decompression sickness, the same principals apply, but the gases involved are different. Instead of employing the gradient to remove carbon monoxide from blood and tissues, the nitrogen (or helium) ongassed to the tissues during the dive is washed out. If the ascent is too rapid, the inert gas will come out of solution and form bubbles. Theoretically, the bubbles and/or remaining inert gas in the tissue will be off-gassed about four times more rapidly breathing oxygen as with breathing air (which is about 80 % nitrogen). With HBO_2, the speed increases to 15 times at pressurization to 3 atmospheres absolute. The other component of the decompression sickness treatment protocol is pressurization to reduce the bubble volume, a primary mechanism of HBO_2 and a direct application of Boyle's law. The result is an immediate decrease in the size of the bubble. This may allow bubbles that were blocking the microcirculation to pass into the venous blood, be carried to the heart, then offloaded when exhaled by the lungs. The combined effect is that bubble volume reduction and gas washout complement each other in the management of decompression sickness.

A corollary of this is the isobaric counter diffusion/isobaric gas sequencing concept. This has been used in technical diving to avoid nitrogen narcosis in deep dives and to speed off-gassing of inert gases by switching gas mixtures while the diver remains at a constant depth. For off-gassing, this enhances removal of the "switched-off" gas. This is due to the gradient effect, and if at a shallow enough depth, allows the breathing of increased percentages of oxygen. Not only does the increased oxygen percentage speed the washout of the remaining inert gas in the tissues, but it also allows oxygen to equilibrate with inert gas in the bubble. Once the inert gas in the bubble is replaced with oxygen, it is expected that the oxygen in the bubble will diffuse into the tissues which have a lower concentration of oxygen (i.e., the gradient effect), be utilized in tissue metabolism, and further dissipate the bubble (Figure 37).

Approved uses of HBO_2 gas offloading (and counter diffusion) to improve outcomes: Carbon monoxide poisoning, cyanide poisoning, decompression sickness, arterial gas embolism.

Off-label considerations for HBO_2 where these effects may improve outcomes: Nonclostridial gas forming infections/necrotizing fasciitis with gas dissecting along tissue planes, open fractures/crush injuries with gas in the soft tissues, neurological deficits (due to gas embolisms) after cardiac and brain surgeries, subcutaneous and mediastinal emphysema.

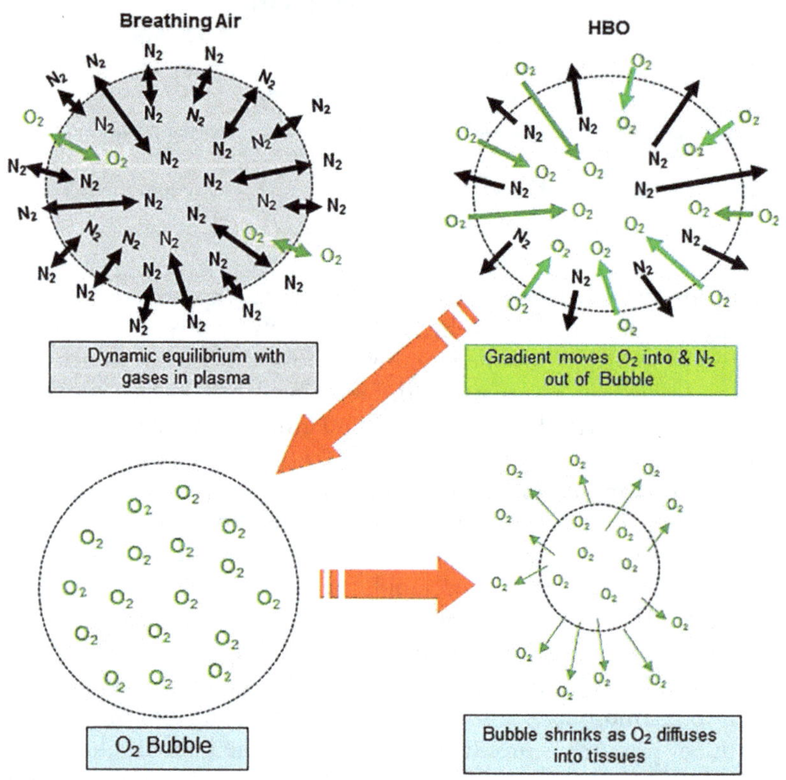

LEGEND: The mechanism of isobaric counter diffusion is potentially an additional benefit of using HBO_2 rather than air alone to reduce bubble volume.

KEY: N_2 = Nitrogen, HBO = Hyperbaric Oxygen, O_2 = Oxygen

Figure 37. Isobaric counter diffusion as a possible mechanism to reduce bubble size in decompression sickness and arterial gas embolism.

OTHER THEORETICAL SECONDARY MECHANISMS OF HYPERBARIC OXYGEN

Red Blood Cell Deformability

Red blood cell (RBC) deformability is a necessary and normal physiological function of the 7.5-micron-diameter RBC. Deformation results in elongation of the RBC so it can pass through the 5-micron-diameter capillary (Figure 38). As RBCs age, they lose their ability to deform. When this occurs, they are filtered out by the reticuloendothelial system in the spleen and other hematopoietic organs where their products (iron, hemoglobin, etc.) are recycled. Sepsis and hypoxia also interfere with the ability for RBCs to deform.[42] Red blood cell deformity is quantified by using a micropore filter to measure how many RBCs pass through it in a finite length of time. This is somewhat analogous to the method to determine a hematocrit. Hurd et al. studied RBC deformability using the micropore filter technique in septic, postoperative, and control patients.[54] The index (i.e., number of RBCs passing through the filter) in septic patients was ⅓ of that observed in the other two patient groups. Red blood cells have oxygen consumption requirements for their metabolic needs like other cell types.[65] Perhaps they, like other cells, need to derive their oxygen supplies from the tissues fluid rather than being able to utilize it directly from the hemoglobin molecule. There is a single report attesting to the beneficial effects of HBO_2 on RBC deformability.[62]

CLINICAL SCENARIO: A 64-year-old patient's septic state secondary to a perforated viscus worsened even after surgical intervention. With progressive deterioration, even with critical care management, triple antibiotics, and intubation during a 30-day period, last rites prayers were being initiated. Serendipitously (the staff surgeon left for a meeting, and a resident surgeon requested a hyperbaric medicine consultation), HBO_2 treatments were initiated, and the patient stopped deteriorating. A few days later, the patient started to improve, gradually recovered fully, and eventually resumed working without restrictions at the same occupation as before becoming ill.

Comment: *See the following text box for comments and a possible explanation for the favorable outcome.*

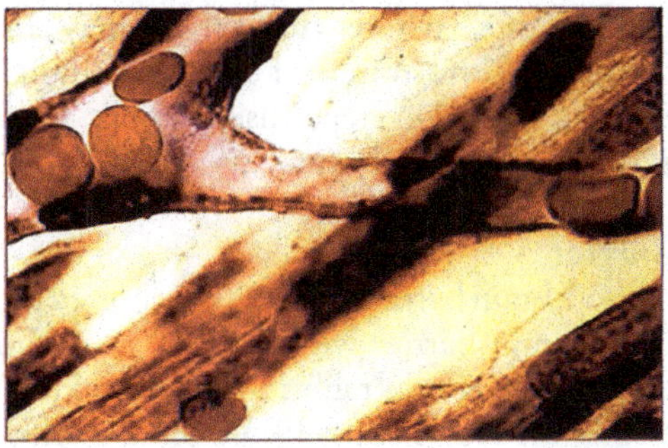

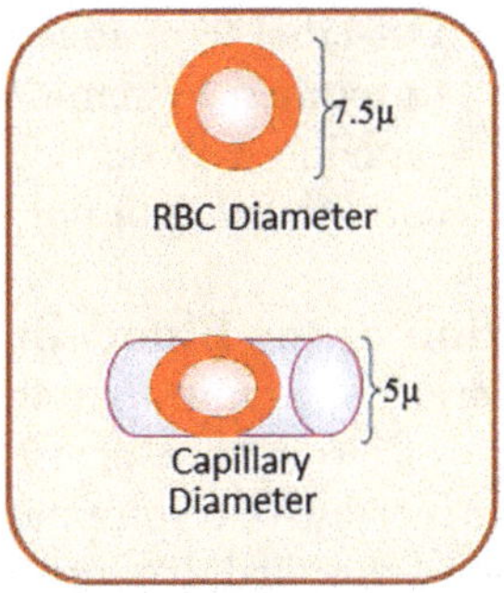

LEGEND: The 7.5μ diameter RBC must deform (elongate) in order to pass through the 5μ diameter capillary. As RBC's age, they loose their ability to deform and are filtered out of the blood stream. Their products are recycled to make new RBC's. In addition to aging, hypoxia (oxygen is necessary for and independent of the hemoglobin carried O_2 in the RBC) and sepsis appear to interfere with RBC deformability.

KEY: O_2 = Oxygen, RBC = Red blood cell, μ = Micron (micrometer)

Figure 38. Red blood cell deformity (elongation) required in order for these cells to pass through the capillary bed and offload their oxygen.

Thom reported marked reductions in mortality using HBO_2 in a polymicrobial sepsis model where he injected feces into the peritoneum of rats.(78) All rats in the study that were managed with room air died. Ten percent of those that were given 100% oxygen at one atmosphere absolute survived, whereas 90% survived in the HBO_2 treatment limb. In addition, and perhaps a more surprising observation, was that those animals that survived had markedly greater bacterial counts in their bloodstreams than those animals that died. Thom offered no explanations for these thought-provoking results.

We proposed an explanation for Thom's findings and the favorable outcome reported in the previous clinical scenario based on RBC deformability. In septic shock, two primary cardiovascular events occur, namely 1) increased cardiac output and 2) decreased peripheral vascular resistance (PVR). We suggest that the decrease in PVR is due to arterial-venous (AV) shunting because the RBCs ability to deform and pass through the capillary bed is severely compromised secondary to sepsis. The decreased PVR then may be due to a decreased pressure head for blood to pass through AV fistulas than would occur if the blood passed through the capillary bed.

The consequences of this are obvious. With RBCs unable to pass through the capillary bed, oxygen can no longer be off-loaded to critical organs. This would be particularly apparent in the liver that is known to have macrophages (e.g., Kupffer cells) to mitigate the effects of the massive bacterial loads from the bowel. If, in fact, HBO_2 improves RBC deformability, a plausible explanation is generated for explaining the outcome in the previous clinical scenario and the findings in Thom's abdominal sepsis laboratory study. The explanation is that HBO_2 restored the ability for RBCs to deform and pass though the capillary bed and thereby offload their oxygen. This restored oxygen to critical tissues and allowed cellular mechanisms to manage the bacterial loads.

Approved uses of HBO_2 where hyperbaric oxygen may improve RBC deformability and improve outcomes: None are specifically approved at this time.

Off-label considerations for HBO_2 where this effect may improve outcomes: Systemic sepsis syndromes, frostbite and other conditions where sludging may occur in the microcirculation, reperfusion injury, vasospastic conditions/ergot poisoning, sickle cell crises, burns.

Alteration of the Blood-Brain Barrier

Hyperbaric oxygen appears to alter the blood-brain barrier. Lance et al. reported increased transport of tetracycline across the blood-brain barrier with HBO_2.(59) We showed a dramatic increase of tryptophan blue into the brains of rabbits exposed to HBO_2 after injection of this vital dye into their carotid arteries (Figure 39).(46) Similar effects were observed if HBO_2 was given up to one hour before the dye injection and as long as four hours after the injection. Burt reported infarct size in a gerbil model decreased from 72% in control animals to 11% in the HBO_2-treated limb.(45) Others have reported in animal studies that HBO_2 reduces ischemic brain injury in animal models.(75,82) This information has obvious clinical implications. First, it contributed to the decision for the Hyperbaric Oxygen Therapy Committee of the Undersea and Hyperbaric Medical Society to include intracranial abscess as an approved indication of HBO_2 therapy.

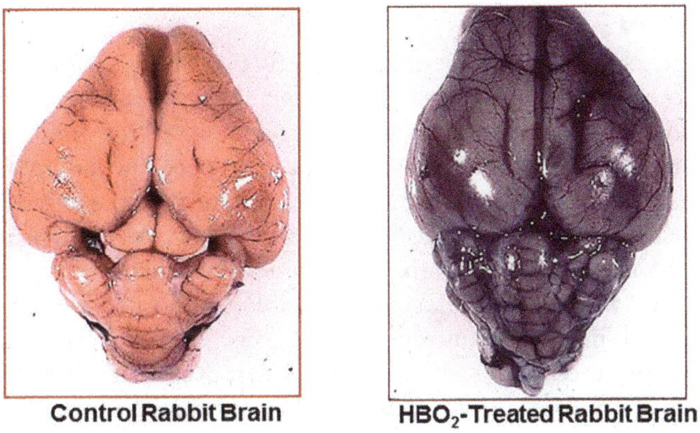

LEGEND: Hyperbaric oxygen markedly altered the amount of tryptophan blue that crossed the blood-brain barrier in our rabbit model.[46]

KEY: HBO_2 = Hyperbaric Oxygen

Figure 39. Permeability of the blood-brain barrier in rabbits improved with HBO_2 after tryptophan blue injection into their carotid arteries.

Although the decision was based on clinical data, the laboratory studies cited above support the decision and help provide the pathophysiology rationale for using HBO_2 for this condition. Second, HBO_2's alteration of the permeability of the blood-brain barrier may improve the delivery of antibiotics for infections and chemotherapeutic agents for tumors in the central nervous system. This consideration, alone, has important ramifications for improving outcomes of these often times difficult-to-treat problems. In addition, this may be the mechanism that improves survival when HBO_2 is used for the intracranial abscess. Third, with acute ischemic injuries of the brain and spinal cord, the preservation of neuro-tissue with HBO_2 (and perhaps coupled with hypothermia) appears promising and could be an important contribution to the management of acute strokes and traumatic brain injuries.[83] Fourth, in patients with established (i.e., chronic and post rehabilitation) neurological impairments such as stroke, Alzheimer's disease, multiple sclerosis, paraplegia/quadriplegia, cerebral palsy, etc., but with changing symptoms, HBO_2 may improve oxygenation of the ischemic penumbra and stop deterioration or even improve function. Finally, HBO_2 may offer "neuroprotection" for high-risk cardiovascular and neurosurgical procedures.[50] In about ⅓ of patients who have these high-risk surgeries, neurological deficits are detectable after the surgery. Although most resolve with time, it can take up to a year's time to do such.

Approved uses of HBO_2 where alterations of the blood-brain barrier may improve outcomes: Intracranial abscess.

Off-label considerations for HBO_2 where this effect may improve outcomes: Chemotherapy and antibiotic delivery to the CNS, enhanced oxygen availability for acute ischemic disorders (stroke, spinal cord injury, near-drowning, carbon monoxide poisoning, etc.), acute management of concussions, neuroprotection for high-risk surgeries, amelioration of the late effects of stroke and degenerative nervous system disorders.

CONCLUSIONS

The secondary mechanisms of hyperbaric oxygen (HBO_2) occur as a consequence of the primary mechanism of breathing pure oxygen at increased partial pressure (i.e., hyperoxygenation). The increased partial pressure is achieved through pressurization in a hyperbaric chamber. The secondary mechanisms occur when hyperoxygenation interacts with tissues and microorganisms. There are four possible outcomes from these interactions. First, tissues that are unable to function because of hypoxia can resume their functions once their environment becomes sufficiently oxygenated. This is especially apparent when HBO_2 makes it possible for host factors to resume their wound-healing and infection-controlling functions. Second, bacterial killing and cessation of toxin production is a secondary effect that occurs in substances that are not normally found in the body that is exogenously produced by bacteria. Third, the secondary mechanisms can augment the normal physiological mechanisms of tissues. The effect is appreciated with vasoconstriction as a mechanism to reduce posttraumatic and vasogenic edema. Fourth, hyperoxygenation provides gradients to tissues for washout of inimical substances that are introduced accidentally or willfully such as in carbon monoxide poisonings and consequentially from inert gas with compressed gas diving. While this might be considered a primary effect of hyperoxygenation, the interactions are secondary to gas gradients introduced to the tissues.

There are noteworthy differences between the primary and secondary mechanisms of HBO_2 (Table 12). Whereas the effects of hyperoxygenation and pressurization occur as soon as pressurization in the hyperbaric chamber is initiated, the secondary mechanisms generally take longer to be realized, are accumulative, and depend on repeated HBO_2 exposures, i.e., "pulses" of HBO_2. Normally, side effects are not associated with the secondary mechanisms of HBO_2, whereas oxygen toxicity and barotrauma are chief concerns of hyper oxygenation and pressurization. Hyperoxygenation as a primary effect is directed at maintaining tissue viability, while the secondary mechanisms focus on tissue viability and repair. As pressures increase with hyperoxygenation, gradients increase and more tissue oxygenation is realized (at the expense of increased oxygenation toxicity risks). The secondary mechanisms appear

TABLE 12. COMPARISON AND CONTRASTS BETWEEN PRIMARY AND SECONDARY MECHANISMS OF HYPERBARIC OXYGEN

	Primary	Secondary
Onset	Immediate	Delayed
Duration	Transient	Long lasting (durable)
Goal	Cell/Tissue survival	Cell/Tissue Function
Effective O_2 pressure	Proportional to ppO_2	~ 2 ATA
Justification	Physics & physiology	Outcomes
Side effects	O_2 toxicity Seizure, pulmonary edema,	Visual acuity changes

to be best realized at 2 to 2.4 atmospheres absolute pressures. Finally, the rationale for justifying the primary hyperoxygenation and pressurization mechanisms is based on verifiable physics and physiological information. In contrast, justifications for the secondary effects are largely based on observed outcomes.

The mechanisms, both primary and secondary, of HBO_2 provide justification for its approved uses. The mechanisms also help to explain why outcomes reported from "off-label" uses of this modality justify further inquiries into their effectiveness. For example, one new possible mechanism that may have important ramifications is that of stem cell mobilization by HBO_2.(77) Consequently, whenever considering using HBO_2 for "off-label" conditions, the mechanisms that may benefit the problem must be a primary consideration. In the future, information of this type will add to the approved uses of HBO_2 therapy.

ACKNOWLEDGMENTS

Dr. George B. Hart, deceased, did much to enlighten the understanding of the HBO_2 mechanisms, and his work greatly contributed to the content of this chapter.

REFERENCES

Part 1:

1. Babior BM. The respiratory burst of phagocytes. J Clin Invest. 1984;73(3):599-601.
2. Dahl-Jorgensen K. Diabetic microangiopathy. Acta Paediatr Suppl. 1998;425:31-4.
3. Guyton AC, Hall JE. O2 and CO2 diffusion. In: Textbook of Medical Physiology, 13th ed. Philadelphia: W.B. Saunders, 13th Ed., 2016. p. 529.
4. Guyton AC, Hall JE, Local and humoral control of tissue blood flow,. Textbook of Medical Physiology, 13th Ed. Philadelphia: W.B. Saunders; 2016. p. 203-214.
5. Hampton MB, Kettle AJ, Winterbourn CC. Inside the neutrophil phagosome: oxidants, myeloperoxidase, and bacterial killing. Blood. 1998;92(9):3007-17.
6. Hansen RO, Lundback K. The basement membrane morphology in diabetes mellitus. In: Ellenberg M, Frikin H, editors. Diabetes mellitus: theory and practice. New York: McGraw-Hill; 1970. p. 178-209.
7. Hohn DC, Hunt TK. Oxidative metabolism and microbial activity of rabbit phagocytes: cells from wounds and peripheral blood. Surg Forum. 1975;26:85-7.
8. Hunt TK, Dunphy JE. Effects of increasing oxygen supply to healing wounds. Br J Surg. 1969;56(9):705.
9. Hunt TK, Linsey M, Sonne M, Jawetz E. Oxygen tension and wound infection. Surg Forum. 1972;23(0):47-9.
10. Hunt TK, Twomey P, Zederfeldt B, Dunphy JE. Respiratory gas tensions and pH in healing wounds. Am J Surg. 1967;114(2):302-7.
11. Hunt TK, Zederfeldt B, Goldstick TK. Oxygen and healing. Am J Surg. 1969;118(4):521-5.
12. Klabunde RE. Oxygen blood flow. In: Cardiovascular physiology concepts. Lippincott Williams & Wilkins; 2011.
13. Moon H, Strauss MB, La SS, Miller SS. The validity of transcutaneous oxygen measurement in predicting healing of diabetic foot ulcers. Undersea Hyperb Med. 2016.
14. Niinikoski J. Effect of oxygen supply on wound healing and formation of experimental granulation tissue. Acta Physiol Scand Suppl. 1969;334:1-72.
15. Nimni ME. Polypeptide growth factors targets delivery systems. Biomaterial. 1997;18:1201-25.
16. Peirce EC Jr. Pathophysiology, apparatus, and methods including the special techniques of hypothermia and hyperbaric oxygen. In: Extracorporeal circulation for open-heart surgery. Springfield (IL): Charles C. Thomas; 1969. p. 84-8.
17. Saiepour D. Glucose and insulin modulate phagocytosis and production of reactive oxygen metabolites in human neutrophil granulocytes. Umea (Sweden) University medical dissertations; 2006. p. 14.
18. Sbarra AJ, Karnovsky ML. The biomechanical basis of phagocytosis I. Metabolic changes during the ingestion of particles by polymorphonuclear leukocytes; II. Incorporation of C14-labeled building blocks into lipid, protein, and glycogen of leukocytes during phagocytosis. J Biol Chem. 1959;234(6):1355-62. 1960;235(8):2224-9.
19. Strauss MB. Diabetic foot and leg wounds: principles, management, and prevention. Prim Care Rep. 2001;7(22):187-98.
20. Strauss MB, Askenov I, Miller S. Challenges of wound healing. Wound Care Hyperb Med. 2011;2(1):28-36.

21. Strauss MB, Askenov I, Miller S. Masterminding wounds. Flagstaff (AZ): Best Publishing Co.; 2010. p. 308-20.

22. Strauss MB, Bryant BJ, Hart GB. Transcutaneous oxygen measurements under hyperbaric oxygen conditions as a predictor for healing problem wounds. Foot Ankle Int. 2002;23(10):933-7.

23. Strauss MB, Chase P, Kustich N, Nation P. Use of the one-two-three- protocol to augment HBO management of dysvascular foot wounds. Annual Scientific Meeting of the Undersea & Hyperbaric Medical Society; 1997.

24. Strauss MB, Miller S, Nhan L. The end-stage wound: its determination and management. Wound Care Hyperb Med. 2013;4(4):19-26.

25. Taylor S, Kalbough C, Balackhurst D, et al. Determinants of functional outcomes after revascularization for critical limb ischemia: an analysis of 1000 consecutive vascular interventions. J Vasc Surg. 2006;44(4):747-56.

26. Wells CH, Goodpasture JE, Horrigan DJ, Hart GB. Tissue gas measurements during hyperbaric oxygen exposure. In: Smith G, editor. Proceedings of the 6th International Congress of Hyperbaric Medicine; 1977. Aberdeen University Press. p. 118-24.

27. Wyss CR, Harrington RM, Burgess EM, Matsen FA. Transcutaneous oxygen as a predictor of success after an amputation. JBJS. 1988;70(2):203-7.

Part 2:

1. Boerema I, Meyne MG, Brummelkamp WK, et al. Life without blood. A study of the influence of high atmospheric pressure and hyperthermia in dilution of the blood. J Cardiovasc Surg. 1960;1:133-46.

2. Cotto-Cumba C, Velez E, Velu SS, et al. Transcutaneous oxygen measurements in normal subjects using topical HBO control module. Undersea Biomed Res. 1991;18(Suppl):109.

3. Fischer BF. Topical hyperbaric oxygen treatment of pressure sores and skin ulcers. Lancet. 1969;2:405-9.

4. Gordillo GM, Roy S, Khanna S, et al. Topical oxygen therapy induces vascular endothelial growth factor expression and improves closure of clinically presented chronic wounds. Clin Exp Pharmacol Physiol. 2008;35(8):957-64.

5. Guyton AC, Hall JE. Carbon dioxide dissociation, Textbook of Medical Physiology, 13th Ed. Philadelphia: W.B. Saunders; 2016. p. 534.

6. Kalliainen LK, Gordillo GM, Schlanger R, Sen CK. Topical oxygen as an adjunct to wound healing: a clinical case series. Pathophysiology. 2003;9(2):81-7.

7. Krogh A. The number of distribution of capillaries in muscle with calculations of the oxygen pressure head necessary for supplying the tissue. J Physiol. 1919;52:409-15.

8. Shandling AH, Ellestad MH, Hart GB, et al. Hyperbaric oxygen and thrombolysis in myocardial infarction: the "HOT MI" pilot study. Am Heart J. 1997;134:544-50.

9. Stavitsky Y, Shandling AH, Ellestad MH, et al. Hyperbaric oxygen and thrombolysis in myocardial infarction: the 'HOT MI' randomized multicenter study. Cardiology. 1998;90:131-6.

10. Strauss MB, Askenov IV, Miller S. Masterminding wounds. Flagstaff (AZ): Best Publishing Co.; 2010. p. 253-85.

11. Thomas MP, Brown LA, Sponseller DR, et al. Myocardial infarct size reduction by the synergistic effect of hyperbaric oxygen and recombinant tissue plasma activator. Am Heart J. 1990;120(4):791-800.

12. Thurston JGB, Greenwood TW. Results of a controlled trial of hyperbaric oxygen in acute myocardial infarction. Quarterly J Med. 1973;168:752-70.

13. Zamboni WA, Persons BL. Hyperbaric oxygen in plastic and reconstructive surgery. In: Bakker DK, Cramer FS, editors. Hyperbaric surgery perioperative care. Flagstaff (AZ): Best Publishing Co.; 2002. p. 397-416.

14. Zamboni WA, Roth AC, Russell RC, et al. Morphologic analysis of the microcirculation during reperfusion of ischemic skeletal muscle and the effect of hyperbaric oxygen. Plast Reconstr Surg. 1993;91(6):1110-23.

Part 3:

1. Baskurt OK, Gelmont D, Meiselman HJ. Red blood cell deformability in sepsis. Am J Respir Crit Care Med. 1988;157(2):421-7.

2. Bird AD, Telfer AB. Effect of hyperbaric oxygen on limb circulation. Lancet. 1965;1(7381):355-6.

3. Bornside GH. Bactericidal effect of hyperbaric oxygen determined by direct exposure. Proc Soc Exp Biol Med. 1969;130(4):1165-7.

4. Burt JT, Kapp JP, Smith RR. Hyperbaric oxygen and cerebral infarction in the gerbil. Surg Neurol. 1987;28(4):265-8.

5. Chambi IP, Ceverha B, Hart GB, Strauss MB. Effect of hyperbaric oxygen in the permeability of the blood-brain barrier. 8th International Congress on Hyperbaric Medicine; 1984; Long Beach, CA. Personal communication.

6. Demello FJ, Haglin JJ, Hitchcock CR. Comparative study of experimental clostridium perfringens infection in dogs treated with antibiotics, surgery, and hyperbaric oxygen. Surgery. 1973;73:936-41.

7. Gottlieb SF. Effect of hyperbaric oxygen on microorganisms. Ann Rev Microbiol. 1971;25:111-52.

8. Hampton MB, Kettle AJ, Winterbourn CC. Inside the neutrophil phagosome: oxidants, myeloperoxidase, and bacterial killing. Blood. 1998;92(9):3007-17.

9. Hang JH, Lo T, Mychaskiw G, Colohan A. Mechanisms of hyperbaric oxygen and neuroprotection in stroke. Pathophysiology. 2005;12(1):63-77.

10. Hart GB, Lamb RC, Strauss MB. Gas Gangrene. J Trauma. 1983;23(11):991-1000.

11. Hart GB, O'Reilly RR, Broussard ND, et al. Treatment of burns with hyperbaric oxygen. Surg Gynecol Obstet. 1974;139(5):693-6.

12. Hopf HW, Gibson JJ, Angles AP, et al. Hyperoxia and angiogenesis. Wound Repair Regen. 2005;13(6):558-64.

13. Hurd TC, Dasmahaparta KC, Rush BF Jr, Machiedo GW. Red blood cell deformability in human and experimental sepsis. Arch Surg. 1998;123(2):217-20.

14. Hyperbaric oxygen therapy. Rev. 48. Effective/Implementation Dates: 06-19-06, CMS Manual System, Pub 100-03 Medicare National Coverage Determinations, Transmittal 48. U.S. Department of Health & Human Services, Centers for Medicare & Medicaid Services; 2006 Mar 17. Change Request 4278.

15. Johnson LC. Kinetics of osteoarthritis. Lab Invest. 1959;8:1223-41.

16. Jones JP Jr, Lewis RH, Lewis T, et al. The effect of hyperbaric oxygen on osteonecrosis. Undersea Biomed Res. 1991;18(Suppl 135):82.

17. Kendall TE, Caniglia RJ. Hyperbaric oxygen in treatment of clinically diagnosed brown recluse spider bites: a review of 48 cases. Undersea Biomed Res. 1989;16:21.

18. Lanse SB, Lee JC, Jacobs EA, Brody H. Changes in the permeability of the blood-brain barrier under hyperbaric oxygen conditions. Aviat Space Environ Med. 1978;49(7):890-4.

19. MacLennan JD. The histotoxic clostridial infections of man. Bact Rev. 1962;26:177-276.

20. Marx RE et al. Relationship of oxygen dose to angiogenesis induction in irradiated tissue. Am J Surg. 1990;160:519-24.

21. Mathieu D, Goget J, Vinkier L. Red blood cell deformity and hyperbaric oxygen therapy [abstract]. HBO Review. 1985;6:280.

22. Maynor ML, Moon RE, Klitzman B, et al. Brown recluse spider envenomation: a prospective trial of hyperbaric oxygen therapy. Acad Emerg Med. 1997;4(3):184-92.

23. Patel V, Chivukula IV, Roy S, et al. Oxygen: from the benefits of inducing VEGF expression to managing the risk of hyperbaric stress. Antioxid Redox Signal. 2005;7(9-10):1377-87. Erratum in: Antioxid Redox Signal. 2005;7(11-12):1783.

24. Powell RJ, Machiedo GW, Rush BF Jr. Decreased red blood cell deformability in sepsis. Ann Surg. 1993;59(1):65-8.

25. Reenstra WR, Buras JA, Svoboda KS. Hyperbaric oxygen increases human dermal fibroblast proliferation, growth factor receptor number and in vitro wound closure. Undersea Hyperb Med. 1998;25(Suppl):35-6.

26. Skyhar MJ, Hargens AR, Strauss MB, et al. Hyperbaric oxygen reduces edema and necrosis of skeletal muscle in compartment syndromes associated with hemorrhagic hypotension. J Bone Joint Surg Am. 1986;68(8):1218-24.

27. Stewart RJ, Mason SW, Taira MT, et al. Effect of radical scavengers and hyperbaric oxygen on smoke-induced pulmonary edema. Undersea Hyperb Med. 1994;21(1):21-30.

28. Strauss MB, Aksenov IV. Diving science. Champaign (IL): Human Kinetics; 2004. p. 51-81.

29. Strauss MB, Askenov I, Miller S. Masterminding wounds. Flagstaff (AZ): Best Publishing Co.; 2010. p. 270-1.

30. Strauss MB, Hargens AR, Gershuni DH, et al. Delayed use of hyperbaric oxygen for treatment of a model anterior compartment syndrome. J Orthop Res. 1986;4(1):108-11.

31. Strauss MB, Hargens AR, Gershuni DH, et al. Reduction of skeletal muscle necrosis using intermittent hyperbaric oxygen in a model compartment syndrome. J Bone Joint Surg Am. 1983;65(5):656-62.

32. Strauss MB, Hart GB, Miller SS, et al. Mechanisms of hyperbaric oxygen, part 1. Wound Care Hyperb Med. 2012;3(3):27-42.

33. Sukoff MH, Lewis D, Nordstrom H, Larson J. Reduction of post-ischemic edema with hyperbaric oxygen. Plast Reconstr Surg. 1985;76(4):596-603.

34. Sunami K, Takeda Y, Hashimoto M, et al. Hyperbaric oxygen reduces [brain] infarct volume in rats by increasing oxygen supply to the ischemic periphery. Crit Care Med. 2000;28(8):2831-6.

35. Svenden FJ. Treatment of clinically diagnosed brown recluse spider bites with hyperbaric oxygen: a clinical observation. J Arkansas Med Soc. 1986;83:199-204.

36. Thom SR, Bhopale VM, Velazquez OC, et al. Stem cell mobilization by hyperbaric oxygen. Exp Biol. 2006;290(4):1378-86.

37. Thom SR, Lauermann MW, Hart GB. Intermittent hyperbaric oxygen therapy for reduction of mortality in experimental polymicrobial sepsis. J Infect Dis. 1986;154(3):504-10.

38. Thom SR, Mendiguren I, Hardy K, et al. Inhibition of human neutrophil beta2-integrin-dependant adherence by hyperbaric O2. Am J Physiol. 1997;272:770-7.
39. Thom SR, Myers RAM, Kindwall EP. Carbon monoxide and cyanide poisoning. In: Kindwall EP, Whelan HT, editors. Hyperbaric medicine practice. 3rd ed. Flagstaff (AZ): Best Publishing Co.; 2008. p. 401-40.
40. Verklin RN, Mandel GL. Alteration of effectiveness of antibiotics by anaerobiosis. J Lab Clin Med. 1977;89:65-71.
41. Wada K, Nishi D, Kitamura T, et al. Hyperbaric oxygenation therapy enhances the protective effective of moderate hypothermia against forebrain ischemia in the gerbil hippocampus. Undersea Hyperbaric Med. 2006;33(6):399-405.
42. Wang GH, Zhang XG, Jiang ZL, et al. Neuroprotective effects of hyperbaric oxygen on traumatic brain injury in the rat. J Neurotrauma. 2010;27(9):1733-43.
43. Weaver LK, editor. Hyperbaric oxygen therapy indications – the Hyperbaric Oxygen Therapy Committee report. Durham (NC): Undersea & Hyperbaric Medical Society; 2014.
44. Zamboni WA, Wong HP, Stephenson LL. Effect of Hyperbaric oxygen on neutrophil concentration and pulmonary sequestration in reperfusion injury. Arch Surg. 1996;131(7):756-60.

SECTION 2 SECTION

Disorders Approved for Hyperbaric Treatment

CHAPTER 13 CHAPTER

Carbon Monoxide

CHAPTER THIRTEEN OVERVIEW

Introduction **303**
Pathophysiology **304**
Clinical Presentation **306**
Neurologic Manifestations 306
Cardiac Manifestations 307
Diagnosis **307**
Management **309**
Prehospital 309
Hospital Treatment 309
Oxygen Therapy 309
Complications of Oxygen Therapy 311
Mechanisms of Action of Hyperbaric Oxygen in CO Poisoning 312
Disposition 313
Special Populations **313**
Pregnancy 313
Pediatrics 314
Conclusion **314**
Acknowledgments **315**
References **316**

Carbon Monoxide

Jillian Theobald

INTRODUCTION

Carbon monoxide is a colorless, tasteless, and odorless gas. It is one of the leading causes of injury and death worldwide. Based on death certificate data, mortality from unintentional, non-fire-related carbon monoxide exposures results in an average of 439 deaths each year in the United States.[117] However, with improved data collection through the Center for Disease Control, estimates may be closer to 2,000 deaths per year.[53] In 2014, the National Poison Data System listed gases/fumes/vapors as the leading cause of death in children five years old or less.[92] Furthermore, carbon monoxide poisoning results in more than 200,000 emergency department visits per year and more than 20,000 hospital admissions.[61]

Carbon monoxide (CO) originates from incomplete combustion of carbon-containing materials. Common external exposure sources include house fires, automobile exhaust, ice resurfacing machines, furnaces, burning of charcoal, wood, and natural gas for heating or cooking, propane-powered equipment, and methylene chloride paint stripper.[29,59,97] Another major source of CO is cigarette smoking. Average carboxyhemoglobin levels (COHb) of 3.0%–7.7% are found in heavy cigarette smokers, compared to 1.3%–2.0% in nonsmokers.[122] Carbon monoxide poisoning can occur occupationally (i.e. firefighters, ice resurfacing machine or forklift operators), unintentionally, and as a means of suicide. The incidence of carbon monoxide poisoning increases during power outages caused by natural disasters.[52] Interestingly, since the introduction of the Clean Air Act in 1970, the mortality rate from motor vehicle–related CO poisoning has declined.[91] Carbon monoxide is also produced endogenously through the degradation of hemoglobin by heme oxidase, resulting in detectable carboxyhemoglobin levels in nonexposed individuals.[142]

In industry, the major factor for carbon monoxide exposure is inadequate ventilation where propane-powered vehicles are used. Exposures from forklifts and ice resurfacing machines have been reported.[29,140] Other work environments that produce large amounts of CO, and therefore heighten the risk of poisoning, are the steel industry, due to coke ovens, and the paint industry, in which inhaled methylene chloride (dichloromethane) is metabolized to CO by the liver.[108] Firefighters and other first responders are also at increased risk for CO poisoning from smoke inhalation and from entering environments with elevated CO levels unknowingly.[37,109-110]

Men have higher rates of death from carbon monoxide poisoning, presumably due to higher risk behaviors and environments.[20,59] The elderly (age ≥ 65) are also at increased risk for death from CO poisoning as they are more likely to dismiss symptoms as being caused by underlying medical conditions more prevalent in this population.[20]

Women and children, however, are more likely to be exposed to carbon monoxide, and most exposures occur in the winter months (November to February).[19]

PATHOPHYSIOLOGY

Carbon monoxide exerts its detrimental effects through multiple mechanisms. These include tissue hypoxia, interference with cellular respiration, inflammatory-mediated damage, and neuronal cell damage. CO typically enters the body through inhalation and is transported to the blood through the alveolar-capillary membrane where it binds hemoglobin. The relative affinity of CO for hemoglobin is approximately 200-fold greater than that of O_2. The dynamics of CO movement across the alveolar-capillary membrane are well described mathematically (e.g., Coburn-Forster-Kane equation).[27] Movement is influenced by the CO and O_2 partial pressures in inspired gas, the content of these two gases in the blood, pulmonary CO diffusivity, alveolar ventilation, duration of exposure, and pulmonary perfusion.

Hypoxia is the most important aspect of CO pathophysiology, and cellular hypoxia occurs by several mechanisms. The oxygen-carrying capacity of blood is decreased due to the formation of carboxyhemoglobin (COHb). Carboxyhemoglobin is CO bound to hemoglobin which renders the involved hemoglobin unable to bind O_2. Furthermore, CoHb causes a leftward shift of the oxyhemoglobin dissociation curve. A leftward shift increases the binding affinity of hemoglobin for oxygen and decreases the delivery to tissues. Early in CO poisoning, hyperventilation-induced respiratory alkalosis also produces leftward shift, further decreasing oxygen delivery to the tissues. Yet the formation of carboxyhemoglobin alone is not enough to fully explain CO's detrimental effects, as dogs transfused with the same concentration of carboxyhemoglobin formed by inhalation of CO displayed no toxic effects.[46] Other mechanisms of CO toxicity are likely mediated by CO binding to myoglobin and cytochrome oxidase. This impairs cellular function and further worsens tissue hypoxia. Several investigators have suggested that the myocardial compromise seen in CO poisoning may be related to CO binding to myoglobin.[26,123] Myoglobin is an intracellular protein which facilitates O_2 transport from hemoglobin to mitochondria; abnormal functioning of the protein is most likely to be seen in muscles with high metabolic demand like the myocardium. Coburn estimated that myoglobin may be the principal protein responsible for extravascular CO binding, which accounts for 10% to 15% of the total body burden.[26] CO can also bind to cytochrome c oxidase, and hypotension and hypoxia augment this process.[13,22] Brown and Piantadosi have shown experimentally that during exposure to 5,000 to 10,000 ppm CO, the COHb level rises, hypotension occurs, and binding of CO to cytochrome c oxidase can be detected.[15] This binding causes cellular stress through mitochondrial dysfunction. ATP synthesis is inhibited and causes mitochondria to generate hydroxyl-like radicals.[13,104] Energy production and mitochondrial function are restored after COHb levels decrease.[13]

Organ blood flow is also altered in CO poisoning and typically rises within minutes following exposure to CO. Brain perfusion increases 47% above normal in lambs exposed to 1,000 ppm CO.[72] Exposure to 3,000 ppm CO can cause brain blood flow to rise 450% in cats,[121] and a dose/response relationship has been observed in rats.[83] Vasodilation in response to high concentrations of CO is linked to extravascular acidosis and hypoxic stimulation of the carotid bodies, leading to increases in ventilation.[75,83] Clinical reports have frequently noted vascular insults to precede or coincide with neurological deficits.[71,88] Although local tissue blood flow is markedly elevated early during exposure to CO, animals sustain a temporary drop in systemic blood pressure as time of exposure becomes prolonged. This change appears to be accentuated in some vascular beds. For example, Song et al. studied the cardiovascular responses of cats to 3,000 ppm CO for 90 to 193 minutes.(121) Brain blood flow increased 200% within minutes while mean systemic blood pressure decreased somewhat, from 150 to 100 mmHg. The animals tolerated this state for approximately 2 hours, and then blood pressure dropped to about 70 mmHg. Although systemic pressure dropped by approximately 30%, blood flow in several areas of the brain dropped by 100% (back to the normal blood flow rate). The sudden relative drop in local blood flow correlated with development of pathology in the globus pallidus.

Cerebral vasodilation is mediated through the release of nitric oxide (NO), and one biochemical mechanism by which CO can damage vascular endothelium is via NO. CO enhances the rate of release of NO from both platelets and endothelial cells.(124) At CO concentrations less than 3,000 ppm, nitric oxide synthase activity is unchanged from control, but CO competes with NO for intracellular hemoprotein-binding sites.(124,129) Therefore, the steady-state concentration of NO rises and allows for alternative reactions. This includes the reaction between superoxide anion and NO, to yield the potent oxidizing and nitrating agent peroxynitrite. Nitrotyrosine, the product of protein tyrosine nitration by peroxynitrite, is increased in aorta, lung, and brain after exposure to CO, and it is found closely associated with the vascular endothelium.(62,131) Endothelial NO-mediated changes are a prerequisite for leukocyte adherence to the cerebral microvasculature following CO poisoning. The sudden alteration in microvascular flow causes leukocytes to adhere to endothelium. Once leukocytes are adherent and activated, they liberate proteases and reactive O_2 species that cause conversion of endothelial xanthine dehydrogenase to xanthine oxidase, and xanthine oxidase activity is required for subsequent brain lipid peroxidation.(127-128) Beta 2 integrin adhesion molecules are required for leukocyte activation and progression of the oxidative stress cascade.(62,126)

Additionally, CO poisoning causes elevations of glutamate, norepinephrine, and dopamine. This has been shown in the brains of experimental animals and in human fatalities.(5,63,96) Enzymatic breakdown, as well as autooxidation of the monoamine neurotransmitters, generates reactive oxygen species.(10) Based on the effects of agents that block the N-methyl-D-aspartate (NMDA) receptor, elevations of glutamate in experimental CO poisoning have been linked to delayed amnesia, the loss of CA1 neurons in the hippocampus of mice, and the loss of glutamate-dependent cochlear ganglion cells of rats.(63,77,96) Antioxidants can protect against CO-mediated cytotoxicity of glutamate-dependent nerve cells.(41) Mechanisms of glutamate neurotoxicity include excessive calcium influx, free-radical production, calcium-calmodulin-dependent activation of cytosolic nitric oxide synthase, and lipid peroxidation. Moderate neuronal stimulation by excitatory amino acids also causes mitochondrial dysfunction with impaired ATP synthesis and production of reactive O_2 species.(9) Neuronal cell death can occur through necrosis or apoptosis, and there may be synergistic injury with other forms of oxidative stress as reactive O_2 species can intensify excitotoxicity.(12,101) Glutamate can also injure cells in the central nervous system that do not have NMDA receptors by competing for cysteine uptake, which inhibits synthesis of glutathione.(98) Overall, the pathophysiology of carbon monoxide–mediated neurotoxicity likely involves CO-mediated primary vascular effects, concurrent hypoxic stress, and excitotoxicity. These mechanisms all work in concert to precipitate one or more of the clinical manifestations of delayed neurological sequelae.

CLINICAL PRESENTATION

Carbon monoxide exposed patients commonly present with nonspecific symptoms that mimic influenza-like illnesses (Table 1).[7,35] Symptoms typically include headache, dizziness, nausea, vomiting, weakness, and fatigue. The most common symptom reported is headache. Because these symptoms are so nonspecific, the treating physician must retain a high level of suspicion for carbon monoxide poisoning as delays in recognition and treatment are common.

TABLE 1. COMMON SYMPTOMS OF CO POISONING[40,137]

SYMPTOMS	
Headache	Visual Disturbances
Nausea	Chest pain
Vomiting	Loss of consciousness
Dizziness	Myalgias
Weakness	Coma
Difficulty concentrating	Death
Shortness of breath	

Similar to the symptoms patients report, physical exam findings also vary greatly in CO-poisoned patients. Physical exam findings depend on the time between exposure and presentation to the hospital. They also depend on the duration and magnitude of exposure. The most common physical findings include tachycardia and tachypnea.[45] However, the majority of patients have normal vital signs upon presentation. Like carboxyhemoglobin levels, vital sign abnormalities do not predict the severity of poisoning.[1] It is extremely rare to find the cherry-red color that is classically described in CO poisoning. This sign represents a true soaking of the tissues with CO over a significant length of time and is typically found at autopsy. Any evidence of smoke inhalation such as soot in the nasal or upper airways, singed nasal hair, or voice changes should be considered as an indicator of exposure to CO. Blistering of the skin over pressure-bearing areas may be present, especially if the patient was unconscious for an extended period of time. This is thought to be due to local tissue ischemia from pressure combined with tissue hypoxia from CO.[56] Retinal hemorrhages can occur, especially after exposures greater than 12 hours.[68]

Neurologic Manifestations

A thorough neurological exam should be performed to establish a baseline and to evaluate for subtle neurological signs as they can be easily missed. Patients with carbon monoxide exposures can develop two neurological syndromes: persistent neurological sequelae and delayed neurological sequelae. Persistent neurological sequelae refers to patients with abnormal neurological findings immediately following exposure. These can improve but may not resolve completely. Any component of the neurologic system can be affected, and there have been reports of damage to the vestibulocochlear system, extrapyramidal system, and even the brachial plexus.[38,70,106]

Delayed neurological sequelae develop days to months after exposure.[138] The reported incidence of developing delayed neurological symptoms ranges widely from 3%

to 47%.[25,120] The true incidence of delayed neurological symptoms is likely higher, because mild changes in personality and cognition are often subtle and overlooked. Some delayed neurological sequelae can be quite dramatic and can have cognitive, motor, and affective qualities. Symptoms can include aphasia, apraxia, apathy, disorientation, hallucinations, nuchal rigidity, gait disturbances, fecal and urinary incontinence, bradykinesia, memory deficits, insomnia, and dementia.[138] There have been reports of personality changes with impulsiveness, violence, verbal aggressiveness, and psychosis.[64] In one prospective study, CO-poisoned patients who received HBO_2 therapy still reported significant anxiety and depression even one year post exposure.[64] There are no clinical indicators that will predict the occurrence of this syndrome; however, many people who later developed delayed neurological sequelae had an initial loss of consciousness.[25] Neuropsychiatric testing may allow earlier detection of subtle neurological changes. In two studies, the degree of impairment on early testing correlated with the number of HBO_2 treatments deemed clinically necessary.[66,87] It is prudent for patients to be referred for testing upon discharge following CO exposure.[89]

Cardiac Manifestations

Many patients who die on scene or upon arrival at the hospital do so from a cardiac etiology. This is often from an arrhythmia or hypotension with severe impairment of tissue perfusion. In a large observational study, nearly half of patients who died of acute CO poisoning showed signs of circulatory failure at autopsy. Histologically, there was evidence of hyperemia of the myocardial stroma, cardiac muscle fiber damage with swelling, and loss of cross striation.[85] Carbon monoxide is well-known to induce arrhythmias and electrocardiographic abnormalities.[18,21,113] This likely occurs through modulation of sodium channels in the heart.[30] The most commonly seen electrocardiogram (ECG) changes are sinus tachycardia and t-wave and ST segment abnormalities.[135] Furthermore, even low levels of COHb can lower the ventricular fibrillation threshold of the myocardium.[32,76] Patients with preexisting heart disease seem to be at greater risk for the cardiotoxic effects of carbon monoxide, and they may have symptoms at lower levels of COHb than patients without heart disease. One study showed that those with known coronary artery disease who were exposed to CO displayed ischemic ECG changes and angina during exercise.[2-3] Even low-level occupational exposures of workers with preexisting coronary artery disease can result in death. For example, two workers died from CO exposure with COHb levels in the 20% to 30% range. Preexisting heart disease and atherosclerosis were documented at autopsy, and it was thought that cardiac arrhythmias were the major factor leading to death.[6]

Myocardial infarction can occur following CO exposure, and there have been many case reports of both non-ST-segment elevation and ST-segment elevation myocardial infarctions.[47,134] Often these patients will have normal coronary arteries on angiography.[65] For those who sustain cardiac injury during an acute episode of poisoning, long-term mortality significantly increases compared to CO-poisoned patients without evidence of myocardial injury.[57] There is also some evidence that exposure to CO may accelerate atherosclerotic vascular disease.[102] However, significant gaps in our understanding of this association persist.[143]

DIAGNOSIS

A high index of suspicion of CO poisoning must be maintained at all times as it is a diagnosis that is easily missed. Diagnosing the acute exposure is relatively simple if the patient has been in a fire, a known exhaust situation, or an industry where the possibility of CO generation is high. In the home, exposure to CO may be more subtle, and clues that should heighten suspicion for CO poisoning include the development of flu-like symptoms in multiple family members, improvement upon leaving the home, or symptomatic pets.

A carboxyhemoglobin level should be obtained on all patients. Pulse oximetry is unreliable in CO poisoning; therefore, patients require a blood sample to determine COHb concentrations.(54) A COHb level measures the load of CO present in red blood cells but does not assess consequent cellular CO-associated effects that may be involved with injuries in the myocardium and brain. Furthermore, COHb levels correlate poorly with symptoms or outcomes and are only an indicator of exposure to CO.(55) There are finger probe pulse co-oximeters that can detect carboxyhemoglobin. Co-oximeters are good noninvasive screening tools; however, they tend to overestimate carboxyhemoglobin levels, especially at lower levels.(111,115) Co-oximeters should not replace obtaining a blood sample for accurate carboxyhemoglobin determination. Alternatively, CO exposure can be measured by detecting CO levels in expired alveolar air and directly in the blood. This method may be used as another indicator of poisoning.

A complete blood count is also important to obtain because the amount of functional hemoglobin is greatly reduced in anemic patients poisoned by CO. A COHb level of 30% is much more significant in a patient who has a hemoglobin of 7g/dL compared to one who has a hemoglobin of 15g/dL. A pregnancy test should be obtained in all women of childbearing age. Because CO poisoning can cause significant cardiotoxicity, there should be a low threshold for obtaining an EKG or cardiac markers of injury. Although patients with known coronary artery disease or those with risk factors are at increased risk for CO cardiotoxicity, even those with normal coronary arteries can sustain cardiac damage from CO poisoning.(65) Patients who have been unconscious for an extended period of time are at risk for rhabdomyolysis, and a creatine kinase level should be done. Rhabdomyolysis can lead to acute tubular necrosis and renal failure.(141)

Secondary to tissue hypoxia, a metabolic acidosis or elevation in lactate may indicate more severe CO poisoning. Higher levels of lactate may correlate with need for treatment or more severe symptoms.(34) Although there is a correlation between high COHb levels and acidosis, patients with normal or alkalotic pH can have equally severe neurologic symptoms. There is greater correlation between abnormal psychometric test results and COHb levels than between abnormal psychometric results and blood gases.(94)

Computed tomography and magnetic resonance imaging may detect brain lesions in CO-poisoned patients. The globus pallidus is the most commonly involved area, although all areas of the brain can show radiologic abnormalities.(78) The incidence of radiographic abnormalities varies widely.(60) However, there is correlation between cognitive impairments and abnormalities on MRI.(100) Recently, more sophisticated neuroimaging techniques have been used to detect abnormalities in patients who, in some cases, exhibited only subtle neurological impairments. Aberrations in resting cerebral blood flow and cerebral vasoactivity to carbon dioxide have been detected by single-photon emission computed tomography (SPECT).(84,116) The perfusion defects seen on SPECT seem to correlate with cognitive deficits found on neuropsychological testing even months after exposure.(44) Abnormalities have also been found on positron emission tomography and fMRI in CO-poisoned patients.(31,33) The primary shortcoming with these imaging techniques is their limited sensitivity and availability.

Hence, neuroimaging has not yet provided a reliable method for assessing the severity of CO poisoning.

MANAGEMENT

Prehospital

Emergency medical service providers should protect themselves with standard-issue personal protective equipment when entering an environment where there is concern for elevated carbon monoxide levels. For the CO-poisoned patient, prehospital care should focus on removing the patient from the source, protecting the airway, and providing respiratory support. Unconscious patients or patients showing evidence of respiratory distress should be intubated as early as possible. Oxygen should be provided in the highest concentration possible during transport. An intravenous (IV) line should be established for potential drug administration should cardiac arrhythmias develop as CO-poisoned patients are at risk for these. Advanced cardiac and trauma life support protocols should be followed to ensure safe and successful transport of the patient.

Hospital Treatment

Initial workup and management of carbon monoxide–poisoned patients should focus on airway and breathing. If the patient is not protecting his or her airway, or there is concern for smoke inhalation, then early intubation should occur. Oxygen delivery is an important component of treatment and should be given at the highest concentration possible (see Oxygen Therapy section below). If not already done, an IV line should be placed, and the patient should be attached to a cardiac monitor. Carbon monoxide–poisoned patients require a thorough physical exam to evaluate for potential traumatic injuries or alternative causes of their condition. Arrhythmias are treated according to advanced cardiac life support protocols. Hypotension should be treated with IV fluids and then vasopressors if need be.

Oxygen Therapy

Oxygen therapy is the most critical component of treatment for carbon monoxide poisoning. It consists of both normobaric oxygen delivery and hyperbaric oxygen (HBO_2) therapy. Oxygen therapy reduces the half-life of COHb. In patients breathing ambient room air, the half-life of carboxyhemoglobin is about 5–6 hours.[103] Carbon monoxide poisoned patients breathing normobaric 100% oxygen exhibit a half-life of 75 ± 25 minutes. HBO_2 treatment further shortens the half-life to approximately 20 minutes with a range of 4–86 minutes.[93] Normobaric oxygen is readily available and should be applied as soon as carbon monoxide poisoning is suspected. In spite of treatment, approximately 12% to 23% of patients treated with normobaric oxygen develop delayed or recurrent sequelae between 1 and 21 days after their original exposure.[95,132] Hyperbaric oxygen has been used with increasing frequency for severe CO poisoning, as clinical recovery seems to be improved beyond that expected with normobaric oxygen therapy.[48,95,132,139] However, significant controversy exists as to whether the optimal method of treatment of CO poisoning is normobaric oxygen as opposed to HBO_2.[17]

The first prospective clinical trial involving hyperbaric oxygen therapy failed to find it superior to normobaric oxygen treatment.[107] However, the HBO_2 therapy given was at a much lower oxygen partial pressure, 2 atmospheres absolute (ATA), versus the more standard pressure of 2.5 to 3 ATA. Furthermore, in nearly half of the study population, hyperbaric treatment was initiated more than six hours after patients were discovered. In 1969, a retrospective study indicated that hyperbaric oxygen reduced mortality and morbidity only if administered within six hours after CO poisoning.[49]

Scheinkestel et al. also reported no benefit from hyperbaric oxygen therapy in a prospective double-blind trial of 191 patients.[114] They randomized patients to 1 HBO_2 treatment at 2.8 ATA versus normobaric oxygen, each for 100 minutes. Unfortunately, the mean delay to treatment was 7.3 hours, and only 46% of patients who entered the study were assessed to determine treatment efficacy at 1-month follow-up. These issues severely diminish the potential impact of the investigation.

A much-larger trial of hyperbaric oxygen therapy for 575 patients with acute symptoms was published as an abstract of an interim analysis of data.[86] The final study data has never been published. Patients were treated with 90 minutes of HBO_2 at 2.5 ATA or 12 hours of normobaric oxygen and were followed up at 1, 3, 6, and 12 months. At one month, there was no statistical difference between patients who were and those who were not treated with hyperbaric oxygen. At 3 months, those treated with normobaric oxygen had a higher incidence of delayed sequelae, 15% versus 9.5%, than those treated with HBO_2. At 6 months, the difference between the groups was less, and at 12 months there was no statistical difference.

Hyperbaric oxygen therapy was found to have a significant benefit in another prospective, randomized trial.[36] However, the end points used in this study were not typical in that they assessed EEG activity and cerebral blood flow and not delayed neurologic sequelae. Twenty-six patients were hospitalized within 2 hours of discovery, and they were equally divided between 2 treatment groups: normobaric oxygen or 2.5 ATA O_2. Three weeks later, patients treated with hyperbaric oxygen had significantly fewer abnormalities on electroencephalogram and SPECT scans than those treated with ambient pressure oxygen.

A prospective, randomized investigation involving 60 patients who appeared to suffer from mild to moderate poisoning showed a positive effect of HBO_2.[132] All patients had symptoms such as headache, nausea, and lethargy, but patients with ischemic changes on electrocardiogram or a history of unconsciousness were excluded. Patients were treated with 2.8 ATA for 30 minutes followed by 90 minutes at 2.0 ATA or normobaric oxygen until symptoms resolved. Delayed neurological sequelae were defined as development of new neurological symptoms and also as reductions from original scores on the standardized psychometric battery. Interestingly, the initial test scores were not helpful in identifying those who went on to suffer delayed sequelae. Twenty-three percent of patients (7 of 30) treated with ambient-pressure oxygen developed neurological sequelae approximately 6 days after poisoning, and sequelae persisted for up to 49 days. No patients treated with hyperbaric oxygen developed sequelae.

Another positive prospective, double-blind, randomized controlled trial by Weaver LK, et al., evaluated 152 CO-poisoned patients at 6 weeks, 6 months, and 1 year following treatment. Patients were randomized to receive 3 HBO_2 treatments (1 session at 3.0 ATA for 1 hour and 2.0 ATA for the second hour, followed by 2 sessions at 2.0 ATA for 2 hours) or a sham treatment of normobaric oxygen for 1 hour. Only 25% of those treated with HBO_2 had cognitive sequelae at 6 weeks, compared to 46.1% of those given normobaric oxygen.[139] Although this study is probably the most rigorous to demonstrate a positive effect of HBO_2 therapy for CO poisoned patients, there are some important flaws in the study to consider. The study was initially designed to assess the outcome of delayed neurologic sequelae (DNS); however, in the final published study, the measured outcome was changed to total cognitive sequelae. The study was terminated early due to demonstration of benefit of HBO_2 on total cognitive sequelae not DNS. Moreover, patients in the normobaric oxygen arm were found to have longer exposure times and greater prevalence of cerebellar abnormalities on initial evaluation. [139]

The most recent study comparing HBO_2 to normobaric oxygen for carbon monoxide–poisoned patients was a prospective, randomized, unblended trial that spanned 11 years.[4] Patients with transient loss of consciousness were randomized to HBO_2 at 2.0 ATA for 2 hours or normobaric oxygen for 6 hours. Patients with more significant impairment, defined as a Glascow Coma Score of less than 8 upon rescue, were randomized to HBO_2 for 1 or 2 sessions at 2.0 ATA for 2 hours. At 1-month follow-up, 42% of HBO_2-treated patients and 39% of normobaric-treated patients were found to have neurologic symptoms. For the more severe group, those treated with two sessions of HBO_2 seemed to do worse than those treated with just one session. Concerns with this study are that 20% were lost to follow-up, and the HBO_2 ATA was lower than customary for CO-poisoned patients.

While a recent Cochrane review found no statistical difference between normobaric oxygen or HBO_2 therapy, the authors cautioned the interpretation of that result. The difficulty in drawing direct conclusions from the review comes from the wide variability in the manner with which the severity of exposure was assessed, the methods used to determine morbidity, and the heterogeneity among the treatments in the included studies.[17]

There is no definition for staging the severity of CO poisoning; thus, it remains difficult to evaluate patients in a prospective manner or compare the efficacy of different treatments. The ultimate decision for the use of surface oxygen versus hyperbaric oxygen treatment should be based on neurologic presentation, rather than the COHb level alone. As there is some evidence of benefit in CO poisoning and minimal adverse effects, HBO_2 therapy should be used when the risk of mortality or morbidity is high. In terms of defining clear guidelines for referral for hyperbaric oxygen treatment, however, the major dilemma appears to be in establishing a threshold for poisoning severity below which clinical outcomes are not favorably affected by hyperbaric oxygen. Thus, until reliable diagnostic tests are identified to prospectively determine the relative risk of carbon monoxide poisoning, a conservative treatment plan is likely to be in the patient's best interest. Overall, the general consensus is to recommend HBO_2 therapy for patients with the characteristics outlined in Table 2.

Complications of Oxygen Therapy

Normobaric oxygen delivery can cause a number of complications even if the duration of treatment is on the magnitude of hours. Hyperoxia can cause atelectasis, mucosal inflammation, generation of reactive oxygen species, and vasoconstriction.[118] Complications among patients treated with normobaric oxygen for carbon monoxide poisoning ranged from 5%–30%. One study of severely poisoned patients admitted to an intensive care unit found that the complication rate was 30.4%, which is higher than typically reported.[74] There is an argument that normobaric oxygen therapy leads to prolonged hospital stays in comparison to HBO_2, and most complications arise from the length of hospital stay.[74,90]

The types of complications seen with hyperbaric oxygen include hyperoxia seizures, barotrauma, pulmonary edema, and claustrophobia. The most common adverse event is middle- and inner-ear barotrauma.[105] Pulmonary edema is more likely to occur in heart failure patients, and HBO_2 therapy should be used with caution in this population.[138] Seizures, although rare, can occur, and patients with uncontrolled seizure disorders are at the most risk.[51,112] Other, less severe symptoms can occur

TABLE 2. PATIENT HISTORICAL, PHYSICAL EXAM, OR LABORATORY FINDINGS THAT WARRANT REFERRAL FOR HBO_2 THERAPY

COHb levels greater than 25%
History of ischemic heart disease and COHb level greater than 20%
COHb levels greater than 15% in a pregnant woman
Angina and/or electrocardiographic evidence of ischemia
Cardiac arrhythmias
Metabolic acidosis
Prolonged (greater than 24 hours) exposure
History of unconsciousness
Altered mental status
Seizure
Abormal neurological examination
Patients who remain symptomatic following 4 hours of 100% oxygen treatment
Those patients arriving moderatly symptomatic, but conscious, and with suspected CD poisoning at a hospital that lacks the ability to test COHb

during HBO_2 therapy and include nausea, vomiting, muscle twitching, anxiety, respiratory changes, vertigo, behavior changes, visual changes, sweating, and auditory changes. Although there are varying reports of the incidence of complications from HBO_2 treatment, it seems as though they are less than 1% per treatment session.[50] A detailed summary of the management of critically ill children in hyperbaric chambers shows that, although complications do occur, most can be managed easily by a skilled clinical team.[67]

Mechanisms of Action of Hyperbaric Oxygen in CO Poisoning

Current knowledge indicates that there are multiple mechanisms of action of hyperbaric oxygen therapy in CO poisoning. Based on the law of mass action, elevated partial pressures of O_2 will accelerate the rate of CO dissociation from hemoglobin. Thus, COHb half-life can be decreased from approximately 5.5 hours when breathing air and to approximately 20 minutes when breathing O_2 at 3 ATA.[99] Indeed, this was the reasoning behind the first clinical implementation of hyperbaric oxygen therapy for CO poisoning.[119] As the COHb level is not associated with clinical risk, it is hard to accept that a more rapid dissociation of CO from hemoglobin could be the central factor for the benefit of hyperbaric oxygen. A fraction of the acute mortality from CO is due to hypoxia, however, and prompt removal of CO from hemoglobin will be of benefit. HBO_2 also promotes normalization of tissue hypoxia.[43] CO binds to cytochrome oxidase, particularly when the COHb level exceeds 40% to 50%. Brown and Piantadosi demonstrated that hyperbaric oxygen at 3 ATA markedly accelerates the dissociation of CO from cytochrome oxidase.[13] Furthermore, it was shown that HBO_2 completely reversed brain mitochondrial electron transport chain inhibition by CO.[14] Hyperbaric oxygen also has effects related to the cascade of vascular injury triggered by CO poisoning.[62,128] Hyperbaric oxygen was found to be effective for preventing brain oxidative injury through increased heme oxygenase and upregulation of antioxidants.[125] The mechanism appears to be associated with denaturation of a membrane-associated guanylate cyclase that plays a role in coordinating the elevated affinity of beta 2 integrins expressed on the cell surface.[8] Given that vascular changes are prominent in clinical CO poisoning, it is feasible that neurological sequelae in patients may involve a perivascular injury mediated by leukocyte sequestration and activation.[62,126] Moreover, HBO_2 reduces neuronal apoptosis and necrosis,[16,82] and it also mobilizes stem cells via a nitric oxide–dependent mechanism.[130] Hence, timely administration of hyperbaric oxygen may ameliorate the cascade leading to brain injury via multiple mechanisms.

Disposition

The critical determination in carbon monoxide–poisoned patients is the severity of the poisoning. The majority of patients seen in emergency departments have a mild exposure to CO and become asymptomatic after receiving 100% oxygen for 3 to 4 hours. These asymptomatic patients may be sent home as long as their place of residence is deemed safe and CO free. Adequate follow-up with a primary care doctor and referral for neuropsychiatric testing should be assured prior to discharge.

The ultimate decision to treat a patient with 100% oxygen at a local hospital or to transfer that patient to a hyperbaric facility will remain a difficult one to make. The community, length of transport, available staff, and severity of symptoms must be considered. However, even in severe poisonings, it can be both advantageous and safe to transport patients for hyperbaric treatment.[11] Each area should establish its own specific criteria prior to a CO emergency, to determine which patients will be transferred. Information about the location of hyperbaric facilities in the continental United States and Canada is available from the Diver's Alert Network (DAN) at Duke University in Durham, North Carolina (919-684-9111). The poison center in each state will also have a list of the closest hyperbaric facilities.

SPECIAL POPULATIONS

Pregnancy

A pregnant woman exposed to CO usually has a 10% to 15% lower steady-state level of COHb than does her fetus.[58] This difference arises following diffusion of maternal blood-borne CO into fetal blood. Fetal hemoglobin has a higher affinity for CO than does hemoglobin in the adult. As fetal weight increases with gestational age, so does placental CO diffusion.[79] Transplacental diffusion occurs at a slow, steady state: the fetal COHb level equals and then exceeds the maternal level after 5–6 hours of exposure.[80-81] Thus, the fetal hemoglobin saturation is dependent on the duration of exposure and the concentration of CO to which the mother is exposed. Fetal PaO_2 is usually 20 to 30 mmHg lower than the normal maternal PaO_2. This level falls in the fetal blood in direct proportion to the increasing COHb concentrations in both the fetal and maternal blood. The normal fetal oxyhemoglobin-dissociation curve is to the left of the adult curve, allowing discharge of oxygen at lower oxygen tensions in fetal tissue. Exposure to CO results in a further leftward shift in both maternal and fetal oxyhemoglobin curves, decreasing oxygen release from the mother to the fetus and from fetal hemoglobin to fetal tissue. During oxygen therapy, the elimination half-life of carboxyhemoglobin in the fetus is much longer in comparison to maternal elimination. It will take approximately five times the normal duration of treatment for a given maternal carboxyhemoglobin level to adequately treat the fetus.[58]

It is common for the mother to survive exposure to CO levels that are lethal for the fetus. Cramer reported a fetal death occurring as a result of accidental maternal CO poisoning. The mother's highest recorded COHb level was 23.7%. In the same exposure, the father had a COHb level of 45%. Both mother and father were treated with 100% oxygen via normal rebreathing mask for 8 hours. After that treatment, their COHb levels were below 3%. Within 48 hours of discharge, the mother returned to the hospital, reporting loss of fetal movement. Sonography confirmed intrauterine death, and after induction of labor, a stillborn male was delivered. The fetus showed the classic signs of cherry red lips and pink nail beds and skin in the nonmacerated areas. A right-ventricle sample of blood indicated a 25% COHb level. Higher levels of COHb (35.1%) were found on analysis of the liver and spleen.(28) Exposure to carbon monoxide in utero not only increases the risk of intrauterine fetal demise, but it can also cause preterm delivery, cerebral palsy, cardiomegaly, limb malformations, and microcephaly.(42) Most cases of mild to moderate CO poisoning in the mother go on to uncomplicated deliveries of healthy children. However, the more severe the maternal exposure, especially those with neurologic impairment, the higher the likelihood of a poor outcome in the infant.(73)

In pregnant females who present following a carbon monoxide exposure, management is the same as nonpregnant females with a few exceptions. In hospitals where carboxyhemoglobin levels are not attainable, it may be prudent to obtain fetal heart rate monitoring. There have been cases of CO poisoning in the third trimester that showed fetal tachycardia and absence of heart rate variability. These changes resolved with normobaric oxygen therapy.(133) Pregnant women should be referred for HBO_2 therapy if they meet the referral criteria of nonpregnant patients. Most agree that, in pregnant patients, HBO_2 therapy should also be considered for carboxyhemoglobin levels of 15%–20% and signs of fetal distress such as abnormal heart rate monitoring. Although almost all the HBO_2 therapy studies described above excluded pregnant patients, HBO_2 therapy has been used safely in pregnancy with no evidence of adverse neonatal outcomes.(39)

Pediatrics

Children seem to be more susceptible to carbon monoxide exposures than adults. They tend to be more symptomatic at lower carboxyhemoglobin levels.(69) Also, children typically have a higher minute ventilation and metabolic rate than adults; thus, for any given ambient carbon monoxide level they are more likely to become symptomatic sooner.(24) Although children will still manifest the same symptoms as adults, it is not uncommon for them to have unusual presentations. The same management and diagnostic principles for adults apply to children. Yet carboxyhemoglobin levels can be difficult to interpret in the very young due to the presence of significant levels of fetal hemoglobin and elevated bilirubin levels.(136) Children who do develop delayed neurological sequelae, however, seem to do better than adults long-term.(25) HBO_2 therapy has been shown to be safe for children.(23)

CONCLUSION

Carbon monoxide poisoning is very common and easily missed. Diagnosis is based on reported symptoms, assessing for signs of end organ damage, and obtaining carboxyhemoglobin levels if possible. Management should focus on removal from the source and oxygen delivery. Because of low risk for adverse events, patients with severe signs of poisoning should be referred for HBO_2 therapy.

ACKNOWLEDGMENTS

The author would like to acknowledge the significant contribution of Roy Myers, Stephen Thom, and Eric Kindwall to the original and subsequent versions of this chapter.

REFERENCES

1. Aksu NM, Akkaş M, Çoşkun F, et al. Could vital signs predict carbon monoxide intoxication? J Int Med Res. 2012;40(1):366-70.
2. Allred EN, Bleecker ER, Chaitman BR, et al. Effects of carbon monoxide on myocardial ischemia. Environ Health Perspect. 1991;91:89-132.
3. Anderson EW, Andelman RJ, Strauch JM, Fortuin NJ, Knelson JH. Effect of low-level carbon monoxide exposure on onset and duration of angina pectoris: a study in ten patients with ischemic heart disease. Ann Intern Med. 1973;79(1):46-50.
4. Annane D, Chadda K, Gajdos P, Jars-Guincestre M, Chevret S, Raphael JC. Hyperbaric oxygen therapy for acute domestic carbon monoxide poisoning: two randomized controlled trials. Intensive Care Med. 2011;37(3):486-92.
5. Arranz B, Blennow K, Eriksson A, Maånsson J, Marcusson J. Serotonergic, noradrenergic, and dopaminergic measures in suicide brains. Biol Psychiatry. 1997;41(10):1000-9.
6. Atkins EH, Baker EL. Exacerbation of coronary artery disease by occupational carbon monoxide exposure: a report to two fatalities and a review of the literature. Am J Ind Med. 1985;7(1):73-9.
7. Baker MD, Henretig FM, Ludwig S. Carboxyhemoglobin levels in children with nonspecific flu-like symptoms. J Pediatr. 1988;113(3):501-4.
8. Banick PD, Chen Q, Xu YA, Thom SR. Nitric oxide inhibits neutrophil β2 integrin function by inhibiting membrane-associated cyclic GMP synthesis. J Cell Physiol. 1997;172(1):12-24.
9. Beal MF. Does impairment of energy metabolism result in excitotoxic neuronal death in neurodegenerative illnesses? Ann Neurol. 1992;31(2):119-30.
10. Bindoli A, Rigobello MP, Deeble DJ. Biochemical and toxicological properties of the oxidation products of catecholamines. Free Radic Biol Med. 1992;13(4):391-405.
11. Bosco G, Garetto G, Rubini A, et al. Safety of transport and hyperbaric oxygen treatment in critically-ill patients from Padua hospitals into a centrally-located, stand-alone hyperbaric facility. Diving Hyperb Med. 2016;46(3):155-9.
12. Bridges RJ, Koh JY, Hatalski CG, Cotman CW. Increased excitotoxic vulnerability of cortical cultures with reduced levels of glutathione. Eur J Pharmacol. 1991;192(1):199-200.
13. Brown SD, Piantadosi CA. Reversal of carbon monoxide-cytochrome c oxidase binding by hyperbaric oxygen in vivo. Adv Exp Med Biol. 1989;248:747-54.
14. Brown SD, Piantadosi CA. Recovery of energy metabolism in rat brain after carbon monoxide hypoxia. J Clin Invest. 1992;89(2):666-72.
15. Brown SD, Piantadosi CA. In vivo binding of carbon monoxide to cytochrome c oxidase in rat brain. J Appl Physiol. 1990;68(2):604-10.
16. Brvar M, Luzar B, Finderle Ž, Šuput D, Bunc M. The time-dependent protective effect of hyperbaric oxygen on neuronal cell apoptosis in carbon monoxide poisoning. Inhal Toxicol. 2010;22(12):1026-31.
17. Buckley NA, Juurlink DN, Isbister G, Bennett MH, Lavonas EJ. Hyperbaric oxygen for carbon monoxide poisoning. Cochrane Database Syst Rev. 2011(4).
18. Canpolat U, Aytemir K, Oto A. Familial brugada syndrome unmasked by carbon monoxide intoxication. Int J Cardiol. 2012;156(1):e18-9.
19. Centers for Disease Control and Prevention (CDC). Carbon monoxide exposures – United States, 2000-2009. MMWR Morb Mortal Wkly Rep. 2011;60(30):1014-7.

20. Centers for Disease Control and Prevention (CDC). Carbon monoxide-related deaths – United States, 1999-2004. MMWR Morb Mortal Wkly Rep. 2007;56(50):1309-12.

21. Cetin M, Ornek E, Murat SN, Cetin ZG, Oksuz F, Gokcen E. A case of carbon monoxide poisoning presenting with supraventricular tachycardia. Intern Med. 2011;50(21):2607-9.

22. Chance B, Erecinska M, Wagner M. Mitochondrial responses to carbon monoxide toxicity. Ann N Y Acad Sci. 1970;174(1):193-204.

23. Chang Y, Lee H, Huang J, Chiu C, Chen C, Wu C. Risk factors and outcome analysis in children with carbon monoxide poisoning. Pediatr Neonatol. 2016. Epub ahead of print.

24. Cho C, Chiu N, Ho C, Peng C. Carbon monoxide poisoning in children. Pediatr Neonatol. 2008;49(4):121-5.

25. Choi S. Delayed neurologic sequelae in carbon monoxide intoxication. Arch Neurol. 1983;40(7):433-5.

26. Coburn RF. The carbon monoxide body stores. Ann N Y Acad Sci. 1970;174(1):11-22.

27. Coburn RF, Forster RE, Kane PB. Considerations of the physiological variables that determine the blood carboxyhemoglobin concentration in man. J Clin Invest. 1965;44(11):1899-910.

28. Cramer CR. Fetal death due to accidental maternal carbon monoxide poisoning. J Toxicol Clin Toxicol. 1982;19(3):297-301.

29. Creswell PD, Meiman JG, Nehls-Lowe H, et al. Exposure to elevated carbon monoxide levels at an indoor ice arena – Wisconsin, 2014. MMWR Morb Mortal Wkly Rep. 2015;64(45):1267-70.

30. Dallas ML, Yang Z, Boyle JP, et al. Carbon monoxide induces cardiac arrhythmia via induction of the late Na+ current. Am J Respir Crit Care Med. 2012;186(7):648-56.

31. De Reuck J, Decoo D, Lemahieu I, et al. A positron emission tomography study of patients with acute carbon monoxide poisoning treated by hyperbaric oxygen. J Neurol. 1993;240(7):430-4.

32. DeBias DA, Banerjee CM, Birkhead NC, Greene CH, Scott SD, Harrer WV. Effects of carbon monoxide inhalation on ventricular fibrillation. Arch Environ Health. 1976;31(1).

33. Dinghua L, Dongbo L, Jianyu Z, Lan P. A resting-state functional magnetic resonance imaging study of acute carbon monoxide poisoning in humans. Cell Biochem Biophys. 2013;67(3):1029-32.

34. Doğan NÖ, Savrun A, Levent S, et al. Can initial lactate levels predict the severity of unintentional carbon monoxide poisoning? Hum Exp Toxicol. 2015;34(3):324-9.

35. Dolan MC, Haltom TL, Barrows GH, Short CS, Ferriell KM. Carboxyhemoglobin levels in patients with flu-like symptoms. Ann Emerg Med. 1987;16(7):782-6.

36. Ducassé JL, Celsis P, Marc-Vergnes JP. Non-comatose patients with acute carbon monoxide poisoning: hyperbaric or normobaric oxygenation? Undersea Hyperb Med. 1995;22(1):9-15.

37. Dunn KH, Shulman S, Stock AL, Naeher LP. Personal carbon monoxide exposures among firefighters at prescribed forest burns in the Southeastern United States. Arch Environ Occup Health. 2013;68(1):55-9.

38. El Murr T, Tohme A, Ghayad E. [Acute deafness after carbon monoxide poisoning. Case report and review of the literature]. Ann Med Interne. 2002;153(3):206-8.

39. Elkharrat D, Raphael JC, Korach JM, et al. Acute carbon monoxide intoxication and hyperbaric oxygen in pregnancy. Intensive Care Med. 1991;17(5):289-92.

40. Ernst A, Zibrak JD. Carbon monoxide poisoning. N Engl J Med. 1998;339(22):1603-8.

41. Fechter LD, Liu Y, Pearce TA. Cochlear protection from carbon monoxide exposure by free radical blockers in the guinea pig. Toxicol Appl Pharmacol. 1997;142(1):47-55.

42. Friedman P, Guo XM, Stiller RJ, Laifer SA. Carbon monoxide exposure during pregnancy. Obstet Gynecol Surv. 2015;70(11):705-12.

43. Fuson RL, Saltzman HA, Boineau JP, Smith WW, Spach MS, Brown IW. Oxygenation and carbonic acidosis in cyanotic dogs exposed to hyperbaric oxygenation. Surg Gynecol Obstet. 1966;122(2):340-52.

44. Gale SD, Hopkins RO, Weaver LK, Bigler ED, Booth EJ, Blatter DD. MRI, quantitative MRI, SPECT, and neuropsychological findings following carbon monoxide poisoning. Brain Injury. 1999;13(4):229-43.

45. Gandini C, Castoldi A, Candura S, et al. Carbon monoxide cardiotoxicity. J Toxicol Clin Toxicol. 2001;39(1):35.

46. Goldbaum LR, Orellano T, Dergal E. Mechanism of the toxic action of carbon monoxide. Ann Clin Lab Sci. 1976;6(4):372-6.

47. Gonullu H, Karadas S, Aydin I, Vuruskan E. ST elevation myocardial infarction due to carbon monoxide poisoning. Eurasian J Med. 2011;43(2):125-8.

48. Gorman DF, Clayton D, Gilligan JE, Webb RK. A longitudinal study of 100 consecutive admissions for carbon monoxide poisoning to the royal adelaide hospital. Anaesth Intensive Care. 1992;20(3):311-6.

49. Goulon M, Barois A, Rapin M, Nouailhat F, Grosbuis S, Labrousse J. [Carbon monoxide poisoning and acute anoxia due to inhalation of coal gas and hydrocarbons: 302 cases, 273 treated by hyperbaric oxygen at 2 ata]. Ann Med Interne. 1969;120(5):335-49.

50. Hadanny A, Meir O, Bechor Y, Fishlev G, Bergan J, Efrati S. The safety of hyperbaric oxygen treatment – retrospective analysis in 2,334 patients. Undersea Hyperb Medicine. 2016;43(2):113-22.

51. Hadanny A, Meir O, Bechor Y, Fishlev G, Bergan J, Efrati S. Seizures during hyperbaric oxygen therapy: retrospective analysis of 62,614 treatment sessions. Undersea Hyperb Med. 2016;43(1):21-8.

52. Hampson NB, Stock AL. Storm-related carbon monoxide poisonings: lessons learned from recent epidemics. Undersea Hyperb Med. 2006;33(4):257-63.

53. Hampson NB. U.S. mortality due to carbon monoxide poisoning, 1999–2014. Accidental and intentional deaths. Annals ATS. 2016;13(10):1768-74.

54. Hampson NB. Pulse oximetry in severe carbon monoxide poisoning. Chest. 1998;114(4):1036-41.

55. Hampson NB, Hauff NM. Carboxyhemoglobin levels in carbon monoxide poisoning: do they correlate with the clinical picture? Am J Emerg Med. 2008;26(6):665-9.

56. He H, Gao Y, Li C, et al. Cutaneous blistering secondary to acute carbon-monoxide intoxication. Clin Exp Dermatol. 2007;32(1):129-31.

57. Henry CR, Satran D, Lindgren B, Adkinson C, Nicholson CI, Henry TD. Myocardial injury and long-term mortality following moderate to severe carbon monoxide poisoning. JAMA. 2006;295(4):398-402.

58. Hill EP, Hill JR, Power GG, Longo LD. Carbon monoxide exchanges between the human fetus and mother: a mathematical model. Am J Physiol Heart Circ Physiol. 1977;232(3):H311-23.

59. Hnatov MV. Non-fire carbon monoxide deaths associated with the use of consumer products. 2013 annual estimates. 2016.

60. Hopkins RO, Fearing MA, Weaver LK, Foley JF. Basal ganglia lesions following carbon monoxide poisoning. Brain Inj. 2006;20(3):273-81.

61. Iqbal S, Law H, Clower JH, Yip FY, Elixhauser A. Hospital burden of unintentional carbon monoxide poisoning in the United States, 2007. Am J Emerg Med. 2012;30(5):657-64.

62. Ischiropoulos H, Beers MF, Ohnishi ST, Fisher D, Garner SE, Thom SR. Nitric oxide production and perivascular nitration in brain after carbon monoxide poisoning in the rat. J Clin Invest. 1996;97(10):2260-7.

63. Ishimaru H, Katoh A, Suzuki H, Fukuta T, Kameyama T, Nabeshima T. Effects of N-methyl-D-aspartate receptor antagonists on carbon monoxide-induced brain damage in mice. J Pharmacol Exp Ther. 1992;261(1):349-52.

64. Jasper BW, Hopkins RO, Duker HV, Weaver LK. Affective outcome following carbon monoxide poisoning: a prospective longitudinal study. Cogn Behav Neurol. 2005;18(2).

65. Kalay N, Ozdogru I, Cetinkaya Y, et al. Cardiovascular effects of carbon monoxide poisoning. Am J Cardiol. 2007;99(3):322-4.

66. Karaman D, Metin S, Kara K, et al. Neuropsychological evaluation of children and adolescents with acute carbon monoxide poisoning. Pediatr Emerg Care. 2016;32(5):303-6.

67. Keenan HT, Bratton SL, Norkool DM, Brogan TV, Hampson NB. Delivery of hyperbaric oxygen therapy to critically ill, mechanically ventilated children. J Crit Care. 1998;13(1):7-12.

68. Kelley JS SG. Retinal hemorrhages in subacute carbon monoxide poisoning: exposures in homes with blocked furnace flues. JAMA. 1978;239(15):1515-7.

69. Klasner AE, Smith SR, Thompson MW, Scalzo AJ. Carbon monoxide mass exposure in a pediatric population. Acad Emerg Med. 1998;5(10):992-6.

70. Kleinert A, Sińczuk-Walczak H, Góraj B. Acute poisoning by carbon monoxide affecting the extrapyramidal system. Med Pr. 1998;49(6):573-7.

71. Koehler RC, Traystman RJ. Cerebrovascular effects of carbon monoxide. Antioxid Redox Signal. 2002;4(2):279-90.

72. Koehler RC, Jones MD, Traystman RJ. Cerebral circulatory response to carbon monoxide and hypoxic hypoxia in the lamb. Am J Physiol Heart Circ Physiol. 1982;243(1):H27-32.

73. Koren G, Sharav T, Pastuszak A, et al. A multicenter, prospective study of fetal outcome following accidental carbon monoxide poisoning in pregnancy. Reprod Toxicol. 1991;5(5):397-403.

74. Krantz T, Thisted B, Strom J, Sørensen MB. Acute carbon monoxide poisoning. Acta Anaesthesiol Scand. 1988;32(4):278-82.

75. Lahiri S, Mulligan E, Nishino T, Mokashi A, Davies RO. Relative responses of aortic body and carotid body chemoreceptors to carboxyhemoglobinemia. J Appl Physiol. 1981;50(3):580-6.

76. Lippi G, Rastelli G, Meschi T, Borghi L, Cervellin G. Pathophysiology, clinics, diagnosis and treatment of heart involvement in carbon monoxide poisoning. Clin Biochem. 2012;45(16-17):1278-85.

77. Liu Y, Fechter LD. MK-801 protects against carbon monoxide-induced hearing loss. Toxicol Appl Pharmacol. 1995;132(2):196-202.

78. Lo C, Chen S, Lee K, et al. Brain injury after acute carbon monoxide poisoning: early and late complications. Am J Roentgenol. 2007;189(4):W205-11.

79. Longo LD, Ching KS. Placental diffusing capacity for carbon monoxide and oxygen in unanesthetized sheep. J Appl Physiol. 1977;43(5):885-93.

80. Longo LD, Hill EP. Carbon monoxide uptake and elimination in fetal and maternal sheep. Am J Physiol Heart Circ Physiol. 1977;232(3):H324-30.

81. Longo LD. The biological effects of carbon monoxide on the pregnant woman, fetus, and newborn infant. Obstet Gynecol. 1977;129(1):69-103.

82. Lou M, Chen Y, Ding M, Eschenfelder CC, Deuschl G. Involvement of the mitochondrial ATP-sensitive potassium channel in the neuroprotective effect of hyperbaric oxygenation after cerebral ischemia. Brain Res Bull. 2006;69(2):109-16.

83. MacMillan V. Regional cerebral blood flow of the rat in acute carbon monoxide intoxication. Can J Physiol Pharmacol. 1975;53(4):644-50.

84. Maeda Y, Kawasaki Y, Jibiki I, Yamaguchi N, Matsuda H, Hisada K. Effect of therapy with oxygen under high pressure on regional cerebral blood flow in the interval form of carbon monoxide poisoning: observation from subtraction of technetium-99m HMPAO SPECT brain imaging. Eur Neurol. 1991;31(6):380-3.

85. Marek Z, Piejko M. Circulatory failure in acute carbon monoxide poisoning. Forensic Sci. 1972;1(4):419-25.

86. Mathieu D, Wattel F, Mathieu-Nolf M, et al. Randomized prospective study comparing the effect of HBO vs. 12 hours NBO in non-comatose CO poisoned patients: results of the preliminary analysis. Undersea Hyperb Med. 1996;23 Suppl(7).

87. McNulty JA, Maher BA, Chu M, Sitnikova T. Relationship of short-term verbal memory to the need for hyperbaric oxygen treatment after carbon monoxide poisoning. Neuropsychiatry Neuropsychol Behav Neurol. 1997;10(3):174-9.

88. Meilin S, Rogatsky GG, Thom SR, Zarchin N, Guggenheimer-Furman E, Mayevsky A. Effects of carbon monoxide on the brain may be mediated by nitric oxide. J Appl Physiol. 1996;81(3):1078-83.

89. Messier LD, Myers RAM. A neuropsychological screening battery for emergency assessment of carbon-monoxide-poisoned patients. J Clin Psychol. 1991;47(5):675-84.

90. Min SK. A brain syndrome associated with delayed neuropsychiatric sequelae following acute carbon monoxide intoxication. Acta Psychiatr Scand. 1986;73(1):80-6.

91. Mott JA, Wolfe MI, Alverson CJ, et al. National vehicle emissions policies and practices and declining US carbon monoxide–related mortality. JAMA. 2002;288(8):988-95.

92. Mowry JB, Spyker DA, Brooks DE, McMillan N, Schauben JL. 2014 annual report of the American Association of Poison Control Centers' National Poison Data System (NPDS): 32nd annual report. Clin Toxicol. 2015;53(10):962-1147.

93. Myers RAM, Jones DW, Britten JS. Carbon monoxide half life study. In: Kindwall E, editor. Proceedings of the 8th International Congress on Hyperbaric Medicine. Flagstaff (AZ): Best Publishing Co.; 1987. p. 263-6.

94. Myers RAM, Britten JS. Are arterial blood gases of value in treatment decisions for carbon monoxide poisoning? Crit Care Med. 1989;17(2):139-42.

95. Myers RAM, Snyder SK, Emhoff TA. Subacute sequelae of carbon monoxide poisoning. Ann Emerg Med. 1985;14(12):1163-7.

96. Nabeshima T, Katoh A, Ishimaru H, et al. Carbon monoxide-induced delayed amnesia, delayed neuronal death and change in acetylcholine concentration in mice. J Pharmacol Exp Ther. 1991;256(1):378-84.

97. Nager EC, O'Connor RE. Carbon monoxide poisoning from spray paint inhalation. Acad Emerg Med. 1998;5(1):84-6.

98. Oka A, Belliveau M, Rosenberg P, Volpe J. Vulnerability of oligodendroglia to glutamate: pharmacology, mechanisms, and prevention. J Neurosci. 1993;13(4):1441-53.

99. Pace N, Strajman E, Walker EL. Acceleration of carbon monoxide elimination in man by high pressure oxygen. Science. 1950;111(2894):652-4. doi: 10.1126/science.111.2894.652.

100. Parkinson RB, Hopkins RO, Cleavinger HB, et al. White matter hyperintensities and neuropsychological outcome following carbon monoxide poisoning. Neurology. 2002;58(10):1525-32.

101. Pellegrini-Giampietro D, Cherici G, Alesiani M, Carla V, Moroni F. Excitatory amino acid release and free radical formation may cooperate in the genesis of ischemia-induced neuronal damage. J Neurosci. 1990;10(3):1035-41.

102. Penn A, Snyder CA. Inhalation of sidestream cigarette smoke accelerates development of arteriosclerotic plaques. Circulation. 1993;88(4):1820-5. doi: 10.1161/01.CIR.88.4.1820.

103. Peterson JE, Stewart RD. Absorption and elimination of carbon monoxide by inactive young men. Arch Environ Health. 1970;21(2):165-71.

104. Piantadosi CA, Tatro L, Zhang J. Hydroxyl radical production in the brain after CO hypoxia in rats. Free Radic Biol Med. 1995;18(3):603-9.

105. Plafki C, Peters P, Almeling M, Welslau W, Busch R. Complications and side effects of hyperbaric oxygen therapy. Aviat Space Environ Med. 2000;71(2):119-24.

106. Rahmani M, Belaidi H, Benabdeljlil M, et al. Bilateral brachial plexus injury following acute carbon monoxide poisoning. BMC Pharmacol Toxicol. 2013;14(1):61.

107. Raphael JC, Elkharrat D, Jars-Guincestre M, et al. Trial of normobaric oxygen and hyperbaric oxygen for acute carbon monoxide intoxication. Lancet. 1989;334(8660):414-9.

108. Rioux JP, Myers RAM. Methylene chloride poisoning: a paradigmatic review. J Emerg Med. 1988;6(3):227-38.

109. Roth D, Krammel M, Schreiber W, Herkner H, Havel C, Laggner AN. Unrecognized carbon monoxide poisoning leads to a multiple-casualty incident. J Emerg Med. 2013;45(4):559-61.

110. Roth D, Bayer A, Schrattenbacher G, et al. Exposure to carbon monoxide for patients and providers in an urban emergency medical service. Prehosp Emerg Care. 2013;17(3):354-60.

111. Roth D, Herkner H, Schreiber W, et al. Accuracy of noninvasive multiwave pulse oximetry compared with carboxyhemoglobin from blood gas analysis in unselected emergency department patients. Ann Emerg Med. 2011;58(1):74-9.

112. Sanders RW, Katz KD, Suyama J, et al. Seizure during hyperbaric oxygen therapy for carbon monoxide toxicity: a case series and five-year experience. J Emerg Med. 2012;42(4):e69-72.

113. Sari I, Zengin S, Ozer O, Davutoglu V, Yildirim C, Aksoy M. Chronic carbon monoxide exposure increases electrocardiographic P-wave and QT dispersion. Inhal Toxicol. 2008;20(9):879-84.

114. Scheinkestel CD, Bailey M, Myles PS, et al. Hyperbaric or normobaric oxygen for acute carbon monoxide poisoning: a randomised controlled clinical trial. Med J Aust. 1999;170(5):203-10.

115. Sebbane M, Claret P, Mercier G, et al. Emergency department management of suspected carbon monoxide poisoning: role of pulse CO-oximetry. Respir Care. 2013;58(10):1614.

116. Shimosegawa E, Hatazawa J, Nagata K, et al. Cerebral blood flow and glucose metabolism measurements in a patient surviving one year after carbon monoxide intoxication. J Nucl Med. 1992;33(9):1696-8.

117. Sircar K, Clower J, Shin MK, Bailey C, King M, Yip F. Carbon monoxide poisoning deaths in the United States, 1999 to 2012. Am J Emerg Med. 2015;33(9):1140-5.

118. Sjöberg F, Singer M. The medical use of oxygen: a time for critical reappraisal. J Intern Med. 2013;274(6):505-28.

119. Smith G, Sharp GR. Treatment of carbon-monoxide poisoning with oxygen under pressure. Lancet. 1960;276(7156):905-6.

120. Smith JS, Brandon S. Morbidity from acute carbon monoxide poisoning at three-year follow-up. Br Med J. 1973;1(5849):318-21.

121. Song SY, Okeda R, Funata N, Higashino F. An experimental study of the pathogenesis of the selective lesion of the globus pallidus in acute carbon monoxide poisoning in cats. With special reference to the chronologic change in the cerebral local blood flow. Acta Neuropathol. 1983;61(3-4):232-8.

122. Stewart RD, Baretta ED, Platte LR, et al. Carboxyhemoglobin levels in American blood donors. JAMA. 1974;229(9):1187-95.

123. Takano T, Miyazaki Y, Shimoyama H, Maeda H, Okeda R, Funata N. Direct effects of carbon monoxide on cardiac function. Int Arch Occup Environ Health. 1981;49(1):35-40.

124. Thom SR, Xu YA, Ischiropoulos H. Vascular endothelial cells generate peroxynitrite in response to carbon monoxide exposure. Chem Res Toxicol. 1997;10(9):1023-31.

125. Thom SR. Functional inhibition of leukocyte B2 integrins by hyperbaric oxygen in carbon monoxide-mediated brain injury in rats. Toxicol Appl Pharmacol. 1993;123(2):248-56.

126. Thom SR. Leukocytes in carbon monoxide-mediated brain oxidative injury. Toxicol Appl Pharmacol. 1993;123(2):234-47.

127. Thom SR. Dehydrogenase conversion to oxidase and lipid peroxidation in brain after carbon monoxide poisoning. J Appl Physiol. 1992;73(4):1584-9.

128. Thom SR. Carbon monoxide-mediated brain lipid peroxidation in the rat. J Appl Physiol. 1990;68(3):997-1003.

129. Thom SR, Kang M, Fisher D, Ischiropoulos H. Release of glutathione from erythrocytes and other markers of oxidative stress in carbon monoxide poisoning. J Appl Physiol. 1997;82(5):1424-32.

130. Thom SR, Bhopale VM, Velazquez OC, Goldstein LJ, Thom LH, Buerk DG. Stem cell mobilization by hyperbaric oxygen. Am J Physiol Heart Circ Physiol. 2006;290(4):H1378-86. doi: 10.1152/ajpheart.00888.2005.

131. Thom SR, Fisher D, Xu YA, Garner S, Ischiropoulos H. Role of nitric oxide-derived oxidants in vascular injury from carbon monoxide in the rat. Am J Physiol Heart Circ Physiol. 1999;276(3):H984-92.

132. Thom SR, Taber RL, Mendiguren II, Clark JM, Hardy KR, Fisher AB. Delayed neuropsychologic sequelae after carbon monoxide poisoning: prevention by treatment with hyperbaric oxygen. Ann Emerg Med. 1995;25(4):474-80.

133. Towers CV, Corcoran VA. Influence of carbon monoxide poisoning on the fetal heart monitor tracing: a report of 3 cases. J Reprod Med. 2009;54(3):184-8.

134. Tucciarone M, Dileo PA, Castro ER, Guerrero M. Myocardial infarction secondary to carbon monoxide poisoning: an uncommon presentation of a common condition. Case report and review of the literature. Am J Ther. 2009;16(5).

135. Van Mieghem C, Sabbe M, Knockaert D. The clinical value of the ECG in noncardiac conditions. Chest. 2004;125(4):1561-76.

136. Vreman HJ, Ronquillo RB, Ariagno RL, Schwartz HC, Stevenson DK. Interference of fetal hemoglobin with the spectrophotometric measurement of carboxyhemoglobin. Clin Chem. 1988;34(5):975-7.

137. Weaver LK. Carbon monoxide poisoning. N Engl J Med. 2009;360(12):1217-25.

138. Weaver LK, Churchill S. Pulmonary edema associated with hyperbaric oxygen therapy. Chest. 2001;120(4):1407-9.

139. Weaver LK, Hopkins RO, Chan KJ, et al. Hyperbaric oxygen for acute carbon monoxide poisoning. N Engl J Med. 2002;347(14):1057-67.

140. Wesley Ely E, Moorehead B, Haponik EF. Warehouse workers' headache: emergency evaluation and management of 30 patients with carbon monoxide poisoning. Am J Med. 1995;98(2):145-55.

141. Wolff E. Carbon monoxide poisoning with severe myonecrosis and acute renal failure. Am J Emerg Med. 1994;12(3):347-9.

142. Wu L, Wang R. Carbon monoxide: endogenous production, physiological functions, and pharmacological applications. Pharmacol Rev. 2005;57(4):585-630. doi: 10.1124/pr.57.4.3.

143. Zevin S, Saunders S, Gourlay SG, Jacob P, Benowitz NL. Cardiovascular effects of carbon monoxide and cigarette smoking. J Am Coll Cardiol. 2001;38(6):1633-8.

CHAPTER 14 CHAPTER

Idiopathic Sudden Sensorineural Hearing Loss

CHAPTER FOURTEEN OVERVIEW

Introduction 327
Etiopathogenesis of ISSHL 328
Early Experiments Investigating a Hypoxic Etiology for ISSHL 328
Circulatory Derangement Theories Regarding ISSHL 328
The Contribution of Comorbid Conditions to the Development of ISSHL 329
Competing Multifactorial Theories for ISSHL 329
The Challenge in Treating ISSHL – Multifactorial Etiopathogenesis 330
Rationale for the Use of Steroids 330
Literature Review of Steroids in the Treatment of ISSHL 331
Rationale for the Use of HBO_2 Therapy 333
Literature Review: The Use of HBO_2 in the Treatment of ISSHL 333
Use of HBO_2 as a Primary Treatment for ISSHL 333
Use of HBO_2 as a Salvage Therapy for ISSHL 334
Use of HBO_2 Therapy for Chronic Hearing Loss 336
Use of HBO_2 with Medical Therapies in the Treatment of ISSHL 336
Use of HBO_2 with Steroids in the Treatment of ISSHL 338
Prognostic Factors for ISSHL 340
Prognostic Factors for Adults 340
Prognostic Factors for Children 342
Literature Summary for the Treatment of ISSHL 342
ISSHL Meta-Analyses of Treatments 343
Use of Vasodilators and Vasoactive Agents for ISSHL 348
Use of Antivirals for ISSHL 349
Use of Steroids for ISSHL 349
Use of HBO_2 for ISSHL 349
Patient Selection Criteria 350
Differential Diagnosis of Acquired Sudden Deafness 350

The Work-Up **351**
Patient Management **351**
Treatment **351**
Steroid Therapy 351
Hyperbaric Oxygen Therapy 352
Other Medical Therapies 352
Follow-Up **352**
Prognosis **352**
Cost Impact **352**
References **353**

Idiopathic Sudden Sensorineural Hearing Loss

Tracy Leigh LeGros, Heather Murphy-Lavoie

INTRODUCTION

Idiopathic sudden sensorineural hearing loss (ISSHL) is a medical emergency that presents with the abrupt onset of an unexpected sudden sensory deficit that is often underappreciated by patients, and at times by clinicians. Approximately 88% of sudden sensorineural hearing loss (SSNHL) has no identifiable etiology and is termed ISSHL.(40) Otolaryngologists have intensely investigated ISSHL since the 1970s. Over the past 30 years, more than 800 articles, or 1 every 2 weeks, have been published in the English medical literature.(89) Idiopathic sudden sensorineural hearing loss is the abrupt onset of hearing loss, typically present upon wakening, usually unilateral, and involving a hearing loss of at least 30 decibels (dB) occurring within 3 days over at least 3 contiguous frequencies.(48,113) As most patients do not present with premorbid audiograms, the degree of hearing loss is usually defined by the presentation thresholds of the unaffected ear.(113) Other associated symptoms include tinnitus, aural fullness, dizziness, and vertigo.(104,113) The reported historical incidence of ISSHL ranges from 5–20 per 100,000 population, with approximately 4,000 new cases per annum in the United States.(18,113) The true incidence is thought to be higher, as ISSHL is perceived to be underreported. Interestingly, the number of cases per annum appears to be an underestimation as well, as 4,000 cases annually calculates to 1.3 cases per 100,000 with a population estimate of approximately 300 million people in the United States. Calculating an ISSHL incidence rate of 5–20 per 100,000 translates to 15,000–60,000 new cases per annum in the United States. A recent study has reported the annual incidence of ISSHL in the United States is currently 27 per 100,000, and the pediatric incidence is 11 per 100,000.(4) Additional literature states that the incidence of ISSHL is increasing, especially in the elderly, with a recent reported incidence of 77 per 100,000.(4,121) Others place the incidence of ISSHL at 160 cases per 100,000 and conclude that ISSHL is no longer rare.(62) In 1984, Byl reviewed the literature and found the mean age of ISSHL presentation to be 46–49 years, with variation of ISSHL incidence with age, and an equal gender distribution.(17-18,49,78,109) The presentation of ISSHL does not appear to have seasonal variations, uneven distributions of presentation throughout the year, or an association with upper respiratory infections, either prior to or following symptom onset.(58) The spontaneous recovery is currently thought to be 30%–60%.(9,24,133)

ETIOPATHOGENESIS OF ISSHL

The first scientific reporting of ISSHL was published in 1944 in *Acta Oto-Laryngologica* by De Kleyn.[32] To this day, otolaryngologists continue to investigate the etiologies and pathogenesis of ISSHL. Many mechanisms have been postulated, including circulatory disturbances, ototoxicity, trauma, neoplasms, vascular occlusions, viral infections, labyrinthine membrane leaks, immune-associated disease, abnormal cochlear stress response, abnormal tissue growth, and cochlear membrane damage.[6,28,40,57]

Early Experiments Investigating a Hypoxic Etiology for ISSHL

Early animal studies by Lamm and colleagues revealed that perilymph pO_2 of the scala tympani fell 50%–80% during noise exposure.[67] Additionally, compound action potential latency times were prolonged, and hair cell function declined by 60%–70%. The authors surmised that during noise exposure, the oxygen-dependent sodium and potassium pumps of the organ of Corti (OOC) decompensate, resulting in intracellular sodium accumulations, causing microstructural damage, manifested as hair cell-cilia fusion, hair cell synaptic and dendritic swelling, hair cell contraction, and sustained depolarization.[69]

Circulatory Derangement Theories Regarding ISSHL

In 1980, Belal discussed the role of occlusive arterial disease (thrombotic, embolic, or spastic) in the development of ISSHL and suggested a vascular etiology of ISSHL.[10] This is the reasoning for the use of vasodilator drugs, stellate ganglion blocks (SGB), anticoagulants and rheological agents in the treatment of ISSHL. Animal studies have shown that labyrinthine artery occlusion results in severe degenerative changes, fibrosis, and new cochlear bone formation. This is similar to what occurs to the human cochlea deprived of its blood supply. There is progressive ossification of the cochlear spaces, loss of cochlear neurons, labyrinthine fibrosis, new bone formation, and endolymphatic hydrops.[138] In 2001, otolaryngologists at Orsola Hospital (University of Bologna, Italy), investigated the blood pressures (BP) of 23 young, untreated and otherwise healthy, ISSHL patients. They were compared with 20 age and sex matched, normotensive control subjects. Both groups underwent 24-hour blood pressure (BP) monitoring. The authors found that both the systolic and diastolic BP measurements were significantly lower in the ISSHL group; the authors concluded that systemic hypotension must be considered as a possible cause in the development of ISSHL in young, healthy subjects.[96] The presence of significant hypotension in ISSHL patients has been reported before, and these studies are important for several reasons.[71,76,97-98] First, they are in contradistinction to a previous theory regarding circulatory disorders and ISSHL, which proffered that sustained increases in BP are responsible for hemorrhagic and thrombotic events that may occur within the cochlea of ISSHL patients. Secondly, they provide plausible reasoning for how young, previously healthy patients, without known comorbidities, acquire ISSHL. Importantly, the implication of hypotension as a causative insult would caution against the use of vasodilators in the treatment of those with lowered BP readings who acquire ISSHL. Importantly, hypotension may be prominently deleterious for the inner ear, which has significantly less circulatory autoregulation when compared to cerebral blood flow.[60] The vascular hypothesis for ISSHL maintains that, as a result of a vascular disruption with resultant ischemia, the cochlear apparatus, cochlear nerve, or other components of the central auditory nervous system are damaged.

The Contribution of Comorbid Conditions to the Development of ISSHL

Interestingly, a recurrence of ISSHL has been observed in those with comorbid conditions, principally diabetes mellitus (DM), hypertension (HTN), and dyslipidemia.[26] In 1996, Brant and colleagues examined the relationship between the development of age-associated hearing loss in the speech frequencies and several cardiovascular (CV) risk factors, including age, BP, alcohol use, and cigarette smoking. They reviewed the records of 531 men participating in the Baltimore Longitudinal Study of Aging that began in 1965. They found that only systolic BP showed a significant relationship with hearing loss in the speech frequencies.[16] Others have theorized that atherosclerosis, and its associated risk factors, may play a role in the etiology of ISSHL.[105] In 2010, Aimoni and coworkers performed an observational case-control study of ISSHL patients (n = 141), matched for age and gender, with a control group (n = 271). They examined CV risk factors, including DM, HTN, smoking history, hypercholesterolemia, and hypertriglyceridemia. They found that DM and hypercholesterolemia were significantly more frequent in the ISSHL group, and that the risk of ISSHL increased with the number of CV risk factors.[3] In 2012, Ciccone and colleagues studied 29 consecutive patients with ISSHL. The control subjects had no history of CV disease and normal hearing. Compared to the control group, the ISSHL patients had significantly higher total cholesterol, low-density lipoprotein cholesterol levels (early markers of atherosclerosis), and flow-mediated dilation of the brachial artery, an early marker of endothelial dysfunction.[26] Moreover, ISSHL has been shown to be an early marker for an increased risk of stroke. Lin et al. followed two cohorts of patients followed for 5 years. One group consisted of all patients admitted for ISSHL (n = 1,423). The control group consisted of all patients admitted with appendicitis (n = 5,692). The authors found a 12.7% stroke rate in the ISSHL group versus 8.7% of the appendicitis cohort. The stroke hazard was 1.64 times greater ($p < 0.001$) for the ISSHL patients, suggesting that ISSHL can be an early warning sign for stroke.[73] In 2014, Ozler investigated the neutrophil-lymphocyte ratio (NLR) levels in 40 ISSHL patients and compared them to 40 control subjects without evidence of auditory pathology. He found that all ISSHL patients, regardless of severity (mild, moderate, or severe), had elevated NLR values compared to controls. The author suggests that high NLR values may be a predictor of other ischemic conditions, such as coronary or cerebral ischemia, and advocates that ISSHL patients be referred to cardiology and neurology specialists in follow-up.[91]

Competing Multifactorial Theories for ISSHL

Gloddek and colleagues reviewed the differing theories regarding the pathogenesis of ISSHL and noted that a viral infection of the stria vascularis, OOC, or spiral ganglion is often alluded to in the American literature, while European scientists favor a vascular pathology with impaired inner-ear perfusion.[45]

A viral association with ISSHL has been suggested before. However, no specific serological profiles or response to antiviral treatment have been reported.[80] Gloddek's group also put forth a theory melding the competing theories of immunologic, viral, and vascular etiologies for ISSHL. They hypothesize that a virally stimulated, immunologically mediated perivasculitis, promoted by endothelial cell secretion of cytokines, results in circulating immunoglobulin deposition perivascularly, cochlear hypoperfusion, and tissue hypoxia.[45] This is the basis of the immunopathological theory of ISSHL, which results in ischemia, stenosis, and atresia. There is additional evidence that ISSHL may be the result of abnormal activation of endocochlear nuclear factor B, a molecular transcription factor that mediates the cellular responses to pathogenic stress, such as infections, mechanical stress, osmotic stress, and other insults.[79]

The Challenge in Treating ISSHL – Multifactorial Etiopathogenesis

More than 60 protocols have been investigated for the treatment of ISSHL, including agents that decrease blood viscosity (osmotic diuretics, volume expanders, hydroxyethyl starch, rheologic agents, dextran, pentoxifylline, plasmapheresis, therapeutic phlebotomy, and normovolemic hemodilution); vasodilator drugs and procedures (histamine, papaverine, verapamil, procaine, cyclandelate, nifedipine, carbogen, dorsal sympathectomy, and SGBs); antiviral agents (acyclovir and valaciclovir); anticoagulants (sodium enoxaparin and heparin); free-radical scavenging vitamins (B, C, and E); antibiotics; gingko biloba; magnesium; benzodiazepines; xanthinonictone; probanthine; lipoprostaglandin E1; intravenous (IV) lidocaine; repeated smallpox vaccinations; interferon alpha; ATP; betahistine; thrombolytics (tissue plasminogen activator, batroxibin); vinpocetine; bed rest; salt restriction; increased fluid intake; modification of CV risk factors; contrast dye (diatrizoate meglumine); steroids; and HBO_2 therapy.[89,121] Of this large number, the use of steroids in combination with HBO_2 has the greatest efficacy.

RATIONALE FOR THE USE OF STEROIDS

The initial rationale for the use of steroids in the treatment of ISSHL was related to their properties in reducing both inflammation and edema. One theory assumes that the cochlear damage in ISSHL results from inflammatory triggers or an insult, and steroids counteract the inflammatory cascade, spare the cochlea further damage, and reverse some of the damage.[114] However, there are additional benefits of steroids in the treatment of ISSHL. Steroids have a primary role in protecting the cochlea from inflammatory mediators, specifically tumor necrosis factor alpha (TNFα) and nuclear factor kappa-light chain enhancer (NF-κB).[45,114] TNFα is a cell signaling protein (cytokine), and one of the initial components of the acute phase reaction of inflammation. It induces fever, apoptotic cell death, cachexia, the inflammatory response to tumorigenesis, viral replication, and the response to sepsis via interleukins. NF-κB is a protein complex that controls DNA transcription, cytokine production, and cell survival. It is produced in times of stress from cytokines, free radicals, and bacterial or viral antigens. Additionally, steroids increase cochlear blood flow and ameliorate cochlear ischemia, favorably altering the inner-ear milieu.[86,110,119] Steroids also regulate protein synthesis within the inner ear. Glucocorticoid and mineralocorticoid receptors have been found within the inner ear, and steroid therapy may be affecting inner-ear electrolyte and fluid balance.[110] It is within the inner ear, specifically at the vascular stria, where both sodium and potassium secretion are regulated to maintain the endocochlear membrane potential. This region is also the most frequent site of injury in those with ISSHL.[72] Systemic steroids improve stria vascularis function, and this may preserve its morphology in those that recover from ISSHL.[123]

LITERATURE REVIEW OF STEROIDS IN THE TREATMENT OF ISSHL

In 2001, Alexiou and colleagues reported their retrospective review showing those with lower, middle, or pancochlear hearing deficits had improved outcomes with steroids and vasoactive agents.[5] In 2005, Slattery and colleagues conducted an unblinded, nonrandomized, open-label clinical trial (n = 20) involving ISSHL patients who received four injections of intratympanice (IT) methylprednisolone within a two-week period, following failure of oral steroid therapy. The authors reported statistically significant improvement in four-frequency pure-tone average (PTA) and speech discrimination score at one-month follow up. Additionally, the improvements in tinnitus were statistically significant.[111] In 2008, Battaglia and colleagues performed a multicenter, double-blinded, placebo-controlled randomized study involving ISSHL patients who received either IT dexamethasone + placebo taper (Group A, n = 17), IT placebo injections + high dose prednisone taper (Group B, n = 18), or both steroid therapies (Group C, n = 16). They enrolled 51 patients with ISSHL with < 6 weeks of symptoms and followed them prospectively for 3 weeks. The combination group had an average improvement in speech discrimination of 44%, with a 40dB improvement in PTA, significant improvement compared to the prednisone-taper-only group ($p < 0.05$ and $p < 0.02$, respectively). Logistic regression analyses revealed the combination group demonstrated better odds of hearing recovery than patients in both of the other groups ($p < 0.05$), and recovered their hearing more quickly than the other groups ($p < 0.05$).[9] In 2011, Dispenza and others performed a prospective randomized trial comparing IT steroids versus systemic steroids in the treatment of ISSHL. They found both treatments resulted in hearing gains above that shown without treatment; however, there were no significant between-group differences.[36] In the same year, Seggas and colleagues performed a comprehensive literature review on the use of IT steroids for ISSHL. They identified the three main protocols for IT steroid administration, including initial treatment, adjunctive treatment in combination with systemic steroids, and as a salvage therapy after failure of systemic steroid (standard) treatment. The purpose of the review was to seek the best delivery technique and the optimal administration schedule. Randomized and nonrandomized case-control studies and case-series studies were reviewed from 1996 to 2009. The authors concluded that IT steroids can be a valuable treatment for ISSHL. However, the use of combination therapy yielded controversial results, and they were unable to determine whether this therapy could yield superior results to systemic steroids, the established first-line treatment. They also remarked upon the need for establishment of standard criteria for hearing recovery.[108] Another systematic review on the use of IT steroids for ISSHL was also published in 2011 by Spears and Schwartz.[112] They identified 176 articles, of which 32 were studies of initial or salvage IT steroids for sudden hearing loss. These studies included six randomized trials and randomized controlled trials (RCTs). The vast majority the IT steroid salvage therapy demonstrated benefit at all levels. The higher-quality studies imparted a statistically significant benefit of 13.3 dB

However, it was unclear to the authors if this difference was clinically significant. Moreover, initial IT steroid therapy was equivalent to standard therapy (systemic steroids) in the existing literature of all qualities. The authors concluded that primary IT steroid therapy for SSHNL is equivalent to high-dose oral prednisone therapy. However, as a salvage therapy, IT steroids offer the potential for some degree of additional hearing recovery.(112) In 2012, Ferri and coworkers investigated the use of IT steroids in ISSHL patients who had failed 10 days of IV steroid therapy. They injected 0.5 mL of IT methylprednisolone up to 7 time over 20 days. This salvage therapy resulted in improvement for 52.7% of patients. The authors surmised that the greatest positive influences on hearing recovery were early IT steroid therapy, hearing losses < 80 dB, and the involvement of low-frequency deficits.(39)

Despite a reported ISSHL spontaneous recovery rate of 30%–60%, the hearing recovery for ISSHL patients is much poorer for those who have failed previous IV steroid therapy.(9,24,27,50,92,111,139) Intratympanic steroid therapy has several advantages over systemic therapy, including increasing intracochlear steroid concentrations and reducing the incidence of possibly toxic side effects. The use of IT steroids leads to much higher perilymphatic concentrations compared to system steroid therapy.(15,24,39) A substantial concentration gradient occurs in the scala tympani perilymph following round window application of IT steroids.(15,100) Currently, the use of systemic steroids is thought to impart a 50%–80% recovery rate in the treatment of ISSHL.(39) However, there is some concern regarding the potential for side effects of systemic steroids, including hyperglycemia (glucose intolerance), HTN, gastrointestinal bleeding, cataracts, adrenal suppression, psychosis, immunosuppression, and altered mental status. Currently, there is a paucity of data regarding the prevalence of these side effects with the relatively short courses of systemic steroid therapy used in the treatment of ISSHL.(131) In 2016, Gao and Liu reported their meta-analysis on the combined use of IT and systemic steroids for ISSHL. They searched the literature databases for all available observational studies. They accepted eight studies for review, including seven prospective and one retrospective study. They reported that combination steroid therapy provides greater benefit than systemic steroid administration alone and that those with severe-profound ISSHL would benefit more with combination therapy than mild-moderate patients for hearing outcomes but not recovery rate. They advocated that IT steroid therapy might serve as an alternative modality for seeking better outcomes.(43) In 2016, Qiang et al. published a meta-analysis, also comparing the use of systemic steroids versus IT steroids as initial therapy for ISSHL. They evaluated six RCTs and concluded that IT steroid groups exhibited better outcomes in PTA improvement and recovery rate than systemic steroid therapy, and that IT steroids might be a potentially more beneficial modality for ISSHL patients regardless of the initial hearing loss severity.(102) Intratympanic steroids have several advantages, including assured compliance, therapy directed to the affected ear, high concentrations of steroids in the perilymph, few side effects and complications, office-based procedure (no anesthesia), well tolerated, and greater suitability for those in whom systemic steroids are contraindicated or refused (DM, immunosuppressed states, and peptic ulcer disease).(2,9,24,50-51,55,61,89,99,108,111,124,135)

Alternatively, there are disadvantages to IT steroid administration, including pain, tympanic membrane perforation, otitis media, vertigo (usually temporary), and hearing loss.(89)

RATIONALE FOR THE USE OF HBO_2 THERAPY

The rationale for the use of HBO_2 therapy in the treatment of ISSHL is supported by an understanding of the rapid metabolism and vascular paucity of the cochlea and the structures within it. The stria vascularis and OOC, in particular, require an extremely high oxygen supply.(21) Moreover, a direct vascular supply to the OOC is minimal.(85) Tissue oxygenation to the cochlea occurs via oxygen diffusion from cochlear capillary networks into the perilymph and the cortilymph.(67) It is the perilymph that serves as the primary oxygen source for structures within the cochlea. In 1983, Nagahara and colleagues studied the perilymph pO_2 in anesthetized humans with hearing loss. The duration of hearing loss varied greatly (13 days–15 years). However, they found that perilymph pO_2 tended to be lower in those with ISSHL than in those with otosclerosis, sudden cochleovestibular loss, or rapidly progressive SSHNL. There was no correlation between the degree of hearing loss and the perilymph pO_2. However, these results led the authors to comment that some cases of ISSHL may be due to ischemia.(85) Later animal studies confirmed that, while normobaric oxygen increases perilymph pO_2 3.4-fold, HBO_2 increases perilymph pO_2 9.4-fold.(67) Although normobaric hyperoxygenation increases intracochlear oxygen tensions, only HBO_2 therapy achieves the extremely high arterial perilymphatic oxygen concentration differences required for efficacy.(67-68,125) Additional benefits of HBO_2 may be related to its obviation of ischemic reperfusion injury, edema reduction, and anti-inflammatory effects.

LITERATURE REVIEW: THE USE OF HBO_2 IN THE TREATMENT OF ISSHL

Use of HBO_2 as a Primary Treatment for ISSHL

For the treatment of ISSHL, HBO_2 is usually an adjunctive therapy with medical therapies or a salvage therapy following failure of medical therapy, and the literature regarding HBO_2 as a primary therapy for ISSHL is sparse. In 1998, Schwab and colleagues reported the results of their RCT of 75 ISSHL patients treated within 14 days, with or without HBO_2 therapy (1.5 ATA for 45 minutes daily for 10–20 sessions). There were 37 patients in the HBO_2 group and 38 in the control group. They found clinical and statistically significant improvement with the use of HBO_2 compared to the control group (15.6 dB versus 10.7 dB, respectively).(107) In 2001, Fatorri et al. published a RCT of 50 ISSHL patients who presented to their otolaryngology offices within 48 hours of symptom onset and were treated with either HBO_2 (2.2 ATA for 90 minutes daily for 10 sessions; n = 30) or medical therapy (IV buflomedil; n = 20). The HBO_2 group showed statistically significant improvement in hearing compared to the medical therapy group (61.3 dB versus 24.0 dB, respectively) as well as significantly greater response to therapy (73% versus 55%, respectively). They also found that those with pantonal hypoacusis responded significantly better than those with a milder presentation.(38) In 2003, Racic and colleagues compared HBO_2 (2.8 ATA) with varying dosages of IV pentoxifylline infusion (n = 64). The HBO_2 group showed statistically significant improvement compared to

IV pentoxifylline in overall hearing (46.35 dB versus 21.48 dB, respectively), attainment of physiological hearing values (47.1% versus 6.2%, respectively), and in moderate hearing gains (41.2% versus 12.5%), respectively.(103) In 2007, Dundar and colleagues prospectively compared ISSHL patients treated primarily with HBO_2 to those treated with medical therapy. The HBO_2 patients had statistically significant hearing gains across all frequencies, with tinnitus patients showing the greatest hearing improvement.(37)

Use of HBO_2 as a Salvage Therapy for ISSHL

The literature supports that a significant number of patients – between 35% and 39% – do not respond to medical or placebo therapies. These patients may benefit from salvage therapy. One of the earliest studies was the 1995 RCT, presented by Hoffman and coworkers, evaluating 20 ISSHL patients treated with HBO_2 therapy 14 days after failing primary medical therapy. The primary medical therapy consisted of treatment with hydroxylethyl starch, pentoxifylline, and cortisone. Half of these patients were then treated with HBO_2 therapy (10–20 sessions, once daily at 1.5 ATA for 45 minutes). The HBO_2 salvage therapy resulted in significant hearing gains compared to the control group (7.5 dB versus 0.7 dB, respectively).(52) In 1998, Lamm and colleagues analyzed more than 50 trials utilizing HBO_2 as an adjunctive therapy for ISSHL, acoustic trauma, noise-induced hearing loss, and tinnitus. They also performed a subset analysis on the patients within these studies that failed to respond to any medical therapies (n = 4,109). In this subset, they found that if HBO_2 was started between 2 and 4 weeks, 50% showed marked hearing gains (at least 3 frequencies of > 30 dB), 33% showed moderate improvement (10–20 dB), and 13% showed no improvement. If adjunctive HBO_2 was utilized between 6 weeks and 3 months, 13% showed definite improvement in hearing, 25% showed moderate improvement, and 62% had no improvement.(70) In 2000, Marchesi and others retrospectively studied 95 patients, 80% of whom had had previous ineffective medical treatment, who were then treated with HBO_2. Following HBO_2 therapy, 78.9% of patients had a mean improvement of 38.3 +/- 8.3 dB, and 41% gained > 20 dB. Complete recovery occurred in 11.6%. HBO_2 was most effective in those patients treated within 14 days.(77) That same year, Murakawa and colleagues reviewed 522 cases of ISSHL, occurring over a 10-year period, in patients unresponsive to medical therapies who then received HBO_2 therapy. Following HBO_2 treatment, complete recovery occurred in 19.7%, with significant improvement in 34.9% and slight improvement in 23.2%. Delay to treatment > 14 days, advanced age, and vertigo were associated with poorer outcomes.(82) In 2010, Muzzi et al. treated 19 ISSHL patients who failed medical therapy with HBO_2. The use of HBO_2 salvage therapy improved PTAs, particularly at the low frequencies. They also found better results with early HBO_2 therapy and in older patients.(84) In the same year, Ohno and colleagues compared ISSHL patients who had failed four weeks of medical treatment and were then treated with HBO_2 to a similar group treated with medical therapy alone. The mean hearing gains were not different between groups. However, those with profound hearing loss did show significantly higher hearing gains.(90) Importantly, in 2012, the American Academy of Otolaryngology – Head and Neck Surgery Foundation published their *Clinical Practice Guidelines for Sudden Hearing Loss.* They recommended HBO_2 therapy for use within three months of symptom onset.(113) In 2013, Cvorovic and colleagues published a randomized prospective trial utilizing IT steroids and HBO_2 as salvage therapies for ISSHL. They enrolled 155 ISSHL patients at their tertiary referral center and treated them with the primary medical therapy of IV dexamethasone. They then enrolled the 50 patients who failed primary therapy (< 10 dB improvement in hearing gains), in a 1:1 fashion, to receive salvage therapy with either IT steroids (4 IT injections in 13 days) or HBO_2 therapy (2.0 ATA for 60 minutes daily for 20 days). They found that HBO_2 salvage therapy resulted in significant improvement in hearing thresholds at all tested frequencies. The IT steroid salvage therapy was found to be significantly beneficial at most frequencies (except 2 kHz). Their subgroup analyzes revealed that those patients with PTAs < 81 dB and those younger than 60 years had a better response to HBO_2 therapy than did those who were profoundly deaf or elderly.[(30)] During this same time, Yang and coworkers published their historical cohort study of ISSHL patients who received primary medical therapy. They then related in detail a smaller subset of this group (n = 103) who, after failing primary systemic therapy, opted to participate in salvage therapy. All patients were initially admitted to the Kaohsiung Chang Gung Memorial Hospital in Taiwan and treated with IV dexamethasone in decreasing dosages. Over the next five days, they also received 30 mg oral prednisolone daily, radiopaque contrast (Hypaque 76, 10 ml IV daily), and a plasma expander (dextran-40, 500 ml IV daily). Patients who were refractory to this regimen were then informed of 4 choices: IT steroids (4 injections of dexamethasone within 2 weeks), HBO_2 therapy (2.5 ATA for 120 minutes for 10 sessions within 2 weeks), combination of IT steroids and HBO_2, and observation only without salvage therapy. The patients chose their treatment arms; IT steroids (n = 35); HBO_2 (n = 22); IT steroid + HBO_2 (n = 19); and control group (n = 27). The authors reported no significant differences between groups regarding baseline characteristic, duration of symptoms, or initial hearing thresholds between the four groups. The hearing gains in PTA were significantly improved in those who received either IT steroids, HBO_2, or both (IT steroids + HBO_2) compared to the control group (p = 0.02, 0.036, and 0.003, respectively). However, the hearing gain in dB between treatment groups was not statistically different. The combined therapy group (IT steroids + HBO_2) also had statistically significant improvement in word recognition scoring (WRS) compared to the control group. The authors concluded that the combination of IT steroids and HBO_2 as salvage therapy may be the most beneficial for the recovery of hearing.[(136)] In 2015, Pezzoli and colleagues reported their study of 135 ISSHL patients treated with primary therapy and their additional investigations on the 23 patients who accepted salvage therapy with HBO_2. Over a roughly 2-year period, they evaluated 168 ISSHL patients and excluded 33 patients. The remaining 135 patients were treated primarily with IV 4 mg betamethasone and osmotic diuretics for 6 consecutive days. Those failing primary therapy were then treated with a 7-day course of oral dexamethasone (25 mg daily) and offered HBO_2 salvage therapy. Twenty-three patients were treated with oral dexamethasone and HBO_2 (2.5 ATA for 60 minutes for 15 treatments) and compared with the 21 patients who accepted oral steroid therapy but refused HBO_2 salvage therapy (nonrandomized control group). There were no reported differences between these groups in baseline characteristics. The patients receiving HBO_2 had a significantly increased mean improvement of 15.6 dB versus the spontaneous mean improvement of the control group of 5.0 dB (p = 0.013).

They also found that those with the worst hearing had the greatest degree of improvement, regardless of treatment onset (within 10 days or 11–30 days).[(94)]

This study was not randomized and had probable selection bias (inability to afford treatment at private facility) and an outcome measure based upon absolute values of hearing gains but not clinical improvement.

Use of HBO_2 Therapy for Chronic Hearing Loss

The strength of evidence is weaker for the use of HBO_2 in the treatment of chronic hearing loss. In 1990, Schumann and colleagues treated 557 chronic hearing loss patients with 10 sessions of HBO_2. An improvement of > 10 dB was found in 27.8% of cases.(106) In 1995, Hoffman and colleagues presented their RCT of 44 ISSHL patients with symptoms lasting greater than 6 months. The HBO_2 group (n = 22) received 15 sessions (1.5 ATA with 100% oxygen for 45 minutes). The control group (n = 22) received 15 sessions of hyperbaric air (1.5 ATA air for 45 minutes). No significant differences were found between groups. The study was limited by unclear randomization and allocation concealment and a lack of a sham true control group.(53) Importantly, this was, in fact, a RCT with two hyperbaric treatment groups and without a true control group. Hyperbaric oxygen therapy is a dual-therapy treatment of both hyperoxygenation and pressure, and pressurized air is not physiologically inert.(34,64) In 1997, Kau and coworkers reported their use of HBO_2 salvage therapy in 359 ISSHL patients who failed primary medical therapy. In those with hearing loss for between 1 and 3 months, noticeable improvement or complete recovery was seen in 13% (> 20 dB in at least 3 test frequencies), and moderate recovery occurred in 25.2% (10–20 dB). Overall, 30% had an improvement of > 10 dB, but only 2% regained normal hearing.(59) The use of HBO_2 for those with chronic hearing loss does show some promise, but the best results occur with the use of early HBO_2 therapy combined with steroid administration.

Use of HBO_2 with Medical Therapies in the Treatment of ISSHL

The use of HBO_2 in combination with various medical and procedural therapies has been extensively investigated. In this section, greater emphasis will be placed on larger and more recent studies that have not been discussed in detail elsewhere. In 1979, Giger published a prospective randomized trial of 55 patients treated with either carbogen inhalation (95% O_2/5% CO_2) or IV infusion of papaverine and dextran. Although immediate differences were not found, audiogram testing at one year showed statistically better audiometric testing in those treated with carbogen, suggesting hyperoxygenation may improve ISSHL outcomes.(44) In the same year, Goto and coworkers compared medical therapy, SGB, and HBO_2. They found that 100% of the patients treated with SGB and HBO_2 achieved > 10 dB PTA improvement, and 40% of these patients recovered to within 20 dB of their baseline hearing.(46) In 1985, Pilgramm and colleagues published a RCT (n = 37) of ISSHL patients treated with medical therapy with or without HBO_2 therapy. All patients presented within 14 days of symptoms onset. The medical therapy group (n = 19) received 500 ml of 10% dextran-40 and sorbitol 5%, 600 mg naphitidrofuryl hydrogenaxalate, and vitamin B orally for 14 days. The HBO_2 therapy included 10 sessions once daily (2.5 ATA for 60 minutes). The HBO_2 group (n = 18) had a significantly increased hearing gains when compared to the medical therapy group (29.2 dB versus 20.2 dB, respectively).(95) In 1993, French investigators conducted several studies evaluating the use of HBO_2 in combination with various medical therapies. They found HBO_2 to be a useful synergistic adjunct, with twice-daily HBO_2 sessions reducing the length of therapy.(31,140) In

1996, Cavallazzi and coworkers published their RCT of 64 patients with ISSHL treated with medical therapy, with or without HBO_2. The authors did not relay the duration of patients' ISSHL symptomatology, so the acuity or chronicity of the ISSHL is unknown. The medical therapy group provided to both groups consisted of multiple drugs, including heparin, betamethasone, nicotinic acid, flunarizine, cytidine, phosphocholine, dextran, vitamins, and neurotropic and antiviral drugs. The doses for these medical therapies were also not provided. The HBO_2 therapy was provided for 15 sessions over 3 weeks (2.5 ATA for 60 minutes daily). The addition of HBO_2 to the medical therapy conferred improvement in hearing gains compared to those treated with medical therapy alone (95% versus 71%, respectively). However, these differences were not statistically significant. This study is limited by the unknown duration of the subjects' hearing loss, unknown specifics regarding multiple medical therapies, possible selection bias (no mention of allocation concealment), and the fact that it was not blinded. Moreover, this study may not have been randomized, as randomization was not described.(22) Most importantly, due to the lack of specifics regarding the acuity or chronicity of the participants' ISSHL symptomatology and the unknown dosages of the 10 drugs used in the medical therapy of both groups, this study cannot be replicated or validated – basic tenets required for ensuring the accuracy and meaningfulness of scientific inquiry. In 2002, Aslan et al. published their experience utilizing medical therapy combined with either SGB or HBO_2. A significant increase in hearing gains was found with the addition of HBO_2 therapy.(7) In 2004, Topuz and others published a RCT of 51 ISSHL patients who presented within 2 weeks of symptomatology and were treated with medical therapy with or without HBO_2. All patients were admitted and given primary medical therapy, which included IV prednisone (1 mg/kg per day for 14 days), IV rheomacrodex (a plasma expander dextran given as a 500 ml infusion over 6 hours daily for 5 days), diazepam (5 mg orally twice daily), IV pentoxiphylline (200 mg twice daily), and salt restriction. The medical control group (n = 21) received no further therapy. Those patients randomized to the HBO_2 group (n = 30) received 25 sessions in total, applied at 2.5 ATA for 90 minutes twice daily for the first 5 days and then once daily for 15 days. For those with mild hearing loss, there was no difference between groups. However, for those with moderate hearing loss, the addition of HBO_2 significantly improved hearing gains compared to the medical control group (35.4 dB versus 16.2 dB, respectively). For those with severe hearing loss, the statistically superior results for the HBO_2 group were more impressive (50.7 dB versus 13 dB, respectively). The HBO_2 group displayed statistically significant improvement in hearing gains over all frequencies tested except 2000 Hz. Within the HBO_2 group, the mean hearing gains for those older than 50 years was greater than for those younger than 50 years.(122) In 2006, Narozny et al. reviewed two historical groups of ISSHL patients treated with combinations of medical therapy, steroids, and HBO_2. The hearing gains were statistically significant for the HBO_2 group over all frequencies and in four ranges of frequencies for both relative and absolute values. Additionally, the combination of steroids and HBO_2 resulted in statistically improved clinical outcomes. The authors found delay to treatment and flat hearing loss to be predictors of poor clinical outcomes. Linear regression analyses were also performed to identify prognostic factors related to hearing improvement.

Favorable prognostic factors included treatment with high-dose steroids + HBO_2 and early treatment (within 10 days). A poor prognosis was found with delayed treatment, labyrinth responsiveness disorders, and decreased thyroid stimulating hormone (TSH) levels.(87) In 2008, Suzuki and coworkers reported on 196 consecutive ISSHL patients, comparing steroid or IV prostaglandin E1 (PGE1) combined with HBO_2. No differences were found between groups, indicating steroids and PGE1 may be equally effective when combined with HBO_2 therapy. Additionally, PGE1 may be a potential alternative for steroid-intolerant patients.(117) In the same year, the same lead author published a similar trial, comparing ISSHL patients treated with IV PGE1 or SGB combined with HBO_2. In those with less severe hearing loss (< 80 dB), the outcomes were similar. However, for those with severe hearing loss (> 80 dB), the hearing rate was statistically superior in those treated with SGB and HBO_2.(116) In 2009, Cekin et al. conducted a RCT study evaluating 57 ISSHL patients treated with medical therapy with prednisolone (1 mg/kg tapering dose over 3 weeks) and famotidine (40 mg once daily) with or without HBO_2. There were 21 patients in the medical therapy group and 36 patients in the HBO_2 group. Hyperbaric therapy was applied with 2.5 ATA O_2 for 90 minutes for 10 sessions. Both groups had recovery rates above 70% (79.0% HBO_2 versus 71.3% medical therapy). However, there were no statistical differences between the groups.(23) The most interesting limitation of this study was that it lacked an intention-to-treat analysis. The lead author of this study was contacted regarding the size disparity between groups. The author responded that some of the patients in the control group were not improving and did not return. An intention-to-treat analysis would have been beneficial. In 2010, Liu and others reviewed their treatment of 120 ISSHL patients treated within 2 weeks with medical therapy, with or without HBO_2. The overall effectiveness was clinically and statistically superior for the HBO_2 patients. The most profound improvement occurred in those with moderate to severe deafness and those with descending and flat types of audiograms.(75) In 2011, Korpinar and coworkers published their treatment of 80 ISSHL patients treated with medical therapy and HBO_2. They sought to identify factors that affect treatment outcomes. They found that hearing gains were significantly improved for those with early HBO_2, a higher number of HBO_2 treatments, the use of steroids, low-frequency ascending and total audiogram configurations, and profound hearing loss.(63) In 2011, Holy and colleagues reviewed the outcomes of 61 ISSHL patients treated with IV vasodilation therapy and HBO_2. Hearing improvement occurred in 59.7% of patients. However, if HBO_2 was started within 10 days, significant or complete recovery was found in 65.9% of patients. In those treated with HBO_2 > 10 days from symptom onset, improvement was noted in only 38.9%.(54) In 2011, Liu and colleagues retrospectively reported their care of 465 ISSHL patients treated with IV and oral steroids, IV and oral steroids plus dextran, or IV and oral steroids, dextran, and HBO_2. The addition of HBO_2 was found beneficial in those with initially profound hearing loss. The addition of dextran did not improve outcomes.(74)

Use of HBO_2 with Steroids in the Treatment of ISSHL

The best outcomes in the literature are found when HBO_2 is combined with steroid therapy in the treatment of ISSHL. In 2007, Fujimura and colleagues published their work with 130 consecutive ISSHL patients treated with steroids, with or without HBO_2. The HBO_2 group showed statistically improved rate of hearing recovery. A subset analysis of those with severe hearing loss (> 80 dB) showed that the HBO_2 groups had a statistically superior rate of hearing improvement.[42] In 2011, Suzuki and colleagues performed simple and multiple regression analysis on 174 consecutive ISSHL patients treated with hydrocortisone and HBO_2. They sought to develop a regression model for predicting hearing outcomes in ISSHL patients. They found significant inverse correlations between hearing improvement and days from onset to treatment, patient age, and the presence of vertigo.[118] In the same year, Alimoglu and others retrospectively reviewed their treatment of 217 ISSHL patients (219 ears) receiving various combinations of oral or IT steroids and HBO_2. The most statistically superior hearing gains (highest mean gain among all groups and the greatest proportion of complete recovery) occurred with the use of both oral steroids and HBO_2 therapy.[6] In 2012, Filipo and colleagues reported their prospective randomized trial of 48 ISSHL patients with < 14 days of symptoms, who were recruited by the ENT emergency room staff of the Department of Sensory Organs of Sapienza University of Rome. The patients were grouped according to initial PTAs. Group I (n = 25) had severe hearing loss (70 dB – 90 dB), while Group II (n = 23) had profound hearing loss (> 90 dB). All patients received HBO_2 therapy (multiplace chamber, 2.4 ATA for 75 minutes daily for 10 sessions). Intravenous steroid (IV methylprednisolone, 1 mg/kg/d for 7 days) was given to 13 patients in the severe group and 13 patients in the profound group. Intratympanic steroids (IT prednisolone, 62.5 mg/ml day for 3 days, injected 2 hours prior to HBO_2 therapy) was given to 12 patients in the severe group and to 10 patients in the profound group. The authors reported positive additional benefit with the addition of HBO_2 therapy. They also found an increase in the success rate in the IT steroid + HBO_2 group; however, the results were not statistically significant.[41] In 2015, Capuano and colleagues published a retrospective 4-year cohort study of 300 patients, divided into 3 groups. Group A (IVS) received the IV steroid metilprednisolone, at decreasing doses of 40 mg for 7 days and 20 mg for another 3 days (n = 100). Group B (HBO_2) received HBO_2 at 2.5 ATA for 90 minutes, weekdays for 16 sessions (n = 100). Group C (IVS + HBO_2) received both therapies (n = 100). There were no statistically significant between-group differences in baseline characteristics. The IVS + HBO_2 group had the highest response rate to therapy, compared to the HBO_2 group or the IVS group (84% versus 70% and 68%, respectively), as well as the highest rate of complete recovery (58% versus 24% and 20%, respectively) regardless of initial hearing levels. In all groups, those who began therapy within the first two weeks had significantly greater mean hearing gains, while those with hypercholesterolemia (> 240 mg/dL) had significantly worse responses.[19] Importantly, the authors concluded that HBO_2 in conjunction with steroid therapy, results in improved recoveries when compared to the use of either treatment alone.[19]

In 2016, Carneiro and coworkers published two case reports of ISSHL occurring following spinal anesthesia. These cases are illustrative in that they opine a mechanistic causation not usually discussed in ISSHL literature. They are considered to be the first cases of spinal-anesthesia-related cases treated with HBO_2 to be published. The first case involved a healthy 27-year-old woman who received spinal anesthesia prior to a cesarean section. Six hours following surgery, the patient complained of left-sided hearing loss, which persisted for three days.

She was diagnosed with profound left-sided ISSHL across the entire spectrum of frequencies and was treated with pentoxifylline and steroids. The patient did not improve and began HBO_2 therapy 14 weeks after symptom onset. Following HBO_2 therapy, the patient showed improvement in audiogram testing. The second case involved a 61-year-old man with HTN, dyslipidemia, hyperuricemia, left nephrectomy due to renal cell carcinoma, adrenal adenoma, and gonarthrosis, who underwent spinal anesthesia for a total knee replacement. Immediately following the surgery, the patient developed severe left-sided hearing loss and mild left-sided tinnitus. Audiogram results confirmed new left-sided moderate SSNHL in the lower frequencies. Speech discrimination was 60% on the left and 80% on the right. The patient was initially treated with conservative measures (bed rest and fluid intake) and steroids. The patient began HBO_2 therapy on the 10th day from symptom onset. Following HBO_2 therapy, the PTA thresholds significantly improved, and speech discrimination was 100% on both sides. The authors discuss the possible etiologies of postoperative SSNHL following noncardiac surgery and conclude that decreases in cerebrospinal fluid (CSF) pressure, more common after spinal anesthesia, were contributory in these cases. The anesthesia literature has been studying this phenomenon for some time and has evaluated the spinal needle design, the type of spinal needle, the size of the spinal needle, and the association of postdural procedural headache (PDPH) and hearing loss. The current prevailing theory is that there is disruption of the endolymph/perilymph balance caused by the decrease in CSF pressure.[20] Cerebrospinal fluid dynamics are integral to auditory function of the inner ear. The puncture of the dura membrane results in a CSF leak and drop in CSF volume and pressure, and that reduced subarachnoid pressure is transmitted to the inner ear through a patent cochlear aqueduct, reducing perilymphatic pressure, resulting in an endolymphatic hydrops, which disrupts the hair cells on the basement membrane. Treatment relies on management of the PDPH and drugs or procedures to ensure adequate oxygenation.[20] In 2017, Hosokawa and others retrospectively reviewed the clinical data of the 334 ISSHL patients presenting to Shizuoka Saiseikai General Hospital in Japan over a 5-year period. All patients were treated with HBO_2 (2.0 ATA for 60 minutes once daily for 10 days) therapy and IV steroids (hydrocortisone 400 mg, tapered over 10 days). They reported that improvement rates varied with the degree of initial hearing loss. Improvement rates for those with Grade 1 hearing loss (< 40 dB) were 44.7%, 60.5% for those with Grade 2 hearing loss (40–60 dB), 81.5% for those with Grade 3 hearing loss (60–90 dB), and 75.6% for those with Grade 4 hearing loss (> 90 dB.). The authors concluded that HBO_2 therapy has a significant additional effect when used in combination with IV steroids for ISSHL. The study was limited by lack of a control group or blinding.[56]

PROGNOSTIC FACTORS FOR ISSHL

Prognostic Factors for Adults

The prognostic factors associated with the treatment of ISSHL have changed considerably as the fields of anesthesiology, otolaryngology, and hyperbaric medicine have advanced. This section will review the positive and negative prognostic factors for ISSHL recovery with treatment not previously discussed in other sections. In 1976, when Shaia and Sheehy reviewed 1,220 cases of ISSHL over a 9-year period and found the favorable prognostic findings to be low tone loss and the absence of vertigo, their main treatment was a vasodilator regimen only, and their positive response rate was 40%.(109) In the last several decades, the etiopathogenesis of ISSHL has been extensively studied, and over 60 protocols have been developed for the treatment of ISSHL. Slattery and colleagues identified the presence of vertigo, persistent or profound hearing loss, and prolonged time from onset to evaluation and treatment as negative prognostic factors for those patients treated with steroids.(111) In 2006, Xenellis and coworkers identified that good predictors of ISSHL recovery included improved PTAs following initial IV steroid therapy, earlier salvage IT steroid therapy, and the absence of vertigo.(135) In 2011, Tsai et al. studied the efficacy of IT steroid therapy in SSHL patients and found that earlier IT steroid administration and patients with low- and mid-frequency hearing loss had improved responses to treatment compared to other groups. Vertigo was also found to be a negative prognostic factor for recovery.(124) In 2015, Yildirim and others retrospectively investigated whether HBO_2 starting times affect outcomes in ISSHL patients. They treated 59 ISSHL patients over a 4-year period with HBO_2 therapy (2.4 ATA for 120 minutes with 3 twenty-minute O_2 periods and 3 twenty-minute breaks daily for 20 sessions). Each patient also received IV piracetam (a cyclic GABA derivative, used in many European, Asian, and South American countries due to its peripheral vascular effects but not Food and Drug Administration approved for any medical use in the United States). Thirty-seven patients also received IV steroid therapy (1 mg/kg methylprednisolone, in a tapered fashion to 10 mg every 2 days). They found significant hearing gains in those HBO_2 patients treated within 14 days from symptom onset. Those treated with HBO_2 after this time (15–28 days) did not have significantly improved outcomes.(137) In 2015, a group of Turkish otolaryngologists published a retrospective study of 96 ISSHL patients who presented to their otolaryngology departments between January 1992 and April 2010. The study aimed to investigate whether the time from symptom onset to time of treatment is a prognostic indicator in ISSHL patients. All patients were treated with dextran-40, pentoxifylline, vitamin B complex, and vitamin C over a 10-day hospitalization with bed rest. Of those patients who presented within 7 days, complete recovery occurred in 60%, partial recovery was obtained in 22.7%, and no recovery occurred in 17.3%. These results were clinically and statistically superior when compared to those patients presenting 8–15 days following symptoms onset (complete recovery 9.5%, partial recovery 33.3%, and no recovery 57.1%). The authors put forth that ISSHL treatment outcomes are improved in those presenting at an early stage of hearing loss.(128) In the same year, Passamonti and colleagues published their prospective study population on 124 patients consecutively referred to their Thrombosis Center (August 2004–June 2013) for a thrombophilia screening following a first episode of ISSHL. Their objective was to evaluate the role of thrombophilia and CV risk factors in those with ISSHL. These study participants were matched with 415 healthy partners or friends of the study group. The study group participants were slightly older than those in the control group. The authors reported that antithrombin deficiencies, protein C and S deficiencies, high factor VIII levels, and hyperhomocyteinemia were significantly associated with ISSHL. Moreover, arterial HTN, hyperlipidemia, DM, and smoking were also associated with an increased risk of ISSHL and poor clinical outcomes.(93) In 2017, Hosokawa and coworkers retrospectively reviewed 344 patients to evaluate the prognosis of ISSHL patients treated with both HBO_2 and IV steroids.

They found that prognosis was more favorable for patients with worse initial hearing losses, patients 60 years or younger when compared to those older than 60 years, and those who presented within 7 days of symptom onset. The presence or absence of vertigo and DM did not affect outcomes.[56]

Prognostic Factors for Children

In 2015, Chung and colleagues reported a multivariate analysis of the prognostic factors for ISSHL in children. The incidence of ISSHL for those younger than 18 years is 11 per 100,000.[4] In children, the possible etiologies of ISSHL are somewhat different from adults; congenital anomalies and nonorganic causes should be explored.[81,120] This group retrospectively analyzed the medical records of 37 pediatric ISSHL patients over a 5-year period (January 2007–December 2013). All patients were admitted for 6 days and received high-dose oral steroid (prednisolone 1 mg/kg/d for 7 days, followed by a 7-day taper) and IV dextran (5 ml/kg/d for 5 days). Median onset to symptoms for these pediatric patients was seven days. These children were then compared to 276 adult ISSHL patients. They found the pediatric patients had an improved recovery compared to the adult subjects (57.4% versus 47.2%, respectively). The complete recovery rate in the pediatric group was also higher than the adult group (46.6% versus 30.8%; $p = 0.04$). The authors concluded that the recovery rate of ISSHL in pediatric patients is higher than in adults, and the presence of tinnitus and earlier treatment onset is associated with improved outcomes.[25]

LITERATURE SUMMARY FOR THE TREATMENT OF ISSHL

The best evidence regarding improvement in hearing for those with ISSHL involves combination therapy with steroids and HBO_2. Table 1 summarizes the retrospective and prospective case-controlled series for the treatment of ISSHL. These 15 studies represent 2,343 patients treated with a variety of medical therapies, HBO_2, or both.[6-7,19,37,42,46,74-75,87,90,94,103,116-117,136] All of these trials are Level 2 evidence; however, most are adequately dosed and treated within 30 days of symptom onset. While acknowledging that Level 1 evidence is preferred, it is important to remember the large number of clinical treatments, in all realms of medicine and surgery, without any RCT support. Surgeons have argued for decades that sham surgeries are unethical, and large amounts of critical care and emergency medicine do not have RCTs for many common and lifesaving interventions. Specific to the application of HBO_2 and RCTs, it is not an overestimation to say that no one has devised an appropriate sham control for the use of HBO_2 therapy. Lack of sham controls is a limitation of every comparative trial in the HBO_2 literature. One of the most beneficial advances that could be made in the field of hyperbaric medicine would be the development of a truly sham control protocol for future studies.

Table 2 highlights eight RCTs on the use of HBO_2 in the treatment of ISSHL.[23,30,38,41,52,95,107,122] This chapter has added several recently published RCTs and removed others. Specifically, the 1996 RCT by Cavallazzi and coworkers is excluded.[22] The study has possible selection bias for two reasons: a lack of information regarding allocation concealment and unclear randomization with possible random sequence generation.[12] It is also unblinded and lacks sham controls. Importantly, the study has flaws involving the authors' exclusion of information. The authors did not report the study groups' duration of ISSHL symptomatology, making the acuity or chronicity of the ISSHL unknown. Additionally, medical therapy given to both groups involved pharmacological treatments with 10 drugs, including heparin, betamethasone, nicotinic acid, flunarizine, cytidine, phosphocholine, dextran, vitamins, and neurotropic and antiviral drugs. However, the doses for these medical therapies were not provided. Both of these exclusions prohibit trial replication or validation, a basic tenet for ensuring the accuracy and meaningfulness of scientific inquiry. The 1995 RCT by Hoffman and coworkers is also excluded.[53] This study is limited by unclear randomization and allocation concealment, and it is unblinded.[12] Importantly, this is a RCT with two hyperbaric treatment groups and without a true control group. The control group was treated with hyperbaric air, which is not physiologically inert.[34,64] Finally, this RCT evaluated patients with chronic ISSHL. This bears mentioning because this RCT has been included and compared to the numerous RCTs performed in those with earlier onset of symptomatology and treatment.[11-14] Patients with chronic hearing loss are not similar to those with acute hearing loss. Numerous studies have shown that the highest significance of benefit is found with early HBO_2 therapy for those with ISSHL.[19,35,54,56,63,70,75,77,84,87,137] It would be prudent to refine meta-analysis criteria to evaluate similar patient groups. Further meta-analyses of the use of HBO_2 for the treatment of chronic hearing loss or tinnitus are not useful. The literature does not support the use of HBO_2 for these patients. However, future meta-analyses evaluating very specifically the use of HBO_2 therapy solely for the treatment of acute hearing loss would be welcomed.

Table 3 delineates the positive and negative prognostic factors in recovery from ISSHL. Assuredly, the table is incomplete, as the literature is prolific. However, it is evident that some conclusions can be drawn. Patients that present early, with moderate-to-profound hearing loss and descending-to-flat audiograms, may do better than others. Additionally, they may also experience improved outcomes if they are 50 years or younger and without BP perturbations, DM, or dyslipidemia. The contribution of vertiginous symptoms, tinnitus, thyroid function, other CV and thrombotic risk factors is less clear. Regarding treatment, many studies have shown that HBO_2 therapy is effective, given as soon as possible. Early steroid therapy is also critical. However, the best outcomes are seen in those patients receiving combination therapy with HBO_2 and steroids.

ISSHL META-ANALYSES OF TREATMENTS

In the realm of otolaryngology, few topics are more controversial than the treatment of ISSHL. Treatment is often regionally specific and may be provided in the outpatient setting or upon hospital admission. Over 60 protocols, with many variations, can be found within the literature. The most common approach in North America is treatment with systemic steroids, which is considered by some to be the gold standard. In 2008, Conlin and Parnes published their systematic review of the prospective RCTs available for the treatment of ISSHL. A total of 20 RCTs were identified, utilizing a variety of treatments, including systemic and IT steroids; antivirals and hemodilution agents; minerals, vitamins, and herbal preparations; batroxibin; carbogen; and HBO_2 therapy. All studies used audiometric outcome measures. Positive results were reported for the use of systemic steroids, IT steroids, batroxibin, magnesium, vitamin E, and HBO_2 therapy. The authors, however, found serious limitations in each study with positive findings. There were no differences in outcomes reported in any studies involving antiviral and hemodilution agents, the use of systemic steroids versus placebo.

TABLE 1. RETROSPECTIVE AND PROSPECTIVE CASE-CONTROLLED STUDIES OF ISSHL AND HBO_2

Reproduced and modified with permission from UHM 2012, Murphy-Lavoie H et al.[83A] and *Hyperbaric Oxygen Therapy Indications, 13th ed.* UHMS; 2014. [83]

Study	Patient Groups	HBO	Hearing Gains
Capuano 2015[19]	**n = 300** IVS (n = 100) HBO (n = 100) IVS + HBO (n = 100)	2.5 ATA 90 minutes 16 sessions	Complete Recovery Regardless of Initial Levels 58% IVS + HBO* 24% HBO 20% IVS Response Rate to Therapy 84% IVS + HBO 70% HBO 68% IVS
Pezzoli 2014[94]	**n = 44** treatment applied after failing MT POS (n = 21) POS + HBO (n = 23) POS group (controls)	2.5 ATA 60 minutes 15 sessions	Hearing Gains 15.6 dB POS + HBO* 5.0 dB POS those with worst hearing had greatest improvement with HBO, regardless of symptom onset
Yang 2013[136]	**n = 103** treatments applied after failing MT ITS (n = 35) HBO (n = 22) ITS + HBO (n = 19) observation-only controls (n = 27)	2.5 ATA 120 minutes 10 sessions	Compared to Controls ITS (p = 0.02)* HBO (p = 0.036)* ITS + HBO (p =0.003)** no between-group differences Word Recognition Scoring ITS + HBO (p = 0.05)*
Alimoglu 2011[6]	**n = 219** HBO (n = 57) POS (n = 58) ITS (n = 43) POS + HBO (n = 61) POS & ITS (control groups)	2.5 ATA 120 minutes 20 sessions	Response to Therapy 86.9% POS / HBO* 63.8% POS 46.5% ITS 43.9% HBO Complete Recovery 42.6% POS / HBO* 19.0% POS 17.5% HBO 11.6% ITS Highest Mean Hearing Gain POS + HBO*
Liu 2011[74]	**n = 465** IVS & POS (n = 76) IVS & POS + Dex (n = 277) IVS & POS + Dex + HBO (n = 112)	2.5 ATA 60 minutes 10–20 sessions	addition of HBO improved good and fair recoveries significantly more than other groups* and is beneficial with profound initial hearing loss
Liu 2010[75]	**n = 120** treated < 14 d MT + HBO (n = 60) MT only (n = 60) MT control (type unknown)	unknown	Overall Effectiveness 83.3% HBO* 60% MT

TABLE 1 (CONTINUED)

Ohno 2010(90)	**n = 92** HBO (n = 48) MT only (n = 44) MT control (IVS, POS, vitamins, ATP) HBO applied (mean 7.4 wks) following MT failure	2.0 ATA 60 minutes mean sessions 13.0	HBO Mean Hearing Gains Initial Profound Loss 18.3 dB* Initial Severe Loss 4.4 dB Initial Moderate Loss 2.1 dB Initial Mild Loss 2.3 dB
Suzuki 2008(117)	**n = 196** POS + HBO (n = 101) PEG1 & HBO (n = 95) hearing loss ≥ 40 dB for ≤ 30 days unaffected ears (controls)	2.5 ATA 60 minutes 10 sessions	no between-group differences PGE1 as an alternative for steroid intolerant
Suzuki 2008(116) acta	**n = 205** PGE1 + HBO (n = 95) SBG + HBO (n = 110) hearing loss ≥ 40 dB for ≤ 30 days unaffected ears (controls)	2.5 ATA 60 minutes 10 sessions	Improvement Rate > 80 dB SGB + HBO 53.0%* PGE1 + HBO 35.3%
Dundar 2007(37)	**n = 80** MT + HBO (n = 55) MT only (n = 25) hearing loss ≥ 40 dB for < 30 days MT type unknown unaffected ears (controls)	unknown	HBO gains across all frequencies* patients with tinnitus showed the highest hearing improvement but only with the addition of HBO
Fujimura 2007(42)	**n = 130** POS + HBO (n = 67) POS only (n = 63) hearing loss ≥ 40 dB for ≤ 30 days unaffected ears (controls)	unknown	Severe Loss (≥ 80 dB) Hearing Rate Improvement 51.1% HBO* 27.1% controls Rate of Recovery 59.7% HBO* 39.7% controls
Narozny 2004(87)	**n = 133** MT + HBO (n = 52) MT only (n = 81) HBO + MT (VD, high-dose steroid, vitamins, & histamine analog) MT = VD, low-dose steroid & vitamins	2.5 ATA 60 minutes 5 days a week unknown # sessions	Hearing Gain In All Frequencies MT + HBO* % Hearing Gain In All Frequencies MT + HBO*
Racic 2003(103)	**n = 115** HBO (n = 51) MT (n = 64) MT control group (varying pentoxifylline infusion dosages)	2.8 ATA	Improvement in Hearing 46.4 dB HBO* 21.5 dB MT Physiologic Hearing Values 47.1% HBO* 6.2% MT Moderate Hearing Gains 41.2% HBO* 12.5% MT

TABLE 1 (CONTINUED)

Aslan 2002[7]	**n = 50** MT + HBO (n = 25) MT only (n = 25) MT (betahistine HCl, prednisone, SGB)	2.4 ATA 90 minutes 20 sessions BID x 7 days daily X 6 days	Hearing Gains 37.9 dB MT + HBO* 20.0 dB MT MT + HBO Mean Hearing Gains (Age) 51.4 dB (< 50 years)* 23.3 dB (> 50 years) 48.9 dB (< 60 years)** 14.5 dB (> 60 years) HBO effective within 14 days
Goto 1979[46]	**n = 91** MT + SGB + HBO (n = 20) SGB + HBO (n = 49) MT (n = 22) MT = VD, steroids, and vitamins	2.4 ATA 90 minutes 20 sessions	Treated < 7 d (PTA > 10 dB) 100% MT + SGB + HBO 83% SGB + HBO* 69% MT only Treated < 14 d (PTA > 10 dB) 100% MT + SGB + HBO** 69% SGB + HBO** 33% MT only Hearing Improvement Initial Profound Hearing Loss 100% MT + SGB + HBO** 83% SGB + HBO* 33% MT only

LEGEND:

MT = Medical Therapy
HBO = Hyperbaric Oxygen
IVS = Intravenous Steroid
ITS = Intratympanic Steroid
POS = Oral Steroid
Dex = Dextran
PGE1 = Prostaglandin E1
SGB = Stellate Ganglion Block
VD = Vasodilator
ATP = Adenosine Tri Phosphate
*($p < 0.05$)
**($p < 0.01$)

TABLE 2. RANDOMIZED CONTROLLED TRIALS OF ISSHL AND HBO_2

Reproduced and modified with permission from UHM 2012, Murphy-Lavoie H et al.[83A] and *Hyperbaric Oxygen Therapy Indications, 13th ed.* UHMS; 2014.[83]

Study	Patient Groups	HBO	Hearing Gains	Study Flaws
Cvorovic 2013[30]	**n = 50** failed MT + salvage HBO failed MT + salvage ITS failed MT = IVS	2.0 ATA 60 minutes 20 sessions	HBO salvage improved hearing thresholds at all 5 frequencies* ITS salvage improved hearing thresholds at 4 frequencies* (except 2 kHz) HBO significantly better* for PTA < 81 dB and in those < 60 years	unblinded patients not matched patients not similar
Filipo 2012[41]	**n = 48** Severe Loss Group (n = 25) (PTA 70 dB – 90 dB) Profound Loss Group (n = 23) (PTA > 90 dB) Severe IVS + HBO (n = 13) Profound IVS + HBO (n = 13) Severe ITS + HBO (n = 12) Profound ITS + HBO (n = 10) treatment within 15 days	2.4 ATA 75 minutes 10 sessions	Severe Hearing Loss Complete/Good Recovery ITS + HBO 83.3% IVS + HBO 53.8% Profound Hearing Loss Complete/Good Recovery ITS + HBO 60% IVS + HBO 52.8% increased success rate with ITS + HBO not statistically significant	unblinded

TABLE 2 (CONTINUED)

Topuz 2004[122]	**n = 51** MT + HBO (n = 30) MT control (n = 21) treated within 14 days without prior therapy MT = prednisone, diazepam, rheomacrodex, salt restriction, and pentoxiphylline	2.5 ATA 90 minutes 25 sessions	Mild Loss no difference Moderate Loss 35.4 dB HBO* 16.2 dB control Severe Loss 50.7 dB HBO* 13 dB control	unblinded unclear randomization
Fattori 2001[38]	**n = 50** MT + HBO (n = 30) MT control (n = 20) treatment within 2 days MT = IV VD (buflomedil)	2.2 ATA 90 minutes 10 sessions	Hearing Gains 61.3 dB HBO* 24 dB controls Good Response 73% HBO* 55% control	unblinded unclear randomization
Schwab 1998[107]	**n = 75** HBO (n = 37) no treatment controls (n = 38) treated within 14 days without prior therapy	1.5 ATA 45 minutes 10–20 sessions	Hearing Gains 15.6 dB HBO* 10.7 dB control	unblinded unclear randomization possible attrition bias proceedings publication
Hoffman 1995[53]	**n = 20** MT + Salvage HBO (n = 10) MT controls (n = 10) Primary MT = hydroxyethyl starch, pentoxifylline, and cortisone	1.5 ATA 45 minutes 10–20 sessions	Acute Hearing Loss Gains 7.5 dB HBO* 0.7 dB control	unblinded unclear randomization proceedings publication
Pilgramm 1985[95]	**n = 37** MT + HBO (n = 18) MT control (n = 19) treatment within 14 days MT = 10% Dex, vitamin B, and naphtidrofuryl hydrogenalalate	2.5 ATA 60 minutes 10 sessions	Acute Loss Hearing Gains 29.2 HBO* 20.2 controls	unblinded possible attrition bias

LEGEND:

MT = Medical Therapy IVS = Intravenous Steroid VD = Vasodilator ITT = Intention to Treat
HBO = Hyperbaric Oxygen ITS = Intratympanic Steroid Dex = Dextra n*($p < 0.05$)

The authors concluded that there is no valid RCT to determine effective treatment of ISSHL.[29] However, the authors failed to consider the voluminous amount of Level 2 evidence supporting the uses of steroids in the treatment of ISSHL. Interestingly, these authors found four RCTs that met inclusion criteria for vasoactive therapies. However, they do not appear to be the same studies evaluated in the 2009 Cochrane Review on the use of vasodilators and vasoactive agents published by Agarwal and Pothier.[1] The authors did identify the two RCTs evaluated by Wei and colleagues in their 2006 Cochrane Review of steroids and the treatment of ISSHL.[27,133] Moreover, they also identified and included six additional RCTs involving the use of steroids that were not included 2006 Cochrane Review by Wei et al.[51,66,115,126-127,132] Of great interest is that these authors could only find one RCT on the use of HBO_2 for the treatment of ISSHL.[122] However, the 2007 Cochrane Review regarding the use of HBO_2 for ISSHL and tinnitus analyzed 6 trials (n = 308).[14]

TABLE 3. ISSHL PROGNOSTIC FACTORS FOR RECOVERY

Positive Prognostic Factors	Negative Prognostic Factors
Low–Mid Frequency Hearing Loss(5,39,63,84,96,124)	
Descending/Flat Audiograms(75,87)	
Moderate to Severe Deafness(30,39,75)	
Profound Hearing Loss (30,42,54,56,63)	Profound Hearing Loss(111)
HBO Therapy(7,31,35,37-38,41-42,74-75,87,95,103,107,116,118,122,140)	
Early HBO Therapy(19,35,54,56,63,70,75,77,84,87,137)	Delayed HBO Therapy(54,56,82,87,137)
HBO Salvage Therapy(30,52,77,82,90,94,136)	
HBO for Chronic ISSHL(59,106)	
HBO + Steroids(6,19, 30, 41, 42, 56, 87, 94,136)	
Absence of Vertigo(109,135)	Presence of Vertigo(82,111,118)
Presence of Tinnitus(25,37)	
Younger Age(30,56,122) Older Age(84)	Older Age(82,118)
	Antithrombin Deficiencies, Protein C & S Deficiencies, Elevated Factor VIII Levels, and Hyperhomocyteinemia(93)
	Diabetes(3,26,93) Decreased TSH(87)
	Hypertension(16,26,93) Hypotension(71, 76, 96-98)
	Hypercholesterolemia/Dyslipidemia(3,19,26)

This was a positive review in which the Cochrane Collaboration found that the use of HBO_2 imparts a statistically significant mean improvement over controls at all frequencies and confirmed that, for people with early presentation of ISSHL, the application of HBO_2 significantly improved hearing loss. Objectively, only the RCTs of Pilgramm, Fattori, and Topuz would have been easily retrieved, as the RCTs of Schwab, Cavallazzi, and the two from Hoffman were proceeding publications. However, they were identified by the Cochrane Reviews, both in 2005 and in 2007, and were possibly accessible from the publisher. Unfortunately, none of the existing meta-analyses thoroughly evaluates all of the published RCTs and Level 2 evidence regarding the treatment of acute ISSHL.

Use of Vasodilators and Vasoactive Agents for ISSHL

In 2009, Agarwal and Pothier published their Cochrane Review on the use of vasodilators and vasoactive substances for ISSHL. They evaluated 3 trials (n = 189) and found that the effectiveness of vasodilators in the treatment of ISSHL remains unproven due to small numbers of patients and heterogeneities regarding the type, dosage, and duration of the vasodilators utilized. The results of these studies could not be combined to reach a conclusion.[1]

Use of Antivirals for ISSHL

In 2012, Awad and colleagues performed a Cochrane Review on the use of antivirals for ISSHL. They evaluated RCTs comparing different antivirals versus placebo (both with or without other treatment). Four RCTs, comprising 257 patients, were included in analyses. All trials evaluated had a low risk of bias, and no serious adverse effects related to antiviral treatment were found. There was also no statistically significant advantage detected in the use of antivirals in the treatment of ISSHL.(8)

Use of Steroids for ISSHL

In 2006, Wei and colleagues published a Cochrane Review on the use of systemic steroids in the treatment of ISSHL. Two trials were reviewed. One showed significant improvement in hearing of ISSHL patients receiving oral steroids compared (61% versus 32%, respectively). The other study showed a lack of effect of steroids on hearing improvement. The authors concluded that the value of steroids in the treatment of ISSHL remains unclear.(130) In 2013, the Cochrane Collaboration performed an update of their 2006 review on the use of systemic steroids for ISSHL.(131) One study was added, and 3 studies (n = 267) were evaluated.(27,88,133) The third study also showed a lack of effect of oral steroids in improving hearing compared to placebo control and was hindered by a lack of strict inclusion criteria, significant exclusion of patients from the final analysis, and lack of patient compliance to the treatment protocol.(88) The authors concluded that the value of steroids in the treatment of ISSHL remains unclear due to the contradictory results of the RCTs and the small number of patients.(131) In 2009, Plontke and others performed a Cochrane Collaboration systematic review on the use of IT steroids for the treatment of ISSHL. The authors found IT corticosteroid treatment to be equivalent to systemic steroids and of unclear clinical significance.(101)

Use of HBO_2 for ISSHL

The only Cochrane Reviews regarding the treatment of ISSHL that show significant benefit of therapy are the meta-analyses involving the use of HBO_2. In the 2005 Cochrane Review, 6 trials were reviewed (n = 304), and it was reported that "HBO_2 did improve hearing."(13) The 2007 Cochrane Review, by the same authors, analyzed 6 trials (n = 308). This review found that the use of HBO_2 imparts a statistically significant mean improvement over controls at all frequencies. Specifically, HBO_2 improves hearing loss by 37.7 dB for those with severe loss, 19.3 dB for those with moderate loss, and 15.6 dB of hearing improvement overall. It also confirmed that "For people with early presentation of ISSHL, the application of HBO_2 significantly improved hearing loss." Moreover, this update defined that the number needed to treat (NNT) for one extra-good outcome was 5.3.(14) This NNT correlates well with the NNT for diabetic foot wounds treated with HBO_2 (NNT = 4) reported in the 2009 Cochrane Review on the use of HBO_2 for chronic wounds.(65) This is an extremely low number that is superior to the vast majority of treatments found on the NNT website, which contains 119 reviews spanning 22 specialties (http://www.the nnt.com/home-nnt/#green). The only treatments with a NNT lower than 5 are the following: defibrillation (1 in 2.5 no RCT); IV magnesium for asthma (1 in 3); and steroids for pain relief in pharyngitis (1 in 3). Both the 2010 and the 2012 Cochrane Reviews for the use of HBO_2 for ISSHL analyzed the same 7 trials (n = 392) and reported the same objective and positive conclusions.(11-12)

PATIENT SELECTION CRITERIA

The Undersea and Hyperbaric Medical Society Committee Report advocates that for patients with moderate to profound ISSHL hearing loss (> 40 dB) who present within 14 days of symptoms onset, HBO_2 therapy should be considered.[(83)] However, the literature shows that patients presenting later than 14 days may show improvement with HBO_2, and the American Academy of Otolaryngology – Head and Neck Surgery advocates for the consideration of HBO_2 therapy for up to three months following symptom onset.[(113)] This statement of advocacy from the American Academy of Otolaryngology is important, in that the *National Guideline Clearinghouse Clinical Practice Guidelines for Sudden Hearing Loss* lists this reference as the entirety of their guidelines (guidelines.gov). However, the majority of the medical literature supports that early intervention is associated with improved outcomes. In Europe, the pattern of use of HBO_2 in the treatment of ISSHL is wider ranging. A recent 2016 survey was conducted by Uzun and colleagues. This questionnaire was comprised of 9 questions and was presented to 192 European hyperbaric centers. The aim of the study was to identify practice differences in the use of HBO_2 for SSNHL in Europe. The response rate was 41.6% (80 centers from 25 countries). Seventy of these centers were utilizing HBO_2 in the treatment of SSNHL. Over a 12-month period, the number of patients treated at each HBO_2 center ranged from 2–150 (mean 34, median 18). The majority of HBO_2 centers (73.3%) were accepting patients if they applied within 30 days of a SSHNL diagnosis. Approximately 43% of these HBO_2 centers were also treating patients with tinnitus symptoms only. The number of HBO_2 treatments ranged from 5–40 (mean 19, median 20). Most HBO_2 centers (76.6%) treated SSNHL patients once daily. However, 23.2% reported using twice-daily sessions, at least for part of the HBO_2 therapy. Treatment duration varied between 60 and 140 minutes, and the treatment pressure between 151 kPa and 253 kPa (1.5–2.5 ATA).[(129)] These rather wide-ranging approaches to the treatment of SSHNL with HBO_2 across Europe illustrate the need for more research to identify an optimal HBO_2 treatment protocol.

DIFFERENTIAL DIAGNOSIS OF ACQUIRED SUDDEN DEAFNESS

The differential diagnosis of acquired sudden deafness is large. Approximately 1% of sudden sensorineural hearing loss is due to retrocochlear disorders (vestibular schwannoma, demyelinating disease, or stroke).[(109)] Another 10%–15% of these cases are to due identifiable causes. Infectious causes include meningitis, mumps, rubeola, rubella, syphilis, Lyme's disease, herpesvirus, Lassa fever, HIV, AIDs, mononucleosis, mycoplasma, toxoplasmosis, and cytomegalovirus. Traumatic causes may be obvious or occult and include temporal bone fracture, acoustic trauma, barotrauma, lumbar puncture perturbations in CSF pressure, and perilymphatic fistula. Possible circulatory etiologies may include sickle cell disease, cardiopulmonary bypass, hypoperfusion states, and vertebrobasilar insufficiency. Neurological etiologies may include stroke, multiple sclerosis, and neurosarcoidosis. Neoplastic causes include acoustic neuroma, vestibular schwannoma, lymphoma, meningioma, leukemia, myeloma and meningeal carcinomatosis, and metastatic disease. Other causes include snake bites, ototoxic drugs, oral contraceptives, Cogan's syndrome, Wegener's granulomatosis, primary immune inner ear disease, cochlear membrane rupture, pseudohypoacusis, hyperostosis cranialis interna,

Meniere's disease, endolymphatic hydrops, metabolic derangements, and cochlear dysfunction.[40,57,78,89,104] Unfortunately for many, even after a thorough search for a cause, approximately 88% of cases of adult-onset hearing loss are idiopathic.[40]

THE WORK-UP

The American Academy of Otolaryngology makes the following recommendations for clinicians:[113]

1. Assess patients with presumptive sudden sensorineural hearing loss for bilateral disease, recurrent episodes of SSNHL, or focal neurologic findings.
2. Diagnose presumptive ISSHL if audiometry confirms a 30 dB hearing loss at 3 consecutive frequencies, and an underlying condition cannot be identified by history and physical examination.
3. Evaluate patients with ISSHL for retrocochlear pathology by obtaining magnetic resonance imaging, auditory brainstem response, or audiometric follow-up.
4. Offer intratympanic steroid therapy when patients have incomplete recovery from ISSHL after failure of initial management.
5. Obtain follow up audiometric evaluation within six months of diagnosis for those patients with ISSHL.

PATIENT MANAGEMENT

The most recent guidelines published by the American Academy of Otolaryngology strongly recommend the following:[113]

1. Complete physical examination, and referral to an otolaryngologist to distinguish sensorineural hearing loss from conductive hearing loss
2. Patient education regarding ISSHL, inclusive of the natural history of the condition, the benefits and risks of medical interventions, and the limitations of existing evidence regarding efficacy of treatment
3. Counseling of patients with incomplete recovery of hearing about the possible benefits of amplifications and hearing assistive technologies and other supportive measures

TREATMENT

Steroid Therapy

Patients without contraindications to steroid therapy should be treated with either IT steroids or systemic oral steroids. It is prudent to begin with oral steroid therapy along with urgent referral to an otolaryngologist for audioimetric testing to confirm the diagnosis. It is reasonable to start oral steroid therapy with prednisone (1 mg/kg/day) with a slow taper over 2–3 weeks.[83] The decision either to switch to IT steroids or to add IT steroids should be made by the patient and the referring otolaryngologist.

For decades, the standard of care has been oral steroids. However, many studies have shown the efficacy of IT steroid therapy, and the use of IT steroids does result in higher steroid concentrations within the perilymph compared with oral steroid therapy.[24,39,92]

Additionally, IT steroids reduce the incidence of possible toxic side effects of systemic steroid regimens. Currently, there is a paucity of data regarding the prevalence of these side effects with the relatively short courses of systemic steroid therapy used in the treatment of ISSHL.[131] However, it may be that IT steroids are a better option for those who are intolerant of or refuse systemic steroid therapy.[2,9,24,50-51,55,61,99,108,111,124,135]

Hyperbaric Oxygen Therapy

Patients diagnosed with ISSHL who meet selection criteria and are without contraindications to HBO_2 therapy may benefit from treatment. The recommended treatment profile is 100% O_2 at 2.0–2.5 ATA for 90 minutes daily for 10–20 sessions.[83]

Other Medical Therapies

The American Academy of Otolaryngology recommends against the routine use of antivirals, thrombolytics, vasodilators, vasoactive substances, or antioxidants for patients with ISSHL.[113] There are more than 60 protocols involving a multitude of medical therapies in the treatment of ISSHL. However, only two therapies have been shown to be efficacious: the use of steroids and HBO_2 therapy. These two therapies have received the highest medical therapy recommendation in the *Guidelines for the Treatment of ISSHL*, published by the American Academy of Otolaryngology. They are also the only two therapies endorsed by the *UHMS Committee Report* on the treatment of ISSHL.[83]

FOLLOW-UP

Continued consultation and follow-up with an otolaryngologist is recommended. Additional testing and therapy may be recommended by the otolaryngologist, and the patient should continue to be followed by the otolaryngology specialist during and following HBO_2 therapy.[83,113]

PROGNOSIS

Hearing loss results in a significant socioeconomic and health burden for those affected. For some, with slight impairment, education and counseling may be all that is needed. However, those with more significant deficits, hearing aids, lip reading and signing are usually required.[47] Importantly, the use of HBO_2 therapy improves hearing function 19 dB in those with moderate deficits. For those with severe hearing loss, the improvement in hearing with the use of HBO_2 therapy is more impressive (37.3 dB.).

COST IMPACT

The World Health Organization has detailed the cost impact of hearing loss worldwide. Hearing loss impairs the ability of a patient to obtain, perform, or retain employment. These patients are often stigmatized and may become socially isolated. The cost of specialized education and lost employment imposes a heavy social and economic burden.[33] Adult-onset hearing loss is the third leading cause of years lost to disability, and the fifteenth leading cause of burden of disease; it is projected to move up to seventh by the year 2030.[134] Remarkably, hearing loss is the most common cause of disability globally, just ahead of refractive errors, and well ahead of depression, cataracts, and accidental injuries, which round out the top five.[134] For those able to afford them, hearing aids cost between $1,500–$3,000 (USD) per pair. Many require replacement every three to five years and may not result in fully functional hearing.

REFERENCES

1. Agarwal L, Pothier Dd. Vasodilators and vasoactive substances for idiopathic sudden sensorineural hearing loss. Cochrane Database Syst Rev. 2009 Oct 7;(4):CD003422.
2. Ahn JH, Han MW, Kim JH, Chung JW, Yoon TH. Therapeutic effectiveness over time of intratympanic dexamethasone as salvage treatment of sudden deafness. Acta Otolaryngol. 2008 Feb;128(2):128-31.
3. Aimoni C, Bianchini C, Borin M, Ciorba A, Fellin R, Martini A, Scanelli G, Volpato S. Diabetes, cardiovascular risk factors and idiopathic sudden sensorineural hearing loss: a case-control study. Audio Neurotol. 2010;15(2):111-4. Alexander TH, Harris JP. Incidence of sudden sensorineural hearing loss. Otol Neurotol. 2013;34:1586-9.
4. Alexander TH, Harris JP. Incidence of sudden sensorineural hearing loss. Otol Neurotol. 2013;34:1586-9.
5. Alexiou C, Arnold W, Fauser C, Schratzenstaller B, Gloddek B, Fuhrmann S, Lamm K. Sudden sensorineural hearing loss: does application of glucocorticoids make sense? Arch Otolaryngol Head Neck Surg. 2001 Mar;127(3):253-8.
6. Alimoglu Y, Inci E, Edizer DT, Ozdilek A, Aslan M. Efficacy comparison of oral steroid, intratympanic steroid, hyperbaric oxygen and oral steroid and hyperbaric oxygen treatments in idiopathic sudden sensorineural hearing loss cases. Eur Arch Otorhinolaryngol. 2011 Dec;268(12):1735-41.
7. Aslan I, Oysu C, Veyseller B, Baserer N. Does the addition of hyperbaric oxygen therapy to the conventional treatment modalities influence the outcome of sudden deafness? Otolaryngol Head Neck Surg. 2002 Feb;126(2):121-6.
8. Awad Z, Huins C, Pothier DD. Antivirals for idiopathic sudden sensorineural hearing loss. Cochrane Database Syst Rev. 2012 Aug 15;(8):1-22.
9. Battaglia A, Burchette R, Cueva R. Combination therapy (intratympanic dexamethasone + high-dose prednisone taper) for the treatment of idiopathic sudden sensorineural hearing loss. Otol Neurotol. 2008 Jun;29(4):453-60.
10. Belal A Jr. Pathology of vascular sensorineural hearing impairment. Laryngoscope. 1980 Nov;90(11 Pt 1):1831-9.
11. Bennett MH, Kertesz T, Matthias P, Yeung P. Hyperbaric oxygen for idiopathic sudden sensorineural hearing loss and tinnitus. Cochrane Database Syst Rev. 2010 Jan 20(1):CD004739.
12. Bennett MH, Kertesz T, Perleth M, Yeung P, Lehm JP. Hyperbaric oxygen for idiopathic sudden sensorineural hearing loss and tinnitus. Cochrane Database Syst Rev. 2012;(10):CD004739.
13. Bennett MH, Kertesz T, Yeung P. Hyperbaric oxygen for idiopathic sudden sensorineural hearing loss and tinnitus. Cochrane Database Syst Rev. 2005 Jan 25;(1):CD004739.
14. Bennett MH, Kertesz T, Yeung P. Hyperbaric oxygen for idiopathic sudden sensorineural hearing loss and tinnitus. Cochrane Database Syst Rev. 2007 Jan 24;(1):CD004739.
15. Bird PA, Begg EJ, Zhang M, Keast AT, Murray DP, Balkany TJ. Intratympanic versus intravenous delivery of methylprednisolone to cochlear perilymph. Otol Neurotol. 2007 Dec;28(8):1124-30.
16. Brant LJ, Gordon-Salant S, Pearson JD, Klein LL, Morrell CH, Metter EJ, Fozard JL. Risk factors related to age-associated hearing loss in the speech frequencies. J Am Acad Audiol. 1996;7:152-60.
17. Byl FM. Seventy-six cases of presumed sudden hearing loss occurring in 1973; prognosis and incidence. Laryngoscope. 1977 May;87(5 Pt 1):817-25.

18. Byl FM Jr. Sudden hearing loss: eight years' experience and suggested prognostic table. Laryngoscope. 1984 May;94(5 Pt 1):647-61.
19. Capuano L, Cavaliere M, Parente G, Damiano A, Pezzuti G, Lopardo D, Lemma M. Hyperbaric oxygen for idiopathic sudden hearing loss: is the routine application helpful? Acta Oto-Laryngologica. 2015 Jul;135(7):692-7.
20. Carneiro SN, Guerreiro DV, Cunha AM, Camacho OF, Aguiar IC. Hyperbaric oxygen therapy in sudden sensorineural hearing loss following spinal anesthesia: case reports. Undersea Hyperb Med. 2016;43(2):153-9.
21. Cavallazzi GM. Relations between O2 and hearing function. In: Marroni A, Oriani G, Wattel F, editors. Proceedings of International Joint Meeting on Hyperbaric and Underwater Medicine; 1996 Sep 4-8; Milano, Italy. p. 633-45.
22. Cavallazzi G, Pignataro L, Capaccio P. Italian experience in hyperbaric oxygen therapy for idiopathic sudden sensorineural hearing loss. Proceedings of the International Joint Meeting on Hyperbaric and Underwater Medicine; 1996; Grafica Victoria, Bologna. p. 647-9.
23. Cekin E, Cincik H, Ulubil SA, Gungor A. Effectiveness of hyperbaric oxygen therapy in management of sudden hearing loss. J Laryngol Otol. 2009;123:609-12.
24. Chandrasekhar SS. Intratympanic dexamethasone for sudden sensorineural hearing loss: clinical and laboratory evaluation. Otol Neurotol. 2001 Jan;22(1):18-23.
25. Chung JH, Cho SH, Jeong JH, Park CW, Lee SH. Multivariate analysis of prognostic factors for idiopathic sudden sensorineural hearing loss in children. Laryngoscope. 2015;125:2209-15.
26. Ciccone MM, Cortese F, Pinto M, Di Teo C, Fornarelli F, Gesualdo M, Mezzina A, Sabatelli E, Scicchitano P, Quaranta N. Endothelial function and cardiovascular risk in patients with idiopathic sudden sensorineural hearing loss. Atherosclerosis. 2012;225:511-6.
27. Cinamon U, Bendet E, Kronenberg J. Steroids, carbogen or placebo for sudden hearing loss: a prospective double-blind study. Eur Arch Otorhinolaryngol. 2001 Nov;258(9):477-80.
28. Cole RR, Jahrsdoerfer RA. Sudden hearing loss: an update. Am J Otol. 1988 May;9(3):211-5.
29. Conlin AE, Parnes LS. Treatment of sudden sensorineural hearing loss. A systematic review. Arch Otolaryngol Head Neck Surg. 2007 Jun;133:573-81.
30. Cvorovic L, Jovanovic MG, Milutinovic Z, Arsovic N, Djeric D. Randomized prospective trial of hyperbaric oxygen therapy and intratympanic steroid injection as salvage treatment of sudden sensorineural hearing loss. Otol Neurotol. 2013;34(6):1021-6.
31. Dauman R, Poisot D, Cros AM, Zennaro O, Bertrand B, Duclos JY, Esteban D, Milacic M, Boudey C, Bebear JP. Sudden deafness: a randomized comparative study of 2 administration modalities of hyperbaric oxygenotherapy combined with naftidrofuryl. Rev Laryngol Otol Rhinol (Bord). 1993;114(1):53-8.
32. De Kleyn A. Sudden complete or partial loss of function of the octavus system in apparently normal persons. Acta Otolaryngologica. 1944;(32):407-29.
33. Deafness and hearing loss fact sheet. World Health Organization [Internet]. World Health Organization. Deafness and hearing loss fact sheet [updated 2017 Feb]. Available from: http://www.who.int/mediacentre/factsheets/fs300/en/index.html
34. Dean JB, Mulkey DK. Continuous intracellular recordings from mammalian neurons exposed to hyperbaric helium, oxygen, or air. J Appl Physiol (1985). 2000 Aug;89(2):807-22.

35. DeHeyn G, Van Opstal M. Comparative study of acoustic trauma caused by blasts, treated by vasodilators or by a combination of vasodilators and hyperbaric oxygenation. Acta Otorhinolaryngol Belg. 1976;30(3):251-9.

36. Dispenza F, Amodio E, De Stefano A, Gallina S, Marchese D, Mathur N, Riggio F. Treatment of sudden sensorineural hearing loss with transtympanic injection of steroids as single therapy: a randomized clinical study. Eur Arch Otorhinolaryngol. 2011 Sep;268(9):1273-8.

37. Dundar K, Gumus T, Ay H, Yetiser S, Ertugrul E. Effectiveness of hyperbaric oxygen on sudden sensorineural hearing loss: prospective clinical research. J Otoloaryngol. 2007 Feb;36(1):32-7.

38. Fattori B, Berrettini S, Casani A, Nacci A, De Vito A, De Iaco G. Sudden hypoacusis treated with hyperbaric oxygen therapy: a controlled study. Ear Nose Throat J. 2001 Sept;80(9):655-60.

39. Ferri E, Frisina A, Fasson AC, Armato E, Spinato G, Amadori M. Intratympanic steroid treatment for idiopathic sudden sensorineural hearing loss after failure of intravenous therapy. ISRN Otolaryngol. 2012:1-6.

40. Fetterman BL, Saunders JE, Luxford WM. Prognosis and treatment of sudden sensorineural hearing loss. Am J Otol. 1996 Jul;17(4):529-36.

41. Filipo R, Attanasio G, Viccaro M, Russo FY, Mancini P, Rocco M, Pietropaoli P, Covelli E. Hyperbaric oxygen therapy with short duration intratympanic steroid therapy for sudden hearing loss. Acta Otolaryngol. 2012 May;132(5):475-81.

42. Fujimura T, Suzuki H, Shiomori T, Udaka T, Mori T. Hyperbaric oxygen and steroid therapy for idiopathic sudden sensorineural hearing loss. Eur Arch Otorhinolaryngol. 2007 Aug;264(8):861-6.

43. Gao Y, Liu D. Combined intratympanic and systemic use of steroids for idiopathic sudden sensorineural hearing loss: a meta-analysis. Eur Arch Otorhinolaryngol. 2016;273:3699-711.

44. Giger HL. Therapy of sudden deafness with O2/CO2 inhalation. HNO. 1979 Mar;27(3):107-9.

45. Gloddek B, Lamm K, Arnold W. Pharmacological influence on inner ear endothelial cells in relation to the pathogenesis of sensorineural hearing loss. Adv Otorhinolaryngol. 2002;59:75-83.

46. Goto F, Fujiita T, Kitani Y, Kanno M, Kamei T, Ishii H. Hyperbaric oxygen and stellate ganglion blocks for idiopathic sudden hearing loss. Acta Otolaryngol. 1979;88(5-6):335-42.

47. Grades of hearing impairment. World Health Organization [Internet]. World Health Organization. Grades of hearing impairment; 2011. Available from: http://www.who.int/pbd/deafness/hearing_impairment_grades/en/index.html

48. Haberkamp TJ, Tanyeri HM. Management of idiopathic sudden sensorineural hearing loss. Am J Otol. 1999 Sept;20:587-92.

49. Hallberg OE. Sudden deafness of obscure origin. Laryngoscope. 1956 Oct;66(10):1237-67.

50. Haynes DS, O'Malley M, Cohen S, Watford K, Labadie RF. Intratympanic dexamethasone for sudden sensorineural hearing loss after failure of systemic therapy. Laryngoscope. 2007 Jan;117(1):3-15.

51. Ho HG, Lin HC, Shu MT, Yang CC, Tsai HT. Effectiveness of intratympanic dexamethasone injection in sudden-deafness patients as salvage treatment. Laryngoscope. 2004 Jul;114(7):1184-9.

52. Hoffman G, Bohmer D, Desloovere C. Hyperbaric oxygenation as a treatment for sudden deafness and acute tinnitus. In: Proceedings of the 11th International Congress on Hyperbaric Medicine. Flagstaff (AZ): Best Publishing Co.; 1995. p. 146-51.

53. Hoffman G, Bohmer D, Desloovere C. Hyperbaric oxygenation as a treatment of chronic forms of inner ear hearing loss and tinnitus. In: Proceedings of the 11th International Congress on Hyperbaric Medicine. Flagstaff (AZ): Best Publishing Co.: 1995. p. 141-5.

54. Holy R, Navara M, Dosel P, Fundova P, Prazenica P, Hahn A. Hyperbaric oxygen therapy in idiopathic sudden sensorineural hearing loss (ISSNHL) in association with combined treatment. Undersea Hyperb Med. 2011 Mar-Apr;38(2):137-42.

55. Hong SM, Park CH, Lee JH. Hearing outcomes of daily intratympanic dexamethasone alone as a primary treatment modality for ISSHL. Otolaryngol Head Neck Surg. 2009 Nov;141(5):579-83.

56. Hosokawa S, Sugiyama K, Takashashi G, Takebayashi S, Mineta H. Prognostic factors for idiopathic sudden sensorineural hearing loss treated with hyperbaric oxygen therapy and intravenous steroids. J Laryngol Otol. 2017;131:77-82.

57. Hughes GB, Freedman MA, Haberkamp TJ, Guay ME. Sudden sensorineural hearing loss. Otolaryngol Clin North Am. 1996 Jun;29(3):393-405.

58. Jourdy DN, Donatelli LA, Victor JD, Selesnick SH. Assessment of variation throughout the year in the incidence of idiopathic sudden sensorineural hearing loss. Otol Neurotol. 2010 Jan;31(1):53-7.

59. Kau RJ, Sendtner-Gress K, Ganzer U, Arnold W. Effectiveness of hyperbaric oxygen therapy in patients with acute and chronic cochlear disorders. ORL J Otorhinolarygnol Relat Spec. 1997 Mar-Apr;59(2):78-83.

60. Kawakami M, Makimoto K, Fukuse S, Takahashi H. Autoregulation of cochlear blood flow. A comparison of cerebral blood flow with muscular blood flow. Eur Arch Otorhinolaryngol. 1991;248:471-4.

61. Kilic R, Safak MA, Oguz H, Kargin S, Demirci M, Samim E, Ozluoglu LN. Intratympanic methylprednisolone for sudden sensorineural hearing loss. Otol Neurotol. 2007 Apr;28(3):312-6.

62. Klemm E, Deutscher A, Mosges R. A present investigation of the epidemiology in idiopathic sudden sensorineural hearing loss. Larygorhinootologie. 2009;88:524-7.

63. Korpinar S, Alkan Z, Yigit O, Gor AP, Toklu AS, Cakir B, Soyuyuce OG, Ozkul H. Factors influencing the outcome of idiopathic sudden sensorineural hearing loss treated with hyperbaric oxygen therapy. Eur Arch Otorhinolaryngol. 2011 Jan;268(1):41-7.

64. Kramer MR, Springer C, Berkman N, Glazer M, Bubil M, Bar-Yishay E, Godfrey S. Rehabilitation of hypoxemic patients with COPD at low altitude at the Dead Sea, the lowest place on earth. Chest. 1998 Mar;113(3):571-5.

65. Kranke P, Bennett MH, Debus SE, Roeckl-Wiedmann I, Schnabel A. Hyperbaric oxygen therapy for chronic wounds. Cochrane Database Syst Rev. 2009 Jul 8;(1):CD004123.

66. Kubo T, Matsunaga T, Asi H, Kawamoto K, Kusakari J, Nomura Y, Oda M, Yanagita N, Niwa H, Uemura T, Komune S. Efficacy of defibrinogenation and steroid therapies on sudden deafness. Arch Otolaryngol Head Neck Surg. 1988;114(6):649-52.

67. Lamm C, Walliser U, Schumann K, Lamm K. Oxygen partial pressure measurements in the perilymph and the scala tympani in normo- and hyperbaric conditions. An animal experiment study. HNO. 1988 Sept;35(9):363-6.

68. Lamm H. Der einfluss der hperbaren sauerstofftherapie auf den tinnitus und horverlust bei akuten und chronischen innenohrschaden. Otorhinolaryngol Nova. 1995;5:161-9. German.

69. Lamm K, Lamm C, Lamm H, Schumann K. Simultaneous determinations of oxygen partial pressure in the scala tympani, electrocochleography and blood pressure measurements in noise stress in guinea pigs. HNO. 1988 Sep;36(9):367-72.

70. Lamm K, Lamm H, Arnold W. Effect of hyperbaric oxygen therapy in comparison to conventional or placebo therapy or no treatment in idiopathic sudden hearing loss, acoustic trauma, noise-induced hearing loss and tinnitus. A literature survey. Adv Otorhinolaryngol. 1998;54:86-9.

71. Lehnhardt E, Hesch RD. Causes of inner ear deafness: a critique of therapy. HNO. 1980;28:73-9.

72. Lin DW, Trune DR. Breakdown of stria vascularis blood-labyrinth barrier in C3H/lpr autoimmune disease mice. Otolaryngol Head Neck Surg. 1997 Nov;117(5):530-4.

73. Lin HC, Chao PZ, Lee HC. Sudden sensorineural hearing loss increases the risk of stroke: a 5-year follow-up study. Stroke. 2008 Oct;39(10):2744-8.

74. Liu SC, Kang BH, Lee JC, Lin YS, Huang KL, Liu DW, Su WF, Kao CH, Chu YH, Chen HC, Wang CH. Comparison of therapeutic results in sudden sensorineural hearing loss with/without additional hyperbaric oxygen therapy: a retrospective review of 465 audiologically controlled cases. Clin Otolyarngol. 2011 Apr;36(2):121-8.

75. Liu Y, Sun D, Shao S, Jiang W, Sun Z, Li Z. The effect of hyperbaric oxygen therapy to different degree of hearing loss and types of threshold curve in sudden deafness patients. Lin Chung Er Bi Yan Hou Tou Jing Wai Ke Za Zhi. 2010 Oct;24(19):890-4.

76. Maass B. Autonomic nervous system and hearing. Adv Otorhinolaryngol. 1981;27:14-25.

77. Marchesi G, Valetti TM, Amer M, Ross M, Tiberti R, Ferani R, Mauro G Di. The HBO2 effective in sudden hearing loss treatment. In: UHMS Meeting abstracts [Internet]. 2000. Available from: http://archive.rubicon-foundation.org/6781

78. Mattox DE, Simmons FB. Natural history of sudden sensorineural hearing loss. Ann Otol Rhinol Laryngol. 1977 Jul-Aug;86(4 Pt 1):463-80.

79. Merchant SN, Adams JC, Nadol JB Jr. Pathology and pathophysiology of idiopathic sudden sensorineural hearing loss. Otol Neurotol. 2005 Mar;26(2):151-60.

80. Merchant SN, Durand ML, Adams JC. Sudden deafness: is it viral? ORL J Otorhinolaryngol Relat Spec. 2008;70:52-62.

81. Morita S, Suzuki M, Iizuka K. Non-organic hearing loss in childhood. Int J Pediatr Otorhinolaryngol. 2010;74:441-6.

82. Murakawa T, Kosaka M, Mori Y, Fukazawa M, Misaki K. Treatment of 533 patients with sudden deafness performed oxygenation at high pressure. Nihon Jibiinkoka Gakkai Kaiho. 2000 May;103(5):506-15.

83. Murphy-Lavoie H et al. Idiopathic sudden sensorineural hearing loss (2014). In: Hyperbaric oxygen therapy indications: the Hyperbaric Oxygen Therapy Committee report. North Palm Beach (FL): Best Publishing Co.

83A. Murphy-Lavoie H, Piper S, Moon RE, Legros T. Hyperbaric oxygen therapy for idiopathic sudden sensorineural hearing loss. Undersea Hyperb Med. 2012; 39(3) May-June. 777-792.

84. Muzzi E, Zennaro B, Visentin R, Soldano F, Sacilotto C. Hyperbaric oxygen therapy as salvage treatment for sudden sensorineural hearing loss: review of rationale and preliminary report. J Laryngol Otol. 2010;124(2):e2.

85. Nagahara K, Fisch U, Yagi N. Perilymph oxygenation in sudden and progressive sensorineural hearing loss. Acta Otolaryngol. 1983 Jul-Aug;96(1-2):57-68.

86. Nagura M, Iwasaki S, Wu R, Mizuta K, Umemura K, Hoshino T. Effects of corticosteroid, contrast medium and ATP on focal microcirculatory disorders of the cochlea. Eur J Pharmacol. 1999 Jan 29;366(1):47-53.

87. Narozny W, Kuczkowski J, Kot J, Stankiewicz C, Sicko Z, Mikaszeweski B. Prognostic factors in sudden sensorineural hearing loss: our experience and a review of the literature. Ann Otol Rhinol Laryngol. 2006 Jul;115(7):553-8.

88. Nosrati-Zarenoe R, Hultcrantz E. Corticosteroid treatment of idiopathic sudden sensorineural hearing loss: randomized triple-blind placebo-controlled trial. Otol Neurotol. 2012 Jun;22(4):523-31.

89. O'Malley MR, Haynes DS. Sudden hearing loss. Otolaryngol Clin N Am. 2008;41:633-49.

90. Ohno K, Noguchi Y, Kawashima Y, Yagishita K, Kitamura K. Secondary hyperbaric oxygen therapy for idiopathic sudden sensorineural hearing loss in the subacute and chronic phases. J Med Dent Sci. 2010;57(2):127-32.

91. Ozler GS. Increased neutrophil-lymphocyte ratio in patients with idiopathic sudden sensorineural hearing loss. J Craniofac Surg. 2014 May;25(3):e260-3.

92. Parnes LS, Sun AH, Freeman DJ. Corticosteroid pharmacokinetics in the inner ear fluids: an animal study followed by clinical application. Laryngoscope. 1999 Jul;109(7 Pt 2):1-17.

93. Passamonti SM, Di Berardino F, Bucciarelli P, Berto V, Artoni A, Gianniello F, Abrosetti U, Cesarani A, Pappalardo E, Martinelli I. Risk factors for idiopathic sudden sensorineural hearing loss and their association with clinical outcome. Thrombosis Res. 2015;135:508-12.

94. Pezzoli M, Magnano M, Maffi L, Pezzoli L, Marcato P, Orione M, Cupi D, Bongioannini G. Hyperbaric oxygen therapy as salvage treatment for sudden sensorineural hearing loss: a prospective controlled study. Eur Arch Otorhinolaryngol. 2015 Jul;272(7):1659-66.

95. Pilgramm M, Lamm H. Schumann K. Hyperbaric oxygen therapy in sudden deafness. Laryngol, Rhinol, Otol. 1985 Jul;64(7):351-4.

96. Pirodda A, Ferri GG, Modugno GC, Borghi C. Systemic hypotension and the development of acute sensorineural hearing loss in young healthy subjects. Arch Otolaryngol Head Neck Surg. 2001 Sep;127:1049-52.

97. Pirodda A, Ferri GG, Modugno GC, Gaddi A. Hypotension and sensorineural hearing loss: a possible correlation. Acta Otolaryngol. 1999;119(7):758-62.

98. Pirodda A, Saggese D, Giausa G, Ferri GG, Nascetti S, Gaddi A. Can hypotension episodes cause cochlear damage in young subjects? Med Hypotheses. 1997;48:195-86.

99. Plaza G, Herraiz C. Intratympanic steroids for treatment of sudden hearing loss after failure of intravenous therapy. Otolaryngol Head Neck Surg. 2007 Jul;137(1):74-8.

100. Plontke SK, Biegner T, Kammerer B, Delabar U, Salt AN. Dexamethasone concentration gradients along scala tympani after application to the round window membrane. Otol Neurotol. 2008 Apr;29(3):401-6.

101. Plontke SK, Meisner C, Caye-Thomasen P, Parnes L, Agrawal S, Mikulee T. Intratympanic glucocorticoids for sudden sensorineural hearing loss. Cochrane Database Syst Rev. 2009 Oct 7;(1):CD0088080.

102. Qiang Q, Wu X, Yang T, Yang C, Sun H. A comparison between systemic and intratympanic steroid therapies as initial therapy for idiopathic sudden sensorineural hearing loss: a meta-analysis. Acta Oto-Laryngologica. 2016 Dec 6:1-8. ISSN: 0001-6489.

103. Racic G, Maslovara S, Roje Z, Dogas Z, Tafra R. Hyperbaric oxygen in the treatment of sudden hearing loss. ORL J Otorhinolaryngol Relat Spec. 2003 Nov-Dec;65(6):317-20.

104. Rauch SD. Idiopathic sudden sensorineural hearing loss. N Engl J Med. 2008 Aug 21;359(8):833-40.

105. Rudack C, Langer C, Stoll W, Rust S, Walter M. Vascular risk factors in sudden hearing loss. Thromb Haemost. 2006;95:454-561.

106. Schumann K, Lamm K, Hettich M. Effect and effectiveness of hyperbaric oxygen therapy in chronic hearing disorders. Report of 557 cases 1989. HNO. 1990 Nov;38(11):408-11.

107. Schwab B, Flunkert C, Heermann R, Lenarz T. HBO2 in the therapy of cochlear dysfunctions – first results of a randomized study. In: EUBS Diving and Hyperbaric Medicine, collected manuscripts of XXIV Annual Scientific Meeting of the European Underwater and Baromedical Society. Stockholm: EUBS; 1998. p. 40-2.

108. Seggas I, Koltsidopoulos P, Bibas A, Tzonou A, Sismanis A. Intratympanic steroid therapy for sudden hearing loss: a review of the literature. Otol Neurotol. 2011 Jan;32(1):29-35.

109. Shaia FT, Sheehy JL. Sudden sensori-neural hearing impairment: a report of 1,220 cases. Layrngoscope. 1976 Mar;86(3):389-98.

110. Shirwany NA, Seidman MD, Tang W. Effect of transtympanic injection of steroids on cochlear blood flow, auditory sensitivity, and histology in the guinea pig. Am J Otol. 1998;19:230 –5.

111. Slattery WH, Fisher LM, Iqbal Z, Friedman RA, Liu N. Intratympanic steroid injection for treatment of idiopathic sudden hearing loss. Otolaryngol Head Neck Surg. 2005 Aug;133(2):251-9.

112. Spear SA, Schwartz SR. Intratympanic steroids for sudden sensorineural hearing loss. A systematic review. Otolaryngol Head Neck Surg. 2011 Oct;145(4): 534-43.

113. Stachler R, Chandrasekhar S, Archer S, Rosenfeld R, Schwartz S, Barrs D, Brown S, Fife T, Ford P, Ganiats T, Hollingsworth D, Lewandowski C, Montano J, Saunders J, Tucci D, Valente M, Warren B, Yaremchuk K, Robertson P. Clinical practice guidelines: sudden hearing loss. Otolayrngol Head Neck Surg. 2012;146:S1-35.

114. Stokroos RJ, Albers FW, Schirm J. The etiology of idiopathic sudden sensorineural hearing loss. Experimental herpes simplex virus infection of the inner ear. Am J Otol. 1998 Jul;19(4):447-52.

115. Stokroos RJ, Albers FWJ, Tenvergert EM. Antiviral treatment of idiopathic sudden sensorineural hearing loss: a prospective, randomized, double-blinded clinical trial. Acta Otolaryngol. 1998;118:488-5.

116. Suzuki H, Fujimura T, Ikeda K, Shiomori T, Udaka T, Ohbuchi T, Nagatani G. Prostaglandin E1 in combination with hyperbaric oxygen therapy for idiopathic sudden sensorineural hearing loss. Acta Otolaryngol. 2008 Jan;128(1):61-5.

117. Suzuki H, Fujimura T, Shiomori T, Ohbuchi T, Kitamura T, Hashida K, Udaka T. Prostaglandin E1 versus steroid in combination with hyperbaric oxygen therapy for idiopathic sudden sensorineural hearing loss. Auris Nasus Larynx. 2008 Jun;35(2):192-7.

118. Suzuki H, Mori T, Hashida K, Shibata M, Nguyen KH, Wakasugi T, Hohchi N. Prediction model for hearing outcome in patients with idiopathic sudden sensorineural hearing loss. Eur Arch Otorhinolaryngol. 2011;268(4):497-500.

119. Tabuchi K, Oikawa K, Uemaetomari I, Tsuji S, Wada T, Hara A. Glucocorticoids and dehydroepiandrosterone sulfate ameliorate ischemia-induced injury of the cochlea. Hear Res. 2003 Jun;180(1-2):51-6.

120. Tarshish Y, Leschinski A, Kenna M. Pediatric sudden sensorineural hearing loss: diagnosed causes and response to intervention. Int J Pediatr Otorhinolaryngol. 2010;74:441-6.

121. Teranishi M, Katayma N, Uchida Y, Tominaga M, Nakashima T. Thirty-year trends in sudden deafness from four nationwide epidemiological surveys in Japan. Acta Otolaryngol. 2007;127:1259-65.

122. Topuz E, Yigit O, Cinar U, Seven H. Should hyperbaric oxygen be added to treatment in idiopathic sudden sensorineural hearing loss? Eur Arch Otorhinolaryngol. 2004 Aug;261(7):393-6.

123. Trune DR, Wobig RJ, Kempton JB, Hefeneider SH. Steroid treatment improves cochlear function in the MRL.MpJ-Fas(lpr) autoimmune mouse. Hear Res. 1999 Nov;137(1-2):160-6.

124. Tsai YJ, Liang JG, Wu WB, Ding YF, Chiang RP, Wu SM. Intratympanic injection with dexamethasone for sudden sensorineural hearing loss. J Laryngol Otol. 2011 Feb;125(2):133-7.

125. Tsunoo M, Perlman MB. Temporary arterial obstruction. Effects on periplymph oxygen and microphonics. Acta Otolaryngol. 1969;67:460-6.

126. Tucci DL, Farmer JC, Kitch RD, Witsell DL. Treatment of sudden sensorineural hearing loss with systemic steroids and valacyclovir. Otol Neurotol. 2002;23:301-8.

127. Uri N, Doweck I, Cohen-Kerem R, Greenberg E. Acyclovir in the treatment of idiopathic sudden sensorineural hearing loss. Otolaryngol Head Neck Surg. 2003;128:544-9.

128. Uysal IO, Muderris T, Polat K, Yuce S, Gulturk S. Is the time from the onset to the treatment a prognostic indicator for hearing recovery in idiopathic sudden sensorineural hearing loss? Kulack Burun Bogaz Ihtis Derg. 2015;25(2):70-6.

129. Uzun G, Mutluoglu M, Metin S. The use of hyperbaric oxygen treatment for sudden sensorineural hearing loss in Europe. Diving Hyperb Med. 2016 Mar;46(1):43-6.

130. Wei BP, Mubiru S, O'Leary S. Steroids for idiopathic sudden sensorineural hearing loss. Cochrane Database Syst Rev. 2006 Jan 25;(1):CD003998.

131. Wei BPC, Stathopoulos D, O'Leary S. Steroids for idiopathic sudden sensorineural hearing loss. Cochrane Database Syst Rev. 2013;(7):CD003998.

132. Westerlaken BO, Stokroos RJ, Dhooge IJ, Wit HP, Albers FW. Treatment of idiopathic sudden sensorineural hearing loss with antiviral therapy: a prospective, randomized, double-blind clinical trial. Ann Otol Rhinol Laryngol. 2003;112:993-1000.

133. Wilson WR, Byl FM, Laird N. The efficacy of steroids in the treatment of idiopathic sudden hearing loss. A double-blind clinical study. Arch Otolaryngol. 1980 Dec;106(12):772-6.

134. World Health Organization. The global burden of disease: 2004 update. Geneva, Switzerland: WHO Press; 2008. ISBN: 9789241563710.

135. Xenellis J, Papadimitriou N, Nikolopoulos T, Maragoudakis P, Segas J, Tzagaroulakis A, Ferekidis E. Intratympanic steroid treatment in idiopathic sudden sensorineural hearing loss: a control study. Otolaryngol Head Neck Surg. 2006 Jun;134(6):940-5.

136. Yang CH, Wu RW, Hwang CF. Comparison of intratympanic steroid injection, hyperbaric oxygen and combination therapy in refractory sudden sensorineural hearing loss. Otol Neurotol. 2013;34:1411-6.

137. Yildirim E, Murat Ozcan K, Palah M, Ali Cetin M, Ensari S, Dere H. Prognostic effect of hyperbaric oxygen therapy starting time for sudden sensorineural hearing loss. Eur Arch Otorhinolaryngol. 2015;272:23-8.

138. Yoon TH, Paparella MM, Schachern PA, Alleva M. Histopathology of sudden hearing loss. Laryngoscope. 1990 Jul;100(7):707-15.

139. Zadeh MH, Storper IS, Spitzer JB. Diagnosis and treatment of sudden-onset sensorineural hearing loss: a study of 51 patients. Otolaryngol Head Neck Surg. 2003 Jan;128(1):92-8.

140. Zennaro O, Dauman R, Poisot A, Esteben D, Duclose JY, Bertrand B, Cros AM, Milacic M, Bebear JP. Value of the association of normovolemic dilution and hyperbaric oxygenation in the treatment of sudden deafness. A retrospective study. Ann Otolaryngol Cir Cervicofac. 1993;110(3):162-9.

CHAPTER 15 CHAPTER

Gas Embolism

CHAPTER FIFTEEN OVERVIEW

Introduction 363
Pathophysiology 363
Excessive Alveolar Stretch 363
Latrogenic Causes 364
Decompression-Induced Bubble Formation 364
Other 364
Mechanisms of Injury 364
Clinical Presentation 365
Diagnostic Tests 365
Treatment 366
Supportive First-Aid Treatment 366
Hyperbaric Treatment 366
Adjunctive Therapy 367
Summary 368
Acknowledgment 368
References 369

Gas Embolism

Richard E. Moon

INTRODUCTION

Gas inside blood vessels in small quantities, such as intravenous injection of ultrasonic imaging contrast material or small bubbles in intravenous solutions, is usually benign. However, larger volumes can occlude arteries and damage endothelium, causing clinical illness that can be fatal. Recognition and appropriate, timely treatment can prevent sequelae and death. Venous gas embolism (VGE), which has different causes, is usually differentiated from arterial gas embolism (AGE). VGE is often benign due to filtration by air by the pulmonary vessels; however, the pulmonary capillary network can be overwhelmed by VGE in sufficient quantity and can allow bubbles to be arterialized, resulting in AGE. VGE can also cross into the left side via intracardiac or intrapulmonary shunts.

PATHOPHYSIOLOGY

Several mechanisms that can result in air within blood vessels are described below.

Excessive Alveolar Stretch

The classic example of this is breath holding during ascent from a scuba dive. In this instance the fixed quantity of gas within the lungs expands and eventually stretches the lung parenchyma beyond its elastic limit, causing disruption of alveoli and blood vessels though which gas can enter the circulation.(111) This can also occur without breath holding when there is focal lung pathology such as a bulla or cyst(105) or in the presence of diffuse airways obstruction such as asthma.(167) Interestingly, despite the lack of pulmonary overpressurization and hyperexpansion, AGE has occurred after breath-hold diving, where the diver holds his or her breath during descent and ascent. In these cases, pulmonary injury probably occurs during descent when the intrapulmonary gas is compressed to a volume less than residual volume. The resulting alveolar-capillary injury then provides a passage via which gas can enter the circulation during lung reexpansion upon ascent.(112)

Hyperexpansion of bullae resulting in AGE has occurred during ascent to altitude, including travel in commercial aircraft.(15,33,78,169) Hyperexpansion of the lung can also be self-induced by glossopharyngeal insufflation, sometimes performed to increase lung volume prior to a breath-hold dive.(96) AGE has also been described without any change in barometric pressure due to penetrating chest trauma.(59) AGE has occurred without any positive pressure in the presence of acute inflammatory lung disease such as pneumonia.(20,27) Gas embolism has been triggered by positive pressure ventilation.(6,69,113) Pulmonary barotrauma and AGE can also occur as a result of blast injury.(52,101) An insidious cause of AGE is inadvertent air entry while flushing a radial arterial line, causing stroke due to retrograde flow of bubbles into the ipsilateral vertebral or carotid artery.[28]

Latrogenic Causes

Causes of gas embolism other than diving include accidental intravenous air injection,[1,81] cardiopulmonary bypass accidents,[125] needle biopsy of the lung,[90] hemodialysis,[8] central venous catheter placement or disconnection,[123,155] gastrointestinal endoscopy,[128] hydrogen peroxide irrigation,[9,77,142] arthroscopy,[48,57] cardiopulmonary resuscitation,[70] and percutaneous hepatic puncture.[62] AGE has occurred as a result of atrioesophageal fistula formation as a complication of radiofrequency ablation for atrial fibrillation.[67] Air embolism can occur during procedures in which a surgical site is under pressure (e.g., laparoscopy,[32,34,55,89,115] transurethral surgery,[143,146] vitrectomy,[91] endoscopic vein harvesting,[95] and hysteroscopy[74,135,147]). Massive VGE can occur due to passive entry of air into surgical wounds that are elevated above the level of the heart (such that the pressure in adjacent veins is subatmospheric),[99] thus allowing passive transfer of air into the bloodstream. This has classically been described in sitting craniotomy,[107] where intraosseous venous lakes are particularly susceptible to air entry because they are not collapsible. However, VGE has also occurred due to this mechanism during cesarean section,[50] prostatectomy using the radical perineal[76] and retropubic[3,129] approaches, spine surgery,[87,168] hip replacement,[4] liver resection,[92] liver transplantation,[122] and insertion of dental implants.[22,35]

Decompression-Induced Bubble Formation

Venous gas embolism (VGE) occurs commonly after compressed gas diving.[37,54,140] VGE bubbles after most dives do not usually cause symptoms because they are mostly trapped by the pulmonary vessels and eliminated via the alveoli. However, in large volumes, VGE can cause cough, dyspnea, and pulmonary edema ("chokes"),[46,53,171] and may overwhelm the capacity of the pulmonary capillary network, allowing bubbles to enter the arterial circulation.[23,157] VGE can also enter the left heart directly via shunts within the heart (atrial septal defect, ASD or patient foramen ovale, PFO)[106,131,158,159] or lungs.[68] High volumes of VGE can increase pulmonary artery pressure and hence right atrial pressure, thereby promoting passage of bubbles through an ASD or PFO.

Another cause of VGE is rapid exposure to low ambient pressure.[7] Without preoxygenation, the typical threshold altitude for VGE formation is 15,000–17,000 ft (4,570–5,180 m).[166] Altitude-induced VGE only occurs at rapid rates of decompression, such as during rapid climb in a military jet, during decompression in an altitude chamber, or accidental loss of pressure during commercial aircraft flight.

Other

Ingestion and systemic absorption of hydrogen peroxide results in oxygen bubble formation due to the effect of catalase.[29,66,116,127,136] Massive VGE has been reported after blowing air into the vagina during orogenital sex[13,19,80] and sexual intercourse.[10,43,132]

MECHANISMS OF INJURY

AGE in sufficiently high volumes can occlude vessels, causing infarction. Small bubbles remain in the circulation only for a short time; however, they can initiate a sustained reduction in local blood flow[64-65] due to endothelial injury.[120-121]

Adherence of leukocytes to damaged vessel walls[41,58,63,94] can also mechanically occlude small vessels. Damaged endothelium results in plasma leak, resulting in edema in both lung and brain,[30,171] leading to elevated intracranial pressure and brain hypoxia.[151-153] Capillary leak can be sufficiently severe to cause hemoconcentration[18,139] and even frank hypovolemia.[21,100] Impaired endothelial-dependent vasoactivity has been documented in an animal model,[120] which can predispose to vasoplegia and attenuated responsiveness to vasoactive agents.

CLINICAL PRESENTATION

AGE typically presents with neurological manifestations typical of stroke. Impaired consciousness, confusion, seizures, hemiparesis, posturing, and cardiac arrhythmias are common in severe cases.[12] In mild cases the signs can be subtle, requiring a detailed neurological exam to confirm the diagnosis. AGE in divers with a preexisting inert gas load due to a dive presents differently, with neurological manifestations typical of decompression sickness, such as paraplegia due to spinal cord damage,[119] versus the typical "stroke pattern" usually seen. In such cases, arterial bubbles presumably trigger decompression sickness manifestations in structures such as the spinal cord that are intrinsically predisposed to in situ bubble formation. While neurological manifestations predominate, other organ systems can be involved such as the heart,[25,79,134,137,160] kidney[56,156] and GI tract.[14] Gas can occasionally be observed in the retinal vessels ("boxcars"). Mottling of the tongue characterized by sharply circumscribed areas of glossal pallor (Liebermeister's sign)[149] is rare but said to be pathognomonic of AGE.

VGE may be asymptomatic but with sufficient intravenous gas load, manifestations can include hypotension, tachypnea, hypocapnia, pulmonary edema, and cardiac arrest.[16,44-45,49,51,86,171] AGE manifestations can occur in parallel due to arterialization of venous gas bubbles.

DIAGNOSTIC TESTS

While imaging studies may reveal intravascular air, which confirms the diagnosis, brain imaging is often normal even in the presence of severe neurological abnormalities.[12,26,130,133,164] Of 11 cases of iatrogenic cerebral AGE reported by Benson, only 3 had visible air on brain CT scan.[12] Imaging is therefore not recommended to make the diagnosis.

Findings that support the diagnosis of AGE include evidence of pulmonary barotrauma such as mediastinal emphysema. Air tends to migrate cephalad in the mediastinum and may enter the soft tissues of the vocal folds, causing a change in the tonal quality of the voice. Subcutaneous emphysema may be palpable in the upper chest or neck. Mediastinal crunch (Hamman's sign) may be audible via stethoscope placed over the heart. Other confirmatory manifestations include evidence of intravascular gas using ultrasound or direct observation (e.g., aspiration of gas from a central venous line).

Lab tests are nonspecific. Hematocrit is often elevated due to plasma leak. Elevated serum CPK has been proposed as a specific marker of AGE;[138] however, the level may not rise above normal for several hours after the embolic event.[169] Thus, CPK level may not be sensitive for acute management decisions early after gas embolism.

The diagnosis of gas embolism must therefore be presumptive, based on the observation of an acute (usually neurological) event in the setting of a scuba dive, central venous line disconnection, or other possible cause of air entry into the circulation. Time spent attempting to demonstrate intravascular air radiographically should be discouraged as it usually results in unnecessary delay in obtaining definitive treatment (see below).

TREATMENT

Supportive First-Aid Treatment

General supportive measures should be initiated immediately to maintain ventilation, treat hypoxia, and maintain isocapnia and blood pressure. Large animal studies support the use of maintaining normal blood pressure and PCO_2; hyperventilation in an attempt to reduce intracranial pressure is not helpful.(40,150,152) Intravenous fluids should be administered as needed to treat hypovolemia. Fluids containing glucose can worsen cerebral injury and should not be administered.(145) Aggressive hydration is recommended for decompression sickness; however, it is unnecessary for isolated AGE and due to increase in cerebral and pulmonary edema could be harmful.(145,154) High inspired oxygen concentration facilitates oxygenation of ischemic tissue. Hyperoxia increases the nitrogen gradient between bubble and tissue, thus accelerating bubble resolution.(71-73) Use of first-aid oxygen in divers with decompression illness often completely relieves the manifestations and increases the effectiveness of hyperbaric oxygen therapy.(97) Using the American Heart Association Guidelines for Clinical Efficacy, first-aid oxygen is a class 1, level C recommendation.(145)

Head-down position has been recommended in the past as part of emergency treatment of AGE, on the grounds that it might prevent further embolization due to buoyancy effects and shrinkage of bubbles due to the increase in vascular pressure.(5) Indeed, there are some anecdotes that support its use.(84) Lateral decubitus position has been recommended for VGE on the grounds that it may help retain gas within the right heart. However, studies have shown that buoyancy has little if any effect upon the distribution of either arterial(24) or venous gas,(104) and head-down position can worsen cerebral edema.(38) Therefore, the supine position is recommended.(111,154)

Hyperbaric Treatment

Indications for hyperbaric treatment

Treatment of patients with gas embolism with hyperbaric oxygen is the definitive treatment and is recommended for all cases with neurological, cardiopulmonary, or other associated clinical abnormalities.(111,118,154) Isolated VGE without AGE or clinical manifestations is not an indication for hyperbaric oxygen (HBO_2). It has been suggested that the decision to treat with HBO_2 therapy should be based upon the presence or absence of air on brain imaging.(36) This is not the recommended decision tool as timely administration of HBO_2 usually results in clinical improvement even when there is no visible air.

Reviews of published cases and case series of AGE reveals superior outcomes with the use of HBO_2 compared to non-recompression treatment.(2,16,19,39,44,47,60,75,93,114,117,148,170) Shorter time between embolism and recompression treatment is associated with better outcome. However, contrary to widespread belief, there is no established "magic interval" after which hyperbaric therapy is ineffective. Gas bubbles have been known to persist for several days, and there are many reports of clinical success when HBO_2 treatments were begun after delays of hours to days.[12,16,19,98,102,141,170] On the other hand, some patients spontaneously resolve shortly after symptoms develop, particularly if first-aid oxygen is administered early. However, because secondary deterioration can occur hours later,[124] HBO_2 is recommended even if initial manifestations are no longer present.

Pneumothorax due to coexisting pulmonary barotrauma could develop into tension pneumothorax during chamber decompression. Therefore, if HBO_2 is to be administered using a monoplace chamber, where "hands-on" patient management is not possible, insertion of a tube thoracostomy is recommended before treatment. For multiplace chamber treatment, careful monitoring is a feasible option. Coexisting pneumomediastinum does not generally require specific therapy and will usually resolve during HBO_2.[111]

If possible, an initial compression to 2.82 atmospheres absolute (ARA) (60 fsw or 18 msw equivalent depth) breathing 100% oxygen is recommended, using USN Treatment Table 6 or equivalent.[118] Although deeper recompression is generally felt not to be necessary in the vast majority of AGE cases, if the clinical response during treatment is judged to be suboptimal, options including deeper recompression or extension of the treatment table can be instituted if the expertise and resources are available.[111,154] Shorter treatment tables have been designed for monoplace use,[60-61,82-83] and appear effective in most cases.[17,31]

Standard recommendations include administration of repetitive hyperbaric treatments daily or twice daily until no further stepwise improvement occurs,[111,154] typically after 1–2 treatments, but occasionally up to 5–10.

Adjunctive Therapy

Adjunctive therapies for AGE have been reviewed by the Undersea and Hyperbaric Medical Society,[145] a summary of which is available online at the UHMS website.[144]

Lidocaine

Lidocaine has been demonstrated to be effective in several animal models of AGE[108] and in some human trials of cardiopulmonary bypass[110,161] but not others.[103,109] Evidence for the use of lidocaine for AGE has therefore been classified by the Undersea and Hyperbaric Medical Society as class 2A, level B.[145] If lidocaine is to be used clinically, an appropriate end point is a serum concentration suitable for an antiarrhythmic effect (2–6 milligrams/liter or micrograms/milliliter). Intravenous dosing of 1 mg/kg and then subsequent boluses of 0.5 mg/kg every 10 minutes to a total of 3 mg/kg, while infusing continuously at 2–4 mg/minute, will typically produce therapeutic serum concentrations. In the field, intramuscular dosing of 4–5 mg/kg will typically produce therapeutic plasma concentration 15 minutes after dosing, lasting for around 90 minutes.

Aspirin

There is published evidence in humans from a randomized, multicenter trial that the nonselective NSAID tenoxicam reduces the number of hyperbaric treatments in decompression illness (including both decompression sickness and AGE).[11] However, to date there are no data on the effectiveness of aspirin for AGE (class 2B, level C).[145]

Corticosteroids

Dexamethasone has been studied in canine AGE without evidence of beneficial effect.[42] Corticosteroid administration in high doses can promote hyperglycemia and predispose to infections. Use of corticosteroids in AGE is not recommended (class 3, level C).[145]

Deep vein thrombosis prophylaxis

Patients who are immobilized due to neurological illness are at increased risk for deep vein thrombosis, and death has occurred from pulmonary embolism after decompression illness. Therefore, it is recommended that for patients who are immobilized for 24 hours or greater due to neurological injury, low molecular weight heparin should be administered for prophylaxis against venous thromboembolism (class I, level A).[145]

Avoidance of hyperthermia

Even mild hyperthermia exerts an adverse effect on outcome after several models of neurological injury.[162-163,165] Therefore, it is recommended that in patients with neurological manifestations, fever should be treated aggressively in order to maintain normothermia.

Avoidance of hyperglycemia

Avoidance of glucose-containing IV fluids has been discussed earlier. Administration of even small amounts of glucose, for example 1 liter of intravenous 5% dextrose solution, may worsen neurological outcome, even in the absence of significant hyperglycemia.[88] Hyperglycemia has been shown to worsen several types of brain injury,[85,88,126,162] and thus it is prudent to prevent and treat hyperglycemia.

SUMMARY

Gas embolism occurs in divers and patients undergoing treatment for various disorders. The diagnosis of AGE can be facilitated by maintaining an index of suspicion when there is an otherwise-unexplained neurological event in a setting where there is a plausible mechanism for gas embolism. Administration of high inspired oxygen fraction and general supportive measures should be instituted as soon as possible, followed by referral for hyperbaric oxygen therapy.

ACKNOWLEDGMENT

This chapter includes significant contributions from the author of the previous edition, the late Dr. Eric Kindwall.

REFERENCES

1. Abernathy CM, Dickinson TC. Massive air emboli from intravenous infusion pump: etiology and prevention. Am J Surg. 1979;137:274-5.
2. Ah-See AK. Review of arterial air embolism in submarine escape. In: Smith G, editor. Proceedings of the Sixth International Congress on Hyperbaric Medicine. Aberdeen (Scotland): Aberdeen University Press; 1977. p. 349-51.
3. Albin MS, Ritter RR, Reinhart R, Erickson D, Rockwood A. Venous air embolism during radical retropubic prostatectomy. Anesth Analg. 1992;74:151-3.
4. Andersen KH. Air aspirated from the venous system during total hip replacement. Anaesthesia. 1983;38:1175-8.
5. Atkinson JR. Experimental air embolism. Northwest Med. 1963;62:699-703.
6. Avanzas P, Garcia-Fernandez MA, Quiles J. Echocardiographic detection of systemic air embolism during positive pressure ventilation. Heart. 2003;89:1321.
7. Balldin UI, Pilmanis AA, Webb JT. Central nervous system decompression sickness and venous gas emboli in hypobaric conditions. Aviat Space Environ Med. 2004;75:969-72.
8. Baskin SE, Wozniak RF. Hyperbaric oxygenation in the treatment of hemodialysis-associated air embolism. N Engl J Med. 1975;293:184-5.
9. Bassan MM, Dudai M, Shalev O. Near-fatal systemic oxygen embolism due to wound irrigation with hydrogen peroxide. Postgrad Med J. 1982;58:448-50.
10. Batman PA, Thomlinson J, Moore VC, Sykes R. Death due to air embolism during sexual intercourse in the puerperium. Postgrad Med J. 1998;74:612-3.
11. Bennett M, Mitchell S, Dominguez A. Adjunctive treatment of decompression illness with a non-steroidal anti-inflammatory drug (tenoxicam) reduces compression requirement. Undersea Hyperb Med. 2003;30:195-205.
12. Benson J, Adkinson C, Collier R. Hyperbaric oxygen therapy of iatrogenic cerebral arterial gas embolism. Undersea Hyperb Med. 2003;30:117-26.
13. Bernhardt TL, Goldmann RW, Thombs PA, Kindwall EP. Hyperbaric oxygen treatment of cerebral air embolism from orogenital sex during pregnancy. Crit Care Med. 1988;16:729-30.
14. Bird N. CT finding of VGE in the portal veins and IVC in a diver with abdominal pain: a case report. Undersea Hyperb Med. 2007;34:393-7.
15. Blaise BJ, Massenavette B, Javouhey E, Delafosse B. In-flight air embolism in a child. Ann Am Thorac Soc. 2014;11:681-3.
16. Blanc P, Boussuges A, Henriette K, Sainty JM, Deleflie M. Iatrogenic cerebral air embolism: importance of an early hyperbaric oxygenation. Intensive Care Med. 2002;28:559-63.
17. Bond JG, Moon RE, Morris DL. Initial table treatment of decompression sickness and arterial gas embolism. Aviat Space Environ Med. 1990;61:738-43.
18. Boussuges A, Blanc P, Molenat F, Bergmann E, Sainty JM. Haemoconcentration in neurological decompression illness. Int J Sports Med. 1996;17:351-5.
19. Bray P, Myers RA, Cowley RA. Orogenital sex as a cause of nonfatal air embolism in pregnancy. Obstet Gynecol. 1983;61:653-7.
20. Brown ZA, Clark JM, Jung AL. Systemic gas embolus: a discussion of its pathogenesis in the neonate, with a review of the literature. Am J Dis Child. 1977;131:984-5.
21. Brunner F, Frick P, Bühlmann A. Post-decompression shock due to extravasation of plasma. Lancet. 1964;1:1071-3.

22. Burrowes P, Wallace C, Davies JM, Campbell L. Pulmonary edema as a radiologic manifestation of venous air embolism secondary to dental implant surgery. Chest. 1992;101:561-2.

23. Butler BD, Hills BA. Transpulmonary passage of venous air emboli. J Appl Physiol (1985). 1985;59:543-7.

24. Butler BD, Laine GA, Leiman BC, Warters D, Kurusz M, Sutton T, Katz J. Effects of Trendelenburg position on the distribution of arterial air emboli in dogs. Ann Thorac Surg. 1988;45:198-202.

25. Cales RH, Humphreys N, Pilmanis AA, Heilig RW. Cardiac arrest from gas embolism in scuba diving. Ann Emerg Med. 1981;10:589-92.

26. Catron PW, Dutka AJ, Biondi DM, Flynn ET, Hallenbeck JM. Cerebral air embolism treated by pressure and hyperbaric oxygen. Neurology. 1991;41:314-5.

27. Ceponis PJ, Fox W, Tailor TD, Hurwitz LM, Amrhein TJ, Moon RE. Non-dysbaric arterial gas embolism associated with chronic necrotizing pneumonia, bullae and coughing: a case report. Undersea Hyperb Med. Forthcoming 2017.

28. Chang C, Dughi J, Shitabata P, Johnson G, Coel M, McNamara JJ. Air embolism and the radial arterial line. Crit Care Med. 1988;16:141-3.

29. Christensen DW, Faught WE, Black RE, Woodward GA, Timmons OD. Fatal oxygen embolization after hydrogen peroxide ingestion. Crit Care Med. 1992;20:543-4.

30. Chryssanthou C, Springer M, Lipschitz S. Blood-brain and blood-lung barrier alteration by dysbaric exposure. Undersea Biomed Res. 1977;4:117-29.

31. Cianci P, Slade JB Jr. Delayed treatment of decompression sickness with short, no-air-break tables: review of 140 cases. Aviat Space Environ Med. 2006;77:1003-8.

32. Clark CC, Weeks DB, Gusdon JP. Venous carbon dioxide embolism during laparoscopy. Anesth Analg. 1977;56:650-2.

33. Closon M, Vivier E, Breynaert C, Duperret S, Branche P, Coulon A, De La Roche E, Delafosse B. Air embolism during an aircraft flight in a passenger with a pulmonary cyst: a favorable outcome with hyperbaric therapy. Anesthesiology. 2004;101:539-42.

34. Cottin V, Delafosse B, Viale JP. Gas embolism during laparoscopy: a report of seven cases in patients with previous abdominal surgical history. Surg Endosc. 1996;10:166-9.

35. Davies JM, Campbell LA. Fatal air embolism during dental implant surgery: a report of three cases. Can J Anaesth. 1990;37:112-21.

36. Dexter F, Hindman BJ. Recommendations for hyperbaric oxygen therapy of cerebral air embolism based on a mathematical model of bubble absorption. Anesth Analg. 1997;84:1203-7.

37. Dunford RG, Vann RD, Gerth WA, Pieper CF, Huggins K, Wachholz C, Bennett PB. The incidence of venous gas emboli in recreational diving. Undersea Hyperb Med. 2002;29:247-59.

38. Dutka AJ. Therapy for dysbaric central nervous system ischemia: adjuncts to recompression. In: Bennett PB, Moon RE, editors. Diving accident management. Bethesda (MD): Undersea and Hyperbaric Medical Society; 1990. p. 222-34.

39. Dutka AJ. Air or gas embolism. In: Camporesi EM, Barker AC, editors. Hyperbaric oxygen therapy: a critical review. Bethesda (MD): Undersea and Hyperbaric Medical Society; 1991. p. 1-10.

40. Dutka AJ, Hallenbeck JM, Kochanek P. A brief episode of severe arterial hypertension induces delayed deterioration of brain function and worsens blood flow after transient multifocal cerebral ischemia. Stroke. 1987;18:386-95.

41. Dutka AJ, Kochanek PM, Hallenbeck JM. Influence of granulocytopenia on canine cerebral ischemia induced by air embolism. Stroke. 1989;20:390-5.

42. Dutka AJ, Mink RB, Pearson RR, Hallenbeck JM. Effects of treatment with dexamethasone on recovery from experimental cerebral arterial gas embolism. Undersea Biomed Res. 1992;19:131-41.

43. Eckert WG, Katchis S, Dotson P. The unusual accidental death of a pregnant woman by sexual foreplay. Am J Forensic Med Pathol. 1991;12:247-9.

44. Elliott DH, Harrison JAB, Barnard EEP. Clinical and radiological features of 88 cases of decompression barotrauma. In: Shilling CW, Beckett MW, editors. Underwater physiology VI proceedings of the Sixth Symposium on Underwater Physiology. Bethesda (MD): FASEB; 1978. p. 527-35.

45. Elliott DH, Moon RE. Manifestations of the decompression disorders. In: Bennett PB, Elliott DH, editors. The physiology and medicine of diving. Philadelphia: WB Saunders; 1993. p. 481-505.

46. Ence TJ, Gong H Jr. Adult respiratory distress syndrome after venous air embolism. Am Rev Respir Dis. 1979;119:1033-7.

47. Ericsson JA, Gottlieb JD, Sweet RB. Closed-chest cardiac massage in the treatment of venous air embolism. N Engl J Med. 1964;270:1353-4.

48. Faure EAM, Cook RI, Miles D. Air embolism during anesthesia for shoulder arthroscopy. Anesthesiology. 1998;89:805-6.

49. Fitchet A, Fitzpatrick AP. Central venous air embolism causing pulmonary oedema mimicking left ventricular failure. BMJ. 1998;316:604-6.

50. Fong J, Gadalla F, Gimbel AA. Precordial Doppler diagnosis of haemodynamically compromising air embolism during caesarean section. Can J Anaesth. 1990;37:262-4.

51. Francis TJR, Mitchell SJ. Manifestations of decompression disorders. In: Brubakk AO, Neuman TS, editors. Bennett & Elliott's physiology and medicine of diving. New York: Elsevier Science; 2003. p. 578-99.

52. Freund U, Kopolovic J, Durst AL. Compressed air emboli of the aorta and renal artery in blast injury. Injury. 1980;12:37-8.

53. Frim DM, Wollman L, Evans AB, Ojemann RG. Acute pulmonary edema after low-level air embolism during craniotomy. Case report. J Neurosurg. 1996;85:937-40.

54. Gardette B. Correlation between decompression sickness and circulating bubbles in 232 divers. Undersea Biomed Res. 1979;6:99-107.

55. Gillart T, Bazin JE, Bonnard M, Schoeffler P. Pulmonary interstitial edema after probable carbon dioxide embolism during laparoscopy. Surg Laparosc Endosc. 1995;5:327-9.

56. Gleeson PJ, Kelly Y, Ni Sheaghdha E, Lappin D. A SCUBA diver with acute kidney injury. BMJ Case Rep. 2015;2015.

57. Habegger R, Siebenmann R, Kieser C. Lethal air embolism during arthroscopy. A case report. J Bone Joint Surg Br. 1989;71:314-6.

58. Hallenbeck JM, Dutka AJ, Tanishima T, Kochanek PM, Kumaroo KK, Thompson CB, Obrenovitch TP, Contreras TJ. Polymorphonuclear leukocyte accumulation in brain regions with low blood flow during the early postischemic period. Stroke. 1986;17:246-53.

59. Halpern P, Greenstein A, Melamed Y, Taitelman U, Sznajder I, Zveibil F. Arterial air embolism after penetrating lung injury. Crit Care Med. 1983;11:392-3.

60. Hart GB. Treatment of decompression illness and air embolism with hyperbaric oxygen. Aerosp Med. 1974;45:1190-3.

61. Hart GB, Strauss MB, Lennon PA. The treatment of decompression sickness and air embolism in a monoplace chamber. J Hyperb Med. 1986;1:1-7.
62. Helmberger TK, Roth U, Empen K. Massive air embolism during interventional laser therapy of the liver: successful resuscitation without chest compression. Cardiovasc Intervent Radiol. 2002;25:335-6.
63. Helps SC, Gorman DF. Air embolism of the brain in rabbits pre-treated with mechlorethamine. Stroke. 1991;22:351-4.
64. Helps SC, Meyer-Witting M, Rilley PL, Gorman DF. Increasing doses of intracarotid air and cerebral blood flow in rabbits. Stroke. 1990;21:1340-5.
65. Helps SC, Parsons DW, Reilly PL, Gorman DF. The effect of gas emboli on rabbit cerebral blood flow. Stroke. 1990;21:94-9.
66. Hendriksen SM, Menth NL, Westgard BC, Cole JB, Walter JW, Masters TC, Logue CJ. Hyperbaric oxygen therapy for the prevention of arterial gas embolism in food grade hydrogen peroxide ingestion. Am J Emerg Med. 2016.
67. Hirji SA, Haney JC, Welsby I, Lombard FW, Berry MF. Hyperbaric oxygen therapy for treatment of neurologic sequela after atrioesophageal fistula. Ann Thorac Surg. 2015;99:681-2.
68. Hsu YL, Wang HC, Yang PC. Desbaric air embolism during diving: an unusual complication of Osler-Weber-Rendu disease. Br J Sports Med. 2004;38:E6.
69. Hung SC, Hsu HC, Chang SC. Cerebral air embolism complicating bilevel positive airway pressure therapy. Eur Respir J. 1998;12:235-7.
70. Hwang SL, Lieu AS, Lin CL, Liu GC, Howng SL, Kuo TH. Massive cerebral air embolism after cardiopulmonary resuscitation. J Clin Neurosci. 2005;12:468-9.
71. Hyldegaard O, Madsen J. Influence of heliox, oxygen, and N_2O-O_2 breathing on N_2 bubbles in adipose tissue. Undersea Biomed Res. 1989;16:185-93.
72. Hyldegaard O, Madsen J. Effect of air, heliox, and oxygen breathing on air bubbles in aqueous tissues in the rat. Undersea Hyperb Med. 1994;21:413-24.
73. Hyldegaard O, Moller M, Madsen J. Effect of He-O_2, O_2, and N_2O-O_2 breathing on injected bubbles in spinal white matter. Undersea Biomed Res. 1991;18: 361-71.
74. Imasogie N, Crago R, Leyland NA, Chung F. Probable gas embolism during operative hysteroscopy caused by products of combustion. Can J Anaesth. 2002;49:1044-7.
75. Ingvar DH, Adolfson J, Lindemark C. Cerebral air embolism during training of submarine personnel in free escape: an electroencephalographic study. Aerosp Med. 1973;44:628-35.
76. Jolliffe MP, Lyew MA, Berger IH, Grimaldi T. Venous air embolism during radical perineal prostatectomy. J Clin Anesth. 1996;8:659-61.
77. Jones PM, Segal SH, Gelb AW. Venous oxygen embolism produced by injection of hydrogen peroxide into an enterocutaneous fistula. Anesth Analg. 2004;99:1861-3, table of contents.
78. Jung S, Wiest R, Frigerio S, Mattle HP, Hess CW. Cerebral air embolism caused by a bronchogenic cyst. Pract Neurol. 2010;10:164-6.
79. Kanter AS, Stewart BF, Costello JA, Hampson NB. Myocardial infarction during scuba diving: a case report and review. Am Heart J. 1995;130:1292-4.
80. Kaufman BS, Kaminsky SJ, Rackow EC, Weil MH. Adult respiratory distress syndrome following orogenital sex during pregnancy. Crit Care Med. 1987;15: 703-4.

81. Khan M, Schmidt DH, Bajwa T, Shalev Y. Coronary air embolism: incidence, severity, and suggested approaches to treatment. Cathet Cardiovasc Diagn. 1995;36:313-8.

82. Kindwall EP. Use of short *versus* long tables in the treatment of decompression sickness and arterial gas embolism. In: Moon RE, Sheffield PJ, editors. Treatment of decompression illness. Kensington (MD): Undersea and Hyperbaric Medical Society; 1996. p. 122-6.

83. Kindwall EP, Goldman RW, Thombs PA. Use of the monoplace *versus* multiplace chamber in the treatment of diving diseases. J Hyperb Med. 1988;3:5-10.

84. Krivonyak GS, Warren SG. Cerebral arterial air embolism treated by a vertical head-down maneuver. Catheter Cardiovasc Interv. 2000;49:185-7.

85. Lam AM, Winn HR, Cullen BF, Sundling N. Hyperglycemia and neurological outcome in patients with head injury. J Neurosurg. 1991;75:545-51.

86. Lam KK, Hutchinson RC, Gin T. Severe pulmonary oedema after venous air embolism. Can J Anaesth. 1993;40:964-7.

87. Lang SA, Duncan PG, Dupuis PR. Fatal air embolism in an adolescent with Duchenne muscular dystrophy during Harrington instrumentation. Anesth Analg. 1989;69:132-4.

88. Lanier WL, Stangland KJ, Scheithauer BW, Milde JH, Michenfelder JD. The effects of dextrose infusion and head position on neurologic outcome after complete cerebral ischemia in primates: examination of a model. Anesthesiology. 1987;66:39-48.

89. Lantz PE, Smith JD. Fatal carbon dioxide embolism complicating attempted laparoscopic cholecystectomy--case report and literature review. J Forensic Sci. 1994;39:1468-80.

90. Lattin G Jr, O'Brien W Sr, McCrary B, Kearney P, Gover D. Massive systemic air embolism treated with hyperbaric oxygen therapy following CT-guided transthoracic needle biopsy of a pulmonary nodule. J Vasc Interv Radiol. 2006;17:1355-8.

91. Ledowski T, Kiese F, Jeglin S, Scholz J. Possible air embolism during eye surgery. Anesth Analg. 2005;100:1651-2.

92. Lee SY, Choi BI, Kim JS, Park KS. Paradoxical air embolism during hepatic resection. Br J Anaesth. 2002;88:136-8.

93. Leitch DR, Green RD. Pulmonary barotrauma in divers and the treatment of cerebral arterial gas embolism. Aviat Space Environ Med. 1986;57:931-8.

94. Levin LL, Stewart GJ, Lynch PR, Bove AA. Blood and blood vessel wall changes induced by decompression sickness in dogs. J Appl Physiol (1985). 1981;50: 944-9.

95. Lin SM, Chang WK, Tsao CM, Ou CH, Chan KH, Tsai SK. Carbon dioxide embolism diagnosed by transesophageal echocardiography during endoscopic vein harvesting for coronary artery bypass grafting. Anesth Analg. 2003;96:683-5, table of contents.

96. Liner MH, Andersson JP. Suspected arterial gas embolism after glossopharyngeal insufflation in a breath-hold diver. Aviat Space Environ Med. 2010;81:74-6.

97. Longphre JM, Denoble PJ, Moon RE, Vann RD, Freiberger JJ. First aid normobaric oxygen for the treatment of recreational diving injuries. Undersea Hyperb Med. 2007;34:43-9.

98. Mader JT, Hulet WH. Delayed hyperbaric treatment of cerebral air embolism: report of a case. Arch Neurol. 1979;36:504-5.

99. Majendie F. Sur l'entree accidentelle de l'air dans les veins. J Physiol Exp (Paris). 1821;1:190. French.

100. Malette WG, Fitzgerald JB, Cockett AT. Dysbarism. A review of thirty-five cases with suggestion for therapy. Aerosp Med. 1962;33:1132-9.

101. Mason WH, Damon TG, Dickinson AR, Nevison TO Jr. Arterial gas emboli after blast injury. Proc Soc Exp Biol Med. 1971;136:1253-5.

102. Massey EW, Moon RE, Shelton D, Camporesi EM. Hyperbaric oxygen therapy of iatrogenic air embolism. J Hyperb Med. 1990;5:15-21.

103. Mathew JP, Mackensen GB, Phillips-Bute B, Grocott HP, Glower DD, Laskowitz DT, Blumenthal JA, Newman MF. Randomized, double-blinded, placebo controlled study of neuroprotection with lidocaine in cardiac surgery. Stroke. 2009;40:880-7.

104. Mehlhorn U, Burke EJ, Butler BD, Davis KL, Katz J, Melamed E, Morris WP, Allen SJ. Body position does not affect the hemodynamic response to venous air embolism in dogs. Anesth Analg. 1994;79:734-9.

105. Mellem H, Emhjellen S, Horgen O. Pulmonary barotrauma and arterial gas embolism caused by an emphysematous bulla in a SCUBA diver. Aviat Space Environ Med. 1990;61:559-62.

106. Messina AG, Leslie J, Gold J, Topkins MJ, Devereux RB. Passage of microbubbles associated with intravenous infusion into the systemic circulation in cyanotic congenital heart disease: documentation by transesophageal echocardiography. Am J Cardiol. 1987;59:1013-4.

107. Michenfelder JD, Martin JT, Altenburg BM, Rehder K. Air embolism during neurosurgery. An evaluation of right-atrial catheters for diagnosis and treatment. JAMA. 1969;208:1353-8.

108. Mitchell SJ. Lidocaine in the treatment of decompression illness: a review of the literature. Undersea Hyperb Med. 2001;28:165-74.

109. Mitchell SJ, Merry AF, Frampton C, Davies E, Grieve D, Mills BP, Webster CS, Milsom FP, Willcox TW, Gorman DF. Cerebral protection by lidocaine during cardiac operations: a follow-up study. Ann Thorac Surg. 2009;87:820-5.

110. Mitchell SJ, Pellett O, Gorman DF. Cerebral protection by lidocaine during cardiac operations. Ann Thorac Surg. 1999;67:1117-24.

111. Moon RE. Hyperbaric oxygen treatment for air or gas embolism. Undersea Hyperb Med. 2014;41:159-66.

112. Moon RE, Gray LL. Breath-hold diving and cerebral decompression illness. Undersea Hyperb Med. 2010;37:1-5.

113. Morris WP, Butler BD, Tonnesen AS, Allen SJ. Continuous venous air embolism in patients receiving positive end-expiratory pressure. Am Rev Respir Dis. 1993;147:1034-7.

114. Moses HL. Casualties in individual submarine escape 1928-1957. Groton (CT): U.S. Naval Submarine Medical Center; 1964.

115. Moskop RJ Jr, Lubarsky DA. Carbon dioxide embolism during laparoscopic cholecystectomy. South Med J. 1994;87:414-5.

116. Mullins ME, Beltran JT. Acute cerebral gas embolism from hydrogen peroxide ingestion successfully treated with hyperbaric oxygen. J Toxicol Clin Toxicol. 1998;36:253-6.

117. Murphy BP, Harford FJ, Cramer FS. Cerebral air embolism resulting from invasive medical procedures. Treatment with hyperbaric oxygen. Ann Surg. 1985;201: 242-5.

118. Navy Department (U.S.). U.S. Navy Diving Manual. Revision 6. Vol 5 : diving medicine and recompression chamber operations. Washington (DC): Naval Sea Systems Command; 2008. NAVSEA 0910-LP-106-0957.

119. Neuman TS, Bove AA. Combined arterial gas embolism and decompression sickness following no-stop dives. Undersea Biomed Res. 1990;17:429-36.

120. Nossum V, Hjelde A, Brubakk AO. Small amounts of venous gas embolism cause delayed impairment of endothelial function and increase polymorphonuclear neutrophil infiltration. Eur J Appl Physiol. 2002;86:209-14.

121. Nossum V, Koteng S, Brubakk AO. Endothelial damage by bubbles in the pulmonary artery of the pig. Undersea Hyperb Med. 1999;26:1-8.

122. Olmedilla L, Garutti I, Perez-Pena J, Sanz J, Teigell E, Avellanal M. Fatal paradoxical air embolism during liver transplantation. Br J Anaesth. 2000;84: 112-4.

123. Ordway CB. Air embolus via CVP catheter without positive pressure: presentation of case and review. Ann Surg. 1974;179:479-81.

124. Pearson RR, Goad RF. Delayed cerebral edema complicating cerebral arterial gas embolism: case histories. Undersea Biomed Res. 1982;9:283-96.

125. Peirce EC 2nd. Specific therapy for arterial air embolism. Ann Thorac Surg. 1980;29:300-3.

126. Pulsinelli WA, Levy DE, Sigsbee B, Scherer P, Plum F. Increased damage after ischemic stroke in patients with hyperglycemia with or without established diabetes mellitus. Am J Med. 1983;74:540-4.

127. Rackoff WR, Merton DF. Gas embolism after ingestion of hydrogen peroxide. Pediatrics. 1990;85:593-4.

128. Raju GS, Bendixen BH, Khan J, Summers RW. Cerebrovascular accident during endoscopy - consider cerebral air embolism, a rapidly reversible event with hyperbaric oxygen therapy. Gastrointest Endosc. 1998;47:70-3.

129. Razvi HA, Chin JL, Bhandari R. Fatal air embolism during radical retropubic prostatectomy. J Urol. 1994;151:433-4.

130. Reuter M, Tetzlaff K, Hutzelmann A, Fritsch G, Steffens JC, Bettinghausen E, Heller M. MR imaging of the central nervous system in diving-related decompression illness. Acta Radiol. 1997;38:940-4.

131. Ries S, Knauth M, Kern R, Klingmann C, Daffertshofer M, Sartor K, Hennerici M. Arterial gas embolism after decompression: correlation with right-to-left shunting. Neurology. 1999;52:401-4.

132. Sadler DW, Pounder DJ. Fatal air embolism occurring during consensual intercourse in a non-pregnant female. J Clin Forensic Med. 1998;5:77-9.

133. Sayama T, Mitani M, Inamura T, Yagi H, Fukui M. Normal diffusion-weighted imaging in cerebral air embolism complicating angiography. Neuroradiology. 2000;42:192-4.

134. Schneeweis C, Fleck E, Gebker R. Myocardial infarction after scuba diving. Eur Heart J. 2012;33:2224.

135. Sherlock S, Shearer WA, Buist M, Rasiah R, Edwards A. Carbon dioxide embolism following diagnostic hysteroscopy. Anaesth Intensive Care. 1998;26:674-6.

136. Smedley BL, Gault A, Gawthrope IC. Cerebral arterial gas embolism after pre-flight ingestion of hydrogen peroxide. Diving Hyperb Med. 2016;46:117-9.

137. Smerz RW. Concomitant cerebral and coronary arterial gas emboli in a sport diver: a case report. Hawaii Med J. 2005;64:12-3.

138. Smith RM, Neuman TS. Elevation of serum creatine kinase in divers with arterial gas embolization. N Engl J Med. 1994;330:19-24.

139. Smith RM, Van Hoesen KB, Neuman TS. Arterial gas embolism and hemoconcentration. J Emerg Med. 1994;12:147-53.

140. Spencer MP. Decompression limits for compressed air determined by ultrasonically detected bubbles. J Appl Physiol (1985). 1976;40:229-35.

141. Takita H, Olszewski W, Schimert G, Lanphier EH. Hyperbaric treatment of cerebral air embolism as a result of open-heart surgery. Report of a case. J Thorac Cardiovasc Surg. 1968;55:682-5.

142. Tsai SK, Lee TY, Mok MS. Gas embolism produced by hydrogen peroxide irrigation of an anal fistula during anesthesia. Anesthesiology. 1985;63:316-7.

143. Tsou MY, Teng YH, Chow LH, Ho CM, Tsai SK. Fatal gas embolism during transurethral incision of the bladder neck under spinal anesthesia. Anesth Analg. 2003;97:1833-4.

144. Undersea & Hyperbaric Medical Society. Adjunctive therapy for decompression illness (DCI): summary of Undersea & Hyperbaric Medical Society guidelines [Internet]. [place unknown]: Undersea & Hyperbaric Medical Society; 2002 [cited 2017 Jan 16]. Available from: https://www.uhms.org/images/Position-Statements/adjunctive_committee_summary.pdf

145. Undersea & Hyperbaric Medical Society. UHMS guidelines for adjunctive therapy of DCI. In: Moon RE, editor. Adjunctive therapy for decompression illness. Kensington (MD): Undersea & Hyperbaric Medical Society; 2003. p. 184-9.

146. Vacanti CA, Lodhia KL. Fatal massive air embolism during transurethral resection of the prostate. Anesthesiology. 1991;74:186-7.

147. Van Dijck C, Rex S, Verguts J, Timmerman D, Van de Velde M, Teunkens A. Venous air embolism during hysteroscopic myomectomy: an analysis of 7 cases. Gynecol Obstet Invest. 2017.

148. Van Genderen L. Study of air embolism and extra-aveolar accidents associated with submarine escape training. Groton (CT): U.S. Naval Submarine Medical Center; 1967.

149. Van Hoesen KB, Lang MA. Diving medicine. In: Auerbach PS, editor. Auerbach's wilderness medicine. 7th ed. Philadelphia: Elsevier; 2017. p. 1583-618.

150. van Hulst RA, Haitsma JJ, Lameris TW, Klein J, Lachmann B. Hyperventilation impairs brain function in acute cerebral air embolism in pigs. Intensive Care Med. 2004;30:944-50.

151. van Hulst RA, Hasan D, Lachmann B. Intracranial pressure, brain PCO2, PO2, and pH during hypo- and hyperventilation at constant mean airway pressure in pigs. Intensive Care Med. 2002;28:68-73.

152. van Hulst RA, Klein J, Lachmann B. Gas embolism: pathophysiology and treatment. Clin Physiol Funct Imaging. 2003;23:237-46.

153. van Hulst RA, Lameris TW, Hasan D, Klein J, Lachmann B. Effects of cerebral air embolism on brain metabolism in pigs. Acta Neurol Scand. 2003;108:118-24.

154. Vann RD, Butler FK, Mitchell SJ, Moon RE. Decompression illness. Lancet. 2011;377:153-64.

155. Vesely TM. Air embolism during insertion of central venous catheters. J Vasc Interv Radiol. 2001;12:1291-5.

156. Viecelli A, Jamboti J, Waring A, Banham N, Ferrari P. Acute kidney injury due to decompression illness. Clin Kidney J. 2014;7:380-2.

157. Vik A, Brubakk AO, Hennessy TR, Jenssen BM, Ekker M, Slordahl SA. Venous air embolism in swine: transport of gas bubbles through the pulmonary circulation. J Appl Physiol (1985). 1990;69:237-44.

158. Vik A, Jenssen BM, Brubakk AO. Paradoxical air embolism in pigs with a patent foramen ovale. Undersea Biomed Res. 1992;19:361-74.

159. Vik A, Jenssen BM, Brubakk AO. Arterial gas bubbles after decompression in pigs with patent foramen ovale. Undersea Hyperb Med. 1993;20:121-31.

160. Villela A, Weaver LK, Ritesh D. Coronary gas embolism during a dive: a case report. Undersea Hyperb Med. 2015;42:613-7.

161. Wang D, Wu X, Li J, Xiao F, Liu X, Meng M. The effect of lidocaine on early postoperative cognitive dysfunction after coronary artery bypass surgery. Anesth Analg. 2002;95:1134-41.

162. Warner DS. Current concepts in neuroprotection. In: Moon RE, editor. Adjunctive therapy for decompression illness. Kensington (MD): Undersea and Hyperbaric Medical Society; 2003.

163. Warner DS, McFarlane C, Todd MM, Ludwig P, McAllister AM. Sevoflurane and halothane reduce focal ischemic brain damage in the rat. Possible influence on thermoregulation. Anesthesiology. 1993;79:985-92.

164. Warren LP, Djang WT, Moon RE, Camporesi EM, Sallee DS, Anthony DC. Neuroimaging of scuba diving injuries to the CNS. AJNR Am J Neuroradiol. 1988;9:933-8.

165. Wass CT, Lanier WL, Hofer RE, Scheithauer BW, Andrews AG. Temperature changes of > or = 1 degree C alter functional neurologic outcome and histopathology in a canine model of complete cerebral ischemia. Anesthesiology. 1995;83:325-35.

166. Webb JT, Pilmanis AA, O'Connor RB. An abrupt zero-preoxygenation altitude threshold for decompression sickness symptoms. Aviat Space Environ Med. 1998;69:335-40.

167. Weiss LD, Van Meter KW. Cerebral air embolism in asthmatic scuba divers in a swimming pool. Chest. 1995;107:1653-4.

168. Wills J, Schwend RM, Paterson A, Albin MS. Intraoperative visible bubbling of air may be the first sign of venous air embolism during posterior surgery for scoliosis. Spine. 2005;30:E629-35.

169. Zaugg M, Kaplan V, Widmer U, Baumann PC, Russi EW. Fatal air embolism in an airplane passenger with a giant intrapulmonary bronchogenic cyst. Am J Respir Crit Care Med. 1998;157:1686-9.

170. Ziser A, Adir Y, Lavon H, Shupak A. Hyperbaric oxygen therapy for massive arterial air embolism during cardiac operations. J Thorac Cardiovasc Surg. 1999;117:818-21.

171. Zwirewich CV, Müller NL, Abboud RT, Lepawsky M. Noncardiogenic pulmonary edema caused by decompression sickness: rapid resolution following hyperbaric therapy. Radiology. 1987;163:81-2.

CHAPTER 16 CHAPTER

Effects of Hyperbaric Oxygen in Infectious Diseases: Basic Mechanisms

CHAPTER SIXTEEN OVERVIEW

Introduction 381

Oxygen Tension in Tissues during Infection 381

General Mechanisms of Action of Oxygen in Infections 382

Oxygen Tensions Alter Pharmacokinetics 383

Oxygen Tensions Alter Pharmacodynamics 384

Effects of Hypoxia and Anaerobiosis on Conventional Antibacterial Agents 384

Interactions between Hyperoxia and HBO_2 with Conventional Antibacterial Agents 385

Effects of Oxygen on the Activity of Antiparasitic Agents 385

Effects of Oxygen on the Activity of Antifungal Agents 385

Bacteriostatic and Bactericidal Effects of Hyperbaric Oxygen 385

Susceptibility of Anaerobic and Aerobic Bacteria to HBO_2 385

Mechanisms of Bacteriostatic Effects of HBO_2 386

Mechanisms of Bactericidal Effects of HBO_2 386

Role of Superoxide and Hydrogen Peroxide in Bacterial Killing by Hyperoxia and Hyperbaric Oxygen 388

Genetic Mechanisms of Bacterial Resistance to Oxygen 388

Effects of Hyperbaric Oxygen in Experimental Bacterial Infections 388

Effects of Hyperbaric Oxygen in Parasitic Infections 389

Susceptibility of Protozoa to Oxygen 389

Susceptibility of Helminths to Oxygen 390

Effects of Hyperbaric Oxygen in Fungal Infections 390

Mechanisms of Antifungal Effects of Oxygen 390

Influence of Oxygen Tensions in Viral Infections 391

Oxygen Tensions and Acute and Chronic Inflammatory Cells 392

Influence of Oxygen on Phagocytosis and Killing of Microorganisms by Polymorphonuclear Neutrophils (PMNs) 392

Influence of Oxygen on Lymphocyte Function 393
Dosing Interval, Duration, and Timing 393
Conclusion 395
Acknowledgments 395
References 396

Effects of Hyperbaric Oxygen in Infectious Diseases: Basic Mechanisms

Rodney E. Willoughby Jr., Charles C. Falzon, Aliyah Keval, Harry T. Whelan

INTRODUCTION

Oxygen Tension in Tissues during Infection

Normoxia (15%–21% O_2) is defined in this review as the fractional inspired oxygen (FiO_2) concentration necessary to maintain aerobic metabolism and homeostasis in the body. Oxygen tensions outside this normal range will be defined as follows: anaerobiosis (less than 0.01% FiO_2), hypoxia (12% FiO_2 or less), hyperoxia (45%–100% FiO_2), and hyperbaric oxygen (any O_2 tension greater than 1 atmosphere absolute pressure [ATA] or 760 mmHg).

Different partial pressures of oxygen (pO_2) are normally found in various body compartments. The pO_2s under normoxia range from approximately 100 mmHg within pulmonary alveoli to 15 mmHg in the liver parenchymal cells. Within individual cells, pO_2s are heterogeneous by organelle and are much lower than extracellular pO_2s. For example, pO_2s in mitochondria are less than 1 mmHg.[165] Tissue oxygen tensions are controlled by the concentration of inspired oxygen, cardiac output, local blood flow, cellular metabolism, and substrate availability. Hemoglobin in erythrocytes is essential for carrying oxygen and also binds the gasotransmitters, nitric oxide (NO), carbon monoxide (CO), and hydrogen sulfide (H_2S) with varying affinities. During hyperbaric oxygen (HBO_2) therapy, hemoglobin is fully saturated, and additional oxygen dissolved in serum is delivered, proportional to fractional inspired oxygen and total absolute pressure. HBO_2 causes vasoconstriction and hypocarbia, so the mass of oxygen delivered to tissues is reduced. HBO_2 also delivers oxygen topically to exposed wounds.[145] Once delivered by the vasculature, oxygen is freely diffusible in tissues, demonstrating a spatial gradient from the vasculature.[145] Tissue-derived gasotransmitters (NO, CO, H_2S) bind to cytochrome c oxidase to down-modulate mitochondrial respiration, controlling diffusion of oxygen through proximal tissues and distally. A relatively sharp spatial gradient also exists in potential anatomic spaces where effusions may form, as well as in microbiome compartments "external" to the body such as the gingival crevice, urethra, vagina, and intestinal tract.

The composition of microbial colonizers (bacteria, fungi, protozoa, and metazoa), or microbiome, orients to this extracorporeal oxygen gradient.[2,144] In the colon, strictly anaerobic, sulfur-reducing bacteria predominate, and the redox potential is strongly reducing (negative) except for the area immediately adjacent to the mucosa.

With disease, oxygen delivery is compromised. Abscesses and infarcted tissues show steep oxygen gradients into avascular spaces or tissues where pO_2s may reach 0 mmHg.[56] The inflammatory response following infection is characterized by capillary leak and vasogenic edema that increases the diffusion distance between the vascular supply of dissolved and bound oxygen and adjacent tissues. Tissue edema also leads to variable degrees of tamponade and venous thrombosis, further compromising perfusion and oxygen delivery. Infection leads to microcirculatory shunting (reducing oxygen extraction) and mitochondrial failure.[66,155] Both NO and H_2S are elaborated by pyogenic bacteria as antioxidants to counter the effects of antimicrobials we administer, further inhibiting nearby mitochondrial respiration and the phagocytic oxidative burst.[51,141]

General Mechanisms of Action of Oxygen in Infections

Increasing oxygen concentrations in infected tissues is generally beneficial during infection, compensating for reduced vascular perfusion, shunting, and increased oxygen diffusion distances. Hyperoxia and HBO_2 also raise oxygen tensions in hypoxic tissues to levels necessary for the killing of bacteria by neutrophils and monocytes.[94] While phagocytosis remains unaffected by low oxygen tensions, killing of microorganisms by the oxidative burst is dependent on oxygen tensions.[54,71,156] In an animal model of osteomyelitis, HBO_2 was as effective as cephalothin therapy.[95] The benefit of HBO_2 in osteomyelitis was postulated to result from decreased edema and restoration of the oxidative burst following improved oxygen tensions.[94]

The effects of hyperoxia and HBO_2 on invasive microbes and the microbiome are mixed, and not always beneficial to the host. Hyperoxia and the use of HBO_2 kill strictly anaerobic pathogens. While this provides benefit during treatment of anaerobic infections, HBO_2 also adversely reduces the colonizing anaerobic symbionts that comprise roughly 90% of the human microbiome.[2,144] It is therefore remarkable that HBO_2-associated diarrhea has not been reported to the same extent as antibiotic-associated diarrhea. In contrast to the effect on anaerobes, hyperoxia and the use of HBO_2 at pressures of 1.5 ATA or less promotes the growth of aerobic bacteria in vitro.[117,123] These effects may be particularly detrimental for lung infections (see below). At higher ATA doses used clinically, HBO_2 is usually bacteriostatic (inhibiting growth without killing aerobic bacteria). The biphasic activity of oxygen against aerobes raises therapeutic concerns for mixed infections when the pO_2 being delivered to the site of infection is uncertain (as it invariably is).[124]

A special situation is the intracellular pathogen, where oxygen tensions are quite low (1 mmHg). Some antimicrobials (cotrimoxazole, rifampicins, macrolides, quinolones) are concentrated intracellularly and can be used to target these organisms. The very low pO_2 intracellularly limits the activity of some intracellular antibacterials (see below).[124]

A second special situation is bacterial biofilm. Bacterial gene expression and metabolic activity in biofilms differ from planktonic (freely living) bacteria, which affects the efficacy of many antibacterials.[38,55] While biofilms are of theoretical concern, it needs to be emphasized that our empirically derived experience over decades of treating infections with antibacterials has long since compensated for biofilms – long before such biofilms were of research interest. Intracellular infections and biofilm-containing infections have generally required prolonged courses of antibacterials. The potential for certain unusual antibacterials – including hyperbaric oxygen – to alter bacterial biofilms and perhaps accelerate the therapeutic response is promising and under investigation.[144]

Ultimately, most infections are treated by a combination of antimicrobial, immunomodulatory, and surgical therapies. Surgical drainage obviates avascular spaces, reestablishing diffusion of oxygen (and HBO_2) from perfused vessels into tissues. Drainage of pus also removes covalently bound H_2S pools that release sulfide under acidic conditions found in abscesses to maintain a toxic, anaerobic environment.[142,162]

As an antimicrobial drug, oxygen has the particular advantage of being freely diffusible across tissue planes. HBO_2 can potentiate the effect of some more traditional antimicrobials. HBO_2 is also immune modulatory and, in contrast to most immunomodulatory drugs, tissue regenerative.

Hyperbaric oxygen indirectly improves patient outcomes after infections by influencing functional recovery, notably repair and regeneration responses in infected necrotic tissues. For example, hypoxia (12% O_2 at 1 ATA) retards healing of skin wounds and thus probably favors bacterial invasion.[80] Hyperbaric oxygen (100% O_2 at 2 ATA, for 2 hours, twice daily) does not affect the healing of vascularized, full-thickness skin wounds, but HBO_2 does enhance wound closure in ischemic wounds.[79]

HBO_2 as a drug has a narrow therapeutic index, particularly in infancy, and is difficult to administer.[145] Oxygen has a markedly short half-life but prolonged antimicrobial effects.[144] In practice, oxygen as an antimicrobial drug is reserved for medically complex or severe infections.

Hyperoxia cannot be used for surgical prophylaxis.[145] The incidence of infection was significantly higher in the group receiving 80% O_2 than the group receiving 35% O_2 (25.0% versus 11.3%; $P = .02$).[127]

OXYGEN TENSIONS ALTER PHARMACOKINETICS

Oxygenation affects both pharmacokinetics (drug delivery and elimination) and pharmacodynamics (antibacterial and postantibacterial effects). Hyperoxia decreases in blood flow in tissues at 100% FiO_2 at 1 ATA.[63] Hyperbaric oxygen (100% FiO_2, between 2–5 ATA) decreases blood flow to liver and splanchnic tissues, muscle, brain, spinal cord, and bone.[94,107] Blood flow to the kidney may increase.[140] The 10% negative inotropic effects on myocardium may also play a role in these changes. As far as can be judged from a model of antibiotic-controlled sepsis, the presence of sepsis, per se, does not cause further hemodynamic change during exposure to HBO_2.[107]

There are relatively few studies of the changes in kinetics of antimicrobials during HBO_2. The effects of decreased antibacterial delivery to underperfused tissues during hyperoxia and HBO_2 do not appear to be clinically recognized so are likely compensated by other effects of hyperoxia. There was no change in renal elimination of aminoglycosides during HBO_2.[100] There was no difference in hepatic elimination of lidocaine, pentobarbital, or xanthines.[132] Wound concentration of linezolid was increased by HBO_2.[83] A hypothesis is that decreased fractional delivery of antibacterials to tissues during hyperoxia or HBO_2 may be offset by increased tissue perfusion from the reduction in tamponade in the tissue as blood volume falls. This mechanism can be especially beneficial for intracranial infections, osteomyelitis, and compartment syndromes. HBO_2 does not affect the function of the blood-brain barrier.[73,135]

OXYGEN TENSIONS ALTER PHARMACODYNAMICS

There are many classes of antibacterials with different mechanisms of action, including cell wall active agents, antimetabolites, DNA-, RNA-, and protein-synthesis inhibitors, and redox cycling agents. The mechanisms of action determine in part whether antibacterials are bacteriostatic (inhibiting growth but not killing the bacterium) or bactericidal (killing the bacterium).

All bactericidal antimicrobials may share a final common pathway resulting in lethal oxidative damage to the bacterial DNA through the Fenton reaction.[40,82,161] A final common pathway for bactericidal antimicrobials may be of high clinical importance because, experimentally, bactericidal drugs were rendered bacteriostatic under anaerobic conditions. Consistent with this hypothesis, bacteria engineered to produce copious volumes of NO or H_2S as antioxidants showed resistance to multiple antimicrobial classes.[51,141] (Anthrax was potentially weaponized by this approach.) The claim that oxidative damage is shared by all bactericidal antibacterials has not been replicated by other groups, and the matter remains unsettled.[75,88]

Effects of Hypoxia and Anaerobiosis on Conventional Antibacterial Agents

Minimal inhibitory concentrations (MIC) and minimal bactericidal concentrations (MBC) assays have been used to study the interactions between oxygen and antimicrobial agents in vitro. MBCs are no longer reported by clinical microbiological laboratories, but the choice between bactericidal and bacteriostatic agents remains important for certain diseases (endocarditis, osteomyelitis) and patient populations (oncologic neutropenia, chronic granulomatous disease). Anaerobiosis did not affect antibacterials targeting cell wall synthesis such as penicillins, cephalosporins, and carbapenems.[53,151] The effect of hypoxia on vancomycin and aztreonam is unsettled.[38,78,114,159] Hypoxia had no effect on rifampin.[114]

The MBC of fluoroquinolones against *E. coli* and *P. aeruginosa* increased (worsened) under anaerobic conditions, but the MIC was unchanged.[78,96] There was no effect on MIC or MBC of quinolones against *S. aureus* under anaerobic conditions.[167-168] The MBC of folate antimetabolites, sulfamethoxazole and trimethoprim, against *S. aureus* markedly worsened (increased) under anaerobic and hypoxic conditions.[53,163] Time-kill curves for *Chlamydia trachomatis* by azithromycin and tetracycline worsened.[143] The MBC effect may be related to the final common pathway of oxidative damage via the Fenton reaction.

In anaerobic environments, the MICs of the aminoglycoside antibiotics were significantly worse (higher) against *Pseudomonas*, *E. coli*, *Enterobacter*, *Klebsiella*, *Salmonella*, *Serratia*, *Staphylococcus*, and *Streptococcus* spp.[38,124] Hypoxia decreases the transport of aminoglycosides into bacteria. One way to circumvent the redox-dependent transport of aminoglycosides is to disrupt the bacterial cell wall. Cefotaxime, targeting the bacterial cell wall, enhanced tobramycin and amikacin uptake in *E. coli* under anaerobic conditions, resulting in enhanced bactericidal activity.[18] The lack of transport intracellularly of aminoglycosides under anaerobiosis may also explain why aminoglycosides are contraindicated for treatment of the intracellular pathogen *Salmonella* particularly during sickle cell crisis and osteomyelitis.

In contrast, the bactericidal activity of metronidazole is optimal under anaerobic conditions and is reduced or almost absent in aerobic conditions.[153] Oxygen-dependent changes in redox potential affect the activation of this antimicrobial and explain the loss of activity in aerobic conditions. It is not necessarily rational to use metronidazole during HBO_2 therapy, although metronidazole has shown additive effect with HBO_2 in animal models.[1,105]

Interactions between Hyperoxia and HBO_2 with Conventional Antibacterial Agents

The effects of hyperoxia and HBO_2 in potentiating antibacterials is generally modest.[124] HBO_2 may normalize the activity of oxygen-dependent antimicrobials by raising the pO_2 of ischemic tissue to normoxia. In addition, HBO_2 may potentiate the activity of certain antimicrobials by inhibiting biosynthetic reactions in bacteria, notably folic acid metabolism.[49,121]

Effects of Oxygen on the Activity of Antiparasitic Agents

Free-radical mechanisms account for parasite killing by many antiparasitic drugs such as antimalarials, quinones, and nitro compounds.[28] By contrast, normoxia reduces the uptake of metronidazole by *Trichomonas vaginalis*, *Trichomonas foetus*, and *Entamaoeba invadens*.[49,108]

Effects of Oxygen on the Activity of Antifungal Agents

Hypoxia protected *C. albicans* protoplasts from amphotericin B–induced lysis.[146] In contrast, the effect of hyperoxia and HBO_2 on the activity of amphotericin B against *Candida* is modest.[50]

BACTERIOSTATIC AND BACTERICIDAL EFFECTS OF HYPERBARIC OXYGEN

Susceptibility of Anaerobic and Aerobic Bacteria to HBO_2

Pathogenic bacteria are classified in terms of the partial pressure of oxygen in which they grow. By definition, anaerobic bacteria cannot survive in normal oxygen tensions. As such, they are susceptible to HBO_2. Bacterial spores are more aerotolerant. For example, hyperbaric oxygen (3 ATA for 18 hours) is completely bactericidal for *Clostridium perfringens* in vitro.[57] Hyperbaric oxygen (100% O_2 at 2 ATA) blocks the germination of *C. perfringens* spores in vitro but is not bactericidal for the spores.[25]

Facultative anaerobic bacteria, which include most cultured human pathogens, are able to grow in normoxia and hyperoxia by increasing the synthesis of antioxidant enzymes.[20] Hyperbaric oxygen is bactericidal for aerobic and facultative anaerobic bacteria but only at pressures and/or durations which are greater than can be used clinically. Caution is advised, because the growth of some aerobic bacteria is biphasic – enhanced by normobaric hyperoxia but inhibited by HBO_2. For example, oxygen tensions up to 1 ATA enhance the growth of *Escherichia coli*, whereas oxygen tensions greater than 2 ATA inhibit growth in vitro.[117] Hyperoxia (100% O_2 at 1 ATA) enhances the growth of P. *aeruginosa* in vitro.[122] A 1-hour intermittent exposure to HBO_2 (100% O_2 at 2 ATA, every 8 hours) has no effect on the growth of *P. aeruginosa* or *S. aureus*.[16]

Mechanisms of Bacteriostatic Effects of HBO_2

Inhibition of Amino Acid and Protein Biosynthesis

Exposure of *E. coli* to HBO_2 (100% O_2 at greater than 3 ATA) causes a rapid inhibition of growth and respiration.[17] Superoxide inactivates bacterial dihydroxyacid dehydratase, which catalyzes the formation of alpha-ketoisovalerate, an intermediate in the formation of valine and leucine. Hyperbaric oxygen (100% O_2, 4.2 ATA) decreases the specific activity of dihydroxyacid dehydratase by destroying the Fe-S cluster of this enzyme; however, this enzyme remains in a form that can be reactivated.[39] The inhibition of amino acid biosynthesis by HBO_2 eventually leads to increased levels of uncharged tRNA, which is responsible for inducing the stringency response by bacteria and cessation of bacterial growth.[139]

The inhibition by HBO_2 of protein synthesis in bacteria may also be caused by a free-radical-induced block in the transport of substrates used in RNA transcription. Hyperoxia or oxygen free radicals oxidize sulfhydryl-containing proteins involved in the transport of lactose, guanosine, and methylglucopyranoside into *E. coli.*[35]

Decreased Levels of Key Cofactors of Metabolic Reactions

HBO_2 inhibits bacterial growth by decreasing the levels of thiamine and both the reduced and oxidized forms of nicotinamide adenine dinucleotide (NAD, NADH). Quinolinate synthetase is the oxygen-sensitive enzyme controlling de novo NAD biosynthesis.[43]

HBO_2 inhibits folate metabolism, potentiating the effects of folic acid antagonists such as trimethoprim-sulfamethoxazole.[49,121]

Decreased Synthesis and Increased Degradation of DNA and RNA

Production of the superoxide anion and hydrogen peroxide in vitro and in vivo has been linked to mutations in bacteria.[26,65,87,133,158] Cells containing high levels of SOD or catalase are more resistant to toxicity and mutagenicity than cells containing normal levels of these enzymes.[154,158] HBO_2 is mutagenic in *E. coli.*[44]

Mechanisms of Bactericidal Effects of HBO_2

Bacterial Defense Mechanisms against Free Radicals

For protection against the free radicals generated during normal aerobic metabolism, prokaryotic and eukaryotic cells have developed antioxidant defense mechanisms. Three main antioxidant enzymes are known. Superoxide dismutase (SOD) is an extremely efficient O_2-scavenger. Catalase is a hydrogen peroxide scavenger. Glutathione peroxidase (GSH peroxidase) catalyzes the reduction of hydrogen peroxide to water and dioxygen and is capable of converting toxic lipid peroxides into nontoxic products.

Superoxide anions may undergo spontaneous dismutation to form hydrogen peroxide. The rate of reaction is enhanced markedly by the presence of SOD. Dismutation of two superoxide radicals results in the formation of one hydrogen peroxide molecule. Catalase subsequently converts hydrogen peroxide to water and oxygen. Studies with SOD- and catalase-deficient mutants of *E. coli* confirm that SOD is more important than catalase in protecting against the growth inhibition caused by hyperoxia.[137] The role of catalase is probably more important during hyperoxia than in normoxia. In the presence of trace amounts of transition metals, particularly iron, hydrogen peroxide may participate in the Fenton reaction to produce the highly reactive hydroxyl radical. The hydroxyl radical damages DNA and leads to lipid peroxidation of membranes.

Free radicals may also be inactivated by reacting with low-molecular-weight substances located in the cellular membranes or in the cytosol. Tocopherol (vitamin E) is an antioxidant located in membranes. Ascorbate, beta-carotene, and sulfhydryl-containing compounds such as cysteine, cysteamine, and glutathione are water-soluble antioxidant compounds. Under normal metabolic conditions, these free-radical scavengers neutralize oxygen free radicals before they can cause cellular injury. In addition, there are enzyme systems to repair proteins with methionine sulfoxide adducts that affect both bacterial adhesion and intracellular survival.[(131;134,166)] However, if host defense mechanisms are overwhelmed, damage to eukaryotic as well as prokaryotic cells will occur.[(70)]

Cellular Utilization of Oxygen and Generation of Oxygen-Based Free Radicals

Oxygen normally undergoes a four-electron reduction to water that is catalyzed by mitochondrial oxidases. This reaction accounts for the greatest proportion of oxygen consumption in the cell. During normal aerobic metabolism, partially reduced oxygen species are also generated within cells. These highly reactive species of oxygen are known as free radicals. The levels of oxygen free radicals and other reactive oxygen molecules formed within cells increase during exposure to hyperoxia.[(67)] These molecules are toxic to cells because they react with and damage cellular proteins, membrane lipids, and DNA.[(67)]

Increased oxygen tensions cause an increase in the conversion of molecular oxygen (O_2) to the free radical superoxide anion (O_2-). Superoxide anion can be converted to another toxic oxygen species, namely hydrogen peroxide (H_2O_2); H_2O_2 in the presence of iron can react with O_2- to form another toxic molecule, the hydroxyl radical (·OH).[(130)]

Cellular Sources of Free Radicals

The production of toxic oxygen species can occur in various cellular compartments (including the cytosol) by enzymatic and nonenzymatic reactions. Flavoproteins and cuproproteins generate H_2O_2, while several types of flavin-containing oxidoreductases can generate O_2-.[(68)]

A cellular source of superoxide of particular relevance in infectious diseases is the NADPH oxidase located in the plasma membrane of polymorphonuclear leukocytes and macrophages. This enzyme converts oxygen to O_2-.[(8)] Phagocytic stimuli induce production of O_2- by NADPH oxidase. The majority of oxygen free radicals produced are directed into the phagosome where they participate in bacterial killing. If the activated NADPH oxidase remains on the external surface of the cell, oxygen products are shed into the surrounding tissues. Soluble substances, such as immune complexes and chemotactic factors, stimulate superoxide anion release from human neutrophils.[(164)] There are multiple pathways of activation of the NADPH oxidase.[(12)] Chemotactic factors, arachidonic acid, and cell-surface binding lectins activate NADPH oxidase by different pathways and with additive effects.

From a quantitative standpoint, an important cellular source of superoxide is the nonenzymatic oxidation of cytochrome intermediates of the electron transport chain in mitochondria. Superoxide is also generated by the cytochrome-P-450 substrate-oxygen complexes in the endoplasmic reticulum. Another cellular organelle producing toxic oxygen species is the peroxisome. Here H_2O_2 production occurs by oxidation of substrates such as long-chain fatty acids. In all these cellular organelles, the generation of toxic oxygen species is dependent on tissue oxygen tensions.[160] Xanthine oxidase is a major source of O_2- in ischemic and hypoxic tissues that undergo re-oxygenation by blood reflow.[98] In summary, the presence of an adequate amount of molecular oxygen is necessary for oxygen-dependent killing by PMNs and macrophages to occur. A variety of enzymatic and nonenzymatic cellular reactions also normally result in the production of O_2- and H_2O_2. The production of these molecules is enhanced by increasing tissue-oxygen tensions. Free radicals are highly reactive and, if not removed by scavengers, may cause extensive cellular injury.

Role of Superoxide and Hydrogen Peroxide in Bacterial Killing by Hyperoxia and Hyperbaric Oxygen

The superoxide anion radical is particularly important in bacterial killing. Several in vitro studies have shown that the absence of the enzyme responsible for the detoxification of superoxide SOD increases the susceptibility of many anaerobic and facultative anaerobic bacteria to oxygen.[99] On the other hand, by raising bacterial levels of SOD, the susceptibility of the bacteria to oxygen can be diminished in vitro.[27]

Bacteria such as *N. gonorrhoeae* are particularly susceptible to a different toxic-oxygen species, namely hydrogen peroxide. In these bacteria, resistance to oxygen-induced killing is associated with high levels of catalase, the enzyme responsible for detoxification of hydrogen peroxide. Additional antioxidant defenses, such as peroxidase and high levels of glutathione, also contribute to survival of these bacteria in aerobic conditions.[5]

Microorganisms with adequate antioxidant defenses are resistant to toxic actions of superoxide and may use the production of reactive oxygen species to injure host cells. For example, virulent strains of *Listeria monocytogenes* exhibit maximal production of hydrogen peroxide and superoxide. Virulence is correlated with survival of *L. monocytogenes* in macrophage monolayers.[46]

The presence of a capsule appears to protect bacteria against oxygen-induced damage. In the case of *Streptococcus pyogenes*, the presence of a hyaluronic acid capsule increases resistance to the bacteriostatic effects of oxygen.[22]

Genetic Mechanisms of Bacterial Resistance to Oxygen

Bacterial resistance to hyperoxia is inducible. Hyperoxia and superoxide induce the synthesis of 30 proteins; approximately 20 of these proteins are regulated by the soxRS, oxyR, and RpoS regulons.[70]

Effects of Hyperbaric Oxygen in Experimental Bacterial Infections

The mortality of infected rats with *Clostridium perfringens* gas gangrene receiving HBO_2 and surgical debridement (12.5%) was significantly less than rats treated with surgery (37.5%) or untreated controls (100%). More strikingly, 82.5% of animals in the HBO_2 and surgery group healed their wounds and ambulated, compared to only 12.5% of animals treated with surgery alone.[59] Two studies demonstrated the lack of enhanced survival when HBO_2 was used alone.[105,147]

In a polymicrobial rat model of gas gangrene involving *C. perfringens*, *B. fragilis*, *E. coli*, and *E. faecalis*, HBO_2 did not significantly enhance survival. However, 84% of the survivors in the HBO_2 and surgery group recovered completely, compared to 15% of the survivors in the surgery-alone group ($p < 0.001$).[60] It is important, therefore, to differentiate effects of HBO_2 on microbiology from wound repair.

In a murine model of *S. pyogenes* myositis, HBO_2 was not beneficial in decreasing mortality or bacterial growth.(169)

The effects of HBO_2 have also been studied in two models of polymicrobial sepsis induced by implanting pooled fecal material contained in gelatin capsules into the peritoneal cavity of rats. Treatment with HBO_2 alone (100% O_2 at 2 ATA for 1.5 hours, every 6 hours) reduced mortality to 8% from the 100% mortality seen in animals maintained in normoxia.(157) Hyperoxia (100% O_2 at 1 ATA) had no effect on mortality.(157) However, a more recent study showed that HBO_2 (100% O_2 at 2.7 ATA) did not significantly decrease mortality in septic rats with a single large, undrained intra-abdominal abscess containing *E. coli* and/or *B. fragilis.*(106) Drainage is fundamental to any successful treatment strategy.

Lung infections behave differently and may be a relative contraindication to HBO_2 therapy. Low inspired oxygen tensions appear to be beneficial in some pneumonias caused by aerobic bacteria. Continuous exposure to 12% O_2 prolonged the survival of mice infected with *D. (Streptococcus) pneumoniae.* On the other hand, continuous hyperoxic exposure (75% O_2 at 1 ATA) shortened survival of infected mice without inducing pulmonary toxicity.(4) Exposure to hyperoxia during the evolution of *Legionella* or *Pseudomonas* pneumonia resulted in a marked increase in lethality in mice in an oxygen concentration and exposure time-dependent manner.(76,111) *Mycoplasma pneumoniae* and other *Mycoplasma* spp. lack SOD and catalase and yet do not appear to be susceptible to hyperoxia.(92) Hyperoxia (80% O_2) increases the percentage of lung cultures positive for *Ureaplasma urealyticum* and mortality in newborn mice.(24) These findings are all in agreement with the increased incidence and more severe course of pneumonias in patients treated for respiratory failure with continuous high FiO_2 (more on this below).

In a rabbit model of bacterial osteomyelitis, HBO_2 (100% O_2 at 2 ATA) is as effective as the antibiotic cephalothin in the treatment of *S. aureus.*(95) In addition, treatment with HBO_2 (100% O_2 at 2.5 ATA for 1.6 hours twice daily) and tobramycin for *P. aeruginosa* osteomyelitis is superior to either tobramycin alone or HBO_2 alone.(93) HBO_2 enhances antibacterial activity in infected bone by restoring oxygen tensions to levels necessary for aminoglycoside activity and oxygen-dependent killing by phagocytes.(94)

Hyperoxia (77% O_2) prevented mortality in mice infected with the intracellular pathogen *C. trachomatis*, while a 65% mortality occurs in the infected, normoxia-exposed group.(47)

EFFECTS OF HYPERBARIC OXYGEN IN PARASITIC INFECTIONS

Susceptibility of Protozoa to Oxygen

Many protist parasites (amoeba, diplomonads, trichomonads, trypanosomatids) are microaerophilic rather than strict anaerobes.(15) The susceptibility of parasites to oxidative stress varies depending upon the stage in the parasite life cycle. Different stages in parasite life cycles are also associated with shifts in levels of antioxidant enzymes.(6,101,115)

Plasmodium falciparum has very low levels of endogenous superoxide dismutase, and its growth in vitro is optimal at 3% O_2 – near intracellular concentrations – whereas growth is slightly reduced (by 15%) at 20% O_2.(21,136) *Plasmodium* converts to anaerobic metabolism within red blood cells, possibly to avoid the interaction of reactive oxygen species with ubiquitous hemoglobin.(116)

Entamoeba histolytica is tolerant to 5% O_2 (venous O_2 pressure).[10] Growth of *Trichomonas vaginalis* is more rapid at 1 uM O_2 than anaerobically.[91]

HBO_2 improved outcome of experimental cerebral malaria.[14] HBO_2 therapy appears effective in a *Leishmania amazonensis* model infection. HBO_2 enhances the effect of amphotericin B in *L braziliensis* infection and imidazoles in *L infantum*. HBO_2 is ineffective in an animal model of *L major* infection.[6,90,101,104]

Susceptibility of Helminths to Oxygen

As is the case for protozoans, the susceptibility of metazoans such as *Schistosoma mansoni*, *Ascaris suum*, *Fasciola hepatica*, and *Trichinella spiralis* to oxygen appears to be dependent upon the levels of antioxidant enzymes present in specific developmental stages.[19,72,103,112] The viability of *Schistosoma* eggs depends on tissue oxygen tensions.[36] *Paragonimus westermani* carries both aerobic and anaerobic mitochondria.[152] *Onchocerca volvulus* is best grown anaerobically.[149]

EFFECTS OF HYPERBARIC OXYGEN IN FUNGAL INFECTIONS

Mechanisms of Antifungal Effects of Oxygen

Oxygen-based free radicals are thought to be responsible for the fungistatic and fungicidal effects of hyperbaric oxygen because mutants lacking antioxidant enzymes are more susceptible to killing by HBO_2. On the other hand, induction of antioxidant defenses may protect fungi from subsequent exposure to hyperoxia.[41,119] Hyperoxia inhibits the growth of some Mucorales fungi. The effects of pressure and oxygen are additive in inhibiting the growth of *Rhizopus oryzae* in vitro.[28,37] An additive antifungal effect of HBO_2 (100% O_2 at 2.5 ATA, 1.5 hours) and amphotericin B has been found in vitro against *C. albicans*.[50] *Pneumocystis jirovecii* has low levels of antioxidant enzymes and is very susceptible to hyperoxia. A 10-minute exposure to 70% O_2 in vitro appears to be lethal for this microorganism.[125] It is notable that this infection presents as relatively pure hypoxemia without ventilatory failure.

Clinical Studies

Studies with animal models of fungal infections are needed to further evaluate the antifungal effects of HBO_2. Two clinical reports have found hyperbaric oxygen to be a useful adjunctive therapy in mucormycosis infections. Price and Stevens [126] used HBO_2 (100% O_2 at 2 ATA, twice daily for two days, then once daily, for 18 days) and amphotericin B to treat a patient with fulminant mucormycosis. The patient eventually died of unrelated causes; lack of fungal growth was documented at autopsy. Couch et al.[23] used HBO_2 to successfully treat a patient diagnosed with rhinocerebral mucormycosis. HBO_2 (100% O_2 at 2.5 ATA for 90 minutes, 6 days a week) was used as an adjunctive treatment to surgical debridement and amphotericin B and ketoconazole.

Ferguson et al.[37] performed a retrospective study of 13 patients with rhinocerebral mucormycosis. All patients were treated with amphotericin B and underwent surgical debridement; six of these patients received HBO_2 treatments (2 ATA O_2 for 2 hours, 2–11 times at 12-hour intervals, then 3–20 times at 24-hour intervals). Two out of six patients receiving HBO_2 therapy died of non-fungus-related causes. In contrast, four out of seven patients not receiving HBO_2 therapy died as a result of the mucormycosis infection.[37]

A more recent randomized controlled trial in a murine model analyzing the efficacy of HBO_2 as an adjunct for treating zygomycosis showed that the addition of hyperbaric oxygen (2.0 ATA) to amphotericin B did not improve survival over that achieved with amphotericin B and placebo air treatments.[11] Another group examined the effects of transient hyperoxia in CD4+ depleted mice with *Pneumocystis pneumonia* where the mice were initially maintained in normoxia, then exposed to a hyperoxic treatment regimen.[120] Despite no difference in organism burden between the two groups, CD4+ depleted mice with *Pneumocystis pneumonia* demonstrated significant mortality after transient exposure to hyperoxia while all uninfected control mice survived the stress.[120]

In summary, hyperbaric oxygen within clinically achievable ranges is either fungistatic or fungicidal for *Pneumocystis carinii* and *Rhizopus oryzae*. In the case of *P. carinii*, as little as a 10-minute exposure to hyperoxia appears to be lethal. However, hyperoxia should not be substituted for current antimicrobial therapy in the treatment of patients infected with *P. carinii*. The mechanism of fungal killing by HBO_2 appears to be caused by oxidative stress, which inhibits protein synthesis and decreases transport of amino acids across fungal membranes.

INFLUENCE OF OXYGEN TENSIONS IN VIRAL INFECTIONS

Presently there is no evidence of direct beneficial effects of HBO_2 in viral infections. However, it appears that oxygen tensions affect the growth and virulence of certain viruses. Hypoxia (3% O_2) causes marked alterations in growth characteristics of some viruses. Plaque diameter and plating efficiency of adenoviruses cultured under hypoxic conditions are markedly reduced.[29] In contrast, polioviruses are not adversely affected by hypoxic conditions.[29] Replication of rubella virus in hamster kidney cells was not altered during exposure to oxygen tensions ranging from 1 to 330 mmHg.[77]

Reactive oxygen species cause single-strand breaks in DNA.[64] Viral DNA may be particularly susceptible to oxidative damage because viruses lack antioxidants and DNA repair mechanisms. Exogenous SOD and catalase combine to confer protection against inactivation of viruses.[34] Therefore, it is possible that antioxidants in the host cells may protect viruses against free radicals. Thus, exogenous antioxidants may account, at least in part, for the viral resistance to hyperoxia.

Effects of various oxygen tensions in murine models of viral infections have been examined. In a model of encephalomyocarditis caused by the MM virus, hypobaric hypoxia (21% O_2 at 0.5 ATA) significantly increased mortality as compared to normoxia.[49] Exposure to hypobaric normoxia (100% O_2 at 0.2 ATA) also increased mortality in mice infected with influenza A virus.[48] However, neither normobaric hypoxia (11% O_2 at 1 ATA) nor hyperoxia (77% O_2 at 1 ATA) altered mortality. Thus, it appears that decreased atmospheric pressure, rather than oxygen tension, influenced mortality due to influenza A virus in that study. In contrast, Ayers et al.[7] found that exposure to hyperoxia (99% O_2 at 1 ATA) resulted in influenza-infected mice dying 3 to 4 days earlier than normoxic controls. One possible explanation is the finding by Naldini et al.[110] that the antiviral activity of interferon-alpha (and interferon-gamma) is decreased in vitro under "normoxic" conditions (140 mmHg O_2) compared to "hypoxic" conditions (14 mmHg O_2). Exposure to hypoxia (11% O_2) increased mortality and viral titers in tissue of mice infected with Coxsackie B-1 virus.[45] Interestingly, hypobaric hypoxia (21% O_2 at 0.5 ATA) increased viral titers, but not mortality.[45] In addition, HBO_2 (100% O_2 at 3 ATA) enhanced mortality in mice infected with Coxsackie B-1 virus.[118] Pretreatment of mice with HBO_2 significantly increased viral titers in heart muscle and brown fat by three days after inoculation of the virus.[118] The effects of HBO_2 may have been mediated through free radicals since, in another model of Coxsackie B3 myocarditis, polyethylene-conjugated SOD reduced cellular infiltration, myocardial necrosis, and calcification scores, compared to the control group at day 14, after intraperitoneal challenge in C3H/He mice.[58] There were no differences in viral titers among the three groups at day 7 and viral titers were no longer detected by day 14 in any of the treatment groups.[58]

Another recent study investigated the basis of treating chronic hepatitis with HBO_2 and to compare the changes in hepatic function, immunity, pathologic morphology, ultrastructure and HBV in hepatic tissues before and after treatment. The experimental group was treated with six courses of HBO_2 while the control group was treated for 60 days with standard therapy.[89] There were significant differences between the experimental and control groups after treatment; for the experimental group, all markers of hepatic function and hepatocyte degeneration or necrosis were decreased, but the fibrosis and fat-storing cells in the liver were not reduced.[89]

In summary, oxygen tensions appear to influence the outcome of viral infections in animal models. Hyperoxia appears to increase mortality in mice infected with influenza A virus or Cocksackie B-1 virus. Hypoxic conditions also increase mortality in Coxsackie B-1 infected mice. Treatment of chronic HBV with HBO_2 appears to be effective, and should be considered as an adjunct to standard pharmacologic therapy. HBO_2 has not been shown to be effective at reversing liver fibrosis.

OXYGEN TENSIONS AND ACUTE AND CHRONIC INFLAMMATORY CELLS

Influence of Oxygen on Phagocytosis and Killing of Microorganisms by Polymorphonuclear Neutrophils (PMNs)

Physiologic functions (e.g., phagocytosis) of PMNs are sustained in hypoxic or near-anaerobic environments of infected tissues by anaerobic glycolysis.[31] In contrast, anaerobiosis (< 1% O_2) inhibits the killing of *Staphylococcus aureus*, *Escherichia coli*, *Serratia marcescens*, *Klebsiella pneumoniae*, *Proteus vulgaris*, and *Salmonella typhimurium* by PMNs.[97]

Studies in vivo have confirmed that hyperoxia and HBO_2 can increase phagocytic killing of bacteria by raising tissue oxygen tensions. Optimal killing of *S. aureus* in subcutaneous lesions occurs when rabbits breathe 45% O_2.[62] Hyperbaric oxygen (100% O_2 at 2 ATA) increases the killing of *S. aureus* by PMNs in osteomyelitis by increasing the pO_2 in infected bone from 21 mmHg to 104 mmHg.[94]

Dosing interval and duration of hyperoxia and HBO_2 are important. Continuous prolonged exposure to high FiO_2, such as is required for severe respiratory failure, can inhibit PMN function within days.[24,30,69,129] Prolonged in vitro exposure (greater than 24 hours) of macrophages to hyperoxia or HBO_2 reduces bacterial clearance by inhibiting phagocytosis, oxidant-mediated killing, cell locomotion, and DNA synthesis.[113,128,150] An in vivo study in mice showed that hyperoxia leads to greatly reduced alveolar epithelial cell GM-CSF expression, a growth factor that is critically involved in the maintenance of normal alveolar macrophage function in mice that are infected with *K. pneumoniae*. Systemic treatment of these mice with recombinant murine GM-CSF during hyperoxia exposure preserved alveolar macrophage function.[9]

Influence of Oxygen on Lymphocyte Function

Resting T-lymphocytes are highly resistant to injury by either hypoxia or hyperoxia.[3] However, mitogen-stimulated lymphocytes are markedly affected by tissue oxygen tensions. DNA synthesis by phytohemagglutinin-stimulated human lymphocytes is reduced or completely inhibited by exposure to hypoxia (3%–9% O_2). Hyperoxia (70%–100% O_2 for longer than 48 hours) also inhibits DNA synthesis in stimulated lymphocytes.[3,87] The growth inhibition is slowly reversible when T-lymphocytes are returned to normoxia.[87] In lymphocytes exposed to hyperoxia, RNA synthesis is inhibited even before DNA synthesis.[61] The growth of unstimulated B-lymphocytes is also completely inhibited by hyperoxia.[102]

Hyperoxia also inhibits the proliferation of T-lymphocytes in vivo. T-lymphocytes from mice exposed daily to 100% O_2 for 8 days (2.4 ATA for 1.5 hours) show a 50% decrease in lymphocyte proliferation.[42] Proliferation returns to normal in the presence of either an antioxidant (2-mercaptoethanol) or macrophages. This suggests that hyperoxia may also inactivate critical macrophage functions necessary for the restoration of lymphocyte proliferation (see reconstitution by GM-CSF above).

The effect of HBO_2 (100% O_2 at 2.5 ATA for 5 hours daily) on T-lymphocytes has been studied using a model of contact sensitivity to the chemical dinitrofluorobenzene (DNFB). Treatment with HBO_2 four days before and five days after DNFB sensitization decreased the amount of tissue swelling compared to normoxia-exposed controls.[52] Another study examined the effect of HBO_2 treatment (1 to 3 ATA for 1 hour daily) five days before and four days after transgenic transfusion of red blood cells. In the treated animals, the humoral responses to the incompatible transfusion (direct hemagglutination) were transiently decreased. The cellular response (delayed hypersensitivity reaction) was not affected. However, the number of HBO_2-treated animals that developed lymphocytic infiltrates was significantly decreased.[33]

DOSING INTERVAL, DURATION, AND TIMING

It is important to differentiate the required oxygen exposure or duration of HBO_2 for antimicrobial effects from those required for modulation of inflammation or tissue repair. Fever, for example, is a marker of inflammation that often persists far longer than pathogen viability. Increasingly, more specific markers of infection or inflammation than fever are used to shorten the duration of antimicrobial therapy.[32,138,148]

Few antimicrobials are dosed for longer than two weeks without clear indication by type of infection (endocarditis, osteomyelitis, multiple abscesses, prosthetic infection) or host compromise (continued oncologic neutropenia, chronic granulomatous disease, poor surgical candidate). Review of functional outcomes following HBO_2 treatment of brain abscesses suggests no clear advantage to prolongation of HBO_2 exposure beyond 55 ATM-hours (Table 1). Assuming treatment at 2.5 ATA, this corresponds to 15 days of 90-minute therapies or 22 days of 60-minute therapies, similar to conventional antimicrobial courses and far shorter than 4–6 weeks of therapy using conventional antibacterials alone. It follows that one of the future advantages of HBO_2 may be in abridging longer courses of conventional antimicrobial therapy, predicated on improved efficacy of HBO_2 as adjunctive therapy in reversing the metabolic and antimicrobial consequences of hypoxia in avascular tissues and abscesses, detoxifying H_2S pools, and disrupting biofilms.[13,84]

On the other hand, an animal model shows advantage to longer courses of HBO_2 therapy in improving functional outcomes.[59] This is likely indicative of improved tissue repair and regeneration past eradication of infection. Tissue repair is likely responsive to different dosing and duration of HBO_2 than treating infections and may show prolonged posttreatment effects lasting days to weeks.

The interaction of oxygen as a drug with conventional antimicrobials requires consideration of timing of administration. For aminoglycosides, folic acid antagonists, macrolides, and tetracyclines that require normoxia for full effect, ideally antibiotic administration would precede HBO_2 therapy by 30–60 minutes for intravenous drugs and 2–3 hours for oral agents. For metronidazole, administration should follow HBO_2 therapy to minimize hyperoxia interfering with drug uptake. For beta-lactams, rifampicins, and likely vancomycin and aztreonam, timing is less important; administration of these drugs following HBO_2 therapy likely minimizes the mismatch between peak blood concentrations and HBO_2-induced vasoconstriction in tissues to optimize tissue delivery of drugs.

TABLE 1. OUTCOME FOLLOWING HBO_2 THERAPY OF BACTERIAL BRAIN ABSCESSES, STRATIFIED BY THE PRODUCT OF ATMOSPHERES AND HOURS OF 100% OXYGEN

N	ATA-HOURS	MODERATE TO SEVERE FUNCTIONAL OUTCOME	ORGANISMS	REFERENCES
2	< 50	50%	*Bacteroides, Listeria, Peptostreptococcus, Streptococcus*	(85,109)
20	53.25	9%	*Actinomyces, Bacteroides, Clostridium, Enterobacter, Fusobacterium, Peptostreptococcus, S. aureus, S. epidermidis, Streptococcus, Veillonella*	(85-86)
20	55+	0%	*Bacteroides, Clostridium, Eikenella, Haemophilus, Peptostreptococcus, Pseudomonas, S. aureus, Streptococcus,* (negative culture)	(84-85,74)

CONCLUSION

The mechanisms of action of hyperbaric oxygen in infectious diseases fall under four main categories: 1) oxygenation of diseased tissue, 2) growth inhibition and viability of microorganisms (favoring benefit when treating anaerobic bacteria and possibly parasites), 3) alteration of activity of antimicrobial agents under different redox conditions (including pharmacokinetic considerations), and 4) immunomodulation. Lung infections and use of metronidazole may be relative contraindications to HBO_2 therapy. Clinical activity against Mucorales fungi should be confirmed in collaborative studies. HBO_2 has various effects on immune cells, potentiating and then decreasing immune responses as exposure accrues.

ACKNOWLEDGMENTS

The author is indebted to the original authors of this chapter: Matthew Park, Charles C. Falzon, and Harry T. Whelan.

REFERENCES

1. Abe K, Nakayama M, Yoshimura M, Nakamura S, Ito T, Yamamuro M, et al. Increase in the transcriptional activity of the endothelial nitric oxide synthase gene with fluvastatin: a relation with the -786T>C polymorphism. Pharmacogenet Genomics 2005 May;15(5):329-36.
2. Albenberg L, Esipova TV, Judge CP, Bittinger K, Chen J, Laughlin A, et al. Correlation between intraluminal oxygen gradient and radial partitioning of intestinal microbiota. Gastroenterology 2014 Nov;147(5):1055-63.
3. Andersen V, Hellung-Larsen P, Sorensen SF. Optimal oxygen tension for human lymphocytes in culture. J Cell Physiol 1968 Dec;72(3):149-52.
4. Angrick EJ, Somerson NL, Weiss HS. Oxygen effects on mortality of mice infected with Diplococcus pneumoniae. Aerosp Med 1974 Jul;45(7):730-4.
5. Archibald FS, Duong MN. Superoxide dismutase and oxygen toxicity defenses in the genus Neisseria. Infect Immun 1986 Feb;51(2):631-41.
6. Arrais-Silva WW, Collhone MC, Ayres DC, de Souza Souto PC, Giorgio S. Effects of hyperbaric oxygen on Leishmania amazonensis promastigotes and amastigotes. Parasitol Int 2005 Mar;54(1):1-7.
7. Ayers LN, Tierney DF, Imagawa D. "Shortened survival of mice with influenza when given oxygen at one atmosphere." Am Rev Respir Dis. 1973;107:955-961.
8. Babior BM. "Oxygen-dependent microbial killing by phagocytes." New Engl J Med. 1978;298:659-668.
9. Baleeiro CE, Christensen PJ, Morris SB, Mendez MP, Wilcoxen SE, Paine R, III. GM-CSF and the impaired pulmonary innate immune response following hyperoxic stress. Am J Physiol Lung Cell Mol Physiol 2006 Dec;291(6):L1246-L1255.
10. Band RN, Cirrito H. Growth response of axenic Entamoeba histolytica to hydrogen, carbon dioxide, and oxygen. J Protozool 1979 May;26(2):282-6.
11. Barratt DM, Van Meter K, Asmar P, Nolan T, Trahan C, Garcia-Covarrubias L, Metzinger SE. Hyperbaric oxygen as an adjunct in zygomycosis: randomized controlled trial in a murine model. Antimicrob Agents Chemother. 2001 Dec;45(12):3601-2.
12. Bender JG, Van Epps DE. "Stimulus interactions in release of superoxide anion (O2-) from human neutrophils." Inflammation. 1985;9:67-79.
13. Bilic I, Petri NM, Krstulja M, Vuckovic M, Salamunic I, Kraljevic KS, et al. Hyperbaric oxygen is effective in early stage of healing of experimental brain abscess in rats. Neurol Res 2012 Dec;34(10):931-6.
14. Blanco YC, Farias AS, Goelnitz U, Lopes SC, Arrais-Silva WW, Carvalho BO, et al. Hyperbaric oxygen prevents early death caused by experimental cerebral malaria. PLoS ONE 2008;3(9):e3126.
15. Bringaud F, Ebikeme C, Boshart M. Acetate and succinate production in amoebae, helminths, diplomonads, trichomonads and trypanosomatids: common and diverse metabolic strategies used by parasitic lower eukaryotes. Parasitology 2010 Aug;137(9):1315-31.
16. Brown GL, Thomson PD, Mader JT, Hilton JG, Browne ME, Wells CH. Effects of hyperbaric oxygen upon S. aureus, Ps. aeruginosa and C. albicans. Aviat Space Environ Med 1979 Jul;50(7):717-20.
17. Brown OR. Reversible inhibition of respiration of Escherichia coli by hyperoxia. Microbios 1972;5:7-16.
18. Bryant RE, Fox K, Oh G, Morthland VH. Beta-lactam enhancement of aminoglycoside activity under conditions of reduced pH and oxygen tension that may exist in infected tissues. J Infect Dis 1992 Apr;165(4):676-82.

19. Chen W, Huang X, Komuniecki PR, Komuniecki R. Molecular cloning, functional expression, and characterization of pyruvate dehydrogenase kinase from anaerobic muscle of the parasitic nematode Ascaris suum. Arch Biochem Biophys 1998 May 1;353(1):181-9.

20. Chiang SM, Schellhorn HE. Regulators of oxidative stress response genes in Escherichia coli and their functional conservation in bacteria. Arch Biochem Biophys 2012 Sep 15;525(2):161-9.

21. Clarebout G, Slomianny C, Delcourt P, Leu B, Masset A, Camus D, et al. Status of Plasmodium falciparum towards catalase. Br J Haematol 1998 Oct;103(1):52-9.

22. Cleary PP, Larkin A. Hyaluronic acid capsule: strategy for oxygen resistance in group A streptococci. J Bacteriol 1979 Dec;140(3):1090-7.

23. Couch L, Theilen F, Mader JT. "Rhinocerebral mucormycosis with cerebral extension successfully treated with adjunctive hyperbaric oxygen therapy." Arch Otolaryngeol Head Neck Surg. 1988;114:791-794.

24. Crouse DT, Cassell GH, Waites KB, Foster JM, Cassady G. Hyperoxia potentiates Ureaplasma urealyticum pneumonia in newborn mice. Infect Immun 1990 Nov;58(11):3487-93.

25. Demello FJ, Hashimoto T, Hitchcock CR, Haglin JJ. The effect of hyperbaric oxygen on the germination and toxin production of Clostridium perfringens spores. In: Wada J, Iwa T, editors. Proceedings of the Fourth International Congress on Hyperbaric Medicine.Tokyo: Igaku Shoin, Ltd; 1970. p. 276-81.

26. DeRose CM, Claycamp HG. Oxidative stress effects on conjugational recombination and mutation in catalase-deficient Escherichia coli. Mutat Res 1991 Sep;255(2):193-200.

27. DiGuiseppi J, Fridovich I. Oxygen toxicity in Streptococcus sanguis. The relative importance of superoxide and hydroxyl radicals. J Biol Chem 1982 Apr 25;257(8):4046-51.

28. Docampo R. Sensitivity of parasites to free radical damage by antiparasitic drugs. Chem Biol Interact 1990;73(1):1-27.

29. Dubes GR, Al-Moslih MI, Sambol AR. "Differential effect of limitation in oxygen supply on plaquing and multiplication of adenovirus and poliovirus." Arch Virol. 1981;70:247-54.

30. Dunn MM, Smith LJ. The effects of hyperoxia on pulmonary clearance of Pseudomonas aeruginosa. J Infect Dis 1986 Apr;153(4):676-81.

31. Egners A, Erdem M, Cramer T. The Response of Macrophages and Neutrophils to Hypoxia in the Context of Cancer and Other Inflammatory Diseases. Mediators Inflamm 2016;2016:2053646.

32. Ehl S, Gering B, Bartmann P, Hogel J, Pohlandt F. C-reactive protein is a useful marker for guiding duration of antibiotic therapy in suspected neonatal bacterial infection. Pediatrics 1997 Feb;99(2):216-21.

33. Eiguchi K, Bertholds M, Grana D, Malteste C, Mareso E, Gomez E, et al. Immunoregulatory effect of HBO2 on rats. J Hyperbaric Med 1990;5:197-1.

34. Farr SB, Natvig DO, Kogoma T. "Toxicity and mutagenicity of plumbagin and the induction of a possible new DNA repair pathway in Escherichia coli." J Bacteriol. 1985;164:1309-1316.

35. Farr SB, Touati D, Kogoma T. Effects of oxygen stress on membrane functions in Escherichia coli: role of HPI catalase. J Bacteriol 1988 Apr;170(4):1837-42.

36. Feldman GM, Dannenberg AM, Jr., Seed JL. Physiologic oxygen tensions limit oxidant-mediated killing of schistosome eggs by inflammatory cells and isolated granulomas. J Leukoc Biol 1990 Apr;47(4):344-54.

37. Ferguson BJ, Mitchell TG, Moon R, Camporesi EM, Farmer J. Adjunctive hyperbaric oxygen for treatment of rhinocerebral mucormycosis. Rev Infect Dis 1988 May;10(3):551-9.

38. Field TR, White A, Elborn JS, Tunney MM. Effect of oxygen limitation on the in vitro antimicrobial susceptibility of clinical isolates of Pseudomonas aeruginosa grown planktonically and as biofilms. Eur J Clin Microbiol Infect Dis 2005 Oct;24(10):677-87.

39. Flint DH, Smyk-Randall E, Tuminello JF, Draczynska-Lusiak B, Brown OR. The inactivation of dihydroxy-acid dehydratase in Escherichia coli treated with hyperbaric oxygen occurs because of the destruction of its Fe-S cluster, but the enzyme remains in the cell in a form that can be reactivated. J Biol Chem 1993 Dec 5;268(34):25547-52.

40. Foti JJ, Devadoss B, Winkler JA, Collins JJ, Walker GC. Oxidation of the guanine nucleotide pool underlies cell death by bactericidal antibiotics. Science 2012 Apr 20;336(6079):315-9.

41. Fujiwara H, Kawai S, Murata K. Significance of sulfiredoxin/peroxiredoxin and mitochondrial respiratory chain in response to and protection from 100% O(2) in Saccharomyces cerevisiae. Mitochondrion 2013 Jan;13(1):52-8.

42. Gadd MA, McClellan DS, Neuman TS, Hansbrough JF. Effect of hyperbaric oxygen on murine neutrophil and T-lymphocyte functions. Crit Care Med 1990 Sep;18(9):974-9.

43. Gardner PR, Fridovich I. Quinolinate synthetase: the oxygen-sensitive site of de novo NAD(P)+ biosynthesis. Arch Biochem Biophys 1991 Jan;284(1):106-11.

44. Gifford GD. Mutation of an auxotrophic strain of Escherichia coli by high pressure oxygen. Biochem Biophys Res Commun 1968 Oct 24;33(2):294-8.

45. Gillmore JD, Gordon FB. "Parabarosis and experimental infection. 5. Effect of altered oxygen tension on Coxsackie B-1 infection in adult mice." Aerospace Med. 1974;45:840-842.

46. Godfrey RW, Wilder MS. Generation of oxygen species and virulence of Listeria monocytogenes. Infect Immun 1985 Mar;47(3):837-9.

47. Gordon FB, Gillmore JD. Parabarosis and experimental infections. 4. Effect of varying 02 tensions on chlamydial infection in mice and cell cultures. Aerosp Med 1974 Mar;45(3):257-62.

48. Gordon FB, Gillmore JD. "Parabarosis and experimental infections. 1. Effect of varying O2 tensions on influenza virus infection in mice." Aerospace Med. 1974;45:241-248.

49. Gottlieb SF, Solosky JA, Aubrey R, Nedelkoff DD. Synergistic action of increased oxygen tensions and PABA-folic acid antagonists on bacterial growth. Aerosp Med 1974 Aug;45(8):829-33.

50. Gudewicz TM, Mader JT, Davis CP. Combined effects of hyperbaric oxygen and antifungal agents on the growth of Candida albicans. Aviat Space Environ Med 1987 Jul;58(7):673-8.

51. Gusarov I, Shatalin K, Starodubtseva M, Nudler E. Endogenous nitric oxide protects bacteria against a wide spectrum of antibiotics. Science 2009 Sep 11;325(5946):1380-4.

52. Hansbrough JF, Piacentine JG, Eiseman B. Immunosuppression by hyperbaric oxygen. Surgery 1980 Jun;87(6):662-7.

53. Harrell LJ, Evans JB. Effect of anaerobiosis on antimicrobial susceptibility of staphylococci. Antimicrob Agents Chemother 1977 Jun;11(6):1077-8.

54. Hassett DJ, Cohen MS. Bacterial adaptation to oxidative stress: implications for pathogenesis and interaction with phagocytic cells. FASEB J 1989 Dec;3(14):2574-82.

55. Hathroubi S, Mekni MA, Domenico P, Nguyen D, Jacques M. Biofilms: Microbial Shelters Against Antibiotics. Microb Drug Resist 2016 May 23.

56. Hays RC, Mandell GL. PO2, pH, and redox potential of experimental abscesses. Proc Soc Exp Biol Med 1974 Oct;147(1):29-30.

57. Hill GB, Osterhout S. Experimental effects of hyperbaric oxgen on selected clostridial species. I. In-vitro studies. J Infect Dis 1972 Jan;125(1):17-25.

58. Hiraoka Y, Kishimoto C, Takada H, Kurokawa M, Ochiai H, Shiraki K, Sasayama S. "Role of oxygen derived free radicals in the pathogenesis of coxsackie B3 myocarditis in mice." Cardiovasc Res 1993;27:957-961.

59. Hirn M, Niinikoski J, Lehtonen OP. Effect of hyperbaric oxygen and surgery on experimental gas gangrene. Eur Surg Res 1992;24(6):356-62.

60. Hirn M, Niinikoski J, Lehtonen OP. Effect of hyperbaric oxygen and surgery on experimental multimicrobial gas gangrene. Eur Surg Res 1993;25(5):265-9.

61. Hofert JF. An acute effect of high oxygen tension on the uptake of 3H-deoxycytidine into thymocyte deoxyribonucleic acid. Biochem Pharmacol 1974 Nov 15;23(22):3216-8.

62. Hohn DC, MacKay RD, Halliday B, Hunt TK. Effect of O2 tension on microbicidal function of leukocytes in wounds and in vitro. Surg Forum 1976;27(62):18-20.

63. Hordnes C, Tyssebotn I. Effect of high ambient pressure and oxygen tension on organ blood flow in conscious trained rats. Undersea Biomed Res 1985 Jun;12(2):115-28.

64. Imlay J, Linn S. "DNA damage and oxygen radical toxicity." Science. 1988;240:1302-1309.

65. Imlay JA, Linn S. Mutagenesis and stress responses induced in Escherichia coli by hydrogen peroxide. J Bacteriol 1987 Jul;169(7):2967-76.

66. Ince C, Mik EG. Microcirculatory and mitochondrial hypoxia in sepsis, shock, and resuscitation. J Appl Physiol (1985) 2016 Jan 15;120(2):226-35.

67. Jamieson D, Chance B, Cadenas E, Boveris A. "The relation of free radical production to hyperoxia." Ann Rev Physiol. 1986;48:703-719.

68. Jones DP. "The role of oxygen concentration in oxidative stress: hypoxic and hyperoxic models. In: Oxidative Stress. (Sies H, Ed.) Academic Press London, 1985;151-195.

69. Kalns J, Lane J, Delgado A, Scruggs J, Ayala E, Gutierrez E, et al. Hyperbaric oxygen exposure temporarily reduces Mac-1 mediated functions of human neutrophils. Immunol Lett 2002 Sep 2;83(2):125-31.

70. Kalyanaraman B. Teaching the basics of redox biology to medical and graduate students: Oxidants, antioxidants and disease mechanisms. Redox Biol 2013;1:244-57.

71. Karnovsky ML. The metabolism of leukocytes. Semin Hematol 1968 Apr;5(2):156-65.

72. Kazura JW, Meshnick SR. Scavenger enzymes and resistance to oxygen mediated damage in Trichinella spiralis. Mol Biochem Parasitol 1984 Jan;10(1):1-10.

73. Kent TA, Sheftel TG, Sutton TE, Morrison LT, Mader JT. Effect of hyperbaric oxygen on the blood: cerebrospinal fluid transfer of tobramycin. Aviat Space Environ Med 1986 Jul;57(7):664-6.

74. Keogh AJ. Clostridial brain abscess and hyperbaric oxygen. Postgrad Med J 1973 Jan;49(567):64-6.

75. Keren I, Wu Y, Inocencio J, Mulcahy LR, Lewis K. Killing by bactericidal antibiotics does not depend on reactive oxygen species. Science 2013 Mar 8;339(6124):1213-6.

76. Kikuchi Y, Tateda K, Fuse ET, Matsumoto T, Gotoh N, Fukushima J, et al. Hyperoxia exaggerates bacterial dissemination and lethality in Pseudomonas aeruginosa pneumonia. Pulm Pharmacol Ther 2009 Aug;22(4):333-9.

77. Kilburn DG, Van Wezel AL. "Rubella virus replication at controlled dissolved oxygen tension." Biotech Bioengin. 1972;14:493-497.

78. King P, Citron DM, Griffith DC, Lomovskaya O, Dudley MN. Effect of oxygen limitation on the in vitro activity of levofloxacin and other antibiotics administered by the aerosol route against Pseudomonas aeruginosa from cystic fibrosis patients. Diagn Microbiol Infect Dis 2010 Feb;66(2):181-6.

79. Kivisaari J, Niinikoski J. Effects of hyperbaric oxygenation and prolonged hypoxia on the healing of open wounds. Acta Chir Scand 1975;141(1):14-9.

80. Knighton DR, Halliday B, Hunt TK. Oxygen as an antibiotic. A comparison of the effects of inspired oxygen concentration and antibiotic administration on in vivo bacterial clearance. Arch Surg 1986 Feb;121(2):191-5.

81. Kohanski MA, DePristo MA, Collins JJ. Sublethal antibiotic treatment leads to multidrug resistance via radical-induced mutagenesis. Mol Cell 2010 Feb 12;37(3):311-20.

82. Kohanski MA, Dwyer DJ, Collins JJ. How antibiotics kill bacteria: from targets to networks. Nat Rev Microbiol 2010 Jun;8(6):423-35.

83. Koomanachai P, Keel RA, Johnson-Arbor KK, Suecof LA, Nicolau DP, Kuti JL. Linezolid penetration into wound tissue of two diabetic patients before and after hyperbaric oxygen therapy. Undersea Hyperb Med 2011 Jan;38(1):11-6.

84. Kutlay M, Colak A, Yildiz S, Demircan N, Akin ON. Stereotactic aspiration and antibiotic treatment combined with hyperbaric oxygen therapy in the management of bacterial brain abscesses. Neurosurgery 2008 Feb;62 Suppl 2:540-6.

85. Lampl LA, Frey G, Diteze T, Trauschel M. Hyperbaric oxygen in intracranial abscesses. J Hyperbaric Med 1989;4(3):111-26.

86. Lampl L, Frey G. Hyperbaric oxygen in intracranial abscess. In: Whelan HT, Kindwall EP, editors. Hyperbaric medicine practice. 3 ed. Flagstaff: Best Publishing; 2006. p. 639-54.

87. Lindahl-Kiessling K, Karlberg I. High oxygen pressure inhibits DNA synthesis in mitogen-activated lymphocytes. Int Arch Allergy Appl Immunol 1979;60(1):97-100.

88. Liu Y, Imlay JA. Cell death from antibiotics without the involvement of reactive oxygen species. Science 2013 Mar 8;339(6124):1210-3.

89. Liu W, Zhao W, Lu X, Zheng X, Luo C. Clinical pathological study of treatment of chronic hepatitis with hyperbaric oxygenation. Chin Med J (Engl). 2002 Aug;115(8):1153-7.

90. Livneh A, Youngster I, El-On Y, Berkovitch M, Abu-Kishk I. The lack of effectiveness of hyperbaric oxygenation as a treatment for Leishmania major in a mouse model. Acta Parasitol 2015 Jun;60(2):345-9.

91. Lloyd D. 'Anaerobic protists': some misconceptions and confusions. Microbiology 2004 May;150(Pt 5):1115-6.

92. Lynch RE, Cole BC. Mycoplasma pneumoniae: a prokaryote which consumes oxygen and generates superoxide but which lacks superoxide dismutase. Biochem Biophys Res Commun 1980 Sep 16;96(1):98-105.

93. Mader JT, Adams KR, Wallace WR, Calhoun JH. Hyperbaric oxygen as adjunctive therapy for osteomyelitis. Infect Dis Clin North Am 1990 Sep;4(3):433-40.

94. Mader JT, Brown GL, Guckian JC, Wells CH, Reinarz JA. A mechanism for the amelioration by hyperbaric oxygen of experimental staphylococcal osteomyelitis in rabbits. J Infect Dis 1980 Dec;142(6):915-22.

95. Mader JT, Guckian JC, Glass DL, Reinarz JA. Therapy with hyperbaric oxygen for experimental osteomyelitis due to Staphylococcus aureus in rabbits. J Infect Dis 1978 Sep;138(3):312-8.

96. Malik M, Hussain S, Drlica K. Effect of anaerobic growth on quinolone lethality with Escherichia coli. Antimicrob Agents Chemother 2007 Jan;51(1):28-34.

97. Mandell GL. Bactericidal activity of aerobic and anaerobic polymorphonuclear neutrophils. Infect Immun 1974 Feb;9(2):337-41.

98. McCord JM. "Oxygen-derived free radicals in postischemic tissue injury." N Engl J Med. 1985;312:159-163.

99. McCord JM, Keele BB, Jr., Fridovich I. An enzyme-based theory of obligate anaerobiosis: the physiological function of superoxide dismutase. Proc Natl Acad Sci U S A 1971 May;68(5):1024-7.

100. Merritt GJ, Slade JB. Influence of hyperbaric oxygen on the pharmacokinetics of single-dose gentamicin in healthy volunteers. Pharmacotherapy 1993 Jul;13(4):382-5.

101. Mesquita JT, da Costa-Silva TA, Borborema SE, Tempone AG. Activity of imidazole compounds on Leishmania (L.) infantum chagasi: reactive oxygen species induced by econazole. Mol Cell Biochem 2014 Apr;389(1-2):293-300.

102. Mizrahi A, Vosseller GV, Yagi Y, Moore GE. The effect of dissolved oxygen partial pressure on growth, metabolism and immunoglobulin production in a permanent human lymphocyte cell line culture. Proc Soc Exp Biol Med 1972 Jan;139(1):118-22.

103. Mkoji GM, Smith JM, Prichard RK. Antioxidant systems in Schistosoma mansoni: correlation between susceptibility to oxidant killing and the levels of scavengers of hydrogen peroxide and oxygen free radicals. Int J Parasitol 1988 Jul;18(5):661-6.

104. Muhvich KH, Anderson LH, Criswell DW, Mehm WJ. Hyperbaric hyperoxia enhances the lethal effects of amphotericin B in Leishmania braziliensis panamensis. Undersea Hyperb Med 1993 Dec;20(4):321-8.

105. Muhvich KH, Anderson LH, Mehm WJ. Evaluation of antimicrobials combined with hyperbaric oxygen in a mouse model of clostridial myonecrosis. J Trauma 1994 Jan;36(1):7-10.

106. Muhvich KH, Myers RA, Marzella L. Effect of hyperbaric oxygenation, combined with antimicrobial agents and surgery, in a rat model of intraabdominal infection. J Infect Dis 1988 May;157(5):1058-61.

107. Muhvich KH, Piano MR, Myers RA, Ferguson JL, Marzella L. Hyperbaric oxygenation decreases blood flows in normal and septic rats. Undersea Biomed Res 1992 Jan;19(1):31-40.

108. Muller M, Lindmark DG. Uptake of metronidazole and its effect on viability in trichomonads and Entamoeba invadens under anaerobic and aerobic conditions. Antimicrob Agents Chemother 1976 Apr;9(4):696-700.

109. Nakahara K, Yamashita S, Ideo K, Shindo S, Suga T, Ueda A, et al. Drastic therapy for listerial brain abscess involving combined hyperbaric oxygen therapy and antimicrobial agents. J Clin Neurol 2014 Oct;10(4):358-62.

110. Naldini A, Carraro F, Fleishmann WR, Bocci V. "Hypoxia enhances the antiviral activity of interferons."J Interferon Res 1993;13:127-132.

111. Nara C, Tateda K, Matsumoto T, Ohara A, Miyazaki S, Standiford TJ, et al. Legionella-induced acute lung injury in the setting of hyperoxia: protective role of tumour necrosis factor-alpha. J Med Microbiol 2004 Aug;53(Pt 8):727-33.

112. Nare B, Smith JM, Prichard RK. Schistosoma mansoni: levels of antioxidants and resistance to oxidants increase during development. Exp Parasitol 1990 May;70(4):389-97.

113. Nerurkar LS, Zeligs BJ, Bellanti JA. Proliferation of alveolar macrophages in hyperoxia. Ann Allergy 1988 Nov;61(5):344-7.

114. Norden CW, Shaffer M. Treatment of experimental chronic osteomyelitis due to staphylococcus aureus with vancomycin and rifampin. J Infect Dis 1983 Feb;147(2):352-7.

115. Novais FO, Nguyen BT, Beiting DP, Carvalho LP, Glennie ND, Passos S, et al. Human classical monocytes control the intracellular stage of Leishmania braziliensis by reactive oxygen species. J Infect Dis 2014 Apr 15;209(8):1288-96.

116. Oliveira PL, Oliveira MF. Vampires, Pasteur and reactive oxygen species. Is the switch from aerobic to anaerobic metabolism a preventive antioxidant defence in blood-feeding parasites? FEBS Lett 2002 Aug 14;525(1-3):3-6.

117. Ollodart RM. Effects of hyperbaric oxygenation and antibiotics on aerobic microorganisms. In: Brown Jr IW, Cox BG, editors. Proceedings of the third international conference on hyperbaric medicine.Washington, D.C.: National Academy of Science; 1966. p. 565-671.

118. Orsi EV, Mancini R, Barriso J. "Hyperbaric enhancement of Coxsackievirus infection in mice." Aerospace Med. 1970;41:1169-1172.

119. Outten CE, Falk RL, Culotta VC. Cellular factors required for protection from hyperoxia toxicity in Saccharomyces cerevisiae. Biochem J 2005 May 15;388(Pt 1):93-101.

120. Paine R 3rd, Preston AM, Wilcoxen S, Jin H, Siu BB, Morris SB, Reed JA, Ross G, Whitsett JA, Beck JM. Granulocyte-macrophage colony-stimulating factor in the innate immune response to Pneumocystis carinii pneumonia in mice. J Immunol. 2000 Mar 1;164(5):2602-9.

121. Pakman LM. Inhibition of Pseudomonas aeruginosa by hyperbaric oxygen. I. Sulfonamide activity enhancement and reversal. Infect Immun 1971 Oct;4(4):479-87.

122. Park MK, Muhvich KH, Myers RA, Marzella L. Hyperoxia prolongs the aminoglycoside-induced postantibiotic effect in Pseudomonas aeruginosa. Antimicrob Agents Chemother 1991 Apr;35(4):691-5.

123. Park MK, Myers RA, Marzella L. Hyperoxia and prolongation of aminoglycoside-induced postantibiotic effect in Pseudomonas aeruginosa: role of reactive oxygen species. Antimicrob Agents Chemother 1993 Jan;37(1):120-2.

124. Park MK, Myers RA, Marzella L. Oxygen tensions and infections: modulation of microbial growth, activity of antimicrobial agents, and immunologic responses. Clin Infect Dis 1992 Mar;14(3):720-40.

125. Pesanti EL. Pneumocystis carinii: oxygen uptake, antioxidant enzymes, and susceptibility to oxygen-mediated damage. Infect Immun 1984 Apr;44(1):7-11.

126. Price JC, Stevens DL. "Hyperbaric oxygen in the treatment of rhinocerebral mucormycosis." Laryngoscope. 1980;90:737-747.

127. Pryor KO, Fahey TJ, III, Lien CA, Goldstein PA. Surgical site infection and the routine use of perioperative hyperoxia in a general surgical population: a randomized controlled trial. JAMA 2004 Jan 7;291(1):79-87.

128. Raffin TA, Simon LM, Braun D, Theodore J, Robin ED. Impairment of phagocytosis by moderate hyperoxia (40 to 60 per cent oxygen) in lung macrophages. Lab Invest 1980 Jun;42(6):622-6.

129. Rister M. Effects of hyperoxia on phagocytosis. Blut 1982;45:157-66.

130. Rosen H, Klebanoff SJ. "Bactericidal activity of a superoxide anion-generating system. A model for the polymorphonuclear leukocyte." J Exp Med. 1979;149:27-39.

131. Rosen H, Klebanoff SJ, Wang Y, Brot N, Heinecke JW, Fu X. Methionine oxidation contributes to bacterial killing by the myeloperoxidase system of neutrophils. Proc Natl Acad Sci U S A 2009 Nov 3;106(44):18686-91.

132. Rump AF, Siekmann U, Kalff G. Effects of hyperbaric and hyperoxic conditions on the disposition of drugs: theoretical considerations and a review of the literature. Gen Pharmacol 1999 Jan;32(1):127-33.

133. Ryder VJ, Chopra I, O'Neill AJ. Increased mutability of Staphylococci in biofilms as a consequence of oxidative stress. PLoS ONE 2012;7(10):e47695.

134. Sansom FM, Tang L, Ralton JE, Saunders EC, Naderer T, McConville MJ. Leishmania major methionine sulfoxide reductase A is required for resistance to oxidative stress and efficient replication in macrophages. PLoS ONE 2013;8(2):e56064.

135. Schaeffer DO, Caprile KA, Strain GM, Bivin WS, Cohn GH. Effect of hyperbaric oxygen on cerebrospinal fluid gentamicin concentrations. J Vet Pharmacol Ther 1992 Mar;15(1):104-6.

136. Scheibel LW, Ashton SH, Trager W. Plasmodium falciparum: microaerophilic requirements in human red blood cells. Exp Parasitol 1979 Jun;47(3):410-8.

137. Schellhorn HE, Hassan HM. Response of hydroperoxidase and superoxide dismutase deficient mutants of Escherichia coli K-12 to oxidative stress. Can J Microbiol 1988 Oct;34(10):1171-6.

138. Schuetz P, Christ-Crain M, Thomann R, Falconnier C, Wolbers M, Widmer I, et al. Effect of procalcitonin-based guidelines vs standard guidelines on antibiotic use in lower respiratory tract infections: the ProHOSP randomized controlled trial. JAMA 2009 Sep 9;302(10):1059-66.

139. Seither RL, Brown OR. Induction of stringency by hyperoxia in Escherichia coli. Cell Mol Biol 1982;28(3):285-91.

140. Sharkey RA, Mulloy EM, O'Neill SJ. Acute effects of hypoxaemia, hyperoxaemia and hypercapnia on renal blood flow in normal and renal transplant subjects. Eur Respir J 1998 Sep;12(3):653-7.

141. Shatalin K, Shatalina E, Mironov A, Nudler E. H2S: a universal defense against antibiotics in bacteria. Science 2011 Nov 18;334(6058):986-90.

142. Shen X, Peter EA, Bir S, Wang R, Kevil CG. Analytical measurement of discrete hydrogen sulfide pools in biological specimens. Free Radic Biol Med 2012 Apr 19;52(11-12):2276-83.

143. Shima K, Szaszak M, Solbach W, Gieffers J, Rupp J. Impact of a low-oxygen environment on the efficacy of antimicrobials against intracellular Chlamydia trachomatis. Antimicrob Agents Chemother 2011 May;55(5):2319-24.

144. Signoretto C, Bianchi F, Burlacchini G, Canepari P. Microbiological evaluation of the effects of hyperbaric oxygen on periodontal disease. New Microbiol 2007 Oct;30(4):431-7.

145. Sjoberg F, Singer M. The medical use of oxygen: a time for critical reappraisal. J Intern Med 2013 Dec;274(6):505-28.

146. Sokol-Anderson ML, Brajtburg J, Medoff G. Amphotericin B-induced oxidative damage and killing of Candida albicans. J Infect Dis 1986 Jul;154(1):76-83.

147. Stevens DL, Bryant AE, Adams K, Mader JT. Evaluation of therapy with hyperbaric oxygen for experimental infection with Clostridium perfringens. Clin Infect Dis 1993 Aug;17(2):231-7.

148. Stolz D, Smyrnios N, Eggimann P, Pargger H, Thakkar N, Siegemund M, et al. Procalcitonin for reduced antibiotic exposure in ventilator-associated pneumonia: a randomised study. Eur Respir J 2009 Dec;34(6):1364-75.

149. Strote G. Successful use of a simple anaerobic system for the in vitro cultivation of infective larvae of Onchocerca volvulus. Trans R Soc Trop Med Hyg 1987;81(1):174-5.

150. Suttorp N, Simon LM. Decreased bactericidal function and impaired respiratory burst in lung macrophages after sustained in vitro hyperoxia. Am Rev Respir Dis 1983 Sep;128(3):486-90.

151. Tack KJ, Sabath LD. Increased minimum inhibitory concentrations with anaerobiasis for tobramycin, gentamicin, and amikacin, compared to latamoxef, piperacillin, chloramphenicol, and clindamycin. Chemotherapy 1985;31(3):204-10.

152. Takamiya S, Fukuda K, Nakamura T, Aoki T, Sugiyama H. Paragonimus westermani possesses aerobic and anaerobic mitochondria in different tissues, adapting to fluctuating oxygen tension in microaerobic habitats. Int J Parasitol 2010 Dec;40(14):1651-8.

153. Tally FP, Sullivan CE. Metronidazole: in vitro activity, pharmacology and efficacy in anaerobic bacterial infections. Pharmacotherapy 1981 Jul;1(1):28-38.

154. Tarassova K, Tegova R, Tover A, Teras R, Tark M, Saumaa S, et al. Elevated mutation frequency in surviving populations of carbon-starved rpoS-deficient Pseudomonas putida is caused by reduced expression of superoxide dismutase and catalase. J Bacteriol 2009 Jun;191(11):3604-14.

155. Taylor CT, Moncada S. Nitric oxide, cytochrome C oxidase, and the cellular response to hypoxia. Arterioscler Thromb Vasc Biol 2010 Apr;30(4):643-7.

156. Thalinger KK, Mandell GL. Bactericidal activity of macrophages in an anaerobic environment. J Reticuloendothel Soc 1971 May;9(5):393-6.

157. Thom SR, Lauermann MW, Hart GB. Intermittent hyperbaric oxygen therapy for reduction of mortality in experimental polymicrobial sepsis. J Infect Dis 1986 Sep;154(3):504-10.

158. Torres-Barcelo C, Cabot G, Oliver A, Buckling A, Maclean RC. A trade-off between oxidative stress resistance and DNA repair plays a role in the evolution of elevated mutation rates in bacteria. Proc Biol Sci 2013 Apr 22;280(1757):20130007.

159. Tsukayama DT, Guay DR, Gustilo RB, Wicklund B, Gruninger R, Peterson PK. The effect of anaerobiosis on antistaphylococcal antibiotics. Orthopedics 1988 Sep;11(9):1285-9.

160. Turrens JF, Freeman BA, Crapo JD. "Hyperoxia increases H2O2 release by lung mitochondria and microsomes." Arch Biochem Biophys. 1982;217:411-419.

161. Vatansever F, de Melo WC, Avci P, Vecchio D, Sadasivam M, Gupta A, et al. Antimicrobial strategies centered around reactive oxygen species--bactericidal antibiotics, photodynamic therapy, and beyond. FEMS Microbiol Rev 2013 Nov;37(6):955-89.

162. Verma S, Landisch R, Quirk B, Schmainda K, Prah M, Whelan HT, et al. Presumed Hydrogen Sulfide-Mediated Neurotoxicity Following Streptococcus Anginosus Group Meningitis. Pediatr Infect Dis J 2012 Sep 25;32(2):189-91.

163. Virtanen S. Antibacterial activity of sulphamethoxazole and trimethoprim under diminished oxygen tension. J Gen Microbiol 1974 Sep;84(1):145-8.

164. Ward PA. "Role of toxic oxygen products from phagocytic cells in tissue injury." Adv Shock Res. 1983;10:27-34.

165. Wilson DF, Erecinska M. The role of cytochrome c oxidase in regulation of cellular oxygen consumption. In: Gottlieb SF, Longmuir IS, Totter JR, editors. Oxygen: An In-Depth Study of its Pathophysiology.Bethesda: Undersea Medical Society; 1984. p. 459-92.

166. Wizemann TM, Moskovitz J, Pearce BJ, Cundell D, Arvidson CG, So M, et al. Peptide methionine sulfoxide reductase contributes to the maintenance of adhesins in three major pathogens. Proc Natl Acad Sci U S A 1996 Jul 23;93(15):7985-90.

167. Wright DH, Gunderson BW, Hovde LB, Ross GH, Ibrahim KH, Rotschafer JC. Comparative pharmacodynamics of three newer fluoroquinolones versus six strains of staphylococci in an in vitro model under aerobic and anaerobic conditions. Antimicrob Agents Chemother 2002 May;46(5):1561-3.

168. Zabinski RA, Walker KJ, Larsson AJ, Moody JA, Kaatz GW, Rotschafer JC. Effect of aerobic and anaerobic environments on antistaphylococcal activities of five fluoroquinolones. Antimicrob Agents Chemother 1995 Feb;39(2):507-12.

169. Zamboni WA, Mazolewski PJ, Erdmann D, Bergman BA, Hussman J, Cooper MD, et al. Evaluation of penicillin and hyperbaric oxygen in the treatment of streptococcal myositis. Ann Plast Surg 1997 Aug;39(2):131-6.

CHAPTER 17 CHAPTER

Gas Gangrene

CHAPTER SEVENTEEN OVERVIEW

Introduction **409**
Bacteriology **410**
Pathophysiology **411**
Clinical Considerations **412**
Clostridial Myonecrosis with Toxicity 412
Localized Clostridial Myonecrosis 413
Clostridial Cellulitis without Toxicity 413
Clostridial Cellulitis with Toxicity 413
Effects of Hyperbaric Oxygen **414**
Diagnosis of Gas Gangrene **414**
Treatment Strategy **415**
Initial Care of High-Risk Patients **415**
Initial Surgical Intervention **416**
Antibiotic Therapy **417**
Polyvalent Gas Gangrene Antitoxin **418**
Tetanus Prophylaxis **418**
Blood and Blood Components **418**
Transfer of Patient for Hyperbaric Therapy **418**
Hyperbaric Oxygen Treatment **418**
Fluids, Electrolytes, and pH **419**
Care of Patients between Hyperbaric Oxygen Treatments **420**
Hyperbaric Oxygen Treatment Prior to Debridement **420**
Complications **421**
ARDS 421
Disseminated Intravascular Coagulopathy (DIC) 421
Oliguria and Acute Renal Failure (ARF) 422
Myocardial Irritability 422
Deep Vein Thrombosis (DVT) 422
Fat Embolism 422
Conclusions **423**
References **424**

Gas Gangrene

Aliyah Keval, Harry T. Whelan

INTRODUCTION

Gas gangrene is a fulminating myonecrotic infection caused by the clostridial species of bacteria which can result in a rapidly fatal outcome when untreated. Historically, the incidence of gas gangrene has paralleled that of armed combat because of contaminated wounds on the battlefield, but in the last 30 years this historical correlation has become less distinct. In 8 years of combat in Vietnam, only 22 cases of gas gangrene were recorded in American casualties, while in a 10-year period in Miami, Florida, there were at least 27 cases of clostridial infection.(26)

Accidental trauma continues to be the leading cause of gas gangrene(33,41,78,86) with 50% of the cases arising as a consequence of contamination of traumatic wounds. Gas gangrene following surgery is an uncommon but devastating complication. The number of major and minor procedures that precede development of gas gangrene is extensive. The disease has been reported following amputation for peripheral vascular disease,(153) intramuscular injection,(34,62,74,96,115,129-131,148,175) abortion,(32,45,116) femoral venipuncture,(46) gastric surgery,(65 91) hernia repair,(127) colon surgery,(82,113) gall bladder and common bile duct surgery,(71,103,149) appendectomy,(66,134) total hip replacement,(142) small bowel surgery,(105) chemotherapy for choriocarcinoma,(105) endoscopy,(70) colonic polypectomy,(24) hip nailing,(54) and vaginal delivery.(137) In addition, the disease has been reported in association with carcinoma of the cecum,(63,128) femoral neck fracture,(186) thermal burns,(125) dissection of the aorta,(138) retroperitoneal rupture of the duodenum,(192) rupture of the humeral artery,(19) diabetes,(20,127) metastatic breast cancer,(122) intracardiac thrombus,(122) and perforation of the esophagus.(124) Hitchcock et al. comment that, compared with gas gangrene secondary to trauma, the disease secondary to elective surgery is usually less suspected, diagnosed later, and therefore associated with a higher mortality rate.(83)

The use of hyperbaric oxygen in the treatment of gas gangrene was first reported by Brummelkamp and his associates in 1961.(27) In this initial series of 26 patients, hyperbaric oxygen was the sole treatment modality used. Clinical series reported later, including a follow-up report on 10 years' experience by Brummelkamp's associates, emphasize the use of surgery, antibiotics, and hyperbaric oxygen adjunctively.(41,78,83,86,141) This has been shown experimentally by Demello et al., who demonstrated greater survival in dogs with experimental gas gangrene when all three treatment modalities were used together as compared with the use of each treatment modality alone or in combinations of two.(42)

BACTERIOLOGY

Clostridial species are gram-positive, spore forming, non-motile, rod-shaped organisms. Although over 90 species of clostridial bacteria have been identified, only six have been implicated in gas gangrene in humans. *Clostridium perfringens* is the most common of these bacteria, being found in close to 80% of contaminated wounds.(114) The other causative clostridial bacteria, in decreasing order of prevalence, in wounds of gas gangrene patients are *C. oedematiens*, 40%; *C. septicum*, 20%; and *C. histolyticum*, *C. bifermentans*, and *C. fallux*, less than 10% taken together.(188)

These 6 clostridial organisms produce over 20 exotoxins, 6 of which are known to be lethal. (114,188) The more severe pathologic scenarios are usually caused by vascular compromise due to local trauma, resulting in an anaerobic environment that fosters the elaboration of exotoxins by clostridial organisms. Since the ensuing inflammatory response is triggered by the elaboration of toxin rather than the bacterium itself, the clinical scenario may be better described as intoxication rather than infection. Despite their remarkable prevalence in contaminated wounds, invasive clostridial organisms stimulate a remarkably minor inflammatory response and produce draining wounds with nonpurulent exudates. Barring superinfection with other organisms, the classic disease process produces a broad range of clinical scenarios, including simple wound contamination, anaerobic cellulitis, and myonecrosis.(7)

As the most common cause of clostridial myonecrosis, which is commonly referred to as "gas gangrene," the *C. perfringens* species has been of interest to clinical investigators for several decades. Since it is not a strict anaerobe, it grows freely in oxygen tensions of 30 mmHg with restricted growth in oxygen tensions up to 70 mmHg and is ubiquitous in nature, particularly found in the normal flora of the gastrointestinal tract as well as in soil throughout the world, except in the North African desert. *C. perfringens* has been identified as having five specific sub-types, A–E, of which type A has been shown to cause the majority of human infections. The species also produces several extracellular toxins, but only two of them are critical to inducing the pathologic state.

Alpha toxin is the defining component of its parent species' virulence, and its detection in tissue samples or blood cultures is ultimately diagnostic for *C. perfringens* infection.(143) Alpha toxin is a phospholipase-C (PLC) compound, which allows it to catalyze the hydrolysis of phosphatidyl choline and sphingomyelin. The PLC activity is essential to the inhibition of the influx of polymorphonuclear leukocytes (PMNL) at the infected site and initiation of local microvascular thrombosis. This creates an environment favorable for tissue necrosis at the inoculation site, which is the hallmark of clostridial wound infections.(7,58,164)

One study demonstrated that a *C. perfringens* mutant lacking the ability to produce alpha toxin was nonvirulent when injected into a mouse model. By complementing the chromosomal mutation with a recombinant plasmid that carried a wild-type PLC gene, the investigators were able to restore *C. perfringens*'s ability to both produce alpha toxin and reestablish lethality in infected mice.(7) Another study showed that vaccination with a part of the C-terminal domain of PLC protected mice from experimental *C. perfringens* infection.(168,189) Finally, intramuscular injection of PLC in experimental animals caused a rapid and irreversible decline in skeletal muscle blood flow due to the formation of intravascular aggregates of activated platelets, leukocytes, and fibrin, which were primarily mediated by PLC activation of the platelet fibrinogen receptor gp-IIb/IIIa.(30,31)

Theta toxin, also known as perfringolysin O (PFO), has been shown in studies to have a synergistic effect on the degree of hemolysis, leukostasis, and necrosis induced by alpha- toxin.[8] Experimental models have shown that exposure to theta toxin increases production of several factors that induce vasodilation, including prostacyclin, platelet activating factor, and various lipid autocoids.[187] Upregulation of these native hematologic factors results in "warm shock," which is defined as a markedly reduced systemic vascular resistance combined with markedly increased cardiac output and rapid expansion of the intravascular blood volume.[5,169]

While alpha toxin is the only truly lethal toxin produced in significant quantities by *C. perfringens*, its effects can be significantly augmented by the presence of other nonlethal toxins, including several varieties of hyaluronidases, hemolysins, and elastases. Among this class of nonlethal clostridial factors, kappa toxin has significant proteolytic activity. In addition, "circulating factor" inhibits phagocytosis, while Mu toxin, neuraminidase, and hemagglutinin function to modify DNA, destroy immunologic receptors, and inactivate group-A factor of erythrocytes.[83] When these accessory toxins are elaborated by the parent clostridial organisms, they act synergistically with alpha toxin to create a rapidly spreading liquefaction necrosis.

The destruction of tissue that characterizes gas gangrene depends upon the continuous production of alpha toxin by clostridial organisms at the site of infection. Even though the infected tissue succumbs to liquefaction necrosis, alpha toxin becomes tissue-fixed and neutralized into a nontoxic form within two hours of being produced.[114] These factors can also be removed from the inoculation site through the bloodstream and transported to the liver and kidneys for detoxification. This means that the overall impact of a clostridial infection is attributable to the severity of the initiating injury and local levels of alpha toxin, which combine to create the increasingly hypoxic, avascular environment that is essential to the survival of *C. perfringens.*

PATHOPHYSIOLOGY

Studies have shown that the mere presence of clostridial organisms is insufficient for gas gangrene to develop at the site of inoculation. While it has been estimated that 30% of traumatic wounds are contaminated with *C. perfringens* spores, clostridial myonecrosis develops in less than 3% of these wounds.[114] DeHaven and Evarts suggested that gas gangrene could be thought of as a disease associated with a particular opportunity rather than with a specific organism.[41] Consequently, two clinical conditions have been established as necessary for this disease to occur: (1) clostridial contamination and (2) a decreased oxidation-reduction potential in the wound.

Since clostridial contamination of wounds is a fairly common event, establishing the necessary oxidation-reduction potential is likely the rate-limiting step in this process. Local circulatory failure at the wound site is the primary cause of below-normal oxidation-reduction potentials, which establishes the ischemic, hypoxic conditions. This is most often caused by trauma to vessels from penetrating foreign bodies that introduce nonnative bacteria and cause hemorrhage or edema. The situation can be exacerbated during the initial management of these patients by applying excessively tight tourniquets, casts, or dressings that create additional necrotic tissue.

Wounds caused by high-velocity missiles, such as bullet fragments and debris in motor vehicle accidents, result in the rapid transfer of high levels of kinetic energy when a projectile initially strikes the tissue. The penetrating object produces a relatively small, superficial entrance wound, while generating significantly more damage by transferring kinetic energy to internal structures as it slows along its path. While the projectile travels within the tissue planes, it forms large cavities by fracturing bones, shearing tissue, and severing blood vessels. Many muscles have small, well-defined arterial supplies with minimal collateral flow, so damage to these principle vessels may eliminate a significant percentage, if not all, of their vasculature. This compromised circulation immediately results in local ischemia and tissue hypoxia and eventually causes necrosis of the affected muscle. The literature indicates that damage to vessels supplying the affected area is found in up to 75%–85% of cases of gas gangrene following trauma.(188)

Even under more controlled conditions, tissue hypoxia remains the primary cause of gas gangrene. In the surgical suite, where every effort is made to eliminate contamination and infection, postoperative clostridial infections following "clean" procedures are most frequently encountered in patients with atherosclerosis or diabetes mellitus.(40) When the gastrointestinal tract is instrumented in patients with these predisposing conditions, gas gangrene of the trunk is seen as convincing evidence of a bowel leak. Postinjection gas gangrene is commonly associated with the use of epinephrine, whose vasoconstrictive properties can last as long as two hours.(69) As a result, the use of epinephrine with local anesthetics is contraindicated during wound debridements and primary closure. Outside the hospital, many intravenous drug users are not educated in the principles of sterile technique and have experienced infection and recurrent trauma at their injection sites. These injection sites contain fibrotic tissue that is relatively hypoxic and predisposes these patients to developing clostridial infections.(6)

It is important to note that not all cases of clostridial myonecrosis are due to either surgical or other penetrating traumas. *C. septicum* is one of the leading causes of occult, atraumatic gas gangrene. Infections from this species usually results from bacterium secondary to lesions of the gastrointestinal tract. This is often seen with colonic malignancies, especially in immunocompromised patients. Several studies have postulated that *C. septicum*'s tolerance to aerobic environments may decrease the efficacy of hyperbaric therapy relative to *C. perfringens*.(81,163)

CLINICAL CONSIDERATIONS

The four forms of necrotizing clostridial disease delineated by Altemeier in 1966 still best describe the clinical picture of gas gangrene.(1)

Clostridial Myonecrosis with Toxicity

The clinical scenario that is classically associated with gas gangrene is characterized by diffuse and rapid spread from the initial site of involvement. Its onset is acute and follows an incubation period with an average range between four hours and three days; however, cases have been reported after incubation periods that have lasted up to six weeks.(184) The first symptom observed in most cases is pain out of proportion to the extent and timing of the correlated injury. The tissue surrounding the wound swells with edema, causing the overlying skin to become tense and blanch to the touch. From this point, the toxic process accelerates rapidly as the skin surrounding the site of involvement appears light bronze within a few hours and progressively darkens as underlying tissue dies, before finally giving way to the blebs and bullae.

Barring additional wound contamination by nonclostridial organisms, patients typically do not develop fevers above 101°F and remain normotensive despite becoming disproportionately tachycardic, between 140–160 beats per minute. When shock develops, it marks the latter stages of the disease and is a grave prognostic sign. Most patients remain oriented to person, place, and time but can exhibit a characteristic flattening of affect and a "la belle indifference" attitude. Drainage from the wound site is usually serosanguinous with a typical "sweetish" or "mousy" odor, unless the wound is superinfected, and may contain gas bubbles, which can be observed on exam, as crepitus within the soft tissue, or demonstrated radiographically, as free air dissecting along fascial planes. Gas in the soft tissue can also be caused by an initiating injury that introduces air into a wound or by non-clostridal organisms contaminating the wound that are associated with gas production, such as E. coli and anerobic streptococci.[41] Since there is no evidence of gas in at least half of the cases diagnosed as clostridial infections, the presence of this finding is not necessary to establish the diagnosis.[78] Most cases of gas gangrene will show some evidence of hemolysis on laboratory analysis, but clinically significant levels are diagnostic for bacteremia, which is a very serious complication. When there is a high index of suspicion for clostridial infections, these patients must be managed and treated appropriately to improve their chances for survival.

Secondary to clostridial gas gangrene as well is arterial gas embolism (AGE). Emboli, or lack of blood supply to vessels or arteries, can cause gangrene, especially in divers, as AGE is associated with air bubbles blocking blood flow.[75,126] Gas gangrene is essentially caused by a lack of blood supply.

Localized Clostridial Myonecrosis

This uncommon form of the disease is usually seen following nonsterile injection of drugs. The infection tends to remain localized, and few, if any, toxic symptoms are manifested. Local incision and drainage with appropriate antibiotic therapy is the appropriate management for this disease, but these patients must be monitored closely to potentially manage the more aggressive, disseminated form of the disease.

Clostridial Cellulitis without Toxicity

The involvement of invasive clostridial disease can also be limited to the subcutaneous tissue without invading the muscle, which creates a benign lesion, commonly referred to as a "gas abscess." Definitive treatment for this issue is incision and drainage, but these patients must be followed closely for the development of toxic symptoms.

Clostridial Cellulitis with Toxicity

A small number of patients with clostridial cellulitis can present with the same clinical picture as patients with spreading, toxic clostridial myonecrosis. If the clinical scenario goes undiagnosed or untreated, the patient has a similarly grave prognosis to those diagnosed with fulminant gas gangrene and requires equally intensive treatment.

EFFECTS OF HYPERBARIC OXYGEN

There is extensive evidence to support the efficacy of hyperbaric oxygen in gas gangrene, based upon in vivo and in vitro studies. Demello et al[42] did a comparative study on an experimental gas gangrene model in dogs by comparing the outcomes of treatment with hyperbaric oxygen, antibiotics, and surgery, both individually and in combination. They found that when all three treatment modalities were used together, the mortality was significantly lower than when they were used individually or in any other combination. In a related study, the Demello group also demonstrated that hyperbaric oxygen reduces the germination rate of heat-activated spores of *Clostridium perfringens*.[45] The combination of such treatments was also reaffirmed by studies including that of Yang et al.[191]

Hill and Osterhout showed a significant increase in survival of mice who were treated with HBO_2 therapy versus those who were left untreated.[81] Similar findings were also published by both Kelley and Pace, and Nora and Associates.[98,135] Van Unnik showed that alpha toxin production by clostridial organisms is inhibited by exposing the organisms to oxygen pressures of three atmospheres absolute (ATA).[178] This finding was expanded upon by Hill and Osterhout, who demonstrated that high concentrations of oxygen can overcome the effects of catalase in necrotizing tissue, and by Kaye, who showed the bactericidal effects of hyperbaric oxygen on clostridial organisms.[80,97] In a similar study, Stevens found that oxygen tensions of 40 mmHg suppress clostridial growth, while oxygen tensions of 80 mmHg suppress toxin synthesis.[161]

From 1961 to 1978, hyperbaric oxygen was used in the treatment of well over 1,200 cases of gas gangrene. There are 117 case reports and comments on the efficacy of hyperbaric oxygen with regards to this disease in the world literature.[1,3,4,7,9,11-18,20-23,25,27-29,36-39,41,44,47-53,55-57,59-61,67,68,72,73,76-79,81,82,84,85-90,92, 93-95,97,99-102,104-111,117-121,123,124 ,132,133,136,139-141,144,145,147-149,152,155,157-161,170-177,180,181,183,184,186] For this series of reports, the approximate cumulative mortality rate is 25%, while the approximate disease-specific fatality rate is 15%. When patients received treatment within 24 hours of the presumptive diagnosis of gas gangrene, the disease-specific fatality rate was reported as 5%.[78]

Many cases have been reported in the world's literature since 1978 proving that HBO_2 has been accepted among clinicians who are aware of its benefits. Despite the evidence supporting HBO_2 therapy as a noninvasive adjunct to proper surgical techniques and antibiotic therapy, gas gangrene patients must continue to be managed as multi-organ, intensive-care problems. Constant vigilance and prompt intervention are essential to the successful prevention and treatment of life-threatening complications.

DIAGNOSIS OF GAS GANGRENE

The most common initial symptom in patients with gas gangrene is pain out of proportion to the extent and timing of the correlated injury at the traumatic or surgical site. Depending on the duration of infection, gas gangrene patients can present with signs of clinical toxicity.[114] The presence of gas in the soft tissue can be detected on physical exam and confirmed with various imaging modalities; however, this finding is not diagnostic for clostridial myonecrosis. Microscopic evaluation of biopsy material demonstrates necrotizing or degenerating muscle tissue, clostridial organisms, and a remarkable paucity of inflammatory cells.[7,58]

While definitive diagnosis is ultimately contingent upon demonstrating large, gram-positive rods, it is essential that proper treatment not be delayed in favor of diagnostic confirmation from the laboratory. Once tissue destruction from clostridial proliferation begins, the patient's outcome depends upon the time that elapses between achieving a working diagnosis and initiating appropriate surgical intervention. The decision to proceed with treatment of clostridial myonecrosis is based primarily on the patient's current clinical status, as described above and summarized in Table 1. If the patient's clinical status does not indicate a need for immediate debridement, then the results of the anaerobic culture and tissue biopsies should be considered.

In reality, the diagnosis of gas gangrene is most often made empirically during surgical exploration in patients who present with less definitive signs and symptoms that are suggestive of gas gangrene. These patients require more aggressive debridement to prevent a more serious wound complication from developing. For patients with a confirmed diagnosis of clostridial myonecrosis, the goal of debridement is to extirpate just enough viable tissue to stop the spread of the disease. Grossly necrotic tissue should always be removed, but it is important that as much viable, well-vascularized tissue be left intact to reduce both the morbidity and the length of postoperative recovery associated with such procedures. By combining the use of early hyperbaric oxygen treatments, it is possible to limit the spread of the clostridial organisms, thereby reducing the tissue destruction associated with the infection and the treatment and improving the patient's final outcome.

TREATMENT STRATEGY

The following strategy emphasizes hyperbaric oxygen as an important adjunctive therapy for the treatment of clostridial myonecrosis. Since the approach for treating both gas gangrene and its complications have changed over time, this text has been updated to reflect the current standard of care, as defined by the world's literature.

INITIAL CARE OF HIGH-RISK PATIENTS

Approximately ⅔ of patients who develop gas gangrene do so postoperatively or after suffering a traumatic wound. The remaining ⅓ of gas gangrene cases are spontaneous in origin and arise most often in patients with chronic medical conditions that induce subclinical ischemia in previously healthy tissue. Patients with preexisting diabetes mellitus or atherosclerosis are at increased risk for developing clostridial myonecrosis following "clean," but occultly contaminated, large bowel or gall bladder procedures. This same class of chronic diseases is often present in the small number of de novo clostridial infections that have been reported.

TABLE 1. COMMON PRESENTING SIGNS AND SYMPTOMS IN TOXIC CLOSTRIDIAL MYONECROSIS AND CELLULITIS

Pain	Low-grade fever
Tachycardia	Bronzing of the skin over involved area
Crepitus	Formation of blebs and bullae
Hemolysis	Obtunded sensorium

Among high-risk patients, traumatic wounds, including minor ones suffered underwater, should be considered contaminated by default and treated accordingly. These wounds should undergo wide debridement to include tissue that shows signs of compromised circulation. Special care must be taken when removing foreign material from the wound. Pulsatile irrigation should be performed, using copious quantities of sterile electrolyte solution or a nonionic surfactant complexed with elemental iodine. Commercially available surgical-scrub solutions should not be used for irrigation because they contain anionic detergents which have been shown to decrease tissue resistance to infection. The wounds should be left open and inspected at least daily; further debridement should be performed as necessary. Delayed primary closure can be performed approximately five days after the injury in wounds showing no evidence of infection and when the wound edges have maintained adequate perfusion for a minimum of 24 hours.

The operative patient with compromised tissue perfusion presents special problems. Such patients undergoing gall bladder or large bowel surgery have the greatest risk of postoperative clostridial infection. Meticulous attention must be paid to ensure the use of both aseptic surgical technique and appropriate instrumentation.

Electrocautery should be used judiciously to avoid inducing necrosis in neigHBO_2ring tissue, thereby creating new potential sites of infection. If electrocautery must be used to achieve hemostasis, the bipolar setting should be used at all times, as it produces ⅔ less necrosis to neighboring tissue when compared with monopolar. Suture ligation should be used to control bleeding in vessels larger than 2 mm in diameter. Tissue should be approximated with minimal tension sutures and closed in layers to avoid unnecessarily compromising perfusion.

During the postoperative period, wound inspections and dressing changes must be performed daily, but the actual schedule can vary according to the rate of wound healing. Consultation with a wound care specialist may be indicated in the immediate postoperative period or to manage more complicated cases, such as nonhealing wounds. The presence of significant edema surrounding the incision, nonserous drainage from the wound, or complaints of increasing pain at the operative site are all signs concerning for an emerging wound infection and demand immediate evaluation by the surgical team.

INITIAL SURGICAL INTERVENTION

Aside from minimal debridement, few surgical procedures are required to make the initial diagnosis. This is not the case, however, for patients with extremity involvement, where thorough fasciotomies must be performed to ensure complete decompression of all anatomic compartments. While there are numerous adjunctive therapies for this disease, rapid diagnosis followed by surgical debridement, including thorough, yet conservative, fasciotomies when indicated, remains the standard of care for the treatment of clostridial myonecrosis. Adherence to these principles helps preserve tissue, prevents complications, improves postoperative function, and increases overall survival.[65,112]

One of the more common characteristics of clostridial infections is massive edema, which can compromise local tissue perfusion, thereby making any therapeutic procedures that are attempted significantly less effective. Without adequate circulation, neither high levels of oxygen nor antibiotics can be delivered to the infected area. By maintaining the hypoxic milieu, the clostridial organisms and their toxins are allowed to proliferate and eventually become intravascularly disseminated, which can result in shock. This makes both the planning and management of patients requiring surgical intervention significantly more challenging.

If the patient shows signs of being in fulminant shock, general anesthesia should be avoided in favor of local or regional blocks. A central venous line and at least one other intravenous line should be introduced by either the catheter or cut-down techniques. Particular care should be taken to keep the end of the central venous line from entering the right atrium. Patients with gas gangrene can easily develop myocardial irritability, and an uncontrollable arrhythmia can be induced by placing a catheter into the right atrium. An arterial line should be placed and secured with a heparin lock to facilitate repeated determinations of arterial blood gases for patients who are either suffering from severe trauma and are in particular danger of developing acute respiratory distress syndrome (ARDS) or are suspected of having underlying pulmonary disease.

ANTIBIOTIC THERAPY

Based upon studies of in vitro susceptibility, penicillin G remains the first-line therapy for antibiotic treatment of clostridial infections. The standard regimen for this medication is a total dose of 10 to 20 million units per day administered intravenously for 2 weeks. Several other antibiotics, including clindamycin, tetracycline, chloramphenicol, metronidazole, and some cephalosporins, are effective in vitro against both *C. perfringens* and other clostridial species.[65,112] In patients with known penicillin allergy, chloramphenicol and metronidazole can potentially be used as alternatives. When the pathology shows mixed infections, specifically with gram-negative bacilli, initial treatment should include aminoglycosides, new-generation cephalosporins, or choramphenicol.

One animal study showed a survival benefit in a treatment group receiving a regimen of both clindamycin and penicillin when compared to treating with penicillin alone. In this same study, another treatment group had an increase in mortality rates while receiving penicillin and metronidazole simultaneously.[165] Studies also indicate that when used alone, clindamycin may have greater efficacy than penicillin in experimental models.[165,166] In experimental models of gas gangrene, clindamycin and penicillin have been shown to be rapidly bactericidal, while clindamycin has the added benefit of suppressing alpha-toxin production. This difference may account for clindamycin's superior performance in experimental models when compared with penicillin.[167] Despite this experimental increase in activity, it is important to consider the combination of clindamycin and penicillin in clinical applications, since a small but significant percentage of clostridial strains show resistance to monotherapy with clindamycin. Tetracycline can also be used alone or in combination with penicillin for the treatment of clostridial infections and has been recommended as an alternative to clindamycin for its ability to rapidly inhibit toxin synthesis.[2,167]

It is important to note that these regimens were designed using evidence from both preclinical trials and anecdotal evidence. Unfortunately, clinical trials have not yet been performed to establish the efficacy of these proposed regimens for the treatment of clostridial myonecrosis in human subjects.

POLYVALENT GAS GANGRENE ANTITOXIN

Even though its efficacy has never been proven, polyvalent equine antitoxin has been used intravenously to treat gas gangrene. Administration of the antitoxin resulted in a significant percentage of patients demonstrating serious allergic reactions, ranging from serum sickness to anaphylactic shock. This treatment is no longer being produced for clinical applications.

TETANUS PROPHYLAXIS

Since the wounds being evaluated are often severe and contaminated, patients with suspected or diagnosed gas gangrene are also at increased risk for tetanus infections. In these cases, an aggressive approach to tetanus prophylaxis is indicated. The regimen for tetanus prophylaxis consists of an intramuscular injection of 500 units of tetanus immune globulin (human) and 0.5 cc of tetanus toxoid injected intramuscularly at another site.

BLOOD AND BLOOD COMPONENTS

Whole blood should be administered to replace acute blood loss, but it should only be used sparingly. Bedridden patients show remarkable improvement when their hematocrits (HCT) fall to between 30%–35%, as long as their intravascular volumes are kept within normal range. Outcome analyses have demonstrated that the overall cardiac workload increases for patients whose hematocrits are maintained above the suggested range, resulting in worsened outcomes.

Whole blood should be administered through a microaggregate filter to prevent patients from developing ARDS. Specific blood components, such as fresh-frozen plasma or platelets, can be used to treat platelet deficiencies or coagulopathies, as needed.

TRANSFER OF PATIENT FOR HYPERBARIC THERAPY

If a hyperbaric chamber is not available at the initial receiving hospital, arrangements must be made quickly to transfer the patient to a facility equipped with a hyperbaric chamber within 24 hours.

The physician covering the chamber at the receiving facility should be contacted to arrange for the transfer of care. Patient transport, which should involve the most expeditious method available, is often performed by air ambulance when the distance between the 2 facilities is greater than 100 miles.

HYPERBARIC OXYGEN TREATMENT

The hyperbaric oxygen treatment schedule used should closely follow the protocol that was originally promulgated by Drs. Brummelkamp and Boerema.[27] The depth-equivalent chamber pressure used is 66 feet of seawater (3 ATA). Some facilities treat gas gangrene patients at a depth-equivalent pressure of 49.5 feet of seawater (2.5 ATA), which is the minimum pressure where oxygen has been found to be effective in the treatment of gas gangrene.

The patient breathes 100% oxygen for 90 minutes per treatment, using a tightly fitting aviator's mask, anesthesia mask, or endotracheal tube. The cuffs of the endotracheal tubes should be inflated with normal saline solution. The 90-minute period of oxygen treatments can be divided into two 45-minute periods or three 25-minute periods with a final 15-minute period. In either case, the oxygen breathing periods should be separated by five-minute air breaks to minimize the potential for oxygen toxicity.

Three oxygen treatments are administered and evenly spaced over the first 24 hours. For seriously ill patients, the first two treatments are given with only two-hour surface interval. After the first 24 hours, two treatments are given every 24 hours, until toxic signs and symptoms have abated. This usually requires seven treatments, but in no case should fewer than five treatments be administered.

Following each treatment, the patient can be decompressed directly to the surface since the excess oxygen that he or she was administered prevented the uptake of excess nitrogen into the bloodstream. Unlike the patient, the attendants inside the chamber must follow a conservative decompression schedule, such as a variant of the standard U.S. Navy Oxygen Decompression Tables, to avoid developing decompression illness.

Should symptoms of central nervous system oxygen toxicity develop during any of the treatments, the patient should be taken off 100% oxygen and allowed to breathe air for 15 minutes. Following this, the oxygen schedule should be resumed at the point of interruption, but the oxygen periods should be shortened to 20 minutes and include five-minute air breaks. The chamber pressure should also be decreased by 5 feet of seawater, but only after any convulsive diathesis has abated. If additional episodes of oxygen toxicity occur, the chamber pressure should be decreased by increments of 5 feet of seawater and the oxygen-breathing periods shortened, as needed.

In no case should the pressure be decreased to less than 49.5 feet of seawater or the oxygen-breathing periods shortened to less than 15 minutes. If these limits have been reached, and symptoms of oxygen toxicity continue, the treatment should be terminated. Any treatments that follow should not be attempted until a surface interval of at least eight hours has elapsed. In the event that anticonvulsive drugs are used to prevent the convulsive diathesis, there must be strict adherence to both time and depth limits, as described in the published protocols, to prevent central nervous system damage from continued oxygen administration.

FLUIDS, ELECTROLYTES, AND pH

The patient's fluid and electrolyte status must be monitored frequently and adjusted accordingly to maintain homeostatic conditions. It is particularly important to maintain a full intravascular volume to avoid peripheral vasoconstriction, optimize adequate circulation, and dilute and promote the elimination of both clostridial toxins and the toxic by-products of tissue breakdown. Since the pulse rate will typically be elevated by clostridial toxins, it cannot be used to evaluate the patient's fluid status. One must rely on the central venous pressure (CVP), urinary output, and clinical signs, such as mucous membrane appearance and skin turgor. Adequate intravenous fluid should be given to maintain the CVP within the normal range and a urinary output of 80cc–100cc per hour.

In choosing the fluids for administration, the following details should be taken into consideration. The ratio of the quantity of crystaloid retained in the intravascular compartment to the quantity administered will approximate 1:4, while colloid will be retained on a 1:1 basis. Following aggressive debridement, particularly of the trunk, insensible fluid losses can increase by a factor of 3 or 4, even exceeding this estimate in the febrile patient. Alternating 0.9% NaCl with a balanced electrolyte solution such as Lactated Ringer's will optimize electrolyte balance while minimizing the chance of iatrogenic lactic acidosis. Finally, 1 liter of 5% glucose should be administered with every other liter of intravenous fluid for patients who do not receive oral nutrition to prevent catabolic metabolism and to stabilize the intravascular pH.

In the seriously ill patient, blood glucose, pH, and electrolyte status should be reevaluated every two hours. Appropriate treatments should be instituted immediately to correct any deviations from normal values. Acidosis, a common issue with critically ill patients, can occur rapidly and should be treated with intravenous bicarbonate. An early blood sugar determination must be performed to identify patients with potentially undiagnosed diabetes mellitus, a comorbidity commonly associated with gas gangrene. Even in patients with diabetes that is diagnosed and controlled, clostridial infections can precipitate diabetic ketoacidosis that must be identified and treated immediately.

Hyperkalemia is another significant issue for these patients and can result from both tissue breakdown and hemolysis. Elevated potassium levels can be controlled by administering an enema containing sodium polystyrene sulfonate cation resin or kayexalate. A single, 30- to 50-gram dose of kayexalate usually lowers the potassium level into the normal range and has a more predictable measurable outcome in the nondiabetic patient with gas gangrene compared to glucose and insulin, which can lower the threshold for central nervous system oxygen toxicity. When treating hyperkalemia, particular care must be taken not to avoid inducing hypokalemia, especially in the digitalized patient.

CARE OF PATIENTS BETWEEN HYPERBARIC OXYGEN TREATMENTS

Patients who are between hyperbaric oxygen treatments demand constant monitoring and frequent evaluation, both of which are best accomplished in an intensive care unit. If ventilatory assistance is required, it is extremely important to avoid treating patients with partial pressures of oxygen above ambient levels. When FIO_2 levels exceed 0.2 between hyperbaric oxygen treatments, patients are at increased risk for developing pulmonary oxygen toxicity. Patients should be maintained at ambient oxygen levels, unless their arterial oxygen tension falls below 65 mmHg, and the FIO_2 should be titrated to ensure adequate tissue oxygenation. Any changes in the patient's fluid, electrolyte, and immunologic status should also be addressed when determining the critically ill patient's oxygen demands, as these issues can significantly alter the blood pH and result in a compensatory shift of the oxygen dissociation curve.

In addition, positive end-expiratory pressure (PEEP) is frequently used to treat gas gangrene patients requiring ventilatory assistance either during or between hyperbaric oxygen treatments. This practice minimizes the chance of atelectasis secondary to a decrease in pulmonary surfactant that may result from pulmonary oxygen toxicity and/or ARDS.

HYPERBARIC OXYGEN TREATMENT PRIOR TO DEBRIDEMENT

Since providing hyperbaric oxygen treatments prior to surgical intervention has been shown to arrest the growth and spread of clostridial myonecrosis, it is recommended that patients receive at least two hyperbaric oxygen treatments before undergoing debridement. The benefits of this preoperative intervention include the improvement of the patient's overall clinical status and a decrease of both the intraoperative and the anesthetic risk. Administering hyperbaric oxygen therapy also establishes the line of demarcation between viable and nonviable tissue, which limits the amount of nonnecrotic tissue that is mistakenly excised. After the debridement is completed, the course of hyperbaric oxygen treatments should be performed along with the routine daily wound inspections. Additional debridement may be required until there is no evidence of necrotic tissue at the wound site. When all toxic signs and symptoms have abated, one final hyperbaric oxygen treatment should be given and the patient followed closely to monitor for reemergence of the clostridial infection. In the rare event of a clostridial reinfection, hyperbaric oxygen treatments should be reinstituted.

COMPLICATIONS

In addition to the physiological and biochemical management issues mentioned above, the following clinical issues are complications frequently experienced by patients with clostridial myonecrosis and require immediate identification and treatment.

ARDS

This complication is commonly seen following severe trauma and is characterized by poor alveolar gas exchange. ARDS is caused by inflammatory injury by damage to pulmonary capillaries or alveolar epithelium, resulting in acute or subacute pulmonary edema. Loss of pulmonary surfactant is part of the syndrome and can be compounded by microemboli from blood transfusions as well as pulmonary oxygen toxicity. As a protective measure, the use of blood transfusions and supplemental oxygen should be minimized between hyperbaric oxygen treatments.

Diagnosis is based upon arterial blood gas determinations that demonstrate inadequate alveolar gas exchange; radiographic abnormalities may be minimal or absent. Treatment consists of correction of the initiating cause, adequate fluid balance, and use of PEEP ventilation or, when necessary, continuous mechanical ventilation (CMV).

Disseminated Intravascular Coagulopathy (DIC)

This complication is the result of dysfunctional fibrinogen and platelet activity. It is often seen concomitantly with serious infections and has two primary clinical manifestations. The hemorrhagic type presents in patients as a bleeding diathesis and is due to a decrease in circulating platelets. The thrombotic type is characterized by the formation of platelet thrombi form in small vessels, leading to significantly decreased tissue perfusion at the arteriolar and capillary level. Generally, elements of both types are present in all cases of DIC since they share a common physiological pathway involving the conversion of fibrinogen to fibrin, fibrinolysis, an increase in platelet adhesion, and thrombocytopenia.

Making the diagnosis of DIC is based upon correlating the patient's history and clinical status with laboratory analysis, including fibrinogen levels, platelet counts (below normal), and the level of fibrin-split products (a fourfold increase is diagnostic). Treatment is based on rapid correction of the underlying disorder. While there are still no controlled studies that have demonstrated an improvement in outcome by directly treating the resulting coagulopathy, heparin may be administered intravenously by infusion pump at a dose of 500 units per hour, if the underlying cause of DIC can be controlled within 48 to 72 hours of onset.

After heparin has been infused for two hours procoagulant replacement can be administered safely. Two to three units of fresh frozen plasma and four to eight units of platelets will provide an adequate amount of procoagulants.

Oliguria and Acute Renal Failure (ARF)

While not commonly seen in gas gangrene, renal impairment can occur and must be adequately managed. In many oliguric patients, the toxic process can be reversed with hyperbaric oxygen, resulting in the reestablishment of normal renal function. If oliguria progresses to acute renal failure, treatment should focus on maintaining fluid and electrolyte balance. Dialysis should be considered when the patient's fluid and electrolyte status cannot be managed conservatively. Acute renal failure is not a contraindication to initiating or continuing hyperbaric oxygen therapy.

Myocardial Irritability

Several clostridial exotoxins have cardiotoxic side effects that can result in significant myocardial irritability, especially in children. Common dysrhythmias that have been seen in both adults and children include wandering atrial pacemaker, atrial tachycardia, nodal rhythms, unifocal and multifocal premature ventricular contractions, ventricular tachycardia, and ventricular fibrillation.

These patients should receive continuous cardiac monitoring during the course of their illness to rapidly identify and treat the arrhythmias, while simultaneously undergoing detoxification to prevent additional complications. Iatrogenically-induced arrythmias have been associated with the introduction of CVP catheters, but this complication can be prevented by not allowing the catheter to enter the right atrium.

The action of hyperbaric oxygen in decreasing the toxin load appears to be adequate treatment for most supranodal arrhythmias. In more severe arrhythmias or scenarios where cardiac function is significantly compromised, specific cardio-pharmacologic agents should be used without hesitation, including rapid digitalization of patients in cardiac failure.

Deep Vein Thrombosis (DVT)

Any patient immobilized for a prolonged period of time is in danger of developing deep vein thrombosis, particularly of the lower extremities. This danger is increased in the patient who has suffered traumatic injury to the lower extremities, recently undergone surgery, or has preexisting inadequate lower-extremity venous drainage.

Low-dose heparin and low-molecular-weight heparin are two commonly used pharmacologic modalities for preventing deep vein thrombosis. A traditional low-dose heparin schedule consists of the subcutaneous administration of 5,000 units of heparin every 8–12 hours. Low-molecular-weight heparin, such as enoxaparin, is administered at a dose of 30 mg subcutaneously every 12 hours, and is shown to be much less likely to induce immune-mediated, or heparin-induced, thrombocytopenia than unfractionated heparin.[182] In addition, injured extremities should be elevated to avoid complications from dependent edema, and all dressings should be carefully applied to ensure that gentle, even pressure is applied from the foot to the thigh.

Fat Embolism

This complication can be seen following injuries involving fractures of long-bones. It is a particular hazard in the gas gangrene patient who is frequently moved from the intensive care unit to the hyperbaric chamber. Immobilization of the involved extremity will minimize the risk of this disorder. There is still no proven treatment for fat embolism, although corticosteroids, maintenance of adequate intravenous fluids, and PEEP are often used as adjunctive therapies.

Secondary to clostridial gas gangrene as well is arterial gas embolism (AGE). Emboli, or lack of blood supply to vessels or arteries, can cause gangrene, especially in divers, as AGE is associated with air bubbles blocking blood flow.[(75,126)]

CONCLUSIONS

While proper care of traumatic and surgical wounds can lessen the incidence of gas gangrene, it has become apparent that the disease is resistant to total eradication. No longer solely a disease of combat, it is now a real and serious threat to patients who suffer injuries in an increasingly violent and high-speed civilian society.

The devastating nature of gas gangrene created a primary need for decisive, aggressive surgical intervention directed toward stopping the potentially rapid spread of an established clostridial process. Early cases could only be treated with radical amputations and mutilating flaying procedures, and despite its profound impact on a wide variety of medical and surgical issues, the advent of antibiotic therapy had very little impact on the surgical approach to treating clostridal myonecrosis. The efficacy of hyperbaric oxygen, as originally demonstrated in the Netherlands in the early 1960s, was destined to ultimately be recognized by the medical community. Despite several decades of dogmatic resistance, the medical and surgical communities have accepted the early use of hyperbaric oxygen as an effective weapon for treating this potentially fatal disease. Though still a surgical disorder, radical surgical intervention is no longer the only tool available for the successful treatment of gas gangrene. The success of hyperbaric oxygen at rapidly detoxifying patients allows surgeons to operate with far less risk while minimizing the morbidity associated with aggressive debridement.

Despite its utility in controlling the proliferation of clostridial organisms and the elaboration of their toxins, hyperbaric oxygen therapy should not be considered a definitive treatment for clostridial myonecrosis. These patients pose multi-organ, intensive-care problems throughout the course of their disease that can test the abilities of the most astute physician. Only a thorough and coordinated approach to diagnosis, maintenance, monitoring, prevention, and therapy, such as the one presented in this chapter, can result in successful treatment of this disease.

REFERENCES

1. Altemeier WA. Diagnosis, classification, and general management of gas producing infections, particularly those produced by *Clostridium perfringens*. In: Brown IW Jr, Cox BG, editors. Proceedings of the Third International Conference of Hyperbaric Medicine. Washington (DC): National Academy of Science-National Research Council Publication 1404; 1966. p. 481.
2. Altemeier WA, Fullen WD. Prevention and treatment of gas gangrene. JAMA. 1971; 217:806.
3. Alvis HJ. Hyperbaric oxygen therapy of gas gangrene. JAMA. 1971;218:445.
4. Alvis HJ. What hyperbaric medicine has to offer the industrial physician. J Occup Med. 1967;9:304-7.
5. Asmuth DA, Olson RD, Hackett SP, et al. Effects of *Clostridium perfringens* recombinant and crude phospholipase C and theta toxins on rabbit hemodynamic parameters. J Infect Dis. 1995;172:1317.
6. Assadian O, Assadian A, Senekowitsch C, et al. Gas gangrene due to *Clostridium perfringens* in two injecting drug users in Vienna, Austria. Wien Klin Wochenschr. 2004 Apr 30;116 (7-8):264-7.
7. Awad MM, Bryant AE, Stevens DL, Rood JI. Virulence studies on chromosomal alpha-toxin and theta toxin mutants constructed by allelic exchange provide genetic evidence for the essential role of alpha-toxin in *Clostridium perfringens*-mediated gas gangrene. Mol Microbiol. 1995;15:191-202.
8. Awad MM, Ellemor DM, Boyd RL, et al. Synergistic effects of alpha-toxin and perfringolysin O in *Clostridium perfringens*-mediated gas gangrene. Infect Immun. 2001 Dec;69(12):7904-10.
9. Baffes TG and Agustsson MH. Changing concepts in hyperbaric oxygen therapy. Dis Chest. 1966;49:83-8.
10. Bagdade JD. Infection of diabetes, predisposing factors. Postgrad Med. 1976;59:160-4.
11. Bahr R and Koslowski L. Hyperbaric oxygenation in gas gangrene therapy. Helv Chir Acta. 1977;44:431-8.
12. Balldin U, Hedstrum SA, Lundgren C. Cases of gas gangrene treated with hyperbaric oyxgen. Nord Med. 1968;79:589-91.
13. Barr PO and Dunner H. Hyperbaric oxygen therapy. Läkartidningen. 1970;67:3538-9.
14. Bayliss GJ and Cass C. Hyperbaric oxygen used in the treatment of gas gangrene. Med J Aust. 1967;2:991-3.
15. Beavis JP and Watt J. Hyperbaric oxygen therapy in the treatment of gas gangrene. J R Nav Med Serv. 1970;56:26-38.
16. Bebenerd J. The hyperbaric oxygen therapy in gas gangrene infections in gynecology. Gynaeckol Rundsch. 1969;7:235-40.
17. Belokurov Yu, Kamennyy AN, Mormytko AS, et al. Treatment of anaerobic infection using hyperbaric oxygenation. Vestn Khir. 1970;105:137-8.
18. Bernhard WF, Filler RM. Hyperbaric oxygenation: current concepts. Am J Surg. 1968;115:661-8.
19. Bes JC, Deidier C, Baulieux J, et al. Gas gangrene after rupture of the humeral artery. Temporary by-pass on the third day. Lyon Chir. 1972;68:198-9.
20. Bhargava SK, Chopdar A. Gas gangrene panophthalmitis. Br J Ophthalmol. 1971;55:136-8.

21. Blaise G, Noel F, Lamy M. Treatment of gas gangrene. Interest in hyperbaric oxygen therapy. Acta Anesthesiol. 1977;28:41-52.

22. Blenkarn GD. Hyperbaric therapy: report of its utilization at the Toronto General Hospital. Can Med Assoc J. 1970;102:951-6.

23. Boccaletti E, Nofrini U, Josi G., et al. Hyperbaric oyxgen therapy and its clinical uses. Policlinico Prat. 1966:1157-70.

24. Boenicke L, Maier M, Merger M, et al. Retroperitoneal gas gangrene after colonoscopic polypectomy without bowel perforation in an otherwise healthy individual: report of a case. Langenbecks Arch Surg. 2006 Apr;391(2):157-60. Epub 2006 Feb 8.

25. Bristow JH, Kassar B, Sevel D. Gas gangrene panophthalmitis treated with hyperbaric oyxgen. Br J Ophthalmol. 1971;55:139-42.

26. Brown PW, Kinman PB. Gas gangrene in a metropolitan community. J Bone Jt Surg. 1974;56:1445-51.

27. Brummelkamp WH, Hoogendijk J, Boerema I. Treatment of anaerobic infections (clostridial myositis) by drenching the tissue with oxygen under high atmospheric pressure. Surgery. 1961;49:299-302.

28. Brummelkamp WH. Treatment of anaerobic infections with hyperbaric oxygen. In: Brown IW Jr, Cox BG, editors. Proceedings of the Third International Conference on Hyperbaric Medicine. Washington (DC): National Academy of Science-National Research Council Publication 1404; 1966. p. 492.

29. Brummelkamp WH. Treatment of infections due to anaerobic germs by inhalation of hyperbaric oxygen. Ann Chir Thorac Cardiovasc. 1966;5:607-10.

30. Bryant AE, Chen RY, Nagata Y, et al. Clostridial gas gangrene. I. Cellular and molecular mechanisms of microvascular dysfunction induced by exotoxins of *Clostridium perfringens*. J Infect Dis. 2000;182:799-807.

31. Bryant AE, Chen RY, Nagata Y, et al. Clostridial gas gangrene. II. Phospholipase C-induced activation of platelet gpIIbIIIa mediates vascular occlusion and myonecrosis in *Clostridium perfringens* gas gangrene. J Infect Dis. 2000;182:808-15.

32. Cantillo W, Rojas L. Postabortion septicemia caused by Clostridium welchii: Report of 4 cases. Rev Colomb Obstet Ginecol. 1971;22:247-55.

33. Caplan ES, Kluge RM. Gas gangrene. Arch Intern Med. 1976;136:788-91.

34. Charon P, Duthois S. Fatal gas gangrene after intramuscular injection. Nouv Presse Med. 1972;1:109.

35. Chowdhury PS, Timmis SB, Marcovitz PA. *Clostridium perfringens* within intracardiac thrombus: a case of intracardiac gas gangrene. Circulation. 1999 Nov 16;100(20):2119.

36. Colwill MR, Maudsley RH. The management of gas gangrene with hyperbaric oxygen therapy. J Bone Joint Surg. 1968;50:732-42.

37. Cooke JN. Hyperbaric oxygen treatment in the Royal Air Force. Proc R Soc Med. 1971;64:881-2.

38. Darke SG, King AM, Slack WK. Gas gangrene and related infection: classification, clinical features and aetiology, management and mortality. A report of 88 cases. Br J Surg. 1977;64:104-12.

39. Davis JC, Dunn JM, Hagood CO, et al. Hyperbaric medicine in the U.S. Air Force. JAMA. 1973;224:205-9.

40. de Virgilio C, Klein S, Chang L, et al. Clostridial bacteremia: implications for the surgeon. Am Surg. 1991 Jun;57(6):388-93.

41. DeHaven KE, Evarts CM. The continuing problem of gas gangrene: a review and report of illustrative cases. J Trauma. 1971;11:983-91.

42. Demello FJ, Haglin JJ, Hitchcock CR. Comparative study of experimental *Clostridium perfringens* infection in dogs treated with antibiotics, surgery, and hyperbaric oxygen. Surgery. 1973;73:936-41.

43. Demello FJ, Hashimoto T, Hitchcock CR, et al. The effect of hyperbaric oxygen on the germination and toxin production of *Clostridium perfringens* spores. In: Wada J, Iwa T, editors. Proceedings of the Fourth International Congress on Hyperbaric Medicine. Tokyo: Igaku Shoin Ltd.; 1970. p. 276.

44. Desfemmes C, Metrot J, Boussignac G, et al. Treatment of gas gangrene with hyperbaric oxygenation. Parenteral hyperalimentation, antibiotic and heparin therapy and surgery. Apropos of 17 cases. Ann Anesthesiol Fr. 1974;15:249-67.

45. Dieminger HJ, Braune M. On the therapy of postabortal gas gangrene infection. Zentralb Gynaekol. 1967;89:484-8.

46. Dikshit SK, Mehrotra SN. Gas gangrene of the lower limb following femoral venepuncture. J Trop Med Hyg. 1968;71:162-4.

47. Dolatkowski A. The necessity for organizing hospital centers dispensing oxygen hyperbaric treatment. Pol Tyg Lek. 1975;30:315-7.

48. Dominguez AA, De Miguel GF, Grande MM, et al. Personal experience in the treatment of gas gangrene using hyperbaric oxygenation. Rev Esp Anestesiol Reanim. 1969;16:545-7.

49. Dominiguez, AA, Garcia FA, Diaz AM. A case of gas gangrene caused by Clostridium treated with hyperbaric oxygen. Rev Esp Anestesiol Reanim. 1968;15:674-6.

50. DuCailar J, Dossa J, Kienlen J, et al. Results of treatment of 20 gas gangrene patients with hyperbaric oxygenation. Ann Anesthesiol Fr. 1974;15:243-8.

51. DuCailar J, Lefebvre F, Roquefeuil B, et al. Indication for hyperbaric oxygen therapy in certain anoxic and infectious conditions. Maroc Med. 1970;50:378-82.

52. Duff JH, Shibata HR, Vanschaik L, et al. Hyperbaric oxygen: a review of treatment in eighty-three patients. Can Med Assoc J. 1967;97:510-5.

53. Durant CJ, Bailey AS. Hyperbaric oxygen in the treatment of gas gangrene. Radiography. 1971;37:61-4.

54. Dykes RG. Gas gangrene after hip nailing. Aust NZ J Surg. 1977;47:790-2.

55. Editorial. Gas gangrene and hyperbaric oxygen. Br Med J. 1972;3:715.

56. Editorial. Gas gangrene and hyperbaric oxygen. Br Med J. 1972;4:174-5.

57. Editorial. Hyperbaric oxygen. Lancet. 1968;1:336-8.

58. Ellemor DM, Baird RN, Awad MM, Boyd RL, Rood JI, Emmins JJ. Use of genetically manipulated strains of *Clostridium perfringens* reveals that both alpha-toxin and theta-toxin are required for vascular leukostasis to occur in experimental gas gangrene. Infect Immun. 1999 Sep;67(9):4902-7.

59. Eraklis AJ, Filler RM, Pappas AM, et al. Evaluation of hyperbaric oxygen as an adjunct in the treatment of anaerobic infections. Am J Surg. 1969;117:485-92.

60. Fowler DL, Evans LL, Mallow JE. Monoplace hyperbaric oxygen therapy for gas gangrene. JAMA. 1977;238:882-3.

61. Frichs G, Klepp G, Gollman K, et al. Hyperbaric oxygenation in the hospital, first experiences. Zentralbl Chir. 1975;100:321-31.

62. Gaylis H. Gas gangrene and intramuscular injection. Br Med J. 1968;3:59-60.

63. Gazzaniga AB. Nontraumatic clostridial gas gangrene of the right arm and adenocarcinoma of the cecum: report of a case. Dis Colon Rectum. 1967;10:298-300.

64. Glenert J. Gas gangrene in the abdominal wall following gastrectomy. Nord Med. 1966;75:623-4.

65. Gorbach, SL. *Clostridium perfringens* and other clostridia. In: Gorbach SL, Bartlett JG, Blacklow NR, editors. Infectious diseases. Philadelphia (PA): WB Saunders; 1992. p. 1587.

66. Greiner PM. Clostridial infection following appendectomy. J Am Osteopath Assoc. 1973;72:909-12.

67. Gunter V. Gas gangrene treated by hyperbaric oxygen. Nurs Times. 1969;65: 526-8.

68. Hahnloser P. Hyperbaric oxygenation. Schweiz Med Wochenschr. 1966;96:1462-3.

69. Hallagan LF, Scott JL, Horowitz BC, Feied CF. Clostridial myonecrosis resulting from subcutaneous epinephrine suspension injection. Ann Emerg Med. 1992 Apr;21(4):434-6.

70. Halpern AA, Jameson RM, Nagel DA, et al. Nontraumatic embolic clostridial gas gangrene: involvement of an extremity associated with endoscopy. West J Med. 1978;129:141-5.

71. Hamburger S, Zaltse H. Early diagnosis of biliary Clostridium welchii during cholecystectomy. Harefuah. 1972;82:553-4.

72. Hart GB, Cave RH, Goodman DB, et al. Clostridial myonecrosis: the constant menace. Milit Med. 1975;140:461-3.

73. Hart GB, O'Reilly RR, Cave RH, et al. The treatment of clostridial myonecrosis with hyperbaric oxygen. J Trauma. 1974;14:712-5.

74. Harvey PW, Purnell GV. Fatal case of gas gangrene associated with intramuscular injection. Br Med J. 1968;1:774-6.

75. Hayden SR, Buford KC, Castillo EM. Accuracy of a SET of screening parameters developed for the diagnosis of arteria gas embolism: the SANDHOG criteria. J Emerg Med. 2015 Nov;49(5):792-8.

76. Hedström SA. Differential diagnosis and treatment of gas producing infections. Acta Chir Scan. 1975;141:582-9.

77. Hedström SA. Ten cases of gas gangrene treated with hyperbaric oxygen. Nord Med. 1970;84:989.

78. Heimbach RD, Boerema I, Brummelkamp WH, Wolfe WG. Current therapy of gas gangrene. In: Davis JC, Hunt TK, editors. Hyperbaric oxygen therapy. Bethesda (MD): Undersea Medical Society, Inc.; 1977. p. 153.

79. Heimbach RD, Davis JG, Davis JC, et al. Hyperbaric medicine in the U.S. Air Force. Aeromed Rev. 1976;6:3-22.

80. Hill GB, Osterhout S. In vitro and in vivo effects of hyperbaric oxygen on *Clostridium perfringens*. In: Brown IW Jr, Cox BG, editors. Proceedings of the Third International Conference on Hyperbaric Medicine. Washington (DC): National Academy of Science-National Research Council Publication 1404; 1966. p. 538.

81. Hill GB, Osterhout S. Experimental effects of hyperbaric oxygen on selected clostridial species. II. In vitro studies in mice. J Infect Dis. 1972;125:26.

82. Hitchcock CR, Bubrick MP. Gas gangrene infections of the small intestine, colon and rectum. Dis Colon Rectum. 1976;19:112-9.

83. Hitchcock CR, Demello FJ, Haglin JJ. Gas gangrene: new approaches to an old disease. Surg Clinics N Amer. 1975;55:1403-10.

84. Hitchcock CR, Haglin JJ, Arnar O. Treatment of clostridial infections with hyperbaric oxygen. Surgery. 1967;62:759-69.

85. Hoffman S, Katz JF, Jacobson JH. Salvage of lower limb after gas gangrene. Bull NY Acad Med. 1971;7:40-9.

86. Holland JA, Hill GB, Wolfe WG, et al. Experimental and clinical experience with hyperbaric oxygen in the treatment of clostridial myonecrosis. Surg. 1975;77: 75-84.

87. Hommelgaard P, Kolind-Sorenson V. Gas gangrene treated with hyperbaric oxygen. Ugeskr Laeger. 1974;136:1073-5.

88. Howell LM. Hyperbaric oxygen in gas gangrene. Northwest Med. 1969;68:1016-9.

89. Hyperbaric oxygen therapy. Med Lett Drugs Ther. 1971;13:29-32.

90. Hyperbaric oxygen therapy. Med Lett Drugs Ther. 1978;20:51-2.

91. Irvin TT, Donaldson AJ, Smith G. Clostridium welchii infection in gastric surgery. Surg Gynecol Obstet. 1967;124:77-81.

92. Irvin, TT. Gas gangrene and hyperbaric oxygen. Br Med J. 1972;4:47.

93. Jackson RW, Waddell JP. Hyperbaric oxygen in the management of clostridial myonecrosis (gas gangrene). Clin Orthop. 1973;96:271-6.

94. Jacobsen A, Secher O. Hyperbaric oxygenation: clinical results and experiences in hyperbaric oxygenation in the individual pressure chamber. Ugeskr Laeger. 1967;129:822-8.

95. Johnson JT, Gillespie TE, Cole JR, et al. Hyperbaric oxygen therapy for gas gangrene in war wounds. Am J Surg. 1969;118:839-43.

96. Kakande I. Gas gangrene following an injection. East Afr Med J. 1977;54:434-7.

97. Kaye D. Effect of hyperbaric oxygen on Clostridia in vitro and in vivo. Proc Soc Exp Biol Med. 1967;124:360-6.

98. Kelley HG Jr, Pace WG 3rd. Treatment of anaerobic infections in mice with high pressure oxygen. Surg Forum. 1962;14:46.

99. Keogh AJ. Clostridial brain abscess and hyperbaric oxygen. Postgrad Med J. 1973;49:64-6.

100. Kindwall EP. Gas gangrene: acute medical emergency: the role of hyperbaric oxygen. Wis Med J. 1970;69:261-3.

101. Kitamoto H. Hyperbaric oxygen therapy. Naika. 1965;16:78-80.

102. Kokame GM, Olinde HD, Krementz ET, et al. Gas gangrene: successful treatment with hyperbaric oxygenation. J La State Med Soc. 1967;119:193-8.

103. Kole W, Mose JR, Ratzenhofer M. Gas gangrene caused by war injury—28 years later fatal gas gangrene following cholecystectomy. Zentralbl Chir. 1973;98:926-31.

104. Kucher R, Riedel W. Treatment of gas gangrene in hyperbaric oxygen chamber. Wien Klin Wochenschr. 1969;81:308-10.

105. Lacey CG, Futoran R, Morrow CP. *Clostridium perfringens* infection complicating chemotherapy for choriocarcinoma. Obstet Gynecol. 1976;47:337-41.

106. Lambertsen CJ. Oxygen in the therapy of gas gangrene. J Trauma. 1972;12:825-7.

107. Lamy M, Lejeune G, Noel FX, et al. Gas gangrene: importance of early diagnosis and hyperbaric oxygen therapy. Rev Med Liège. 1977;32:589-93.

108. Lamy ML, Hanquet MM. Hyperbaric oxygen therapy in a monoplace chamber with pure oxygen. Experience in 700 clinical cases. Maroc Med. 1971;51:602-10.

109. Larcan A, Laprevote-Heully, Lambert H, et al. Gas gangrene on the basis of 19 observations. Advantages of combining surgery with hyperbaric oxygen therapy. Mater Med Pol. 1974;6:116-9.

110. Larcan A, Laprevote-Huelly MC, Fieve G, et al. Gas gangrene, apropos of 24 cases. Value of combined surgical and hyperbaric oxygen therapy. Ann Chir. 1974;28:445-54.

111. Long WB 3rd, Howatson A, Gill W. Marlex mesh in gas gangrene. J Trauma. 1976;16:948-53.

112. Lorber B. Gas gangrene and other Clostridium-associated diseases. In: Mandell GL, Bennett JE, Dolin R, editors. Principles and practice of infectious diseases. 6th ed. Philadelphia (PA): Churchill Livingstone; 2005. p.2828.

113. MacGregor KH. Gas gangrene complicating surgery of the colon: report of two cases. Dis Colon Rectum. 1965;8:431-6.

114. MacLennan JD. The histotoxic clostridial infections in man. Bacteriol Rev. 1962;26:177-276.

115. Maguire WB, Langley NF. Gas gangrene following an adrenaline-in-oil injection into the left thigh with survival. Med J Aust. 1967;1:973-5.

116. Maretic Z, Kuze-Capar Z, Srketic M, et al. Gas gangrene following criminal abortion. Med Klin. 1969;64:2186-9.

117. Maudsley RH, Arden GP. Gas gangrene and hyperbaric oxygen. Br Med J. 1972;4:362.

118. Maudsley RH. Proceedings: post-operative gas gangrene managed by hyperbaric oxygen. J Bone Joint Surg Br. 1975;57:251.

119. McDonald DF. Adjunctive treatment of life-threatening emergencies with oxygen under high pressure. Tex Med. 1976.

120. Meijne NG, Mellink HM, Kox C. The main present-day indications for clinical treatment in a hyperbaric chamber. Pneumonologie. 1973;149:173-80.

121. Meijne NG. Hyperbaric oxygen, increased pressure and the activities in this field in Boerema's department in the period 1956-1972. Arch Chir Neerl. 1973;25:195-213.

122. Momm F, Schafer O, Henke M. Metastatic breast cancer causing gas gangrene. J Pain Symptom Manage. 2006 May;31(5):385.

123. Monafo WW, Brentano L, Gravens DL, et al. Gas gangrene and mixed clostridial infections of muscle complicating deep thermal burns. Archives of Surgery. 1966;92:212-21.

124. Monies-Chass I, Altman, Joachims HZ, et al. Treatment of gas gangrene of the neck by hyperbaric oxygen. Harefuah. 1973;84:538-40.

125. Monies-Chass I, Joachims HZ, Altman MM. Hyperbaric oxygen in anaerobic infection of the mediastinum. J Laryngol. 1975;89:1147-50.

126. Moon RE. Hyperbaric oxygen treatment for air or gas embolism. Undersea Hyperb Med. 2014 Mar-Apr;41(2):159-66.

127. Morton A. Testicular gas gangrene after hernia repair with cord division. Med J Aust. 1967;2:605-6.

128. Mukai T, Nishoika T, Uyama A. Acute peritonsillitis followed by gas phlegomon in the neck in a diabetic. J Otolaryngol JPN. 1975;78:1177-83.

129. Mzabi R, Himal HS, Maclean LD. Gas gangrene of the extremity: the presenting clinical picture in perforating carcinoma of the caecum. Br J Surg. 1975;62:373-4.

130. Nahir AM, Hasmonai M, Merzbach D, et al. Gas gangrene: following intramuscular injection of aqueous solution. N.Y. State J Med. 1978;78:1948-9.

131. Nahir AM, Scharf J, Merzbach D, et al. Gas gangrene following intramuscular injection. Harefuah. 1971;81:502.

132. Nali MN. Fatal gas gangrene after intramuscular injection; apropos of a case. Union Med Can. 1977;1400-1.

133. Ney R, Podlesch I, Buchard A, et al. "ndications for active surgical procedures within the area. Hyperbaric oxygen therapy for gas edema. Experiences with 42 gas edema infections. Tidsskr Nor Laegeføren. 1971;91:766-71.

134. Nichols RL, Smith JW. Gas in the wound: what does it mean? Surg Clin North Am. 1975;55:1289-96.

135. Nier H, Sailer R, Palomba P. Hyperbaric oxygen treatment in gas gangrene. Dtsch Med Wochenschr. 1978;103:1958-60.

136. Nini W, Nini N, Assouad I. A case of fatal fulminating gas gangrene complicating surgery of acute appendicitis. Chirurgie. 1970;96:174-7.

137. Nora PF, Bransfield J, Cheslak F, et al. H.P.O. in clostridial toxicity and strangulation obstruction. Arch Surg. 1966;93:236.

138. Patchell RD. Clostridial myonecrosis of the postpartum uterus with radiologic diagnosis. Obstet Gynecol. 1978;51(Suppl):145-55.

139. Prabhakar MJ, Redding ME, Anagnostopoulos CE, et al. Gas gangrene complicating aortic dissection. Report of a case. Arch Surg. 1971;103:96-7.

140. Ratner GL, Nenashev AA, Svechnikova EL, et al. Treatment of anaerobic infection by hyperbaric oxygenation. Khirurgiya. (Moscow) 1971;47:39-44.

141. Rifkind D. The diagnosis and treatment of gas gangrene. Surg Clin N Amer. 1963;43:511-7.

142. Roding B, Groenveld PHA, Boerema I. Ten years of experience in the treatment of gas gangrene with hyperbaric oxygen. Surg Gynecol Obstet. 1972;134:579-85.

143. Rood JI. Virulence genes of *Clostridium perfringens*. Annu Rev Microbiol. 1998;52:333-60.

144. Rush JH. Clostridial infection in total hip replacement; a report of two cases. Aust NZ J Surg. 1976;46;45-8.

145. Sailer R, Juneman A, Ghazwinian R. Therapy of gas gangrene. Comparison of results of the standard and hyperbaric oxygen therapy. Med Klin. 1974;69:1620-5.

146. Saltzman HA. Hyperbaric oxygen. Med Clin North Am. 1967;51:1301-14.

147. Schaupp KL Jr, Pinto D, Valentine RJ. Hyperbaric oyxgen in therapy of gas gangrene: report of a case following induced abortion. Calif Med. 1966;105:97-101.

148. Schautz R. Hyperbaric oxygen therapy for gas gangrene. Dtsch Med Wochenschr. 1968;93:1328-30.

149. Schmauss AK, Bahrmann E. Gas and oedema producing infections today—still a challenge. Zentralbl Chir. 1977;102:120-9.

150. Schmauss AK, Bahrmann E, Fabian W. Gas gangrene therapy and hyperbaric oxygenation. Zentrabl Chir. 1973;98:912-25.

151. Schmauss AK. Gas gangrene following intramuscular injections. Z Aertzl Fortbild. 1974;68:41-7.

152. Schonfelder M. Gas gangrene after common bile duct exploration. Zentralbl Chir. 1971;96:96-9.

153. Schraibman IG. Gas gangrene after amputation for peripheral vascular disease. Postgrad Med J. 1968;44:551-3.

154. Schulte JH. The use of hyperbaric oxygen in clinical medicine. J Occup Med. 1969;11:462-5.

155. Schuppisser JP. Gas gangrene. Langenbecks Arch Chir. 1979;348:1-5.

156. Schweigel JF, Shim SS. A comparison of the treatment of gas gangrene with and without hyperbaric oxygen. Surg Gynecol Obstet. 1973;139:969-70.

157. Skiles MS, Covert GK, Fletcher HS. Gas-producing clostridial and nonclostridial infections. Surg Gynecol Obstet. 1978;147:65-7.

158. Slack WK, Hanson GC, Chew HE. Hyperbaric oxygen in the treatment of gas gangrene and clostridial infection. A report of 40 patients treated in a single-person hyperbaric oxygen chamber. Br J Surg. 1969;56:505-10.

159. Slack WK. Hyperbaric oxygen therapy in anaerobic infections: gas gangrene. Proc R Soc Med. 1976;69:326-7.

160. Slack WK. Hyperbaric oxygen therapy in anaerobic infections. Med Times. 1978;06:15D(82)-16D(82), 21D(82).

161. Srivolocki WP, Nick WV, Pace WG. Gas gangrene treated by isolated perfusion with hyperbaric oxygenation. Surg Forum. 1970;21:231-2.

162. Stevens DL. Personal Communications.

163. Stevens DL, Musher DM, Watson DA, et al. Spontaneous, nontraumatic gangrene due to Clostridium septicum. Rev Infect Dis. 1990;12:286-96.

164. Stevens DL, Tweten RK, Awad MM, Rood JI, Bryant AE. Clostridial gas gangrene: evidence that alpha and theta toxins differentially modulate the immune response and induce acute tissue necrosis. J Infect Dis. 1997 Jul;176(1):189-95.

165. Stevens DL, Laine BM, Mitten JE. Comparison of single and combination antimicrobial agents for prevention of experimental gas gangrene caused by *Clostridium perfringens*. Antimicrob Agents Chemother. 1987; 31:312.

166. Stevens DL, Maier KA, Laine BM, Mitten JE. Comparison of clindamycin, rifampin, tetracycline, metronidazole, and penicillin for efficacy in prevention of experimental gas gangrene due to *Clostridium perfringens*. J Infect Dis. 1987;155:220.

167. Stevens DL, Maier KA, Mitten JE. Effect of antibiotics on toxin production and viability of *Clostridium perfringens*. Antimicrob Agents Chemother. 1987; 31:213.

168. Stevens DL, Titball RW, Jepson M, et al. Immunization with the C-Domain of alpha-toxin prevents lethal infection, localizes tissue injury, and promotes host response to challenge with *Clostridium perfringens*. J Infect Dis. 2004;190:767.

169. Stevens DL, Troyer BE, Merrick DT, et al. Lethal effects and cardiovascular effects of purified alpha- and theta-toxins from *Clostridium perfringens*. J Infect Dis. 1988;157:272.

170. Szekely O, Szanto G, Takats A. Hyperbaric oxygen therapy in injured subjects. Injury. 1973;4:294-300.

171. Tarbiat S. Results of combined surgical-antibiotic and hyperbaric oxygenation therapy in gas gangrene. Chirurg. 1970;41:506-11.

172. Taylor AR, Maudsley RH. Post-operative gas gangrene managed by early hyperbaric oxygen therapy (two cases). Proc R Soc Med. 1968;61:661.

173. Tenev K. Hyperbaric oxygen therapy and the treatment of anaerobic infections. Khirurgiia. (Sofia) 1975;28:154-9.

174. Thunold J, Gjengsto H, Smith-Silvertsen J. Hyperbaric oxygenation in the treatment of anaerobic gas forming infections. Tidsskr Nor Laegeføren. 1974;94:1069-73.

175. Thurston JG. Place of hyperbaric oxygen in intensive care. Proc R Soc Med. 1971;64:1287-8.

176. Tooley AH, Watt J. Hyperbaric oxygen therapy: review of the present position and experiences in the management of naval patients. J.R. Nav Med Serv. 1968;54:101-28.

177. Trippel OH, Ruggie AN, Stanley CJ, et al. Hyperbaric oxygenation in the management of gas gangrene. Surg Clin North Am. 1967;47:17-27.

178. Van Hook R, Vandervelde AG. Gas gangrene after intramuscular injection of epinephrine: report of fatal case [letter]. Ann Intern Med. 1975;83:669-70.

179. Van Unnik AJM. Inhibition of toxin production in *Clostridium perfringens* in vitro by hyperbaric oxygen. Antonie von Leeuwenhoek. 1965;31:181-6.

180. Van Zyl JJ. Gas gangrene, the modern therapeutic approach. S Afr J Surg. 1973;11:181-5.

181. Van Zyl JJW. Discussion of hyperbaric oyxgen. In: Brown IW Jr, Cox BG, editors. Proceedings of the Third International Conference on Hyperbaric Medicine. Washington (DC): National Academy of Science-National Research Council Publication 1404; 1966. p. 552.

182. Warkentin, TE, Levine, MN, Hirsh, J, et al. Heparin-induced thrombocytopenia in patients treated with low-molecular-weight heparin or unfractionated heparin. N Engl J Med. 1995; 332:1330.

183. Watt J. Surgical applications of hyperbaric oxygen therapy in the Royal Navy. Proc R Soc Med. 1971;64:877-81.

184. Wattel F, Gosselin B, Chopin C, et al. Current aspects of gas gangrene, apropos of 47 cases collected over a 3-year period (1974-1976). Ann Anesthesiol Fr. 1977;18:825-30.

185. Weinstein L, Barza MA. Medical intelligence: current concepts, gas gangrene. New Engl J Med. 1973;289:1129-31.

186. Wernitsch W. Technic and administration of hyperbaric oxygenation. Med Welt. 1969;49:2668-71.

187. Whatley RE, Zimmerman GA, Stevens DL, et al. The regulation of platelet activating factor production in endothelial cells. The role of calcium and protein kinase. C. J Biol Chem. 1989; 264:6325.

188. Williams JM. Fractured neck of femur and subsequent gas gangrene. Proc Pap Annu Conf Calif Mosq Control Assoc. 1966;34:63-4.

189. Williamson ED, Titball RW. A genetically engineered vaccine against the alpha-toxin of *Clostridium perfringens* protects mice against experimental gas gangrene. Vaccine. 1993;11:1253.

190. Willis AT. Clostridia of wound infection. London: Butterworth; 1969.

191. Yang Z, Hu J, Qu Y, Sun F, Leng X, Li H, Zhan S. Interventions for treating gas gangrene [review]. Cochrane Database Syst Rev. 2015 Dec 3;(12):CD010577.

192. Yeo CK, McNamara JJ. Retroperitoneal rupture of duodenum with complicating gas gangrene. Arch Surg. 1973;106:856-7.

193. Zierott G, May E, Harms H. Changes in the evaluation of therapy of gas edema through the administration of hyperbaric oxygenation. A clinical comparative study of 31 cases of gas edema. Bruns Beitr Klin Chir. 1973;220:292-6.

CHAPTER 18 CHAPTER

Selected Aerobic and Anaerobic Soft-Tissue Infections

CHAPTER EIGHTEEN OVERVIEW

Introduction 435
History 435
Classification 438
Etiology 438
Diagnosis 440
Clinical Picture and Bacteriology 441
Progressive Bacterial Gangrene 441
Necrotizing Fasciitis 443
Nonclostridial Myonecrosis 446
Therapy 447
Introduction 447
Progressive Bacterial Gangrene 448
Necrotizing Fasciitis 450
Nonclostridial Myonecrosis 454
References 456

Selected Aerobic and Anaerobic Soft-Tissue Infections

R. A. van Hulst, D. J. Bakker

INTRODUCTION

Necrotizing soft-tissue infections (NSTI) caused by aerobic, anaerobic, and mixed bacterial floras are an increasing problem in surgical and medical practice. They occur with increasing frequency and seriousness, especially in immune-compromised patients. The suppression of the immune system may be caused by underlying systemic diseases, mainly diabetes mellitus, malignancies, vascular insufficiency, and alcoholism; by the use of immunosuppressive drugs as in transplant recipients; and in drug addicts and in neutropenic patients.

These infections occur after trauma (sharp and blunt), around foreign bodies in surgical wounds, or even "spontaneously" as is seen sometimes in scrotal and penile necrotizing fasciitis (Fournier's gangrene). A large number of these infections have even been reported after a volcanic cataclysm[108] and also in children.[15,38,67,118,149,150]

Necrotizing fasciitis (NF) is also seen postoperatively, for example, after cesarean delivery in young women without risk factors (no diabetes or peripheral vascular disease),[56] after such "sterile" operations such as suction lipectomy, [61,139] and in Crohn's disease.[104] As in gas gangrene, every operation can be followed by necrotizing fasciitis, and a high index of suspicion is necessary for the diagnosis, especially after so-called "sterile" operations.

The clinical picture can vary considerably from patient to patient. Treatment is difficult, often irrational, and very often "one step behind the facts," because early recognition is difficult and etiology, bacteriology, and the clinical course are sometimes not well understood or are expected to evolve in a different and more favorable way.

Considerable morbidity occurs, and mortality can be very high, from 20% up to 70% or 80%. The highest mortality is found in the group of older, debilitated, diabetic patients with synergistic necrotizing cellulitis.[134]

HISTORY

For a proper understanding of these infections, a short historical review is necessary. In 1883, Jean Alfred Fournier, a French venereologist, described five cases of "gangrène foudroyante de la verge," later called Fournier's gangrene. Five healthy young men (ages 24–30 years) developed penile and/or scrotal gangrene, "spontaneously or after a superficial erosion, and despite large incisions and eschar excision, mortality was 60%."[52]

Even before that time, descriptions of the same clinical entity can be found in the works of Hippocrates from the fifth century BC. He described "erysipelas, which was at its worst when it reached the private parts, the pubes and the genitals. Flesh, sinews and bones fell away in large quantities."[64] After Hippocrates the first description of a possible case of necrotizing fasciitis came from Baurienne in 1764[16] in an adult, and thereafter a case in a young baby boy reported by Hebler in 1848.[59] Also the work by the Confederate Army Surgeon Joseph Jones must be mentioned, who described a variant of this disease in 1869 and 1870 during the Civil War in the United States, which he called "hospital gangrene."[69,114]

Extensive reviews of the literature on necrotizing soft-tissue infections including Fournier's gangrene have been published by McCrea,[94] Jones,[70] and Stevens,[124] as well as by Loudon,[87] Sutherland,[136] Chapnick and Abter,[28] Weiss and Lavardière,[145] Smith et al.,[123] Eke,[47] Capelli-Schellpfeffer and Gerber,[27] and also by Wienecke and Lobenhoffer.[148]

Meleney, in 1924, found the cause of this gangrene to be "a pure invasion of hemolytic streptococci."[97] Fournier's gangrene could thus be considered as a special form of hemolytic *streptococcus* gangrene. In the same article Meleney described this hemolytic *streptococcus* gangrene, or "Meleney's ulcer," also caused by hemolytic streptococci.[97] This publication was based on Meleney's experience in the Imperial Hospital in Peking (Beijing).

Cullen, also in 1924, gave a description of the so-called "postoperative progressive bacterial synergistic gangrene," in a patient after an appendectomy.[34]

At first a confusing variety of microorganisms was found. But in studying the spreading periphery of the lesion, both clinically and experimentally (in guinea pigs), the interaction of a microaerophilic nonhemolytic *streptococcus* and a hemolytic *staphylococcus aureus* was found to be synergistic.[21] The confusion in the nomenclature started here, because Meleney described Cullen's ulcer, and since then Meleney's and Cullen's ulcer were often regarded in the literature as the same disease. Sometimes this was even considered to be a variant of Fournier's gangrene. This confusion is clearly shown by Kingston and Seal, who stated that "this animal model of Brewer and Meleney (anaerobic *streptococcus* and *staphylococcus aureus*) was unrelated to the disease Meleney's postoperative synergistic gangrene, which it was developed to explain."[74]

From this historical review, it must be clear that Kingston and Seal refer to "Cullen's postoperative progressive bacterial synergistic gangrene" and call that "Meleney's gangrene." Brewer and Meleney described very clearly for the first time the very important mechanism of bacterial synergy for these infections. By "bacterial synergy" we mean that mixtures of organisms (two or more) can cause more severe infections than each of the organisms alone. This must be differentiated from the term "mixed infections," often with different aerobes and anaerobes, meaning that the net pathogenic effect is no greater than the sum of the damage caused by infection with each of the organisms alone.[21]

This bacterial synergism was the reason for Meleney to propose the first classification for these necrotizing soft-tissue infections with special reference to this phenomenon.[98-99] Meleney distinguished acute (for example hemolytic streptococcal gangrene) and chronic infectious skin gangrene, an example of the latter being postoperative progressive bacterial synergistic gangrene. Kingston and Seal base the conclusions in their article on the division of these infections into three different categories based on the rates of progression (from slow to rapid).(74)

Since 1926 a great variety of synergistic microorganisms both in humans and in animals have been found.(9)

The bacteriology of these diseases has apparently changed considerably through the years. Meleney mentioned "associated organisms next to streptococci, concomitants, not adding to the development of the disease, in a minority of cases."(97) Wilson found streptococci in 58% of his patients,(149) Crosthwait in 57%,(33) Ledingham and Tehrani in 8.5%,(81) and in our series we initially found streptococci in 13.3% of our patients.(9) When necrosis of the deep fascia was recognized as essential in hemolytic streptococcal gangrene or Meleney's ulcer in 1948 by Wilson, the disease was renamed "necrotizing fasciitis" in 1952.(149)

Giuliano et al.(55) thought that two bacteriologic types of necrotizing fasciitis could be recognized, and Lamerton(80) even suggested three bacteriologic groups whose clinical pictures, however, largely overlap. Also, many microorganisms were suggested as causing postoperative progressive bacterial synergistic gangrene throughout the years.(9)

The problem is that we seldom see patients at the onset of the disease. Time elapsed since the onset and initial treatment, for example antibiotics given and possible surgical interventions, are of course very important to explain later findings, especially later bacteriological culture results. Remarkably this is never mentioned in the literature either about necrotizing fasciitis or about progressive bacterial gangrene. Stone and Gorbach give a very detailed description of the microbiological findings without mentioning what we stated above.(135) Smith et al. wonder why normal urethral, rectal, and cutaneous flora of otherwise low to moderate virulence are able to cause severe infections of this type.(123) Maybe they do not. Is it possible that Meleney was right after all when he mentioned "concomitants, not adding to the development of the disease"?(97) Not every microorganism that is cultured is automatically causative to the disease. Another thing that is seldom mentioned is the location from where the cultures are taken. It can make a big difference if one takes a swab from the center of the wound or cultures tissue biopsies at the spreading periphery of the disease. Brewer and Meleney had already mentioned that in their first experiments on bacterial synergy.(21)

Interestingly a case of Fournier's gangrene was described where only *Candida* was cultured as the primary organism from the urine and later from perianal debrided tissues.(68)

In the spring of 1994, a cluster of seven cases of invasive group A streptococcal (GAS) infections, including four cases of necrotizing fasciitis, occurred in Gloucestershire, England. When the British media reported this outbreak, the stories resembled Edgar Allan Poe's horror stories at their best. Expressions like "flesh-eating bacteria or virus," "galloping gangrene," and "killer bugs" were used to describe the process, and the impression was given that a whole new disease was discovered there. From the historical review given above, it should be clear that this was not the case. A description of this outbreak can be found by Efstratiou et al.(46) and Monnickendam et al.(101) Kujath and Eckmann(79) state that only a minority of necrotizing fasciitis cases are caused by streptococci (three to four times less than cases caused by a polymicrobial flora). Podbielski et al(111) found 10%–18% group A streptococci and 51% "other" *streptococci* in their cultures of necrotizing fasciitis. In 75%–85%, peptostreptococci were isolated (peptostreptococci cause a gas-forming infection). Group A streptococci and staphylococci were cultured when only a monoculture was found. All other microorganisms that were found were part of a polymicrobial flora. In both articles, nothing is mentioned about the time of culture in relation to the time of onset of the disease and if the patients were previously treated already. This makes it very difficult to show what the real causative microorganisms are.

A historical review of streptococcal infections with special emphasis on necrotizing fasciitis and the use of hyperbaric oxygen is given by Bakker.(12) Our conclusion is that interpretation and misinterpretation of historical facts and microbiological culture results have caused confusion and have added to the present difficulty in understanding the bacteriology, etiology, and clinical findings in these soft-tissue infections.

CLASSIFICATION

An exact classification of necrotizing soft-tissue infections is difficult because the distinctions between many of the clinical entities are blurred, and a great variety of names have historically been given to the same clinical entity.

Classification of these infections is usually made on the following bases:

- The assumed causative microorganism(s)(51,55,57,80,97,113)
- The kind of tissue involved(2-3,51,81,84-85,149)
- The kind of required therapy(51)
- The rate of progression(74)
- The initial clinical findings(50)

Each of these classifications has its advantages and its disadvantages because each is based on only one part of the problem. It is difficult to determine the causative microorganism(s) out of the wide variety of aerobes and anaerobes that can be cultured in these infections, and it can be equally difficult to diagnose the tissue primarily involved in the advanced stages of these infections when we usually see the patients. The best therapy is almost always a combination of surgery, antibiotics, and adjunctive hyperbaric oxygen.

Also, in our experience the rate of progression of these infections can change considerably from patient to patient and seems to be more dependent on the associated diseases of the patient and/or other systemic or local factors that affect the immune status, metabolism, and local vascularisation than on other factors.(9,89)

Following Ledingham and Tehrani(81) we proposed the Amsterdam classification of soft-tissue infections (Figure 1), based on whether the infections are superficial (as in progressive bacterial gangrene) or involving deeper tissues (as in necrotizing fasciitis and myositis and myonecrosis).

ETIOLOGY

In these infections, anaerobic microorganisms are often found in combination with aerobic gram-negative organisms. With causes such as traumatic crush injury in the surgically or medically compromised patient, local tissue hypoxia and a decreased oxidation-reduction potential (Eh) is usually present, thus promoting the growth of anaerobic microorganisms. The vast majority of these necrotizing soft-tissue infections have an endogenous anaerobic component.

Hypoxic conditions also allow the proliferation of facultative aerobic organisms since polymorphonuclear leukocytes function poorly under decreased oxygen tensions. The growth of aerobic microorganisms further lowers the Eh; more fastidious

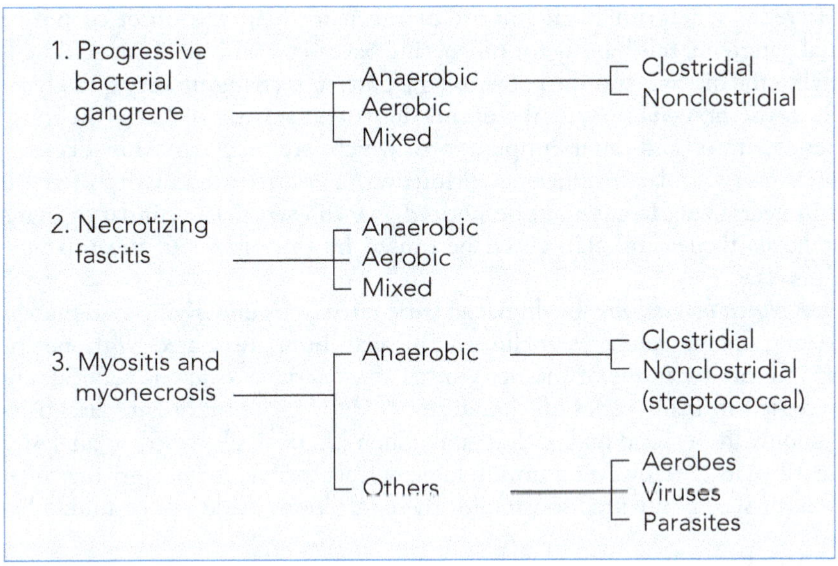

Figure 1. Amsterdam classification of soft-tissue infections. In order to systematize the classification (following Ledingham and Tehrani),[81] we divided these infections into three groups: (1) progressive bacterial gangrene, (2) necrotizing fasciitis, and (3) myositis and myonecrosis.

anaerobes become established, and the disease process can rapidly accelerate. Clinically the most important signs of these infections are tissue necrosis, a putrid discharge, gas production, the tendency of the process to burrow through fascial planes, and in many cases the absence of the classical signs of tissue inflammation.[89]

The variable quantity of gas in the tissues can be used in the differential diagnosis of these infections.[10,105-106] Carbon dioxide and water are the end products of aerobic metabolism; carbon dioxide rapidly dissolves and rarely accumulates in tissues. The major tissue gases found in mixed aerobic and anaerobic soft-tissue infections are probably H_2 and CH_4, less-water-soluble end products of incomplete oxidation of energy sources. Nitrogen and hydrogen sulfide can also be found.[106] Presence of these gases indicates a rapid bacterial multiplication at a low Eh. [82,106]

The etiology, in summary, in necrotizing soft-tissue infections is multifactorial and includes local and systemic factors as well as aerobic and anaerobic microorganisms. Even fungi have been found.[68,108]

1. *Local tissue trauma and bacterial invasion* follow operations such as abdominal surgery for intraperitoneal infections, drainage of ischiorectal and perianal abscesses, and minor and major traumatic lesions (blunt and sharp), and are also seen after intramuscular injections and intravenous infusions.

Initially, streptococci play an important role in necrotizing fasciitis, but very soon the bacteriologic pattern changes by colonization of the infected area and the use of antibiotics.

Much of the recent work by Stevens describes the rediscovered importance of streptococci, especially the invasive group A streptococci (GAS) in these diseases.[128-129] Also, Morantes mentions the return of an old nemesis in connection with streptococcal infections, when these infections are sometimes "rediscovered."[102] Bisno and Stevens[18] and Stevens[130] reviewed the streptococcal infections of skin and soft tissues.

Bacterial synergism is an important mechanism in the onset of progressive bacterial gangrene, but here again no specific bacterial combination could be found underlying the disease, and the bacteriologic pattern is changing very quickly as well.

2. *Local ischemia* frequently occurs in patients with diabetes mellitus and/or arteriosclerosis and after amputations which are necessary for diabetic and arteriosclerotic vascular insufficiency. Moreover, a relative avascularity of the fascial planes in necrotizing fasciitis can be noticed. We showed that secondary gangrene of subcutaneous tissues and skin could be caused by thrombosis of the subcutaneous blood vessels.[5]

3. *Reduced host defense*. In almost all patients, serious underlying systemic diseases are present, mainly diabetes mellitus. This has been associated with necrotizing fasciitis in other locations of the body other than perianal, such as cervical, and has been reported in many series of literature. [30,55,80-81,116,146] Necrotizing fasciitis occurs uncommonly in the head and neck region. Chen Lin et al. described an analysis of 47 cases in 12 years.[86] However, immunologic defects specific for necrotizing soft-tissue infections or specifically predisposing for these infections could not be found.[11]

DIAGNOSIS

The diagnosis of these infections must primarily be made on the macroscopic appearance of the diseased area which will be described below. The general condition of the patient, the clinical course of the disease, and the bacteriologic findings, unless in a very early stage, are not decisive in this respect. One has to realize that the classical local signs of tissue inflammation (rubor, calor, dolor, and tumor) are often absent. There are however, general signs including evidence of fever, elevated white blood cell count, and a severe systemic reaction.

Wall et al.[143] tried to develop a simple model to help distinguish necrotizing fasciitis from nonnecrotizing soft-tissue infections. They found that a white blood cell count (WBC) at admission above 15.4 x 10^9/l or a serum sodium Na lower than 135 mmol/l were useful parameters to distinguish between both infections. However, since 70% of their patients were intravenous (IV) drug users, an evaluation in other settings to prove the value of their model remains necessary.[95] A high index of suspicion and careful clinical examination is always necessary.

Locally, bulla, severe pain, rapid spread, and eventually gas formation can be seen. Gas-forming infections can be caused by both aerobic and anaerobic soft-tissue infections. A very useful algorithm or decision tree on gas-producing infections has been published by Nichols.[106] The initial diagnosis must be followed by immediate antibiotic and, if necessary, surgical therapy, with adjunctive hyperbaric oxygen in selected cases (see Therapy section of this chapter).

A gram stain is taken initially but provides less information than is necessary or hoped for, because the real causative microorganisms can only be found by culturing tissue biopsies from the spreading periphery of the lesion or from the deeper tissues that are reached only when surgical debridement is performed. An interesting publication by Ault et al. mentions a rapid streptococcal diagnostic kit, with which the authors were able to identify group A ß-hemolytic *Streptococcus pyogenes* as the presumptive causative microorganism in cases of NF.[5]

If the anatomic site of involvement is not clear, computed tomography (CT) scanning can provide this information[10] as well as sonography.[102] One must, however, not lose too much time in diagnosis before surgical therapy is started. The same goes for magnetic resonance imaging. Some find this useful for an early diagnosis;[42] others found the images by MRI nonspecific and conclude that the preoperative diagnosis must be based on the clinical picture and the evolution of the clinical status.[4]

In most patients, direct inspection or inspection of the fascia after an incision to the level of the deep fascia under local anesthesia is sufficient for determining the diagnosis; exploration and debridement under general anesthesia can follow immediately.

For a differential diagnosis on clinical signs, see Table 1. In rapidly spreading "closed" infections, needle aspiration and gram stain can provide more reliable information on the microbiological cause of the infection. It is a well-known fact that hemolytic bacteria (for example, streptococci) play an important role in these disease processes and do not grow in open wounds.[129,149]

CLINICAL PICTURE AND BACTERIOLOGY

Progressive Bacterial Gangrene

Progressive bacterial gangrene, originally described as postoperative progressive bacterial synergistic gangrene or Cullen's ulcer[34] and as chronic infectious skin gangrene,[98-99] is generally a slowly advancing infectious process involving the epidermis, the dermis, the subcutaneous tissue including lymphatic channels,[14,17] and hair follicles, but never the deep fascia (the fascial plane that envelops the muscle compartment).

Progressive bacterial gangrene includes

- anaerobic crepitant or clostridial cellulitis,[96]
- pyoderma gangrenosum,[26]
- erysipelas,[64]
- gangrenous or necrotizing erysipelas,[110]
- symbiotic gangrene,[108] and
- phagedena geometrica.[18]

Progressive bacterial gangrene is directly related to skin infection. Around the site of an injury or infection, cellulitis occurs with redness, edema, and a slight swelling, followed by a centrifugal necrosis of skin and subcutaneous tissues. This frequently capricious extension of necrosis is preceded by patchy, purplish discoloration of the skin. It is highly characteristic that the deep fascia, which envelops the muscle compartment, is never involved. Around the afflicted area, a 1–2 cm wide erythematous, raised border zone is present. The speed of the extension may vary from weeks or even months to a few hours. Fresh granulation tissue with re-epithelialization may occur in the center while the centrifugal spread of necrosis still proceeds. The area is always very painful.

Bacteriologically the cause can be anaerobic, as in crepitant *Clostridial cellulitis*, aerobic or mixed. Bacterial synergism plays an important role, but no specific combination can be held responsible for this disease. In order to find the causative microorganisms, one has to culture from the spreading periphery, preferably tissue biopsies, and not from the necrosis or the granulating center, where a great variety of concomitant microorganisms can be found that do not cause or add to the infection. The usual primary pathogens are group A streptococci (GAS) and *Staphylococcus aureus* (alone or in synergism). We found streptococci in 92% in needle aspirates or tissue biopsies in progressive bacterial gangrene followed by multiple other aerobic and anaerobic microorganisms such as *Bacteroides* species, *Clostridium* species, Enterobacteriaceae, coliforms, *Proteus*, and *Pseudomonas*.

Bacteroidaceae as *Bacteroides fragilis* are rarely seen as a single pathogen but always as part of a mixed polymicrobial flora. The role of Bacteroidaceae is not a direct one in causing soft-tissue infections, but it influences the immunology of the host in diminishing the interferon production and the phagocytic capacity of macrophages and polymorphonuclear neutrophil granulocytes. Clinically *Bacteroides fragilis* is often seen in combination with *Escherichia coli*.[100]

Anaerobic crepitant cellulitis involves clostridial and nonclostridial cellulitis and has often been misdiagnosed as gas gangrene. In general it is a more benign disease than gas gangrene. *Clostridia* can be found in pure culture, and there can be marked tissue necrosis but no involvement of the deep fascia or muscles is seen until it is in a very advanced stage. There can be abundant soft-tissue gas.

In cases of extensive soft-tissue damage or marked vascular insufficiency of an extremity, clostridial cellulitis can change into a true clostridial myositis with myonecrosis.

TABLE 1. CLINICAL SIGNS IN DIFFERENTIAL DIAGNOSIS OF NECROTIZING SOFT-TISSUE INFECTIONS

PARAMETERS ASSESSED	PROGRESSIVE BACTERIAL GANGRENE	
	PROGRESSIVE BACTERIAL SYNERGISTIC GANGRENE	ANAEROBIC CREPITANT OR CLOSTRIDAL CELLULITIS
Incubation	1-3 weeks	1 week
Onset	gradual	gradual/acute
Systematic toxicity	(plus or minus)	(plus or minus)
Pain	severe	moderate
Exudate	none or slightly serous	slight serous
Odor of exudate	foul	foul
Gas	may be present	abundant
Muscle	no change	no change
Skin	ulcer and gangrene	gangrene
Mortality	5-15%	5%
Treatment: [5,7,33,66]		
• **Surgery**	necrotomy and skin grafting	incision and drainage
• **Antibiotics**	yes (not always)	yes
• **Adjunctive hyperbaric oxygen (HBO2$_2$)**	yes (compromised host and systemic toxicity)	yes (compromised host and systemic toxicity)

Multiple aerobic and anaerobic organisms have been cultured including *Enterobacteriaceae*, *Clostridium* species, *Bacteroides* species, and *Peptostreptococcus* species.

In our experience, in over 90% of cases of progressive bacterial gangrene there are serious underlying systemic diseases, most frequently diabetes mellitus. Malignancies and arteriosclerosis were also found, but less frequently.

Necrotizing Fasciitis

Necrotizing fasciitis,[149] originally called hemolytic streptococcal gangrene, Meleney's ulcer, or acute dermal gangrene[97-98] is a progressive, generally rapidly spreading, inflammatory process located in the deep fascia with secondary necrosis of subcutaneous tissues and skin.

The speed of skin involvement is directly related and proportional to the thickness of the subcutaneous tissue layer. The infection tends to spread very rapidly along the deep fascial plane.

TABLE 1 (CONTINUED) *LeFrock and Molavi [82] and Mader [89]*

NECROTIZING FASCIITIS		MYOSITIS/MYONECROSIS
STREPTOCOCCAL AND MIXED (FOURNIER)	SYNERGISTIC NECROTIZING CELLULITIS	NON-CLOSTRIDIAL STREPTOCOCCAL
1-4 days	1-2 days	1-4 days
acute	acute	acute
+ +	+ + +	+
moderate to severe	severe	severe
profuse serosanguinous	dishwater pus profuse	none or slight
foul	foul	none
usually not present	may be present	not present
viable	viable to marked change later	change later
cellulitis + secondary gangrene	cellulitis + secondary gangrene	minimal change
35%	75%	25%
"fillet" procedure	"fillet" procedure	muscle removal
yes	yes	yes
yes (compromised host)	yes (compromised host)	yes (compromised host)

Necrotizing fasciitis includes

- Hospital gangrene,[69]
- Suppurative fasciitis,[93]
- Fournier's gangrene or disease,[52]
- Synergistic necrotizing cellulitis,[134] and
- Hemolytic streptococcal gangrene or Meleney's ulcer.[97]

Necrotizing fasciitis may start in a surgical wound, postoperatively; or may start after a trivial injury like an insect bite, an abrasion, or contusion; and may even show up spontaneously, in children.[15,38,81,97-98,150] Usually there is a sudden onset of pain and swelling at the site of or at a certain distance from the injury with a nonspecific redness, swelling, and edema. Initially the area may be very painful but later becomes numb and anesthetic. During the next hours and/or days, the redness rapidly spreads and the margins fade out into the normal skin but are not raised or very sharply outlined as seen in erysipelas.

These signs and symptoms are already secondary to the most pathognomonic feature, the fascial and subcutaneous necrosis. This necrosis manifests itself as an extensive undermining of the skin and subcutis. If there is an opening in the skin, probes or gloved fingers can be passed under the skin and subcutis. In case of intact skin, the only way for diagnosis is incision into the deep fascia. This can be done at the bedside under local anesthesia.

Once the incision is made, the yellowish-green necrotic fascia becomes visible, and after removal of this fascia, healthy, red, normal, bleeding muscle tissue is seen. If the fascia is left untouched, secondary involvement of the muscles with myositis and myonecrosis can be seen in a later phase. This must be prevented, if possible, by early incision and excision of all necrotic fascia ("fillet procedure").

Without treatment, a dusky discoloration of the skin appears as a small purple patch with irregular and initially ill-defined margins. This may occur at a certain distance from the injury or the operative wound. Identical patches may develop in the neighborhood which ultimately fuse and form a large plaque of gangrenous skin while the diffuse redness continues to spread. As a rule the patient is seriously ill: septic with a high fever.[131]

It is highly characteristic that the spread of the fascial necrosis is more extended than the visible changes of the skin. The apparently normal skin and subcutaneous tissue are loosened from the underlying necrotic fascia over a great distance from the original wound. Skin necrosis occurs secondary to thrombosis of subcutaneous blood vessels, and the whole area may become anesthetic by necrosis of nerve fibers.

In our series, the site of necrotizing fasciitis showed an equal distribution between trunk and extremities.[11] The head and neck were less frequently involved as described by Whitesides in a series of patients.[146]

Fournier's gangrene, or Fournier's disease,[52] in its original form as scrotal gangrene, is a form of necrotizing fasciitis. Careful observation shows that the process starts with necrosis of the scrotal fascia, tenderness, local edema, and redness of the scrotal skin. Very soon thereafter the skin becomes necrotic, and the diagnostic "black spot" can be seen. When the infectious process extends from the penal-scrotal region to the abdomen or upper legs, the characteristic picture of necrotizing fasciitis is seen. The scrotal subcutaneous layer is so thin that the majority of the patients are seen when the skin is already necrotic. In women, "Fournier's gangrene" is recognized less easily as necrotizing fasciitis because of the thicker subcutaneous layer. In the literature, however, Fournier's gangrene in women is more and more recognized.[44] Stephenson et al. describe 29 female patients with necrotizing fasciitis of the vulva. Twenty patients, or 69%, were diabetic, and the mortality in the diabetic patients was 78.6%.[133]

Synergistic necrotizing cellulitis has been described as a different clinical entity.[134] Because of the wide involvement of deeper tissues (necrosis of fascia and, in a later stage, but very rapidly thereafter, involvement of subcutaneous tissue and muscles as well) together with severe systemic toxicity, we consider this to be a form of necrotizing fasciitis. Mader considers this disease to be a nonclostridial myonecrosis.[89]

In our opinion the disease is the same, necrotizing fasciitis, but the clinical course of the disease differs from patient to patient, dependent on general condition, the immune status, age, associated systemic diseases, and the time elapsed from the beginning of the disease to the moment when the patient is first examined.

These infections are frequently located in the perianal region following improperly treated perianal and ischiorectal abscesses. About 75%–80% of the mainly elderly patients have diabetes mellitus. Diabetes mellitus, age, malnutrition, hypertension, and intravenous drug abuse have been recognized as considerable risk factors for mortality in necrotizing fasciitis.[53]

The simple facts that the patients were mainly elderly and that a high percentage of systemic sepsis was present in the series of Stone and Martin[134] may explain the unusually high mortality of 75%, compared with the mean mortality of 38.5% in a review of 15 reports including 272 patients [3] and 3% to 45% in the large review of 1,726 patients by Eke.[47]

There is confusion and uncertainty about the exact bacteriologic cause of NF. Meleney[97] described the disease as hemolytic streptococcal gangrene and considered the cause to be "a pure invasion of hemolytic streptococci." This bacteriologic pattern seems to have changed as described before.[9,33,81,149] Wilson was the first to consider the name "hemolytic streptococcal gangrene" inappropriate because in his patients hemolytic staphylococci were frequently cultured.[149]

Mader has stated that better culture techniques have demonstrated that *Streptococcus pyogenes* only occasionally causes these infections. This, however, cannot alter the fact that Meleney indeed found only streptococci, strongly suggesting at least an important role for this organism. Mader explains this by saying that although most infections are mixed aerobic and anaerobic, a type of necrotizing fasciitis caused solely by *Streptococcus pyogenes* has been reported.[89]

Careful bacteriologic techniques have shown anaerobes and aerobes: *Peptostreptococcus* species, *Bacteroides* species, *Fusobacterium* species together with *Streptococcus pyogenes, Staphylococcus aureus, Klebsiella pneumoniae, Pseudomonas aeruginosa, Enterobacteriaceae*. and even fungi.[14,30,48,55,68,80-82,151] Also *Clostridia* have been described in 90% of cases where Fournier's disease was accompanied by myositis. Again, from the description it is not clear if gas gangrene was involved. The same authors describe a large variety of microorganisms which, apparently, they all consider causal.[141] Even a very rare case of NF after blunt trauma caused by a penicillin-resistant *Streptococcus pneumoniae* is reported.[13] It is, however, still very difficult to distinguish the real causative microorganisms from the concomitants. Giuliano described two bacteriologic types of necrotizing fasciitis,[55] and Lamerton even suggested three different groups.[80] We could not confirm their findings in our patients.[11]

In our experience, a pure and very early case of Fournier's gangrene, still without skin necrosis, showed streptococci in pure culture after needle aspiration. We found the same in other early cases of necrotizing fasciitis.

The bacteriologic pattern changes during the clinical course of the disease and seems to be more dependent on the previous use of antibiotics, the extent and frequency of debridements, the use (or nonuse) of diverting colostomies, the age and immune status of the patient, and associated systemic diseases. These pattern changes make it difficult to show that the cultured bacteria can, with certainty, be declared to be causative.

Brunet et al.(132) published a study on a total of 81 patients with perineal gangrene. They advocate very systematic microbiological investigations from specific locations and repeat that after every operative debridement. They start with an antibiotic regimen directed against anaerobes, gram-positive cocci, and gram-negative bacilli. This regimen is changed when later culture results so indicate. They stress the importance of a systematic exploration of the ischiorectal fossae. We are convinced that for the onset of necrotizing fasciitis, streptococci play a very important role and that the reported changes in the bacteriologic pattern are mainly caused by other factors mentioned above.

Stevens gave a review of invasive group A streptococcal infections both clinically(126,130,132) and historically(127) where he also describes the ongoing research in streptococcal virulence factors—important for eventual development of new vaccines. Recent work on streptococcal virulence factors and their possible influence on the onset of soft-tissue infections can be found in Unnikrishnan et al.(140) and Norrby-Teglund et al.(107)

Dele Davies and Schwarz reviewed these infections in children.(38) Stevens(131) also underlined the importance of a rapidly progressive streptococcal toxic shock syndrome that can accompany necrotizing fasciitis (strep TSS). Mortality, even with adequate therapy, is 30%–60% of patients in 72–96 hours.

The bacteriology of synergistic necrotizing cellulitis is largely the same as in other forms of necrotizing fasciitis.(89,134)

Nonclostridial Myonecrosis

The most frequent and devastating anaerobic myositis and myonecrosis is clostridial myonecrosis or gas gangrene. We saw that some forms of synergistic necrotizing cellulitis have been categorized as nonclostridial myonecrosis(82,89,134) and other forms as necrotizing fasciitis. We consider muscle involvement to be a later stage of true necrotizing fasciitis.(11) Other forms of nonclostridial myonecrosis caused by anaerobic streptococci(96) are found mainly in drug addicts in our patient series. Differential diagnosis between gas gangrene and streptococcal myositis can be very difficult. The muscles in streptococcal myositis have in general a more inflamed appearance than in gas gangrene. Muscle necrosis is seen later than in gas gangrene, and the necrotic muscles are more greenish in color than the black muscle necrosis in gas gangrene. Also, gas production is less abundant and differently situated in streptococcal myositis. Severe systemic toxicity, however, can be the same in both diseases.

Myositis caused by aerobic microorganisms, viruses, or certain parasites are known and described but very rare and will not be discussed here.(121)

THERAPY

Introduction

Treatment of aerobic, anaerobic, and mixed necrotizing soft-tissue infections is a combination of surgical debridement (timely, limited, or aggressive), appropriate antibiotics, good nutritional support, and optimal oxygenation of the infected tissues. In selected cases where ambient oxygen is insufficient, hyperbaric oxygen must be used.

Surgical treatment can vary in these infections from simple incision and drainage procedures to very aggressive "fillet" procedures, and even amputations can become necessary. Essential in the management is the administration of appropriate antibiotics.

The problem with this is twofold:

1. Late culture results
2. Treating the causative and not the concomitant microorganisms

Our policy is to initially choose those antibiotics that cover the suspected causative pathogens (aerobic and anaerobic). Usually we start in the early stages with penicillin G (or clindamycin or both), metronidazole, and gentamycin or tobramycin.(9) Sometimes a third-generation cephalosporin is indicated.(89)

As early as 1952, Eagle already described the problem of treatment failure with penicillin in streptococcal infections in mice.(43) Stevens repeated this phenomenon in 1988 in streptococcal myositis in a mouse model.(125) Group A streptococci at the site of inoculation remained highly sensitive to penicillin only as long as the streptococci continued to grow at a rapid rate. The same was found to be true for erythromycin but not for clindamycin.

Zamboni and coworkers found penicillin therapy to be ineffective when started more than two hours after onset of a myositis in a mouse model. Although erythromycin resulted in higher survival rates, survival after clindamycin was still 70% even when treatment was started 16.5 hours after onset of the myositis (80% after 6 hours).(152) It is important to keep these data in mind when choosing a particular antibiotic treatment scheme. It seems that clindamycin is nowadays more appropriate than penicillin G.

Hyperbaric oxygen is indicated when other measures (ambient oxygen) fail to oxygenate the infected tissues sufficiently. This must be monitored by transcutaneous or, even better, by direct intraphlegmonous and/or intramuscular PO_2-measurements.(75,120)

The rationale for the use of adjunctive hyperbaric oxygen and the mechanisms have been outlined extensively by Mader and Thom.(88-89,137) The main goals are (a) improvement of tissue PO_2, necessary for normal wound healing, (b) improvement of phagocytic function by stimulating the oxygen-dependent killing mechanisms, either directly or indirectly, (c) diminishment of edema and improvement of the circulation in the affected areas, (d) stimulation of fibroblast growth, and (e) increased collagen formation. This can be roughly summarized as stimulation of the host defense and repair mechanisms. A useful algorithm or decision tree concerning the possible use of hyperbaric oxygen in soft-tissue infections has been published by Bell.(17)

Because of multiple variables, clinical studies using adjunctive hyperbaric oxygen are very difficult to evaluate. The wide variety in patients makes a randomized controlled trial virtually impossible. No patient is the same or presents him- or herself with the same symptoms. The variety in the bacteriological findings has been outlined sufficiently in this chapter. Almost all patients are compromised hosts. From some of the descriptions it is very difficult, if not impossible, to know which of the different clinical entities is involved. In this way, it is very difficult to respond to the criticism of Tibbles and Edelsberg in their review stating that more prospective trials are necessary in order to prove the value of hyperbaric oxygen in necrotizing fasciitis.[138] Maybe clinical evidence based on large numbers is sufficient to convince our adversaries. Even in gas gangrene, other gas-producing infections are mixed with the true clostridial myonecrosis. The rationale for adjunctive hyperbaric oxygen, however, is clear and based on animal studies, case reports, retrospective studies, and a few prospective studies.[66,116]

Korhonen[77-78] showed in animal experiments, in healthy volunteers, and in patients with necrotizing soft-tissue infections that hyperbaric oxygen raised arterial oxygen tensions sevenfold and that oxygen tensions in the vicinity of the infected area were generally higher than in healthy tissues, thus establishing a hyperoxygenated zone around the infection. The CO_2 tensions rose only slightly during exposure to hyperbaric oxygen. Combining early and extensive surgery, broad spectrum antibiotics, hyperbaric oxygen, and surgical intensive care gave the best results in the treatment of Fournier's disease with a mortality of 9%.

In three publications the use of honey to improve the rate of wound healing is advocated in NF. [45,47,63]

Progressive Bacterial Gangrene

Prognosis in progressive bacterial gangrene is generally better than in necrotizing fasciitis and is mainly determined by associated systemic diseases.

Surgery: Surgery can be limited to necrotomies, limited excisions in the margin of the process, the necessity of which must be judged on a day-to-day basis. Normal wound care, including temporary artificial skin substitution (for example, with a polyvinyl alcohol foam) may be necessary.[103] When a good granulating surface is obtained, split-skin grafting can be performed. We have never been forced to more extensive excisions. If the gangrene is not responsive to the combined treatment scheme, amputation of an extremity may be necessary.

Heinle et al.[60] claim superior results postgrafting, with a trend to lower mortality and morbidity, by the use of 5% mafenide acetate solution.

Antibiotics: These should be directed to the causative and not to concomitant microorganisms. This can be very difficult because a wide variety can usually be cultured from these infections.

In one of the author's patients, a 43-year-old male with a progressive bacterial synergistic gangrene of the abdominal wall postoperatively, a flora with *E. coli, Pseudomonas aeruginosa, Enterobacter cloacae,* enterococci, *Bacteroides* species, and *Acinetobacter anitratum* was cultured. The clinical picture, however, professed that none of the microorganisms needed any treatment. With only local care, wound healing was uneventful. This underlines the significance of close cooperation between the clinical bacteriologist and surgeon.

Since in 92% of the tissue biopsies taken from the margin of the process, streptococci were cultured followed by staphylococci, coliforms, *Proteus, Pseudomonas,* and Clostridia, we usually start with penicillin G, one million IU every three to four hours intravenously and change this regimen only when indicated by the clinical course supported by bacteriologic evidence. Because of unresponsiveness of streptococci depending on the stage of the process, we use more and more clindamycin.[125]

Hyperbaric oxygen: In 1975 Ledingham and Therani reported for the first time in literature that the adjunctive use of hyperbaric oxygen contributed to the arrest of the infection in four out of five of their patients.[81] Experience with hyperbaric oxygen is reported more and more in the literature. The working mechanism makes it clear why it is useful in treating necrotic soft-tissue infections. All our patients reacted favorably when hyperbaric oxygen was added to the therapeutic regimen of surgery and antibiotics. We added hyperbaric oxygen when other treatment modalities failed. No proper prospective randomized trials are known which is a definitive disadvantage when advocating hyperbaric oxygen. From 1978–1987, 89 patients were treated with progressive bacterial gangrene.[9] The mortality was 5.6%. All patients had serious associated diseases, diabetes mellitus being the most frequent (74 patients or 83.1%). Some patients had been treated for as long as 4–6 months with all known treatment modalities. Despite this, the gangrene extended progressively although slowly. At the time that amputation was considered to be unavoidable, the addition of hyperbaric oxygen stopped the progression and resulted in a clean, granulating wound suitable for grafting after approximately three weeks of daily treatments (14–42 days in 84 patients).

We recommend the adjunctive use of hyperbaric oxygen in progressive bacterial gangrene in cases where other treatment modalities fail, in cases with serious underlying systemic diseases and symptoms of general toxicity, and in other immune-compromised patients.

Treatment protocol for progressive bacterial gangrene

- 1st day: 3 x 90 minutes 3 ATA 100% O_2 in a multiplace or a monoplace chamber
- (appropriate air-breaks as mentioned before)
- 2nd day: 2 times
- 3rd day: 2 times

From the fourth day on, continue with one treatment per day. Maximal treatment time is 10 days.

The question if the same results can be reached with lower oxygen pressures is difficult to answer since we do not have a clear definition of a dose of oxygen. In our experience these protocols are safe, and side effects are absent or minimal. The most important thing is to establish in an oxygen challenge test that the PO_2 at the wound margin and/or in the wound itself is too low to expect normal wound healing; the next step is to show that this PO_2 can be raised by hyperbaric oxygen and not by 100% oxygen at 1 bar.

Anaerobic clostridial cellulitis, sometimes misdiagnosed as gas gangrene, is a more benign disease than gas gangrene. Clostridia can be found in pure culture, and there can be marked tissue necrosis. The deep fascia and the muscles, however, are not affected. With extensive tissue damage and/or in a seriously compromised host, a true clostridial myositis with myonecrosis can arise. Surgical treatment can be limited to incision and drainage followed by excision of the necrotic tissue.

Antibiotics: Penicillin G, 8–12 million IU per day intravenously

Hyperbaric oxygen: Adjunctive hyperbaric oxygen is recommended in immunocompromised patients and in patients with systemic toxicity. In these patients, the gas gangrene scheme is used.

- 1st day: 3 x 90 minutes 3 ATA 100% O_2 in a multiplace or a monoplace chamber

- (appropriate air-breaks as mentioned before)
- 2nd day: 2 times
- 3rd day: 2 times

From the fourth day on, continue with one treatment per day until the wound starts granulating. Maximal treatment time is 10 days. We then found normal oxygen tissue tensions for wound healing when breathing normal air at sea level. This is the sign that hyperbaric treatment can be discontinued.

Necrotizing Fasciitis

Surgery: Primary and aggressive surgical debridement is the cornerstone in the management of this disease. Early and extensive incision of skin and subcutaneous tissue wide into healthy tissue, followed by excision of all necrotic fascia and nonviable skin and subcutaneous tissue, is necessary. This has to be repeated as often as necessary. Within the first 24 hours, repeated inspection of the whole infected area under general anesthesia is obligatory, with excision of further necrotized fascia, if present.

These progressive necrotizing surgical infections need a unified approach as soon as possible. It is of no use trying to determine the type of infection first by culturing the infected tissue because every delay in the start of treatment causes a significant higher mortality.(32,35,37,48,53,62,72,142) In most of our patients with a necrotizing fasciitis of the peniscrotal and perianal area, we performed a diverting colostomy.

The extent of fascial necrosis can easily be determined by blunt finger dissection over the deep fascial plane through the incision and by direct inspection. Viable skin flaps need not be excised and can be saved. If no further fascial necrosis is seen, the process can be considered arrested. Usually, at least in our experience, from 1–5 debridements are necessary with a mean of 3 (in 40 patients between 1985–1990). A systematic exploration of the ischiorectal fossa in every case of a perianal soft-tissue infection is very important.(25)

Antibiotics: Antibiotic treatment has an important place in the combined management of necrotizing fasciitis, although second to surgery. Recommendations of drugs have changed with the development of new antibiotics and the risk of resistance. Colonization and selection of microorganisms by a former therapeutic or prophylactic regimen play an important role (for example, antibiotic prophylaxis in large bowel surgery or treatment of a perianal abscess).

If at the time of clinical diagnosis, a polymicrobial flora is present, one has to be very careful not to treat a concomitant agent instead of the causative microorganisms. The present confusing bacteriologic findings in soft-tissue infections are in part caused by the unnecessary, misdirected use of antibiotics.

Streptococci have been identified as a major pathogen in these diseases. Kaul et al. gave a recent review on the incidence of necrotizing fasciitis in Ontario, Canada,(73) as did Smith et al.(123) and Corman et al.;(32) the largest review, on 1,726 cases, is published by Eke.(47) Five cases in trauma patients were reported by Schwarz et al.(118)

The drug of choice is penicillin G, 8–10 million IU/24 hours intravenously, with clindamycin more and more as the alternative. The other pathogens can be treated by metronidazole (anaerobes) and/or third-generation cephalosporins (anaerobes, Enterobacteriaceae).(50) *Bacteroides fragilis* can be treated with clindamycin or metronidazole (or covered by a third-generation cephalosporin). A useful scheme for the initial choice of antibiotics is given by Mader.(89)

Hyperbaric oxygen: Clinical reports indicate an adjunctive role for hyperbaric oxygen in necrotizing fasciitis. Although no large controlled randomized series have been published so far, hyperbaric oxygen provides a valuable adjunct in the overall treatment management.(27,37,65,109) An interesting discussion on the value of adjunctive hyperbaric oxygen can be found in the Deutsche Medizinische Wochenschrift by Bock et al. and Kujath et al.(19,79) Kujath(79) underestimates the advantages and greatly exaggerate the disadvantages of hyperbaric oxygen in necrotizing fasciitis. A useful discussion follows in a later issue of the same journal.(41) The overall mortality figures in this disease range from 20%–75%.

The overall results of hyperbaric oxygen therapy on patients with necrotizing fasciitis or necrotizing soft-tissue infections are as follows:

1. Only Ledingham reported poor results with hyperbaric oxygen (overall mortality 8/12 = 67%, in the hyperbaric oxygen group 8/9 = 89%). However, his initial surgical management is suspect and was probably not extensive enough. Adjunctive hyperbaric oxygen cannot be successful if surgery is inappropriate.(81)

2. Riegels-Nielsen reported five patients with a mortality of 1/5 = 20%. All five patients had necrotizing fasciitis of the external genitals and the lower abdominal wall and were treated with aggressive surgery, appropriate antibiotics, and adjunctive hyperbaric oxygen.(115)

3. We treated 27 patients before 1985 with necrotizing fasciitis, including seven patients with Fournier's disease. Mortality was 5/27 = 18%. In another 40 patients (1985–1990) mortality was 5/40 = 12.5%. Patients were treated with a combination of surgery, antibiotics, and hyperbaric oxygen.(9)

4. Eltorai et al. reported no mortalities in nine patients in which hyperbaric oxygen was added to the standard therapy.(49)

5. Mader reported on a retrospective evaluation of 33 patients, of which 22 had involvement of the scrotum and perianal region. Of the 22, mortality in the hyperbaric oxygen group was 25% compared with a mortality of 67% in the nonhyperbaric oxygen group. All patients were seriously compromised hosts, and 14 had diabetes mellitus.(89)

6. Zamboni et al. treated six patients with one late death due to complications of pneumonia.(151)

7. Riseman et al. reported on 29 patients with necrotizing fasciitis treated between 1980 and 1988. Group I (n = 12) received standard therapy and in group II (n = 17) hyperbaric oxygen was added. Although group II patients were more seriously ill at admission, the mortality in this group was significantly lower (23%) than in group I patients (66%). Their conclusion was that the addition of hyperbaric oxygen to the surgical and antimicrobial treatment of necrotizing fasciitis significantly reduced mortality and wound morbidity (number of necessary debridements). In their view, hyperbaric oxygen should be used routinely in the treatment of necrotizing fasciitis. Following their results, they conclude that withholding hyperbaric oxygen to patients when it is available will cause unnecessary deaths and is thus unethical.(116)

8. Brown et al. reported on a retrospective review of the efficacy of hyperbaric oxygen. They looked only at truncal necrotizing fasciitis and identified 54 patients (30 in the HBO_2 group and 24 without HBO_2). There was a trend to better survival in the HBO_2-treated group but without statistical significance.[23]

9. Shupak et al. in a retrospective study of 37 patients over a rather long period, from 1984–1993, also did not find statistical difference between treatment with and without hyperbaric oxygen.[122]

10. Hirn presented 11 patients treated with HBO_2 in a clinical and experimental study and found a mortality of 1 patient (9%). He advocates HBO_2 as an adjunct in the overall treatment of necrotizing soft-tissue infections.[65]

11. Korhonen et al., in a retrospective study of 33 patients with Fournier's gangrene, found a mortality of 3 patients or 9%. They found that adjunctive hyperbaric oxygen reduced systemic toxicity, prevented extension of the necrotizing infection, and increased demarcation, thereby improving the overall outcome.[76]

12. Hollabaugh et al. reported 7% mortality in a group of patients with Fournier's gangrene when treated with adjunctive hyperbaric oxygen (n = 14). In the group without hyperbaric oxygen, the mortality was 42% (n = 12). This difference was statistically significant. A total of 38% of their patients had diabetes mellitus; 35% had alcohol abuses. Hyperbaric oxygen was given to patients solely on the basis of institution availability. Although the number of patients is still limited, there is a good statistical paragraph concerning survival chances with and without hyperbaric oxygen.[66]

    Also, Clark and Moon[29] underline the importance of adjunctive hyperbaric oxygen in the treatment of life-threatening soft-tissue infection. Dahm et al.[36] found that the extent of the infection as measured by the BSA (body surface area) involved was a highly statistically significant independent predictor of outcome and that Fournier's gangrene with an extension of 5% BSA or greater appeared to be an indication for adjunctive hyperbaric oxygen. Their results in 50 patients did not, however, reach statistical significance.

    Compromised hosts with necrotizing fasciitis have extreme morbidity and mortality. From these reports, it is clear that adjunctive hyperbaric oxygen in these patients is a very valuable therapeutic tool.

13. Devaney[40] described a retrospective series of 34 NF patients in a single center (2002–2014). A total of 341 patients with NF were included in the study, of whom 275 received HBO_2 therapy and 66 did not. The most commonly involved sites were the perineum (33.7%), lower limb, (29.9%) and trunk (18.2%). The commonest predisposing factor was diabetes mellitus (34.8%). Polymicrobial NF (type 1 NF) occurred in 50.7%, and group A streptococcal fasciitis (type 2 NF) occurred in 25.8% of patients. Mortality was 14.4% overall, 12% in those treated with HBO_2 therapy, and 24.3% in those not treated with HBO_2 therapy. Mortality was linked to illness severity at presentation; however, when adjusted for severity score and need for intensive care management, HBO_2 therapy was associated with significant reduction in mortality.

14. Shaw[119] queried 14 hyperbaric centers; 1583 cases of NSTI were identified; 117 cases were treated with HBO_2. Univariate analysis showed that there was no difference between HBO_2 therapy and control groups in hospital length of stay, direct cost, complications, and mortality across the 3 less severe severity of illness (SOI) classes (minor, moderate, and major).

    However, for extreme SOI, the HBO_2 therapy group had fewer complications (45% versus 66%; $p < 0.01$) and fewer deaths (4% versus 23%; $p < 0.01$). Multivariable analysis showed that patients who did not receive HBO_2 therapy were less likely to survive their index hospitalization. They concluded that the use of HBO_2 therapy in conjunction with current practices for the treatment of NSTI can be both a cost-effective and a life-saving therapy, in particular for the sickest patients.

15. Proud et al.[112] described a retrospective study on 219 patients with NSTI in a 10–year period. HBO_2 was administered to 82.65% of patients with a median number of 7 treatments (IQR = 3–10 treatments). The overall mortality rate for the patient group was 16%. It was concluded that, based on current evidence, the role of HBO_2 in treatment of NSTIs is at best as an adjunct to aggressive debridement and antibiotic therapy.[2,14-15]

16. Martinschek[90] analysed 55 patients with Fournier's gangrene, and almost all patients (96.4%) received supportive HBO_2 therapy. The average number was 7.5 treatments. They concluded that, although there are no randomized controlled data, HBO_2 could be an important adjunctive therapy in NSTI and Fournier's gangrene.

17. Massey performed a retrospective study on 80 cases of NSTI.[91] In-hospital mortality was not different between groups (16% in the HBO_2 group versus 19% in the non-HBO_2 group. In patients with extremity NSTI, the amputation rate did not differ significantly between patients who did not receive HBO_2 and those who did (17% versus 25%). In this study, it was found that hyperbaric oxygen therapy does not appear to decrease in-hospital mortality or amputation rate in patients with NSTI. In addition, they mentioned that there may be a role for HBO_2 in treatment of NSTI; nevertheless, consideration of HBO_2 should never delay operative therapy.

18. George et al.[53] did not find differences in favor of the patients treated with HBO_2 ($n = 40$). In a retrospective series of 78 patients, mortality rate, duration of the hospital stay, and antibiotics use does not differ significantly between the HBO_2 group and the non-HBO_2 group.

19. Wilkinson, Doolette[148]conducted a study in which 44 NSTI patients were reviewed. Survival was less likely in those with increased age, renal dysfunction, and idiopathic etiology of infection and in those not receiving HBO_2 therapy. Logistic regression determined the strongest association with survival was the intervention of HBO_2 therapy ($p = .02$). Hyperbaric oxygen therapy increased survival with an odds ratio of 8.9 (95% confidence interval, 1.3–58.0) and a number needed to treat of 3. For NSTI involving an extremity, HBO_2 therapy significantly reduced the incidence of amputation. Survival analysis revealed an improved long-term outcome for the HBO_2 group.

In conclusion, there are many published studies on hyperbaric oxygen therapy as an adjunctive therapy for NF and NSTI. Most of the studies were retrospective series of patients with contradictory results and different outcomes of the use of HBO_2 therapy. Use of hyperbaric oxygen therapy, or HBO_2 therapy, in addition to surgery and antibiotics has been suggested as a way to minimize tissue loss, decrease the number of limb amputations, and reduce death.

However, the Cochrane review from 2015 found no high-quality trials to support or refute the use of HBO_2 therapy in the treatment of individuals with necrotizing fasciitis. They mentioned that HBO_2 therapy may very rarely result in serious adverse effects. Further studies are required to address the effectiveness of HBO_2 therapy because currently it is provided as routine practice in some centers.(83)

Treatment Protocol for Necrotizing Fasciitis. Proper, early, and aggressive surgical debridements remain the cornerstone of the treatment. These are surgical diseases that can only be treated with appropriate surgery first.(6,20,35) Hyperbaric oxygen cannot compensate for bad surgery. However, the best results can only be obtained with a combination of surgery, antibiotics, and hyperbaric oxygen. The same conclusion was reached at a Consensus Conference in 2000 by the French Society of Dermatology – however, without the use of hyperbaric oxygen which was still considered controversial.(6,20,35) Mathieu,(92) answering, stated that the controversy on the use of hyperbaric oxygen as a treatment for necrotizing fasciitis is more caused by the difficulty to dispose of hyperbaric equipment that is suited for the treatment of critical patients than by doubt on its real efficiency.

HBO_2 treatment scheme (necrotizing fasciitis): After the first surgical debridement, 3 treatment sessions are given in the first 24 hours.

- 1st day: 3 x 90 minutes 3 ATA 100% O_2 in a multiplace or a monoplace chamber
- (appropriate air-breaks as mentioned before)
- 2nd day: 2 times
- 3rd day: 2 times

If the improvement of the patient permits this, once daily until granulation is obtained (10–15 treatments in total).

Nonclostridial Myonecrosis

Synergistic necrotizing cellulitis: The name "cellulitis" suggests progressive bacterial gangrene, but the disease is categorized by some as myonecrosis, while, in fact, it is a necrotizing fasciitis. This clearly demonstrates the difficulty of classification of this disease in its advanced stages when literally every kind of tissue is involved.

The therapy is the same as described under necrotizing fasciitis, but because more tissue is involved, and the infection is especially fulminant, mortality reaches 75% without hyperbaric oxygen.(134) This is not so much the result of the necrotizing fasciitis itself, but of the extremely serious immune compromise of the patients, secondary to age, renal failure, arteriosclerosis, diabetes mellitus, malignancies, deficient nutrition, and so on. These factors determine the danger and the rapid spread of this soft-tissue infection.

In light of the above and the grim prognosis of this disease, it is only logical to give adjunctive hyperbaric oxygen where possible.

Treatment Protocol for Non-Clostridial Myonecrosis. Again, hyperbaric oxygen has to be adjunctive to appropriate antibiotics (clindamycin or penicillin) and surgical incision and drainage, followed by excision of necrotic muscle.

Prognosis worsens progressively when muscle tissue is involved. Aggressive surgery, appropriate antibiotics, and adjunctive hyperbaric oxygen is important following the "gas gangrene protocol."

- 1st day: 3 x 90 minutes 3 ATA 100% O_2 in a multiplace or a monoplace chamber
- (appropriate air-breaks as mentioned before)
- 2nd day: 2 times
- 3rd day: 2 times

Because the myositis started in most of our patients as a "closed" disease (after drug injection in addicts), there is an early need for decompressing fasciotomy and hyperbaric oxygen.

Anaerobic streptococcal myositis and myonecrosis: This infection is rare. The author has seen only seven patients since 1978. The mortality was 2/7 = 28.6%. The disease can be very fulminant, mimicking clostridial myonecrosis. Because we have demonstrated hypoxia through intramuscular PO_2 monitoring,[75] we recommend the use of adjunctive hyperbaric oxygen. In cases of fulminant disease, systemic toxicity, and a compromised host, the gas gangrene protocol may be used. Other recent reviews of invasive streptococcal disease, including streptococcal myositis, are given by Stevens. The incidence, reading his report, is clearly much higher than in our experience.[129,132]

Adams et al.[1] described 19 cases from the literature and added 2 own cases. In all cases the infection was caused by group A ß-hemolytic streptococci. Despite aggressive surgical and medical treatment, 18 out of 21 patients (85.7%) died.

Demey et al. reported another two cases from Belgium.[39] Zamboni et al. found in a mouse myositis model using *Streptococcus pyogenes* that HBO_2 alone did not decrease mortality or bacterial proliferation in vivo significantly, but the combined treatment of penicillin with HBO_2 exerts at least additive effects in both decreasing bacterial counts in vivo and increasing survival in this model.[152]

REFERENCES

1. Adams EM, Gudmundsson S, Yocum DE, Haselby RC, et al. Streptococcal myositis. Arch Int Med. 1985;145:1020-3.
2. Ahrenholz DH. Necrotizing soft tissue infections. Surg Clin North Am. 1988;68:199-214.
3. Ahrenholz DH. Physicians world communications [monograph]. West Point (PA): Merck, Sharpe and Dohme; 1988. Surgical spectrum. Clinical skin and soft tissue infection. p. 16-24.
4. Arslan A, Jerome CP, Borthne A. Necrotizing fasciitis: unreliable MRI findings in the preoperative diagnosis. Eur J Radiol. 2000;36:139-143.
5. Ault MJ, Geiderman J, Sokolov R. Rapid identification of group A streptococcus as the cause of necrotizing fasciitis. Ann Emerg Med. 1996;28:227-30.
6. Baier VP, Imdahl A. Nekrotisierende fasciitis. Hier hilft nur radikales debridement. MMW-Fortschr Med. 2001;143:332-3. German.
7. Bakker DJ. De hyperbare zuurstofbehandeling van acuut huidgangreen (necrotiserende fasciitis en progressief bacterieel gangreen). Ned Tijdschr Geneeskd. 1980;124:2164-70. Dutch.
8. Bakker DJ. Proc VIIth Int Congr Hyperbaric Medicine. Moscow: Publishing Office "Nauka"; 1983. The treatment of acute dermal gangrene with hyperbaric oxygen. p. 238-40. Russian.
9. Bakker DJ. The use of hyperbaric oxygen in the treatment of certain infectious diseases especially gas gangrene and acute dermal gangrene. Wageningen. University of Amsterdam: Drukkerij Veenman BV; 1984. p. 74-90.
10. Bakker DJ. The use of hyperbaric oxygen in the treatment of certain infectious diseases especially gas gangrene and acute dermal gangrene. Wageningen. University of Amsterdam: Drukkerij Veenman BV; 1984. p. 42-4.
11. Bakker DJ, Kox C. Classification and therapy of necrotizing soft tissue infections: the role of surgery, antibiotics and hyperbaric oxygen. Curr Probl Gen Surg. 1988;5:489-500.
12. Bakker DJ. Streptococcal infections and hyperbaric oxygen. In: Gennser M, editor. Diving and hyperbaric medicine. Proc XXIV Ann Meeting of the EUBS; 1998 Aug 12-15; Stockholm. Stockholm (Sweden): Print Elanders-Gotab. p 140-5. FOA report: FOA-B-98-00342-721-SE.
13. Ballon-Landa GR, Gherardi G, Beall B, et al. Necrotizing fasciitis due to penicillin-resistant Streptococcus pneumoniae: case report and review of the literature. J Infect. 2001:272-90.
14. Bartlett JG. Necrotizing soft tissue infections. In: Nichols RL, Hyslop NE, Bartlett JG, editors. Decision making in surgical sepsis. Philadelphia: Decker; 1991. p. 62-3.
15. Barton LL, Jeck DT. Necrotizing fasciitis in children. Report of two cases and a review of the literature. Arch Pediatr Adolesc Med. 1996;150:105-8.
16. Beaurienne M. Observation sur une plaie du scrotum. J de Med Chir Pharm. 1764;20:251-6. French.
17. Bell WH. Use of hyperbaric oxygen in anaerobic soft-tissue infection. In: Nichols RL, Hyslop NE, Bartlett JG, editors. Decision making in surgical sepsis. Philadelphia: Decker; 1991. p. 78-81.
18. Bisno AL, Stevens DL. Streptococcal infections of skin and soft tissues. New Eng J Med. 1996;334:240-5.

19. Bock KH, Lampl L, Frey G. Diagnose und therapie der nekrotisierende fasziitis. Hyperbare oxygenation als ergänzende therapieform. Deutsche Med Wochenschr. 1996;121:116-7. German.

20. Brandt MM, Corpron CA, Wahl WL. Necrotizing soft tissue infections: a surgical disease. Am Surg. 2000;66:967-70.

21. Brewer GE, Meleney FL. Progressive gangrenous infection of the skin and subcutaneous tissues, following operation for acute perforative appendicitis. Ann Surg. 1926;84:438-50.

22. Brocq L. Nouvelle contribution à l'étude du phagedenisme geometrique. Ann Dermatol Syph (Paris). 1916-1917;6:1-39. French.

23. Brown DR, Davis NL, Lepawsky M, Cunningham J, Kortbeek J. A multicenter review of the treatment of major truncal necrotizing infections with and without hyperbaric oxygen therapy. Am J Surg. 1994;167:485-9.

24. Brun-Buisson C. Stratégie de prise en charge des fasciites nécrosantes. Conference de consensus. Texte des experts:quatrième question. Ann Dermatol Venereol. 2001;128:394-403. French.

25. Brunet C, Consentino B, Barthelemy A, et al. Gangrènes périnéales: nouvelle approche bactériologique. Résultats du traitement médicochirurgical (81 cas). Ann Chir. 2000;125:420-7. French.

26. Brunsting LA, Goeckerman WH, O'Leary PA. Pyoderma gangrenosum (ecthyma). Clinical and experimental observations in five cases. Arch Dermatol Syph (Paris). 1930;22:655-80.

27. Capelli-Schellpfeffer M, Gerber GS. The use of hyperbaric oxygen in urology. J Urol. 1999;162:647-54.

28. Chapnick EK, Abter EI. Necrotizing soft-tissue infections. Inf Dis Clin N Am. 1996;10:835-55.

29. Clark LA, Moon RE. Hyperbaric oxygen in the treatment of life-threatening soft-tissue infections. Resp Care Clin N Am. 1999;5:203-19.

30. Clayton MD, Fowler JE Jr, Sharifi R, Pearl RK. Causes, presentation and survival of fifty-seven patients with necrotizing fasciitis of the male genitalia. Surg Gynecol Obstet. 1990;170:49-55.

31. Conférence de consensus de la Société Française de Dermatologie. Erysipèle et fasciite nécrosante:prise en charge. Text court. Ann Med Int. 2000;151:465-70. French.

32. Corman JM, Moody JA, Aronson WJ. Fournier's gangrene in a modern surgical setting: improved survival with aggressive management. BJU Int. 1999;84:85-8.

33. Crosthwait RW Jr, Crosthwait RW, Jordan GL. Necrotizing fasciitis. J Trauma. 1964;4:149-57.

34. Cullen TS. A progressively enlarging ulcer of abdominal wall involving the skin and fat, following drainage of an abdominal abscess apparently of appendiceal origin. Surg Gynecol Obstet. 1924;38:579-82.

35. Cunningham JD, Silver L, Rudikoff D. Necrotizing fasciitis: a plea for early diagnosis and treatment. Mount Sinai J Med. 2001;68(4-5):253-61.

36. Dahm P, Roland FH, Vaslef SN, et al. Outcome analysis in patients with primary necrotizing fasciitis of the male genitalia. Urol. 2000;56:31-5.

37. Dellinger EP. Severe necrotizing soft tissue infections. Multiple disease entities requiring a common approach. JAMA. 1981;246:1717-21.

38. Dele Davies H, Schwartz B. Advances in pediatric infectious diseases. Vol 14. Mosby, Inc.; 1999. Chapter 6, Invasive group A streptococcal infections in children; p. 129-145.

39. Demey HE, Goovaerts GC, Pattyn SR, Bossaert LL. Streptococcal myositis. A report of two cases. Acta Clin Belgica. 1991;46(2):82-8.

40. Devaney B, Frawley G, Frawley L, Pilcher DV. Necrotising soft tissue infections: the effect of hyperbaric oxygen on mortality. Anaesth Intensive Care. 2015;43:685-92.

41. Diskussion: Schmidt H, Welslau W, Hencke J, Siekmann U, Scharfe U, Tirpitz D, Kujath P, Eckmann C. Die nekrotisierende fasziitis und schwere weichteilinfektionen durch gruppe-A-streptokokken. Dt Artztebl. 1998;95(39):A-2395-401. German.

42. Drake DB, Woods JA, Bill TJ, et al. Magnetic resonance imaging in the early diagnosis of group A ß streptococcal necrotizing fasciitis: a case report. J Em Med. 1998;16:4403-7.

43. Eagle H. Experimental approach to the problem of treatment failure with penicillin. I. Group A streptococcal infection in mice. Amer J Med. 1952;13:389-99.

44. Ecker KW, Derouet H, Omlor G, Mast GJ. Die Fournier'sche gangrän. Chirurg. 1993;64:558-62. German.

45 Efem SEE. Recent advances in the management of Fournier's gangrene: preliminary observations. Surg. 1993;113:200-4.

46. Efstratiou A, George RC, Tanna A, et al. Characterisation of group A streptococci from necrotizing fasciitis cases in Gloucestershire, United Kingdom. Adv Exp Med Biol. 1997;418:91-3.

47. Eke N. Fournier's gangrene: a review of 1726 cases. Br J Surg. 2000;87:718-28.

48. Elliott D, Kufera JA, Myers RAM. The microbiology of necrotizing soft tissue infections. Am J Surg. 2000;179(5):361-6.

49. Eltorai IM, Hart GB, Strauss MB, Montroy R, Juler GL. The role of hyperbaric oxygen in the management of Fournier's gangrene. Int Surg. 1986;71:53.

50. Fildes J, Bannon MP, Barrett J. Soft tissue infections after trauma. Surg Clin North Am. 1991;71:371-84.

51. Finegold SM, Bartlett JC, Chow AW, et al. Management of anaerobic infections. Ann Intern Med. 1975;83:375-89.

52. Fournier A. Gangrène foudroyante de la verge. Semaine Medicale. 1883;3:345-7. French. 1884;4:69-70. French.

53. Francis KR, Lamaute HR, Davis JM, et al. Implications of risk factors in necrotizing fasciitis. Am Surg. 1993;59:304-8.

54. George ME, Rueth NM, Skarda DE, Chipman JG, Quickel RR, Beilman GJ. Hyperbaric oxygen does not improve outcome in patients with necrotizing soft tissue infections. Surg Infect (Larchmt). 2009;10:21-8.

55. Giuliano A, Lewis F Jr, Hadley K, Blaisdell FW. Bacteriology of necrotizing fasciitis. Am J Surg. 1977;134:52-7.

56. Goepfert AR, Guinn DA, Andrews WW, Hauth JC. Necrotizing fasciitis after cesarean delivery. Obst Gynec. 1997;89:409-12.

57. Gorbach SL, Bartlett JG, Nichols RL. Manual of surgical infections. Boston: Brown; 1984. Chapter 9, Skin and soft tissue infections.

58. Green RJ, Dafoe DC, Raffin TA. Necrotizing fasciitis. Chest. 1996;110:219-29.

59. Hebler. Brand des hodensackes und vollständiger wiederersatz. Med Zeitung. 1848;41:188. German.

60. Heinle EC, Dougherty WR, Garner WL, Reilly DA. The use of 5% mafenide acetate solution in the postgraft treatment of necrotizing fasciitis. J Burn Care Rehab. 2001;22:35-40.

61. Heitmann C, Czermak C, Germann G. Rapidly fatal necrotizing fasciitis after aesthetic liposuction. Aesth Plast Surg. 2000;24:344-7.

62 . Heitmann C, Pelzer M, Bickert B, et al. Chirurgisches konzept und ergebnisse bei nekrotisierender fasciitis. Chirurg. 2001;72:168-73. German.

63. Hejase MJ, Simonin JE, Bihrle R, Coogan CL. Genital Fournier's gangrene: experience with 38 patients. Urology. 1996:47:734-9.

64. Hippocrates. Hippocratic writings. In: Lloyd GER, editor. Translated. Epidemics. Vol. I. Middlesex (England): Penguin Classics; 1983. p. 108-9. Vol. III. p. 121-2.

65. Hirn M. Hyperbaric oxygen in the treatment of gas gangrene and perineal necrotizing fasciitis. A clinical and experimental study [dissertation]. Eur J Surg (Acta Chir). 1993;(Suppl 570).

66. Hollabaugh RS, Dmochowski RR, Hickerson WL, Cox CE. Fournier's gangrene: therapeutic impact of hyperbaric oxygen. Plast Reconstr Surg. 1998;101(1):94-100.

67. Hsieh T, Samson LM, Jabbour M, Osmond MH. Necrotizing fasciitis in children in eastern Ontario: a case-control study. CMAJ. 2000;163(4):393-6.

68. Johnin K, Nakatoh M, Kadowaki T, et al. Fournier's gangrene caused by candida species as the primary organism. Urol. 2000;56(1):153.

69. Jones J. Investigations upon the nature, causes and treatment of hospital gangrene as it prevailed in the Confederate armies 1861-1865, New York. U.S. Sanitary Commission; 1871. (Surgical memoirs of the war of rebellion).

70. Jones RB, Hirschmann JV, Brown GS, Tremann JA. Fournier's syndrome: necrotizing soft tissue infection of the male genitalia. J Urol. 1979;122:279-82.

71. Käch K, Kossman T, Trentz O. Nekrotisierende weichteilinfekte. Unfallchirurg. 1993;96:181-91. German.

72. Kaiser RE, Cerra FB. Progressive necrotizing surgical infections—a unified approach. J Trauma. 1981;21(5):349-53.

73. Kaul R, McGeer A, Low DE, et al. Population-based surveillance for group A streptococcal necrotizing fasciitis: clinical features, prognostic indicators and microbiologic analysis of seventy-seven cases. Am J Med. 1997;103:18-24.

74. Kingston D, Seal DV. Current hypotheses on synergistic microbial gangrene. Br J Surg. 1990;77:260-4.

75. Kleij (van der) AJ, Bakker DJ, Lubbers MJ, Henny CP. Skeletal muscle pO^2 in anaerobic soft tissue infections during hyperbaric oxygen therapy. Adv Exp Med Biol. 1992;317: 125-9.

76. Korhonen K, Hirn M, Niinikoski J. Hyperbaric oxygen in the treatment of Fournier's gangrene. Eur J Surg. 1998;164(4):251-5.

77. Korhonen K. Hyperbaric oxygen therapy in acute necrotizing infections. Ann Chir Gyn. 2000;(Suppl 214):7-36.

78. Korhonen K, Kuttila K, Niinikoski J. Tissue gas tensions in patients with necrotizing fasciitis and healthy controls during treatment with hyperbaric oxygen: a clinical study. Eur J Surg. 2000;166:530-4.

79. Kujath PE, Eckmann C. Die nekrotisierende fasziitis und schwere weichteilinfektio-nen durch gruppe-A-streptokokken. Diagnose, therapie und prognose. Dt Artztebl. 1998;95(8):A-408-13. German.

80. Lamerton AJ. Fournier's gangrene: non-clostridial gas gangrene of the perineum and diabetes mellitus. J R Soc Med. 1986;79:212-5.

81. Ledingham IM, Tehrani MA. Diagnosis, clinical course and treatment of acute dermal gangrene. Br J Surg. 1975;62:364-72.

82. Lefrock JL, Molavi A. Necrotizing skin and subcutaneous infections. J Antimicrob Chemother. 1982;9(Suppl A):183-92.

83. Levett D, Bennett MH, Millar I. Adjunctive hyperbaric oxygen for necrotizing fasciitis. Cochrane Database Syst Rev. 2015;(1):007937

84. Lewis RT. Necrotizing soft tissue infections. In: Meakins JL, editor. Surgical infection in critical care medicine. 20th ed. London: Churchill Livingstone; 1985. p. 153-71.

85. Lewis RT. Soft tissue infection. In: Wilmore DW, Brennan MF, Harken AH, et al., editors. Care of the surgical patient. 21st ed. New York: Scientific American; 1989. p. 1-15.

86. Lin C, Yeh FL, Lin JT, et al. Necrotizing fasciitis of the head and neck: an analysis of 47 cases. Pals Reconstr Surg. 2001;107:1684-93.

87. Loudon I. Necrotizing fasciitis, hospital gangrene, and phagedena. Lancet. 1994;344:1416-9.

88. Mader JT, Adams KR, Sutton TE. Infectious diseases: pathophysiology and mechanisms of hyperbaric oxygen. J Hyp Med. 1987;2:133-40.

89. Mader J. Mixed anaerobic and aerobic soft tissue infections. In: Davis JC, Hunt TK, editors. Problem wounds: the role of oxygen. New York: Elsevier; 1988. p. 153-72.

90. Martinschek A, Evers B, Lampl L, Gerngross H, Schmidt R, Sparwasser C. Prognostic aspects, survival rate and predisposing risk factors in patients with Fournier's gangrene and necrotizing soft tissue infections: evaluation of clinical outcome of 55 patients. Urol Int. 2012;89:173-9.

91. Massey PR, Sakran JV, Mills AM, Sarani B, Aufhausser DD Jr, Sims CA, Pascual JL, Kelz RR, Holena DN. Hyperbaric oxygen therapy in necrotizing soft tissue infections. J Surg Res. 2012;177:146-51.

92. Mathieu D. Place de l'oxygénotherapie hyperbare dans le traitement des fasciites nécrosantes. Conférence de consensus de la Société Française de Dermatologie. Ann Dermatol Venereol. 2001;128:411-8. French.

93. McCafferty EL, Lyons C. Suppurative fasciitis as the essential feature of hemolytic streptococcus gangrene. Surgery. 1948;24:438-42.

94. McCrea LE. Fulminating gangrene of the penis. Clinics. 1945;4(3):796-829.

95. McGreer AJ. Commentary on Wall et al. A 2 factor model helped to rule out early stage necrotizing fasciitis. Evidence Based Med. 2001;6:96.

96. McLennan JD. The histotoxic clostridial infections of man. Bact Rev. 1962;26:177-276.

97. Meleney FL. Hemolytic streptococcus gangrene. Arch Surg. 1924;9:317-64.

98. Meleney FL. A differential diagnosis between certain types of infectious gangrene of the skin, with particular reference to hemolytic streptococcus gangrene and bacterial synergistic gangrene. Surg Gynecol Obstet. 1933;56:847.

99. Meleney FL. Bacterial synergism in disease process, with confirmation of the synergistic bacterial etiology of a certain type of progressive gangrene of the abdominal wall. Ann Surg. 1933;94:961-81.

100. Modai J. Empiric therapy of severe infections in adults. Am J Med. 1990;88(Suppl 4A):12S-17S.

101. Monnickendam MA, McEvoy MB, Blake WA, et al. Necrotizing fasciitis associated with invasive group A streptococcal infections in England and Wales. Adv Exp Med Biol. 1997;418:87-9.

102. Morantes MC, Lipsky BA. Flesh-eating bacteria: return of an old nemesis. Int J Dermat. 1995;34:461-3.

103. Mutschler W, Bakker DJ. Temporärer Hautersatz [temporary skin replacement]. Z für Allg.med. 1988;64:714-20. German.

104. Neuber M, Rieger H, Brüwer M, et al. Fulminante fasciitis necroticans bei morbus crohn-assoziiertem verlauf. Chirurg. 2000;71:1277-80. German.

105. Nichols RL, Smith JW. Gas in the wound: what does it mean? Surg Clin North Am. 1975;55:1289-96.

106. Nichols RL. Gas-producing infections. In: Nichols RL, Hyslop NE, Bartlett JG, editors. Decision making in surgical sepsis. Philadelphia: Decker; 1991. p. 60-1.

107. Norrby-Teglund A, Thulin P, Gan BS, et al. Evidence for superantigen involvement in severe group A streptococcal tissue infections. J Infect Dis. 2001;184:853-60.

108. Patino JF, Castro D, Valencia A, Morales P. Necrotizing soft tissue lesions after a volcanic cataclysm. World J Surg. 1991;15:240-7.

109. Paty R, Smith AD. Gangrene and Fournier's gangrene. Urol Clin N Am. 1992;19(1):149-62.

110. Pfanner W. Zur kenntnis und behandlung des nekrotisierenden erysipels. Kriegschirurgische mitteilungen aus dem Vülkerkrieg 1914/1918, nr 81. Dtsch Z Chir. 1918;144:108-19. German.

111. Podbielski A, Rozdzinski E, Wiedeck H, Lütticken R. Gruppe-A-streptokokken und die nekrotisierende fasziitis. Dt Artztebl. 1998;95(8):A-414-20. German.

112. Proud D, Bruscino Raiola F, Holden D, Paul E, Capstick R, Khoo A. Are we getting necrotizing soft tissue infections right? A 10-year review. ANZ J Surg. 2014;84:468-72.

113. Pruitt BA. Burns and soft tissues. In: Polk HC Jr, editor. Infection in the surgical patient. London: Churchill Livingstone; 1982. p. 113-31. (Clinical surgery international; 4)

114. Quirk WF, Sternbach G. Joseph Jones: infection with flesh eating bacteria. J Em Med. 1996;14:747-53.

115. Riegels-Nielsen P, Hesselfeldt-Nielsen J, Bang-Jensen E, Jacobsen E. Fournier's gangrene: five patients treated with hyperbaric oxygen. J Urol. 1984;132:918-20.

116. Riseman JA, Zamboni WA, Curtis A, Graham DR, Konrad HR, Ross DS. Hyperbaric oxygen therapy for necrotizing fasciitis reduces mortality and the need for debridements. Surg. 1990;108:847-50.

117. Rodloff AC, Montag TH, Gurtz G, Harnoss B-M, Ehlers S. Mikrobiologische aspekte von anaerobierinfektionen. In: Hau T, editor. Anaerobierinfektionen in der chirurgie. Upjohn Heppenheim (Germany); 1991. German.

118. Schwarz N, Redl H, Grasslober H, Krebitz B. Necrotizing soft tissue infection—an increasing problem in orthopedic trauma. Eur J Trauma. 2000;2:62-8.

119. Shaw JJ, Psionos C, Emhoff TA, Shah SA, Santry HP. Not just full of hot air: hyperbaric oxygen therapy increases survival in cases of necrotizing soft tissue infections. Surg Infect (Larchmt). 2014;399:333-41

120. Sheffield PJ. Tissue oxygen measurements. In: Davis JC, Hunt TK, editors. Problem wounds: the role of oxygen. New York: Elsevier; 1988. p. 37-44.

121. Sherris JC. Skin and wound infection. In: Sherris JC, editor. Medical microbiology. New York: Elsevier; 1984. p. 555-61.

122. Shupak A, Shoshani O, Goldenberg I, Barzilai A, Moskuna R, Bursztein S. Necrotizing fasciitis: an indication for hyperbaric oxygen therapy? Surgery. 1995;118:873-8.

123. Smith GL, Bunker CB, Dinneen MD. Fournier's gangrene. Brit J Urol. 1998;81:347- 55.

124. Stevens BJ, Lathrop JC, Rice WT, Gruenberg JC. Fournier's gangrene: historic (1764-1978) versus contemporary (1979-1988) differences in etiology and clinical importance. Am Surg. 1993;59:149-54.

125. Stevens DL, Gibbons AE, Bergstrom R, Winn V. The Eagle effect revisited: efficacy of clindamycin, erythromycin and penicillin in the treatment of streptococcal myositis. J Inf Dis. 1988;158:23-8.

126. Stevens DL. Invasive group A streptococcus infections. Clin Inf Dis. 1992;14:2-13.

127. Stevens DL. Invasive group A streptococcal infections: the past, the present and future. Pediatr Inf Dis J. 1994;13:561-6.

128. Stevens DL. Streptococcal toxic shock syndrome: spectrum of disease, pathogenesis and new concepts in treatment. Em Inf Dis. 1995;1:69-78.

129. Stevens DL. Invasive group A streptococcal disease [review]. Infec Agents and Dis. 1996;5:157-66.

130. Stevens DL. The flesh-eating bacterium: what's next?" J Infect Dis. 1999;179(Suppl 2):S366-74.

131. Stevens DL. Streptococcal toxic shock syndrome associated with necrotizing fasciitis. Ann Rev Med. 2000;51:271-88.

132. Stevens DL. Invasive streptococcal infections. J Infect Chemother. 2001;7:69-80.

133. Stephenson H, Dotters DJ, Katz V, Droegemueller W. Necrotizing fasciitis of the vulva. Am J Obstet Gynecol. 1992;166(5):1324-7.

134. Stone HH, Martin JG Jr. Synergistic necrotizing cellulitis. Ann Surg. 1992;175:702-11.

135. Stone DR, Gorbach SL. Necrotizing fasciitis. The changing spectrum.. Dermatol Clin. 1997;15:213-20.

136. Sutherland ME, Meyer AA. Necrotizing soft-tissue infections. Surg Clin N Am. 1994;74:591-607.

137. Thom SR. Hyperbaric oxygen therapy in septicemia. J Hyp Med. 1987;2:141-6.

138. Tibbles PM, Edelsberg JS. Hyperbaric oxygen therapy. N Eng J Med. 1996;334:1642-8.

139. Umeda T, Ohara H, Hayashi O, et al. Toxic shock syndrome after suction lipectomy. Plast Reconstr Surg. 2000;106:204-7; discussion Mladick RA 208-9.

140. Unnikrishnan M, Cohen J, Sriskandan S. Complementation of a speA negative Streptococcus pyogenes with speA: effects on virulence and production of streptococcal pyrogenic exotoxin A. Microb Pathogen. 2001;31:109-14.

141. Vick R, Carson CC. Fournier's disease. Urol Clin N Am. 1999;26:841-51.

142. Voros D, Pissiotis C, Georgantas D, et al. Role of early and extensive surgery in the treatment of severe necrotizing soft tissue infections. Br J Surg. 1993;80:1190-1.

143. Wall DB, Klein SR, Black S, Virgilio de C. A simple model to help distinguish necrotizing fasciitis from nonnecrotizing soft tissue infection. J Am Coll Surg. 2000;191:227-31.

144. Webb R, Berg E. Symbiotic gangrene due to Pseudomonas pyocyanea and E. coli. Austr NZ J Surg. 1966;36:159-60.

145. Weiss KA, Lavardière M. Group A streptococcus invasive infections: a review. Can J Surg. 1997;40:18-25.

146. Whitesides L, Cotto-Cumba C, Myers RAM. Cervical necrotizing fasciitis of odontogenic origin: a case report and review of 12 cases. J Or Max Surg. 2000;58:144-51.

147. Wienecke H, Lobenhoffer P. Nekrotisierende weichteilinfektionen. Chirurg. 2001;72:320-37. German.

148. Wilkinson D, Doolette D. Hyperbaric oxygen treatment and survival from necrotizing soft tissue infections. Arch Surg. 2004;139:1339-45.

149. Wilson B. Necrotizing fasciitis. Am Surgeon. 1952;18:426-31.

150. Wilson DH, Haltalin KC. Acute necrotizing fasciitis in childhood. Am J Dis Child. 1973;125:591-5.

151. Zamboni WA, Riseman JA, Kucan JO. Management of Fournier's gangrene and the role of hyperbaric oxygen. J Hyp Med. 1990;5:177-86.

152. Zamboni WA, Mazolewski PJ, Erdmann D, et al. Evaluation of penicillin and hyperbaric oxygen in the treatment of streptococcal myositis. Ann Plast Surg. 1997;39:131-6.

CHAPTER 19 CHAPTER

Hyperbaric Oxygen in Intracranial Abscess

CHAPTER NINETEEN OVERVIEW

Introduction **467**
Morbidity/Mortality 467
Rationales for HBO_2 . . . . **469**
Bacteriology 469
Perifocal Cerebral Edema 472
Enhanced Host Defense 472
Concomitant Osteomyelitis of the Skull 472
Other Effects 472
An Exemplary Case Report **473**
International Case Series Treated by Adjunctive HBO_2 . . . . **474**
Current Therapy and Indications for Adjuvant HBO_2 . . . . **477**
Our Most Recent Case **478**
References **480**

Hyperbaric Oxygen in Intracranial Abscess

Lorenz A. Lampl, Guenter Frey, Dietmar Fischer, Enrico Staps

INTRODUCTION

Based upon considerations similar to the rationale for the use of HBO_2 in gas gangrene as well as management of necrotizing soft-tissue infections, the treatment of intracranial abscess with adjunctive HBO_2 has been approved by the Undersea and Hyperbaric Medical Society (UHMS) since 1994,[16] followed by the European Committee for Hyperbaric Medicine (ECHM) in its Consensus Conference 2004 in Lille, France.[41]

The first review of the bacteriologic and pathophysiologic rationale for HBO_2 treatment of intracranial abscesses was published in the Journal of Hyperbaric Medicine in 1989.[33] However, at that time as well as today, data from animal series are scarce,[5] and the number of case series as well as anecdotal case reports has been increasing just slowly over the years.[2,25,28-29,63]

Inasmuch as the clinical course, diagnosis, and treatment of subdural or epidural empyemas have similarities, these are all included along with intracerebral abscesses. All these disorders are discussed under the term "intracranial abscesses."

As a consequence of the nature of intracranial abscesses, prospective randomized trials (RCTs) on HBO_2's therapeutic effectiveness in humans are not to be expected. For this reason, collecting as many case reports as possible was of first priority in the past. Today, in 2016, case series from 7 hyperbaric centers are available internationally, involving 230 patients. So the comparison between adjuvant HBO_2 therapy and standard management in those patients has become possible.

Morbidity/Mortality

Intracranial abscesses account for only three to five admissions per year even at a large medical center.[17] Thus, the incidence is roughly in the same range or a little higher than that of gas gangrene and necrotizing soft-tissue infections.

However, the overall mortality in numerous series from various countries averages 19.2% over 35 years (Table 1). In spite of a significantly reduced death rate in recent years to below 10%, mortality still remains unacceptably high. Permanent sequelae such as epileptic disorders are frequently reported in the survivors.

TABLE 1A - C: MORTALITY RATES FROM INTRACRANIAL ABSCESSES DURING DIFFERENT STUDY PERIODS (1981–1985/1986–1995/1996–2005)

1a: 1981–1985

Author	Yr.of. Publ.	Country of Origin	No. Px	Px died	Mortality	[Ref.]
Yang	1981	PR China	400	91	23%	[74]
Alderson	1981	Great Britain	90	9	10%	[1]
Dohrmann	1982	Australia	28	10	36%	[11]
Britt	1983	USA	14	5	36%	[7]
Cowie	1983	Great Britain	89	24	27%	[10]
Harris	1985	USA	15	3	20%	[17]
			636	**142**	**22.3%**	

1b: 1986–1995

Author	Yr. of Publ.	Country of Origin	No. Px	Px Died	Mortality	[Ref.]
Ferriero	1987	USA	17	1	6%	[12]
Pattisapu	1987	USA	8	0	0%	[53]
Miller	1988	Great Britain	100	20	20%	[44]
Schliamser	1988	Sweden	54	17	31%	[58]
Basit	1989	Saudi Arabia	21	5	24%	[4]
Szuwart	1989	Germany	38	10	26%	[70]
Witzmann	1989	Austria	38	7	18%	[73]
Pathak	1990	India	41	10	24%	[52]
Kratimenos	1991	Great Britain	14	2	14%	[27]
McIntyre	1991	Australia	14	3	21%	[43]
Bagdatoglu	1992	Turkey	78	16	20%	[3]
Seydoux	1992	Switzerland	39	5	13%	[61]
Bok	1993	South Africa	21	5	24%	[6]
Stapleton	1993	Great Britain	11	3	27%	[64]
Yang	1993	PR China	140	11	8%	[75]
Sharma	1995	India	38	12	32%	[62]
			672	**127**	**18.9%**	

1c: 1996–2005

Author	Yr. of Publ.	Country of Origin	No. Px	Px died	Mortality	[Ref.]
Takada	1998	Japan	13	0	0%	[71]
Stephanov	1999	Switzerland	17	2	12%	[65]
Mamatova	2000	Uzbekistan	13	1	8%	[37]
Liliang	2001	Taiwan	15	4	27%	[34]
Marchiori	2003	Italy	20	1	5%	[38]
Jansson	2004	Sweden	66	3	5%	[21]
Ozkaya	2005	Turkey	25	4	16%	[51]
			169	**15**	**8.9%**	

RATIONALES FOR HBO_2

In 1983, we had favorable results in an anecdotal case in which HBO_2 was initiated as a last-ditch attempt to save a young mother's life.[31] A thorough literature research then led to a better understanding of HBO_2's potential usefulness in the treatment of intracranial abscess. Our group was able to combine this with the clinical experience in a series of 25 own patients treated to date, as well as with the data of 6 other hyperbaric centers.

Bacteriology

Over the past 30 years, knowledge of the bacteriology of intracranial abscess has become better defined in the literature. Anaerobes account for up to 90% of the bacteria isolated from intracranial foci. This, of course, depends on the culturing technique used.

Nevertheless, the predominance of anaerobic organisms in intracranial abscesses has been well documented in the world literature for decades.[1,7,8,11,23,32,74]

The fact that in the past, several studies (for example, Yang), found a high percentage of sterile cultures may be deceptive.[74] One explanation is that anaerobic culturing either had not been done or that it had not been done correctly.

TABLE 2: BACTERIAL ISOLATES (OWN PATIENT SERIES, N = 25): IN 18 PATIENTS EXCLUSIVELY ANAEROBIC/MICROAEROPHILIC PATHOGENS. IN 10 PATIENTS, MORE THAN 1 GERM ISOLATED.

STRICTLY ANAEROBIC		
Peptostreptococci	7	
Bacteroides spp.	4	
Fusobacteria	2	
Clostr. perfringens	1	59.5%
Veillonella	1	
Streptococci (anaerobic)	4	
Actinomyces spp.	2	
Prevotella oralis	1	
INTERMEDIATE		
Streptococci (microaerophilic)	9	27.0%
Enterobacter	1	
AEROBIC		13.5%
Staphylococci spp.	5	

These results coincide with our own (Table 2). In 25 consecutive, nonselected patients, 37 different organisms were identified. In 18 patients, cultures were purely anaerobic, including microaerophilic streptococci. In five patients, staphylococci were found, combined with enterobacter, microaerophilic streptococci, and fusobacteria, respectively. In one septic patient with a small subdural empyema treated without surgery, only peptostreptococci were harvested from a blood culture, suggesting them to be the empyema's underlying cause. In a five-year-old boy, *Clostridium perfringens* was cultured from the cerebrospinal fluid after a penetrating skull injury; probably due to antibiotic therapy, cultures from the cerebral abscess, which emerged some days later, were sterile (Table 3).

TABLE 3: DATA AND DIAGNOSIS, UNDERLYING DISORDERS AND BACTERIOLOGICAL FINDINGS (SEE TABLE 2) IN 25 UNSELECTED PATIENTS WITH INTRACRANIAL ABSCESSES (OWN CASES)

No.	Age	Sex	Diagnosis	Underlying Disorder	Bacterial Isolate
1	31	f	multiple abscesses left hemisphere	septic tonsillectomy	*Bacteroides fragilis*, pep-to-streptococci
2	22	m	epidural empyema	pansinusitis	*Fusobacteria*, streptococci (microaerophilic)
3	34	m	parietal abscess	pulmonary angioma	*Bacteroides fragilis*, pepto-streptococci, streptococci (microaerophilic)
4	13	m	frontal abscess	sinusitis frontalis	streptococci (microaerophilic)
5	15	f	frontal abscess	pansinusitis	pepto-streptococci
6	26	m	frontal abscess	sinusitis frontalis	*Veillonella parv., Bacteroides spp.*
7	47	m	parietal abscess	apical ostitis tooth 3/5	pepto-streptococci
8	36	m	frontal abscess	???	*Staph. epidermidis*
9	27	m	subdural empyema	sinusitis maxillaris	pepto-streptococci (blood culture)
10	42	f	frontal abscess	progressive osteomyelitis	*Enterobacter, Staph. aureus*
11	48	m	multiple abscesses left hemisphere	sinusitis frontalis	*Staph. epider-midis*, strepto-cocci (microaero-philic)
12	52	m	frontal abscess	sinusitis maxil-laris?	streptococci (anaerobic)
13	21	m	multiple abscesses right hemisphere	pansinusitis	streptococci (microaerophilic)
14	5	m	frontal abscess	penetrating injury	*Clostr. perfringens*
15	45	m	subdural empyema	pansinusitis	----

TABLE 3 (CONTINUED)

No.	Age	Sex	Diagnosis	Underlying Disorder	Bacterial Isolate
16	47	f	subdural empyema	osteomyelitis femur (?)	*Fusobacteria, Staph. Sp.*
17	17	m	epi-/subdural empyema	open skull base fracture	*Staph. epidermidis* Streptococci (anaerobic) Streptococci (microaerophilic)
18	57	f	subdural empyema	mastoiditis	Streptococci (microaerophilic)
19	22	m	subdural empyema	pansinusitis	*Bacteroides* sp. Pepto-streptococci
20	4	m	multiple abscesses both hemispheres	pulmonary abscess	Streptococci (anaerobic) Streptococci (microaerophilic)
21	19	m	multiple abscesses	sinusitis maxillaris	Streptococci (microaerophilic)
22	40	m	parietal abscess	unknown	Pepto-streptococci *Actinomyces spp.* Streptococci (anaerobic)
23	59	m	solitary abscess thalamus left side	unknown	----
24	59	m	subdural abscesses frontotemporal right side	otitis externa maligna	*Prevotella oralis*
25	32	m	subdural empyema frontal, solitary abscess capsula interna right side	pansinusitis	*Actinomyces spp.*

Most astonishing to us was the fact that anaerobes were the predominant organisms in four patients with rhinogenic intracranial abscesses when only aerobes were cultivated from the inflamed nasal sinuses, the infection's source. We do not fully understand this selection phenomenon yet. Lampl et al. has provided case reports for further examination.[33]

The bacteriologic results quoted above are mostly from patients with endogenous intracranial abscesses. No data have been found in the literature to indicate whether the same is true in exogenous abscesses following penetrating head injuries.

The therapeutic effect of HBO_2 on anaerobic and miscellaneous flora is well known and has been widely documented for many years.[15,18,50,55,60]\

Perifocal Cerebral Edema

The expansive growth of an intracranial abscess and the formation of its perifocal edema may result in either secondary lesions to surrounding brain tissue or, at worst, may lead to a life-threatening increase in intracranial pressure (ICP). The beneficial influence of HBO_2 on increased ICP has been documented for more than 50 years.[45-49,54,66-67]

HBO_2 acts directly on autoregulated small blood vessels. Elevated arterial oxygen tension results in a vasoconstriction leading to a decrease in cerebral blood flow; consequently this leads to a reduction of the intracranial vascular volume. In turn, this results in the reduction of ICP. HBO_2 additionally guarantees sufficient oxygen delivery to potentially hypoxic brain areas.[60] This mechanism may be of major importance in the prevention or treatment of secondary brain damage.[14,19-20]

The therapeutic impact of these physiologic effects of HBO_2 is expected to be even more pronounced in cases of perifocal brain swelling due to intracranial abscess. HBO_2 acts specifically against anaerobic microorganisms as the predominant cause of intracranial abscess and the consequent brain swelling. Therefore, HBO_2's influence on the edema, and on elevated ICP, should tend to be curative, secondary to its attack on the underlying bacteriology. It is not just a reversible symptomatic effect, as seen with other agents used to lower intracranial pressure.

At present, there is only one anecdotal case report describing the favorable influence of adjunctive HBO_2 on a critically elevated ICP[31] in an intracranial abscess patient.

Enhanced Host Defense

The effects of HBO_2 in enhancing leukocyte-mediated host defense mechanisms are well known to the hyperbaric community. Therefore, they need not to be described in detail here.

Nevertheless, potentiation of leukocyte microbial killing seems to be of twofold importance:

1. as the predominant defense mechanism at the abscess site
2. as an adjunct in cases of concomitant osteomyelitis

Concomitant Osteomyelitis of the Skull

Rhinogenic as well as otogenic intracranial abscesses are frequently combined with more or less pronounced osteomyelitic processes involving the skull's bony structure. HBO_2 is a powerful adjuvant to surgery and antibiotics in infections of this kind. Despite its potency, however, as in other infectious diseases, it remains an adjunctive treatment.

Other Effects

At present, the influence of HBO_2 on the abscess membrane formation has not been clearly assessed in humans. However, in a randomized study published in 2012 involving 80 female Wistar rats, Bilic et al. investigated the effects of HBO_2 in the early healing stage of experimental brain abscesses.[5] HBO_2 proved to be beneficial either alone or in combination with antibiotics. This was mainly manifested on days three and five and was evident as a statistically significant increase of blood vessel formation, increase in mean vascular densitiy, and lower abscess necrotic score.

Since frequently there is either only a slight inflammatory reaction of the meninges, or none at all in the case of intracerebral abscesses, achieving effective antibiotic treatment may easily pose major problems in terms of antibiotic penetration. For this reason, studies showing a reversible opening of the blood-brain barrier by HBO_2, leading to an improved penetration of antibiotics through noninflamed meninges,[9] might be promising. Additionally, improved tissue oxygenation due to HBO_2 is able to potentiate the antimicrobial effects of antibiotics such as aminoglykosides.

AN EXEMPLARY CASE REPORT

History: Presenting the nonspecific history of a flu for a few days, a four-year-old old boy was admitted to the pediatric university hospital because of progressive vigilance disturbances.

Diagnosis ***Multiple cerebral abscesses*** predominantly in the left hemisphere (Figure 1, Figure 2).

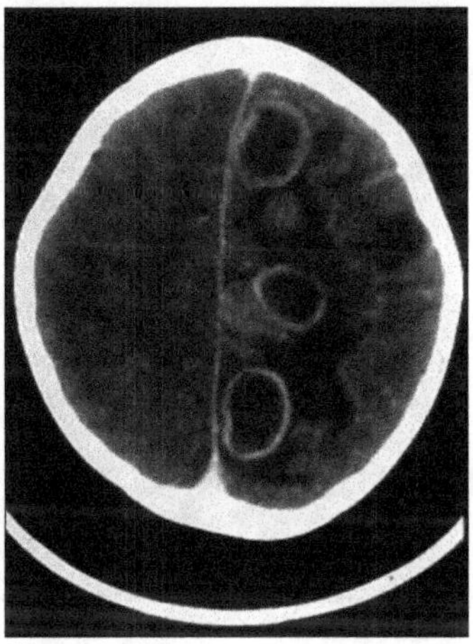

Figure 1.

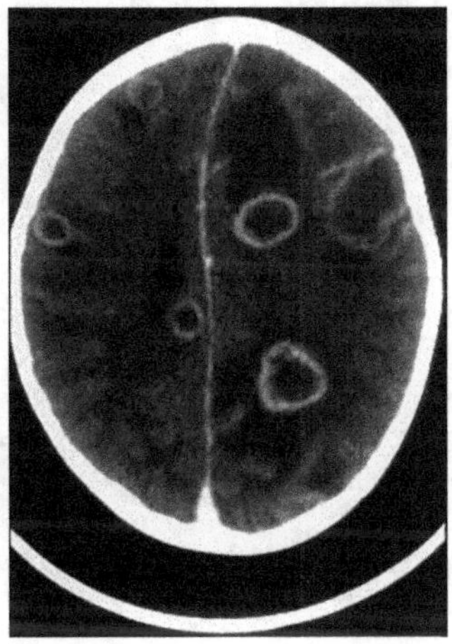

Figure 2.

Source: ***Pulmonary abscess*** right lower lobe (Figure 3).

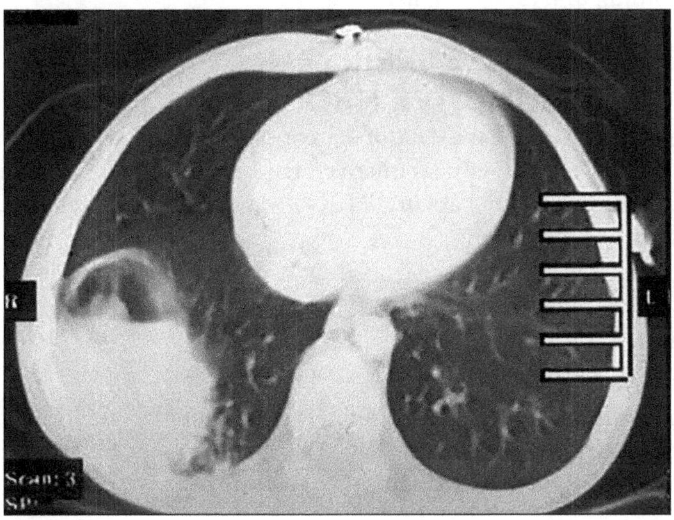

Figure 3.

Bacteriology: Streptococci (anaerobic/microaerophilic).

Course: Neurosurgery limited to drainage (➔) of the most space-occupying abscess only (Figure 4). Repeated fine-needle aspirations of all abscess formations within stereotactic reach over the following days. Comprehensive intensive care including controlled ventilation and adequate antibiosis, completed by immediate HBO_2 therapy. Because of open lung surgery after six days (lobectomy of the right lower lobe) and a favorable neurological course seen at that time already, limitation of HBO_2 to six sessions altogether before thoracotomy (Figure 5, before HBO_2 session 6, mind the thoracic abscess drainage).

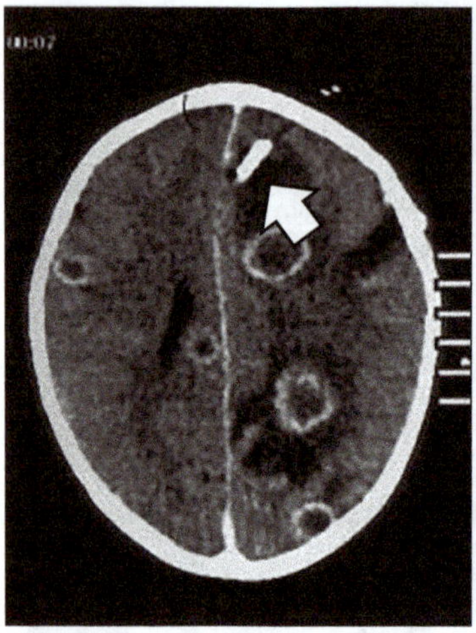

Figure 4.

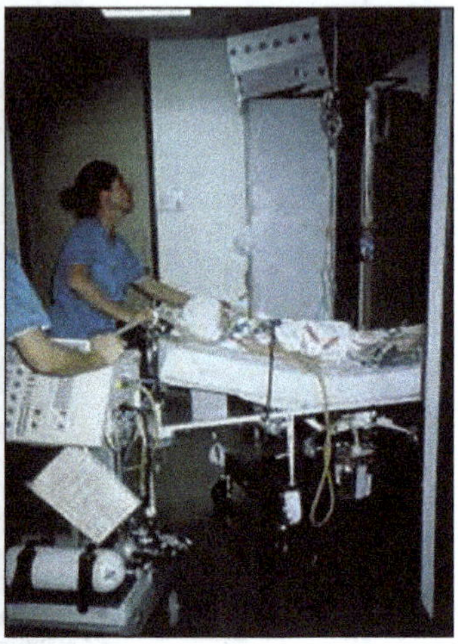

Figure 5.

Outcome: With no neurological deficit remaining, the boy was put to school at the age of six, according to national regulations.

INTERNATIONAL CASE SERIES TREATED BY ADJUNCTIVE HBO_2

To date (August 2016), we have data of 25 consecutive and unrelated patients with intracranial abscesses treated with adjunctive HBO_2 at our facility in Ulm from 1983 to 2016 (Table 3). In all our patients, HBO_2 was started when at least one of the following criteria was met:

- Anaerobic or mixed pathogens
- Multiple abscesses
- Abscess in a deep or dominant location

When the infection was life threatening, treatment was performed twice daily; otherwise there was one treatment per day at 2.5 ATA, except for patient 1 (Table 3) who was treated at 2.8 ATA. The duration of each treatment was between 60 and 90 minutes.

Time will tell whether 2.5 ATA is the optimal pressure for this disorder; therefore, the ultimate protocol is open to discussion. However, in the entire series of 25 patients managed with 348 hyperbaric treatments, no signs of cerebral oxygen toxicity were observed nor were other adverse effects of pressurization seen. In our opinion, when choosing the appropriate treatment pressure, treatment of the infection should be considered primary, before concerns about possible side effects.

The number of HBO_2 sessions varied from 4 to 30 and averaged 13.9 in our patients. Usually, the number of HBO_2 treatments depended on the patient's response, which included neurosurgical evaluation as well as radiological findings from repeated head scans. In two cases, patient cooperation proved to be a major problem, probably secondary to psychic derangements attendant to their disease. In these two cases, fewer HBO_2 treatments than desired were administered.

The mortality observed with our patients was 0.0 % with a complete recovery in 72%, and 76% were able to resume their former occupational work and life (Table 4).

TABLE 4: NUMBER OF HBO SESSIONS AND OUTCOME IN 25 PATIENTS WITH INTRACRANIAL ABSCESSES (OWN CASES)

No.	Age	Sex	HBOs	Outcome	
1	31	f	14	slightly disabled	*
2	22	m	4	complete recovery	*
3	34	m	10	severely disabled (lost follow-up)	
4	13	m	16	complete recovery	*
5	15	f	10	complete recovery	*
6	26	m	10	complete recovery	*
7	47	m	6	brachio-facial hemiparesis (in recovery, lost follow-up)	
8	36	m	27	complete recovery	*
9	27	m	7	moderate motor-dysphasia, minimal brachial hemiparesis (in recovery, lost follow-up)	
10	42	f	19	complete recovery	*
11	48	m	12	complete recovery	*
12	52	m	13	complete recovery	*
13	21	m	12	complete recovery	*
14	5	m	17	complete recovery	*
15	45	m	22	complete recovery	*
16	47	f	16	persistent aphasia	
17	17	m	20	complete recovery	*
18	57	f	7	complete recovery	*
19	22	m	20	complete recovery	*
20	4	m	6	complete recovery	*
21	19	m	14	complete recovery	*
22	40	m	**30	lost follow-up	
23	59	m	17	complete recovery	*
24	59	m	8	brachial hemiparesis, dysphasia (lost follow-up)	
25	32	m	11	complete recovery	*

* patient has returned to his / her former occupational work or school

** with kind support by BG-Unfallklinik Murnau, Germany

The favorable results that we have seen in our own patients could be confirmed by other investigators (Figure 6).

This is true for the patients treated by Mathieu in France:[40,42] His inclusion criteria was deterioration of the patient´s neurological condition, due to lack of response to standard therapy – which, without doubt, primarily means a very poor prognosis: only 4 out of 20 have been lost.

The same is true for a series from Graz, Austria:[69] these investigators achieved a 0% mortality in their 18 patients, beginning in the 1970s at a time when, in the international literature, the mortality of intracranial abscess patients still was up to 36% (Table 1).

The unpublished data from Murnau Trauma Center in Germany[24,59] completely match with these results, as do the observations of Kindwall and Whelan, United States,[26,72] and quite a number of single anecdotal case reports.[2,25,28,63]

Furthermore, these findings are confirmed by another study from Turkey,[29] once more demonstrating a 0% mortality in a series for 13 brain abscess patients treated by adjuvant HBO_2.

Also, the data from Mathiesen and Lind (Karolinska Hospital, Stockholm, Sweden) not only show again a 0 mortality in 56 patients but especially report a markedly reduced permanent residual disability in a 6-months' follow-up: no severe morbidity, 1 case of moderate handicap only, and no severe disability.[35,39]

So, at present (summer 2016), data from 7 series with an overall mortality of 4.3% are available, enrolling 230 patients in whom HBO_2 was used as an adjunctive component in intracranial abscess management during the years 1976 to 2016 (Figure 6).

During the same time span, 29 studies enrolling 1,477 patients treated conventionally with an average mortality of 19.2% were found in the literature (Table 1).

Taking mortality as the criterion, the results are significantly superior ($p < 0.01$) when HBO_2 is applied as an adjuvant component to the standard therapeutic principles of intracranial abscess management [30](Figure 7).

HBO in intracranial abscess

Series Available

Author	Year	Origin	No. Px	Px died	Mortality
Kindwall & Whelan	2016	Wisconsin / USA	24	1	4 %
Kutlay et al.	2005	Istanbul / Turkey	13	0	0 %
Lampl et al.	2016	Ulm / Germany	25	0	0 %
Mathiesen et al.	2009	Stockholm / Sweden	56	0	0 %
Mathieu	2016	Lille / France	20	4	20 %
Murnau Trauma Center	2016	Murnau / Germany	74	5	7 %
Sutter et al.	1996	Graz / Austria	18	0	0 %
			230	10	4.3 %

HBO-patient series compiled with assistance by UHMS

Timespan 1974 - 2016

Figure 6.

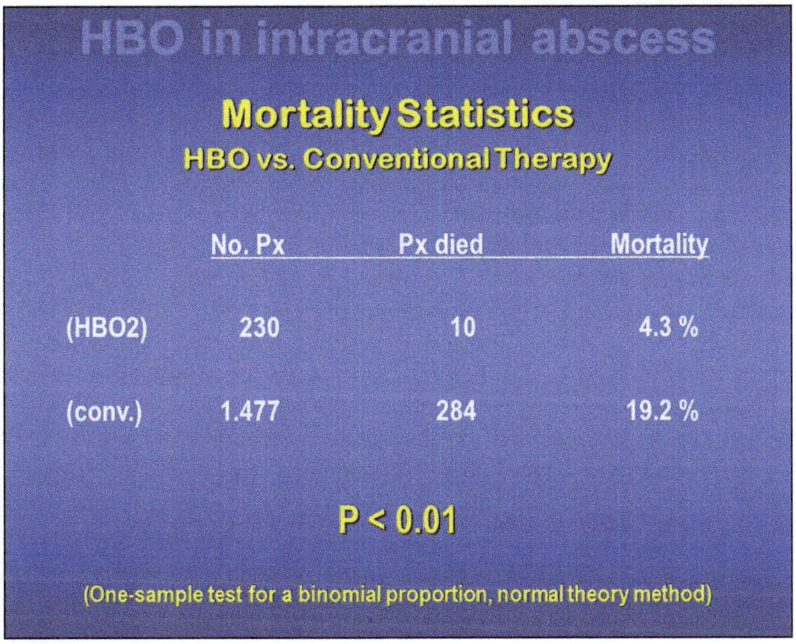

Figure 7.

CURRENT THERAPY AND INDICATIONS FOR ADJUVANT HBO_2

As with other life-threatening conditions such as necrotizing soft-tissue infections, it is mandatory to apply HBO_2 in intracranial abscesses only in combination with currently accepted standard procedures or as a complement to them. Above all, treatment must include appropriate neurosurgical management (e.g., fine-needle aspiration, drainage, or resection, depending on the individual situation) and the administration of adequate antibiotics, as well as steroids.

The benefit of steroid medication in intracranial abscess management has been a controversial topic in the international literature for decades.(13) The influence of steroids on the perifocal edema in intracranial abscess may prove beneficial, but the impairment of host defense in infectious disorders must be seriously considered.

In this context, HBO_2 certainly is a beneficial therapeutic component with proven antibiotic as well as edema-reducing efficacy. Its use is approved in the following conditions:(16)

- Anaerobic or mixed pathogens
- Multiple abscesses
- Abscess in a deep or dominant location
- Compromised host
- In situations where surgery is contraindicated or where the patient is a poor surgical risk
- No response, or further deterioration, in spite of standard surgical care (e.g., 1–2 fine-needle aspirations) and adequate antibiotic treatment

The **early** administration of HBO_2 seems to be of utmost importance. To delay the onset of HBO_2, or to start it as a last-ditch attempt when everything else has failed, will obscure the true potential benefit and may also cause avoidable brain damage.

Since the infectious component of the intracranial abscess has to be considered primary, we recommend a treatment pressure of 2.5 ATA, 1 or 2 sessions a day, depending on the clinical status of the patient. The number of HBO_2 treatments given has to be assessed on an individual basis, in accordance with the patient's clinical response, as well as with the radiological findings.

As the mortality and long-term sequelae of intracranial abscesses are substantial, HBO_2 treatment is warranted, even in the absence of rigid double-blind, randomized, and controlled trials. The number of treatments required is relatively small, and the costs of hyperbaric treatment are trivial in comparison to the total costs of managing these critically ill patients.

In view of the high morbidity and mortality of cerebral abscess and the fact that HBO_2 is relatively noninvasive and carries an extremely low complication rate, the risk-benefit ratio is not arguable.The full benefit of an HBO_2-based protocol is expected to become even more significant once study criteria such as epileptic sequelae and permanent handicap and parameters such as the ability to return to former occupational life are properly documented in addition to the surveillance of pure mortality rates.[35,39]

OUR MOST RECENT CASE

History: Male patient, 32 years old, admitted to the emergency department of a general hospital because of persistent headache for 2 weeks. Medical history was uneventful aside from a tooth extraction 5 months before.

Findings: CT scans are revealing a pansinusitis and an epidural frontal empyema (Figure 8). Onset of antibiosis (clindamycin and metronidazole), transfer to our facilities.

Neurosurgery: Immediate craniotomy and evacuation of the frontal empyema.

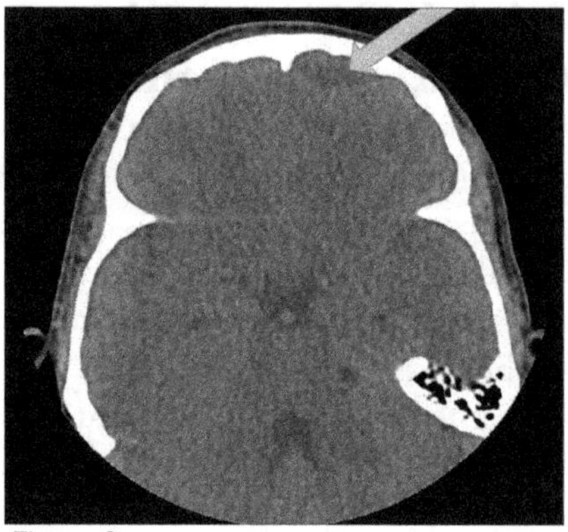

Figure 8.

Course: MRI scan the following day shows no frontal empyema remaining, but now a new septic focus at the capsula interna right side (Figure 9).

Bacteriology from the epidural empyema: **Actinomyces spp.**

HBO_2: In spite of an adaption of antibiotics, the septic focus at the capsula interna still is to be seen 12 days later. Initiation of HBO_2 because of

- abscess in a deep or dominant location,
- anaerobic/microaerophilic pathogens, and
- no response to standard therapy.

11 HBO_2 sessions at 2.5 bar, 90 minutes each, 1 session per day.**Outcome:** On the MRI scan 1 month later the abscess formation had disappeared (Figure 10).

Complete recovery, patient has resumed his former work.

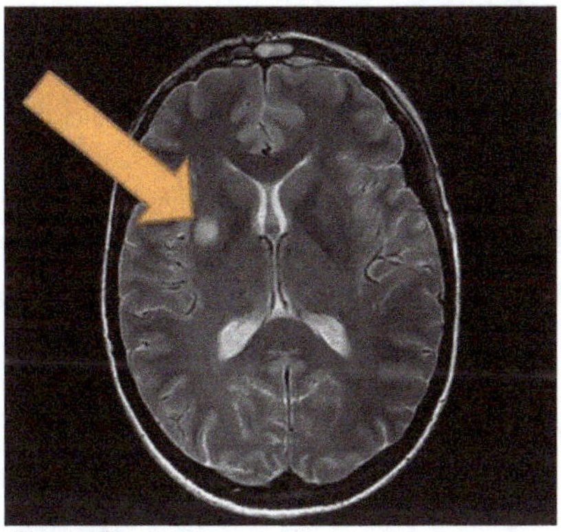

Figure 9.

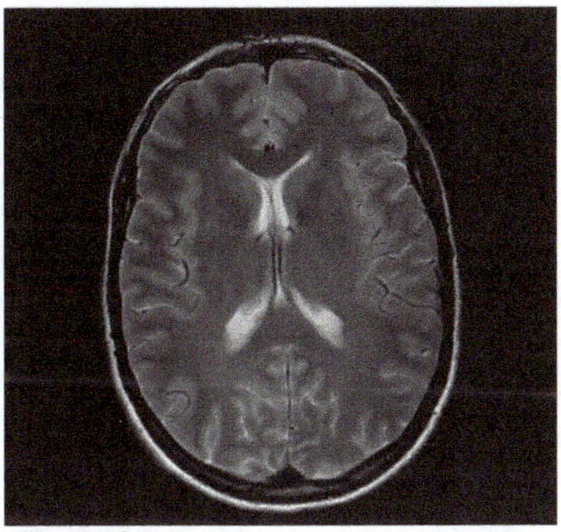

Figure 10.

REFERENCES

1. Alderson D, Strong AJ, Ingham HR, Selkon JB. Fifteen-year review of the mortality of brain abscesses. Neurosurgery. 1981; 8:1-6.
2. Baechli H, Schmutz J, Mayr J. Hyperbaric oxygen therapy (HBO2) for the treatment of an epidural abscess in the posterior fossa in an 8-month-old infant. Pediatr Neurosurg. 2008;44(3):239-42.
3. Bagdatoglu H, Ildan F, Cetinalp E, et al. The clinical presentation of intracranial abscesses. A study of seventy-eight cases. J Neurosurg Sci. 1992;36:139-43.
4. Basit AS, Ravi B, Banerji AK, Tandon PN. Multiple pyogenic brain abscesses: an analysis of 21 patients. J Neurol Neurosurg Psychiatry. 1989;52:591-4.
5. Bilic I et al. Hyperbaric oxygen is effective in early stage of healing of experimental brain abscess in rats. Neurol Res. 2012;34(10):931-6.
6. Bok AP, Peter JC. Subdural empyema: burr holes or craniotomy? A retrospective computerized tomography era analysis of treatment in 90 cases. J Neurosurg. 1993;78:574-8.
7. Britt RH, Enzmann DR. Clinical stages of human brain abscesses on serial CT scans after contrast infusion. Computerized tomographic, neuropathological, and clinical correlations. J Neurosurg. 1983;59:972-89.
8. Brook I. Bacteriology of intracranial abscess in children. J Neurosurg. 1981;54:484-8.
9. Chambi IP, Ceverha MD, Hart GB, Strauss MB. Effect of hyperbaric oxygen in the permeability of the blood-brain-barrier. 8th International Congress on Hyperbaric Medicine; 1984; Long Beach (CA). Abstract.
10. Cowie R, Williams B. Late seizures and morbidity after subdural empyema. J Neurosurg. 1983;58:569-73.
11. Dohrmann PJ, Elrick WL. Observations on brain abscesses. Review of 28 cases. Med J Austr. 1982;2:81-3.
12. Ferriero DM, Derechin M, Edwards MS, Berg BO. Outcome of brain abscess treatment in children: reduced morbidity with neuro-imaging. Pediatr Neurol. 1987;3:148-52.
13. Garvey G. Current concepts of bacterial infections of the central nervous system. J Neurosurg. 1983;59:735-44.
14. Götte U, Holbach KH. Hyperbare sauerstofftherapie bei neuro-chirurgischen patienten. Anaesthesist. 1969;18:139-45. German.
15. Gottlieb SF. Oxygen under pressure and microorganisms. In: Davis JC, Hunt TK, editors. Hyperbaric oxygen therapy. Bethesda (MD): Undersea Medical Society; 1977. p. 79-99.
16. Hampson NB, editor. Hyperbaric oxygen therapy: 1999 committee report. Kensington (MD): Undersea and Hyperbaric Medical Society; 1999.
17. Harris LF, McCubbin DA, Triplett JN Jr, Haws FP. Brain abscess: recent experience at a community hospital. South Med J. 1985;78:704-7.
18. Heimbach RD, Boerema I, Brummelkamp WH, et al. Current therapy of gas gangrene. In: Davis JC, Hunt TK, editors. Hyperbaric oxygen therapy. Bethesda (MD): Undersea Medical Society; 1977. p. 153-76.
19. Holbach KH, Wassmann K, Kolberg T. Verbesserte reversibilität des traumatischen mittelhirn-syndroms bei anwendung der hyperbaren oxygenation. Acta Neurochir. 1974;30:247-56.
20. Holbach KH, Wassmann K, Hohelüchter KL, Jain KK. Differentiation between reversible and irreversible post-stroke changes in brain tissue: its relevance for cerebro-vascular surgery. Surg Neurol. 1977;7:325-31.

21. Jansson AK, Enblad P, Sjoelin J. Efficacy and safety of cefotaxime in combination with metronidazole for empirical treatment of brain abscess in clinical practice: a retrospective study of 66 consecutive cases. Eur J Clin Microbiol & Inf Dis. 2004;23:7-14.

22. Kaide CG, Khandelwal S. Hyperbaric oxygen: applications in infectious disease. Emerg Med Clin North Am. 2008;26(2):571-95.

23. Kaplan K. Brain abscess. Med Clin N Am. 1985;69:345-60.

24. Kemmer A. (Murnau Trauma Center, Germany). Personal communication. 2006.

25. Kilic O, Kafadar A, Camcioglu Y, Akcakaya N, Cokugras H, Hasiloglu ZI. Primary intracranial abscess localized in the basal ganglia: a case report. J Trop Pediatr. 2012;58(1):71-3.

26. Kindwall EP. (Medical College of Wisconsin). Personal communication. 2001.

27. Kratimenos G, Crockard HA. Multiple brain abscess: a review of fourteen cases. Br J Neurosurg. 1991;5:153-61.

28. Kurschel S, Mohia A, Weigl V, Eder HG. Hyperbaric oxygen therapy for the treatment of brain abscess in children. Child's Nerv Syst. 2006;22(1):38-42.

29. Kutlay M, Colak A, Yildiz S, Demircan N, Akin ON. Stereotactic aspiration and antibiotic treatment combined with hyperbaric oxygen therapy in the management of bacterial brain abscesses. Neurosurgery. 2005;57(6):1140-6.

30. Lampl LA. Intracranial abscess management: are the results of adjunctive HBO2 therapy superior to conventional treatment? In: Cramer FS, Sheffield PJ, editors. Proceedings of the Fourteenth International Congress on Hyperbaric Medicine. Flagstaff (AZ): Best Publishing Company; 2003. p. 120-4.

31. Lampl L, Frey G, Miltner FO, Wörner U. Multiple anaerobic brain abscesses—life saving HBO2 therapy, integrated with comprehensive intensive care. In: Kindwall EP, editor. Proceedings of the Eighth International Congress on Hyperbaric Medicine. San Pedro (CA): Best Publishing; 1987. p.107-11.

32. Lampl LA, Frey G. Intra-cranial abscess. In: Mathieu D, editor. Handbook on hyperbaric medicine. Dordrecht (NL): Springer; 2006. p. 291-304.

33. Lampl L, Frey G, Dietze T, Trauschel M. Hyperbaric oxygen in intracranial abscesses. J Hyperbaric Med. 1989;4(3):111-26.

34. Liliang PC, Lin YC, Su TM, et al. Klebsiella brain abscess in adults. Infection. 2001;29:81-6.

35. Lind F. HBO2 Treatment Strategy for CNS infections: Registry Research Needed. In:
Pignel R, Gelsomino M, Reymond L, Germonpré P, editors. EUBS Geneva 2016 Abstract & Conference Book. 42nd Annual Scientific Meeting of the European Underwater & Baromedical Society; 2016 Sep 13-16; Geneva (CH). 2016. p. 11.

36. Mader JT. Bacterial osteomyelitis: adjunctive hyperbaric oxygen therapy. In: Bakker DJ, Schmutz J, editors. Hyperbaric Medicine Proceedings. Basel (CH): Foundation for Hyperbaric Medicine; 1988. p. 65-70.

37. Mamatova TS, Rasulova AK. Otogenic cerebellar abscesses. Vestn Otorinolaringol. 2000;4:47-50.

38. Marchiori C, Tonon E, Boscolo Rizzo P, et al. Hirnabszesse nach extrakraniellen infektionen im kopf-hals-bereich. HNO. 2003;51:813-22. German.

39. Mathiesen T, Larsson A, Lind F. Brain abscesses—spontaneous and traumatic abscesses and empyema. ECHM Conference Oxygen and Infection; 2009 May 7-9; Stockholm, Sweden. Available from: www.hyperbaricoxygen.se.

40. Mathieu D, Wattel F, Neviere R, Bocquillon N. Intracranial infections and hyperbaric oxygen therapy: a five year experience. Undersea Hyperb Med. 1999;26(Suppl):67. Abstract.
41. Mathieu D, editor. 7th European Consensus Conference on Hyperbaric Medicine, European Committee for Hyperbaric Medicine; 2004 Dec 3-4; Lille, France.
42. Mathieu D. (CHRU Lille, France). Personal communication. 2016.
43. McIntyre PB, Lavercombe PS, Kemp RJ, McCormack JG. Subdural and epidural empyema: diagnostic and therapeutic problems. Med J Aust. 1991;154:653-7.
44. Miller ES, Dias PS, Uttley D. CT scanning in the management of intracranial abscess: a review of 100 cases. Br J Neurosurg. 1988;2:439-46.
45. Miller JD, Fitch W, Ledingham IM. The effect of hyperbaric oxygen on experimentally increased intracranial pressure. J Neurosurg. 1970;33:287-96.
46. Miller JD, Ledingham IM. Reduction of increased intra-cranial pressure—a comparison between hyperbaric oxygen and hyperventilation. Arch Neurol. 1971;24:210-6.
47. Mogami RA, Hayakawa T, Kanai N. Clinical application of hyperbaric oxygenation in the treatment of acute cerebral damage. J Neurosurg. 1969;31:636-43.
48. Moody RA, Mead CO, Ruamsuke S. Therapeutic value of oxygen at normal and hyperbaric pressure in experimental head injury. J Neurosurg. 1970;32:51-4.
49. Ohta H, Yasui N, Kitami K. Intracranial pressure and hyperbaric oxygen. In: Kindwall EP, editor. Proceedings of the Eighth International Congress on Hyperbaric Medicine. San Pedro (CA): Best Publishing; 1987. p. 68-72.
50. Ollodart RM. Effects of HBO2 on aerobic microorganisms. In: Brown IW, Cox BG, editors. Proceedings of the 3rd International Congress on Hyperbaric Medicine; Duke University, Durham NC. 1966. p. 565-71. Abstract. Publ No 1404.
51. Ozkaya S, Bezircioglu H, Sucu HK, Ozdemir I. Combined approach for otogenic brain abscess. Neurologia medico-chirurgica. 2005;45:82-5.
52. Pathak A, Sharma BS, Mathuriya SN, et al. Controversies in the management of subdural empyema. A study of 41 cases with review of the literature. Acta Neurochir. 1990;102:25-32.
53. Pattisapu JV, Perent AD. Subdural empyemas in children. Pediatr Neurosci. 1987;13:251-4.
54. Peirce EC Jr, Jacobson JH Jr. Cerebral edema. In: Davis JC, Hunt TK, editors. Hyperbaric oxygen therapy. Bethesda (MD): Undersea Medical Society; 1977. p. 287-301.
55. Petrovsky BV, Tsatsanidi K, Bogomolova N, et al. Treatment of peritonitis caused by non-spore-forming anaerobic bacteria. In: Kindwall EP, editor. Proceedings of the 8th International Congress on Hyperbaric Medicine. San Pedro (CA): Best Publishing; 1987. p. 100-6.
56. Rockswold GL, Ford SE, Anderson DC, Bergmann TA, Sherman RE. Results of a prospective randomized trial for treatment of severely brain-injured patients with hyperbaric oxygen. J Neurosurg. 1992;76:929-34.
57. Schaan M et al. Die behandlung des hirnabszesses. Trauma und Berufskrankheit. 2003;5(Suppl 2):305. German.
58. Schliamser SE, Baeckmann K, Norrby SR. Intracranial abscess in adults: an analysis of 54 consecutive cases. Scand J Infect Dis. 1988;20:1-9.
59. Schöppenthau H. (Murnau Trauma Center, Germany). Personal communication. 2016.

60. Schreiner A, Tonjun S, Digranes A. Hyperbaric oxygen therapy in Bacteroides infections. Acta Chir Scand. 1974;140:73-6.

61. Seydoux C, Francioli P. Bacterial brain abscesses: factors influencing mortality and sequelae. Clin Infect Dis. 1992;15:394-401.

62. Sharma BS, Khosla VK, Kak VK, et al. Multiple pyogenic brain abscesses. Acta Neurochir. 1995;133:36-43.

63. Shimogawa T, Sayama T, Haga S, Akiyama T, Morioka T. [Cerebellar abscess due to infection with the anaerobic bacteria fusobacterium nucleatum: a case report]. No Shinkei Geka. 2015;43(2):137-42.

64. Stapleton SR, Bell BA, Uttley D. Stereotactic aspiration of brain abscesses: is this the treatment of choice? Acta Neurochir. 1993;121:15-9.

65. Stephanov S. Brain abscesses from neglected open head injuries: experience with 17 cases over 20 years. Swiss Surg. 1999;5:288-92.

66. Sukoff MH, Hollin SA, Espinosa OE, Jacobson JH Jr. The protective effect of hyperbaric oxygenation in experimental cerebral edema. J Neurosurg. 1968;29:236-41.

67. Sukoff MH, Ragatz RE. Hyperbaric oxygen for the treatment of acute cerebral edema. Neurosurgery. 1982;10:29-38.

68. Sun J, Sun J. Intracranial complications of chronic otitis media. Eur Arch Otorhinolaryngol. 2014;271(11):2923-6.

69. Sutter B, Legat JA, Smolle-Juettner FM. Brain abscess before and after HBO2. 12th Proceedings Sc Soc Physiol; Styria. 1996.

70. Szuwart U, Brandt M, Bennefeld H, Tewes G. Hirnabszess und subdurales empyem aus bakteriologischer sicht. Zentralbl Chir. 1989;114:534-44.

71. Takada Y, Ohno K, Wakimoto H, Hirakawa K. Treatment of intracranial abscess in the era of neuroimaging: an analysis of 13 consecutive cases. J Med Dent Sci. 1998;45:69-76.

72. Whelan HT. (Medical College of Wisconsin). Personal communication. 2016.

73. Witzmann A, Beran H, Boehm-Jurkovic H, et al. Der hirnabszess. Prognostische faktoren. Dtsch Med Wochenschr. 1989;114:85-90.

74. Yang SY. Brain abscess: a review of 400 cases. J Neurosurg. 1981;55:794-9.

75. Yang SY, Zhao CS. Review of 140 patients with brain abscess. Surg Neurol. 1993;39:290-6.

CHAPTER 20 CHAPTER

Hyperbaric Oxygen for the Management of Chronic Refractory Osteomyelitis

CHAPTER TWENTY OVERVIEW

Introduction 487

Pathophysiology of Chronic Refractory Osteomyelitis 491

Justification for Hyperbaric Oxygen: Lab and Animal Studies 494

Justification for Hyperbaric Oxygen: Clinical Experiences 498

Evaluation 503

Management 506

Compromised Host Presentation 506

Septic Nonunion Presentations 508

Diffuse Sclerosing Osteomyelitis Presentation 509

Reimbursement Considerations 510

Conclusions 512

Acknowledgments 516

References 517

Hyperbaric Oxygen for the Management of Chronic Refractory Osteomyelitis

Michael B. Strauss, Stuart S. Miller, Lientra Q. Lu

INTRODUCTION

Chronic refractory osteomyelitis (CROM) is an infection of bone that involves both its cortical and medullary components which has persisted or recurred after appropriate management (Figure 1). With this fundamental definition, three presentations of chronic refractory osteomyelitis occur: 1) CROM in the **compromised host**, 2) CROM associated with a nonhealing fracture (**septic nonunion**), and 3) CROM of the **diffuse sclerosing** type. Since hyperbaric oxygen (HBO_2) was first used as an adjunct for the management of chronic refractory osteomyelitis, its utilization and role have changed. Contemporary utilization of HBO_2 for chronic refractory osteomyelitis is much different than when its benefits were first reported over 40 years ago.[66,80] The reasons are twofold: First, initially the benefits of HBO_2 were largely thought to be due to the direct effects of HBO_2 on microorganisms and bone responses. Now the contemporary thinking is that CROM is a problem of ischemia/avascularity of bone.

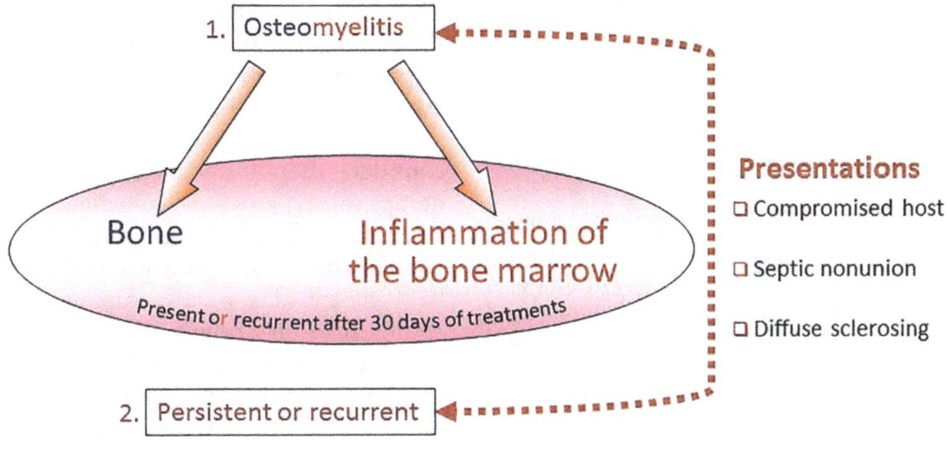

LEGEND: A bone infection is considered by CMS/Medicare to be refractory if it persists or recurs with "appropriate" treatment after a 30-day period. Three presentations account for almost all expressions of chronic refractory osteomyelitis.

Figure 1. Definition of refractory osteomyelitis.

The contemporary use of hyperbaric oxygen for chronic refractory osteomyelitis is paradoxical. Only rarely, in contrast to the past, is hyperbaric oxygen used for this problem in long bones. However, hyperbaric oxygen now is used more than ever because of refractory bone infections in the feet (Figure 2). This is observed especially in the compromised host group, which is largely composed of patients with diabetes mellitus.

The reason HBO_2 is rarely used for chronic refractory osteomyelitis of the long bones of the appendicular skeleton is threefold: first, the incidence of this problem has decreased due to the improvement of open-fracture management, the use of organism-specific antibiotics, the performance of primary amputations for mangled extremities, and staging dead-space management of exposed and/or infected bone with use of antibiotic-laden bone cement.

Second, the use of microvascular free flaps to provide both early coverage and augmented perfusion to the fracture site has been very effective in converting open fractures to "closed" types.[20,54,97]

Third, the Ilizarov technique has added a new dimension to the management of infected, ununited fractures. In this technique, the diseased bone segment is resected after placement of a special external fixation frame to align and rigidly stabilize the extremity. Next, healthy bone is osteotomized at one or both metaphyseal levels. Rather than allowing the iatrogenic fracture to heal, the callus forming at the fracture site(s) is stretched out until the bone is lengthened enough to obliterate the segment that was resected.

Second, whereas in the past HBO_2 was used almost exclusively for the long bones of the extremities and the jaw, today the majority of the use of HBO_2 for CROM is in the small bones of the foot where contemporary orthopaedic and plastic surgery interventions generally are not applicable.

Since the indications for HBO_2 were delineated by the Undersea [and Hyperbaric, added to designation in 1987] Medical Society in 1977, CROM has been an approved use for this modality. Regardless of the change in focus, as described above, CROM remains an important indication for HBO_2. As effective as these techniques are, there are predictable complication rates including nonunion, persistence of infection, and lower limb amputation. However, when the bone infection is not arrested and/or the fracture remains unhealed after these interventions, and the decision is made to avoid a lower limb amputation, HBO_2 should be utilized in conjunction with the other limb salvage interventions.

The underlying causes of failure to arrest the infection are tissue ischemia-hypoxia including dead bone at the injury site, compromised host status, or combinations of these. Cierney and Mader appreciated the significance of host status and incorporated this important consideration in their classification of osteomyelitis (Table 1).[12,46] Not only does this classification consider the host status, but by doing so, it provides guidelines for when hyperbaric oxygen should be considered in the management. We have generated a more contemporary approach to quantifying host status by using a 0-to10 (with 10 being best) Wellness Score based on 5 assessments each graded from 2 (best) to 0 (worst) (Table 2). Judgment is required for making management decisions for patients with CROM. Hyperbaric oxygen and surgery may not always be the best decision when the severity of the problem and

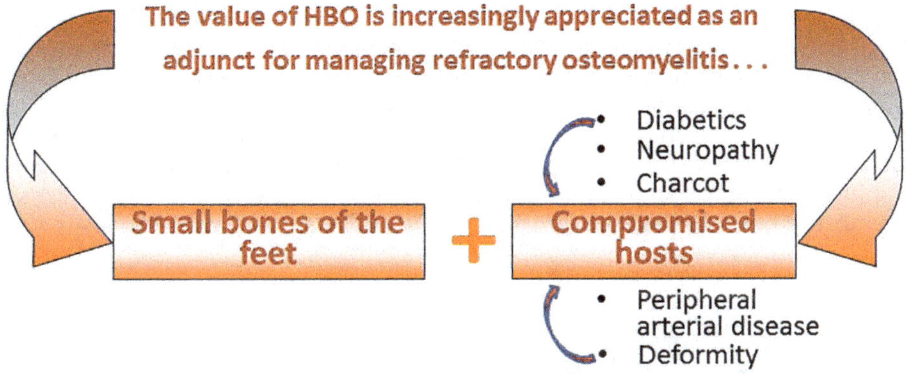

LEGEND: A bone infection is considered by CMS/Medicare to be refractory if it persists or recurs with "appropriate" treatment. The use of HBO$_2$ for CROM has largely shifted from posttraumatic long bone osteomyelitis to small bones in the feet in patients who are compromised hosts.

Figure 2. New Horizons for HBO$_2$ with chronic refractory osteomyelitis.

the patient's functional status are considered. The mating of the Wellness Score with the three different presentations of chronic refractory osteomyelitis provides a useful guide for deciding whether to recommend salvage of the limb with adjunctive HBO$_2$, major limb amputation, or the withholding of treatment interventions for the patient (Figure 3)

TABLE 1. CIERNEY & MADER CROM CLASSIFICATION AND RECOMMENDATIONS FOR HBO$_2$[12,46]

Anatomic Type	Physiological Class
1 Medullary (hematogenous)	A Host (healthy)
2 Contiguous focus	B Host (compromised)
☐ Osteitis (infected bone surface)	☐ Systemic (B_S)
☐ Bone at pressure sore base	☐ Local (B_L)
3 Discrete sequestrum	☐ Systemic & local (B_{SL})
4 Diffuse sclerosing	C Treatment worse than the disease

Systemic and local factors that affect immune surveillance, metabolism, and local vascularity:

B_S = Diabetes mellitus, renal/hepatic insufficiency, malnutrition, chronic hypoxia, immunosuppression, malignancy, immune deficiency, extremes of age, tobacco abuse

B_L = Major vessel compromise, small and medium vessel disease, arteritis, radiation fibrosis, chronic lymphedema, venous stasis, neuropathy

HBO Indications: 3-B and 4 (regardless of host status)

Hyperbaric oxygen (as well as other management interventions) is not always indicated for patients with chronic refractory osteomyelitis. In fact, major limb amputation or the withholding of all care may be the better choices for some patients. Patients with low Wellness Scores, debilitation confining the patient to bed rest, intractable pain associated with the infection, and deformities preventing functional ambulation as well as the treatment being worse than the disease are relative contraindications for using HBO_2 for CROM.

TABLE 2. WELLNESS SCORE

Criteria	2 Points	1 Point	0 Points
ADLs Ability to do activities of daily living	Full	Some	None
Ambulation	Community	Household	None
Comorbidities Except neuro; include obesity	Normal	Impaired	Decompensated
Tobacco/Steroid Use	None	Past	Current
Neuro Function	Normal	Impaired	Decompensated

NOTE: The "Wellness Score" is a quick-to-obtain evaluation tool to assess how functional a patient is. If scores are less than 4.5 points, the likelihood of functional use of a chronically infected extremity wound is low, and lower limb amputation becomes justified based on this tool.

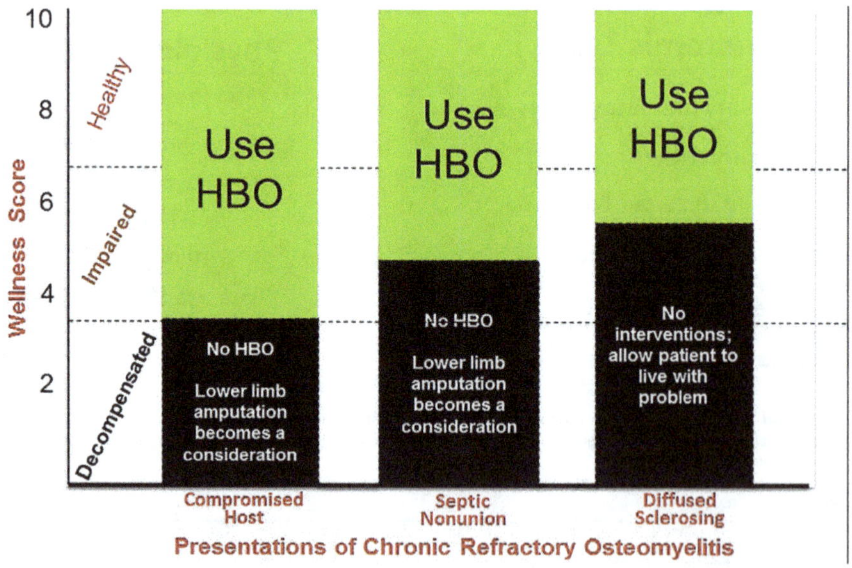

LEGEND: Judgment is required when making a decision to salvage versus recommend a major limb amputation when dealing with the different presentations of chronic refractory osteomyelitis. The Wellness Score helps in the decision-making process.

Figure 3. Wellness Score as a tool to decide when to use HBO_2 for the different presentations of chronic refractory osteomyelitis.

PATHOPHYSIOLOGY OF CHRONIC REFRACTORY OSTEOMYELITIS

The factor that makes chronic refractory osteomyelitis difficult to eradicate is the impaired vascularity at the site of infection.(46,62) The consequences are threefold: 1) hypoxia, 2) development of an impermeable, avascular barrier between intact, healthy tissues and the focus of infection in the bone (i.e., the interface), and 3) necrotic bone (Figure 4). These interfere with the body's responses for dealing with the infection as well as the delivery of antibiotics to the septic focus. Causes of hypoxia are usually a combination of infected thrombi in arteries supplying the infection focus and/or obstruction at the microcirculation level (Figure 5). Without an adequate blood supply, the environment around the infection site becomes hypoxic. This interferes with the body's responses for dealing with infection, namely neutrophil oxidative killing of bacteria and angiogenesis to improve perfusion and deliver antibiotics to the infection site.

Oxygen tensions in the tissue fluids need to be in the 30-to-40 mmHg range in order for neutrophils to generate superoxides and peroxides during the oxidative burst required for bacteria killing and for fibroblasts to elaborate a matrix for angiogenesis to proceed.(32,34) For wounds to heal and infections to be controlled, blood flow and metabolic activity at the infection-wound site must

> Impaired blood supply to the site of infection is the factor that makes osteomyelitis refractory. The majority of factors Cierny and Mader consider in the compromised host group (B Host) are conditions, both systemic and local, that interfere with blood supply to the infection site (Table 1).
>
> Dr. George Hart, as early as the 1970s, expounded on the fact that osteomyelitis is an ischemic disorder. This information helped justify the use of HBO$_2$ for CROM and explains why failures to arrest the infection occur.

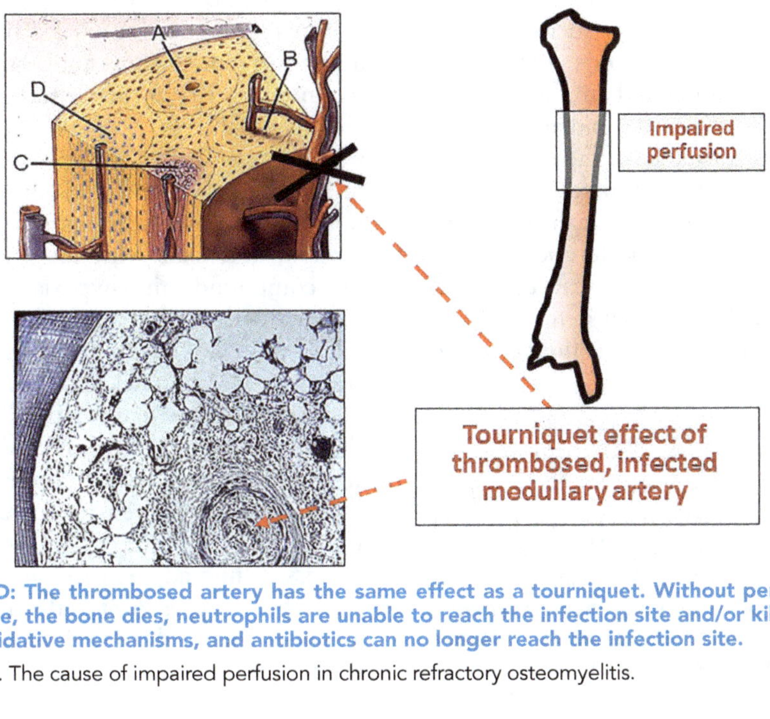

LEGEND: The thrombosed artery has the same effect as a tourniquet. Without perfusion to the bone, the bone dies, neutrophils are unable to reach the infection site and/or kill bacteria with oxidative mechanisms, and antibiotics can no longer reach the infection site.

Figure 4. The cause of impaired perfusion in chronic refractory osteomyelitis.

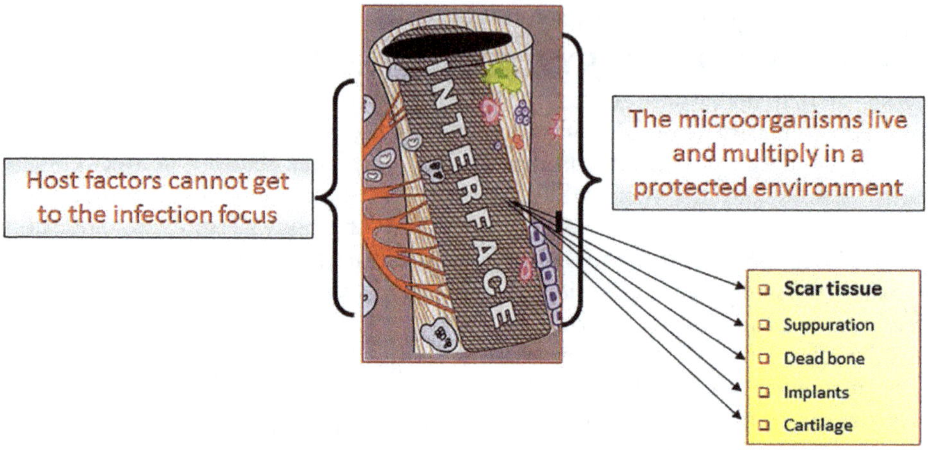

LEGEND: The interface acts as a barrier between the "intact" host tissues and the focus of infection. It is the abortive attempt by the body to isolate the infection from the remainder of the body.

Figure 5. The Interface as a barrier between healthy host tissues and the focus of infection.

increase an estimated 20-fold.[84] Vasodilatation and channeling of blood (the reverse of shunting) to the infected area are the mechanisms that increase blood flow and account for the rubor, calor, and tumor (swelling) associated with infection. Compromise of an already-impaired circulation at the infection site because of calcified vessels and autosympathectomy effects from diabetic neuropathy may not allow perfusion to increase enough to meet the metabolic and mobilization demands needed to manage the infection. Diabetes mellitus is probably the leading comorbidity associated with this latter cause of refractory osteomyelitis and one for which HBO_2 is often used as a management adjunct. Another cause of hypoxia at the infection site is the premature thickening of the capillary basement membrane, a frequent consequence of diabetes.[26] The thickened basement membrane becomes a diffusion barrier for oxygen from the capillary to the tissue fluids. A hypoxic environment also renders some antibiotics such as aminoglycosides and amphotericin ineffective since they require active transport by bacteria, an oxygen-dependent process, across their cell walls.[95]

The significance of the interface cannot be overemphasized in chronic wounds in general and CROM in particular (Figure 5). The interface is the body's response to the inflammatory reaction that the infected bone initiates. The response begins with edema, continues with leukocyte and fibroblast infiltration, and ends with the formation of almost-impenetrable scar tissue. Each stage compounds the hypoxia problem mentioned above. Other items that may be associated with the interface include dead bone (sequestra), cartilage, fluid collections including pus, and foreign materials such as bone cement, shrapnel, and orthopaedic hardware. Edema increases the diffusion distance that oxygen molecules must traverse through tissue fluids from capillaries to target cells. It decreases by the square root of the oxygen tension of the tissue fluid adjacent to the capillary and is only 1/20th as great as the diffusion ability of carbon dioxide through tissue fluids.[22,65]

Each stage (edema, inflammatory cell infiltration, fibroblast activity, cicatrix formation) in the evolution of the interface compounds the hypoxia problem at the infection focus. Thus, each stage further protects the organisms causing the bone infection from the body's mechanisms to arrest the infection and its ability to deliver antibiotics.

Neutrophils and osteoclasts (to reabsorb dead, infected bone) have the potential to arrest the infection. In the presence of hypoxia, metaplasias of fibroblast generated tissues form cicatrix. This makes the interface essentially an impermeable barrier. This has undesirable consequences. First, the interface isolates chronically infected bone from adjacent healthy tissues and the host factors that can mitigate it. Second, the interface thwarts vascular invasion and vascularity of the focus of infection so a "stand-off" situation arises with persistence of the infection. Third, the interface isolates the necrotic bone (i.e. sequestrum). When the sequestrum volume is small, it may remain relatively asymptomatic or periodically drain through a sinus tract from the bone through the skin. Once the cicatrix is removed with surgery and/or its vascularity improved with hyperbaric oxygen, the remodeling/bone resorbing function of the osteoclast can resume.

> The interface, as a host response, is paradoxical. It keeps the infected focus from extending to healthy host tissues. Conversely, it acts as a barrier for leukocytes, other host factors, and antibiotics to get to the site of infection.

The remodeling process is a normal, ongoing physiological function of bone. Osteoclasts remodel, create vascular ingress channels, and remove dead bone while osteoblasts lay down new bone. This differential in activity explains why stress fractures occur. Bone remodeling is a response to stresses transmitted to the bone. Ultimately strengthening of the bone occurs as the osteoblast generates new bone as a response to the stresses. However, osteoclastic reabsorption of bone is 100 times faster than osteoblastic formation of new bone.[37] As expected, the intense metabolic activity of the osteoclasts proportionately increases its oxygen requirements. The metabolic activities of osteoclasts are 100 times greater than that of osteocytes.[37] In the hypoxic environment, the osteoclast stops functioning. Remodeling and removal of dead bone is halted. When bone is infected, as well as dead, and the environment around the osteoclast is hypoxic, this host "debridement" mechanism ceases to function. The consequence is CROM.

> The hyperbaric oxygen effect is often observed in infected metatarsal heads associated with diabetic malperforans ulcers. X-rays typically appear normal until HBO_2 treatments are given. Then bone reabsorption of the metatarsal head occurs. This reflects the osteoclast's bone resorbing ability that now becomes possible with the improved oxygen environment from the HBO_2 treatments.

There are several reasons bone loses its vascularity and becomes necrotic. Traumatic disruption of blood vessels associated with fractures and crush injuries is an obvious cause (see Chapter 26: The Roles of Hyperbaric Oxygen in Crush Injury and Other Acute Traumatic Ischemias). Both nontraumatic intrinsic and extrinsic causes lead to avascularity of bone. When edema, confirmed by magnetic resonance imaging, occurs in bone, it may increase the intraosseous pressure. If the tensions are higher than the capillary perfusion pressure, the bone is rendered avascular. This mechanism is analogous to the pathophysiology of the skeletal muscle-compartment syndrome. External pressure from pus and edema formation in tightly compacted areas such as tissues adjacent to joint capsules, neurovascular compartments, and tendon sheaths may also exceed the capillary filling pressure and render more distal tissues ischemic (Figure 6).[89] This problem is likely to be compounded by flow that is already impeded by peripheral artery disease, hypoxia secondary to impaired oxygen diffusion through thickened capillary basement membranes, and anatomical considerations where perfusion to the target tissue is an end artery or single bone-perforating vessel. This latter consideration is undoubtedly the cause of refractory osteomyelitis of distal tufts of toes and metatarsal heads as so often seen in diabetic feet with sepsis adjacent to these areas.

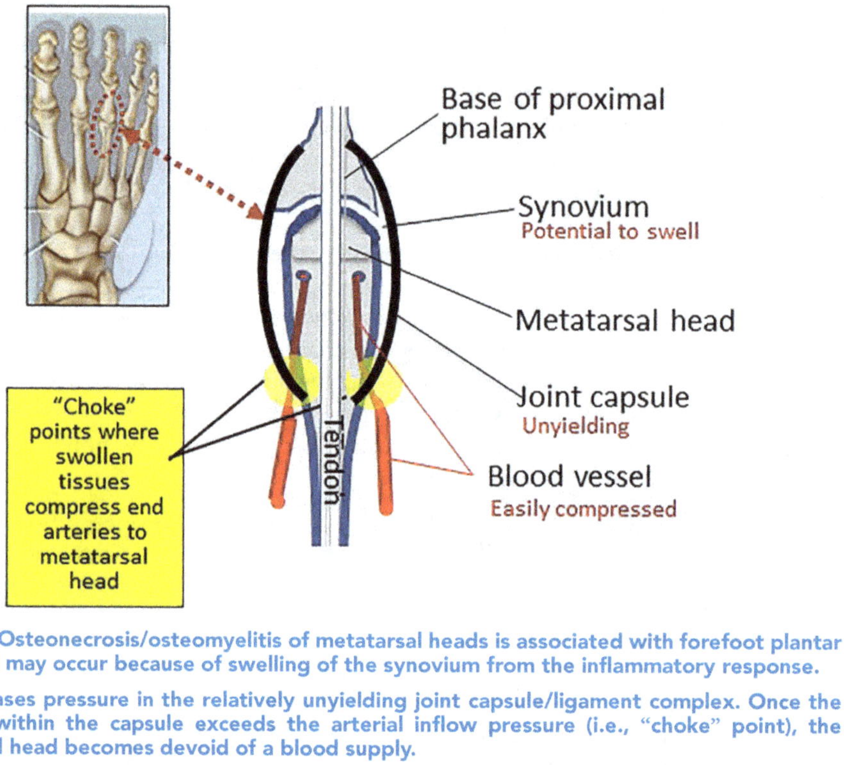

Figure 6. Metatarsal head ischemia from "choke" point at capsular attachment.

JUSTIFICATION FOR HYPERBARIC OXYGEN: LAB AND ANIMAL STUDIES

Much benchwork has been done to demonstrate the value of HBO_2 for refractory osteomyelitis. The oxygen tension in osteomyelitic bone is low, rarely exceeding 25 mmHg of oxygen.(62) Using animal models, Hunt et al., Kivisaari et al., and Mader et al. have shown that the oxygen tension in normal, as well as infected, tissue is increased with HBO_2.(33,40,49) Values ranging from 30 mmHg to as high as 1,200 mmHg have been measured in infected tissue under HBO_2 conditions. Esterhai et al. studied oxygen tensions in infected and uninfected tibias in a rabbit model and observed that HBO_2 elevated the oxygen tension in the infected bone.(19) Under ambient conditions, the oxygen tension in an uninfected tibia was 32 mmHg; the oxygen tension in the infected tibia was only 17 mmHg. By exposing the rabbit to HBO_2 at 2 atmospheres absolute (ATA), the oxygen tension in both tibias rose to over 190 mmHg. In the Mader et al. studies, a rabbit model, with *Staphylococcus aureus* osteomyelitis of the tibia, was used (Figure 7).(49) The animals were treated at 2 ATA with 100% oxygen for 2 hours daily, 5 times per week, for a total of 20 treatments. With mass spectrometry,

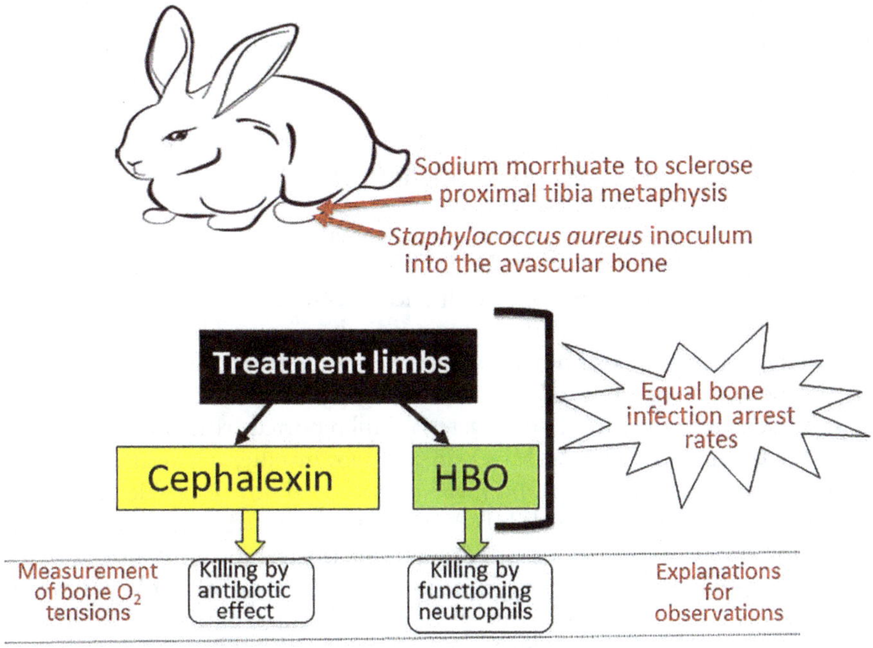

LEGEND: Hyperbaric oxygen was as effective as an antibiotic in arresting osteomyelitis in a rabbit model. Oxygen tension measurements showed that with HBO_2, the oxygen tensions in the sclerosed bone improved enough that the neutrophil could kill bacteria through its oxidative killing mechanisms.

Figure 7. Mader's osteomyelitis rabbit studies.[49]

oxygen tensions were measured in normal and infected tibias, before and during HBO_2 treatment. Hyperbaric oxygen increased the oxygen tensions in both the uninfected (45 to 322 mmHg) and infected (23 to 104 mmHg) bone. In both the Esterhai and Mader studies, the low oxygen tensions in infected bone were secondary to ischemia, but inflammation secondary to infection may have increased the intramedullary pressure in the bone and contributed to the ischemia (Figure 6). Increased pressure and resultant ischemia occur when purulent material and other debris fill the Haversian system and medullary canal.[96]

The neutrophil (polymorphonuclear leukocyte) is the white cell primarily responsible for combatting bacterial infections. Mandell showed that phagocytic killing of aerobes is diminished under low oxygen tensions.[52] Since a majority of aerobic organisms can also function as facultative anaerobes, hypoxic tissue is especially at risk for infection. Using a *Staphylococcus aureus* model, Mader showed a proportional relationship between oxygen tensions and phagocytic killing ability.[48] At the 23 mmHg oxygen tension measured in infected bone, there was a reduced capacity of phagocytes to kill bacteria, as compared to bacteria killing at normal bone oxygen tensions of 45 mmHg. Increasing the oxygen tension to 109 mmHg, the oxygen tension found in osteomyelitic bone under HBO_2 conditions, further augmented the ability of the phagocytes to kill bacteria. Mader also showed that increasing the oxygen tension to 760 mmHg resulted in even greater killing rates of *S. aureus.* Hamblen observed that HBO_2 did not reduce the initial infection rate of experimentally introduced osteomyelitis in the rat tibia model. However, it caused a significant increase in the healing of the established infection. Hamblen also noted that HBO_2 eliminated sequestra. He did not detect a difference in outcomes when the animals were treated with 2 ATA or 3 ATA with HBO_2.[24] In a rabbit tibia model, Mader observed improvement of *S. aureus* osteomyelitis with HBO_2 and subsequently determined that it was due to enhanced oxygen-dependent neutrophil killing.[49] Similar effects in lab studies were reported with HBO_2 exposures for *Staphylococcus epidermidis, Pseudomonas aeruginosa,* and *Escherichia coli,* again attributed to HBO_2 improving the environment for neutrophil oxidative killing.[32,62,96]

Superoxide dismutase and catalase are enzymatic mechanisms used by aerobic bacteria to degrade toxic oxygen radicals.[96] Anaerobic and many microaerophilic organisms do not produce these oxygen radical–degrading enzymes. This results in killing of anaerobic organisms by the oxygen radicals generated by neutrophils. In the hypoxic environment, as is so often associated with anaerobic infections, HBO_2 can raise the tissue oxygen tensions to levels that make it possible for neutrophils to generate the oxygen radicals needed to kill the bacteria. Hill reported reductions in abscess size and number in animals receiving HBO_2 in a mouse intrahepatic liver abscess model inoculated with *Bacteroides fragilis* and *Fusobacterium sp* (both anaerobic organisms).[31]

Another mechanism by which HBO_2 may assist in the treatment of osteomyelitis is in the promotion of fibroblastic activity. Fibroblasts do not synthesize collagen or migrate to the affected area when oxygen tensions are less than 30 mmHg. Tissue-fluid oxygen tensions greater than 40 mmHg support fibroblast function.[34,65] Therefore, increasing oxygen tensions in hypoxic environments with HBO_2 therapy supports fibroblastic functions. With respect to chronic refractory osteomyelitis the benefits are twofold (Figure 8). First, HBO_2 provides a sufficiently oxygenated environment so host factors can function. Second, the oxygen environment allows the fibroblast to generate

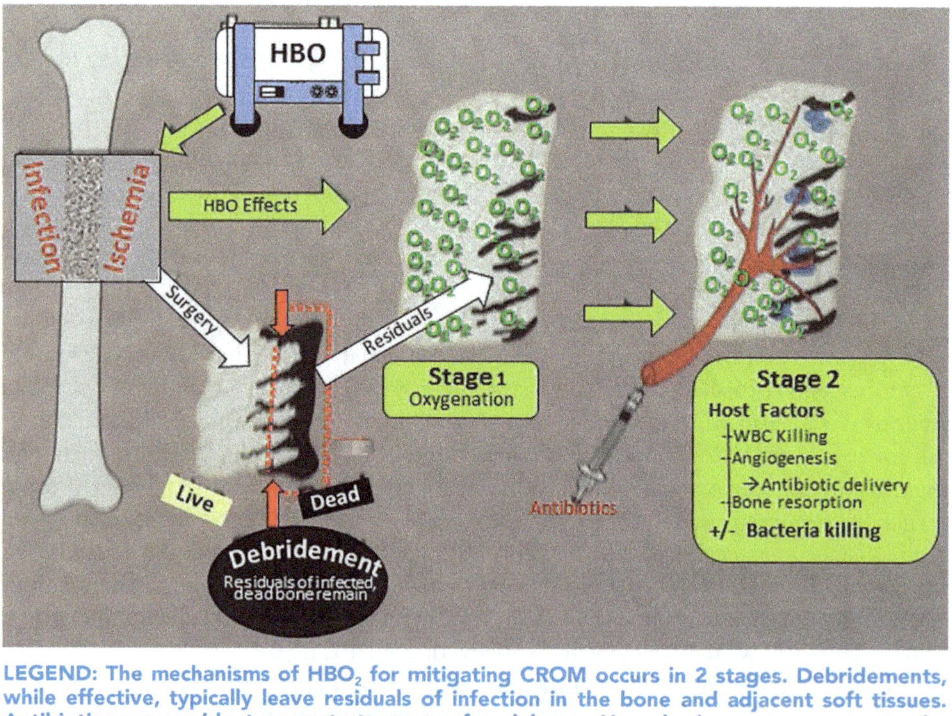

LEGEND: The mechanisms of HBO_2 for mitigating CROM occurs in 2 stages. Debridements, while effective, typically leave residuals of infection in the bone and adjacent soft tissues. Antibiotics are unable to penetrate nonperfused bone. Hyperbaric oxygen supports the bodyÕs "clearing mechanisms" for managing the residuals.

Figure 8. Roles of HBO_2 for chronic refractory osteomyelitis.

a matrix so angiogenesis can occur into the ischemic-hypoxic focus. This provides the environment so the osteoclast can resorb dead, infected bone and a conduit for antibiotics and white blood cells to enter the focus of infection.

The effect of HBO_2 therapy provided during concomitant antibiotic therapy has also been studied. The aminoglycoside class of antibiotics is often used in the treatment of gram-negative aerobic infections. The class includes gentamycin, tobramycin, amikacin, etc. An important therapeutic limitation, however, is their inability to penetrate pus and their decreased activity under low oxygen tensions.(64,95) Verklin et al. demonstrated that HBO_2 helps aminoglycosides enter bacteria, especially in hypoxic environments.(95) Mader showed that with HBO_2 therapy, the bactericidal activity of tobramycin is enhanced.(47) The Mader study compared tobramycin effectiveness against *Pseudomonas aeruginosa* under anaerobic, aerobic, and stimulated HBO_2 conditions in a rabbit model.(47) With tobramycin alone, HBO_2 alone, and the two combined, Mader demonstrated that adjunctive HBO_2 enhanced eradication of the *P. aeruginosa* from infected bone. Other antibiotics, including vancomycin, quinolones, trimethoprim/sulfamethoxazole, and nitrofurantoin have also been shown to be far less active in a hypoxic environment.(64) Such conditions are readily found in ischemic tissues and nonhematogenous types of osteomyelitic environments. Mendel et al. used a rat model to study *Staphylococcus aureus* osteomyelitis and compared the results of treatment with HBO_2, cefazolin, a combination of both, or no treatment.(57) They demonstrated that HBO_2 alone compared to no treatment reduced the number of colony-forming units (CFU) in tibial bone. Antibiotic therapy alone resulted in further reduction in the number of CFUs in the bone. The most marked improvement occurred with a four-week course of combination therapy utilizing HBO_2 and antibiotics.

Subsequently, Mendel et al. evaluated the synergy of HBO_2 and a local antibiotic carrier for osteomyelitis due to *S. aureus* in a rat tibia bone model.(58) They demonstrated significant reductions in colony-forming units (CFUs) in tibia bone in both the HBO_2 and the antibiotic carrier limbs. A synergistic effect with the most marked reductions in CFUs was observed when both agents were used in combination. In fact, 82% of the animals had undetectable organisms after combination therapy.

The consensus of the animal and lab data is that HBO_2 is a useful adjunct for the management of osteomyelitis. These studies consistently demonstrated improved outcomes when HBO_2 was used in conjunction with antibiotic therapy.

In summary, laboratory studies demonstrate that hyperbaric oxygen increases oxygen tensions in infected bone. While hyperbaric oxygen has a direct effect on strict anaerobic organisms through the production of toxic oxygen radicals, it has indirect effects on aerobic organisms. Hyperbaric oxygen increases oxygen tension in infected tissues to promote oxygen-dependent killing mechanisms by neutrophils. Hyperbaric oxygen also augments the bactericidal activity of the aminoglycosides and likely has similar effects on other antibiotics. Finally, hyperbaric oxygen provides adequate oxygen for fibroblastic activity, leading to angiogenesis, antibiotic delivery, and wound healing in hypoxic tissues.

JUSTIFICATION FOR HYPERBARIC OXYGEN: CLINICAL EXPERIENCES

The first report that hyperbaric oxygen (HBO_2) was useful in refractory osteomyelitis was published by Slack in 1965. He reported good results with using this modality in five patients.[80] A year later, Perrins reported a 71% arrest rate of refractory osteomyelitis cases when HBO_2 was used an adjunct in the management after surgery, and antibiotics failed.[66] Subsequently, additional reports attesting to the benefits of HBO_2 in managing refractory osteomyelitis of long bones have appeared (Table 3).[1-3,5-11,13-17,21,25,29-30,35,38,41,43-44,50-51,53,55,60-61,63,67,69, 72-75,77-79,91-94,98-99] Most are reports dealing with the use of HBO_2 as an adjunct to surgery and antibiotics after previous failures with these latter two interventions. In total, there are over 2,000 cases cited.[38] The largest series, 689 patients, was reported by Kawashima (Table 3). Arrest rates with the adjunctive use of HBO_2 ranged from 61% to almost 100%. In those reports where the infection was not arrested, there was almost 100% unanimity in observations that the patients' infections were improved. In an earlier review of chronic refractory osteomyelitis case reports, follow-ups ranged from 12 to 53 months.[83] It is noteworthy that there have been no new published series using hyperbaric oxygen treatment for osteomyelitis of long bones for almost 20 years. This is attributed to the surgical advancements that include the use of microvascular muscle flaps and/or employ Ilizarov principles for managing chronic refractory osteomyelitis (see introduction).

In 1980, the first author published a review of HBO_2 experiences with chronic refractory osteomyelitis.[98] The non-hyperbaric reports which included over 30 publications were typically prospective series of outcomes with surgical techniques utilized by the primary author of each article. The hyperbaric oxygen experiences in the review consisted of 17 reports. Several were ongoing series by the same authors. The largest percentage of reports involved osteomyelitis of the mandible. Many of the outcomes were reported as "favorable," "effective," "successful," and similar observational terms. When actual numbers were provided, favorable results with HBO_2 were reported in about 80% of the cases.

Esterhai, et al., reported in a retrospective study of chronic refractory osteomyelitis that undermines the effectiveness of HBO_2 on initial inspection.[17] After studying a group of 14 patients who received HBO_2 with a 78.6% arrest rate (3 of 14 patients failed), the authors retrospectively reviewed a similar number of patients who did not receive HBO_2. A 93% arrest rate (1 of 14 patients failed) was reported. An analysis of the failures disclosed that all occurred in patients who refused surgical management: three in the HBO_2 limb and one in the control limb. Several questions arose as to the validity of this study, including the question of whether the control group with a 90% arrest rate met the definition of chronic refractory osteomyelitis. Furthermore, the outcomes were only based on the initial arrest of the infection and not the durability of the results. In a subsequent publication from the same institution, a 66% arrest rate was reported in a group of patients who did not receive HBO_2 in their management but appeared to have similar treatment as used for the patients in the 1987 report.[18] How this latter outcome differs so much from the control group in the HBO_2 study raises suspicions about the validity of these patients' HBO_2 experiences.

TABLE 3. SUMMARY OF REPORTS USING HBO_2 FOR CHRONIC REFRACTORY OSTEOMYELITIS

Name	Patients	Outcomes	Comments/ Study Type
LONG BONE OSTEOMYELITIS AND MISCELLANEOUS SITES			
Perrins[66] 1966	24	79% resolved, 8.3% improved, 12.5% failed.	Case study. Four healed cases relapsed. Concurrent debridement was not uniformly provided. All cases were previous failures.
Bingham[5] 1977	70	61% healed, 39% improved or arrested. 80% healed if < 2 years duration; 50% healed if > 2 years duration.	Case study. All patients received concurrent antibiotic therapy.
Morrey[60] 1979	40	85% resolved infection for 2 years or longer where previous treatments failed.	Prospective study. Follow-ups after 7 to 10 years showed 75% remain healed.
Welsh[98] 1980	5	80% arrested of infection.	Retrospective case study. Refractory nature and concurrent treatment were not defined.
Davis[14] 1986	38	89% arrested of infection.	Case studies. All patients had previously failed to heal at least once with combined surgery and antibiotics.
Esterhai[17] 1987	28	21% arrested in control group, 79% arrested in HBO_2 group. All failures refused surgery.	Prospective HBO_2 and retrospective control cohort.
Maynor[55] 1998	34	Infection controlled for 3 mo.: 82%; 24 mo.: 81%; 60 mo.: 80%; 84 mo.: 63% drainage free.	Prospective study. Combining HBO_2 with autogenous microsurgical muscle transplantation.
C. G. Hosp.[7-8,10] 1998, 2003–04	15, 13	86% of 15 patients and 92% of 13 patients arrested of infection; subsequent 2 reports.	Three prospective studies. All patients had had infections for > 6 mo. and failed surgical and antibiotic therapy 3 times.
Barili[3] 2007	32	Infection relapses, duration of IV antibiotic use, and total hospital stay ($p = 0.024$) were significantly lower in HBO_2-treated group.	Prospective trial.
Chen[9] 2008	10	80% healed, 20% limb-amputated.	Retrospective study. All patients were hemodialysis dependent.

TABLE 3 (CONTINUED)

Kawashima [38] 2008	689	Control group: 88.3% good, 2.7% fair, 9% poor. HBO_2 group: 91.9% good, 2.3% fair, 5.8% poor. Both groups utilized debridement and suction irrigation.	Cohort study; $p < 0.01$. But there was not statistical uniformity of the 2 cohorts.
Roje[73] 2008	388	Control group: 74% developed osteomyelitis. HBO_2 group: 63% developed osteomyelitis. Both groups used antibiotics.	Retrospective study; $p = 0.030$. Patients with Gustilo type III A, B, and C open fracture, crush injuries.
Yu[99] 2011	12	Significant decreases in (1) length of ICU stay, (2) duration of mechanical ventilation, and (3) overall mortality.	Case-matched study; $p < 0.05$ for all those criteria in HBO_2 limbs; 6 were controls.
Delasotta[15] 2013	1	Resolution of infection in each limb.	Case study. A recurrent posttraumatic osteomyelitis patient with multiple comorbidities.
Skeik[79] 2015	23	82.6% healed or improved.	Retrospective study.
MANDIBULAR OSTEOMYELITIS			
Slack[80] 1965	5	80% cleared of infection. First recorded use of HBO_2 for refractory osteomyelitis.	Case study. A mix of patients with chronic and refractory disease and varied concurrent treatment.
Mainous[51] 1977	24	96% resolution of infection.	Case report. Combined debridement, antibiotics, and HBO_2 therapy.
Van Merkesteyn [94] 1984	16, 7	11% of 16 patients treated with HBO_2 and antibiotics arrested; 100% of 7 patients treated with additional decortication arrested.	Case study. Demonstrates the necessity of surgery with antibiotics and HBO_2 (as trimodal therapy).
Carragee[6] 1997	44	73% arrest of infection, 27% failed.	Case study. HBO_2 used as monotherapy: shows the need for surgery & antibiotic with HBO_2.
Aitasalo[2] 1998	33	79% resolved infection as early as 5 months; postop HBO_2 treatments	Case study. Only 5–7 postop HBO_2 treatments – below typical HBO_2 protocol totals.
Jamil[35] 2000	16	37% arrest with only HBO_2.	Case study. Patients with treatment-resistant infections.
Talmi[91] 2000	6	66% resolved with HBO_2 alone; no additional benefit with trimodal therapy.	Case study.

TABLE 3 (CONTINUED)

Chen[11] 2005	36	89% resolved, 11% recurred with trimodal therapy and continuous irrigation treatment.	Case reports.
Priest[69] 2005	29	83% arrested, but 50% suffered infection-related sequelae.	Case study.
Hand-schel[26] 2007	22	Primary osteomyelitis: 54% resolved. Refractory osteomyelitis: 44% resolved.	Case study. Younger patients had improved results (75% healed).
Lentrodt[43] 2007	3	100% arrested.	Case report. All patients were children.
OSTEOMYELITIS OF THE AXIAL SKELETON			
Eltorai[16] 1984	44	68% arrested.	Case study. No surgical debridement. Spinal cord injury with osteomyelitis secondary to pressure sores.
Larsson[41] 2002	31	Resolution of infection in 80% of patients without risk factors and in 97% of patients who had risk factors.	Case report. 71% of patients had spinal fixation material in situ.
Ahmed[1] 2009	6	83% resolution of infection.	Case report. No recurrence at 5-month to 3-year follow-ups.
Sandner[75] 2009	10	80% resolution of infection.	Case report. 100% of the 2 failures refused further HBO_2 treatment.
Onen[63] 2015	19	100% improved. Average: 20.1 sessions (10–40).	Retrospective study. Unclear whether it was osteomyelitis, soft tissue infection, or both.
MAGLINANT EXTERNAL OTITIS			
Lucente[44] 1982	16	Only 30% arrested with trimodal therapy.	Case reports.
Mader[50] 1982	1	100% resolution of infection.	Case report. *P. aeruginosa* resistant patient.
Pil-gramm[67] 1986	4	100% improved. Seriousness varied from Stages I to III.	Case reports. Patients were reported to be allergic to broad-spectrum antibiotics.
Shupak[78] 1989	2	100% resolved without recurrences.	Case reports. One patient with facial nerve palsy and 1 with skull base involvement.

TABLE 3 (CONTINUED)

Davis[13] 1992	16	100% resolution.	Case reports. No recurrence at 1- to 4-year follow-ups.
Gilain[21] 1993	1	100% resolution.	Case report. Insulin-dependent patient.
Martel[53] 2000	22	95% arrest rate.	Case reports. Nonsurgically managed cases.
Tisch[92] 2003	22	73% resolved without recurrence.	Case reports. Trimodal therapy with specific immunoglobulins.
Narozny[61] 2006	8	87.5% resolution.	Case reports. One failed case due to fungal etiology.
Tisch[93] 2006	22	95% resolution.	Case reports. 59% of patients had either Stage III or IV involvement.
Heiden[29] 2010		100% improved or resolved of infection.	Case reports. Some patients with facial nerve palsy.
Saxby[77] 2010	17	88% symptom free with apparent resolution of infection.	Case reports. 12% withdrew from HBO_2. 70% of symptom-free patients were cured while the remainder died of other causes.
Sabra [74] 2015	43	Cohort (15 patients): 93.3% pain free and no ear discharge after 2 mo. Control limb (28 patients): 28.5% pain free and no ear discharge after 2 mo.	Cohort study; $p < 0.001$. All patients were treated with antibiotic ciprofloxacin.
STERNAL OSTEOMYELITIS			
Higuchi[30] 2006	4	50% resolution of infection.	Case report. 50% of success cases required a skin graft.
Riddick[72] 2008	27	12 controls and 15 HBO_2 treated. Benefits with HBO_2 in hospital days (65 versus 84), days of IV antibiotics (49 versus 68), and readmissions (0 versus 3).	Retrospective study.

In the 1980s, Barr began displaying his experiences using clinical photographs at hyperbaric medicine meetings using extended HBO_2 treatments for seemingly impossible-to-salvage diabetic foot wounds.[4] Incredible improvements were shown in wounds where osteomyelitis and osteonecrosis were obvious components. This initiated a new important focus for hyperbaric medicine; its use in the management of the diabetic foot wound. In many of the combined hyperbaric medicine wound care programs in the United States, treatment of diabetic foot wounds has become a predominant indication. Criteria for using hyperbaric oxygen in this group of patients are no measurable signs of healing after a 30-day period using standard wound care, antibiotics, and surgical intervention with either the presence of osteomyelitis or deep abscess.[56] Chronic refractory osteomyelitis is undoubtedly present in almost all of those patients where the infection persists after debridement surgery and use of antibiotics. Further discussion of this indication is found in Chapter 21: Strategic Approach to Diabetic Foot Wounds, but from the first author's own review, healing is almost doubled and amputations more than halved versus control groups where HBO_2 was not used.[87-88]

> Dr. Barr should be credited for his almost single-handed perseverance in demonstrating the usefulness of hyperbaric oxygen in the management of seemingly incurable, limb-threatening diabetic foot infections in which chronic refractory osteomyelitis was an obvious component.

EVALUATION

Evaluation of chronic refractory osteomyelitis (CROM) is a four-step process (Figure 9). It starts with establishing the diagnosis of CROM which begins with the history. The essential information in the history is that the bone infection has persisted or recurred after treatment. Secondary information from the history will establish whether the patient's symptoms are related to his/her compromised host status (Table 1), a septic nonunion, or diffuse sclerosing osteomyelitis. By utilizing a simple-to-derive Goal Score coupled with the Wellness Score, quantifiable information becomes available as to whether the infection should be managed with a lower limb amputation, the patient

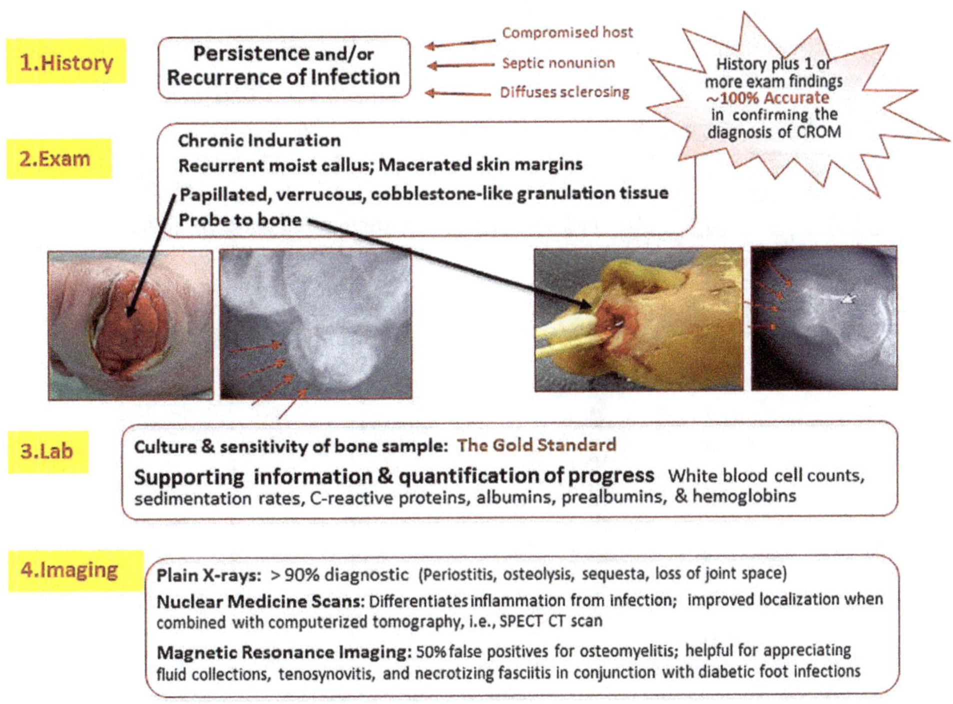

LEGEND: There are four components to the evaluation of CROM. The history and exam determine what additional studies are needed. Images studies help to specify the location and extent of surgery required.

Figure 9. Evaluation and confirmation of the diagnosis of chronic refractory osteomyelitis.

should live with a chronic stable wound, or all efforts to salvage the limb should be done (Table 2, Table 4). The functional status of the patient and his or her aspirations are crucial when making decisions whether to invest resources and time to arrest the infection or to proceed directly to a major limb amputation.

The examination helps to confirm the diagnosis, define the extent of the infection, and plan the strategies for managing CROM. Any time a chronic wound persists over a deformity with exposed bone at the base, osteomyelitis is the diagnosis until proven otherwise. Osteomyelitis of the toe is confirmed in a digit when a wound tracks to bone or joint, there is induration/erythema of the toe, and fusiform swelling is present. A toe with the latter finding has been referred to as a "sausage" toe.[70] Other clinical findings suggestive of CROM in the nonhealing wound include 1) induration, a tense, erythematous swelling; 2) exuberant callus formation especially with underlying maceration of the marginal tissues; and 3) a papillated, verrucous, cobblestone-like appearance of the wound base. The recurrent formation of a well-delineated fibrinous membrane or fibrinous granulation tissue over the wound base, even after repetitive debridements, is often associated underlying bone, bursa, or cicatrix infection. The quantity and character of the exudate in the wound base is an unreliable sign of underlying osteomyelitis and is probably more a function of the diligence of the wound care in the chronic wound than underlying deep infection. Often especially in warm, moist environments, exudate grows profusely on dressings when they are done infrequently. *Pseudomonas* is especially prone to proliferate on exudate in a dressing.

> The "CROM Triad" (1. persistent wound, 2. deformity, and 3. tracking to bone) is invariably present in chronic refractory osteomyelitis associated with diabetic foot wounds.

Laboratory studies are useful for several reasons. The primary reason is that bone cultures not only confirm the diagnosis of osteomyelitis but also are instrumental in

TABLE 4. GOAL SCORE

Assessment	Full 2 Points	Some 1 Point	None 0 Points
	Use half points if mixed or intermediate between 2 grades		
Comprehension			
Motivation			
Compliance			
Support Family, caregiver, institutional			
Insight			

NOTE: The "Goal Score" is another useful tool to determine how successful and how intent the patient and the family are in healing a wound and avoiding a major amputation. Goal Scores greater than 4 points support the decision to avoid lower limb amputation and do everything possible for wound salvage. This score coupled with the Wellness Score (Table 2) provides objectivity to recommend management of limb-threatening wounds.

determining antibiotic selection.[39] They are the gold standard in confirming the diagnosis of osteomyelitis. Other laboratory tests serve several purposes. They provide supporting evidence for the diagnosis and its seriousness such as white blood cell counts and erythrocyte sedimentation rates, provide benchmarks for measuring progress (e.g., decreasing WBCs, ESRs), and justify additional medical interventions (e.g., nutrition management and transfusions if anemia is significant).

Accurate bacteriological diagnosis from the bone causing CROM is important. If the infection is severe enough to cause systemic sepsis (e.g., leukocytosis, nausea, vomiting, fever, and/or chills), blood cultures and sensitivities are sufficient for antibiotic selection. If the infection is of the chronic indolent type, superficial or sinus tract cultures may be obscured by secondary contaminants.[45] If organisms other than *Staphylococcus* are cultured, there is a 60% chance they represent a contamination. Generally, tract or wound base cultures supplemented with judgment are sufficient to initiate appropriate antibiotic therapy. Methicillin-resistant *Staphylococcus aureus* (MRSA) is so commonly observed in the compromised host that appropriate antibiotics to deal with this pathogen are invariably indicated in the absence of actual culture and sensitivity results from bone. For example, 15% to 74% of community-acquired purulent skin and soft-tissue infections in patients without other intercurrent problems culture MRSA.[59]

> The terms methicillin-resistant *Staphylococcus aureus* (MRSA) and oxacillin-resistant *Staphylococcus aureus* (ORSA) can be used interchangeably. For all practical purposes, the antibiotics are identical. Perhaps ORSA is the more precise term since antibiotic sensitivity testing is done with oxacillin rather than with methicillin.

In our experience, approximately 40% of patients presenting to our medical facility with *Staphylococcus* wound infections are positive for MRSA. In those with previous hospitalizations or transferring from assisted care living facilities, the frequency of MRSA infections is doubled. When the response to antibiotics is not as anticipated and/or the bacteriological diagnosis remains in doubt, bone cultures should be obtained.[39] This can be done with needle biopsy preferably under computer tomography control, samples of bone debrided from the wound base, or in the operating room associated with surgical debridement and/or resection of the infected bone. The results may be obscured if the patient is already on antibiotics. In the presence of avascular bone (osteonecrosis), it is unlikely that antibiotics will have much effect on the organisms residing in the bone. Consequently, the culture and sensitivity results are expected to reflect accurately the bacterial flora of the bone. If the bone is perfused, cessation of antibiotics for 24 hours before the biopsy or the planned surgical procedure may improve the accuracy of the bacterial diagnosis. However, with the clinical presence of osteomyelitis, antibiotic management is indicated even if the bone cultures show no growth. Consequently, the use and selection of antibiotics for CROM must be tempered with clinical judgment.

Imaging studies are also helpful in confirming the diagnosis of osteomyelitis. Signs of osteomyelitis on plain X-rays include one or more of the following findings: 1) erosion of cortical bone, 2) periosteal new bone formation (i.e., periostitis), and 3) bone resorption. Other findings that may be observed include sequestra, involucra, and cloacae. The absence of plain X-ray confirmation of osteomyelitis does not rule out this diagnosis. If the infected bone is avascular and/or exists in a hypoxic environment, the above findings, which reflect host responses for dealing with the osteomyelitis, will not be observed. Nuclear medicine imaging is a useful adjunct in this latter situation. Bone scans (technetium pyrophosphate) reflect bone metabolic activity and hence can be positive in a variety of conditions including trauma/fracture healing, infection, metabolic disorders (gout), arthridities, and neuropathic (Charcot) osteoarthropathy. When "cold," that is, no activity is observed, the bone is avascular. This does not rule out infection as explained above. To add specificity to the evaluation, a concomitant white blood cell–labeled (indium) scan will differentiate infected bone from the other conditions which generate the inflammatory response in bone. The combination of computerized tomography with nuclear medicine imaging (i.e., SPECT-CT (single photon emission computed tomography) scanning) add increased discrimination and localization of the infection.[68] Post-acquisition fusion of the CT component of the study with SPECT enables more precise anatomical localization of radiopharmaceutical uptake, This can be very helpful in making decisions about the surgical management of CROM. Magnetic resonance (MR) imaging has over a 90% sensitivity for diagnosing osteomyelitis.[42] Unfortunately, MR imaging studies tend to be over-read in suspected osteomyelitis cases with specificities in the 50% range due to interpretations being based on bone edema. However, the magnetic resonance study is unparalleled in its ability to diagnosis necrotic bone (osteonecrosis), soft-tissue fluid collections such as abscesses, septic arthritis, infected bursa, tract wounds, osteitis (cortical bone involvement), and tenosynovitis.

MANAGEMENT

Once osteomyelitis meets the criteria of chronic refractory, that is the infection persists or recurs after treatment, three presentations become obvious, namely 1) refractory osteomyelitis in a compromised host, 2) osteomyelitis associated with the septic nonunion fracture and 3) diffuse sclerosing osteomyelitis (Figure 1).[87] Each has features that require special considerations for management and different protocols for using hyperbaric oxygen. This approach supplements and is more encompassing than the two anatomic types (namely, localized osteomyelitis in the compromised host and diffuse osteomyelitis) that Mader et al. proposed for using HBO_2 in osteomyelitis (Table 1).[46] In order to make appropriate management decisions, information about patient wellness and goals with respect to the management of CROM and avoidance of a lower limb amputation must be considered (Table 2, Table 4).

Compromised Host Presentation

Of the three presentations of CROM (that is the compromised host, septic nonunion, and diffuse sclerosing types), the major indication for using HBO_2 is in the compromised host. In our experiences over 90% of the use of HBO_2 for CROM is for this presentation type. It is characterized by three features, namely, 1) wound hypoxia, 2) mixed flora frequently with aerobes and anaerobes, and 3) impaired ability by the host to develop a healing response other than a "frustrated type" of granulation tissue. This is distinguished by a pale, anemic appearance of the wound base, failure for epithelialization of the wound margins to occur, persistent biofilm/fibrous membrane formation after debridements, and often cobblestone-like appearance of the granulation tissue.

Treatment requires a fivefold strategic approach including 1) prudent surgical (bedside and/or operating room) management of the wound base and the infected bone, 2) sensible immobilization and protection of the wound site, 3) optimal attention to medical problems/comorbidities, 4) pragmatic selection of dressing materials, and [5] use of appropriate measures to augment wound oxygenation (Figure 10). The

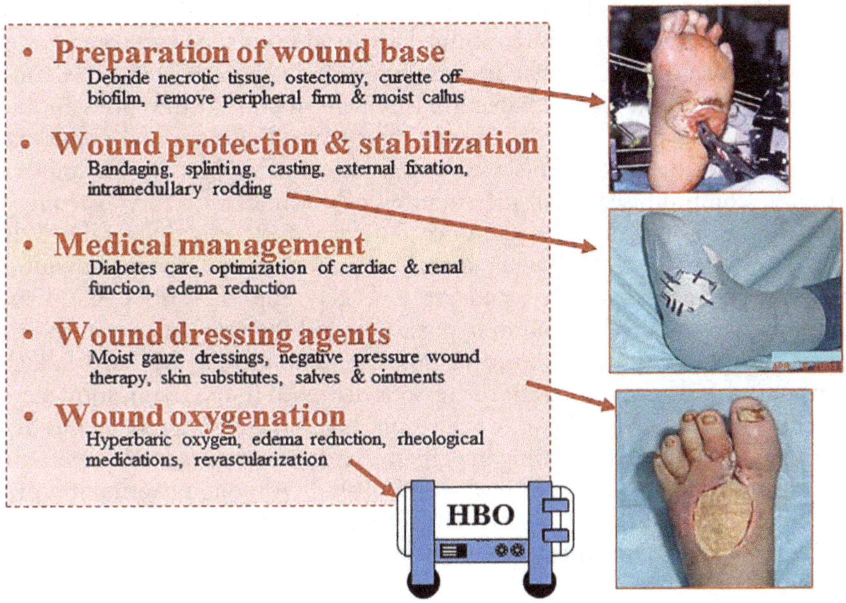

LEGEND: Five strategies are utilized to manage problem wounds in general and chronic refractory osteomyelitis in particular. Preparation of the wound base may require operative room surgeries for bone and soft tissue debridement, amputations, flap management, osteotomies to realign bone deformities, and bone fixation.

Figure 10. The 5 elements of strategic management of CROM.

Wellness and Goal Scores support decision-making for using the strategic approach versus proceeding directly to a major lower limb amputation (Table 2, Table 4). If the host is decompensated and the Goal Score is low, the better choice is a lower limb amputation. Salvage of the limb, in such situations, is unlikely to affect the patient's level of function.

Once the evaluation is completed (see previous section), surgical management is usually required for the wound base strategy. The reason for this is that there is a high probability the infected bone is necrotic, and without removal, the infection will burgeon as soon as the course of antibiotics has been completed. If a significant deformity is present, the wound and bone infection will inevitably recur as soon as activity is resumed even with the selection of appropriate protective footwear. Surgical management may require debridement/ostectomy, partial/complete ray resection, or partial foot amputation. Usually, what needs to be done surgically becomes apparent after examination and imaging studies are completed. Oftentimes surgery to prepare the wound base can be done in the clinic or at the bedside in deference to being done in the operating room. Nonetheless, resourcefulness is required in order to remove the infected bone and generate flaps that will cover the wound but still preserve a structurally stable and functionally sound lower extremity.

If the soft-tissue margins are of questionable viability and/or not clinically free of infection, the operative site should be left open with healing by secondary intention or later returned to the operating room for delayed coverage. A cost-effective alternative that may be appropriate is follow-up at the bedside or in the clinic (where serial partial wound approximations can be done) for delayed closure. Antibiotic selection and duration should be done in conjunction with an infectious disease consultant. If there are reasonable expectations that the bone infection has been eradicated with surgery, postoperative antibiotics should be continued for an additional two weeks after wound closure to assure that the soft tissues adjacent to the infected bone become infection free. When concerns exist that residual infection is present in bone, intravenous antibiotics should be continued for six to eight weeks after wound closure, and consideration should be given for the long-term (six months or more) of suppressive oral antibiotics.

For the compromised host presentation of chronic refractory osteomyelitis, hyperbaric oxygen is indicated as an adjunct to management, especially if the Wellness and Goal Scores justify attempts to eradicate the infection and salvage the limb. The effects of HBO_2 are well defined and are especially applicable to CROM in the compromised host (Figure 8). Wound hypoxia is a predominant concern in this group of patients. Without augmentation of tissue oxygenation levels, wound healing and infection control will be stymied. For the reasons discussed in the justification sections, HBO_2 predictably improves wound oxygenation. Juxta-wound transcutaneous oxygen measurements in room air and during hyperbaric oxygen exposures predict, with nearly a 90% accuracy, which wounds will heal with HBO_2.[81] Although treatment protocols need to be individualized, the recommended approach is to provide this group of patients 10 to 14 HBO_2 treatments to initiate angiogenesis and other host mechanisms before debridement surgery. After surgery, an additional 7 to 14 treatments are recommended to optimize healing of the flaps and potentiate host mechanisms during the very crucial (and oxygen-dependent) immediate postoperative period. Our experiences indicate that almost 90% of patients with CROM who are compromised hosts will avoid lower limb amputation when HBO_2 is used as an adjunct to surgical and antibiotic management in those patients who meet functional and motivation criteria to preserve the limb.[90]

> For wound healing, infection control, and postoperative flap survival, oxygen requirements may need to increase 20-fold or more for successful healing as compared to steady-state oxygen requirements for noncritical tissues.[89] Inability to meet these demands result in wound healing failures. When these requirements are partially met, the wound may initially fail, slough, or dehisce, but then go onto eventual healing, especially when HBO_2 is used in the perioperative period.

Septic Nonunion Presentations

Hyperbaric oxygen is indicated for septic nonunions when other treatment measures such as debridements and courses of antibiotics have failed, and there is justification to preserve the limb as supported by Wellness and Goal Scores (Table 2, Table 4). Two considerations are fundamental before initiating a salvage attempt with adjunctive HBO_2: first, there is the potential for useful function if healing is achieved, and second, intractable pain is not present. Hyperbaric oxygen will only be successful in conjunction with appropriate orthopedic interventions such as debridement, stabilization, bone grafting, and soft-tissue management as well as the use of suitable antibiotics. The recommended HBO_2 treatment protocol for the septic nonunion presentation of CROM includes two weeks of daily preoperative treatments to promote angiogenesis and improve the wound environment as much as possible prior to surgery. After surgery, 20 to 40 postoperative sessions should be done to promote bone remodeling, clearing of any residuals of infection, and osteogenesis. This more extensive course of HBO_2 treatments (as compared to the protocol for CROM in the compromised host) is needed in order to enhance the more slowly responding host factors, especially those associated with bone formation and remodeling. In about of our patients, we have observed stress fractures with resumption of walking activity after healing and eradication of infection. This is attributed to the effect of the well-oxygenated environment for stimulation of the osteoclast and the resultant zealous remodeling of bone. Our limited experiences in patients with septic nonunions reveal almost 100% fracture healing rates when HBO_2 is used in conjunction with appropriate orthopaedic and antibiotic management even after initial failures with these latter two interventions alone.

Diffuse Sclerosing Osteomyelitis Presentation

This is the third presentation of bone infections for which hyperbaric oxygen may be indicated. In this presentation, the bone infection involves the diaphysis and is usually extensive, poorly demarcated (in contrast to the discrete appearance of a sequestrum), and refractory to antibiotic treatment. Surgical management can be challenging since eradication of the infection by this means may compromise the structural integrity of the bone so much that useful function is unlikely. Conversely, residual infection at the margins of the debridement, which is likely to occur unless segmental resection of the diffuse, sclerosed infected bone is done, allows the infection to persist and be labeled refractory. As mentioned in the introduction, dead-space management with antibiotic-impregnated bone cement beads, use of microvascular free flaps, and Illizarov healing principles have been a great asset in managing this type of refractory osteomyelitis.

When these measures fail or the extension is too extensive for the above interventions to be fully utilized, HBO_2 treatments should be considered, especially if the patient's Wellness and Goal Scores merit salvaging the extremity. Saucerization (the debridement technique of creating an undersurface of a saucer-shape defect in the skin and soft-tissue level followed by generating a trough in the cortical bone to the medullary canal) is helpful in debulking the amount of infected bone. Although this technique is not likely to remove all the infected bone, when it is done in conjunction with hyperbaric oxygen treatments, host responses to the infection plus additional antibiotic therapy are often sufficient to eradicate the infection. Once the wound base has

> Rarely the situation occurs where the patient is too ill (this corresponds to the Cierney-Mader type C host; Wellness Score less than 4.5 points) or is unwilling to comply with the requirements needed for postoperative management and convalescence of his or her CROM, typically of the diffuse sclerosing type. In these situations, the "cure may be worse than disease" (from *Don Quixote, the Ingenious Gentleman…* of La Mancha – 1605, 1615 – who loses his sanity while in a fugue state where he imagines he is reviving chivalry, but promptly dies when his sanity is restored – as quoted by his quick-witted squire, Poncho Sanchez).
>
> Typically, these patients present with one or more chronically infected, intermittently or continuously draining sinus tracts. If this is the situation, a course of hyperbaric oxygen and antibiotics becomes an option. A minimum of 21 HBO_2 treatments is recommended in this protocol for managing CROM.
>
> Drainage has been observed to stop and/or markedly decrease with the HBO_2 treatments. The patient should be informed to anticipate future recurrences of drainage, and, if severe enough, consider additional courses of hyperbaric oxygen and antibiotic when this occurs.

granulated, healing by secondary intention or coverage with a flap can be done. If the wound base is observed to have residual focuses of avascular and/or infected bone, the patient can be returned to the operating room for second-stage debridement of these focuses. Hyperbaric oxygen treatment protocols for this presentation of refractory osteomyelitis are similar to those for the septic nonunion. However, postoperative hyperbaric oxygen treatments are usually continued until a total of 60 treatments have been completed.

Chronic refractory osteomyelitis of the axial skeleton such as the mandible, spine, skull, and sternum is also benefited by HBO_2 (Table 3). For the spine and skull, arrest of the infection can usually be achieved with antibiotics and hyperbaric oxygen without major debridement surgery. This may be due to the relatively improved perfusion to these bones as compared to those of the appendicular skeleton. Imaging studies and bone biopsies under CT guidance should be done in order to verify the diagnosis, appreciate the extent of the infection, and optimize the selection of antibiotics. Hyperbaric oxygen treatments should be given for a three-week period for optimizing host responses for infections in these locations. After this, peer review should be done to recommend continuing or stopping HBO_2 treatments at that time.

REIMBURSEMENT CONSIDERATIONS

Reimbursement for the use of hyperbaric oxygen as an adjunct in the management of chronic refractory osteomyelitis is approved by the Centers for Medicare and Medicaid Services (CMS)/Medicare) and is covered by most third-party insurance carriers.(56) In order to justify the use of HBO_2 therapy in CROM, documentation that the condition is chronic and refractory is required prior to initiation of HBO_2. Although CMS does not provide a specific definition for the words "chronic" and "refractory" as they relate to osteomyelitis, it is assumed that the initial acute osteomyelitis has been treated appropriately and has persisted for a 30-day period or longer. In the event that the osteomyelitis remains or recurs despite appropriate therapy, a diagnosis of chronic refractory osteomyelitis is appropriate. For reimbursements from CMS, exact diagnostic codes must be used in accordance with the new ICD-10-CM (International Classification of Diseases, 10th Revision, Clinical Modification) (Table 5).

Since indications on the use of hyperbaric oxygen were first formulated by the Undersea and Hyperbaric Medical Society (UHMS), chronic osteomyelitis has been included in the *Hyperbaric Oxygen Therapy Committee Report* as an approved indication.(27) The U.S. Food and Drug Administration (FDA) uses the UHMS HBO_2 Committee Report as a primary source document when inquiries are made regarding the use of HBO_2 therapy. If the condition is not specifically listed in the UHMS HBO_2 Committee Report, the FDA responds to inquiries by stating the condition, in question, is an "off-label" use of HBO_2.

The ICD-10-CM codes include many permutations for chronic osteomyelitis, each with their own specific code (Table 5). Physician supervision of HBO_2 treatment for CROM is reimbursed by CMS and third-party insurers with appropriate documentation.

According to several CMS/Medicare fiscal intermediaries' Local Coverage Determinations, Medicare covers the adjunctive use of HBO_2 therapy for CROM that has been unreactive to conventional medical and surgical management. Inherent in the statement is that the osteomyelitis must be chronic and refractory to usual standard-of-care management (i.e., an appropriate course of antibiotic therapy – preferably selected from appropriate culture and sensitivity information, drainage of abscesses, suitable

TABLE 5. POSSIBLE ICD-10-CM* CODES FOR HYPERBARIC OXYGEN USED WITH CHRONIC REFRACTORY OSTEOMYELITIS

Site	Side Right	Side Left	ICD-9-CM	ICD-10-CM
Chronic Multifocal Osteomyelitis Category				
Pelvic region and thigh	X		730.15	M86.351
"		X	730.15	M86.352
Lower leg [tibia]	X		730.16	M86.361
"		X	730.16	M86.362
Ankle and foot	X		730.17	M86.371
"		X	730.17	M86.372
Chronic Osteomyelitis with Draining Sinus Category				
Femur	X		730.15	M86.451
"		X	730.15	M86.452
Tibia and fibula	X		730.16	M86.461
"		X	730.16	M86.462
Ankle and foot	X		730.17	M86.471
"		X	730.17	M86.472
Other site			730.18	M86.48
Multiple sites			730.19	M86.49
Other Chronic Osteomyelitis Category				
Pelvic region and thigh	X		730.15	M86.561 / M86.661
"		X	730.15	M86.562 / M86.662
Lower leg [tibia]	X		730.16	M86.561 / M86.661
"		X	730.16	M86.552 / M86.662
Ankle and foot	X		730.17	M86.571 / M86.671
"		X	730.17	M86.572 / M86.672
Other specified sites	X		730.18	M86.58 / 68
Multiple sites In Selected Locations			730.19	M86.59 / 69

ICD-10-CM* International Classification of Disease-10 [10th edition] – Clinical Modification

immobilization of the affected part, and debridement with removal of infected bone). Hyperbaric oxygen that is not documented to be chronic and refractory to conventional treatment, and HBO$_2$ not provided in an adjunctive fashion, is not covered.

In summary, HBO$_2$ therapy is an adjunctive treatment to be used with appropriate antibiotics and surgical debridement (to eliminate necrotic bone, i.e., a sequestrum, acting as a foreign body). When the site of the bone infection is not amendable to debridement or resection, HBO$_2$ may be utilized to enhance systemic therapy but is not to be used as the primary therapy only. This permutation may be justified in the Mader and Cierny type C host or patients with low Wellness Scores, but treatment justified by good Goal Scores (Table 1, Table 2, Table 4).

Hyperbaric oxygen treatments are usually delivered daily for a period of 90 to 120 minutes. Treatments often immediately follow debridement surgeries when concerns are raised by the surgeon that residual infection may exist and/or the loss of structural integrity of the extremity would exist if all infected bone is removed. The number of treatments varies with clinical presentation, i.e., CROM in the compromised host, the septic nonunion and the diffuse sclerosing presentations (Table 6). A maximum of 60 HBO$_2$ treatments within a 12-month period as designated by the CMS/ Medicare preauthorization project is acknowledged, although in most situations (i.e.,

TABLE 6. HYPERBARIC OXYGEN PROTOCOLS FOR THE THREE PRESENTATIONS OF CHRONIC REFRACTORY OSTEOMYELITIS

Presentation (and findings)	Recommended HBO Txs		Total HBO Txs*	Comments
	Pre-Op	Post-Op		
Compromised Hosts 1. Wound hypoxia 2. Mixed flora 3. Impaired host responses	0–14	7–14	28	If infection is erdicated, HBO_2 is stopped. HBO_2 Txs may need to be extended if flaps are threatened after surgery.
Septic Nonunion 1. Chronic infection 2. Instability 3. Avascular interface	14	14–28	40	Surgeries may be staged; first debridement + stabilization; then bone grafting + closure.
Diffuse Sclerosing 1. Diffuse distribution 2. Poor demarcation	14–21	21–40	60	Extended HBO Txs needed to maximize bone resorption and angiogenesis effects.

COMMENTS: HBO treatments are usually for 90 to120 minutesÕ durations at 2.0 to 2.4 atmospheres absolute pressure once a day if an outpatient and twice a day if an inpatient. HBO = hyperbaric oxygen, Op = operation (surgery), Txs = treatments, *Txs = maximum number of HBO_2 treatments

compromised host presentations) the number of treatments to arrest the infection is much less than this number (Table 6).

The Undersea and Hyperbaric Medical Society Hyperbaric Oxygen Therapy Committee Report recommends peer review after 40 treatments for CROM but should be modified in accordance with the type of CROM presentation. Coding and reimbursement information is an ongoing, ever-changing process. Even though information as we present it may change in the future, we feel it provides the justification and rationale for accommodating future changes and making appropriate decisions with regard to using HBO_2 for CROM.

CONCLUSIONS

The role of hyperbaric oxygen treatments in the management of chronic refractory osteomyelitis becomes objective when the definition of this problem and the three clinical presentations as provided in this chapter are employed. During almost 40 years of experience using HBO_2 therapy as an adjunct to manage refractory osteomyelitis, the following salient observations about the usefulness of this modality are summarized below:

1. **Pretreatment with HBO_2 improves the environment around the CROM site.** This is the rationale for recommending two weeks of HBO_2 before surgery and starting antibiotics, especially in the septic nonunion and diffuse sclerosing CROM presentations. Effects observed include 1) decreased wound edema, induration and drainage, 2) improved quality of the skin around the wound, and 3) better demarcation of infected from noninfected tissues.
2. **Hyperbaric oxygen helps demarcate live from dead, infected bone.** This is attributed to angiogenesis and osteoclast stimulation effects of HBO_2. Observations in the operating room support the assumption that

the vascularity of the tissues adjacent to the interface and dead bone are preferentially affected by preoperative HBO_2 treatments even though HBO_2 may not influence the avascular infected bone itself. This assists in establishing viable, infection-free margins at the time of the debridement.

3. **Hyperbaric oxygen preferentially stimulates the osteoclast.** The osteoclast, a derivative of the macrophage line of blood cells, generates acids and phosphatases to dissolve bone. Its metabolic activity and its ability to absorb bone is 100 times greater than the osteoblast's ability to form bone.[37] Osteoclast function is stymied in the hypoxic environment. Evidence to support the osteoclast's role in bone resorption after HBO_2 treatments is twofold: 1) X-ray changes of bone resorption and 2) occurrences of stress fractures when patients resume ambulation after CROM has been arrested in long bones after a course of HBO_2 treatments.
4. **Optimal protocols using HBO_2 must be followed to achieve successful outcomes.** Protocols are guided by the clinical presentation, that is, compromised host, septic nonunion, or diffuse sclerosing types of CROM (Table 6). For the latter two presentations, presurgical, preantibiotic HBO_2 treatments are given, usually during a two-week period, to improve the vascularity and to reduce edema in the infection site. After this, surgical debridement, fracture stabilization, if indicated, and starting antibiotics is done. Redebridements may be required if granulation tissue formation fails to cover the exposed bone after the initial debridement. Once the infection is arrested, and the wounds are covered/closed in septic nonunions and diffuse sclerosing CROM, organism-specific antibiotics should be continued for a minimum of six additional weeks. Usually 2 additional weeks of HBO_2 treatments, up to a total of 60, are given after the last debridement in these 2 presentations to enhance host factor removal of the remaining vestiges of dead, infected bone.
5. **The duration of CROM does not have an adverse effect on the outcomes.** When HBO_2 is used as an adjunct to both surgery and antibiotic therapy, the outcomes appear independent of the duration of the problem. This observation takes exception to a previous report where arrest rates decreased from 80% to 50% if CROM was present for longer than 2 years (Table 3).[5] When the protocols previously described are followed, outcomes appear to be independent of the duration the bone infection has existed.
6. **Advanced age is not a cause for poorer outcomes when HBO_2 is used for the management of CROM.** Advancing age is recognized as a negative predictor for good outcomes, especially in trauma and fracture management.[36] If the bone infection meets the definition of CROM, and the decision is made to avoid amputation based on the patient's Wellness and Goal Scores, outcomes appear to be independent of age especially in the compromised host presentations. Hyperbaric oxygen has been reported to act as a signaling device to stimulate fibroblast activity and reconcile the effects that advancing age has on slowing fibroblast doubling times.[71,76]

When making decisions about limb salvage versus amputation, physiological age is a more important consideration than chronological age. Chronological age is a person's actual age and does not consider cognitive function, comorbidities, experience, physical fitness, judgment, mobility, and strength.[82] Physiological age is more akin to the functional (physical and mental) activities that the average person would be doing at an age that is different than the person's chronological age.

If infirm, for example, the physiological age may be older than the chronological age; if more active and fit, the physiological age may be younger than the chronological age.

The Wellness Score is a quick and easy tool to quantify physiological age. When coupled with the patient's Goal Score, the decision for limb salvage versus amputation becomes more objective (Table 2, Table 4).

7. **Outcomes with HBO_2 are equally good whether the bone infection is caused by synergistic and/or mixed aerobic and anaerobic organisms.** This contrasts to a previous report where failures were observed in over 60% of the patients who had bone infections culturing both aerobic and anaerobic bacteria.[23]

8. **Once CROM has been arrested using HBO_2, the results are durable.** This observation is ascribed to the "jump start" effects HBO_2 has on host factors and the continuation of these effects after surgery and antibiotics have been completed. For the compromised host with arrested CROM, strategies to prevent new or recurrent infections must be followed.[85] A seemingly negative effect that supports the observation that the effects of HBO_2 continue even after treatments have been completed is the delayed appearance of stress fractures after CROM is arrested in septic nonunion and diffuse sclerotic presentations of CROM. Especially strong evidence supporting the durability of the arrest of infection in CROM was reported in Morey's and Davis's studies (Table 3).[14,60]

9. **If the decision is made to arrest CROM, management may require using interventions that were done before but were unsuccessful in the absence of HBO_2.** The protocols for the managing the three presentations of CROM must be followed. Antibiotics should be selected based on bone cultures from the debridement surgery regardless of what had been cultured before. The extent of debridements must be based on clinical findings and imaging studies regardless of previous surgeries. Hyperbaric oxygen needs to be given according to the described protocols.

10. **Not every case of CROM will be arrested with the adjunctive use of HBO_2.** Failures, that is, the need for lower limb amputations, have occurred in several, somewhat predictable, circumstances including 1) methicillin-resistant *Staphylococcus aureus* infections in a subset of diabetics whose infections recur even after ending prolonged courses of antibiotics, 2) patients with collagen vascular diseases, especially those requiring steroids and/or immunosuppressors, 3) new vascular occlusive events, 4) intractable pain, 5) residual structural problems of the arrested infection site that prevent useful function, and 6) insufficient patient compliance to follow the required treatment protocols.

TABLE 7. USING RATIONAL-BASED INDICATIONS TO JUSTIFY HBO$_2$ FOR CROM

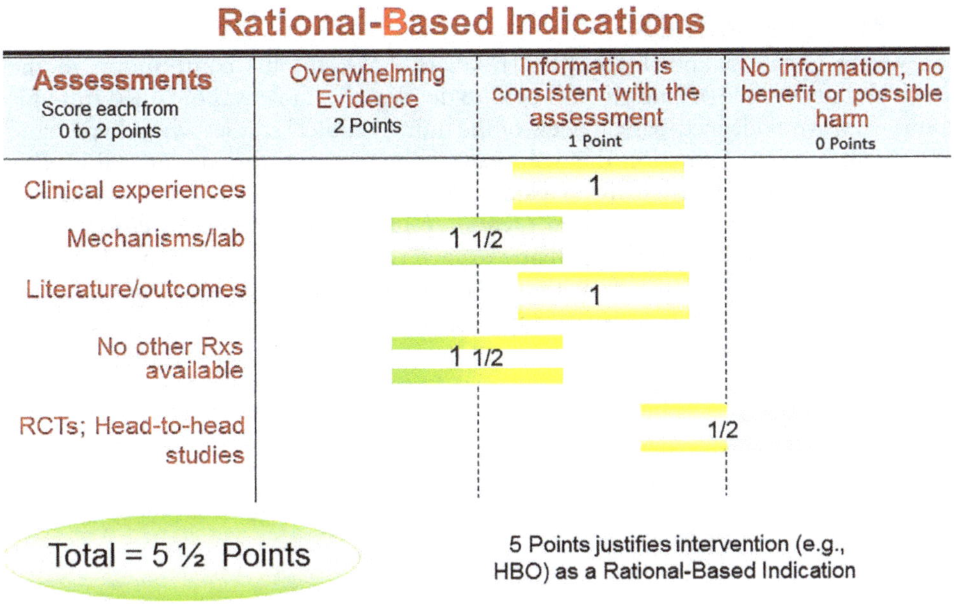

How does hyperbaric oxygen measure up as an evidence-based indication for chronic refractory osteomyelitis? Since it is used as an adjunct to surgery and antibiotics and is used when these managements fail, perhaps it needs to be judged differently than a primary treatment modality. Nonetheless, when the American Heart Association 1999 Guidelines are used, HBO$_2$ meets the criteria of Class-II indication.[28] That is, it is useful and effective with a favorable risk/benefit ratio. The absence of a randomized control trial keeps HBO$_2$ from being classified at a higher level for CROM.

It is apparent that factors other than the criteria used for Evidence Based Indications need to be considered when making decisions about selecting treatment interventions. This is true for the use of HBO$_2$ in CROM. We propose five assessments for justifying a decision on a treatment selection (Table 7).[86] To quantify this approach, each assessment is graded on a 0-to-2 scale with 2 points indicating overwhelming information to support the decision to use the treatment intervention, 1 point to indicate that the information is consistent with the selection, and 0 points if there is no information, no benefit, or possible harm if the treatment is used. By adding up the points of each of the 5 assessments, a 0-to-10 score (with 10 being best) is determined. If the total is 5 or greater, a rational basis for using the treatment is established. For the use of HBO$_2$ in CROM, the score is 5½ (Table 7), thereby qualifying it as a rational-based indication for this condition.

In summary, hyperbaric oxygen has a defined role in the management of chronic refractory osteomyelitis. Laboratory studies and clinical experiences confirm its benefit in this condition. "Chronic refractory" can be precisely defined. Since there are three predominant presentations, HBO$_2$ treatment protocols and other interventions need to be selected based on the type of presentation. The patient's Wellness and Goal Scores (which can be quantified; Table 2, Table 4) need to be factored into the decision whether to attempt to arrest the infection or recommend a limb amputation. Evidenced-based and rational-based criteria exist to support the decision-making process for using HBO_2 in CROM.

ACKNOWLEDGMENTS

We would like to acknowledge Brett B. Hart, MD, for his contribution to the development of Table 3. Information used to develop this table was obtained from his comprehensive evidenced-based review of the human clinical studies where hyperbaric oxygen therapy was utilized in the treatment of chronic refractory osteomyelitis. This information appeared originally in paragraph summary form in the *Undersea and Hyperbaric Medical Society Hyperbaric Oxygen Therapy Indications, 13th Edition.*

No review on the use of hyperbaric oxygen therapy in the treatment of chronic osteomyelitis would be complete without the acknowledgment of the work of the late Jon T. Mader, MD. We are especially appreciative to Dr. Mader for the information he presented in the osteomyelitis chapter on in vitro and in vivo studies in the second edition of this text.

REFERENCES

1. Ahmed R, Severson MA, Traynelis VC. Role of hyperbaric oxygen therapy in the treatment of bacterial spinal osteomyelitis. J Neurosurg Spine. 2009;10(1):16-20.
2. Aitasalo K et al. A modified protocol for early treatment of osteomyelitis and osteoradionecrosis of the mandible. Head Neck. 1998;20(5):411-7.
3. Barili F, Polvani G, Topkara VK, et al. Role of hyperbaric oxygen therapy in the treatment of postoperative organ/space sternal surgical site infections. World J Surg. 2007;31(8):1702-6.
4. Barr PO, Perrins DJD. Prolonged use of hyperbaric oxygen (HBO) in indolent ulcers of the legs. In: Proceedings of the 8th International Congress on Hyperbaric Medicine. Long Beach (CA): Best Publishing Co.; 1984. p. 217-22.
5. Bingham EL, Hart GB. Hyperbaric oxygen treatment of refractory osteomyelitis. Postgrad Med. 1977;61(6):70-6.
6. Caragee EJ et al. The clinical use of erythrocyte sedimentation rate in pyogenic vertebral osteomyelitis. Spine. 1997;22(18):2089-93.
7. Chen CE et al. Hyperbaric oxygen therapy in the treatment of chronic refractory osteomyelitis: a preliminary report. Chang Gung Med J. 2003;26(2):114-21.
8. Chen CE et al. Results of chronic osteomyelitis of the femur treated with hyperbaric oxygen: a preliminary report. Chang Gung Med J. 2004;27(2):91-7.
9. Chen CY et al. Adjuvant hyperbaric oxygen therapy in the treatment of hemodialysis patients with chronic osteomyelitis. Ren Fail. 2008;30(2):233-7.
10. Chen CY et al. Chronic refractory tibia osteomyelitis treated with adjuvant hyperbaric oxygen: a preliminary report. Changgeng Yi Xue Za Zhi. 1998;21(2):165-71.
11. Chen F et al. The treatment of deep wound infection after posterior thoracic and lumbar instrumentation. Zhonghua Wai Ke Za Zhi. 2005;43(20):1325-7.
12. Cierny G, Mader JT. Adult chronic osteomyelitis. Orthopedics. 1984;7:1557-64.
13. Davis JC et al. Adjuvant hyperbaric oxygen in malignant external otitis. Arch Otolaryngol Head Neck Surg. 1992;118(1):89-93.
14. Davis JC et al. Chronic non-hematogenous osteomyelitis treated with adjuvant hyperbaric oxygen. J Bone Joint Surg Am. 1986;68(8):1210-7.
15. Delasotta LA, Hanflik A, Bicking G, Mannella W. Hyperbaric oxygen for osteomyelitis in a compromised host. Open Orthop J. 2013;7 114-7.
16. Eltorai I, Hart GB, Strauss MB. Osteomyelitis in the spinal cord injured: a review and a preliminary report on the use of hyperbaric oxygen therapy. Paraplegia. 1984;22(1):17-24.
17. Esterhai JH, Pisarello J, Brighton CT, et al. Adjunctive hyperbaric oxygen therapy in the treatment of chronic refractory osteomyelitis. J Trauma. 1987;27:763-8.
18. Esterhai JL et al. Treatment of chronic osteomyelitis complicating nonunion and segmental defects of the tibia with open cancellous bone graft, posterolateral bone graft, and soft-tissue transfer. J Trauma. 1990;30(1):49-54.
19. Esterhai JL Jr et al. Effect of hyperbaric oxygen exposure on oxygen tension within the medullary canal in the rabbit tibial osteomyelitis model. J Orthop Res. 1986;4(3):330-6.
20. Fitzgerald RH Jr, Ruttle PE, Arnold PG, et al. Local muscle flaps in the treatment of chronic osteomyelitis. J Bone Joint Surg. 1985;67A:175.
21. Gilain L, Labroue M, Aidan D, et al. Value of hyperbaric oxygen therapy in the treatment of malignant otitis externa. Apropos of a case. Ann Otolaryngol Chir Cervicofac. 1993;110:50-4.

22. Guyton AC, Hall JE. Textbook of medical physiology. Philadelphia: WB Saunders; 2000. p. 144-94.

23. Hall BB, Fitzgerald RH Jr, Rosenblatt JE. Anaerobic osteomyelitis. J Bone Joint Surg. 1983;65(A):30-5.

24. Hamblen DL. Hyperbaric oxygenation: its effect on experimental staphylococcal osteomyelitis in rats. J Bone Joint Surg. 1968;50:1129-41.

25. Handschel J et al. Evaluation of hyperbaric oxygen therapy in treatment of patients with osteomyelitis of the mandible. Mund Kiefer Gesichtschir. 2007;11(5):285-90.

26. Hansen RO, Lundback K. The basement membrane morphology in diabetes mellitus. In: Ellenberg M, Rifkin H, editors. Diabetes mellitus: the theory and practice. New York: McGraw Hill; 1970. p. 178-209.

27. Hart BB. Refractory osteomyelitis. In: Weaver LK, editor. Hyperbaric oxygen therapy indications. 13th ed. North Palm Beach (FL): Best Publishing Co.; 2014. p. 179-207.

28. Hazinski ME, Cummins RD, editors. Handbook of emergency cardiovascular care for health care providers. American Heart Association; 1999. p. 3.

29. Heiden C. Malignant otitis externa: experience with hyperbaric oxygen therapy. Diving Hyperb Med. 2010;40:182.

30. Higuchi T et al. Preliminary report of the safety and efficacy of hyperbaric oxygen therapy for specific complications of lung transplantation. J Heart Lung Transplant. 2006;25(11):1302-9.

31. Hill GB. Hyperbaric oxygen exposure for intrahepatic abscesses produced in mice by non-spore-forming anaerobic bacteria. Antimicrob Agents Chemother. 1976;9:312-7.

32. Hohn DC, MacKay RD, Halliday B, et al. The effect of oxygen tension on the microbial function of leukocytes in wounds and in vitro. Surg Forum. 1976;27:18-20.

33. Hunt TK, Niinikoski J, Zederfelt BH, et al. Oxygen in wound healing enhancement; cellular effects of oxygen. Davis JC, Hunt TK, editors. Hyperbaric oxygen therapy. Bethesda (MD): Undersea Medical Society Inc; 1977. p. 111-2.

34. Hunt TK, Pai MP. The effect of varying ambient oxygen tensions on wound metabolism and collagen synthesis. Surg Gynecol Obstet. 1972;135:756-8.

35. Jamil MU, Eckardt A, Franko W. Hyperbaric oxygen therapy. Clinical use in treatment of osteomyelitis, osteoradionecrosis and reconstructive surgery of the irradiated mandible. Mund Liefer Gesichtschhir. 2000;4(5):320-3.

36. Johansen K, Daines M, Howey T, et al. Objective criteria accurately predict amputation following lower extremity trauma. J Trauma. 1990;30:568-73.

37. Johnson LC. Kinetics of osteoarthritis. Lab Invest. 1959;8:1223-41.

38. Kawashima M. Bone disease with pain. Osteomyelitis in the long bone. Clin Calcium. 2008;18(6):836-43.

39. Khatri G, Wagner DK, Sohnle PG. Effect of bone biopsy in guiding antimicrobial therapy for osteomyelitis complicating open wounds. Am J Med Sci. 2001;321:367-71.

40. Kivisaari J, Niinikoski J. Effects of hyperbaric oxygenation and prolonged hypoxia on the healing of open wounds. Acta Chirurgica Scandinavica. 1975;141:14-9.

41. Larsson A et al. Hyperbaric oxygen treatment of postoperative neurosurgical infections. Neurosurgery. 2002;50(2):287-95; discussion 295-6.

42. Ledermann HP, Schweitzer ME, Morrison WB. Nonenhancing tissue on MR imaging of pedal infection: characterization of necrotic tissue and associated limitations for diagnosis of osteomyelitis and abscess. AJR Am J Roentgenol. 2002;178:215-22.

43. Lentrodt S et al. Hyperbaric oxygen for adjuvant therapy for chronically recurrent mandibular osteomyelitis in childhood and adolescence. J Oral Maxillofac Surg. 2007;65(2):186-91.

44. Lucente FE et al. Malignant external otitis: a dangerous misnomer? Otolaryngol Head Neck Surg. 1982;90(2):266-9.

45. Mackowiak PA, Jones SR, Smith JW. Diagnostic value of sinus-tract cultures in chronic osteomyelitis. J Am Med Assoc. 1978;239:2772-5.

46. Mader J. Osteomyelitis (Refractory). In: Hampson NB, editor. Hyperbaric oxygen therapy: 1999 committee report. Kensington (MD): Undersea and Hyperbaric Medical Society; 1999. p. 47-50.

47. Mader JT, Adams KR, Couch LA, et al. Potentiation of tobramycin by hyperbaric oxygen in experimental Pseudomonas aeruginosa osteomyelitis. Paper presented at: 27th Interscience Conference on Antimicrobial Agents and Chemotherapy; 1987; New York.

48. Mader JT, Brown GL, Guckian JC, et al. A mechanism for the amelioration by hyperbaric oxygen of experimental staphylococcal osteomyelitis in rabbits. J Infect Dis. 1980;142:915-22.

49. Mader JT, Guckian JC, Glass DL, et al. Therapy with hyperbaric oxygen of experimental osteomyelitis due to Staphylococcus aureus in rabbits. J Infect Dis. 1978;138:312-8.

50. Mader JT, Love JT. Malignant external otitis. Cure with adjunctive hyperbaric oxygen therapy. Arch Otolaryngol. 1982;108:38-40.

51. Mainous EG. Hyperbaric oxygen in maxillofacial osteomyelitis, osteoradionecrosis, and osteogenesis enhancement. In: Davis JC, Hunt TK, editors. Hyperbaric oxygen therapy. Bethesda (MD): Undersea Medical Society; 1977. p. 191-203.

52. Mandell GI. Bactericidal activity of aerobic and anaerobic polymorphonuclear neutrophils. Infec Immunity. 1974;9:337-41.

53. Martel J et al. Malignant or necrotizing otitis externa: experience in 22 cases. Ann Otolaryngol Chir Cervicofac. 2000;117(5):291.

54. Mathes SJ. The muscle flap for management of osteomyelitis. N Engl J Med. 1985;294-5.

55. Maynor ML et al. Chronicosteomyelitis of the tibia: treatment with hyperbaric oxygen and autogenous microsurgical muscle transplantation. J South Orthop Assoc. 1998;7(1):43-57.

56. Medicare Coverage Issues Manual National Coverage Determination (NCD) for Hyperbaric Oxygen Therapy (20.29). U.S. Department of Health and Human Services (DHHS), Centers for Medicare and Medicaid Services (CMS); 2006.

57. Mendel V, Reichert B, Simanowski HJ, et al. Therapy with hyperbaric oxygen and cefazolin for experimental osteomyelitis due to Staphylococcus aureus in rats. Undersea Hyperb Med. 1999;26(3):169-74.

58. Mendel V, Simanowski HJ, Scholz H CH. Synergy of HBO and local antibiotic carrier for experimental osteomyelitis due to Staphylococcus aureus in rats. Undersea Hyperb Med 2004;31(4):407-16.

59. Moran GJ, Krishnadasan A, Gorwitz R, et al. Methicillin-resistant S. aureus infections among patients in the emergency department. New Engl J Med. 2006;355:666-74.

60. Morrey BF et al. Hyperbaric oxygen and chronic osteomyelitis. Clin Orthop Relat Res. 1979;(144):121-7.
61. Narozny W et al. Value of hyperbaric oxygen in bacterial and fungal malignant external otitis treatment. Eur Arch Otorhinolaryngol. 2006;263(7):680-4.
62. Niinikoski J. Oxygen tensions in healing bone. Surg Gynecol Obstet. 1972;134:746-50.
63. Onen MR, Yuvruk E, Karagoz G, Maderi S. Efficiency of hyperbaric oxygen therapy in iatrogenic spinal infections. Spine. 2015;40(22):1743-8.
64. Park MK, Muhvich KH, Myers RA, et al. Effects of hyperbaric oxygen in infectious diseases: basic mechanisms. In: Kindwall EP, ed. Hyperbaric medicine practice. Flagstaff (AZ): Best Publishing Co; 1994.: p. 141-64.
65. Peirce EC Jr. Pathophysiology, apparatus, and methods, including the special techniques of hypothermia and hhyperbaric oxygen. In: Extracorporeal circulation for open heart surgery. Springfield (IL): Charles C. Thomas; 1969. p. 84-8.
66. Perrins DJD, Maudsley RH, Colwill MW, et al. OHP in the management of chronic osteomyelitis. In: Brown IW, Cox BG, editors. Proceedings of the 3rd International Conference on Hyperbaric Medicine. Washington (DC): National Research Council, National Academy of Sciences; 1966. p. 578-584.
67. Pilgramm M, Frey G, Schumann K. Hyperbaric oxygenation – a sensible adjunctive therapy in malignant external otitis. Laryngol Rhinol Otol (Stuttg). 1986;65:26-8.
68. Poirier JY, Garin E, et al. Diagnosis of osteomyelitis in the diabetic foot with a 99m TC-HMPAQ leukocyte scintigraphy combined with a 99m TC-MDP bone scintigraphy. Diabetes Metab. 2002;28:485-90.
69. Priest D, Peacock JE Jr. Hematogenous vertebral osteomyelitis due to Staphylococcus aureus in the adult: clinical features and therapeutic outcomes. South Med J. 2005;98(9):854-62.
70. Rajbhandari SM, Sutton M, Davies C, et al. "Sausage toe": a reliable sign of underlying osteomyelitis. Diabet Med. 2000;17:74-7.
71. Renstra WR, Buras JA, Svoboda KS. Hyperbaric oxygen increases human dermal fibroblast proliferation, growth factor receptor number and in vitro wound closure. Undersea Hyperb Med. 1998;25(Suppl):53(#164).
72. Riddick M. Acute and delayed infection and dehiscence. In: Kindwall EP, Whelan H, editors. Hyperbaric oxygen medicine. 3rd ed. Flagstaff (AZ): Best Publishing Co.; 2008. p. 655-76.
73. Roje Z, Eterovic D, Druzijanic N, et al. Influence of adjuvant hyperbaric oxygen therapy on short-term complications during surgical reconstruction of upper and lower extremity war injuries: retrospective cohort study. Croat Med J. 2008;49(2):224-32.
74. Sabra RM, Taha MS, Khafagy AG, Elsamny T. Value of hyperbaric oxygen therapy in the management of malignant otitis externa patients. Egyptian J Otolaryngol. 2015;31(3):143-8.
75. Sandner A et al. Value of hyperbaric oxygen in the treatment of advanced skull base osteomyelitis. Laryngorhihnootologie. 2009;88(10):641-6.
76. Saulis AS, Davidson JD, Mustoe TA, Moford JE. Hyperbaric oxygen modulators PDGF receptor B expression and ERK ½ activation in human dermal fibroblasts in vitro. Plastic Surgery Research Council, 45th Annual Meeting. Seattle (WA); 2000. p. 143.
77. Saxby A, Barakate M, Kertesz T, et al. Malignant otitis externa: experience with hyperbaric oxygen therapy. Diving Hyperb Med. 2010;40:195-200.

78. Shupak A, Greenberg E, Hardoff R, et al. Hyperbaric oxygenation for necrotizing (malignant) otitis externa. Arch Otolaryngol Head Neck Surg. 1989;115:1470-5.

79. Skeik N, Porten BR, Isaacson E, et al. Hyperbaric oxygen treatment outcome for different indications from a single center. Ann Vasc Surg. 2015;29(2):206-14.

80. Slack WK, Thomas DA, Perrins DJD. Hyperbaric oxygenation in chronic osteomyelitis. Lancet. 1965;1:1093-4.

81. Strauss MB, Bryant BJ, Hart GB. Transcutaneous oxygen measurements under hyperbaric oxygen conditions as a predictor for healing of problem wounds. Foot Ankle Int. 2002;23(10):933-7.

82. Strauss MB, Busch JA, Miller SS. SCUBA in older aged divers. Wound Care Hyperb Med. 2013; 4(3):27-37.

83. Strauss MB. Chronic refractory osteomyelitis: review and role of hyperbaric oxygen. HBO Review. 1980;1:231-55.

84. Strauss MB. Diabetic foot and leg wounds: principles, management, and prevention. Prim Care Rep. 2001;7(22):187-97.

85. Strauss MB. Diabetic foot problems: keys to effective, aggressive prevention. Consultant. 2001;31(13):1693-705.

86. Strauss MB. Evidence review of HBO for crush injury, compartment syndrome and other traumatic ischemia. Undersea Hyperb Med. 2001;28(Suppl):35-6.

87. Strauss MB. Hyperbaric oxygen as an adjunct to surgical management of the problem wound. In: Bakker DJ, Cramer FS, editors. Hyperbaric surgery, perioperative. Flagstaff (AZ): Best Publishing Co.; 2002. p. 383-96.

88. Strauss MB. Hyperbaric oxygen as an intervention for managing wound hypoxia: its role and usefulness in diabetic foot wounds. Foot Ankle Int. 2005;26:15-8.

89. Strauss MB, Manji KA, Miller SS, Manji AA. Bursa and callus: friend or foe. Wound Care Hyperb Med. 2013;4(2):13-28

90. Strauss MB. Refractory osteomyelitis. J Hyperbaric Med. 1987;2(3):147-59.

91. Tamil YP et al. Postsurgical prevertebral abscess of the cervical spine. Laryngoscope. 2000;110(7):1137-41.

92. Tisch M, Lorenz KJ, Harm M, et al. The treatment of necrotizing otitis externa with a combination of surgery, antibiotics, specific immunoglobins and hyperbaric oxygen therapy. Results of the Ulm Treatment Concept. HNO. 2003;51:315-20.

93. Tisch M, Maier H. Malignant external otitis. Laryngorhinootologie. 2006;85(10):763-9; quiz 770-3.

94. Van Merkesteyn JP et al. Hyperbaric oxygen treatment of chronic osteomyelitis of the jaws. Int J Oral Surg. 1984;13(5):386-95.

95. Verklin RN, Mandell GL. Alteration of effectiveness of antibiotics by anaerobiosis. J Lab Clin Med. 1977;89:65-71.

96. Waldvogel FA, Medoff G, Swartz MN. Osteomyelitis: a review of clinical features, therapeutic considerations, and unusual aspects. N Eng J Med. 1970;282:198-206, 260-266, 316-322.

97. Weiland AJ, Moore JR, Daniel RK. The efficacy of free-tissue transfer in the treatment of osteomyelitis. J Bone Joint Surg. 1984;66A:181-93.

98. Welsh FML, Matos LU, deTreville TP. Medical hyperbaric oxygen therapy: 22 cases. Aviat Space Environ Med. 1980;51(6):611-4.

99. Yu WK et al. Hyperbaric oxygen therapy as an adjunctive treatment for sternal infection and osteomyelitis after sternotomy and cardiothoracic surgery. J Cardiothorac Surg. 2011;6:141.

CHAPTER 21 CHAPTER

Strategic Approach to Diabetic Foot and Other Wounds

CHAPTER TWENTY-ONE OVERVIEW

Introduction 525

Troublesome Triad of Diabetic Foot Wounds 526

Deformities 528

Evaluation of Diabetic Foot Wounds Using the Long Beach Wound Score 529

Strategies for Management of Diabetic Foot and Other Problem Wounds 531

First Strategy: Management of the Wound Base 531

Second Strategy: Protection and Stabilization 533

Third Strategy: Appropriate Medical Management 534

Fourth Strategy: Selection of Optimal Wound Dressing Agents 536

Fifth Strategy: Wound Perfusion and Oxygenation 538

The Roles of Hyperbaric Oxygen in Diabetic and Other Wounds 539

Prevention of New and Recurrent Diabetic Foot as Well as Other Wounds 545

Education 546

Skin and Toenail Care 547

Protective Footwear 548

Proactive Surgeries 549

Ten "Pearls" to Remember about Diabetic Foot and Related Wounds 549

Conclusion 550

References 552

Strategic Approach to Diabetic Foot and Other Wounds

Michael B. Strauss, Anna M. Tan, Lientra Q. Lu

INTRODUCTION

Diabetic foot wounds (DFWs) are a common cause of morbidity, and a multidisciplinary approach is required to achieve successful healing outcomes. DFWs pose an ongoing challenge to health-care providers due to cycles of recurrent breakdown with accompanying neuropathy, peripheral vascular disease, and/or foot deformity. About 1 in 15 diabetics will develop a foot wound sometime during his or her lifetime.[28] The cost of care imposes significant financial burdens on our health-care system. It adds an additional USD$9 to USD$13 billion to the annual USD$245 billion spent on the care of patients with diabetes mellitus in the United States.[7] Diabetic ulcers are also a major risk factor for lower extremity amputations.[27] Approximately 85% of lower limb amputations are preceded by nonhealing foot wounds.[24] Diabetes results in more deaths in the United States than breast cancer and AIDS combined, and 60% of nontraumatic lower limb amputations in the United States are done in diabetics.[30] Although the progression from preulcer to ulceration to an infected, nonhealing wound is a common course of events and often leads to lower limb amputation, the majority of DFWs are easily managed and resolve completely in their initial stages. These DFWs heal uneventfully with a comprehensive approach to management that includes the appropriate wound dressing, debridement, and offloading. What is appropriate for management of the DFW is also appropriate for managing wounds in other locations and in patients without diabetes.

The traditional definition of wounds and ulcers was based on etiology. A wound is defined as a trauma to tissue caused by physical means with loss of continuity of the tissue, and an ulcer as a lesion through the skin resulting from loss of tissue.[17] However, we feel that this nomenclature is misleading as we define a "wound" to be a generic term to encompass all types of disruptions in the integrity of the skin and underlying tissues. It can vary in depth from superficial, involving only the epithelium, to deep, involving bone and joint structures. The term "ulcer" implies a superficial wound associated with abnormal foot mechanics with deformities and muscle imbalances, neuropathy, inability to address shear forces, attenuated skin and subcutaneous tissues, peripheral artery disease, pressure overload, or combinations of these.

The chapter describes the pathophysiology of diabetic foot wounds, their evaluation management and prevention, and the roles of hyperbaric oxygen for them, along with dispelling some of their common misconceptions.

TROUBLESOME TRIAD OF DIABETIC FOOT WOUNDS

A thorough history and examination explain why almost all diabetic foot ulcers (DFW) occur. The history provides information as to the onset, duration, symptoms, prior management, and why the patient is seeking the current evaluation (Table 1). The examination confirms the seriousness of the wound problem and can be quantified with our user-friendly 0-to-10 Wound Score (Figure 1). From this information, the seriousness of the wound is categorized, and logical decisions can be made as to what needs to be done next such as imaging studies, vascular assessment, hyperbaric oxygen with or without juxta-wound transcutaneous oxygen measurements, wound dressing agent selection, and surgical interventions (Table 2).

Assessment	2 points	1 point	0 points
Appearance of the wound	Red	White/Yellow	Black
Size	< Thumb-print	Thumbprint to fist	> Fist
Depth	Skin coverage ← SC*	→ Muscle/tendon	Bone/joint
Infection/ Bioburden	Colonized	Cellulitis, maceration, or osteomyelitis	Sepsis Leukocytosis, fever, chills, nausea, vomiting, bacteremia, dysglycemia
Perfusion	Palpable pulses	Doppler pulses	Imperceptible pulses

Wound Categories

Healthy 7 ½–10 Points

Problem 3 ½–7 points

Futile 0–3 points

SC* = Subcutaneous tissue

LEGEND: The Long Beach Wound Score is a user-friendly 0-to-10-point (best possible) scoring system that quantifies the seriousness/category of the wound. Five assessments, each graded from 2 points (best) to 0 points (worst), are summated using objective criteria for each grade. Half points may be used if findings are intermediate or mixed between two grade points.

Perfusion, infection/bioburden, and depth are the essential features of the Wagner, Infectious Diseases Society of America, and National Pressure Ulcer Advisory Panel systems, respectively, and are supplemented with wound size and appearance to generate a 5-assessment, 10-possible-point system.

Figure 1. Long Beach Wound Score.

Three problems almost always contribute to the development and persistence of DFWs. They are deformity, deep infection, and/or ischemia-hypoxia (Figure 2).[39] We label these the "Troublesome Triad" of the "problem" type (i.e., those with Wound Scores of 3 ½ to 7 points) of DFW or other wounds. While neuropathy is almost always associated with DFWs, it is only an indirect contributor to the DFW. Sensory impairment often delays the patient seeking care for the DFW in its incipient stages when management is most likely to be the easiest.

TABLE 1. HISTORY CONSIDERATIONS FOR EVALUATION OF THE DIABETIC FOOT ULCER AND RELATED WOUNDS

Item	Questions	Significance
Reason for evaluation and by whom	Why were patients referred and by whom?	Gives clues to aggressiveness of prior management.
Onset	What type of onset: sudden, gradual, only noted by others (drainage or odor)?	Injury and/or vascular problems suggest sudden onset; delayed recognition suggests neuropathy.
Duration	How long: days, weeks, months?	Usually, the longer the duration, the less need for immediate interventions.
Symptoms	How do symptoms interfere with activities of daily living?	Neuropathy often obscures symptoms and delays diagnosis.
Prior management	What care has been given? Wound dressings, antibiotics, surgery; when and where?	Did care address bioburden, biomechanics, wound characteristics?
Course	Has the wound problem improved/not changed/worsened with time?	If the wound has rapidly worsened, immediate medical care is needed.

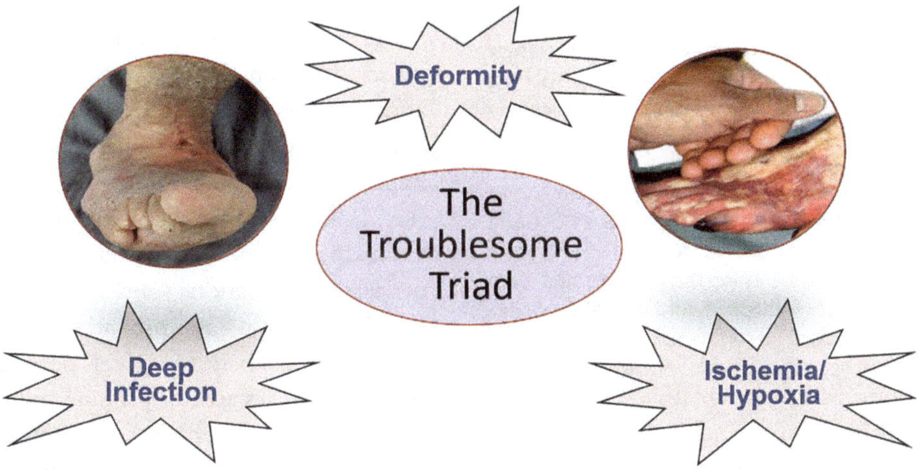

LEGEND: The above three problems are the predominant reasons wounds fail to improve. Each component of the Triad requires specific evaluations to and appropriate interventions for management.

Figure 2. The "Troublesome Triad" reasons wounds don't improve.

TABLE 2. USING THE WOUND SCORE TO CATEGORIZE WOUNDS

Category	Wound Scores	'Equivalent' Wagner Grade	Management	Comments
Healthy	7 ½–10 points	0, 1, 2	Ointments, salves, meshed dressings, possibly biologics	Healing in almost 100 % of cases; failures for reasons other than a nonwound problem (e.g., pain, deformity)
Problem	3 ½–7 points	3, 4	**Five treatment strategies** 1. Management of the wound base 2. Protection/immobilization 3. Medical management 4. Selection of wound dressing agents 5. Augmentation of perfusion-oxygenation	Protection and immobilization is the most overlooked strategy. Except for revascularization, other perfusion-oxygenation interventions are also often overlooked.
Futile	0–3 points	5	Amputation, revascularization if feasible	The wound score quantifies the decision to amputate.

The role of neuropathy in DFW is paradoxical. It is unquestionably a risk factor for DFWs. This is principally because of delays in diagnosis and its contributions to motor neuropathies. However, it is not a direct cause of the DFW unlike components of the "Troublesome Triad."

Another aspect of the paradox is that the diabetic sensory neuropathy contributes to wound management.[9] It allows for debridements and dressing changes to be done effectively without discomfort.

A third aspect of the neuropathy is that motivated and compliant patients with sensory neuropathies are usually very successful in avoiding new and/or recurrent wounds, thus supporting our opinion that sensory neuropathy need not be the cause of a wound.

Finally, diabetic patients often have painful sensory neuropathies, usually in the legs proximal to the feet, severe enough that narcotic analgesics and neuromodulators such as gabapentin (Neurontin) are required. However, their feet are numb enough that debridements are painless.

Motor imbalances from neuropathy cause deformities such as clawing of toes, equinus contractures, and abnormal foot posturing. These problems, when associated with loss of proprioception, cause abnormal stresses on bone and ligamentous structures, which is an important contributing factor to the development of Charcot neuroarthropathy. With time the constricted joints structures become rigidly deformed, which is the hallmark of contractures.

Deformities

These problems occur at all levels of the lower extremity from the hip to the toes. There are two causes: contractures from muscle imbalances and bony structure abnormalities. At the toe levels, mallet, hammer, and metatarsophalangeal joint hyperextensions are the common axial (i.e., in line with the foot) deformities. Other toe abnormalities include medial or lateral deviations and rotational problems such as pronation and supination. Diabetic foot ulcers occur at the toe levels because of pressure injury over the apexes of the deformities, shear stresses, or increased contact pressures. Bone deformities include spurs, which usually develop as a consequence of ligament traction stresses or arthritic changes, malalignments associated with fracture healing or bone collapse, hypertrophied scar and bursa, and bone extrusion as observed with Charcot neuroarthropathy.

Hallux wounds are good examples of how abnormal biomechanics contribute to deformities and cause wounds. They have analogies to other deformity-related wounds in the foot and ankle. Ulcers at the tip of hallux arise because of hyperflexion of the interphalangeal joint, i.e., hammer toe. This pushes the toe tip into the bottom of the shoe and, with repeated contact stresses, leads to an ulcer. If the ulcer penetrates to the distal tuft of the hallux, osteomyelitis is likely to develop.

Ulcers along the medial aspects of the interphalangeal joint arise because of traction spurs from ligaments and joint capsule due to repeated stresses across the site from abnormal biomechanics. The result is a malperforans ulcer, an ulceration that arises because of an underlying bony deformity. Plain X-rays, especially rotational views, verify the bony abnormality.

Bunion deformities as a result of eburnation (hypertrophy of bone around joints) of the medial aspect of the first metatarsal head are associated with hallux valgus and hyperpronation deformities of the hallux. Ulcerations develop at the apex of the deformity with repeated shear stresses, or the deformity exceeds the elasticity of the skin over the defect.

Deformities are addressed by offloading and surgical interventions and will be discussed later.

As in the toe deformities, other locations in the lower extremity develop ulcers with analogous biomechanical abnormalities. The combinations of shear (tangential to the skin surface) stresses in conjunction with deformities or bony prominences are particularly prone to ulcer development. Aging skin with loss of elasticity, attenuated skin from healing by secondary intention, and attenuated subcutaneous tissue from ischemia, malnutrition, or neuropathy associated with the mildest of shear stresses lead to ulcerations. Failure to feel pain with the shear stresses allows them to continue until an ulcer develops and the patient seeks medical advice.

The other two components of the "Troublesome Triad," deep infection and ischemia-hypoxia, have their own pathophysiology and will be discussed later.

A heel blister associated with hiking with less-than-optimal footwear or stockings often causes blisters over the apex of the heel. The deformity is the prominence of the heel bone. The repeated shear stresses with the hiking activity generate a blister. Even with normal sensation, the appreciation of pain may be delayed because of concentration on and exertion of the hike (possibly from endorphins) until the hiker rests or the pain becomes so severe that it overrides the endorphins. This example represents a microcosm of the shear stresses the insensate diabetic foot can experience.

EVALUATION OF DIABETIC FOOT WOUNDS USING THE LONG BEACH WOUND SCORE

In association with obtaining the history and examination of the wound, grading systems are used to assess the severity and provide a basis for treatment.(31) Our review of the literature indicates that four DFU scoring systems are used predominantly for evaluating diabetic foot ulcers.(38) They are the Wagner Grades, the National Pressure Ulcer Advisory Panel (NPUAP) stages, the University of Texas Health Sciences Center San Antonio Diabetic Wound Classification (UTDWC), and the Infectious Disease Society Clinical Classification of Diabetic Foot Infections (IDSA). Each has its own special features and focuses on a particular (or, in the case of the UTDWC, several) of the wound characteristics (Table 3).(2,4-6,21-22,26,42-43) Concerns are raised with these scoring systems because mainly they focus only on a single assessment, consider only whether or not the assessment is present, and do not grade the severity of the assessment on a continuum. In addition, except for face validity (i.e., appear to sample superficially that which is to be measured and are accepted because of their widespread use) for the Wagner and NPUAP systems, none have documented outcome studies or reports on their reliability (that is, similarity of scoring between two or more observers).

TABLE 3. PREDOMINANTLY USED DIABETIC FOOT ULCER CLASSIFICATIONS

Name (Reference)	Date/ Revision	Predominant Feature	Concerns	Comments
Wagner Grades[38,43]	1979/ 1981	**Perfusion** based on ankle-brachial indices	Provides algorithms for management based on a single observation	Widely used giving it face validity
NPUAP[2]	1989/ 2007	**Depth** (four stages and unstageable and suspected deep-tissue injuries)	Does not consider exudate, size, or perfusion	Especially used for sacral, ischial, and trochanteric pressure sores
UTDWC[26]	1996	Combines Perfusion (Wagner) + Infection (IDSA) on one axis and Depth (NPUAP) on other	Classification does not consider severity, only presence or absence of findings	Worse outcomes as wounds move down and to the right of 16-square matrix
IDSA[6]	2004	INFECTION Grades severity	Does not consider other features	Provides guidelines for antibiotics and surgery management

LEGEND: NPUAP = National Pressure Ulcer Advisory Panel, UTDWC = Texas Health Sciences Center San Antonio Diabetic Wound Classification, IDSA = Infectious Disease Society of America

For these reasons, we generated the Long Beach Wound Score (LBWS), which addresses the concerns (Figure 1). It takes the essential elements of the predominantly used wound scores, namely perfusion (Wagner), depth (NPUAP), and infection (IDSA), and what we consider the two next most important assessments in evaluating and managing the wound, the appearance of the wound base and the size of the wound. These five assessments are integrated into a 0-to-10 LBWS, with each assessment graded on a 2-(best)-to-0-(worst) continuum with objective criteria for each 0-to-2 grade of the assessment. The derived LBWS becomes intuitively obvious with respect to the seriousness of the wound and what management is indicated. Finally, the LBWS is user-friendly, taking fewer than a couple of minutes to determine. All assessments are apparent with a glance at the wound except for perfusion, which requires palpation and possibly Doppler-obtained information. The LBWS agreements between two observers was over 80% reliable in nearly 100 studied patients.[41]

> Validation (i.e., prediction of outcomes) of our LBWS is in progress. Preliminary examination of our data as well as data from a previous study indicates that, from the initial LBWS, it is accurate in predicting good outcomes for healthy wounds and in predicting amputations for futile wounds. For the problem wound cohort, the initial Wound Score is about 80% accurate in predicting good outcomes.[41]

Since objectivity is inherent in the continuum grading of each assessment, the LBWS is an ideal tool for Comparative Effectiveness Research (CER), i.e., comparing like with like wounds and demonstrating the effectiveness of interventions such as wound dressing agents and hyperbaric oxygen therapy. It also makes it easy to quantify Minimal Clinically Important Improvement (MCII) by re-grading the wounds and upgrading the scores with the progression of wound healing. We recommend using both the LBWS for the evaluation and management of wounds and the Wagner grades for reimbursement purposes when using HBO_2 treatment for diabetic foot ulcers.

The LBWS makes it easy to categorize wounds as "healthy," "problem," or "futile" (Table 2). Healthy wounds (LBWS of 7 ½ to 10 points) heal with minimal interventions. Almost all wound dressing agents are effective. Negative-pressure wound therapy is not indicated for this category, but if epithelialization is sluggish, biologic wound covering agents might be considered. Problem wounds (LBWS of 3 ½ to 7 points) require comprehensive management using five treatment strategies as will described in the next section. The futile wounds (0 to 3 points) require amputation unless reperfusion is feasible and, if done successfully, improves perfusion. The LBWS is applicable to all wounds whether diabetic or not and whether in the foot (as specified by Wagner, UTDWC, and IDSA systems) or in other locations in the body.

It is noteworthy that Dr. Wagner modified his original 1979 article (which considered only diabetic foot ulcers) with a succeeding article published in 1981 that included all foot wounds whether the patient was diabetic or not. The only difference between the two was that for the diabetic an ankle-brachial index (ABI) of 0.45 or higher was used to justify salvage and management according to his treatment algorithms versus 0.35 for the nondiabetic foot wound.[34,38,43] If the ABIs are less than 0.45/0.35, Dr. Wagner referred his patients to the vascular service for revascularization or lower limb amputation.

In a subsequent article, Dr. Wagner acknowledged that the ABI is unreliable in the calcified vessel (because of a transmitted signal), and other techniques should be used to evaluate perfusion to the foot.[29]

STRATEGIES FOR MANAGEMENT OF DIABETIC FOOT AND OTHER PROBLEM WOUNDS

Five strategies are required to optimally treat diabetic foot and other wounds (Table 4). All five strategies should be employed for the initial management of the wound as well as for all succeeding evaluations. This is especially applicable to the problem wound (Wound Scores of 3 ½ to 7 points/Wagner Grades 3 and 4) category. Again, the Wound Score is applicable not only to the DFW but to all wounds regardless of their location and whether the patient is a diabetic. The management strategies include the following:

First Strategy: Management of the Wound Base

This strategy is performed either at the bedside/in-office or in the operating room.[37] Debridement is the hallmark of wound base management. There are five types of debridements. **Sharp debridements** of superficial wounds are suitable for outpatient and in-hospital bedside management. Debridement equipment includes scalpels, scissors, curettes, and rongeurs. Bedside (in-office, clinic, or hospital) debridements are appropriate for removing calluses and crusts around the wound periphery, necrotic skin edges, superficial debris in the wound base, and biofilms.

Autologous debridement relies on two factors. First, the wound generates enzymes such as matrix metalloproteinases to dissolve debris in the wound base. Second, dressing changes with moist gauze dressings remove the debris and exudative material in the wound and thereby help clean the wound. This is a very useful and cost-effective technique for wound care between sharp debridements.

TABLE 4. THE FIVE TREATMENT STRATEGIES FOR MANAGING THE PROBLEM WOUND

Strategy	Comments/Interventions
Management of the Wound Base	**Debridement** (sharp, enzymatic, autologous, pulsatile lavage, and biological/maggots) **Correction of deformities** (osteotomies, ostectomies, tenotomies) **Amputations** (conventional versus creative)
Protection and Stabilization	Padded dressings, splinting, removable walker boots, casting, external fixation
Medical Management	Optimize diabetes control (Glu, HbA1c), cardiac (BNP), renal (BUN, creatinine), nutrition (albumin, prealbumin), edema reduction, and hematological parameters (antibiotics, hemoglobins, INRs)
Wound Dressing Agents	Over 3000 choices; categories include 1. Moist gauze 2. Impervious/semi-impervious coverings; biologic dressings 3. Absorbants including negative-pressure wound therapy 4. Ointments and salves with or without additives (enzymatic debride, antibiotics, moisturizing, etc.)
Perfusion-Oxygenation	Revascularization (bypass, stent, angioplasty), edema reduction and improve cardiac function, hyperbaric oxygen, vasodilators and rheological agents (improve flow, reduce platelet adhesion, anticoagulate, enhance RBC deformability)

LEGEND: Glu = Glucose, HbA1c = Hemoglobin A1c, BNP = brain/B-type natriuretic peptide, BUN = blood urea nitrogen, INRs = international normalized ratios

For those experienced in doing such, protruding bone, exposed, necrotic tendon and ligaments as well as dystrophic, fungus-infected ingrown toenails may also be debrided in the clinic.

Another advanced technique is use of sutures to partially approximate the wounds after debridement. This is an expedient method to reduce the wound surface area and depth without sequestering infected material if the wound were closed completely.

Often the sutures are under tension, but when the patient returns for follow-up, the sutures are loose. This is because of stretching, that is, plastic deformation, of the tissues (viscoelasticity/stress relaxation) that occurs with time. In a serial fashion, healthy wounds with pliable margins can be greatly reduced in size with this technique.

Enzymatic debridement utilizes a collagenase enzyme to help degrade necrotic tissue in the wound base and is marketed under the Santyl® trade name. The enzyme also promotes the generation of granulation tissue. Like autologous debridement, it is a useful wound dressing agent between sharp debridements.

Pulsatile lavage debridement is the fourth debridement technique. It is a technique that uses hydrotherapy to loosen, soften, and remove debris from the wound as well as plaques and scaling from the adjacent skin. It is hospital based and requires trained physical therapy personnel to exudate properly.

Two papain urea agents, Accuzyme® and Panafil®, were previously available for enzymatic debridements but have been removed from the market. This was due to manufacturers' concerns about a small number of allergic reactions that were reported from these agents and the decision to promote Santyl®.

Because of the splatter of debris and infected material, protective garments, gloves, and eyewear must be used by the therapist.

Biological debridement employs maggots (fly larvae) to remove dead, infected material from the wound. It is not generally utilized in the United States in favor of the above techniques, but it is unquestionably beneficial in developing countries that lack the resources for the other types of debridements. Patients who arrive in a medical facility with squirming, robust-appearing, well-fed maggots in a poorly managed wound generate a lot of excitement. In the United States, refined techniques for maggot therapy are available. In 2004, the U.S. Food and Drug Administration (FDA) approved maggot therapy for debridements.

Monarch Labs (17875 Sky Park Circle, Suite K, Irvine, CA 92614, e-mail: Sales@MonarchLabs.Com) supplies medically approved, commercially available maggots. The maggots in a state of hibernation are provided in individual pockets in a Styrofoam container. They are placed on the wound in a meshed, opaque polymer bag that contains the maggots but allows them to feed on the necrotic tissues and secretions though the mesh in the bags. After removal, the maggots are counted to ensure none are left in the wound.

Debridement in the operating room is often needed and is the second wound base management tactic. Procedures include exploration and debridement of necrotic, infected tissue in association with ostectomies to remove bony deformities and infected bone, osteotomies to realign the foot and ankle, capsulotomies to correct joint contractures, and tenotomies to relieve muscle imbalances. Frequently, temporary external fixation is utilized to maintain the correction and optimize the environment for wound healing. The fixator is removed when a soft-tissue mantle has developed to maintain the correction. Casting followed by protective footwear is then utilized to maintain the foot in the plantigrade position. The CROW (Charcot Restraint Orthotic Walker) boot is a custom-made orthotic designed to accommodate the severest of deformities and is utilized permanently or at the minimum for one year until the soft-tissue mantle has matured enough to maintain the correction and allow the patient to walk with less restrictive footwear. Another operating room wound management technique is the use of skin grafts and flaps. These techniques are usually done as staged procedures after the wound has been debrided and a healthy granulating wound base develops.

Amputation is another wound base management technique. Amputation with respect to grading outcomes of digits and the forefoot are considered "minor," and, with successful healing, it is appropriate to classify the results as "good" with respect to overall limb salvage and functional capacity. We classify more proximal lower limb amputations as "poor" or "failed." Often, after debridements, non-textbook descriptions for amputation surgeries must be employed, such as rotating laterally based forefoot flaps medially to provide coverage over exposed bone, using dorsal flap skin to cover plantar wounds, and making diagonal or spear-shaped osteotomies of the metatarsals to most effectively utilize the skin remaining after the debridement is completed.

Second Strategy: Protection and Stabilization

This strategy is crucial for healing of the problem wound. It is probably the most overlooked of the five wound management strategies. Protection and stabilization is achieved through a hierarchy of interventions ranging from well-padded soft dressings (such as the classic Robert Jones knee wrap), splints, removable walker (CAM – controlled ankle motion) boots, casts, and external fixation. Internal fixation is a double jeopardy intervention in many foot wounds. This is because of hardware failure in osteopenic bone and juxta-hardware infection in open wounds. The protection and stabilization strategy requires the most creativity since it necessitates decision-making to decide what is most appropriate, how to effectively immobilize wounds of varying complexities, and, when necessary, how to provide adequate access for wound care.

The protected, stabilized wound provides the best possible environment for the challenging wound to heal. Motion in a problem wound promotes disruption of fibroblastic bridging across the wound and causes shearing-off of new blood vessels resulting in bleeding. The extravasated blood then becomes an ideal medium for bacteria growth. The protected wound will be resistant to damage from external sources such as bumping, falls, and the stresses of loading as occurs with transfers and ambulation.

Micromotion, as associated with using negative-pressure wound therapy, is reported to improve angiogenesis and fibroblast activity.[15]

Unfortunately, this strategy is the most prone to cause iatrogenic complications. Complications include blisters and ulcers from wraps and bindings slipping and causing pressure concentrations in skin that is already compromised by aging and atrophy. Other problems include pressure injuries from casts and splints over bony prominences and skin breakdown from shear when the protective devices do not control motion adequately. Any time a protection, stabilizing device is used, utmost diligence must be used in preventing complications and informing patients to seek immediate medical attention for any newly recognized problem.

The total contact cast (TCC) is considered by many to be the ultimate management for DFWs. Although there are many variations in application of the TCC, the unifying feature is it is a leg cast that totally encloses the foot and is padded and molded to distribute loading forces evenly to the entire plantar surface of the foot. It requires rigid protocols such as weekly then biweekly cast changes and it may require months to heal a forefoot malperforans ulcer.

Because the foot is totally enclosed, dressing changes are not possible. If the ulcer seals off, ascending infection may go unnoticed in the patient with a sensory neuropathy and place the limb in jeopardy for an amputation especially if removal of the cast is delayed to the next biweekly visit. A more common concern with the TCC is that, since the underlying deformity is not addressed, 50% recurrence rates of the DFW occur once protective footwear is resumed.[12]

Third Strategy: Appropriate Medical Management

This strategy is done in collaboration with the primary care physician as well as specialists. Almost all patients with DFWs or ischemia-related foot wounds have comorbidities that must be optimized in order to facilitate wound healing. Diabetes management is at the top of the list for medical conditions that are associated with foot wounds. Diabetes is managed with medications to optimize glucose control and use of hemoglobin A1c blood checks to reflect compliance.

Cardiac and renal issues must also be addressed. A large percentage of patients with diabetes have coronary disease and are in borderline heart failure. The BNP

(Brain/B-type natriuretic peptide) blood test identifies and quantifies congestive heart failure. Other testing such as echo (echocardiogram) to reflect heart wall motion and the MIBI (myocardial infusion scan) to reflect cardiac perfusion may be necessary before a patient with heart disease is cleared for surgery. Optimizing heart function will not only improve perfusion to the wound but will also compliment edema reduction.

Kidney function is another major organ that may require medical management in the patient with foot or other wounds. Blood urea nitrogen (BUN), creatinine, and creatinine clearance studies quantify the severity of renal disease and direct what interventions are needed. Diabetics account for 44% of patients with end-stage kidney disease, and 10%–40% patients with diabetes develop kidney failure.[8] Chronic kidney disease adds increased challenges to wound healing. Problems include a less-than-ideal environment for host factor functions in wound healing and infection control due to azotemia, anemia due to deficient erythropoietin production, and wound hypoxia due to accelerated atherosclerosis.

Other comorbidities that interfere with wound healing and management of infection include collagen vascular and pulmonary diseases. Often steroids and other immunosuppressors are used to manage these diseases which interfere with wound healing and complicate already compromised perfusion and hypoxia that result from the underlying pathophysiology of these diseases. Gastroesophageal reflex disease (GERD) and gastroparesis, which is especially associated with diabetes, are often present in patients who have wound healing challenges. They contribute to malnutrition and malabsorption syndromes. The comorbidities of smoking and obesity need to be addressed. Another user-friendly 0-to-10 score, the Wellness Score, makes it easy to quantify normal to impaired to decompensated conditions (Table 5).[3] If the Wellness Score is 7 ½ to 10 points, it

> Information indicating a "healthy" host includes regular exercise, no smoking or street drug use, minimal-to-moderate alcohol consumption, nearly ideal weight range, and use of only off-the-shelf medications (e.g., multivitamins and food supplements as well as the occasional self-directed use of non-steroid anti-inflammatory, peptic disease, asthmatic, birth control, and similar medications).

TABLE 5. WELLNESS SCORE

Criteria	2 Points	1 Point	0 Points
ADLs Ability to do activities of daily living	Full	Some	None
Ambulation	Community	Household	None
Comorbidities	Normal	Impaired	Decompensated
Tobacco/Immuno-suppressors	None	Past	Current
Neuro Function	Normal	Impaired	Decompensated

NOTE: **Subtract 1/2 point if mixed or between two point grades.**

Subtract 1/2 point if use aids for ambulation (e.g., canes, crutches, walkers, wheelchair, motorized scooters).

Do not consider neurological deficits in the comorbidities assessment since neuro function is a separate assessment in itself.

Malnutrition and obesity should be included in the comorbidities assessment.

indicates a "healthy" host, and management of medical problems, if any, of can be the continuation of present care.[33] Collaboration, in these situations, need not be obtained for management of wounds or in preparations for surgery. Wellness Scores of 3 ½ to 7 points quantify the patient as an "Impaired" host, and primary care physician collaboration is advisable in conjunction with wound management and surgical preparations. Finally, if the score is 0 to 3 points, collaboration with specialists such as nephrologists, cardiologists, critical care specialists, etc. is needed in order to optimally care for the patient and prepare the patient for surgery.

A final medical condition to consider is that of malnutrition. The clinical nutritionist should always be a member of the wound team. Often patients who are obese are protein deficient. This is confirmed by albumin and prealbumin blood tests. Special expertise is required to initiate diets that promote building of protein while reducing weight. Nutrition is one condition that can be mitigated in a four-level hierarchy and for which something can always be done to mitigate the problem regardless of the severity (Figure 3).

For mild problems, diet supplements and appetite stimulants are used. If anorexia interferes with nutrition, intermittent or sustained feeding with nasogastric tubes can be done. For dysphagia, percutaneous endoscopic gastrostomies (PEG) are utilized. Finally, with malabsorption syndromes, parenteral hyperalimentation is the intervention.

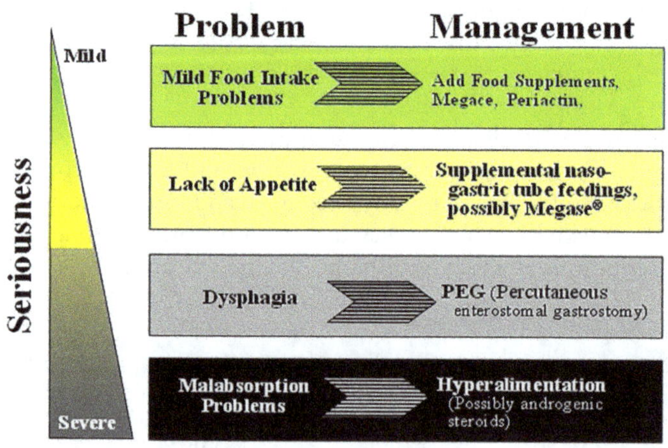

Figure 3. Hierarchy of nutrition interventions.

Fourth Strategy: Selection of Optimal Wound Dressing Agents

The choices for this strategy are considerable with over 3,000 agents from which to choose. By lumping the agents into four groups, appropriate decisions can be made for the dressing agent selection (Table 6).[33] No single agent is ideal for every wound type, although the moisturized gauze dressing comes the closest to achieving this goal. As a wound improves, the wound dressing agent choices increase (Figure 4). For example, after a debridement with remaining questionably viable and/or infective material remaining, the moist gauze dressing is preferred. As the wound improves, other agents can be used for efficiency, cost-effectiveness, and patient comfort. When the wound is not improving, consider switching to a different agent type or an agent with a different additive.

The gauze dressing moisturized with normal saline, acetic acid solution, Dakin's solution, metronidazole solution, or mild, moisturizing, possibly bacteriostatic agents is the fundamental and comparison standard for all other dressings. It can be used for almost all wound types and complexities. It is inexpensive but, to be effective, requires two or three dressing changes a day, which adds to caregiver time.

The second groups of wound dressing agents are the impervious or semi-impervious wound coverings and biologic skin coverings. These are useful for healthy (LBWS of 7.5 to 10 points), superficial, vascular-based wounds. Although more expensive than the gauze dressings, they require less frequent or one-time-only applications. The donor site of a split-thickness skin graft is an example where this type of dressing is particularly applicable. Biologic dressings can be costly, and some require application in the operating room, usually done in conjunction with debridements.

Agents and techniques to absorb secretions is the third "lumper's approach" to wound dressing agents. Sponges, alginates, foams, meshes, hydrophilic/hyperosmolar agents (e.g., sugar mixed with povidone-iodine and honey) are examples of this type of wound dressing agent. Negative-pressure wound therapy/subatmospheric pressure wound therapy (NPWT/SPWT) dressing is the ultimate in dressings to absorb secretions. With intermittent fluid instillations, the wound can be lavaged to soften and clean debris. Antimicrobials can be added to the instillation fluid.

Salves and ointments with or without additives are the fourth type of wound dressings. These are most useful for the healthy, superficial wound that has a vascular base but has yet to epithelialize. The simplest and least expensive are the hydrophilic wound-base moisturizing gels. Other agents have antimicrobial, enzymatic debridement, anti-inflammatory, protease inhibitors, desiccating, and/or growth factor additives to address specific wound-base healing concerns. The costs range from a few dollars for moisturizing and antimicrobial agents to USD$500 or more for a 15-gram tube with the growth factor agent.

TABLE 6. "LUMPERS" APPROACH OF WOUND DRESSING AGENTS

Agent	Benefits	Examples	Comments
Gauze	Availability Inexpensive Facilitates autologous debridement	Gauze moistened with normal saline, acetic acid solution, Dakin's solution, etc.	Sets standards and comparisons for all other wound dressing agents Applicable for all wound types Requires frequent dressing changes – adds to caregiver time with patients
Wound covering agents	Single application Facilitates epithelialization of healthy wounds	Impervious films Semi-impervious films Meshed dressings Biologic dressings	More expensive but single or infrequent application +/– more cost-effective Applicable for the most healthy wounds
Absorbent agents	Removes secretions from wound bases	Sponges, alginates, foams, meshes, hydrophilic/hyperosmolar agents Negative-pressure wound therapy	Requires reapplication periodically Often combines with other agents to handle bioburden or promote healing
Salves and ointments	Moisturize wounds Active ingredients to handle bioburden, reduce inflammation, promote wound healing	Agents with antimicrobials Enzymatic debriding agents Drying agents Steroids, growth factors Protease inhibitors	Multiple choices Prices range from inexpensive to hundreds of dollars for a 15-gram tube containing growth factors

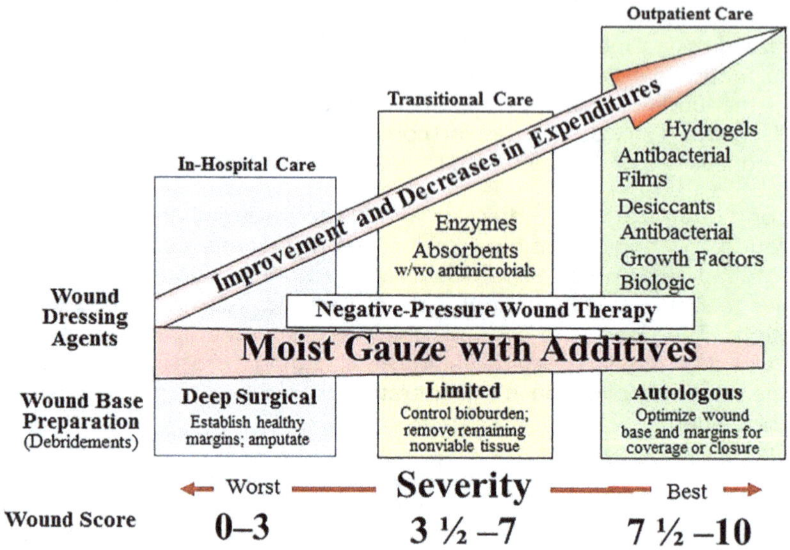

LEGEND: As the wound improves, options for management become simpler, and the choices of wound dressing agents increase. Transitional care may be at home or in a skilled nursing facility while outpatient care is almost always at home.

Figure 4. Dressings and wound base management options as wounds improve.

Fifth Strategy: Wound Perfusion and Oxygenation

This strategy is crucial for healing and controlling infection. Whereas the other four strategies almost always utilize single interventions, this strategy employs tactics that complement each other. Interventions to improve perfusion include enhancing cardiac function, reducing edema, using local vasodilatation, revascularization, hyperbaric oxygen (HBO_2) therapy, and using pharmacological agents (Table 7). Cardiac function and edema reduction were just discussed in the Medical Management strategy. Revascularizations can be achieved by bypass surgery, angioplasty, and stenting. Hyperbaric oxygen therapy is an adjunct to other managements and is especially indicated when wound hypoxia persists after the revascularization, or the vessels are so diseased that revascularization is not possible. Further information on HBO_2 is provided in the next section and its mechanisms fully explained in Chapter 13: The Role of Oxygen and Hyperbaric Oxygen Mechanisms

Pharmacological agents benefit perfusion in low-flow states. Agents such as heparin and warfarin reduce the potential for thrombus formation. Aspirin, clopidogrel (Plavix®), and celostazol (Pletal®) reduce prevent red blood cell (RBC) adhesion and sludging. Low-molecular-weight dextran improves blood rheology, and pentoxifylline (Trental®) improves RBC deformability to facilitate their passage through the capillary. Finally, local vasodilators such as nitroglycerin can be applied locally over the vessels supplying threatened flaps. Since the mechanisms are so different for each of the groups of agents, it is easy to understand why two or more of these agents may be used simultaneously and be combined with other perfusion and oxygen-enhancing techniques.

TABLE 7. METHODS TO IMPROVE WOUND PERFUSION AND OXYGENATION

Interventions	Examples	Mechanisms
Cardiotonic medications	Dobutamine, digoxin	Increase strength of muscle contractions to improve cardiac output
Edema reduction	Diuretics	Reduce edema; decrease oxygen's limited diffusion distance from the capillary to the cell
Revascularizations	Bypass surgery; angioplasty or stenting	Improve perfusion
Hyperbaric oxygen	Treatments at 2 atmospheres absolute	Increases plasma and tissue oxygen tension 10-fold and diffusion distance 3-fold
Pharmacological agents		
-Antiplatelet	Aspirin, clopidogrel (Plavix®), cilostazol (Pletal®)	Especially used after revascularizations to maintain perfusion
-Anticoagulant	Heparin, warfarin (Coumadin®), apixaban (Eliquis®), dabigatran (Praxada®), and rivaroxaban (Xarelto®)	Warfarin requires monitoring
-Plasma expander	Low-molecular-weight dextran (Rheomacrodex®)	Also reduces RBC sludging and improves flow in the microcirculation
-RBC deformation	Pentoxifylline (Trental®)	The 7.5 µm diameter RBC must deform to enter the 5 µm wide capillary to offload its oxygen
-Local vasodilation	Nitroglycerin (Nitro-Bid®, Nitro-Dur®)	Applied to bases of ischemic flaps

THE ROLES OF HYPERBARIC OXYGEN IN DIABETIC AND OTHER WOUNDS

For wounds to heal and infection to be controlled, perfusion and oxygen availability must increase manifold. When the increased demands are not reached, the third component of the "Treacherous Triad," wound ischemia-hypoxia, must be addressed. There is no published scientific data on how much blood flow and oxygen delivery need to be increased for wound healing and control of infection. However, we hypothesized that it could be as much as 20-fold based on blood volume versus total capacity of the cardiovascular system (Table 8).[16] If the increased metabolic demands are not met, wound healing stalls. Blood flow in the circulatory system is very carefully

TABLE 8. BLOOD VOLUME VERSUS POTENTIAL VOLUME OF THE CARDIOVASCULAR SYSTEM

Structure	Mechanism to increase volume	Factor (Ref.)	Comments
Heart	Increased filling	2.5-fold	Increased filling and/or rate
Arteries	Vasodilation	3-fold[30]	Over 60 miles of end-to-end length; over 80% of length in capillaries. Through sympathetic nervous system control and chemical mediations, there is minimal flow through noncritical tissues at rest. Because of the complete capillary bed filling, it would require an enormous volume of blood.
Veins	Expansion	5-fold or more[30]	
Capillaries	Filling	100-fold or more (estimate)	
Arteriovenous shunting	Bypass capillary bed	10-fold (estimate)	Possible explanation for septic shock – i.e., blood and oxygen bypass capillary bed, and no oxygen or nutrient exchange occurs.
Sinusoids and reservoirs (liver, spleen, bone marrow, erectile tissue)	Storage	3-fold (estimate)	Emptying of reservoirs significantly increases blood volume in hypovolemic shock

NOTE: Potential blood capacity of the cardiovascular system is at a minimum 20-fold but probably many folds more than the actual blood volume.

regulated (by the sympathetic nervous system and chemical mediators). At any one time, minimal perfusion goes to noncritical tissues, and their metabolic activity is negligible (i.e., almost a state of hibernation) at rest. With activity, wound healing, tissue repair, infection control, food digestion, heat dissipation, etc., blood flow must be redirected to the active tissues. Clinically, this is observed as activity (such as with muscle), classic signs of inflammation (calor, rubor, dolor, tumor), diaphoresis (sweating), and food digestion as well as wound healing.

The brain, a critical tissue, requires a constant 20% of the resting cardiac output. If this requirement is not met, impaired cognitive function, syncope, stroke, or other signs and symptoms of brain dysfunction occur.

In contrast, muscles and the gastrointestinal system require minimal blood supply at rest. Muscle blood flow can increase as much as 50-fold with maximal activity.[16] Comparable increases in blood flow in the gut are likely required for digestion of food. This is why the adage, "don't swim vigorously immediately after eating a big meal" has a physiological basis.

Transcutaneous oxygen measurements (TCOMs) provide information as to oxygen availability to superficial tissues, but do not reflect their metabolic activity or oxygen requirements. Hunt et al. showed that 30 to 40 mmHg transcutaneous oxygen tensions are needed for wounds to heal.[19] Wound healing is unlikely if the measurement is less than 30 mmHg and likely if greater than 40 mmHg. In the intermediate range of 30 to 40 mmHg, healing may or may not occur and usually is related to how the other components of the Treacherous Triad (i.e., deep infection and underlying deformity) are handled as well as considerations for nutrition, comorbidities, and patient compliance (Table 5, Table 9).

TABLE 9. GOAL SCORE

Assessment	Full 2 Points	Some 1 Point	None 0 Points
	Use half points if mixed or intermediate between 2 grades		
Comprehension			
Motivation			
Compliance			
Support Family, caregiver, institutional			
Insight			

NOTE: The "Goal Score" is another useful tool to determine how successful and how intent the patient and the family are In healing a wound and avoiding a major amputation. Goal Scores greater than 4½ points support the decision to avoid lower limb amputation and do everything possible for wound salvage. This score, coupled with the Wellness Score (Table 5), provides objectivity for recommending management of limb-threatening wounds.

Carbon-dioxide-carrying capacity in blood and diffusability in tissue fluids is 20 times that of oxygen. Elevated juxta-wound transcutaneous carbon dioxide tensions are a reflection of inadequate perfusion inasmuch as the ability to deliver oxygen to tissues is 1⁄20 that of removing carbon dioxide. Hardly ever are elevated tissue carbon dioxide levels a reason for amputations, and, if elevated, oxygen tensions are correspondingly low.

Inhaled oxygen percentage while breathing room air is approximately 21%, while the exhaled oxygen is 18% – i.e., only 3% of inhaled oxygen diffuses through the lung alveoli and into the hemoglobin molecule; 97% of the inhaled oxygen is exhaled. Normal offloading of oxygen at the capillary is only a quarter of the hemoglobin oxygen-carrying capacity (Henderson-Hasselbalch curve), i.e., 20 vol% on the arterial side of the capillary and 15 vol% on the venous side resulting in a 5 vol% oxygen extraction. Finally, inhaled air contains about 0.05% carbon dioxide, while exhaled air contains 5% or a hundredfold increase in carbon dioxide. This physiological information explains why oxygen delivery to wound healing tissues is about 1⁄20 as efficient as carbon dioxide removal.

Since transcutaneous oxygen measurements (TCOMs) provide information as to wound perfusion and tissue oxygenation, it is a diagnostic test. When coupled with carbon dioxide tensions, it offers parameters as to whether HBO_2 treatments will be a useful adjunct in managing the problem wound (Table 10). When juxta-wound oxygen tensions are over 40 mmHg and carbon dioxide tensions are 40 +/- 5 mmHg, the ischemia-hypoxia component of the "Troublesome Triad" is not an issue (Table 10).[32,40] Low oxygen tensions coupled with normal carbon dioxide tensions indicate adequate perfusion to offload carbon dioxide, but insufficient to meet oxygen demands. This permutation is the indication for HBO_2 treatments.

When making decisions whether HBO_2 treatments are needed for the ischemia-hypoxic wound component of the "Troublesome Triad," juxta-wound TCOMs in room air and with HBO_2 are a validated tool for making decisions for using HBO_2

TABLE 10. USE OF JUXTA-WOUND TRANSCUTANEOUS OXYGEN AND CARBON DIOXIDE MEASUREMENTS TO MAKE ISCHEMIC/HYPOXIC WOUND MANAGEMENT DECISIONS

		Oxygen	
		Normal (> 40 mmHg)	**Low** (< 30 mmHg)
Carbon Dioxide	**Normal** (40 ± 5 mmHg)	Adjunctive HBO not needed	Use HBO
Carbon Dioxide	**Elevated** (> 45 mmHg)	Look for other causes of impaired outflow or utilization - venous stasis disease - compartment syndrome - impaired tissue O_2 uptake (hibernation) - hypothermia	Revascularize or, if not possible, amputate

NOTE: If transcutaneous oxygen measurements are between 30 and 40 mmHg, use information from the Wellness and Goal Scores to justify limb salvage versus amputation.

Serial fluorescence angiography is an imaging technique that can view perfusion of superficial structures and is described as useful in assessing viability of flaps as a visual means to augment the clinical exam. It does not have the predictability and scope of use as TCOMs and is not adaptable for use in the monoplace hyperbaric chamber. Its role in justifying HBO_2 is indeterminate at this time.

Near-infrared spectroscopy (NIRS) is related to fluorescence angiography. It uses the near-infrared region of the electromagnetic spectrum to penetrate the superficial layers of tissues. NIRS is able to measure venous oxygen saturation. We are not aware of its use in problem wounds even though it has been studied as a possible diagnostic technique in in acute skeletal muscle-compartment syndromes. [14]

and predicting healing in this group of patients. We reported that 88% healing rates were observed in a prospective series of almost 100 patients with problem wounds whose TCOMs exceeded 200 mmHg with HBO_2 regardless of the room air readings.[11] When this data was combined with a retrospective series of nearly the same number of papers, the 200 mmHg benchmark with HBO_2 becomes a strong indication confirming which ischemic-hypoxic problem wounds will be benefited by using HBO_2 as an adjunct for wound management even if the room air TCOMs are less than 30 mmHg.[11,25]

Several other wound types and etiologies have strong ischemia-hypoxia components and justify the use of HBO_2 as an adjunct for their management. These include clostridial myonecrosis, necrotizing fasciitis, chronic refractory osteomyelitis, crush injuries and acute compartment syndromes, wounds associated with acute peripheral artery ischemia, survival of threatened grafts/flaps after surgeries, nonhealing wounds in patients with vasculitis secondary to collagen vascular diseases, thermal burns, frostbite, Fournier's gangrene, purpura fulminans, radiation injuries of soft tissue/bone, and infiltrations from medications or street drugs (skin "popping"). Most of these problems are discussed in other chapters of this text. Generally, the clinical evaluation provides sufficient justification for including HBO_2 in the management regimen, but TCOMs can provide additional justification and help in making decisions regarding the need for major amputations and when to stop HBO_2.

When HBO_2 is used as an adjunct for managing the ischemic-hypoxic component of problem wounds, well-defined stages of healing are observed (Figure 5).[35-36] After the deterioration phase, or there is no objective improvement in the wound, a latency period of 10 days to 3 weeks or more occurs after HBO_2 is started. Although the wound may not show visible signs of improvement during this time, reduction in pain, exudate, surrounding cellulitis, odor, and edema may be noted. During the latency period, the precursors for angiogenesis are generated as well as mobilization of host factors and growth factors that are necessary for healing to proceed. During the next phase, angiogenesis occurs, with the end point being a healthy-appearing, vascular-based, granulating wound. Finally, the wound transitions into the epithelialization stage and ultimate healing. Even though stages of healing are identifiable, wound healing is a continuum of responses, so elements of two or more stages may be present at any single observation time. The LBWS, being a dynamic grading system, can quantify improvement for each stage of wound healing.

The use of HBO_2 as an adjunct for the management of diabetic foot ulcers and other wounds makes sense in the context of the ischemia-hypoxia component of the "Troublesome Triad." A recently published clinical practice guideline that meticulously

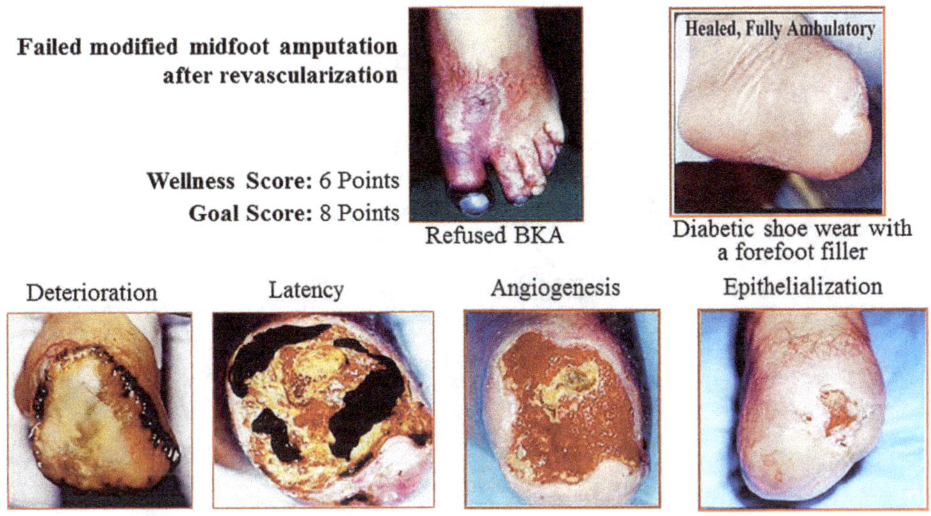

LEGEND: Well-defined stages of healing of a failed, sloughed, dehist amputation. Note how one stage transitions to another; that is, there is a continuum of responses with elements of two or stages at any one observation time. The stage, however, is determined by the predominant appearance of the wound at the time of the observation. The Wellness and Goal Scores supported the decision to do everything possible to avoid a below knee amputation. (BKA = below knee amputation)

Figure 5. Stages of wound healing.

analyzed the randomized control literature using GRADE criteria concluded that HBO_2 is beneficial in preventing amputation and promoting complete healing in patients with Wagner Grade 3 or greater DFWs who have just undergone surgical debridement of the foot as well as in patients with Wagner Grade 3 or greater DFWs that have shown no significant improvement after 30 or more days of treatment. In patients with Wagner Grade 2 or lower DFWs, there was inadequate evidence to justify the use of HBO_2 as an adjunctive treatment.(18) Two recent articles tended to debunk the benefit of HBO_2 in DFWs.(10,23) However, obvious problems with methodologies tend to discredit the results in the publications – among them using populations that consisted of nearly half the patients having Wagner Grade 2 DFWs (with higher percentages of Wagner Grade 2 DFWs being in the non-HBO_2 treated limbs of the study), not taking into consideration DFWs with components of the "Troublesome Triad," using photos by an outside observer to predict failures (needs for amputation), solely using retrospective data from multiple treatment facilities, and employing scoring systems that do not reflect the degree of ischemia-hypoxia of the DFW.

In summary, HBO_2 should be considered for problem wounds in which the ischemia-hypoxia component is a contributing reason why the wound is not improving. The perfusion assessment of the LBWS provides objective criteria (that is, grades of ½ point or less which somewhat corresponds to Wagner Grades 4 and 5 wounds) for which wounds have impaired perfusion. Likewise, if the LBWS is between 2 ½ points ("futile" category) and 4 points ("problem" category), we categorize it as an "end-stage wound" and use Wellness and Goal Scores to justify salvage attempts or to proceed immediately to amputations. Regardless of which indication exists, HBO_2 should be used in the management in an algorithmic approach (Figure 6a, Figure 6b). For the acute wound (with the patient in the hospital) and LBWS in the 3 ½ to 7-point range (Wagner Grades 3 and 4), HBO_2 treatments should be given twice a day to augment host factors such as fibroblast activity, angiogenesis, bone resorption, and neutrophil oxidative

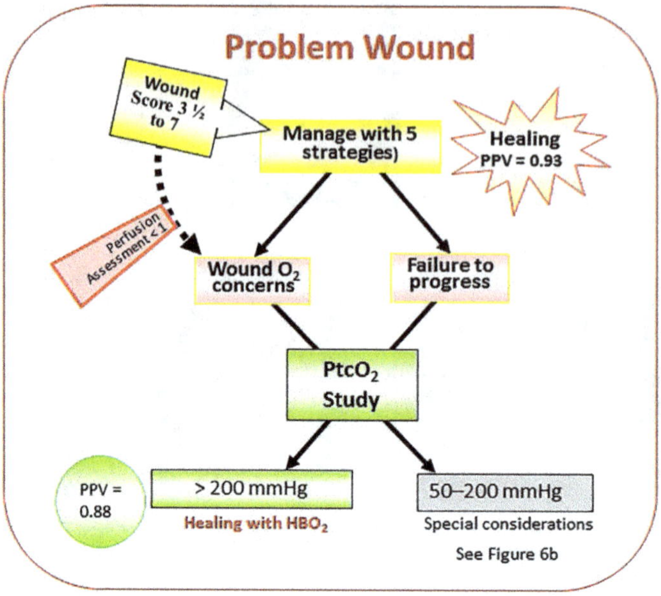

LEGEND: An algorithm approach aids in making decisions for using HBO_2 in the problem wound where the ischemic-hypoxia component of the Treacherous Triad is an important consideration.

Figure 6a. Algorithm for use of transcutaneous oxygen in the problem wound.

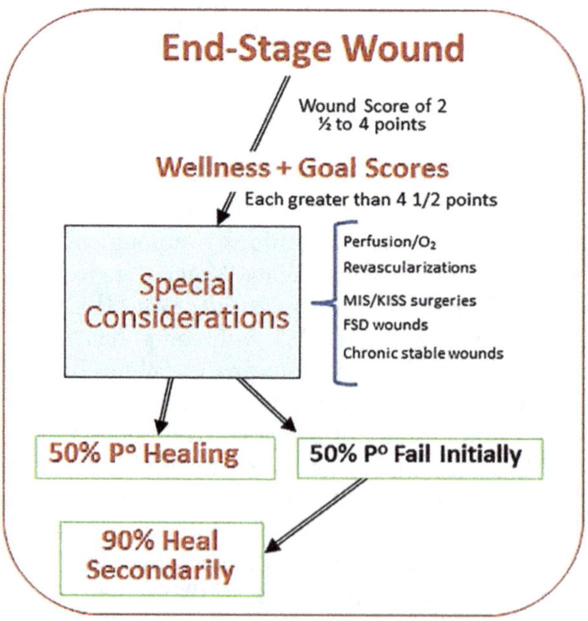

LEGEND: For the "End-stage" wound, Wellness and Goal Scores are needed to make a decision whether to salvage or proceed to a lower limb amputation. If salvage is the option, five considerations are used to supplement the five wound healing strategies and include optimizing perfusion/oxygen availability to the wound, "last resort" revascularizations, MIS/KISS (minimally invasive/keep it simple and speedy surgeries), obtaining secondary healing of initial FSD (failed, sloughed, dehisced postoperative wounds), and allowing the patient to live with a small, easily managed, chronic, stable wound.

Figure 6b. Algorithm for use of transcutaneous oxygen in the end-stage wound.

killing as well as to preserve the viability of as much tissue as possible. Juxta-wound TCOMs help justify the use of HBO_2 for these purposes. Treatment pressures of 2.0 to 2.4 atmospheres absolute should be used for 90-minute periods of hyperoxia. Once systemic sepsis is controlled and tissue viability or demarcation established, HBO_2 can be reduced to daily treatments and, with suitable arrangements, be done as an outpatient. Fourteen to 21 HBO_2 treatments for wounds is recommended in order to achieve angiogenesis and support other host factors in promoting healing and durability of the wound.

Wagner, in his articles on foot wounds, described Grade 3 wounds as acute and limb threatening with associated sepsis, deep abscess, and/or osteomyelitis that require immediate antibiotics and surgery.[38,43] This contrasts with CMS/Medicare requirements for HBO_2 to be only used as an adjunct in DFW management for Wagner Grade 3 and higher foot wounds when the problem has not improved after 30 days.

Immediate use of HBO_2 can be justified in diabetic foot wounds and other wounds that have components of necrotizing fasciitis – usually with mixed aerobic and anaerobic organisms, threatened flap/grafts, and/or acute peripheral artery ischemia.

PREVENTION OF NEW AND RECURRENT DIABETIC FOOT AS WELL AS OTHER WOUNDS

Once a wound is healed, prevention of recurrent or new wounds becomes of paramount importance. Five risk factors formulated by diabetic foot ulcer consortiums are highly predictive of wound development in the diabetic foot.[13] The risk factors include 1) peripheral artery disease, 2) history of a previous foot wound, 3) previous foot amputation, 4) deformity, and 5) neuropathy. The risks of new or recurrent wounds increase proportionally as the number of risk factors increase.[13] These five risk factors are mitigated by four strategies: education, foot skin and toenail care, selection of appropriate protective footwear, and proactive surgeries (Figure 7).

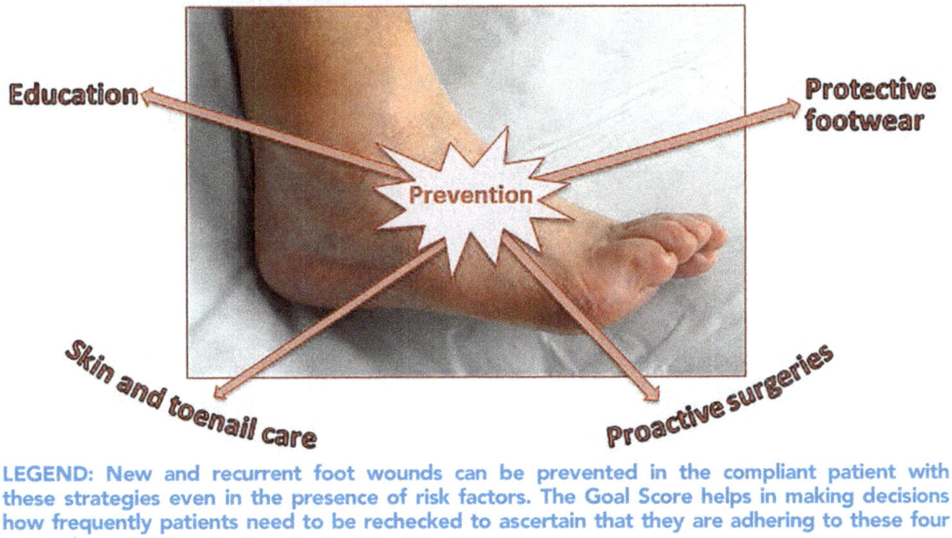

LEGEND: New and recurrent foot wounds can be prevented in the compliant patient with these strategies even in the presence of risk factors. The Goal Score helps in making decisions how frequently patients need to be rechecked to ascertain that they are adhering to these four strategies.

Figure 7. Four strategies to prevent new and recurrent diabetic and other wounds.

Education

The importance of education cannot be overstated. Education is involved at all levels of the patient care spectrum. The primary physician and associated care providers (i.e., nurse practitioners and physician assistants) should be aware of the risk factors for diabetic foot wounds and, when present, always include the foot exam in their patient evaluations. If risk factors are significant, the patient should be referred to specialists such as the vascular surgeon for peripheral artery disease and the foot and ankle specialist for nail care, protective footwear, and proactive surgeries.[1] Other education for the patient should include weight management, smoking cessation, and adherence to diabetes control as well as appropriate activity level for the patient's functional capacity. The other component of education is for the patient and/or those who provide day-to-day care for the patient. These include dos and don'ts with regard to protecting the feet, skin cleansing and lubrication, and the immediate report of pre-ulcerative skin attenuation or new wounds (Table 11).

Assessments from the Wellness and Goal Scores can assist in patient education. For example, the ambulation assessment of the Goal Score is ideally suited to define appropriate activity for the patient, e.g., community ambulation, household ambulation, no ambulation, with provisions whether or not aids such as canes, wheelchairs, etc. should be used. The compliance and insight assessments of the Goal Score provide guidance how often the patient needs to return for follow-up medical checks for their healed wound conditions – for example, biweekly if totally noncompliant with poor insight and yearly if especially diligent with regard to compliance and good insight about preventing new and recurrent wounds in the feet.

TABLE 11. DIABETIC FOOT CARE DOS AND DON'TS

Items	Comments
Dos	
Be aware of foot conditions	Alert care providers immediately if a problem is noted
Inspect feet after removing shoes	Wear white socks if at risk for wounds
Daily foot hygiene and lubrication	Regular toenail care
Be fitted with proper footwear	Regularly check shoes/orthotics for wear
Select appropriate activities	Optimize body weight/body mass index
Don'ts	
Walk barefoot	Use dry heat on the feet
Soak feet in hot water	Use chemicals or sharp objects to remove calluses
Trim ingrown, embedded toenail edges	Use nail polish
Wear new shoes without frequent checks	Wear socks with constricting bands
Wear inappropriate shoes	Smoke tobacco

Skin and Toenail Care

Attention to these matters serve two purposes. First, they are useful in keeping the skin and toenails as healthy as possible. Diabetics, because of autonomic neuropathy, often have dry, scaly skin that is subject to plaque formation, maceration, and ulceration. Healthy, clean, moist, pliable skin is resistant to injury and breakdown. When the skin is atrophic and dry and the underlying padding is lost, minor stresses can lead to ulcerations. A user-friendly tool to assess skin and toenail care is the use of a 0-to-2-point (worst to best) assessment scale (Table 12). Toenail care in the diabetic with sensory neuropathy, fungus-infected toenails, or agility and visual problems is best done by those skilled in toenail care such as podiatrists, and appropriately trained nurse practitioners and physician assistants. How the patient (and the caregiver) manages the skin and toenails is another measure of patient compliance. Second, how patients manage their skin and toenail care between office visits reflects compliance and is a measure to judge compliance on this assessment of the Goal Score.

A subset of diabetic patients continue to re-form thick, firm, keratinized callus at the healed wound site whether healed or not. This requires periodic sharp debridements with a scalpel and sometimes a curette. The callus is thought to be due to the wound healing process activating noncoded DNA (i.e., epigenes) to induce the tissues in the wound site to continue to form exuberant callus at the wound side. The process may have started because the body was trying to isolate healthy tissues from the infected wound in an ischemic-hypoxic environment. Scar tissue is notorious for forming in hypoxic tissue because of activation of the β1 transforming growth factor.

Skin care is easily done by simply cleansing the foot and leg skin with a mild soap and water. After drying, a skin lubricant should be applied. Lubricants include petroleum-based, silicon, coconut oil, hydrogels, glycerol, and lanolin-containing agents. Probably no lubricant is better suited while being the least expensive for skin lubrication than petrolatum. However, care must be given to remove all greasy residues with a soft cloth so as to not leave a medium for desquamated skin to form scales, plaques, and trap moisture.

TABLE 12. SKIN CONDITION AND TOENAIL ASSESSMENTS

Grade	Findings Use ½ points if intermediate between 2 grades	Management
	Skin	
2	Healthy, moisturized	Compliment, continue present care
1	Dry, scaly	Clean and lubricate with skin lotion
0	Plaques, debris, dirty	Cleanse, debride plaques, lubricate
	Toenails	
2	Healthy	Compliment, continue present care
1	Long	Trim
0	Thick, dystrophic, ingrown, fungus-infected	Debride, file, contour, disinfect with antiseptic

For those patients who cannot do their own toenail care, filing the toenails to keep them thin and smooth-edged can safely be done with disposable nail files by the patient's family or caregivers.

Protective Footwear

The selection of appropriate footwear is the third strategy to prevent new and recurrent foot wounds. Like HBO_2 therapy, CMS/Medicare provides payment for protective footwear for diabetic patients, but not for non-diabetic foot wounds.[20]

> The CMS/Medicare diabetic protective footwear bill provides for one pair of new shoes a year plus insert replacements every four months. Reimbursement is such that CMS/Medicare pays 80% of the "agreed upon" price, and the patients and/or their secondary insurance pay the remaining 20%, as is the practice for other CMS/Medicare medical and surgical benefits.

There is a hierarchy of protective footwear options from off-the-shelf quality walking shoes to CROW boots (Figure 8). The price for each doubles or triples as each level of the hierarchy is reached. Regardless of the level of protective footwear used, diligence must be exercised in their use. The patients and their caregivers must inspect their feet for any pre-ulcerative conditions with using the footwear. If any are observed, they need to be brought to the immediate attention of the physician ordering the footwear. Often, adjustments by the orthotist need to be made for each new set of protective footwear to relieve pressure areas and offload weight-bearing concentrations.

> After complex realignment surgery for limb-threatening Charcot neuroarthropathy deformities with associated wounds, convalescence takes a year or more. This can include up to three months in an external fixator, three months in a cast, and a year in a CROW boot, before considering less complicated, more attractive protective footwear.

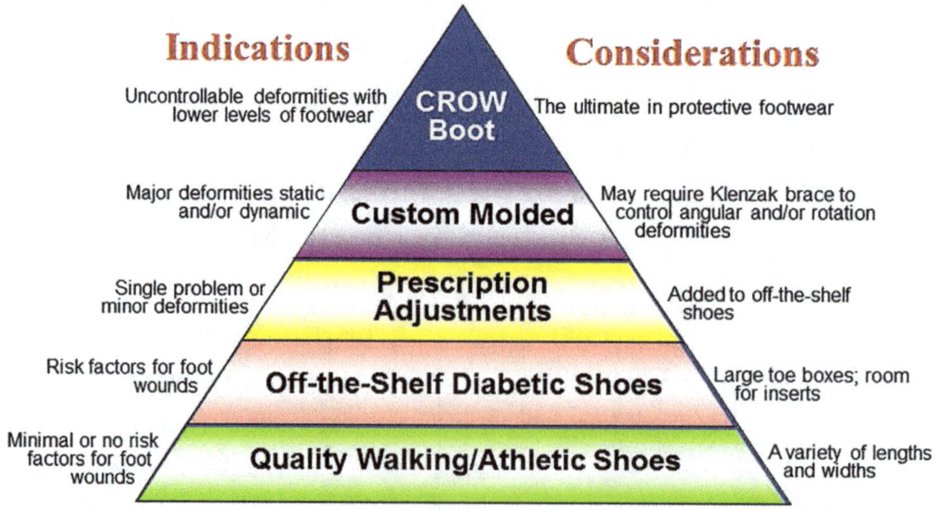

Note: 1. Medicare attestation statement indicating the patient is receiving comprehensive care for his or her diabetes is required for reimbursements for level 2–5 footwear.
2. Charges approximately double for each level of protective footwear (i.e., USD$150 for level 1 to USD$2,400 for level 5).

LEGEND: Specific indications exist for each level of protective footwear. Consequently, practitioners familiar with diabetic foot problems need to make the decisions as to the appropriate protective footwear that needs to be prescribed.

Figure 8. Hierarchy of protective footwear.

Proactive Surgeries

This is the fourth strategy for the prevention of new and recurrent foot wounds. Deformities, especially in conjunction with shear stresses, are subject to developing wounds. Proactive surgeries are done before wounds occur. Most are minimally invasive such as tenotomies, realignment of metatarsal heads with a single drill hole, scoring the bone with the drill and creating a fracture to angle the metatarsal head upward, debridement of protruding bone, and skin grafting. More complicated procedures include Achilles tendon lenghthenings, osteotomies to correct deformities and temporary applications of external fixators, unconventional partial ray and foot amputations, and forefoot narrowings with external fixation to close remaining defects after partial middle ray resections of the foot. This component of the foot care and prevention team needs to be done by the surgeon experienced in these types of procedures. However, it is the primary caregivers who must be diligent in alerting the surgeons for the need for proactive surgeries.

TEN "PEARLS" TO REMEMBER ABOUT DIABETIC FOOT AND RELATED WOUNDS

1. Diabetic foot ulcers in general and wounds in particular that are not improving typically have one or more of the Troublesome Triad problems of deformity, deep infection (bone, bursa or cicatrix), or ischemia-hypoxia.
2. The Wagner system which is required for CMS/Medicare reimbursements for Grade 3, 4, or 5 DFWs generates paradoxes. First, the score consists of six management algorithms where the decision to salvage or amputate is based on ankle-brachial indexes. Then, if salvage is the option, the grade is determined by single disparate observations. Second, Wagner's Grade 3 DFW is described as associated with systemic sepsis requiring immediate intravenous antibiotics and surgery. This is incongruous with the outpatient who has a DFW with deep abscess or osteomyelitis, which has not improved in 30 days. CMS/Medicare accepts this description as a Wagner Grade 3 DFW and reimburses for HBO_2 treatments. Third, in Wagner's follow-up article (1981), he gave equivalence for using his system for foot ulcers in patients without diabetes as for patients with diabetes, but this expanded use has not been approved for HBO_2 treatments.
3. The LBWS combines the salient features (i.e., perfusion, depth, and infection) of the most commonly used DFW scoring systems but amplifies them by adding two additional assessments (appearance of the wound base and size) to generate a user-friendly 0-to-10-point (best) scoring system with objective criteria for grading each assessment. The LBWS quantitatively categorizes wounds as "healthy," "problem," or "futile." The LBWS's objectivity facilitates CER (i.e., comparing like with like with respect to interventions such as biologic dressings, negative-pressure wound therapy, and HBO_2). It is adaptable to all types of wounds and in all locations in contrast to the DFW ulcer evaluation systems.
4. Five strategies (management of the wound base, protection and stabilization of the wound, optimal medical management, selection of appropriate wound dressings, and optimization of perfusion-oxygenation) should always be incorporated in the treatment plan for all wounds whether at the time of the initial evaluations as well as for follow-up visits.

5. Debridement is the essential feature for managing the wound base, and techniques include sharp surgical, enzymatic, autologous, hydrotherapeutic, and biological approaches. Ostectomies, explorations, and operating room debridements and amputations are the surgical end of the continuum for managing the wound base.
6. With over 3,000 choices for wound dressing agents, the dressing selection needs to be based on the characteristics of the wound. The moist gauze dressing is the universal dressing agent, but other agents have advantages in terms of ease of use and properties to address specific wound conditions. As wounds improve, the choices increase, and the wound care becomes simpler.
7. Methods to increase wound perfusion-oxygenation not only include revascularization but also edema reduction, improving cardiac function, use of pharmacological agents, and HBO_2. In contrast to the other treatment strategies, two or more of these tactics may be used simultaneously.
8. Objectivity for using HBO_2 as an adjunct to managing the ischemia-hypoxia component of the Troublesome Triad can be determined with juxta-wound transcutaneous oxygen measurements. If measurements exceed 200 mmHg with HBO_2, almost 90% of problem wounds heal with using HBO_2 as an adjunct.
9. The Wellness and Goal Scores are two additional user-friendly 0-to-10-point evaluation grading tools to help make decisions of salvage versus amputation of wounds in the transition zone between "problem" and "futile," which we label the "end-stage" wound.
10. Four strategies (patient education, skin and toenail care, protective foot wear selection, and proactive surgeries) are essential in preventing new and recurrent diabetic foot and other lower extremity wounds. While neuropathy is a risk factor for DFWs, it does not prevent healing and may, in fact, help with perfusion such as in the Charcot neuroarthropathy patient and make wound care painless.

CONCLUSION

Clinical evaluation is essential in formulating the decision to use HBO_2 as an adjunct for managing DFWs and other foot wounds. The Wagner grading system, which has not been validated other than by use, is not a good tool for appreciating the perfusion-oxygenation status of the wound. Our LBWS evaluates this assessment in a continuum fashion so absolute criteria can be used to use HBO_2 for DFWs and other wound problems. Further justification is provided by using juxta-wound transcutaneous oxygen measurements to show which wounds are hypoxic and then using a HBO_2 exposure to show if the wound hypoxia responds (i.e., exceeds 200 mmHg). This type of information is almost 90% predictive for healing of the "problem" wound.

We appreciate that the Wagner grading system is currently used to receive payment from CMS/Medicare when utilizing HBO_2 as an adjunct for managing DFWs. Nonetheless, we recommend using our LBWS for evaluating the wound, quantifying its seriousness into "healthy," "problem," and "futile" categories, deciding which interventions are needed for management, and measuring outcomes. The LBWS helps justify using HBO_2 for wounds other than DFWs. It is a paradox that Wagner included such foot wounds in his later publication, but insurance payers are reluctant to use this information for justifying HBO_2 treatments. However, in some situations such as necrotizing fasciitis, chronic refractory osteomyelitis, threatened flaps/grafts, and acute peripheral ischemia, HBO_2 is an approved indication notwithstanding that diabetics comprise a large percentage of the patients with these conditions.

In summary, there is a specific role for HBO_2 treatments in the management of DFWs and other wounds. This chapter has demonstrated the indications for such using both the LBWS and TCOM. It shows how perfusion and hypoxia are integrated into the evaluation, management, and prevention of DFWs with the information being equally appropriate for nondiabetic patients with similar wounds.

REFERENCES

1. Abbott CA, Carrington AL, Ashe H, et al. The North-West Diabetes Foot Care Study: incidence of, and risk factors for, new diabetic foot ulceration in a community-based patient cohort. Diabet Med. 2002;19(5):377-84.
2. Agency for Health Care Policy and Research Guidelines. Pressure ulcers in adults: prediction and prevention clinical practice guideline. Rockville (MD): AHCPR; 1992. No. 92-0047.
3. Aksenov IV, Strauss MB, Miller SS. Medical management of the patients with problem wounds. Wound Care Hyperb Med. 2011;2(4):13-32.
4. Armstrong DG, Lavery LA. Diabetic foot ulcers: prevention, diagnosis and classification. Am Fam Physician. 1998;57(6):1325-32, 1337-8.
5. Armstrong DG, Lavery LA, Harkless LB. Treatment-based classification system for assessment and care of diabetic feet. J Am Podiat Med Assoc. 1996;86(7):311-6.
6. Armstrong, Lavery LA, Harkless LB. Validation of a diabetic wound classification system. The contribution of depth, infection, and ischemia to risk of amputation. Diabetes Care. 1998;21(5):855-9.
7. Boyko EJ, Ahroni JH, Stensel V, Forsberg RC, Davignon DR, Smith DG. A prospective study of risk factors for diabetic foot ulcer. The Seattle Diabetic Foot Study. Diabetes Care. 1999;22(7):1036-42.
8. Brownlee M, Aiello LP, Cooper ME, et al. Complications of diabetes mellitus. In: Melmed S, Polonsky KS, Larsen PR, Kronenberg HM, editors. Textbook of endocrinology. 12th ed. Philadelphia: Saunders Elsevier; 2011. p. 1462-551.
9. Craig AB, Strauss MB, Daniller A, Miller SS. Foot sensation testing in the patient with diabetes: introduction of the quick & easy assessment tool. Wounds. 2014;26(8):221-31.
10. Fedorko L, Bowen JM, Jones W, et al. Hyperbaric oxygen therapy does not reduce indications for amputation in patients with diabetes with nonhealing ulcers of the lower limb: a prospective, double-blind, randomized controlled clinical trial. Diabetes Care. 2016;39:392-9.
11. Fife CE, Buyukcakir C, Otto GH, et al. The predictive value of transcutaneous oxygen tension measurement in diabetic lower extremity ulcers treated with hyperbaric oxygen therapy: a retrospective analysis of 1,144 patients. Wound Repair Regen. 2002;10(4):198-207.
12. Frigg A, Pagenstert G, Schafer D, et al. Recurrence and prevention of diabetic foot ulcers and total contact casting. Foot Ankle Int. 2007;28(1):64-9.
13. Frykberg RG, Zgonis T, Armstrong DG, et al. Diabetic foot disorders. A clinical practice guideline (2006 revision). J Foot Ankle Surg. 2006;45(5 Suppl):1-66.
14. Giansotti G, Cohn SM, Brown M, et al. Utility of near-infrared spectroscpoy in the diagnosis of lower extremity compartment syndrome. J Trauma. 2000;48(3):396-401.
15. Greene AK, Puder M, Roy R, et al. Microdeformational wound therapy effects on angiogenesis and matrix metalloproteinases in chronic wounds of 3 debilitated patients. Ann Plast Surg. 2006;56(4):418-22.
16. Guyton AC, Hall JE. Muscle blood flow and cardiac output during exercise. In: Textbook of medical physiology. 13th ed. Philadelphia: WB Saunders; 2016. p. 179.
17. Hermans MH. Wounds and ulcers: back to the old nomenclature. Wounds. 2010;22(11):289-93.
18. Huang ET, Mansouri J, Murad MH, et al. A clinical practice guideline for the use of hyperbaric oxygen therapy in the treatment of diabetic foot ulcers. Undersea Hyperb Med. 2015;42(3):205-47.

19. Hunt TK, Linsey M, Grislis H, et al. The effect of differing ambient oxygen tensions on wound infection. Ann Surg. 1975;181(1):35-9.

20. Janisse DJ. The therapeutic shoe bill: Medicare coverage for prescription footwear for diabetic patients. Foot Ankle Int. 2005;26(1):42-5.

21. Lavery LA, Armstrong DG, Harkless LB. Classification of diabetic foot wounds. J Foot Ankle Surg. 1996;35(6):528-31.

22. Lipsky BA, Berendt AR, Cornia PB, et al. Infectious Diseases Society of America. 2012 Infectious Diseases Society of America clinical practice guideline for the diagnosis and treatment of diabetic foot infections. Clin Infect Dis. 2012;54(12):e132-73.

23. Margolis DJ, Gupta J, Hoffstad O, et al. Lack of effectiveness of hyperbaric oxygen therapy for the treatment of diabetic foot ulcer and the prevention of amputation: a cohort study. Diabetes Care. 2013;36(7):1961-6.

24. Mayfield JA, Reiber GE, Sanders LJ, et al. Preventative foot care in people with diabetes. Diabetes Care. 1998;21(12):2161-77.

25. Moon H, Strauss MB, La SS, Miller SS. The validity of transcutaneous oxygen measurements in predicting healing of diabetic foot ulcers. Undersea Hyperb Med. 2016.

26. National Pressure Ulcer Advisory Panel [Internet]. National Pressure Ulcer Advisory Panel. Available from: http://www.npuap.org/resources/educational-and-clinical-resources/noise-pressure-injury-stages

27. Pecoraro RE, Reiber GE, Burgess EM. Pathways to diabetic limb amputation. Basis for prevention. Diabetes Care. 1990;13(5):513-21.

28. Reiber GE, Ledous WE. Epidemiology of diabetic foot ulcers and amputations: evidence for prevention. The evidence base for diabetes care. London: John Wiley & Sons; 2002. p. 641-65.

29. Siegel ME, Stewart CA, Wagner FW Jr, Sakimura I. An index to measure the healing potential of ischaemic ulcers using thallium 201. Prosthet Orthot Int. 1983;7(3):67-8.

30. Statistics about diabetes: overall numbers, diabetes and prediabetes. American Diabetes Association [Internet]. American Diabetes Association. Statistics about diabetes: overall numbers, diabetes and prediabetes [cited 2016 Aug]. Available from: www.diabetes.org

31. Strauss MB, Aksenov IV, Miller SS. Classification system for the diabetic foot wound. In: Masterminding wounds. Flagstaff (AZ): Best Publishing Co.; 2010. p. 57-83.

32. Strauss MB, Bryant BJ, Hart GB. Transcutaneous oxygen measurements under hyperbaric oxygen conditions as a predictor for healing of problem wounds. Foot Ankle Int. 2002;23(10):933-7.

33. Strauss MB. Diabetic foot and leg wounds: principles, management and prevention. Prim Care Rep. 2001;7(22):187-97.

34. Strauss MB, Lew DC, Miller SS. The Wagner Wound Grading System. Wound Care Hyperb Med. 2012;3(4):38-44.

35. Strauss MB, Miller SS, Aksenov IV. Challenges of wound healing. Wound Care Hyperb Med. 2011;2(1):28-36.

36. Strauss MB, Miller SS, Nhan L. The end-stage wound: its determination and management. Wound Care Hyperb Med. 2013;4(4):19-26.

37. Strauss MB, Miller SS. Preparation of the wound base. The science and art of debridement. Wound Care Hyperb Med. 2011;2(2):14-30.

38. Strauss MB, Moon H, Busch JA, et al. Reliability assessment of an innovative wound score. Wounds. 2016;28(6):206-13.

39. Strauss MB, Moon H, La S, et al. The incidence of confounding factors in patients with diabetes mellitus hospitalized for diabetic foot ulcers. Wounds. 2016.

40. Strauss MB, Strauss AB, Borer KM. Do transcutaneous carbon dioxide measurements predict healing of problem wounds? Undersea Hyperb Med. 2000;27(Suppl):40.

41. Strauss MB, Strauss WG. Wound scoring system streamlines decision-making. Biomechanics. 1999;VI(8):37-43.

42. Wagner FW Jr. A classification and treatment program for diabetic, neuropathic, and dysvascular foot problems. Instructional course lectures: the American Academy of Orthopaedic Surgeons. Vol. 28. Saint Louis (MO): Mosby; 1979.

43. Wagner FW Jr. The dysvascular foot: a system of diagnosis and treatment. Foot Ankle. 1981;2(2):64-122.

CHAPTER 22 CHAPTER

Evaluation and Management of the Diabetic Foot Ulcer

CHAPTER TWENTY-TWO OVERVIEW

Introduction **557**
Pathophysiology of the Diabetic Foot **558**
Vascular 558
Neuropathy 558
Dermatologic 561
Cellular 563
Examination of the Diabetic Foot **564**
History Taking 564
Physical Examination 564
Imaging Studies **569**
Probe-to-Bone Test 570
Laboratory Studies **571**
Classification of DFU **571**
Wagner 572
University of Texas 572
IDSA 575
IWGDF 575
Long Beach Wound Score 576
WIfI 576
Wound Healing Index (WHI) 577
Management of the Diabetic Foot **577**
The Multidisciplinary Limb Salvage Team **580**
References **582**

Evaluation and Management of the Diabetic Foot Ulcer

Enoch Huang, Marvin Heyboer III

INTRODUCTION

Diabetes mellitus is an epidemic of global proportion with a steadily rising prevalence of disease. There were an estimated 28.9 million (21 million diagnosed, 8.1 million undiagnosed) adults with diabetes mellitus in the United States in 2012.(84) The prevalence of diabetes mellitus among adults has quadrupled from 1980 to 2014.(84) This rate continues to rise, with 1.7 million new cases reported in 2012.(84) Globally, it is estimated that there are 422 million adults with diabetes mellitus.(50)

Patients with diabetes mellitus develop multiple types of end organ damage including retinopathy leading to blindness, nephropathy leading to renal failure, and vascular disease leading to stroke and heart attack. In addition, peripheral neuropathy, with or without concomitant peripheral arterial disease (PAD), leads to lower extremity ulcers and limb loss. It is believed at least 15% of diabetics will develop a lower extremity foot ulcer during their lifetimes.(70-71) The annual incidence of foot ulcer development is 5%–6% among diabetics.(17,70-71) The component causes associated with ulcer formation are approximately 20% primary peripheral arterial disease, 50% primary peripheral neuropathy, and 30% combination of both.(70-71) Risk factors identified for development of a foot ulcer include a longer duration of diabetes mellitus, poorer blood glucose control (higher HbA1c), peripheral neuropathy, history of previous foot ulcer, and history of previous amputation.(17)

The total cost associated with diabetes mellitus was estimated at USD$245 billion with a direct cost of USD$176 billion in 2012.(7) The estimated cost of treatment of diabetic foot ulcers (DFUs) and associated amputations was USD$11 billion in 2001.(51) Among Medicare beneficiaries, diabetics with a foot ulcer have associated costs three times higher than those without a foot ulcer. The estimated annual cost for the care of a single patient's diabetic foot ulcer was USD$1,900 in 2008.(69)

Diabetics who develop a foot ulcer are at high risk of nonhealing, major amputation (above the ankle), and death. Approximately 60% of nontraumatic lower limb amputations in the United States occur in those with diabetes mellitus. There were approximately 73,000 nontraumatic lower limb amputations in adults with diabetes mellitus in 2010.(84) There is an approximate 10% mortality rate associated with incident development of a foot ulcer, which increases to 20%–47% following an incident major lower extremity amputation.(39,69-71) These are significant numbers when comparing these rates to breast cancer and prostate cancer survival rates, which are better.[83]

This has led to the development of multidisciplinary teams and established standard wound care practices. Even with appropriate wound care, including local debridement, off-loading, and local wound dressings, the published healing rates are only 30% at 20 weeks.[72] Diabetics treated for a foot ulcer by a multidisciplinary team with a standard wound care regimen, in the absence of advanced treatment modalities, were still found to require amputation in 25% of cases.[8]

PATHOPHYSIOLOGY OF THE DIABETIC FOOT

The diabetic foot ulcer is the result of multiorgan system dysfunction linked to hyperglycemia and its myriad downstream effects. A detailed pathophysiologic description of all of the effects is beyond the scope of this chapter, but there are several overarching processes that should be understood and appreciated by the wound care and hyperbaric physician. Hyperbaric medicine has become more sophisticated than just identifying patients that would benefit from hyperbaric oxygen (HBO_2). Most hyperbaric centers are integrated into wound healing centers, necessitating more than a passing familiarity with the pathophysiology of this ubiquitous disease. On a cellular level, diabetes mellitus affects certain cell subtypes that are unable to downregulate glucose transport into the cell in the face of hyperglycemia, specifically capillary endothelial cells in the retina and peripheral vasculature, mesangial cells in the renal glomerulus, and neuronal and Schwann cells in peripheral nerves.[19]

Vascular

Diabetes mellitus has long been associated with atherosclerotic disease of both the central and peripheral vasculature, leading to higher than normal rates of coronary artery disease, stroke, renal disease, and critical limb ischemia (CLI). In addition to this more traditional understanding of macrovascular disease, there is a component of microvascular disease that is poorly understood and is used as a catchall term to explain the inability of diabetics to heal wounds. Increases in circulating reactive oxygen species (ROS) secondary to hyperglycemia lead to suppression of endothelial nitrogen oxide synthase, a potent vasodilator, and result in decreased perfusion to the capillary beds of the retina and peripheral tissues. Hyperglycemia also leads to thickening of capillary basement membranes, reducing oxygen diffusion from capillary beds to surrounding tissues.[32] Autonomic neuropathy reduces the diabetic patient's ability to mount a hyperemic response to injury, leading to a functional ischemia on top of anatomical ischemia.[32]

Neuropathy

Neuropathy in all of its forms (i.e., sensory, motor, and autonomic) is responsible for the majority of the pathology of the diabetic foot. In a multicenter study of more than 6,000 diabetic patients, neuropathy was present in 28.5% of patients, with a slightly higher percentage in type 2 diabetes mellitus (32.1%) versus type 1 diabetes mellitus (22.7%). It is more prevalent in the older population (44.2% in the 70–79 age group versus 5% in the 20–29 age group) and in those who have had the disease for a longer period of time (20.8% for those diagnosed 5 years ago versus 36.8% for those diagnosed 10 or more years ago). The incidence of neuropathy increases over time, with 50% of type 2 patients over 60 years old having peripheral neuropathy.[112]

Sensory Neuropathy

Sensory neuropathy is perhaps the most obvious manifestation of neuropathic disease as diabetic patients who have loss of protective sensation (LOPS) run the risk of unrecognized injury to soft and bony tissues that are subjected to excessive pressure, friction, or repetitive stress. Patients with neuropathic pain may also be at higher risk of unrecognized injury because their baseline pain masks new injuries.

Motor Neuropathy

Motor neuropathy has commonly been postulated to be the cause of foot deformities as a result of decreased enervation of the small musculature in the foot, allowing larger muscle groups in the lower leg to unbalance the normal anatomic alignment of the foot,[32] but a recent meta-analysis of the literature did not support this theory.[4]

- A clawfoot or hammertoe deformity (Figure 1a, Figure 1b, Figure 2) is characterized by a hyperextension and subluxation of a metatarsophalangeal joint, with flexion deformity of the interphalangeal joints and transfer of weight bearing to the metatarsal heads. When combined with sensory neuropathy, these are high-risk areas for diabetic foot ulcer formation. The management of either of these can include surgery[15,95] or nonsurgical offloading shoes.[41] Failure to address these mechanical deformities is the primary reason for ulcer recurrence.
- Charcot arthropathy (Figure 3) is the result of progressive demineralization of the foot as a result of, ironically, hyperperfusion secondary to autonomic dysregulation of blood flow. This demineralization weakens the bones of the foot and, in conjunction with sensory neuropathy, results

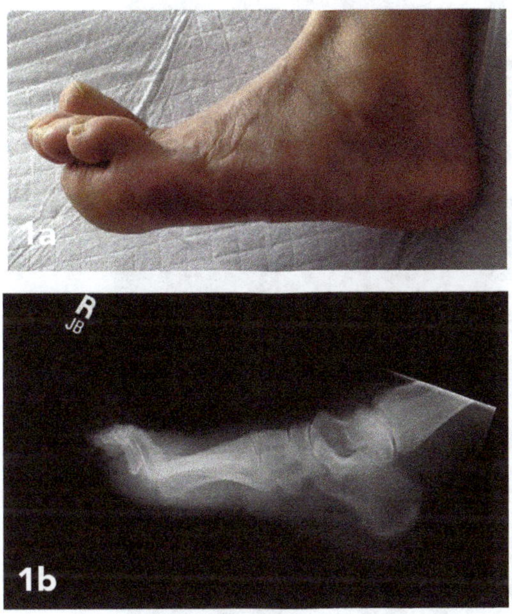

Figures 1a–1b. Clawfoot deformity.
(photos by Enoch Huang, MD)

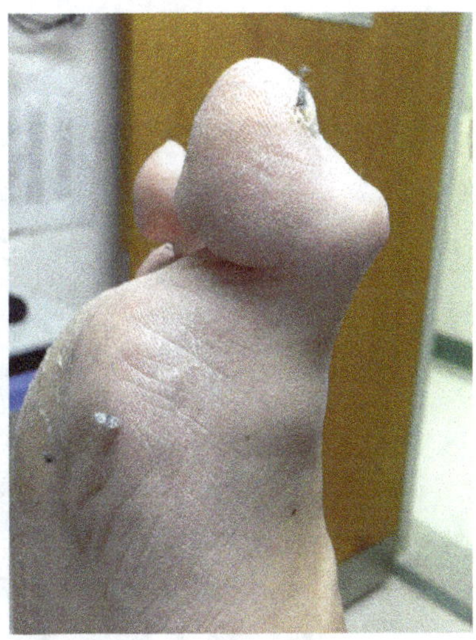

Figure 2. Hammertoe deformity.
(photo by Marvin Heyboer, MD)

in fractures and dislocations of the weight-bearing bones, often in the absence of trauma, with progression into a substantial collapse of the arch of the foot. This results in a foot with a rocker-bottom deformity, putting excessive pressure on the center of the midfoot and increasing the chance of ulceration. In the acute phase, the foot is hot, swollen, and erythematous, leading many to make the diagnosis of infection when there is none. Treatment priorities of Charcot arthropathy depend upon the stage of disease. In acute Charcot arthropathy, off-loading weight from the foot is critical in preventing further bony destruction. A total contact cast can be used to immobilize the foot while reducing pressure on the weakened architecture of the foot. Once the foot has moved out of the acute inflammatory stage, and remodeling without further progression has occurred, long-term orthotic devices such as the Charcot Removable Orthotic Walker (CROW) boot and custom-molded shoes can be used. A total contact cast may also be indicated for healing a plantar foot ulcer that may be the result of Charcot arthropathy. The osseous deformities that occur with Charcot arthropathy can create areas of focal pressure, especially on the plantar surface of the affected foot. Surgical

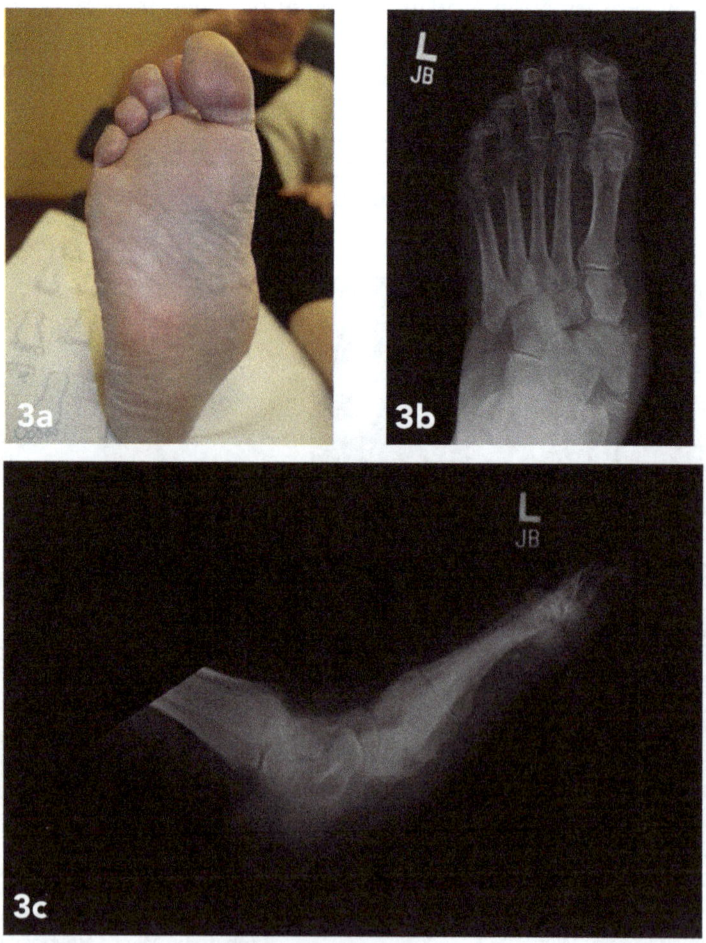

Figures 3a–3c. Charcot arthropathy. (photos by David Greenberg, DPM)

correction of Charcot arthropathy, either by extensive reconstruction or the resection of bony prominences, are options once irreversible bony deformity has occurred, but there have been no published randomized controlled trials investigating surgical techniques. A recent systematic review showed that the amputation rate was 8.9%, and the need for surgical intervention rises if there is proximal ankle involvement. The overall goal of surgical or nonsurgical approaches is to achieve a plantigrade foot that remains ulcer free.[94] Early diagnosis and prevention should be the goal of the clinician.

- Restriction of joint mobility is more prevalent in diabetics as a result of collagen glycosylation, resulting in the periarticular thickening of tendons, ligaments, and joint capsules. The subtalar joint is unable to function as a shock absorber when the heel hits the ground while walking, resulting in higher plantar foot pressures, and the Achilles tendon has decreased resiliency, creating an equinus deformity with redistribution of body weight to the plantar forefoot.[32]

Autonomic Neuropathy

In addition to the vascular effects mentioned above, autonomic neuropathy can have associated dermatologic changes leading to dry, cracking, callused skin that is a gateway for bacterial invasion. Increased pressure from the callus, paired with sensory neuropathy, is a deadly combination of symptoms initiating the diabetic foot ulcer.[108]

Dermatologic

While a diabetic ulcer is an obvious manifestation of disease, there are many nonulcerative dermatologic conditions that are associated with diabetes mellitus. While none of these are exclusive to diabetes mellitus, the wound/hyperbaric physician should be highly suspicious of undiagnosed diabetes mellitus if these conditions are present. In general, nonulcerative dermatologic conditions can be broken into noninfectious or infectious conditions.[18]

Noninfectious Dermatologic Conditions

- Diabetic dermopathy – This benign condition can result in hyperpigmented, atrophic macules of the anterior lower leg. They are usually a few millimeters in diameter and are also known as "shin spots" or "spotted leg syndrome." It is one of the most common lesions associated with diabetes mellitus, occurring in between 7% of young patients[111] and 55% of older patients.[73] It is most often a spontaneous occurrence without a history of trauma. There is no treatment nor is there significant pathology.
- Necrobiosis lipoidica diabeticorum – Necrobiosis lipoidica diabeticorum (NLD) is a rare finding in diabetic patients with an incidence of only 0.3%.[80] It can also be present in patients with rheumatoid arthritis (dropping diabeticorum from its syntax) and is three times more prevalent in women. It can present as bilateral red-brown papules that develop gradually on the anterior lower legs, although it can present in other locations as well. These can then turn into translucent, yellow atrophic plaques that result in ulceration. In 25% of cases, lesions develop before the onset of diabetes mellitus.[33] The etiology is unknown, but histologic diagnosis shows disorganized degeneration of collagen with basement membrane

thickening and inflammation of the underlying subcutaneous fat. The management is challenging and may include topical and systemic corticosteroids as well as aspirin and dipyridamole.[18]

- Diabetic bullae – In rare cases, diabetic patients may develop spontaneous blistering of the feet in the absence of any precipitating trauma, friction, or infection. This unexplained phenomena is rare and can result in tense blistering over the toes, heels, or the anterior surface of the shins. This can be frustrating for patients who will insist that they are doing everything they can to adhere to instructions to avoid trauma and friction, but it is most likely still the underlying etiology in patients with a lower-than-normal threshold for tissue injury.[25,66] Once diagnosed, treatment should include prophylactic drainage of the bullae if spontaneous rupture is imminent, increased off-loading of the ulcer, and precautions to prevent infection.
- Anhydrosis – As mentioned above, autonomic neuropathy is a significant contributor to anhydrosis, leading to fissuring and cracking of the epidermis. Anhydrosis should be treated with regular application of an emollient lotion or cream to maintain hydration of the diabetic foot.[108]
- Nail discoloration – While nail discoloration is a fairly benign process, it is a potential indicator of undiagnosed disease and should heighten clinical suspicion of diabetes mellitus. Onychomycosis must be ruled out, as it is the most common cause of discolored nails.[18]
- Nail hypertrophy – Thickening of the nails, either in the presence or absence of fungal organisms, may indicate a decrease in tissue perfusion, a sign consistent with advanced peripheral arterial disease.
- Granuloma annulare – Another benign dermatologic condition that is associated with diabetes mellitus is granuloma annulare, a self-resolving inflammatory eruption characterized by erythematous plaques and nodules. These typically can be found on the dorsal aspect of the hands and feet. While this does not typically lead to ulcerations or pathology, recognizing this condition allows the clinician to reassure patients that they will resolve on their own.[18]

Infectious Conditions

- Fungal foot infections – This catchall category includes tinea pedis and onychomycosis as the most common form of fungal infection of the foot. Infection usually spreads from the plantar surface of the foot to other parts of the foot, hands, nail, and groin. The infection itself is usually minor, but it can reduce skin integrity, creating fissures and cracks that allow more virulent infections to take hold. Histologically proven dermatomycosis was a significant risk factor for bacterial cellulitis with an odds ratio ranging from 1.7 for tinea plantaris to 3.2 for tinea pedis interdigitalis.[91]
- Bacterial infections – Diabetic foot infections are a significant problem. The most recent guidelines by the Infectious Disease Society of America (IDSA) are quite extensive and thorough, and an infectious disease specialist should be part of the multidisciplinary team caring for the patient.

- The highlights of their guideline[68] include the following:

    1. Aerobic gram-positive cocci (*Staph aureus*) are the predominant pathogens, although wound chronicity and previously treated infections may have gram-negative organisms. Gangrene and ischemia may also include obligate anaerobic bacteria.
    2. Wound infections should be diagnosed clinically on the basis of local signs and symptoms. Laboratory testing, including cultures, is of limited use in diagnosing infections except in the case of osteomyelitis.
    3. Cultures should be sent prior to initiating empiric antibiotics. Cultures obtained by biopsy, curettage, or aspiration are preferable to swabs of open wounds.
    4. Imaging studies may be helpful in diagnosing deeper soft-tissue purulent collections. MRI is superior to isotope scanning for detection of soft-tissue lesions.
    5. Antibiotics are not indicated for clinically uninfected wounds. Antibiotic therapy alone for infected wounds may not be sufficient without concomitant wound care.
    6. Empiric therapy should be based on the most likely etiological organism and the severity of infection. Definitive therapy should be based on culture results and susceptibility data.
    7. Continue antibiotic therapy until there is evidence the infection has resolved but not necessarily until the wound has healed: one to two weeks for mild infections, two to four weeks for moderate to severe infections, and four to six weeks for osteomyelitis.
    8. Spread of infection to the bone may be difficult to distinguish from noninfectious osteoarthropathy, and bone biopsy is valuable for establishing the diagnosis of osteomyelitis and determining a causative organism and antibiotic selection.

Cellular

Diabetes mellitus causes many changes to human physiology that are difficult to categorize. Hyperglycemia causes a chronic increase in ROS, namely superoxide. Elevation of superoxide reduces the production of endothelial nitrogen oxygen synthase, a potent vasodilator, leading to vasoconstriction and peripheral hypoxia.[19] Tissue hypoxia as a result of peripheral arterial disease compounded with cellular hypoxia becomes a fundamental driver of wound healing capacity.

Among the myriad changes to cellular processes involved in wound healing are several cell types that are essential to wound healing. Oxygen delivery is a critical cofactor in many cellular processes from collagen deposition to antimicrobial activity.[5,96]

Fibroblast

Fibroblast activity is a key component in wound healing, specifically collagen synthesis. Human fibroblast activity reduces with age and also in the presence of diabetes mellitus. Decreased fibroblast activity translates to decreased collagen deposition and slower wound healing.

Neutrophil
Neutrophil bacterial killing activity is through an oxygen-dependent respiratory burst, where neutrophils convert oxygen to superoxide.[11] This is depressed in patients with local wound ischemia, commonly found in diabetics. Superoxide production showed a half-maximal rate of production with pO_2 between 80 and 150 mmHg and a maximal rate over 300 mmHg.[5]

EXAMINATION OF THE DIABETIC FOOT

There are many components to the evaluation of the diabetic foot – anatomy, vascular status, and neurological function.

History Taking

The history of the diabetic foot ulcer will provide invaluable information when developing a comprehensive treatment plan. While there are a limited number of etiologies for developing a DFU (e.g., trauma, pressure, friction), there are numerous permutations for how a particular ulcer developed. The presence or absence of key historical markers can guide the clinician in prioritizing diagnostic or therapeutic interventions.

- Pain – While many patients may have sensory neuropathy, they may not be completely insensate. This information can help the clinician determine how likely the patient will be able to adhere to treatment plans, as patients who retain some pain feedback may be able to recognize inadequate off-loading of an ulcer.
- Timing – Unless patients are consistently doing daily foot checks, many may not recall the exact onset of their injury. On the other hand, many patients have a complicated history of recurrent ulcerations. The number of recurrences is an important piece of information. Recurrent ulceration in the face of nonsurgical interventions may suggest a need for more aggressive intervention to correct underlying deformities. Off-loading strategies alone are often unsuccessful, with a 40% recurrence rate within 12 months of a previous ulcer healing.[23]
- Antecedent events – Spontaneous ulcerations are a more significant issue than ulcers that are the result of a traumatic event. There are myriad stories of patients who have worn shoes with keys, rocks, and other objects inside. These obvious causes of injury can be anticipated and avoided with caution and inspection, but ulcers that form because of mechanical deformities of the foot are more difficult to avoid.

Physical Examination

Examination of the foot should include a gross inspection of the anatomy of the foot, cataloging any obvious deformities or previous amputations. One should not focus solely on the ulcer that triggered the clinic visit but should inventory all potential trouble areas. The first thing to do is examine *both* feet, as it can be tempting to focus only on the complaint at hand. Do not miss subtle or even glaringly obvious changes that affect your diagnosis.

Physical examination of the diabetic foot should include the following:

- Monofilament testing – The Semmes-Weinstein monofilament examination (SWME) is the most commonly used method for testing sensory neuropathy, although nerve conduction studies are the gold standard.

The SWME uses a 5.07/10g nylon monofilament (so named because the buckling force of the monofilament is 10 grams – 5.07 refers to the gauge of the monofilament that is calculated by the log base 10 of the force expressed in gram-force then plus 4) that is pressed perpendicularly against the plantar aspect of the foot until there is deflection of the monofilament for a duration of 1 second.(16)

- » Testing protocol – There are many variations to locations ranging from 3 to 10 sites. If a patient fails to sense the monofilament after it bends, the site is declared insensate. A recent protocol found the greatest sensitivity (93%) in diagnosing diabetic sensory neuropathy when 3 sites (plantar aspect of great toe and 3rd metatarsal and 5th metatarsal heads) were used. Insensitivity at any one of those sites constituted a positive SWME test.(42) A meta-analysis of the predictive value of SWME with regard to foot ulceration and lower extremity amputation showed that a positive SWME showed a relative risk of developing a diabetic foot ulcer of 2.5–7.9 and a relative risk of lower extremity amputation between 1.7 and 15.1.(43) All patients with a diabetic foot ulcer should get SWME testing as part of their initial assessment. An abnormal test should alert the clinician to counsel the patient on the importance of daily foot inspections and proper podiatric hygiene.

- Vibration – A 128 Hz tuning fork can be used to test vibration sensation by placing the tuning fork on the tip of the great toe. Loss of vibration sensation while the examiner still perceives vibration is an abnormal test. This is an alternative to the SWME for diagnosing peripheral neuropathy.(16)
- Pinprick sensation – The inability to sense pinprick sensation to the dorsum of the hallux is another test of sensory neuropathy. In this test, a disposable pin is placed just proximal to the toenail of the dorsal aspect of the hallux until the skin is deformed. If the patient is unable to detect the pinprick on either hallux, this is abnormal.(16)

Vascular assessments for any patient with a lower extremity wound are mandatory, although interpretation of screening studies may be different for diabetic patients. No single screening study is reliable in identifying or excluding peripheral arterial disease in diabetics.(87) Abnormal screening studies should trigger a vascular surgery consultation, more definitive investigations, and potential interventions prior to, or in conjunction with, initiating HBO_2.

- Pulses – Palpation of the peripheral pedal pulses are only the beginning of the vascular assessment. There are many instances where a palpable pulse is present with significant limb ischemia. Conversely, absence of a pulse does not always identify critical limb ischemia. Pulse palpation has a statistical accuracy of around 60% diagnosing PAD in diabetics without ulceration.(87) The patient should be examined in a warm room, as cold temperatures may cause vasoconstriction. Palpation should be done using the fingertips. Pulses are traditionally rated on a scale of 0–4+, where 0 indicates no pulse, 1+ indicates a faint pulse, 2+ indicates a slightly diminished pulse, 3+ indicates a normal pulse, and 4+ indicates a bounding pulse.(57)

- » Dorsalis pedis (DP) pulse – The dorsal arch of the foot runs in a loop across the distal third of the foot and is an extension of the anterior tibial artery. It is best palpated by standing at the foot of the examination table with fingertips in line with the long axis of the foot.
- » Posterior tibial (PT) pulse – The posterior tibial artery runs just posterior to the medial malleolus. It is best palpated by placing the fingertips in the hollow between the Achilles tendon and the malleolus.
- » Popliteal pulse – A complete lower extremity evaluation will include palpation of the popliteal pulse. The popliteal pulse is best palpated with the knee placed in a relaxed position and wrapping both hands around the knee and placing the fingertips in the popliteal fossa. This may be difficult to appreciate in obese patients.
- » Femoral pulse – The femoral pulse is located in the inguinal region and can be best palpated with the patient in a recumbent position. The tips of the fingertips should be placed in the groin about ⅓ of the distance between the pubic symphysis and the anterior iliac crest. This may be difficult to appreciate in obese patients.

- Doppler pulses – In additional to palpation of pulses, all patients should have auscultation of their pedal pulses using a continuous wave Doppler ultrasound vascular probe in the 8–9 MHz range. Not all pulses are easily auscultated, and approximately 10% of patients have a congenitally absent posterior tibial artery pulse.[57]
    - » To locate the DP artery, start on the mid-dorsum of the foot and track the probe in a proximal-distal axis, crossing the dorsal arch perpendicularly.
    - » To locate the PT artery, start behind the medial malleolus and track the probe in an anterior-posterior axis in order to transect the artery. The pulse is best auscultated when sufficient conduction gel is used and the probe is tilted at a 60° angle so that the ultrasound waves are directed against the oncoming blood flow.
    - » When describing the ausculated pulse, a *triphasic* pulse describes pattern of antegrade, retrograde, then secondary antegrade flow allowed by an elastic arterial wall. A *biphasic* pulse lacks the secondary antegrade phase and is more likely to be found with progressive atherosclerotic changes associated with aging. A *monophasic* waveform indicates progressive disease as inelastic arterial walls limit the speed of the arterial pulses, and further diagnostic testing for peripheral arterial disease is required.
- Ankle-brachial index (ABI) – ABI is a common screening study that is rapidly becoming a lost art in the clinic and hospital setting. It is inexpensive and easily performed with a minimum of equipment (i.e., a continuous wave Doppler ultrasound with vascular probe, ultrasound gel, and a sphygmomanometer with blood pressure cuff) but requires practice and some time. The sensitivity and specificity of ABI in diagnosing PAD is highly variable (sensitivity 29%–100%, specificity 42%–97%) and lowered with concomitant neuropathy and ulceration.

If the ankle pressure is used independently, a threshold of 80 mmHg predicted ulcer healing with 70% sensitivity and 74% specificity.[87]

- » Testing protocols
  - ◊ Resting ABI – The patient is placed in a recumbent position so that the arms and legs are at the same position relative to the heart, and the patient should ideally be in this position for about 10 minutes before testing begins. The blood pressure of the brachial artery, dorsalis pedis artery, and posterior tibial artery should be measured on both extremities using the Doppler ultrasound. The ABI is documented at each pedal pulse by dividing the measured blood pressure by the *higher* of the two brachial artery measurements as the denominator.[54] While traditional reporting of the ABI is to note only the highest pedal pulse on each side, an appreciation of the different angiosomes of the leg may allow better diagnosis and treatment of infrapopliteal disease if both DP and PT ABIs are considered.
  - ◊ Exercise ABI – An ABI with exercise is an option when resting noninvasive studies are normal, but a high suspicion of PAD remains. A general protocol is to have the patient walk on a treadmill at a predetermined speed for up to five minutes. The patient is instructed to inform the technician when he or she starts to feel pain in the legs, but the patient is encouraged to finish the test. The exercise ABI is calculated immediately after completing the treadmill portion of the test. A drop in the ABI to a value ≤ 0.9 is indicative of a hemodynamically significant arterial obstruction. Other criteria include a drop of 30 mmHg or 20% of the baseline ABI with exercise and a delayed (> 3 minutes) recovery.[99]
- » Interpretation – A normal resting ABI ranges from 0.91–1.30. Measurements over 1.30 suggest incompressible arterial walls secondary to calcifications. This is commonly seen in diabetic patients, leading some clinicians to question the ABI as a decision indicator. Measurements between 0.41 and 0.90 indicate mild-moderate disease, and values < 0.40 indicate severe PAD.[54] An ABI of ≤ 0.90 has been demonstrated to have high sensitivity and specificity for the identification of PAD with a sensitivity ranging from 79% to 95% with a specificity of > 95%.[99] The Society for Vascular Surgery Clinical Practice Guideline (CPG) on the management of PAD recommends using the ABI as the initial noninvasive screening test for PAD if there are symptoms or signs of disease. An exercise ABI is recommended if there are symptoms of claudication with borderline or normal ABI > 0.9.[99]
- » Contraindications – The only contraindication for ABI testing is the presence of a deep venous thrombosis (DVT), as compression of the legs may dislodge a thrombus. If DVT is suspected, one should exclude the possibility by obtaining a venous ultrasound of the limb prior to ABI testing.

- » Toe brachial index (TBI) – The arteries of the toes are not subject to the effects of arterial calcifications, and many advocate using TBI as a screening tool in the presence of diabetes mellitus.[58] The sensitivity of using absolute toe pressures of < 30 mmHg to predict wound healing was low (15%–60%), but specificity is high (90%–97%). A TBI of < 0.75 had a sensitivity > 90% and specificity > 60% in diagnosing PAD.[87]
- Skin perfusion pressure (SPP) – SPP uses a laser Doppler for measurement of microvascular perfusion to the skin. A laser probe placed on the skin surface detects the movement of red blood cells in the capillaries of the skin. A blood pressure cuff is placed over the probe and inflated until pulsatile flow ceases. As the cuff is deflated, the laser probe is able to detect the return of perfusion to the skin. SPP has been used as a diagnostic tool for critical limb ischemia with an overall sensitivity of diagnosing critical limb ischemia of 80%.[26] Measurements of 30 mmHg are used as the threshold below which wounds are not expected to heal, and SPP has a positive predictive value (PPV) that a wound will not heal of 75% and a negative predictive value (NPV) that a wound will heal of 83%. Using a cutoff of 30 mmHg, the NPV for healing minor (e.g., forefoot or toe amputation) and major amputation (e.g., amputation at the knee or above) was 75% and 100% respectively for measurements < 30 mmHg. The PPV for healing minor and major amputations was 66.7% and 83% respectively for SPP values > 30 mmHg.[2] Postintervention SPP has been shown to correlate with amputation free survival, freedom from major adverse limb event (i.e., major amputation or reintervention), and wound healing one year following endovascular therapy for CLI, while postintervention ABI did not.[85]
- Transcutaneous oxygen measurement ($TcPO_2$) – Direct measurement of tissue oxygenation with a transcutaneous probe gives a measurement of wound oxygenation. A value of 30 mmHg is generally accepted as the cutoff for a diagnosis of CLI and triggers a more aggressive vascular evaluation. When using a threshold of 30 mmHg, $TcPO_2$ was 60% sensitive and 87% specific in predicting CLI. If this threshold is dropped to 25 mmHg, the sensitivity and specificity increase to 85% and 92% respectively.[87] When used in conjunction with adjunctive HBO_2, room air measurements do not predict who will or will not respond to HBO_2, whereas a $TcPO_2$ measurement greater than 200 mmHg under hyperbaric conditions correlated with healing almost 90% of diabetic foot ulcers.[77]
- Fluorescence angiography – Indocyanine green fluorescence angiography (ICFA) is a technology that shows some promise in evaluating wound healing potential. Global microvascular flow is visualized directly rather than estimated through surrogates like the $TcPO_2$ or SPP. Although there are no objective cutoff values that accurately predict wound healing or failure, the technology can be used to identify areas of wound ischemia, allowing more rapid and appropriate clinical decision-making. Serial use of ICFA allows objective demonstration of healing and perfusion improvement, as well as demonstrating clinical efficacy of various interventions (e.g., HBO_2, reperfusion, and debridement).

No single vascular screening assessment is effective in predicting wound healing. The International Working Group on the Diabetic Foot (IWGDF) published a 2016 systematic review for patients with DFU. Measuring skin perfusion pressures, toe pressures, and $TcPO_2$ appears to be more useful in predicting ulcer healing than ankle pressures or the ABI. Conversely, an ankle pressure of < 50 mmHg or an ABI < 0.5 is associated with a significant increase in the incidence of major amputation.(20)

IMAGING STUDIES

Imaging studies may also be needed as part of the work-up of the DFU. Not all of these studies are required, but individual studies should be considered if there is sufficient clinical suspicion to warrant them. Making the diagnosis of osteomyelitis may sometimes turn into a Melvillian obsession for practitioners, as some payers require radiographic documentation before authorizing HBO_2.

- Plain Radiographs – Patients presenting de novo to the hyperbaric physician need radiographs of the foot to rule out foreign bodies and occult fractures and to establish a baseline for comparison. If a wound is not healing, repeat imaging may show changes such as an evolving Charcot arthropathy or bony erosions suggesting osteomyelitis. Plain radiographs have a sensitivity of 54%, a specificity of 68%, and an odds ratio of 2.84 of diagnosing osteomyelitis,(31) but interobserver and intraobserver reliability is dependent on the experience of the clinician reading the X-ray.(6)
- MRI – If osteomyelitis is suspected, an MRI is the test of choice. With modern MRI technology, however, MRI can overestimate the incidence of osteomyelitis. MRI has a sensitivity of 90%, a specificity of 79%, and an odds ratio of 24.36 of diagnosing osteomyelitis.(31)
- Bone Scan – Nuclear medicine has been largely replaced by MRI in making the diagnosis of osteomyelitis, but it is sometimes the only option if patients have contrast allergies or other contraindications for MRI. Bone scan has a sensitivity of 81%, a specificity of 28%, and an odds ratio of 2.10 of diagnosing osteomyelitis. This can be improved by using a tagged leukocyte bone scan, which has a sensitivity of 74%, a specificity of 68%, and an odds ratio of 10.07 of diagnosing osteomyelitis.(31)

TABLE 1. META-ANALYSIS OF THE ACCURACY OF DIAGNOSTIC TESTS FOR OSTEOMYELITIS IN DIABETIC PATIENTS WITH FOOT ULCERS(31)

EVALUATION	SENSITIVITY	SPECIFICITY	ODDS RATIO
Probe-to-Bone	0.60	0.91	49.45
Radiography	0.54	0.68	2.84
MRI	0.90	0.79	24.36
Bone Scan	0.81	0.28	2.10
Leukocyte Scan	0.74	0.68	10.07

Probe-to-Bone Test

The probe-to-bone (PTB) test deserves special discussion. It has been a controversial tool that has the potential of being abused in the interest of establishing a diagnosis of osteomyelitis to qualify patients for HBO_2. It is generally accepted that the PTB test is conducted using a sterile, blunt-tipped metal probe to explore the wound, but there is surprising inter-rater disagreement on a positive PTB depending on the level of experience of the clinician. When first introduced in 1995, Grayson reported a sensitivity of 66%, specificity of 85%, PPV of 89%, and NPV of 56%.(53) According to Grayson, palpable bone was detected if a rock-hard, gritty surface was discovered upon gentle probing of the base of the ulcer without any intervening soft tissue.(53) A 2006 study, however, noted significantly worse sensitivity of 38%, similar specificity of 91%, worse PPV of 53%, and superior NPV of 85%.(97) This was followed by Lavery's study in 2007 that showed the PTB test was highly sensitive (87%) and specific (91%), but with PPV of only 0.57 and a NPV of 0.98. He suggested that a negative PTB was more significant than a positive PTB in the diagnosis of osteomyelitis.(63) A 2008 meta-analysis showed that a positive PTB test had a sensitivity of 60%, a specificity of 91%, and an odds ratio of 49.45 of diagnosing osteomyelitis, superior to all imaging studies.(31) A 2016 systematic review of 7 studies was less enthusiastic, concluding that pooled sensitivity and specificity for the PTB test was 87% and 83%, respectively. They also concluded that the PTB test can accurately rule in diabetic foot osteomyelitis in the high-risk patients and rule out osteomyelitis in low-risk patients.(62) Indeed, the prevalence of osteomyelitis in the study population varied from a low of 60% to a high of 85%, corresponding with higher and lower sensitivity and specificity numbers.

TABLE 2. SUMMARY OF PROBE TO BONE STUDIES

STUDY	SENS (%)	SPEC (%)	PPV	NPV	INCIDENCE OF OM
Grayson (1995)(52)	66	85	0.89	0.56	61.5
Shone (2006)(94)	38	91	0.53	0.85	23.5
Lavery (2007)(62)	87	91	0.57	0.98	75.9
Morales-Lozano (2010)(78)	98	78	0.95	0.91	79.5
Aragon-Sanchez (2011)(9)	97	92	0.97	0.93	85.2
Mutlouglu (2012)(81)	66	84	0.87	0.62	60

Sens – Sensitivity, Spec – Specificity, PPV – Positive Predictive Value, NPV – Negative Predictive Value, OM – Osteomyelitis

While the diagnosis of osteomyelitis is an important objective, making the diagnosis should trigger a comprehensive approach that includes surgical debridement, culture-directed antibiotics, and good wound care prior to considering HBO_2. Association between the PTB test and osteomyelitis as described is restricted to the diabetic foot with a chronic ulcer (versus acute postoperative foot or sacral pressure ulcers), although its presence in other ulcers is not likely a good prognostic sign. A meta-analysis of diagnostic criteria concluded that the following criteria were helpful in diagnosing lower extremity osteomyelitis in diabetics:

- an ulcer > 2 cm^2,
- a positive probe-to-bone test,
- an elevated erythrocyte sedimentation rate > 70 mm/h, and
- an abnormal plain radiograph.

A negative MRI makes the diagnosis much less likely, especially when all of the above findings are absent. There is no single historical feature or physical finding that reliably excludes osteomyelitis, and there is no data on the utility of combinations of the above findings in making a diagnosis of osteomyelitis.(24)

LABORATORY STUDIES

A complete laboratory workup should include the following:

- Complete Blood Count – This allows for screening of acute infection and leukocytosis, as well as determining the oxygen-carrying capacity of the available hemoglobin in the blood. Hemoglobin levels less than 10 grams and hematocrit less than 30% have corresponded with decreased ability to oxygenate tissue, and some have advocated transfusions in this situation.
- Hemoglobin A1c – While one should always strive for good metabolic control, it is not always possible to maintain optimal blood sugar concentrations. Attempts to deny therapeutic modalities to patients because of high HbA1c are misguided, as there is no evidence to suggest that patients with high HbA1c are unable to heal wounds or respond to therapy.(75)
- Estimated Average Glucose – Although there are many objections to the validity of this mathematically derived estimate of average glucose,(27,56,64,89,114) this conversion of the hemoglobin A1c to an average glucose in mg/dl is thought to be more relatable to patients. It is commonly provided automatically with HgA1c levels – the formula to determine the eAG is 28.7 x HbA1c – 46.7.(82)
- Albumin – This has been used in the past as a marker of *chronic* nutritional support, with the thinking that albumin levels reflected the available protein for wound healing over the last several months. Recent findings suggest that this is an acute negative phase reactant that can be falsely low in the acute inflammatory phase of disease.(34,46,61,98,104)
- Prealbumin – This has been used in the past as a marker of *acute* nutritional support, suggesting that prealbumin levels reflected the available protein for wound healing over the last several weeks. Like albumin, recent findings show that prealbumin may not be accurate in the setting of acute inflammation.(3,30)
- Erythrocyte Sedimentation Rate and C-Reactive Protein – These have been used for making the diagnosis and monitoring resolution of osteomyelitis.(24) The utility of the testing is usually better for monitoring resolution than making the diagnosis of osteomyelitis.(106-107)

CLASSIFICATION OF DFU

There are many scales that attempt to classify diabetic foot ulcers, but few have been validated and none have demonstrated prognostic reliability or accuracy with regard to healing a DFU.(76) Some scales focus on anatomy (depth of ulcer), some include vascular assessment, and others include the presence or absence of infection.

Each scale has its strengths and weaknesses, trading ease of use for clinically relevant categories for decision-making. Additionally, it is often unclear if the classification scale was developed for research, audit, or clinical care.[47] Here is a look at the most commonly used classification scales currently in use.

Wagner

Wagner created his eponymous grading system in 1981 in conjunction with Bernard Meggitt through observation of the progress of wounds from callus to ulcer, abscess, gangrene, and finally surgical ablation. The system uses 6 grades from 0–5 based on the depth of the skin lesion and the absence or presence of infection (Table 3).[110] Wagner has been criticized for ignoring vascular status in his grading system, but many users of the Wagner grade are unaware that Wagner's treatment algorithms incorporated vascular assessment using ABI to determine the management of the DFU. In fact, he spends 12 of the 61 pages of his original manuscript describing the evaluation and management of vascular disease as a key component of treatment of the dysvascular foot.[101] Despite this, the fact that there is no inclusion of PAD in the actual grading system means most DFUs are clinically classified into Wagner Grade 2 or 3 ulcers, which is insufficiently precise to separate most lesions.[47] In hyperbaric medicine, however, Wagner's grading system is the only one that has been used in clinical research and has been incorporated into the requirements for reimbursement. This leaves the clinician with no other choice at this time.[60] The unintended consequence of linking reimbursement for HBO_2 with the Wagner scale is the application of the Wagner Grade 3 grade to wounds in order to qualify a patient for HBO_2 versus using the Wagner Grade 3 in accordance with the original Wagner management algorithm. For instance, CMS lists a Wagner Grade 3 ulcer as a requirement to receive HBO_2 only when the wound has failed to respond to 30 days of conservative therapy. According to the definition of a Wagner 3 ulcer, this could be a patient with an ulcer that has been present for over 30 days and has radiographically documented osteomyelitis of a phalanx or metatarsal head, or a fluctuant, acutely infected foot needing acute surgical intervention. While both conditions have been shown to respond to HBO_2, they are different clinical entities that are not adequately represented by Wagner's grading system or original description. Wagner wrote that the Grade 3 foot almost always had more deep infection than was apparent from external examination, and careful dissection of ray and midfoot amputations was required to ensure there was no diseased or necrotic tissue left behind. [110]

This mismatch has led to both overutilization and underutilization of HBO_2 in the treatment of DFU.[60,101] When used as a predictor of wound healing, both amputation and wound healing failure increased with grade (Table 4).[86]

University of Texas

The University of Texas classification system (Table 5) combines the presence or absence of infection and perfusion in a vertical scale and the depth of the wound on a horizontal scale to generate a 16-choice matrix.[10] As depth of the wound and the severity of infection and ischemia increase, both amputation and wound healing failure increase. A comparison of the UT versus the Wagner system shows that the UT system is more descriptive and shows a greater association with wound healing and amputation prediction.[86]

TABLE 3. WAGNER GRADING SYSTEM(60)

Classic Wagner Grading System	6 grades based on anatomy and presence of infection	Grade 0. No open lesion, may have healed lesions Grade 1. Superficial ulcer without penetration to deeper layers Grade 2. Deeper ulcer, reaching tendon, bone, or joint capsule Grade 3. Deeper tissues are involved, and there is abscess, osteomyelitis, or tendonitis Grade 4. There is gangrene of some part of the toe, toes, and/or forefoot Grade 5. Gangrene involves the whole foot or enough of the foot that no local procedures are possible and BKA is indicated

TABLE 4. CORRELATION OF WAGNER GRADE WITH CLINICAL OUTCOME(86,110)

GRADE	DESCRIPTION[1]	N/AMP/ UNHEALED[2]
0	Intact skin, may have bony deformities	NA
1	Superficial ulcer, base may be necrotic or viable with granulation tissue	131, 8%, 11%
2	Deeper ulcer and extends to bone, ligament, tendon, joint capsule or deep fascia. There is no abscess or osteomyelitis	25, 24%, 20%
3	Progression of the previous lesions to deep abscess, osteitis, or osteomyelitis	36, 36%, 20%
4	Some portion of forefoot or toes is gangrenous	2, 50%, 50%
5	Complete involvement such that no healing or local procedure is possible	NA

[1] Wagner FW. Orthopedics. 1987;10:163-72.
[2] Oyibo SO et al. Diabetes Care. 2001;24:84-8.

TABLE 5. UNIVERSITY OF TEXAS GRADING SYSTEM(60)

University of Texas Health Science Center at San Antionio	4 stages based on absence or presence of ischemia and infection	Stage A: no infection Stage B: infection Stage C: ischemia Stage D: infection and ischemia
	4 grades based on extent and depth of wound	Grade 0: epithelialized wound Grade 1: superficial wound Grade 2: wound penetrating tendon or capsule Grade 3: wound penetrating bone or joint

TABLE 6. CORRELATION OF UT GRADE WITH CLINICAL OUTCOME[10,86]

STAGE	GRADE	0 Pre- or Post-ulcerative lesion	1 Superficial into dermis	2 Through dermis to SQ, muscle, tendon, or capsule	3 Penetrates to Bone
A	Not infected Not Ischemic	NA	87, 3%, 9%*	3, 0%, 0%	1, 0%, 0%
B	Infected	NA	12, 17%, 0%	14, 14%, 14%	25, 40%, 20%
C	Ischemic	NA	18, 17%, 17%	4, 0%, 25%	0, 0%, 0%
D	Infected & Ischemic	NA	14, 14%, 29%	8, 50%, 25%	8, 50%, 38%

*n, amp, unhealed

TABLE 7. RISK OF AMPUTATION USING UT SYSTEM[90]

STAGE	GRADE	0 Pre- or Post-ulcerative lesion	1 Superficial into dermis	2 Through dermis to SQ, muscle, tendon, or capsule	3 Penetrates to Bone
A	Not infected Not Ischemic	0%	0%	0%	N/A
B	Infected	12.50%	8.50%	28.60%	92%
C	Ischemic	25%	20%	25%	100%
D	Infected & Ischemic	50%	50%	100%	100%

TABLE 8. INFECTIOUS DISEASE SOCIETY OF AMERICA GRADING SYSTEM[60]

IDSA (Infectious Disease Society of America)	4 grades 4 IDSA levels of severity based on severity of infection	Grade 1. Infection with at least two of following criteria: swelling, erythema, pain, warmth, purulent discharge; PEDIS 1; IDSA infection severity: uninfected Grade 2. Local infection involving skin and subcutaneous tissue with erythema >0.5 cm and < 2 cm around ulcer; PEDIS 2; IDSA infection severity: mild Grade 3. Local infection with > 2 cm or involving structures deeper to skin and subcutaneous tissue with no signs of systemic inflammation; PEDIS 3: IDSA infection severity: moderate Grade 4. Local infection with systemic inflammation response signs (SIRS) with two or more of the following criteria: temp. > 38 degrees or < 36 degrees, heart rate > 90 beats/min, $PaCO_2$ < 32 mmHg, white blood count (WBC) > 12,000 or < 4000 cells/microliter or > 10% immature band forms; PEDIS 4: IDSA infection severity: severe

IDSA

The Infectious Disease Society of America (IDSA) bases its classification system (Table 8) on the severity of diabetic foot infections and shows an increasing trend for more frequent and higher levels of amputation compared with the seriousness of infection.[68]

IWGDF

The International Working Group on the Diabetic Foot (IWGDF) attempted to address all of the relevant comorbidities contributing to the pathology of a diabetic foot ulcer by developing a classification system (Table 9) for research purposes based on five key categories: perfusion, extent/size, depth/tissue loss, infection, and sensation (PEDIS).[93] While this has been used in research, it has been infrequently applied in daily clinical practice.

TABLE 9. IWGDF GRADING SYSTEM[60]

International Working Group on the Diabetic Foot	Five categories, scored based on different criteria	**Perfusion** Grade 1: no signs/symptoms of PAD Grade 2: Symptoms or signs of PAD, but not of critical limb ischemia (CLI) Grade 3: Critical limb ischemia as defined by systolic ankle blood pressure <50 mmHg or systolic toe blood pressure <30 mmHg or $tcpO_2$< 30 mmHg.
		Extent/size No scoring system was provided. Recommendations were that wounds should be measured after debridement and that the frequency distribution of the size of the ulcers should be reported in each study as quartiles.
		Depth/tissue loss Grade 1: Superficial full-thickness ulcer, not penetrating any structure deeper than the dermis. Grade 2: Deep ulcer, penetrating below the dermis to subcutaneous structures, involving fascia, muscle or tendon Grade 3: All subsequent layers of the foot involved, including bone and/or joint (exposed bone, probing to bone)
		Infection Grade 1: No symptoms or signs of infection Grade 2: Infection involving the skin and the subcutaneous tissue only (without involvement of deeper tissues and without systemic signs) Grade 3: Erythema >2 cm plus one of the items described above (swelling, tenderness, warmth, discharge) or infection involving structures deeper than skin and subcutaneous tissues such as abscess, osteomyelitis, septic arthritis, fasciitis. No systemic inflammatory response signs, as described below Grade 4: Any foot infection with the following signs of a systemic inflammatory response syndrome. This response is manifested by two or more of the following conditions: Temperature >38 or <36°C; Heart rate >90 beats/min; Respiratory rate >20 breaths/min; $PaCO_2$ <32-mmHg; White blood cell count >12,000 or<4,000/cu mm; 10% immature (band) forms.
		Sensation Grade 1: No loss of protective sensation on the affected foot detected, defined as the presence of sensory modalities described below. Grade 2: Loss of protective sensation on the affected foot is defined as the absence of perception of one of the following tests in the affected foot: • Absent pressure sensation, determined with a 10-g monofilament, on two out of three sites on the plantar side of the foot, as described in the International Consensus on the Diabetic Foot. • Absent vibration sensation, (determined with a 128-Hz tuning fork) or vibration threshold >25 V (using semi-quantitative techniques), both tested on the hallux

Long Beach Wound Score

In an attempt to combine the most important features from multiple scoring systems, Dr. Michael B. Strauss described a system (Table 10) using an easy-to-derive, intuitive 0-to-10 scoring system in order to make logical decisions between limb salvage or major amputation. While not widely used, it demonstrates good inter-rater reliability and is easy to apply – both essential elements of a useful wound score.[102-103] Studies validating its use in predicting wound healing are underway.

TABLE 10. LONG BEACH WOUND SCORE[60]

Long Beach Wound Score	Five assessments, each graded from 0 – 2 points (half points used for mixed or intermediate findings) **Healthy Wound** 7-½ – 10 points **Problem Wound** 3-½– 7 points **Futile Wound** 0 – 3 points	**Appearance (Wound Base)** 2 points for Red 1 point for White (biofilm-fibrous membrane)/Yellow (exudate) 0 points for Black (necrotic, wet gangrene or fluctuant eschar)
		Size 2 points for Less than the surface area of patient's thumbprint 1 point for Thumbprint to fist-size 0 points for Larger than fist size
		Depth (including maximum depth of probe) 2 points for Skin coverage and 1-½ points for Subcutaneous tissue 1 point for Muscle and/or Tendon 0 points for Bone and/or Joint
		Bioburden 2 points for Colonized 1 point for Cellulitis, maceration, and/or deep infection (bone, joint, bursa, or cicatrix) 0 points for Septic (unstable blood sugars, leukocytosis, positive blood cultures, fever, chills)
		Perfusion (use secondary findings of color, temperature & capillary refill if exam obscured by edema, scar, hidebound skin and/or previous surgery) 2 points for Palpable pulses 1 point for Biphasic or Triphasic Dopplerable pulses (cool, pale or dusky, capillary refill 2-5 seconds) 0 points for Monophasic or Imperceptible pulses (cold, black/cyanotic/purplish, capillary refill >5 seconds)

WIfI

The Society for Vascular Surgery (Table 11) published risk stratification based on three major factors that impact amputation risk and clinical management – wound, ischemia, and foot infection (WIfI) – to generate a matrix of 32 permutations of wound categories that generally have worse outcomes as one moves down and to the right.[74]

TABLE 11. WIFI WOUND SYSTEM[60]

Society for Vascular Surgery Wound Ischemia foot Infection (WIfI) System	4 grades for each of three criteria of wound, ischemia, and foot infection (WIfI)	**Wound** Grade 0: no ulcer or gangrene Grade 1: shallow ulcer; no gangrene Grade 2: deeper ulcer with exposed joint or tendon; gangrene limited to digits Grade 3: deep ulcer involving forefoot, midfoot, heel; extensive gangrene involving forefoot, midfoot, or heel
		Ischemia Grade 0: ABI ≥ 0.80; Arterial Systemic Pressure >100 mmHg; and/or $TcPO_2$ ≥ 60 mmHg Grade 1: ABI 0.6-0.79; Arterial Systemic Pressure 70-100 mmHg; and/or $TcPO_2$ 40-59 mmHg Grade 2: ABI 0.4-0.59; Arterial Systemic Pressure 50-70 mmHg; and/or $TcPO_2$ 30-39 mmHg Grade 3: ABI ≤ 0.39; Arterial Systemic Pressure 50-70 mmHg; and/or $TcPO_2$ <30 mmHg
		Infection Grade 0: Uninfected no signs or symptoms Grade 1: Local infection erythema > 0.5 cm and ≤ 2 cm with pain, warmth, purulent discharge (mild) Grade 2: Local infection with > 2 cm erythema, involves deeper structures (moderate) Grade 3: Local infection with signs of SIRS (refer to IDSA definition) (severe)

Wound Healing Index (WHI)

A different approach to generating a wound score involves mining a wound care registry for factors associated with healing. Data from over 50,000 wounds in the U.S. Wound Registry were analyzed to identify 10 factors that were associated with wound healing in DFUs.[59] These were then used to calculate a WHI between 0 and 100 and tested prospectively to predict healing of the diabetic foot ulcer. In an analysis of over 5000 diabetic foot ulcers, the percentage of wounds that healed with a WHI of < 33, 34–67, or > 67 were 35.3%, 50.1%, and 72.8% respectively.[45] This was calculated at the time of first presentation without considering any treatment modalities employed. The score is only calculable by using an integrated EHR. In a world where EHRs, Meaningful Use, quality measures, and outcomes reporting are becoming requirements for reimbursement, we may see that this is the wave of the future with regard to resource allocation for advanced therapies.

TABLE 12. QUESTIONS TO PRODUCE DIABETIC FOOT ULCER WOUND HEALING INDEX[45] used with permission of Dr. Caroline Fife

NUMBER	QUESTION
1	Patient age in years (calculated from date of birth) at first treatment
2	Wound age (duration) in days (calculated from wound onset) at first encounter
3	Wound area in cm^2 (calculated from length x width) at first encounter
4	What is the patient's primary ambulatory method? (walks unaided, cane, crutches, walker, roll about, scooter, wheelchair bound, bed bound)
5	Was the patient admitted to the hospital or the emergency department on the date of service?
6	How many total wounds or ulcers of any type does the patient have?
7	Does this wound have evidence of infection or bioburden? (evidenced by purulent, green, malodorous drainage, periwound induration, tenderness to palpation, warmth)
8	Is the patient on dialysis or status post renal transplant?
9	What is the Wagner grade of the ulcer (1-5)?
10	Does the patient have peripheral vascular disease (claudication, rest pain, abnormal arterial vascular studies, loss of pulses)?

Given the wide variety of wound scoring scales available, one must consider the reason for using them in the first place. Some allow the clinician to risk-stratify patients to determine who is at greatest risk of wound healing failure or amputation, while others have been relegated as a justification for employing therapeutic modalities that would otherwise be denied reimbursement. At this time, there is no single grading system that meets both needs. Future hyperbaric research using specific grading criteria are required before we can see alternatives to the Wagner grading system with regard to utilization of HBO_2.

MANAGEMENT OF THE DIABETIC FOOT

Patients who develop a DFU have a significant risk of major amputation and have an increased mortality rate.[39] The etiology of the diabetic foot ulcers can be neuropathic, neuroischemic, or both. The reasons for nonhealing are multifactorial, involving both local and systemic factors. As such, management must address all of these factors and requires a multidisciplinary approach. Important team members include the wound care specialist, primary care physician, endocrinologist, podiatrist, orthotist, vascular interventionalist, foot and ankle surgeon, infectious disease specialist, and hyperbaric medicine specialist. Algorithms for the systematic evaluation and treatment of patients with DFU and CLI are essential elements for a successful limb salvage program.[39]

Vascular intervention is an important part of management when PAD is present. Multiple diagnostic tools have been discussed in order to identify PAD. When vascular disease is identified, patients should be referred to a vascular surgeon or interventionalist for further evaluation and revascularization. This may be through either endovascular approach or open surgical bypass approach. The type of revascularization is dependent on severity of arterial disease and ischemia, ulcer severity and presence of infection, and level of expertise.[58] Revascularization in patients with a DFU and PAD has been shown to improve healing rates and decrease amputation rates.[20,58,109] While this is especially true in the case of CLI (critical limb ischemia), there is also evidence this is true in the case of less severe PAD.[109] The Society for Vascular Surgery WIfI score (Table 6)[74] has been validated as a predictor of amputation and nonhealing. Both Zahn et al. and Cull et al. published data demonstrating higher WIfI scores had statistically significant correlation with higher amputation rates and prolonged nonhealing.[29,113] As such, the WIfI score may be useful in assisting the vascular surgeon with determining if and what type of revascularization is necessary.

Off-loading the diabetic foot ulcer is a cornerstone of wound care management. There are several options available to off-load a plantar neuropathic diabetic foot ulcer. Nonremovable off-loading devices have been shown to be more effective than removable devices.[21-23,28] As such, patients with plantar neuropathic diabetic foot ulcers who are without ischemia or uncontrolled infection need a nonremovable knee-high device.[22] Devices recommended in this category include the total contact cast (TCC) and irremovable fixed ankle walking boot.[58] There was a significantly higher relative risk ratio of 1.43 for nonremovable devices to promote healing compared with removable devices (95% CI 1.11–1.84, $p = 0.001$).[79] A Cochrane Systematic Review by Lewis and Lipp also found that nonremovable devices were superior to removable devices. There was a significantly higher relative risk ratio of 1.17 for nonremovable devices compared to removable devices (95% CI 1.01–1.36, $p = 0.04$).[65] When a nonremovable device cannot be worn, the most effective of removable devices was found to be a knee-high cast walker followed by a half or heel shoe, the least effective being a therapeutic postoperative shoe.[55] Another option that has not been studied but may be an option for a patient who cannot wear a nonremovable device is the "soft total contact cast" developed by Desmond Bell, DPM.[13-14]

When patients have non-plantar neuropathic foot ulcers it is recommended that one use whichever modality will relieve pressure at the site of the ulcer.[58] Finally, prevention is important in patients who have a history of a DFU. They should receive custom molded diabetic shoes fit by a pedorthist.[23]

Infection control is another important aspect in the management of the diabetic foot ulcer. Diabetics are more prone to serious infection due to a blunted immune response, and their presentation may not have the classical signs of inflammatory response. Infection develops in over half of diabetic foot ulcers and is a factor most often leading to lower extremity amputation.[105] All patients should receive a probe-to-bone test upon initial evaluation and serial radiographic studies. MRI (white blood cell scan and bone scan when MRI not possible) should be performed only as deemed necessary by the wound care specialist.[58,67] Primary treatment typically includes both bone debridement with bone culture/histology in addition to a course of antibiotic therapy.[58,67] When there is no bone debridement, there is a strong recommendation for bone biopsy if there is inadequate culture information or failure to response to empiric antibiotics.[58, 67] A systematic review of treatment for diabetic foot infection (DFI) by Peters et al. looked at 37 randomized controlled trials (RCTs) and 3 cohort studies. It found that "systematic review revealed little evidence upon which to make recommendations for treatment of DFI. There is a great need for further well designed trials."[88] There was no strong evidence of support for topical treatment with antiseptics. In the case of skin and soft-tissue infections, the antibiotic treatment regimens compared were broadly equivalent. Studies that looked at osteomyelitis found no definitive studies on which to base an ideal treatment regimen. There are studies that suggest equivalence of surgery and short-course antibiotics compared to prolonged antibiotic treatment course. No significant difference has been demonstrated between different antibiotic regimens or comparing oral versus parenteral route. Finally, there was evidence of better outcomes with bone biopsy culture over soft-tissue culture.[88]

Promotion of tight glycemic control is considered another important component in the treatment of the diabetic foot ulcer. Tight glycemic control decreases risk of diabetic complications such as peripheral neuropathy and vascular disease.[100] Intuitively, this is also thought to apply to the successful treatment of diabetic foot ulcers. Nonetheless, a 2016 Cochrane Review did not find any completed RCT's supporting this. They were unable to conclude whether intensive glycemic control was superior to conventional glycemic control in promoting healing of diabetic foot ulcers.[44] The authors did note there was evidence that intensive glycemic control had been shown to reduce the risk of amputation from various causes in those with type 2 diabetes mellitus. A study by Boyko et al. in 2006 demonstrated an increased risk of diabetic foot ulcer occurrence over 1 and 5 year intervals with each 1% increase in HgbA1c. Those with no ulcer had a mean HgbA1c of 9.5% ± 3.0 versus those with incidence ulcer who had a mean of 11.8% ± 3.4.[17] In addition, another study found an increased risk of ulcer recurrence with poorer glycemic control (mean 7.6% ± 1.2 without recurrence versus 8.5% ± 1.7 with recurrence). While control of blood sugar is a laudable goal, recent regulatory proposals sought to limit access to HBO_2 only for patients with good glycemic control even though there is evidence that patients with elevated blood sugar can go on to heal.[12,75] Furthermore, tight glucose control is not necessarily a benign act – the ACCORD study showed that intensive control of blood sugar to get HbA1c < 7 was associated with a higher incidence of death.[1] Clearly there are significant psychological and socioeconomic factors that impact a provider's ability to promote tight glycemic control in many patients with a diabetic foot ulcer. Sequential counseling and appropriate treatment team members including the primary care physician, endocrinologist, and possibly nutritionist play an important role.

Another hallmark in the management of the diabetic foot ulcer is serial debridement. This allows removal of nonviable tissue, reducing bioburden and risk of infection and leading to promotion of wound healing.[40,58] DFUs should undergo serial bedside surgical debridement at intervals of 1–4 weeks based on provider clinical judgment.[58] A systematic review and meta-analysis found 11 RCTs and

3 nonrandomized studies.[40] Studies support the efficacy of serial debridement, but the comparative effectiveness evidence was of low quality. As a result, the type of debridement is at the physician's discretion.[40,52,58] There were 3 RCTs that showed autolytic debridement significantly increased healing rates. There were four studies (one RCT) that showed larval debridement reduced amputation rates but did not improve healing rates. Finally, there was one RCT that showed surgical debridement shortened healing time compared to conventional wound care.[40,58]

Good local wound care involves the use of wound care products that maintain a moist wound bed while managing excessive exudates and avoiding maceration and damage to the surrounding periwound skin.[49,58] An optimal local wound dressing provides autolytic debridement, prevents infection, and promotes wound healing.[49,58] Wet-to-dry dressings with saline-soaked gauze are not recommended as they cause nonselective debridement harming viable tissue and impeding healing.[49,58] Four Cochrane Reviews in 2013 found no superior benefit to hydrogels, hydrocolloids, foams, or alginates in the treatment of DFUs.[35-38] A 2016 systematic review and meta-analysis found moderate-quality evidence that hydrogels were more effective in healing DFUs compared to basic wound contact dressings. Comparison of other dressing types did not show any statistically significant difference in healing DFUs. Nonadherent dressings were more cost effective than hydrofiber dressings.[92] NPWT is recommended for DFUs that fail to progress despite four to eight weeks of advanced wound dressings; a systematic review reported one multicenter RCT that demonstrated DFUs healed faster, had less home care, and had fewer secondary amputations with NPWT.[58] The final recommendation is that the choice of dressing should be tailored to the patient and wound.[49,58,92]

Adjunctive therapies should be considered if the DFU has failed to improve at least 50% after all previously described standard-of-care practices have been implemented for a minimum of four weeks.[48,58] These may include NPWT (previously discussed), biologics, and HBO_2 (discussed in Chapter 23: Adjunctive Hyperbaric Oxygen Therapy for Diabetic Foot Ulcer). Biologics include topical growth factor PDGF, skin substitute products derived from autologous skin (single-layer and bilayered), placental-derived products, porcine-derived products, and cadaveric-derived products. Human-derived products from neonatal foreskin have been shown in RCTs to increase healing rates in recalcitrant diabetic foot ulcers despite standard wound care.[48,58] While split-thickness skin grafting is used for nonhealing diabetic foot ulcers, there are no strong methodological studies to support their general use in the treatment of diabetic foot ulcers.[48]

THE MULTIDISCIPLINARY LIMB SALVAGE TEAM

Limb salvage centers have come en vogue as hospitals recognize the high costs associated with treating diabetic patients with lower extremity wounds. Cynics would argue that limb salvage centers were created to realize the increased revenue from additional interventions performed, while supporters argue that prevention of an amputation using evidence-based decisions improves long-term quality of life and reduces overall costs.[39] A 2016 retrospective cohort review of 159 patients with DFU who were managed with an evidence-based limb salvage protocol (Figure 4) including HBO_2 showed that 91.7% of patients who received the limb salvage protocol had intact extremities after a year with a cost of USD$33,100 and mortality rate of 35.4%, while those who had primary amputation without the limb salvage protocol had a cost ranging from USD$66,300 (minor amputation) to USD$73,000 (major amputation) and a mortality rate of 47.2%.(39) Experienced clinicians recognize the importance of a stepwise approach to addressing the ischemic, diabetic lower extremity wound and have built multidisciplinary teams for key components of care in an organized, thoughtful algorithm.(39) These teams should include wound specialists, vascular interventionalists, and podiatry, endocrinology, infectious disease, and hyperbaric medicine specialists. This approach should focus on vascular assessment and intervention (endovascular or open) when indicated, off-loading (total contact cast or removable cast walker), infection control, blood sugar control, surgical debridement, and local care that attains an appropriate moist wound healing environment. These fundamental components of limb salvage can be remembered using a simple **V**ascular, **O**ff-loading, **I**nfection control, **D**iabetes control, and **S**urgical debridement (VOIDS) mnemonic. Serial wound measurements allow for objective decision-making regarding treatment options by analyzing the wound trajectory and reduction of the wound surface area. Systematic reviews of wound trajectory have led to recommendations that patients whose ulcer surface area reduces by < 50% at 4 weeks should receive adjunctive therapy that may include negative-pressure wound therapy, cellular tissue products, and HBO_2.(58)

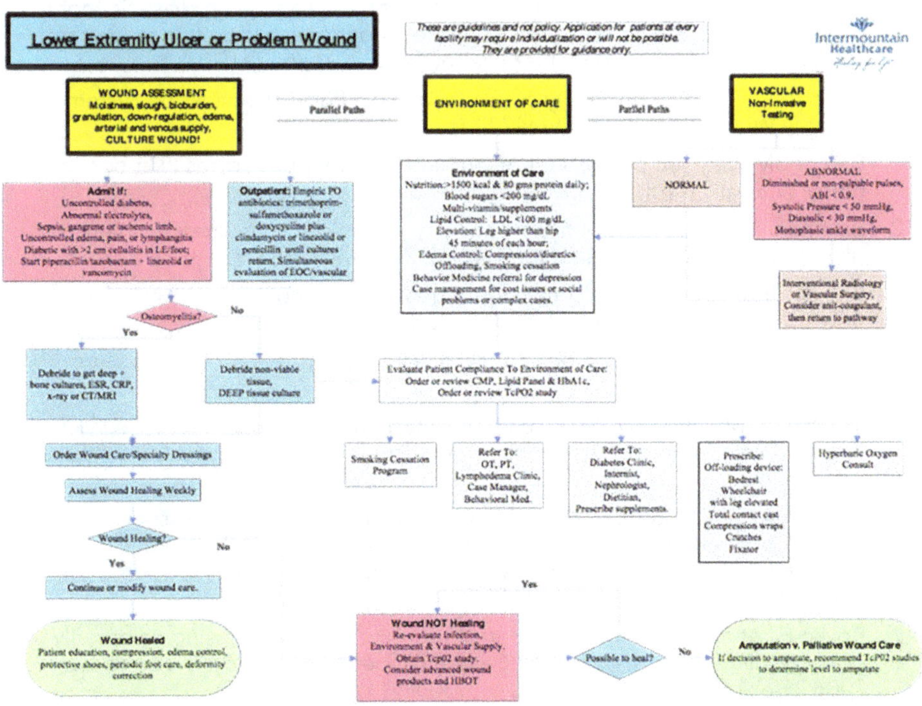

Figure 4. Algorithm courtesy of Eggert JV, Worth ER, Van Gils CC. Cost and mortality data of a regional limb salvage and hyperbaric medicine program for Wagner Grade 3 or 4 diabetic foot ulcers.(39)

REFERENCES

1. Action to Control Cardiovascular Risk in Diabetes Study Group et al. Effects of intensive glucose lowering in type 2 diabetes. N Engl J Med. 2008;358(24):2545-59.
2. Adera HM et al. Prediction of amputation wound healing with skin perfusion pressure. J Vasc Surg. 1995;21(5):823-8; discussion 828-9.
3. Agilli M, Ekinci S. Value of prealbumin in assessment of nutrition for critically ill patients. Turk J Med Sci. 2015;45(4):991.
4. Allan J, Munro W, Figgins E. Foot deformities within the diabetic foot and their influence on biomechanics: a review of the literature. Prosthet Orthot Int. 2016;40(2):182-92.
5. Allen DB et al. Wound hypoxia and acidosis limit neutrophil bacterial killing mechanisms. Arch Surg. 1997;132(9):991-6.
6. Alvaro-Afonso FJ et al. Interobserver and intraobserver reproducibility of plain X-rays in the diagnosis of diabetic foot osteomyelitis. Int J Low Extrem Wounds. 2013;12(1):12-5.
7. American Diabetes Association. Economic costs of diabetes in the U.S. in 2012. Diabetes Care. 2013;36(4):1033-46.
8. Apelqvist J, Larsson J, Agardh CD. Long-term prognosis for diabetic patients with foot ulcers. J Intern Med. 1993;233(6):485-91.
9. Aragon-Sanchez J, Lipsky BA, Lazaro-Martinez JL. Diagnosing diabetic foot osteomyelitis: is the combination of probe-to-bone test and plain radiography sufficient for high-risk inpatients? Diabet Med. 2011;28(2):191-4.
10. Armstrong DG. The University of Texas Diabetic Foot Classification System. Ostomy Wound Manage. 1996;42(8):60-1.
11. Babior BM. Oxygen-dependent microbial killing by phagocytes (first of two parts). N Engl J Med. 1978;298(12):659-68.
12. Bakhtiani P et al. Impact of hyperbaric oxygen on diabetic ulcers is unaffected by glycemic control. Undersea Hyperb Med. 2015;42(3):183-90.
13. Bell DP Jr. Diabetic foot ulcers: current treatment options and new developments. Surg Technol Int. 2010;20:97-105.
14. Bell D. Evidence-based rationale for offloading treatment modalities. Surg Technol Int. 2008;17:113-7.
15. Botezatu I, Marinescu R, Laptoiu D. Minimally invasive-percutaneous surgery – recent developments of the foot surgery techniques. J Med Life. 2015;8(Spec Issue):87-93.
16. Boulton AJ et al. Comprehensive foot examination and risk assessment: a report of the task force of the foot care interest group of the American Diabetes Association, with endorsement by the American Association of Clinical Endocrinologists. Diabetes Care. 2008;31(8):1679-85.
17. Boyko EJ et al. Prediction of diabetic foot ulcer occurrence using commonly available clinical information: the Seattle Diabetic Foot Study. Diabetes Care. 2006;29(6):1202-7.
18. Bristow I. Non-ulcerative skin pathologies of the diabetic foot. Diabetes Metab Res Rev. 2008;24 Suppl 1:S84-9.
19. Brownlee M. The pathobiology of diabetic complications: a unifying mechanism. Diabetes. 2005;54(6):1615-25.
20. Brownrigg JR et al. Performance of prognostic markers in the prediction of wound healing or amputation among patients with foot ulcers in diabetes: a systematic review. Diabetes Metab Res Rev. 2016;32 Suppl 1:128-35.

21. Bus SA et al. Footwear and offloading interventions to prevent and heal foot ulcers and reduce plantar pressure in patients with diabetes: a systematic review. Diabetes Metab Res Rev. 2016;32 Suppl 1:99-118.

22. Bus SA et al. IWGDF guidance on footwear and offloading interventions to prevent and heal foot ulcers in patients with diabetes. Diabetes Metab Res Rev. 2016;32 Suppl 1:25-36.

23. Bus SA. The role of pressure offloading on diabetic foot ulcer healing and prevention of recurrence. Plast Reconstr Surg. 2016;138(3 Suppl):179S-87S.

24. Butalia S et al. Does this patient with diabetes have osteomyelitis of the lower extremity? JAMA. 2008;299(7):806-13.

25. Cantwell AR Jr, Martz W. Idiopathic bullae in diabetics. Bullosis diabeticorum. Arch Dermatol. 1967;96(1):42-4.

26. Castronuovo JJ Jr et al. Skin perfusion pressure measurement is valuable in the diagnosis of critical limb ischemia. J Vasc Surg. 1997;26(4):629-37.

27. Chalew SA, Hempe JM, McCarter R. Clinically significant disagreement between mean blood glucose and estimated average glucose in two populations: implications for diabetes management. J Diabetes Sci Technol. 2009;3(5):1128-35.

28. Crews RT et al. Role and determinants of adherence to off-loading in diabetic foot ulcer healing: a prospective investigation. Diabetes Care. 2016;39(8):1371-7.

29. Cull DL et al. An early validation of the Society for Vascular Surgery lower extremity threatened limb classification system. J Vasc Surg. 2014;60(6):1535-41.

30. Davis CJ et al. The use of prealbumin and C-reactive protein for monitoring nutrition support in adult patients receiving enteral nutrition in an urban medical center. JPEN J Parenter Enteral Nutr. 2012;36(2):197-204.

31. Dinh MT, Abad CL, Safdar N. Diagnostic accuracy of the physical examination and imaging tests for osteomyelitis underlying diabetic foot ulcers: meta-analysis. Clin Infect Dis. 2008;47(4):519-27.

32. Dinh TL, Veves A. A review of the mechanisms implicated in the pathogenesis of the diabetic foot. Int J Low Extrem Wounds. 2005;4(3):154-9.

33. Dissemond J. Images in clinical medicine. Necrobiosis lipoidica diabeticorum. N Engl J Med. 2012;366(26):2502.

34. Don BR, Kaysen G. Serum albumin: relationship to inflammation and nutrition. Semin Dial. 2004;17(6):432-7.

35. Dumville JC et al. Alginate dressings for healing diabetic foot ulcers. Cochrane Database Syst Rev. 2013;(6):CD009110.

36. Dumville JC et al. Foam dressings for healing diabetic foot ulcers. Cochrane Database Syst Rev. 2013;(6):CD009111.

37. Dumville JC et al. Hydrocolloid dressings for healing diabetic foot ulcers. Cochrane Database Syst Rev. 2013;(8):CD009099.

38. Dumville JC et al. Hydrogel dressings for healing diabetic foot ulcers. Cochrane Database Syst Rev. 2013;(7):CD009101.

39. Eggert JV, Worth ER, Van Gils CC. Cost and mortality data of a regional limb salvage and hyperbaric medicine program for Wagner Grade 3 or 4 diabetic foot ulcers. Undersea Hyperb Med. 2016;43(1):1-8.

40. Elraiyah T et al. A systematic review and meta-analysis of debridement methods for chronic diabetic foot ulcers. J Vasc Surg. 2016;63(2 Suppl):37S-45S e1-2.

41. Elraiyah T et al. A systematic review and meta-analysis of off-loading methods for diabetic foot ulcers. J Vasc Surg. 2016;63(2 Suppl):59S-68S e1-2.

42. Feng Y, Schlosser FJ, Sumpio BE. The Semmes Weinstein monofilament examination as a screening tool for diabetic peripheral neuropathy. J Vasc Surg. 2009;50(3):675-82, 682 e1.

43. Feng Y, Schlosser FJ, Sumpio BE. The Semmes Weinstein monofilament examination is a significant predictor of the risk of foot ulceration and amputation in patients with diabetes mellitus. J Vasc Surg. 2011;53(1):220-6 e1-5.

44. Fernando ME et al. Intensive versus conventional glycaemic control for treating diabetic foot ulcers. Cochrane Database Syst Rev. 2016;(1):CD010764.

45. Fife CE et al. A predictive model for diabetic foot ulcer outcome: the Wound Healing Index. Adv Wound Care (New Rochelle). 2016;5(7):279-87.

46. Fuhrman MP. The albumin-nutrition connection: separating myth from fact. Nutrition. 2002;18(2):199-200.

47. Game F. Classification of diabetic foot ulcers. Diabetes Metab Res Rev. 2016;32 Suppl 1:186-94.

48. Game FL et al. Effectiveness of interventions to enhance healing of chronic ulcers of the foot in diabetes: a systematic review. Diabetes Metab Res Rev. 2016;32 Suppl 1:154-68.

49. Game FL, Jeffcoate WJ. Dressing and diabetic foot ulcers: a current review of the evidence. Plast Reconstr Surg. 2016;138(3 Suppl):158S-164S.

50. Global report on diabetes. World Health Organization; 2016.

51. Gordois A et al. The health care costs of diabetic peripheral neuropathy in the US. Diabetes Care. 2003;26(6):1790-5.

52. Gordon KA et al. The role of surgical debridement in healing of diabetic foot ulcers. Skinmed. 2012;10(1):24-6.

53. Grayson ML et al. Probing to bone in infected pedal ulcers. A clinical sign of underlying osteomyelitis in diabetic patients. JAMA. 1995;273(9):721-3.

54. Grenon SM, Gagnon J, Hsiang Y. Video in clinical medicine. Ankle-brachial index for assessment of peripheral arterial disease. N Engl J Med. 2009;361(19):e40.

55. Healy A, Naemi R, Chockalingam N. The effectiveness of footwear and other removable off-loading devices in the treatment of diabetic foot ulcers: a systematic review. Curr Diabetes Rev. 2014;10(4):215-30.

56. Hempe JM, Soros AA, Chalew SA. Estimated average glucose and self-monitored mean blood glucose are discordant estimates of glycemic control. Diabetes Care. 2010;33(7):1449-51.

57. Hill RD, Smith RB 3rd. Examination of the extremities: pulses, bruits, and phlebitis. In: Walker HK, Hall WD, Hurst JW, editors. Clinical methods: the history, physical, and laboratory examinations. Boston: 1990.

58. Hingorani A et al. The management of diabetic foot: a clinical practice guideline by the Society for Vascular Surgery in collaboration with the American Podiatric Medical Association and the Society for Vascular Medicine. J Vasc Surg. 2016;63(2 Suppl):3S-21S.

59. Horn SD et al. Development of a wound healing index for patients with chronic wounds. Wound Repair Regen. 2013;21(6):823-32.

60. Huang ET et al. A clinical practice guideline for the use of hyperbaric oxygen therapy in the treatment of diabetic foot ulcers. Undersea Hyperb Med. 2015;42(3):205-47.

61. Ishida S et al. Serum albumin levels correlate with inflammation rather than nutrition supply in burns patients: a retrospective study. J Med Invest. 2014;61(3-4):361-8.

62. Lam K et al. Diagnostic accuracy of probe to bone to detect osteomyelitis in the diabetic foot: a systematic review. Clin Infect Dis. 2016;63(7):944-8.

63. Lavery LA et al. Probe-to-bone test for diagnosing diabetic foot osteomyelitis: reliable or relic? Diabetes Care. 2007;30(2):270-4.

64. Leslie RD, Kilpatrick ES. Translating the A1C assay into estimated average glucose values: response to Nathan et al. Diabetes Care. 2009;32(1):e11; author reply e12.

65. Lewis J, Lipp A. Pressure-relieving interventions for treating diabetic foot ulcers. Cochrane Database Syst Rev. 2013;(1):CD002302.

66. Lipsky BA, Baker PD, Ahroni JH. Diabetic bullae: 12 cases of a purportedly rare cutaneous disorder. Int J Dermatol. 2000;39(3):196-200.

67. Lipsky BA et al. IWGDF guidance on the diagnosis and management of foot infections in persons with diabetes. Diabetes Metab Res Rev. 2016;32 Suppl 1:45-74.

68. Lipsky BA et al. 2012 Infectious Diseases Society of America clinical practice guideline for the diagnosis and treatment of diabetic foot infections. Clin Infect Dis. 2012;54(12):e132-73.

69. Margolis DK, Hoffstad OJ. Economic burden of diabetic foot ulcers and amputations. Diabetic foot ulcers. Data points #3 (prepared by the University of Pennsylvania DEcIDE Center, under contract no. HHSA29020050041I). Agency for Healthcare Research and Quality; 2011.

70. Margolis DK, Hoffstad OJ. Incidence of diabetic foot ulcer and lower extremity amputation among Medicare beneficiaries, 2006 to 2008. Data points #2 (prepared by the University of Pennsylvania DEcIDE Center, under contract no. HHSA29020050041I). Agency for Healthcare Research and Quality; 2011.

71. Margolis DK, Hoffstad OJ. Prevalence of diabetes, diabetic foot ulcer, and lower extremity amputation among Medicare beneficiaries, 2006 to 2008. Diabetic foot ulcers. Data points #1 (prepared by the University of Pennsylvania DEcIDE Center, under contract no. HHSA29020050041I). Agency for Healthcare Research and Quality; 2011.

72. Margolis DJ, Kantor J, Berlin JA. Healing of diabetic neuropathic foot ulcers receiving standard treatment. A meta-analysis. Diabetes Care. 1999;22(5):692-5.

73. Melin H. An atrophic circumscribed skin lesion in the lower extremities of diabetics. Acta Med Scand. 1964;176:SUPPL 423:1-75.

74. Mills JL Sr et al. The Society for Vascular Surgery Lower Extremity Threatened Limb Classification System: risk stratification based on wound, ischemia, and foot infection (WIfI). J Vasc Surg. 2014;59(1):220-34 e1-2.

75. Moffat AD, Worth ER, Weaver LK. Glycosylated hemoglobin and hyperbaric oxygen coverage denials. Undersea Hyperb Med. 2015;42(3):197-204.

76. Monteiro-Soares M et al. Classification systems for lower extremity amputation prediction in subjects with active diabetic foot ulcer: a systematic review and meta-analysis. Diabetes Metab Res Rev. 2014;30(7):610-22.

77. Moon H et al. The validity of transcutaneous oxygen measurements in predicting healing of diabetic foot ulcers. Undersea Hyperb Med. 2016;43(6).

78. Morales Lozano R et al. Validating the probe-to-bone test and other tests for diagnosing chronic osteomyelitis in the diabetic foot. Diabetes Care. 2010;33(10):2140-5.

79. Morona JK et al. Comparison of the clinical effectiveness of different off-loading devices for the treatment of neuropathic foot ulcers in patients with diabetes: a systematic review and meta-analysis. Diabetes Metab Res Rev. 2013;29(3):183-93.

80. Muller SA. Dermatologic disorders associated with diabetes mellitus. Mayo Clin Proc. 1966;41(10):689-703.

81. Mutluoglu M et al. Performance of the probe-to-bone test in a population suspected of having osteomyelitis of the foot in diabetes. J Am Podiatr Med Assoc. 2012;102(5):369-73.

82. Nathan DM et al. Translating the A1C assay into estimated average glucose values. Diabetes Care. 2008;31(8):1473-8.

83. NIH cancer fact sheet. National Institute of Health; 2010.

84. Number (in millions) of civilian, noninstitutionalized adults with diagnosed diabetes, United States, 1980–2014. Centers for Disease Control and Prevention, National Center for Health Statistics, Division of Health Interview Statistics; 2015. Data from the National Health Interview Survey.

85. Okamoto S et al. Postprocedural skin perfusion pressure correlates with clinical outcomes 1 year after endovascular therapy for patients with critical limb ischemia. Angiology. 2015;66(9):862-6.

86. Oyibo SO et al. A comparison of two diabetic foot ulcer classification systems: the Wagner and the University of Texas wound classification systems. Diabetes Care. 2001;24(1):84-8.

87. Ozdemir BA et al. Systematic review of screening investigations for peripheral arterial disease in patients with diabetes mellitus. Surg Technol Int. 2013;23:51-8.

88. Peters EJ et al. Interventions in the management of infection in the foot in diabetes: a systematic review. Diabetes Metab Res Rev. 2016;32 Suppl 1:145-53.

89. Rodriguez-Segade S et al. Translating the A1C assay into estimated average glucose values: response to Nathan et al. Diabetes Care. 2009;32(1):e10; author reply e12.

90. Rogers L, Driver V, Armstrong D. Assessment of the diabetic foot. In: Krasner D, editor. Chronic wound care. Malver (PA): HMP Communications; 2007.

91. Roujeau JC et al. Chronic dermatomycoses of the foot as risk factors for acute bacterial cellulitis of the leg: a case-control study. Dermatology. 2004;209(4):301-7.

92. Saco M et al. Comparing the efficacies of alginate, foam, hydrocolloid, hydrofiber, and hydrogel dressings in the management of diabetic foot ulcers and venous leg ulcers: a systematic review and meta-analysis examining how to dress for success. Dermatol Online J. 2016;22(8).

93. Schaper NC. Diabetic foot ulcer classification system for research purposes: a progress report on criteria for including patients in research studies. Diabetes Metab Res Rev. 2004;20 Suppl 1:S90-5.

94. Schneekloth BJ, Lowery NJ, Wukich DK. Charcot neuroarthropathy in patients with diabetes: an updated systematic review of surgical management. J Foot Ankle Surg. 2016;55(3):586-90.

95. Scott JE, Hendry GJ, Locke J. Effectiveness of percutaneous flexor tenotomies for the management and prevention of recurrence of diabetic toe ulcers: a systematic review. J Foot Ankle Res. 2016;9:25.

96. Sen CK. Wound healing essentials: let there be oxygen. Wound Repair Regen. 2009;17(1):1-18.

97. Shone A et al. Probing the validity of the probe-to-bone test in the diagnosis of osteomyelitis of the foot in diabetes. Diabetes Care. 2006;29(4):945.

98. Slattery E, Patchett S. Albumin as a marker of nutrition: a common pitfall. Ann Surg. 2011;254(4):667-8; author reply 668.

99. Society for Vascular Surgery Lower Extremity Guidelines Writing Group et al. Society for Vascular Surgery practice guidelines for atherosclerotic occlusive disease of the lower extremities: management of asymptomatic disease and claudication. J Vasc Surg. 2015;61(3 Suppl):2S-41S.

100. Stratton IM et al. Association of glycaemia with macrovascular and microvascular complications of type 2 diabetes (UKPDS 35): prospective observational study. BMJ. 2000;321(7258):405-12.

101. Strauss MB. The Wagner wound grading system. Wound Care Hyperb Med. 2012;3(4):38-45.

102. Strauss MB, Aksenov IV. Evaluation of diabetic wound classifications and a new wound score. Clin Orthop Relat Res. 2005;439:79-86.

103. Strauss MB et al. Reliability assessment of an innovative wound score. Wounds. 2016;28(6):206-13.

104. Sugino H et al. Relation between the serum albumin level and nutrition supply in patients with pressure ulcers: retrospective study in an acute care setting. J Med Invest. 2014;61(1-2):15-21.

105. Uckay I et al. Diabetic foot infections: state-of-the-art. Diabetes Obes Metab. 2014;16(4):305-16.

106. Van Asten SA et al. Erythrocyte sedimentation rate and C-reactive protein to monitor treatment outcomes in diabetic foot osteomyelitis. Int Wound J. 2017;14(1):142-8.

107. Van Asten SA et al. The value of inflammatory markers to diagnose and monitor diabetic foot osteomyelitis. Int Wound J. 2017;14(1):40-5.

108. Vinik AI et al. Diabetic autonomic neuropathy. Diabetes Care. 2003;26(5):1553-79.

109. Vouillarmet J et al. Lower-extremity arterial revascularization: is there any evidence for diabetic foot ulcer-healing? Diabetes Metab. 2016;42(1):4-15.

110. Wagner F. The dysvascular foot: a system for diagnosis and treatment. Foot Ankle. 1981;2(2):64-122.

111. Yosipovitch G et al. The prevalence of cutaneous manifestations in IDDM patients and their association with diabetes risk factors and microvascular complications. Diabetes Care. 1998;21(4):506-9.

112. Young MJ et al. A multicentre study of the prevalence of diabetic peripheral neuropathy in the United Kingdom hospital clinic population. Diabetologia. 1993;36(2):150-4.

113. Zhan LX et al. The Society for Vascular Surgery lower extremity threatened limb classification system based on wound, ischemia, and foot infection (WIfI) correlates with risk of major amputation and time to wound healing. J Vasc Surg. 2015;61(4):939-44.

114. Zhu Y, Williams LM, Horne BD. Disparity in estimated average glucose due to different hemoglobin A1c methods and hemoglobin S trait. Clin Chem Lab Med. 2010;48(4):571-2.

CHAPTER 23 CHAPTER

Adjunctive Hyperbaric Oxygen Therapy for Diabetic Foot Ulcers

CHAPTER TWENTY-THREE OVERVIEW

Introduction **591**

Hyperbaric Literature Review **592**

The Early Studies 593

The Italian Studies 593

The Early Randomized Controlled Trials 594

Criteria for Patient Selection 596

Recent Randomized Controlled Trials 599

The Negative Studies 601

Systematic Reviews and Meta-Analyses 604

Clinical Practice Guidelines 604

Future Research 610

Policy and Politics of Hyperbaric Oxygen Therapy for Diabetic Foot Ulcers **610**

Case Presentations **611**

Case 1 611

Case 2 612

Case 3 613

Case 4 614

Case 5 615

Case 6 616

Conclusion **617**

References **618**

Adjunctive Hyperbaric Oxygen Therapy for Diabetic Foot Ulcers

Enoch Huang, Marvin Heyboer III

INTRODUCTION

The multifactorial causes of a diabetic foot ulcer and necessary global approach (Table 1) to treatment have been discussed in Chapter 22: Evaluation and Management of the Diabetic Foot Ulcer, including a comprehensive multidisciplinary limb salvage protocol.[17] Advanced therapies are implemented when there is a lack of healing in spite of standard care. Diabetic foot ulcers (DFUs) are prone to hypoxia and infection. Local tissue microangiopathy and host endothelial progenitor stem cell mobilization dysfunction are present in diabetics with nonhealing DFUs.[27] Hyperbaric oxygen (HBO_2) directly addresses these deficiencies. HBO_2 impacts wound healing through both local and systemic effects (Figure 1).

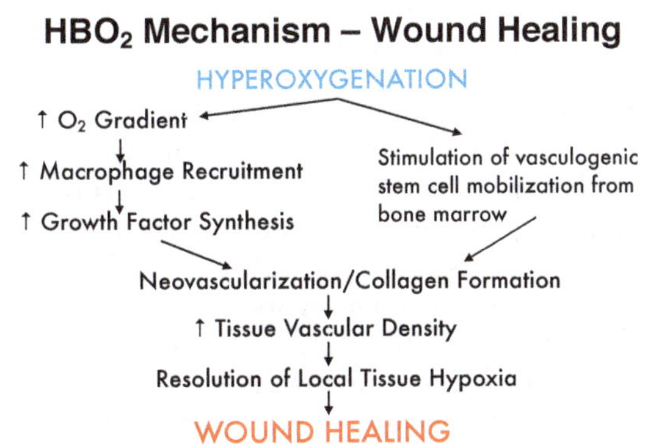

Figure 1. HBO_2 mechanisms in wound healing. (Marvin Heyboer, MD)

Locally, HBO_2 causes a steepened oxygen gradient resulting in elevated levels of multiple growth factors and recruitment of cells involved in wound healing. Elevated growth factors that have been measured include vascular endothelial growth factor (VEGF), basic fibroblast growth factor (FGF), transforming growth factor beta 1 (TGF-B), nitric oxide (NO-), and platelet derived growth factor (PDGF). Systemically, HBO_2 stimulates mobilization of endothelial progenitor stem cells (EPC) through endothelial nitric oxide synthase (eNOS), increasing NO- without the need for the cytokine and receptor complex. This bypasses the missing step in diabetics, resulting in elevated levels of serum endothelial progenitor cells (EPCs) (CD 34+ and CD45-dim) and improved homing to the site of injury.

TABLE 1. GLOBAL APPROACH TO THE DIABETIC FOOT ULCER

VASCULAR ASSESSMENT AND INTERVENTION	ENDOVASCULAR, OPEN SURGICAL BYPASS
Off-Loading	TCC, Irremovable Fixed-Ankle Walking Boot, Removable Knee-High Cast Walker, Half or Heel Shoe, Therapeutic Shoe, Soft TCC
Infection Control	Soft Tissue, Osteomyelitis
Glycemic Control	PCP/Endocrinologist: Oral Agents, Insulin (short-acting, long-acting)
Serial Debridement	Surgical Instrumentation (weekly, biweekly)
Local Wound Care	Moist Wound Healing
Advanced Therapies	CTP, Biologics, NPWT, HBO_2

TCC – Total Contact Cast, PCP – Primary Care Provider, CTP - Cellular Tissue Products, NPWT – Negative-Pressure Wound Therapy, HBO – Hyperbaric oxygen

These EPCs result in de novo neovasculogenesis and collagen formation at the site of the DFU. Clinically, HBO_2 enhances granulation tissue formation and wound bed preparation.[10,32,59,85-86]

HYPERBARIC LITERATURE REVIEW

When looking at study design, the body of literature can be broken down into three blocks:

- nonrandomized, observational studies (prospective and retrospective)
- randomized controlled trials (RCTs)
- systematic reviews and meta-analyses

Some studies had comparison groups that either did not receive a hyperbaric exposure at all (referred to as a control group) or received a combination of increased pressure and lower fraction of inspired oxygen ($FiO_2 \leq 0.21$) to simulate HBO_2 and preserve blinding of the study group (referred to as a sham group).

While the International Working Group on the Diabetic Foot (IWGDF) and the European Wound Management Association (EWMA) have published a 21-point checklist for researchers and readers to assess the quality of published work,[50] these were unavailable for historical studies. The UHMS *Hyperbaric Oxygen Therapy Committee Report* does an excellent job of reviewing the body of literature that has investigated the use of HBO_2 in the treatment of DFUs,[90] but we will be looking at the literature through a slightly different lens.

In this chapter, we will use a simple set of best practice management principles of DFUs *prior* to utilization of HBO_2 (i.e., VOIDS criteria described in in Chapter 22: Evaluation and Management of the Diabetic Foot Ulcer - **V**ascular, **O**ff-loading, **I**nfection control, **D**iabetes control, and **S**urgical debridement.) in order to extract the most relevant takeaway messages from each study. A chronological breakdown of the literature allows us to put each of the lessons learned into a historical perspective and to appreciate how each piece of the puzzle fits into the big picture. Because the inclusion/exclusion criteria of the previous trials differ, it is important to understand which population of DFU was studied and what question each study was designed to answer. Although there are many grading systems in use, all of the studies that categorized the severity of the ulcer used the Wagner grading system for patient selection, requiring us to utilize this classification system above others when considering patient risk stratification.

The Early Studies

The earliest mention of treating diabetic ulcers with HBO_2 was in a 1979 retrospective report of 35 patients with previously refractive skin ulcerations by Hart and Strauss. Ten out of 11 DFUs improved (73%) or healed (18%), but there was no mention of severity of the ulcers or the hyperbaric protocol employed.(44) It is not surprising that reporting standards at that time fall short of what is expected from researchers today, but the evolution of our understanding of DFUs guides us to ask more informed questions in the future.

The first case series that focused on response of DFUs to HBO_2 was by Davis et al. in 1987.(14) They reported 168 patients who underwent HBO_2 for a nonhealing DFU, but there was no information about the severity of ulcers. They recognized that revascularization was a priority and recommended HBO_2 post revascularization in order to support wound healing. They reported a healing rate of 70% with a major amputation rate (above ankle) of 30%, but these results are of limited value because there was no comparison group. Most treatment failures were in older diabetic patients without palpable pedal pulses and angiographic demonstration of large-vessel occlusion at or above the ankle. They did not mention anything about off-loading the extremity, and their HBO_2 protocol was not specified. The generalizability of this study to modern patient care is only of moderate utility. This study suggested a 70% limb salvage rate with HBO_2 and that HBO_2 is usually futile in elderly diabetics with large-vessel occlusion.(14)

The Italian Studies

A group of Italian researchers (including Baroni, Oriani, and Faglia) published both prospective and retrospective series as well as a seminal RCT looking at the effects of HBO_2 on the healing of DFUs. The first was a prospective study published by Baroni et al. in 1987.(5) This prospective cohort trial admitted 28 patients with DFUs to the hospital. Twenty-three had gangrene – most closely corresponding to a Wagner Grade 4 DFU – while 5 had a perforating ulcer, which most closely corresponds to a Wagner Grade 2 or 3 DFU. Eighteen patients were assigned to the HBO_2 group, while 10 patients declined to have HBO_2 because of psychological reasons such as confinement anxiety and fear of earache. These were assigned to the control group and received the same wound care treatment. HBO_2 was delivered for 90 minutes at 2.5–2.8 ATA. Interestingly, Baroni et al. used 2.8 ATA initially for antibacterial effect before switching to 2.5 ATA for reparative effect. The HBO_2 group received a mean of 34 ± 21 treatments and had a healing rate of 89% (16/18) compared to 10% (1/10) in the control group ($p = 0.001$). In addition, the amputation rate in the HBO_2 group was 11% (2/18) compared to 40% (4/10) in the control group ($p = 0.001$). The study noted faster healing and a decreased hospital length of stay (62 days versus 82 days, p = NS) in the HBO_2 group. When considering the VOIDS criteria, this group paid special attention to daily debridement of necrotic tissue with wound cultures to identify infectious pathogens, tight metabolic control with subcutaneous insulin and seven-point daily blood glucose profiles, and assessing macrovascular disease using ultrasound. They did not, however, report the severity of macrovascular disease, direct any revascularization based on the ultrasound results, or specify whether patients off-loaded their ulcers in any systematic way. Their thesis was that there was alteration of the microcirculation (i.e., arteriovenous shunts, obstruction of small vessels by platelet plugs, red blood cell thrombi or albumin deposits in basement membranes) even with normal macrovascular function. Some degree of off-loading may be inferred, however, as their patients were admitted to the hospital for 60–80 days instead of ambulating at home.(5) They provided the first suggestion that HBO_2 had a role in limb salvage, a term that had not yet been popularized. They noted a historical above knee amputation (AKA) rate from 1979–1981 (before utilization of HBO_2) at 40%, while their AKA rate from 1982–1984 was 8.4% for patients receiving HBO_2 and 40% for the control group.

Building on the 1987 data, Oriani et al. published a retrospective review that included 80 patients (62 HBO_2, 18 controls) that were admitted to the hospital with advanced ulcers with gangrene beginning in 1982.(78) They maintained their protocol of lengthy hospital admissions, strict glycemic control, aggressive daily surgical debridement, and culture-driven antibiotics as the 1987 study. The comorbidities and wound care treatment were reported as similar. The HBO_2 group was treated at 2.5–2.8 ATA x 90 minutes for 72 ± 29 treatments. They reported a healing rate of 95% (59/62) in the HBO_2 group versus 67% (12/18) in the control group ($p < 0.001$). There was a major amputation rate of only 5% (3/62) in the HBO_2 group versus 33% (6/18) in the control group ($p < 0.001$). They bolstered their previously reported statistics on limb salvage, noting only a 4.8% (3/62) AKA rate in the HBO_2 group and a 33% (6/18) AKA rate in the non-HBO_2 group between 1983–1987.(78)

A third report from this group in 1992 summarized their 10-year experience, now numbering 172 patients treated between 1982–1992.(77) By this time, they were treating patients earlier, for longer periods of time, and using HBO_2 as part of a systematic effort to assist demarcation, improve debridement, and repair damaged tissue rather than a last-ditch effort to halt wet gangrene. Importantly, they defined a success as complete wound healing, or whether amputation of the leg or the thigh was not required. A transmetatarsal amputation that allowed weight bearing would not be considered a treatment failure. Out of 151 patients who completed at least 12 HBO_2 sessions, they reported an 86% success rate. They also reported several tenets of therapy that are promulgated today: that HBO_2 should be used as early as possible, that a multidisciplinary team be involved in the care of the patient, and that there is periodic reevaluation of the response to therapy. They recommended HBO_2 be stopped if there were no signs of improvement on the basis of clinical or oximetric testing.(77)

The Early Randomized Controlled Trials

It was at this time that the first randomized controlled trial of HBO_2 for DFU was published, although one would be hard pressed to find similarities with HBO_2 protocols commonly used at the time or since. In 1992, Doctor et al. studied 30 hospitalized patients with chronic DFU. They did not report on the severity of the DFUs, but some had gangrene requiring immediate amputation above the ankle, and all of their patients were admitted to the hospital. All patients had periodic surgical debridement and had glucose management with three-times-daily insulin injections. While they did not specify the patient enrollment process, one assumes that there was an even distribution of 15 patients who received HBO_2 and 15 who served as controls. Their only attempt at addressing vascular status was documenting the presence or absence of distal pulses. The research question was whether HBO_2 decreased infections pre- versus post-HBO_2 and whether there was improved healing of wounds or amputation flaps. Their HBO_2 protocol – 3 ATA of 100% oxygen x 45 minutes for a total of 4 treatments over a 2-week period – had not been previously described, yet the major amputation rate was only 13% in the HBO_2 group compared to 47% in the control group ($p < 0.05$). They also showed a decrease of positive wound cultures (19 pre-HBO_2 versus 2 post-HBO_2, $p < 0.05$), compared to the control group (16 versus 12, p = NS).[15] While the strength of evidence was moderate, the generalizability of this data is low due to the atypical HBO_2 protocol used. It does raise the question, though, of whether a prolonged course of HBO_2 for DFU is required, or whether a shortened course of HBO_2 immediately after surgery might be beneficial.

Faglia et al. published a nonblinded randomized controlled trial of 68 hospitalized patients with DFUs in 1996.[18] All patients that presented to their center with Grade 3 or 4 DFU were admitted to the hospital, as were those with Wagner Grade 2 ulcers that were large and infected and showed a defective healing in 30 days of outpatient therapy. There were 35 HBO_2 patients and 35 in the control group. The HBO_2 group received treatment at 2.2–2.5 ATA x 90 minutes (reduced from the 2.5–2.8 ATA used in previous publications) for 38 ± 8 treatments. All patients were given orthotic devices to off-load their ulcers, glucose control was aggressively treated using 7 times/day blood glucose checks with an intravenous (IV) insulin infusion to maintain blood sugar was <9.9 mol/L (178 mg/dL), and wounds were cultured to determine antibiotic sensitivity. Rather than excluding patients with significant PAD, Faglia et al. included them as part of the study population. This was the first time an aggressive pre-HBO_2 revascularization protocol was described – all patients with an ABI < 0.9 or a $TcPO_2$ < 50 mmHg were subjected to arteriography and underwent percutaneous angioplasty if the stenosis was > 50% of the vessel lumen. Those with complete occlusion of the vessel or > 10 cm of stenosis were taken for bypass. Both groups had patients that required angioplasty (25.7% of HBO_2 group versus 24.2% of controls) and bypass grafts (11.4% of HBO_2 group versus 15.1% of controls). Postrevascularization ABI and $TcPO_2$ measurements on the dorsum of the foot showed that both groups still exhibited PAD and wound hypoxia (ABI of 0.65 ± 0.28 and 23.25 ± 10.6 mmHg in the HBO_2 group versus 0.64 ± 0.25 and 21.29 ± 10.7 mmHg in controls). It must be pointed out that this study highlighted the role of aggressive revascularization and glycemic control and included vasculopaths that other studies regularly exclude – essentially showing that HBO_2 was effective for the diabetic *and* ischemic/hypoxic foot. With this protocol, they found that HBO_2 reduced major amputations (9% in HBO_2 group versus 33% in controls, p = 0.002) and increased tissue oxygenation as measured by $TcPO_2$ (increase of 14 mmHg in the HBO_2 group versus 5 mmHg in the controls, p = 0.002). When broken down by Wagner grade, the major amputation rate for those with a Wagner 4 diabetic foot ulcer in the HBO_2 group was 9.1% compared to 55% in the control group (p = 0.002), but there was no statistically significant difference between the 2 groups when comparing Wagner 2 or Wagner 3 ulcers.[18] This marks the first time that a study explicitly reported wound demographics using the Wagner classification, and it is because of this study that the Centers for Medicare and Medicaid Services (CMS) approved the use of HBO_2 for DFU in the United States.[24] It is unfortunate that the CMS criteria did not mirror the Faglia inclusion criteria, as the current (as of 2017) coverage determination restricts HBO_2 to patients with a Wagner 3 or higher DFU that has failed to respond to 30 days of standard wound care,[75] when Faglia actually used HBO_2 on all Wagner 3 or 4 DFUs immediately (showing greatest benefit with HBO_2) and included Wagner 2 DFUs only if there was no response to therapy for 30 days (showing least benefit with HBO_2).[18] The CMS criteria also inexorably tied the use of the Wagner classification with the treatment of DFUs, even though other classifications may be superior in predicting wound healing potential.[29]

Criteria for Patient Selection

In 1991, Wattel et al. recognized that selection criteria for HBO_2 did not exist, and they published a case series of 59 patients with DFUs who underwent HBO_2 in hopes of identifying factors that would predict which patients would heal and which would not.(89) Although they did not use the Wagner Grading Scale by name, it can be inferred that 83% (49/59) of patients (27 perforating ulcers, 21 gangrenous toes, and 6 arteriosclerotic ulcers) were Wagner Grade 2–4 DFUs. They treated all patients with HBO_2 at 2.5 ATA for 90 minutes, and there was no control group. They managed blood glucose with three-times-daily subcutaneous insulin or with an insulin pump, performed surgical debridement as needed, and used antibiotics for cellulitis and abscess although it was not specified whether cultures of the wound were taken or not. They did not address off-loading, and they did not address vascular assessment other than measuring $TcPO_2$ while breathing 1 ATA air, 1 ATA of 100% oxygen, and 2.5 ATA of 100% oxygen. Their reported amputation rate was 18.6% (11/59) with a healing rate of 81.4%. Among the various predictive factors they measured (i.e., age, gender, insulin requirement, large-vessel alteration, microangiopahy, neuropathy, nephropathy, or retinopathy), the only factor that they found associated with a healed DFU was the wound $TcPO_2$ while breathing oxygen under pressure. They found that patients who healed had an in-chamber $TcPO_2$ of 786 +/- 258 mmHg compared with 323 +/- 214 mmHg in those who did not heal ($p < 0.005$).(89)

Faglia et al. published a retrospective cohort in 1998 that attempted to determine prognostic determinants for major amputation.(19) They presented data on 115 patients admitted to their unit from 1990–1993 and compared these results with data from 1979–1981 and 1986–1987. In the most recent period, 51 patients received HBO_2 and 64 patients did not. Using the same aggressive methodology previously described, they reported a major amputation rate of 14% in the HBO_2 group and 31% in the control group ($p = 0.012$). They determined that independent variables associated with major amputation were prior major amputation (OR 1.06, CI 1.01–1.12), higher Wagner grade (OR 7.69, CI 1.58–37.53), prior stroke (OR 35.05, CI 3.14–390.53), ABI (OR 4.35, CI 1.58–12.05), and $TcPO_2$ level (OR 1.06, CI 1.58–12.05). They found that HBO_2 had an independent protective role (OR 0.15, CI 0.03–0.64). When comparing the three time periods, the major amputation rate decreased from 40.5% (1979–1981) to 33.3% (1986–1987) to 23.5% (1990–1993), in spite of a population with statistically significant greater PAD, Wagner grade, and infection. They concluded the decreasing rate was due to evaluation by a foot team and a new dedicated foot clinic.(19) Treating complicated DFUs with a multidisciplinary foot team cannot be overlooked.

Zamboni et al. published a small, nonrandomized, prospective cohort trial on 10 consecutive patients with DFU in 1997.(92) There were only 5 patients in the HBO_2 group, and the 5 patients in the control group were those who refused HBO_2 because of claustrophobia or inconvenience. The HBO_2 group received treatment at 2 ATA x 120 minutes for 30 treatments. All patients had surgical debridement including removal of any infected bone. Antibiotics were based on deep-tissue cultures at the time of debridement. There was no classification of the types of DFU, although one ulcer was on the ankle and the remainder were on the foot. There was no mention of methods to address off-loading or glycemic control, and the only mention of vascular screening was that two patients in the control group underwent lower extremity bypass while the rest had no significant macrovascular disease amenable to surgical intervention.

There was no mention of the criteria for surgical intervention, but $TcPO_2$ measurements showed that the baseline room air tissue oxygenation was lower in the HBO_2 group compared to control (12.0 ± 2.91 mmHg versus 35.3 ± 2.30 mmHg). The change in ulcer size – described as percent area reduction (PAR) – was greater in the HBO_2 group compared to the control group at all time points in the study ($p < 0.05$). In addition, the healing rate at 4–6 month follow-up in the HBO_2 group was 80% compared with 20% in the control group but failed to reach statistical significance ($p = 0.0578$) because of the small sample size. Although their endpoint was *spontaneous* healing of the ulcer, the one patient in the HBO_2 group who did not spontaneously heal ended up healing the wound with a calcaneal flap. There was no mention as to whether any of the control group healed with further surgery. There were no amputations in either group. Although this was a nonrandomized, nonblinded trial with small sample size, the HBO_2 group started with a lower $TcPO_2$ and had superior healing rates and greater PAR. This supports its use for DFU patients with critical limb ischemia (CLI) even if revascularization is not possible.(92)

Two case series reported by Fife et al. in 2002 and 2007 also attempted to answer the question of patient selection.(23,25) The 2002 study focused on the use of $TcPO_2$ to predict healing response with HBO_2. There were 774 patients, of which 629 had adjunctive HBO_2. They reported a success rate of 65% (healed or improved) but did not report an actual healing rate. They found patients with an in-chamber $TcPO_2$ of < 100 mmHg had a low likelihood of healing, while a $TcPO_2$ > 200 mm Hg provides the best single discriminator (reliability of 74% and PPV of 58%).(25) Combining 1 ATA air $TcPO_2$ < 15 mmHg and in-chamber $TcPO_2$ < 400 mmHg predicts wound healing failure (reliability of 75.8% and PPV of 73.3%).(25) The subsequent study published in 2007 analyzed 971 patients who had adjunctive HBO_2 for a DFU. The end point of this study was improvement rather than an actual healing rate and again found that an in-chamber $TcPO_2$ < 100 mmHg had a response rate of only 14% while an in-chamber $TcPO_2$ > 200 mmHg had a response rate of 84%. In addition, factors significantly impacting outcome included renal failure with dialysis, pack-year smoking history, number of HBO_2 treatments, and interruption of the treatment regimen. There was such a large difference between the wound demographics (i.e., severity, outcome) of renal failure patients (n = 136) from non-renal-failure patients (n = 835) that it was necessary to separate the renal failure patients for statistical analysis.(23)

Strauss also published work in 2002 on the use of $TcPO_2$ to predict response to HBO_2.(84) His work revealed that $TcPO_2$ measurements > 200 mmHg under hyperbaric conditions defined a responder group (healing of wound) with 80% sensitivity and 88% specificity regardless of room air $TcPO_2$.(84) A recent analysis of the Fife and Strauss data confirmed that nearly 90% of DFUs with a $TcPO_2$ > 200 mmHg under hyperbaric conditions progressed to healing.(72) A full discussion of the UHMS recommendations on the use of $TcPO_2$ can be found in a clinical practice guideline on the topic published in 2009.(26)

In 2002, Kalani et al. published a prospective cohort trial on 38 patients with chronic diabetic foot ulcer with hypoxia.(51) This was the first prospective study to define a chronic ulcer as one that had been present for more than two months, whereas previous studies had treated patients on a more acute basis. In this study, none of the patients had a deep infection or full-thickness gangrene, so one could infer that this included only Wagner Grade 1 or 2 patients.

This is different than the previously studied patient populations from the prior studies that generally included more severe Wagner Grade 2–4 DFUs.[5,15,18-19,78,89,92] Soft-tissue infections were cultured and treated based on any identified organisms. All patients had angiography and were evaluated by a vascular surgeon. None of the patients were eligible for reconstructive surgery or angioplasty, and all had a dorsal foot $TcPO_2$ < 40 mmHg that tripled in value while breathing 100% oxygen at 1 ATA. All patients were treated with a foot care team consisting of a diabetologist, diabetic nurse, podiatrist, and orthotist to provide off-loading footwear. Glycemic control was achieved through administration of insulin, but there was no description of the parameters for treatment. In a testament to the difficulty of conducting randomized clinical trials, only the first 14 were randomized before the hyperbaric facility became unavailable for a 2-year period. The final 14 patients only received HBO_2 when the hyperbaric facility was available. By the conclusion of the study, 17 patients were enrolled in the HBO_2 group and 21 patients in the control group. The HBO_2 group received a typical treatment at 2.5 ATA x 90 minutes for 40–60 treatments. At the 3-year follow-up period, the HBO_2 group had a superior healing rate and lower major amputation rate than controls (76% healing and 12% amputations versus 48% and 33%), but it was not statistically significant. When comparing the demographics between healed patients and amputated patients, the only difference was in the $TcPO_2$ while breathing oxygen at 2.5 ATA, which was nearly 60% higher in the group that healed (234 ± 110 mmHg in the healed group versus 142 ± 65 mmHg in the major amputation group, $p = 0.3$).[51] Despite a lack of statistical significance and an incomplete randomization, this study showed that HBO_2 was helpful for Wagner Grade 1 and 2 DFUs that had hypoxia even after 3 years.

In 2008, Kaya et al. published a study of 209 consecutive patients that presented to their center between 2005 and 2008 with Wagner Grade 2–5 DFUs.[53] All patients received HBO_2 at 2.4 ATA x 90 minutes of oxygen breathing once or twice daily, six days a week for a mean of 39 sessions. They controlled diabetes mellitus with insulin, directed antibiotics based on wound cultures, and debrided wounds aggressively. They protected feet from uncontrolled mechanical stress but had no specific details of how this was done. Wounds were present between 1 and 260 weeks (mean of 25.27 ± 44.72 weeks), but there was no stated criterium of how long a patient needed to have a wound before adjunctive HBO_2 was used. Their cohort included 31% Wagner Grade 2, 41.3% Wagner Grade 3, 22.3% Wagner Grade 4, and 5.4% Wagner Grade 5 DFUs. This was the first study to report any patients with Wagner Grade 5 DFUs, but a review of the photographic evidence that they provided of two Wagner 5 DFUs looked more like Wagner 4 DFUs, potentially skewing their statistical analysis. They excluded any patient with PAD that required surgical intervention. They were unable to record $TcPO_2$ because of a lack of equipment, so one cannot assess to what degree this patient population had wound hypoxia. In the end, 184 patients were included in the study. Although they collected data at 3, 6, and 12 months following completion of HBO_2, they only reported results at the end of HBO_2 that 115 (62.5%) patients were completely healed, 31 (16.8%) showed no improvements, and 38 (20.7%) underwent amputation, 29 (15.7%) of which were minor amputations and 9 (4.9%) major amputations. Higher Wagner grade, age of the patient, and age of the wound were all associated with major amputation.[53] Despite the limitations of this study, the overall reported major amputation rate with HBO_2 (4.9%) was on par with what was reported by Faglia et al. in 1996 (9%).[18]

Recent Randomized Controlled Trials

After the pioneering work done by Faglia in the 1990s, recent researchers began to apply more rigorous study design methodology in answering questions about adjunctive HBO_2 for DFU. There was, however, a distinct change in the type of patient that was being investigated. All of these more recent studies instituted a screening period of at least four weeks before entering the patient into the study. As a result, this excluded the more serious DFUs that had been investigated by the Italian researchers a decade prior and focused on the more clinically stable outpatient population. This reflects a global shift in focus from the acute, inpatient, limb salvage setting to the outpatient, wound clinic model as these non-U.S.-based researchers were not restricted by CMS reimbursement guidelines.

Abidia et al. published the first randomized, double-blinded, placebo controlled study on 18 patients with DFU and concomitant PAD in 2003.[1] Like Kalani et al., they included only Wagner Grade 1 or 2 patients that had not healed for at least six weeks. These patients were evenly distributed between HBO_2 and control groups. The HBO_2 group received 100% oxygen at 2.4 ATA x 90 minutes for 30 treatments, while the control group received 21% oxygen (air) at 2.4 ATA x 90 minutes for 30 treatments. All patients were screened for PAD, and occlusive arterial disease was confirmed if their ABI was < 0.8 or great toe TBI was < 0.7. Anyone for whom vascular intervention was planned was excluded from the study. Off-loading, infection control, debridement, and glycemic control were nominally addressed with standard care, but there were no additional details given. The primary endpoint of the study was whether there was a significant reduction in ulcer size six weeks after completion of HBO_2, but they also looked at healing rates six months and one year after healing. Their results showed that healing rate at six weeks was not significantly improved in the HBO_2 group, but the healing rate at one-year follow-up was 63% in the HBO_2 group compared to 0% in the control group ($p = 0.027$). There was no statistically significant difference in minor or major amputation rates. There was documented evidence of progression of healing following completion of HBO_2 that suggested persistent benefit following completion of treatment.[1] This supports the theory that HBO_2 initiates the process of healing, which can then continue under normoxic conditions.

Kessler et al. published an unblinded randomized controlled trial on 27 patients with Wagner Grade 1–3 diabetic foot ulcers in 2003.[54] These ulcers had to have been present for at least three months despite stabilization of blood sugars, off-loading of the ulcers, and control of infection. Interestingly, this group excluded 22 patients because they had a dorsal foot $TcPO_2 < 30$ mmHg (there was a baseline dorsal foot $TcPO_2$ of 45.6 ± 18.1 mmHg in the HBO_2 group and 45.2 ± 24.2 mmHg in the control group), but periwound $TcPO_2$ in the enrolled patients did show hypoxia (21.9 ± 12.2 mmHg prior to starting HBO_2 and 25.6 ± 12.8 mmHg after the 20th treatment). There were 14 patients in the HBO_2 group and 13 patients in the control group. Both groups were hospitalized for the first two weeks and were then discharged after the treatment period. The HBO_2 group received treatment at 2.5 ATA x 90 minutes twice daily for 20 treatments during the two-week hospitalization, while the control group received no additional therapy. During the study period after discharge, all patients were given an off-loading shoe to wear, antibiotics based on cultures, and glycemic control using insulin. Measurements were taken at the time of enrollment, at two weeks (immediately after the hospitalization period) and at four weeks (two weeks after discharge).

At the time of discharge (two weeks), the HBO_2 group had a significantly larger reduction in wound size than the control group (41.8% versus 21.7%, $p = 0.037$), but, by the four-week follow-up, there was no significant difference (61.9% versus 55.1%). There was no statistically significant difference in healing rate or amputation rate, but the follow-up period was only two weeks after HBO_2 completion.[54] This is a very short time frame based on the nature of the disease, as most other studies were considering healing durability at the one-year mark. The design of the study also allowed both groups to be discharged home after two weeks, where they would have been able to ambulate with an off-loading shoe. It is possible that the early gains in the HBO_2 group may have been blunted if the deleterious effects of inadequate off-loading outweighed the benefits of HBO_2.

Duzgun et al. published an un-blinded randomized controlled trial on 100 patients with Wagner Grade 2–4 DFUs that had not healed with at least four weeks of appropriate care.[16] They used a modified Wagner grading scale, where a Wagner Grade 2 DFU reached the level of tendon or joint, and a Wagner Grade 3 DFU reached bone but did not have a requirement for infection. There were 50 patients in the HBO_2 group and control group, respectively. While the demographics of the wounds were the same in each group, the HBO_2 group had a higher percentage or males, obesity, and smokers – all high-risk factors for poor wound healing. The HBO_2 group received 100% oxygen at 2–3 ATA x 90 minutes either once or twice daily for 20–30 treatments. There was no description of how vascular status or off-loading was addressed, and there was no prescriptive management of glycemic control or wound infection (although osteomyelitis was diagnosed based on bone biopsy). The HBO_2 group had a higher rate of healing without surgery (66% versus 0%, $p < 0.05$), fewer major amputations (0% versus 34%, $p < 0.05$), and fewer minor amputations (8% versus 48%, $p < 0.05$), although the decision to perform an amputation was made by an unblinded surgeon, leaving room for selection bias.[16] The definition of healing in this study was spontaneous healing without surgical intervention in the operating room, which is different than what most clinicians would consider a relevant statistic and brings into question why the healing rate of the control group was so low. If we look at the actual reported figures, we can extrapolate that there were nine patients in the control group that healed with surgery but without amputation, while four patients in the HBO_2 group healed with surgery but without amputation. This gives a more realistic "healing rate" of 74% in the HBO_2 group versus 18% in the control group.

Löndahl et al. published what is probably the most rigorous randomized, double-blinded, placebo-controlled trial on 75 patients with chronic Wagner Grade 2–4 DFUs in 2010.[62] All patients had a DFU > 3 months' duration and had been treated at a diabetic foot clinic for > 2 months. There were 38 patients in the HBO_2 group and 37 patients in the control group. The HBO_2 group received 100% oxygen at 2.5 ATA x 90 minutes for up to 40 treatments. Like Abidia before him, the control group received treatment on air at 2.5 ATA x 90 minutes for up to 40 treatments. Only patients with adequate distal perfusion or nonreconstructable PAD were included in the study with randomization stratified on a toe blood pressure cutoff of 35 mmHg (33 in HBO_2 group had pressure ≤ 35 mmHg versus 29 in control group). While this protocol excludes anyone who had been revascularized < 2 months before study, it did not prevent patients from being revascularized after inclusion (no patient received open bypass after inclusion, but percutaneous angioplasty was performed in six HBO_2 patients and four control patients). Off-loading, infection control, metabolic control, and wound debridement were performed according to a standard protocol for both groups. The one-year healing rate based on intention-to-treat analysis was significantly higher in the HBO_2 group than in the control group (52% versus 29%, p = 0.03, NNT 4.2) and was even higher using on per protocol analysis for patients who received > 35 treatments (61% versus 27, p = 0.009, NNT 3.1). Of note, the HBO_2 had a nonsignificant increase in major amputation rate (5% versus 2%).[62] Subgroup analysis of $TcPO_2$ showed that baseline $TcPO_2$ correlated with healing rates following HBO_2.

- $TcPO_2$ < 25 mm Hg – 0% healed
- $TcPO_2$ 26–50 mm Hg – 50% healed
- $TcPO_2$ 51–75 mm Hg – 73% healed
- $TcPO_2$ > 75 mm Hg – 100% healed

This suggests that HBO_2 should be reserved for patients whose baseline $TcPO_2$ measurement exceeds 25 mmHg.[63] Long-term health-related quality of life using a Short Form (SF)-36 assessment 12 months after treatment was improved for patients who received HBO_2 (presumably because of ulcer healing) in these categories: role limitation due to physical health, role limitation due to emotional health, and social function.[65]

Ma et al. published a prospective, nonblinded randomized controlled trial of 36 hospitalized patients with Wagner 1–3 diabetic foot ulcers in 2013.[66] There were 18 patients in the HBO_2 group and 18 patients in the control group. Patient had to have a DFU for > 3 months' duration and have received standard care for > 2 months. Like Kessler, they excluded patients with dorsal foot $TcPO_2$ < 30 mmHg. The HBO_2 group received 100% oxygen at 2.5 ATA x 90 minutes twice daily for only 20 treatments (2 weeks), and both groups had strict off-loading with custom-molded footwear and strict non-weight-bearing instructions, treatment of infection with culture-directed antibiotics, and glycemic control (< 8 mmol/L or 144 mg/dL) using subcutaneous insulin. There was a greater reduction in ulcer size at day 14 (42% in the HBO_2 group versus 18% in the control group, $p < 0.05$) but there was no long-term reporting past day 14.[66]

The Negative Studies

Margolis et al. published a study in 2013 that called into question the effectiveness of adjunctive HBO_2 in the treatment of diabetic foot ulcers.[68] The authors reported a large, longitudinal, observational cohort study of 6,259 patients with a plantar DFU. The data came from a clinical database used by National Healing Corporation that included roughly 11,000 subjects with a DFU of all Wagner grades. Eighty-three percent of the patients in the database were excluded from analysis because they had healed or had an amputation within 28 days. Of the remaining patients, 6,259 had < 40% healing at 4 weeks and were included in the study (793 patients HBO_2 group versus 5,466 non-HBO_2 group). The HBO_2 group received 100% oxygen at 2–2.4 ATA for 90 minutes for an undefined number of treatments. Because the groups were not prospectively randomized into treatment groups, Margolis used propensity scoring to determine the propensity that an individual was selected to receive HBO_2 in order to compensate for the lack of randomization.[68] All analysis was dependent upon the assumption that providers had strictly adhered to National Healing Corporation recommendations in these areas, although this could not be independently verified and turned out to be erroneous with regard to restriction of HBO_2 for patients with Wagner Grade 3 or higher DFUs.[11]

For instance, the database reported only whether patients had adequate lower extremity perfusion and standard care, neither of which were defined. While the clinical practice of the participating facilities using the database at the time followed CMS guidelines for use – restricting HBO_2 for Wagner Grade 3 or higher DFUs – 54.3% of patients who received HBO_2 were classified as Wagner Grade 2 DFUs.(68) The HBO_2 group had 45.7% with Wagner 3–5 compared to only 18.4% in the non-HBO_2 group. There were only two outcomes that were of interest: a fully epithelialized (healed) wound and any lower extremity amputation (LEA). The results at 16 weeks comparing the HBO_2 group to the non-HBO_2 group showed that the patients who received HBO_2 had a lower healing rate (42.3% versus 49.6%), higher overall amputation rate (6.7% versus 2.1%), and higher major amputation rate (3.3% versus 1.3%). The hazard ratio for patients receiving HBO_2 was higher for amputation (2.37) and lower for healing (0.68) when compared to patients who did not receive HBO_2. Looking only at patients with Wagner Grade 3 or higher DFUs, the hazard ratio for amputation was still higher (1.41).

There were several confounders in the Margolis study. First, the authors claim this is a prospective, longitudinal, observational cohort study when in reality it is a retrospective case series analysis of data previously collected. Second, the HBO_2 group had more advanced DFUs, increasing the likelihood of nonhealing and amputation. In addition, any DFU in the HBO_2 group was already less likely to heal compared to ulcers in the non-HBO_2 group as they had to be refractive to standard care for four weeks before starting HBO_2. The authors describe propensity scoring in their statistical analysis to adjust for these factors, but, if performed inappropriately, it leads to increased rather than decreased bias.(11) A detailed discussion of the statistical methodology of propensity scoring is beyond the scope of this chapter, but Margolis clarified in response to criticism that this paper was a study of the effectiveness of HBO_2 in clinical practice opposed to the efficacy studies that had previously been performed.(1,15-16,18,61,66) When contacted directly, Margolis stated that a confounder in patient selection of sufficient magnitude could invalidate propensity scoring if it was not taken into account,(67) but secondary analyses that were performed showed that the likelihood of an unaccounted confounder was unlikely.(69) We have already described multiple studies that demonstrate the efficacy of HBO_2 in the treatment of a DFU under standardized conditions, yet the results of this study call into question whether this can be translated into clinical practice. While many hyperbaric medicine proponents recommend discarding this study in its entirety, the lesson from this study emphasizes the importance of proper patient selection and avoiding HBO_2 overuse in cases that are futile, cases where the DFU will heal without HBO_2, or cases with inadequate wound care prior to initiation of HBO_2. Clinical judgment – not payment policy – should drive patient selection. Indeed, it may not be coincidence that the data from a for-profit health-care corporation leads to a closer inspection of the financial drivers of medical decision-making. This raises the possibility that a financial motivation for overtreatment of patients with HBO_2 (e.g., over 50% of patients were Wagner 2 DFUs that should not have received HBO_2) could be that unaccounted confounder that biased the results against finding a benefit.

As the propagation of the outpatient wound center model developed in the late 1990s, adjunctive use of HBO_2 in the treatment of DFU ballooned at the turn of the century.[12] Payers for medical services began to take a more critical look at resource utilization. Government payers began restricting reimbursement based on narrow interpretations of the literature, and the Ontario Ministry of Health and Long-Term Care sponsored a randomized controlled trial looking at the use of HBO_2 for DFU. Fedorko et al. published the results of this double-blinded, placebo-controlled randomized controlled trial analyzing 107 patients with Wagner 2–4 diabetic foot ulcers in 2016.[20] There were 51 patients in the HBO_2 group and 56 patients in the control group. Like Kessler, Löndahl, and Ma, they excluded patients with PAD who were candidates for revascularization or had undergone revascularization within the prior three months. DFUs had to have been present for at least four weeks. The HBO_2 group received 100% oxygen at 2.4 ATA x 90 minutes, while the control group received air at 1.2 ATA x 90 minutes. Both groups received a total of 30 treatments, although only 61% of the HBO_2 group completed all 30 treatments (20% had < 11 treatments). Patient outcome was assessed at completion of HBO_2 and at one one-week follow-up after completion of treatment.[20] Unfortunately, this study deviates from previous studies in its defined outcomes, making it difficult to compare. They did not consider actual amputation rates as end points; instead, their primary end point was the efficacy of HBO_2 in reducing the *indications for amputation* as determined by the vascular surgeon. Furthermore, while it was the surgeon's prerogative to examine the patient, none of the subjects underwent physical examination to make the determination of whether a patient met preset criteria for amputation. All decisions were made using chart review and a photograph of each subject's DFU. The criteria for amputation included a lack of significant progress in wound healing, persistent deep infection in bone and tendon, inability to bear weight on the affected limb, or pain causing significant disability. They reported that 22.4% (11/49) of the HBO_2 group met criteria for amputation compared to 24% (13/54) in the control group. Importantly, there was no reporting of the percent of patients meeting amputation criteria in each group prior to intervention – something that could be done by using chart review and photographs since the subjects' final outcomes were also determined using chart review and photographs. In Canada, there was no requirement that patients have a Wagner Grade 3 or higher DFU for treatment, so it is no surprise that the majority of treated patients were lower Wagner Grade (Wagner Grades 2, 3, and 4 ulcers in HBO_2 group: 47%, 45%, 8% versus control group: 43%, 54% and 4%). As expected, there was much additional criticism of the study[47,64,73] and allegations of irregularities with the research protocol.[56] The fact that this was a government-funded project that did not report actual amputation rates (there is evidence that at least one patient in the "amputation group" is walking around on healed feet without amputation)[22] raises the specter that there was an ulterior motive in overreporting amputations in the HBO_2 group.[47] While it is tempting to disregard this study in its entirety, the takeaway lesson is that HBO_2 may potentially be overused in the treatment of DFUs. In their conclusion, Fedorko et al. acknowledged that there may be a subset of DFU patients that would benefit from HBO_2 but did not recommend its use until that subset could be elucidated with further research.[20] Despite those who were concerned about a government conspiracy to deny access to HBO_2 for this patient population, the 2016 draft Ontario Health Technology Advisory Committee recommended continuing to publicly fund HBO_2 for DFU but restricted it to Wagner Grade 3 or higher DFUs – mirroring the policies of CMS.[48]

Systematic Reviews and Meta-Analyses

In the last decade, systematic reviews and meta-analyses have become en vogue with clinicians as they try to assimilate numerous studies of small sample size and methodology in order to answer important clinical questions. In the area of adjunctive hyperbaric oxygen therapy for DFUs, there have been almost twice as many systematic reviews[6,28,31,46,55,58,61,74,76,79,81,87,91] than randomized clinical trials.[1,15-16,18,20,54,62,66] It is tempting to pool data to make up for multiple small studies, but heterogenous study characteristics make it difficult to match up studies exactly. As can be expected, early reviews had fewer studies for consideration than later reviews, the sophistication of the research protocols improved over time as researchers better understood both the questions to ask and the relevance of the answers, and the methodology for systematic review itself evolved over time. There was a common theme among the early reviews – there was a paucity of quality research of sufficient numbers to convincingly answer whether HBO_2 was effective at either healing DFUs or preventing major lower limb amputation – and they recommended further high-quality studies of the diabetic foot.[88,91] Later reviews that had the benefit of randomized clinical trials were a little more positive, with some showing a reduction in major lower extremity amputations,[79] some showing improved healing of DFUs,[55,81] and some showing both.[6,28,31,58] In contrast, the systematic review generated by the Canadian Programs for Assessment of Technology in Health (PATH) came to a different conclusion when reviewing the same literature. Their review found that even though a pooled analysis of both RCTs and observational studies showed that HBO_2 reduced the risk of major amputation by about 60%, the data from the RCTs was not strong enough to conclusively establish the benefits and harms of treating DFUs with HBO_2.[76] One of the biggest variables in the literature was the heterogeneity of the patient population with DFUs and the perspective of the organization conducting the review. When looking at the types of patients included, some studies included vasculopaths, while others excluded them; some included patients who were revascularized, while others did not; some had acute surgical wounds and others had ulcers that had been present for months. It is clear that all DFUs are not equal, and the approach to analyze this data becomes difficult.

Clinical Practice Guidelines

Along with systematic reviews, clinical practice guidelines (CPGs) have also appeared with greater frequency in the literature and have been promoted by the Institute of Medicine.[13] CPGs can be submitted to the National Guideline Clearinghouse (www.guidelines.gov), a database of evidence-based clinical practice guidelines and related documents maintained as a public resource by the Agency for Healthcare Research and Quality (AHRQ) of the U.S. Department of Health and Human Services. While many guidelines on the management of the diabetic foot ulcer exist, only a few briefly mention hyperbaric oxygen therapy.

The 2012 Infectious Disease Society of America (IDSA) had one recommendation:

- Studies have not adequately defined the role of most adjunctive therapies for diabetic foot infections, but systematic reviews suggest that granulocyte colony-stimulating factors and systemic hyperbaric oxygen therapy may help prevent amputations (B-I).[57]

The National Institute for Health and Care Excellence (NICE) in 2015 updated their singular recommendation *against* hyperbaric oxygen therapy:

- Do not offer the following to treat diabetic foot ulcers, unless as part of a clinical trial – Hyperbaric oxygen therapy.[(49)]

The International Working Group on the Diabetic Foot (IWGDF) published a single recommendation in 2016:

- Consider the use of systemic hyperbaric oxygen therapy, even though further blinded and randomized trials are required to confirm its cost effectiveness, as well as to identify the population most likely to benefit from its use. (weak; moderate)[(30)]

The Society of Vascular Surgery CPG in 2016 had two recommendations (although somewhat redundant) that included hyperbaric oxygen therapy:

- For DFUs that fail to demonstrate improvement (> 50% wound area reduction) after a minimum of 4 weeks of standard wound therapy, we recommend adjunctive wound therapy options including hyperbaric oxygen therapy (Grade 1B).[(45)]
- In patients with DFU who have adequate perfusion that fails to respond to 4 to 6 weeks of conservative management, we suggest hyperbaric oxygen therapy (Grade 2B).[(45)]

For all of the CPGs above, DFUs were considered en masse as a single diagnostic entity, and the recommendations are tepid at best. What they did not do was recognize that the patient population covered by their systematic review homogenized all of the different types of DFU into a single entity. Given that not all DFUs are of the same severity, these recommendations were inadequate for clinicians to make informed clinical decisions. The Undersea and Hyperbaric Medical Society (UHMS), in an effort to take a more hyperbaric-centric analysis, completed a systematic review and generated its own set of CPGs regarding the use of HBO_2 for DFU. The UHMS chose the Grading of Recommendations Assessment, Development and Evaluation (GRADE) methodology for its systematic review. This methodology has been adopted by over 70 organizations including the Cochrane Collaboration, the World Health Organization (WHO), the Centers for Disease Control (CDC), and the AHRQ.

The GRADE methodology of analyzing literature and generating recommendations is based on:

- the clear separation between quality of evidence and strength of recommendations,
- an explicit evaluation of the importance of outcomes or alternative management strategies,
- explicit and comprehensive criteria for downgrading and upgrading the quality of evidence rating,
- a transparent system of moving from evidence to recommendations, explicit acknowledgment of values and preferences of patients, and
- clear, pragmatic interpretation of strong versus conditional recommendations for clinicians, patients, and policy-makers.[(2-4,9,33-43)]

The UHMS CPG analyzed the same body of literature and attempted to homogenize the literature based on severity of the DFUs. While we attempted to include any classification system other than the Wagner Grade, none of the analyzed studies used an alternative system. We attempted to stratify patients into groups based on observations that were made when analyzing the previous literature. These observations included the following:

- Not every study addressed each of the VOIDS criteria (Table 2).
- Most of the patients included in the studies had mild DFUs that many would not have treated with HBO_2 (Table 2).[1,16,20,23,25,51,54,62,68]
- Many studies excluded vasculopaths,[1,54,66] but some included them (Table 3).[1,18,51,92]
- $TcPO_2$ could be used to predict healing or response to HBO_2.[25-26,72,84]
- Earlier studies that included more acute DFUs requiring urgent surgical intervention had decreased major amputations,[5,15,18-19,77-78] while later studies only including chronic DFUs in an outpatient setting did not (Table 4).[1,16,20,51,53-54,60,66,68,92]
- A forest plot of reported major amputation rates for HBO_2 versus control/sham groups demonstrated a heterogenous estimate of effect of HBO_2 (Table 5) but largely corresponded with the observation that earlier intervention was associated with limb salvage.

TABLE 2. OVERVIEW OF STUDIES INVESTIGATING HBO_2 FOR DFU

Study	Study Design	N	Study Population	Co-Morbidities Addressed					HBO_2 Protocol	Strength of Evidence	Generalizable Results
				V	O	I	D	S			
Hart 1979	RCaS	11	NS	0	0	0	0	0	NS	Low	Low
Davis 1987	RCaS	168	NS	1	0	1	1	0	NS	Low	Moderate
Baroni 1987	PCoT	18 vs 10	2 3 4	1	0	1	2	2	2.5-2.8 Daily	Low	Moderate
Oriani 1990	RCoT	62 vs 18	4	1	0	1	2	2	2.5-2.8 Daily	Low	Moderate
Wattel 1991	PCaS	59	2 3 4	1	0	1	2	1	2.5 BID	Moderate	High
Doctor 1992	RCT	15 vs 15	3 4	1	0	2	2	2	Atypical	Moderate	Low
Faglia 1996	RCT	35 vs 33	2 3 4	2	2	2	2	2	2.2-2.5 Daily	High	Moderate
Zamboni 1997	PCoS	5 vs 5	3 4	1	0	2	2	2	2.0 Daily	Moderate	Moderate
Faglia 1998	RCoT	51 vs 64	2 3 4	2	2	2	2	2	2.2-2.5 Daily	Moderate	Moderate
Kalani 2002	PCoT	17 vs 21	1 2	1	1	2	1	1	2.5 Daily	Moderate	Moderate
Fife 2002	RCaS	774	1 2 3 4 5	1	0	0	0	0	2-2.5 Daily	Moderate	Moderate
Abidia 2003	RCT	9 vs 9	1 2	1	1	1	1	1	2.4 Daily	High	Moderate
Kessler 2003	RCT	14 vs 13	1 2 3	1	1	1	1	0	2.5 BID	Moderate	Low
Fife 2007	RCaS	971	1 2 3 4 5	1	0	0	0	0	2-2.5 Daily	Moderate	Moderate
Duzgun 2008	RCT	100	2 3 4	0	0	1	1	1	Atypical	Moderate	Moderate
Kaya 2008	RCaS	184	2 3 4 5	1	1	1	1	1	2.4 Daily/BID	Moderate	Moderate
Löndahl 2010	RCT	38 vs 37	2 3 4	2	1	1	2	1	2.5 Daily	High	High
Ma 2013	RCT	18 vs 18	1 2 3	1	2	2	2	2	2.5 BID	High	Moderate
Margolis 2013	RCoT	793 vs 5466	2 3 4	1	0	0	0	0	2-2.5 Daily	Low	Low
Fedorko 2016	RCT	51 vs 56	2 3 4	1	1	1	0	1	2.4 Daily	Low	Low

0 = not discussed/addressed, 1 = minimally discussed/addressed, 2 = extensively discussed/addressed

RCT - Randomized Controlled Trial PCoT – Prospective Cohort Trial PCaS - Prospective Case Series
RCoT - Retrospective Cohort Trial RCoS - Retrospective Case Series

TABLE 3. HYPERBARIC/DFU STUDIES THAT INCLUDED OR EXCLUDED VASCULOPATHS

Study	Study Design	% Healed ∅ Major Amp	Include or Exclude PAD	Increases Healing Percentage	Decreases Major Amputations	↑$TcPO_2$ after HBO_2
Baroni 1987	PCoT	89 vs 10	Include	Yes	Yes	NS
Oriani 1990	RCoT	96 vs 67	Include	Yes	Yes	NS
Doctor 1992	RCT	87 vs 53	Include	Yes	Yes	NS
Faglia 1996	RCT	91 vs 67	Include	Yes	Yes	Yes
Zamboni 1997	PCoS	80 vs 20	Include	Maybe	No[c]	NS
Faglia 1998	RCoT	86 vs 69	Include	Yes	Yes	NS
Kalani 2002	PCoT	76 vs 48	Include	Maybe	Maybe	NS
Abidia 2003	RCT	63[a] vs 0	Include	Yes	No[d]	No
Kessler 2003	RCT	14[b] vs 0	Exclude	Maybe	No[d]	No
Duzgun 2008	RCT	66 vs 0	NS	Yes	Yes	NS
Löndahl 2010	RCT	52 vs 29	Include	Yes	No[d]	NS
Ma 2013	RCT	NS	Exclude	NS	NS	Yes
Margolis 2013	RCoT	43 vs 50	Exclude	No	No[d]	NS
Fedorko 2016	RCT	51 vs 56	Exclude	No	No[e]	NS

[a]only at 1 year follow-up [b]4 week follow-up [c]neither group had any amputations [d]no statistical difference between groups [e]did not report actual amputations, only those who met criteria for amputations

RCT - Randomized Controlled Trial PCoT – Prospective Cohort Trial PCaS - Prospective Case Series
RCoT - Retrospective Cohort Trial RCoS - Retrospective Case Series

We were unable to find any studies that stratified patients into treatment and control groups based on $TcPO_2$, vascular status, or severity of infection (the Wagner Grade only used osteomyelitis or deep space abscess to define a Wagner Grade 3 ulcer, but Wagner Grade 4 ulcers did not need to have infection, only gangrene). We were able to define patients by the following three criteria:

- Wagner Grade ≤ 2 DFU with wounds older than 30 days
- Wagner Grade ≥ 3 DFU with wounds older than 30 days
- Wagner Grade ≥ 3 DFU with acute wounds that required urgent surgery

Based on these patient populations, the UHMS CPG was able to generate three recommendations. We did not find enough evidence to support the use of HBO_2 in patients with mild DFUs. This is in keeping with many of the other systematic reviews and leads to the first recommendation.

- Recommendation 1: In patients with Wagner Grade 2 or lower DFUs, we suggest against using HBO_2 (very low-level evidence in support of HBO_2, conditional recommendation) (Table 6, Table 7).[(46)]

When looking at chronic Wagner Grade 3 or higher DFU, we found better evidence in support of adjunctive HBO_2.

TABLE 4. HYPERBARIC/DFU STUDIES WITH OR WITHOUT A DELAY IN STARTING HBO_2 AFTER DIAGNOSIS AND TREATMENT OF DFU

Study	Study Design	% Healed ∅ Major Amp	Delay before HBO_2?	Increases Healing Percentage	Decreases Major Amputations
Baroni 1987	PCoT	89 vs 10	No	Yes	Yes
Oriani 1990	RCoT	96 vs 67	No	Yes	Yes
Doctor 1992	RCT	87 vs 53	NS	Yes	Yes
Faglia 1996	RCT	91 vs 67	No	Yes	Yes
Zamboni 1997	PCoS	80 vs 20	Yes > 6mo	Maybe	No[c]
Faglia 1998	RCoT	86 vs 69	No	Yes	Yes
Kalani 2002	PCoT	76 vs 48	Yes > 8 wks	Maybe	Maybe
Abidia 2003	RCT	63[a] vs 0	Yes > 6 wks	Yes	No[d]
Kessler 2003	RCT	14[b] vs 0	Yes > 3 mos	Maybe	No[d]
Duzgun 2008	RCT	74 vs 18	Yes > 4 wks	Yes	Yes
Löndahl 2010	RCT	52 vs 29	Yes > 3 mos	Yes	No[d]
Ma 2013	RCT	n/a	Yes > 8 wks	n/a	n/a
Margolis 2013	RCoT	43 vs 50	Yes > 8 wks	No	No[d]
Fedorko 2016	RCT	51 vs 56	Yes > 4 wks	No	No[e]

[a]only at 1 year follow-up [b]4 week follow-up [c]neither group had any amputations [d]no statistical difference between groups [e]did not report actual amputations, only those who met criteria for amputations

RCT - Randomized Controlled Trial PCoT – Prospective Cohort Trial PCaS - Prospective Case Series RCoT - Retrospective Cohort Trial RCoS - Retrospective Case Series

TABLE 5. FOREST PLOT OF MAJOR AMPUTATIONS FOR ALL DFUs

Study or Subgroup	Experimental Events	Experimental Total	Control Events	Control Total	Weight	Peto Odds Ratio Peto, Fixed, 95% CI	Year
Doctor 1992	2	15	7	15	17.2%	0.22 [0.05, 1.00]	1992
Faglia 1996	3	36	11	34	30.0%	0.23 [0.07, 0.73]	1996
Abidia 2003	1	9	1	9	5.0%	1.00 [0.06, 17.41]	2003
Duzgan 2008	0	50	17	50	37.6%	0.09 [0.03, 0.26]	2008
Londahl 2010	3	49	1	45	10.2%	2.58 [0.35, 18.94]	2010
Total (95% CI)		**159**		**153**	**100.0%**	**0.22 [0.12, 0.42]**	
Total events	9		37				

Heterogeneity: Chi² = 9.64, df = 4 (P = 0.05); I² = 59%
Test for overall effect: Z = 4.64 (P < 0.00001)

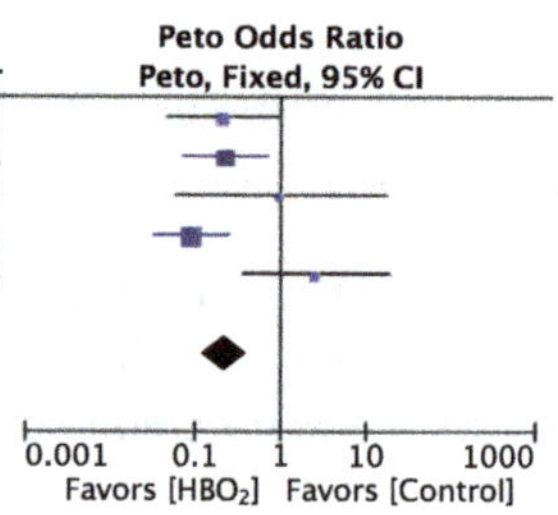

- Recommendation 2: In patients with Wagner Grade 3 or higher DFUs that have not shown significant improvement after 30 days of treatment, we suggest adding HBO_2 to the standard of care to reduce the risks of major amputation and incomplete healing (moderate-level evidence, conditional recommendation) (Table 8, Table 9).(46)

When looking at the acute DFU requiring emergent surgery, we found that there was a benefit in starting HBO_2 immediately rather than waiting an arbitrary 30 days. Whether this is a cost-effective therapy is not known because the majority of the patients in this analysis remained inpatients for between 60 and 90 days.(18)

TABLE 6. FOREST PLOT OF MAJOR AMPUTATIONS FOR WAGNER GRADE 2 OR LOWER DFUs

Study or Subgroup	HBO_2 Events	HBO_2 Total	Control Events	Control Total	Weight	Peto Odds Ratio Peto, Fixed, 95% CI	Year
Faglia 1996	0	4	0	5		Not estimable	1996
Abidia 2003	1	9	1	9	100.0%	1.00 [0.06, 17.41]	2003
Duzgan 2008	0	6	0	12		Not estimable	2008
Total (95% CI)		**19**		**26**	**100.0%**	**1.00 [0.06, 17.41]**	
Total events	1		1				
Heterogeneity: Not applicable							
Test for overall effect: Z = 0.00 (P = 1.00)							

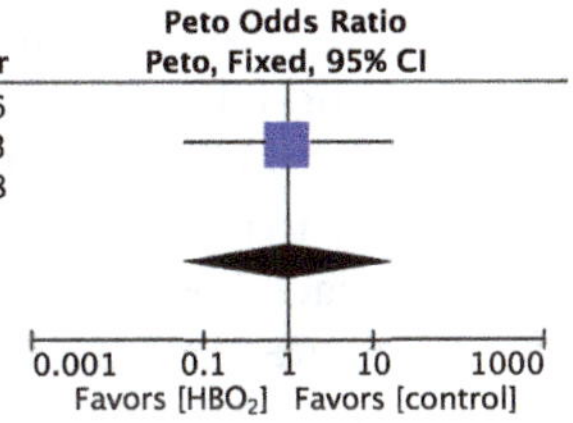

TABLE 7. FOREST PLOT OF INCOMPLETE HEALING FOR WAGNER GRADE 2 OR LOWER DFUs

Study or Subgroup	HBO_2 Events	HBO_2 Total	Control Events	Control Total	Weight	Peto Odds Ratio Peto, Fixed, 95% CI	Year
Duzgan 2008	0	6	12	12	100.0%	0.01 [0.00, 0.11]	2008
Total (95% CI)		**6**		**12**	**100.0%**	**0.01 [0.00, 0.11]**	
Total events	0		12				
Heterogeneity: Not applicable							
Test for overall effect: Z = 4.12 (P < 0.0001)							

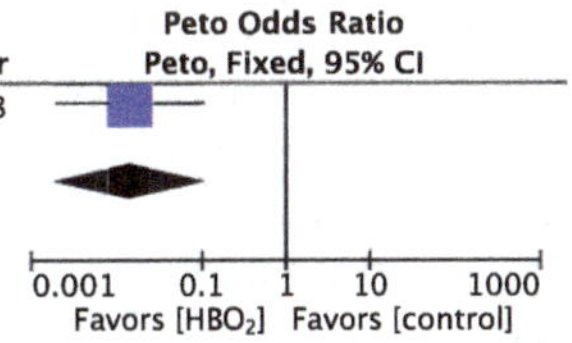

TABLE 8. FOREST PLOT OF MAJOR AMPUTATION FOR WAGNER GRADE 3 OR HIGHER DFUs THAT HAVE NOT RESPONDED AFTER 30 DAYS OF TREATMENT

Study or Subgroup	HBO_2 Events	HBO_2 Total	Control Events	Control Total	Weight	Peto Odds Ratio Peto, Fixed, 95% CI	Year
Duzgan 2008	0	44	17	38	100.0%	0.07 [0.02, 0.20]	2008
Total (95% CI)		**44**		**38**	**100.0%**	**0.07 [0.02, 0.20]**	
Total events	0		17				
Heterogeneity: Not applicable							
Test for overall effect: Z = 4.95 (P < 0.00001)							

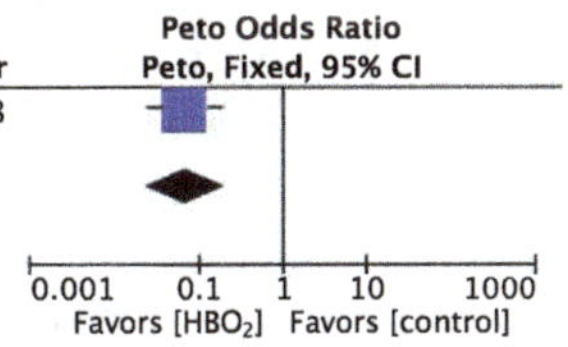

TABLE 9. FOREST PLOT OF NONHEALING WOUNDS FOR WAGNER GRADE 3 OR HIGHER DFUs THAT HAVE NOT RESPONDED AFTER 30 DAYS OF TREATMENT

Study or Subgroup	HBO_2 Events	HBO_2 Total	Control Events	Control Total	Weight	Risk Ratio M-H, Random, 95% CI	Year
Duzgan 2008	13	44	38	38	100.0%	0.30 [0.19, 0.48]	2008
Total (95% CI)		**44**		**38**	**100.0%**	**0.30 [0.19, 0.48]**	
Total events	13		38				
Heterogeneity: Not applicable							
Test for overall effect: Z = 5.21 (P < 0.00001)							

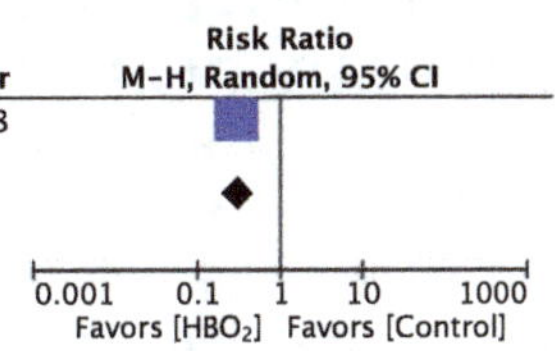

TABLE 10. FOREST PLOT OF MAJOR AMPUTATION FOR WAGNER GRADE 3 OR HIGHER DFUs THAT HAVE REQUIRED URGENT SURGERY

Study or Subgroup	HBO_2 Events	HBO_2 Total	Control Events	Control Total	Weight	Risk Ratio M-H, Random, 95% CI	Year
Doctor 1992	2	15	7	15	41.9%	0.29 [0.07, 1.16]	1992
Faglia 1996	3	36	11	34	58.1%	0.26 [0.08, 0.84]	1996
Total (95% CI)		**51**		**49**	**100.0%**	**0.27 [0.11, 0.67]**	
Total events	5		18				
Heterogeneity: $Tau^2 = 0.00$; $Chi^2 = 0.01$, df = 1 (P = 0.91); $I^2 = 0\%$							
Test for overall effect: Z = 2.84 (P = 0.004)							

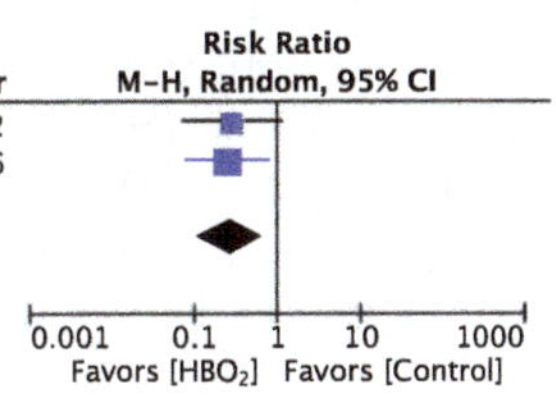

A shorter, concentrated course of HBO_2 may be beneficial,[15,54] but this would have to be proven in a future randomized controlled trial.

- Recommendation 3: In patients with Wagner Grade 3 or higher DFUs who have just had a surgical debridement of an infected foot (e.g., partial toe or ray amputation; debridement of ulcer with underlying bursa, cicatrix or bone; foot amputation; incision and drainage (I&D) of deep space abscess; or necrotizing soft-tissue infection), we suggest adding acute postoperative HBO_2 to standard wound care in order to reduce the risk of major amputation (moderate level evidence, conditional recommendation) (Table 10).[46]

Future Research

In parsing the various study designs, the variables that we suspect are of greatest significance for wound healing and limb salvage are the degree of ischemia/wound hypoxia and the acuity of the DFU. If we could direct future research, it would be to look at the population of patients with wound hypoxia rather than depth and to investigate the acute use of HBO_2 in an inpatient setting rather than the chronic wound clinic setting. We are aware of an ongoing, multicenter randomized clinical trial in the Netherlands looking at the use of HBO_2 for ischemic DFUs (Wagner Grade 2–4 DFUs of the leg with ankle SBP < 70 mmHg, toe SBP < 50 mmHg, or $TcPO_2$ < 40 mmHg). This study does not deal with the acute DFU, however, as all DFUs had to have been present for at least four weeks.[82] We are eagerly awaiting the results.

In summary, adjunctive HBO_2 is a useful therapy in the treatment of advanced DFUs that have failed to respond to standard care alone. It is important to attempt to address the standard care issues previous discussed including macrovascular status, off-loading, infection control, glycemic control, serial debridement, and good local wound care. When the DFU fails to progress despite this care paradigm, one should consider use of adjunctive HBO_2 for advanced Wagner Grade 3–5 DFUs. One should attempt to avoid overuse in cases that are futile, cases where the wound will heal without HBO_2, or cases with inadequate standard care. Furthermore, $TcPO_2$ may be used to assist in selection of appropriate patients.

POLICY AND POLITICS OF HYPERBARIC OXYGEN THERAPY FOR DIABETIC FOOT ULCERS

As alluded to earlier, there is a syndrome of both overutilization and underutilization of HBO_2 for the DFU. The for-profit wound care model prioritizes outpatient HBO_2 and has leveraged the documentation and diagnosis of osteomyelitis in the diabetic foot as a reason to treat the patient with HBO_2.[12] The fact is that not all patients with a DFU require HBO_2, and it is our responsibility to ascertain for which patient HBO_2 should be used. Decisions to treat should not be dictated by reimbursement criteria, but should be based on the best available evidence. The rapid increase in utilization of hyperbaric medical services in the treatment of DFUs has attracted the attention of multiple governmental agencies of the United States and Canada. Third-party systematic reviews have been published to drastically limit the conditions for which they feel HBO_2 is effective, and government-sponsored studies[20] may be biased against finding efficacy for HBO_2.[21,47]

CASE PRESENTATIONS

It may be helpful to utilize clinical cases to illustrate the decision-making process for and against the use of HBO_2. Careful analysis of the case using VOIDS criteria, rather than matching up a patient's history with reimbursement criteria, should help to decrease inappropriate utilization of HBO_2.

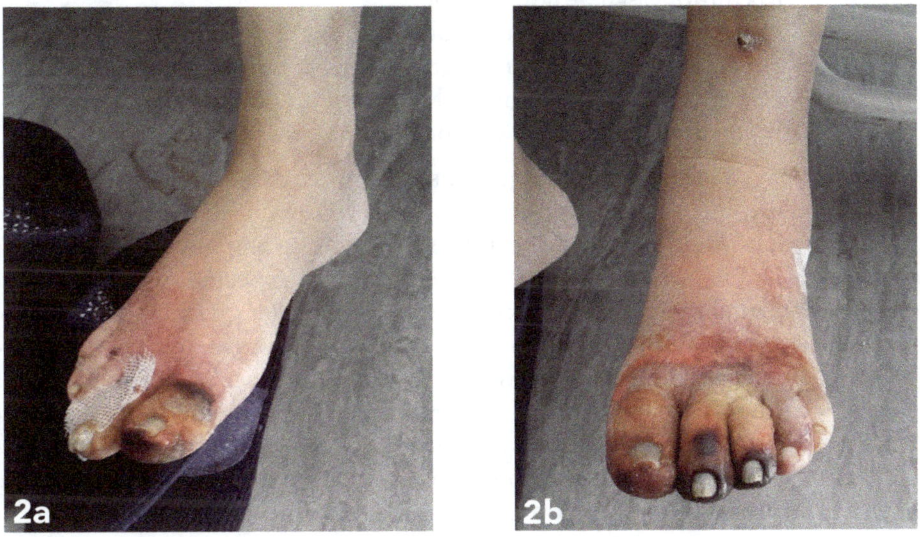

Figure 2a - 2b. Case 1.

Case 1

The patient is a 79-year-old male with a history of diabetes mellitus (DM) and end-stage renal failure. Within the last two weeks, he has had rapid onset of gangrene of the forefoot on the left foot and the first and second toes on the right. He has moderately well-controlled DM with a HbA1c of 6.4% and severe peripheral arterial disease. He has nonpalpable pulses that are monophasic on Doppler. He has mild pain in the foot. He has one-vessel runoff (posterior tibial artery) on the left with minimal runoff to the dorsal foot. He has two-vessel runoff (posterior tibial and peroneal arteries) to the right. His $TcPO_2$ on the left dorsal foot is 12 mmHg and on the right dorsal foot is 34 mmHg.

When considering whether HBO_2 is indicated in this case, one has to consider all of the following VOIDS criteria:

- Vascular – The patient has severe PAD and needs to be evaluated by a vascular specialist to try and obtain maximal perfusion to the foot.
- Off-loading – The patient does not have any plantar ulcers, so weight bearing is not an issue. The patient should not be wearing tight fitting shoes, however.
- Infection – There is no sign of infection.
- Diabetic control – The patient's HbA1c is well controlled.
- Surgery – The question in this case is whether one knows exactly where to operate. In this case, it is not entirely clear where the line between viable and nonviable tissue is located, so there may be some benefit in starting HBO_2 before debridement/amputation of toes. Is there access to fluorescence angiography to help determine whether there is perfusion to the forefoot? If the forefoot is ischemic, then this might indicate that a TMA may be a better way to go than local debridement.

Medical Decision-Making: Wagner's original treatment algorithm combined the DFU Grade with the ABI to help make decisions. Wagner didn't have HBO_2 included in his algorithm, but Faglia[(18)] used a more aggressive surgical approach to deal with Wagner Grade 3 and 4 DFUs than we are currently seeing in wound care practice.[(83)] So, the priorities in this case are the following:

1. Maximize vascular flow to foot
2. HBO_2 to help demarcate viable from nonviable tissue,
3. Surgical debridement of gangrene (fluorescence angiography would be a good tool to determine the level of amputation required)
4. Postoperative HBO_2 to support healing.

Some may want to avoid surgery altogether, as they would see that as a treatment failure, but a BKA is the only treatment failure in this scenario. A healed TMA on the left would be a win. Having only minor toe amputations would be a huge victory, and no amputations at all would be an unexpected "upset" if we are to take the sporting metaphor to its conclusion. The bigger question, and one for which we have no definite answer, is how many preoperative and postoperative HBO_2 treatments are needed. While many treatment protocols are based on data gleaned from the Marx protocol for osteoradionecrosis,[(70-71)] one must recognize that there are different mechanisms and disease states in play and modify the treatment plan based on clear outcome measures (i.e., return of $TcPO_2$ to levels > 40 mmHg, return of fluorescence angiography to baseline levels, etc.).

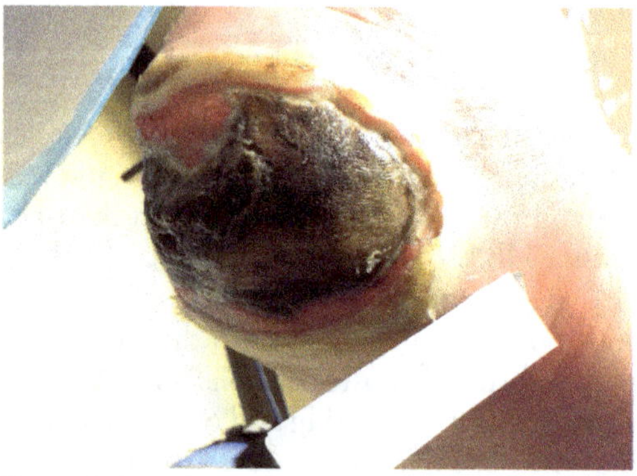

Figure 3. Case 2.

Case 2

The patient is a 67-year-old, morbidly obese, bedbound patient who has had a prior right-sided BKA. The patient has gangrene of the heel and osteomyelitis of the calcaneus (Wagner Grade 4 DFU). He has nonpalpable pulses with monophasic Doppler signals. His ABI on the left leg is 0.65. He has a HbA1c of 7.3% with fluctuating daily blood glucose between 130 and 180 mg/dL. The patient has had a stroke and has decreased mobility. Heel off-loading attempts over the last 30 days have been unsuccessful despite trying both soft and rigid heel protection devices as well as heel flotation pillows.

We once again consider the VOIDS criteria before ordering HBO_2.

- Vascular – The patient has evidence of PAD, but the interventionist deferred angiography until after the patient's off-loading could be effectively be accomplished.

- Off-loading – The patient is not ambulatory, but his left heel could not effectively be off-loaded at home.
- Infection – There is no sign of infection.
- Diabetic control – The patient's HbA1c is moderately controlled.
- Surgery – There is osteomyelitis of the calcaneus and gangrene of the heel. The foot and ankle surgeon did not feel that local debridement was an option as there was too much of the calcaneus that would have to be removed to preserve a weight-bearing surface, plus the fact that the patient was nonambulatory.

Medical Decision Making: While this patient met all of the criteria to receive HBO_2, common sense dictates that one consider a primary amputation of the leg below the knee as the most proper course of action. The patient is nonambulatory, and HBO_2 would not solve his underlying problem – the inability to off-load his heel. It was for this reason that the vascular interventionist did not feel that revascularization alone was sufficient for this patient and why HBO_2 is not warranted.

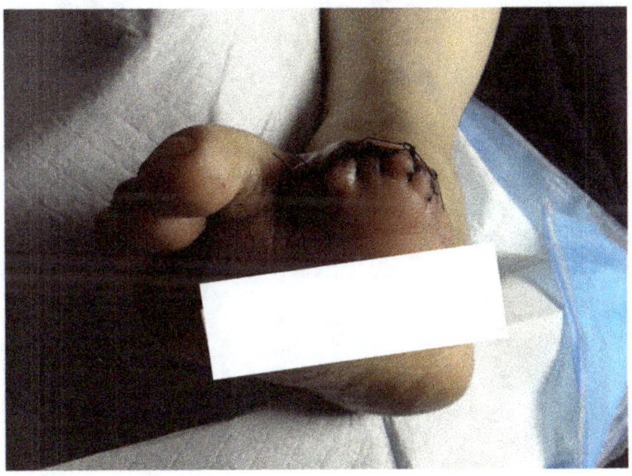

Figure 4. Case 3.

Case 3

The patient is a 58-year-old male with a history of well-controlled DM with neuropathy. He states that he works as a plumber and spent several hours in a kneeling position while wearing a new pair of boots. After coming home from work, he noticed that his right great toe was red and swollen. Within a week it had turned black with purulent drainage. He had amputation of the gangrenous toe and primary closure of the wound. He was referred for HBO_2 because of the diagnosis of a Wagner Grade 4 DFU (gangrene of the toe). The patient's HbA1c is 6.2%. The patient has normal 2+ dorsalis pedis pulses bilaterally. He has normal color of the distal foot, and the surgical wound has not dehisced after three days. A $TcPO_2$ was normal at 52 mmHg on the dorsum of the foot on the first webspace. An SPP was 60 mmHg on the dorsal foot proximal to the toe.

We once again consider the VOIDS criteria before ordering HBO_2.

- Vascular – The patient has no evidence of PAD with palpable pulses, normal $TcPO_2$, and normal SPP.
- Off-loading – The patient is ambulatory, but the issue is most likely related to a poorly fitting boot and not from ambulation.
- Infection – There is no sign of infection.

- Diabetic control – The patient's HbA1c is moderately controlled.
- Surgery – The devitalized and gangrenous tissue has been removed. There is no evidence of surgical wound dehiscence or need for further debridement.

Medical Decision-Making: While it is tempting to start HBO_2 for this gangrenous toe, the patient's vascular status is completely normal. The third recommendation from the UHMS CPG would advocate that HBO_2 be started in the acute postoperative phase to enhance wound healing, but one has to question whether HBO_2 would add anything but additional expense and patient inconvenience in the face of normal perfusion.

In this case, the patient was offered the choice to undergo HBO_2 or manage the wound expectantly. The patient chose to reserve HBO_2 as an option in case the wound did not heal, but it was not needed as the wound healed without any difficulty.

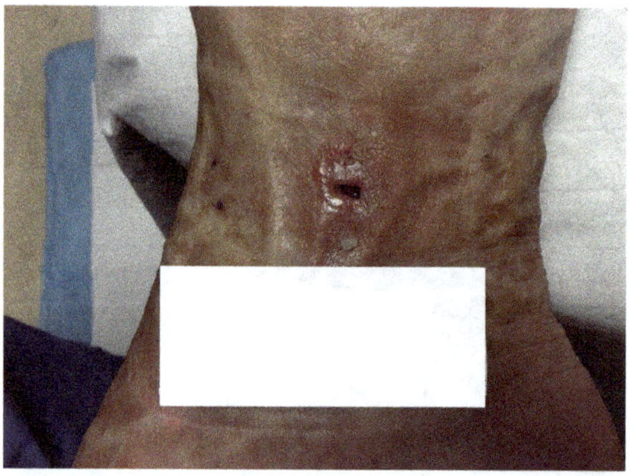

Figure 5. Case 4.

Case 4

A 54-year-old female with a history of poorly controlled Type II DM who developed two cutaneous abscesses on the right leg associated with cellulitis about three months ago. She had incision and drainage of each wound at another hospital. The cellulitis resolved with antibiotics, but the wounds have failed to heal. She has been going to another wound clinic and was told she needed HBO_2 for Wagner Grade 3 equivalent diabetic lower extremity ulcers. She did not live close to that clinic and looked for a facility closer to her home, prompting a second opinion.

An X-ray of the tibia and fibula one month ago was negative for osteomyelitis. She has not had an MRI, nor does she believe the wounds ever probed to bone. She admits to chronic leg edema bilaterally for several years but has not been treated with any compression therapy.

Before even considering the use of the VOIDS criteria, one has to question the diagnosis of a Wagner Grade 3 "equivalent" DFU. There is no such diagnosis defined in the literature, and the proper diagnosis of this ulcer is a venous stasis ulcer. HBO_2 was not recommended, to the delight of the patient, and we were able to heal the ulcer with one month of compression wraps and control of her venous insufficiency.

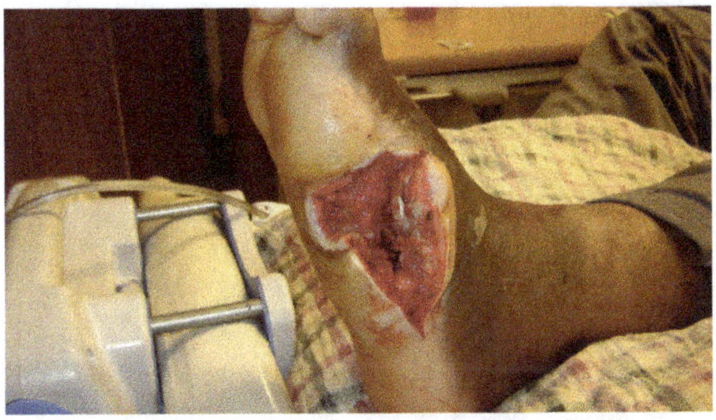

Figure 6. Case 5.

Case 5

The patient is a 32-year-old African-American male with a history of type 1 DM, peripheral neuropathy, Charcot arthropathy, and left fifth toe amputation. The patient is followed by endocrinology and podiatry. The patient initially presented with a left foot plantar lateral ulcer over the fifth metatarsal shaft that had been present for three months. The wound was malodorous and probed deep with purulent drainage. Spot glucose was 325 mg/dL. The patient was admitted to the hospital. An MRI showed a deep space abscess. The patient underwent debridement in the operating room by vascular surgery. He was started on IV antibiotics and local NWPT. Hyperbaric medicine is consulted regarding adjunctive HBO_2. The patient is currently using a wheelchair and transitioning to crutches. His most recent HbA1C was 9% prior to current hospitalization. The patient has ABIs of 1.1 (RLE) and 1.2 (LLE) with palpable 2+ PT and DP pulses. Room air $TcPO_2$ is 32 mmHg.

We again consider the VOIDS criteria before ordering HBO_2.

- Vascular – He has normal ABIs and pulses without evidence of PAD. He is referred by vascular surgery.
- Off-loading – The patient is currently non-weight-bearing on the left.
- Infection – The patient is followed by infectious disease and is on IV antibiotics.
- Diabetic control – The patient's HbA1c was moderately controlled prior to hospitalization followed by endocrinology. Most recent elevation was secondary to acute infection.
- Surgery – The patient had deep space infection and underwent intraoperative debridement.

Medical Decision-Making: The patient has a nonhealing Wagner Grade 3 DFU due to deep space infection requiring intraoperative debridement. The DFU has persisted for greater than 30 days although it is not clear the patient has received standard care for at least 30 days. While the patient may not strictly meet CMS criteria, he is a hospitalized patient with an acute Wagner Grade 3 diabetic foot ulcer. This is a patient who has received hospitalization and aggressive surgical debridement along the same lines as patients in the 1996 Faglia study.[18] He has no evidence of significant PAD. He is receiving adequate off-loading. Infection and glycemic control have been addressed. His $TcPO_2$ indicates local tissue hypoxia is an impediment to healing. The patient will benefit from immediate initiation of HBO_2. One should additionally complete an in-chamber $TcPO_2$ to better guide management.

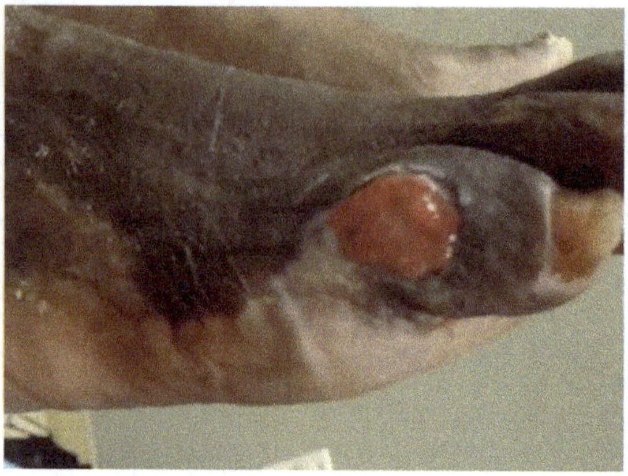

Figure 7. Case 6.

Case 6

The patient is a 65-year-old African-American male with type 2 DM who had previously been under the care of the wound clinic for a nonhealing fifth toe amputation incision secondary to osteomyelitis. The patient was discharged in January with a healed fifth-toe amputation site (without requiring HBO_2), but reports a new DFU on the right fourth toe caused by an ill-fitting shoe that occurred in mid-February, several months after the previous wound had healed. The patient returned to the wound clinic at the end of February and had an X-ray that was suspicious for osteomyelitis. An MRI done four days later was positive for osteomyelitis, and the patient was referred to podiatry but not seen for another week. The podiatrist scheduled an amputation of the fourth toe in 3 days (30 days after DFU was noticed). The patient's $TcPO_2$ is 55 mmHg on the dorsal foot. The fluorescence angiogram shows normal perfusion of the wound bed without any focal ischemia. The ABI was 1.09 on the right foot. The patient's HbA1c was 7.0% in January, and he states his blood glucose has been between 150 and 170 mg/dL on a regular basis.

We again consider the VOIDS criteria before ordering HBO_2.

- Vascular – The patient has normal ABIs, $TcPO_2$ and fluorescence angiogram without evidence of PAD. There are no objective signs of wound ischemia/hypoxia.
- Off-loading – The ulcer is not on a weight-bearing surface, and the patient is wearing open-toed shoes, so there is no pressure on the ulcer.
- Infection – The patient has osteomyelitis, and amputation of the toe is planned but not yet accomplished. No antibiotics have been ordered, but intraoperative cultures are planned.
- Diabetic control – The patient's HbA1c was moderately controlled (7.0%) prior to the development of the ulcer, and his daily glucose has been a little higher than his estimated average glucose (154 mm/Hg).
- Surgery – Surgical debridement (amputation) of the infected bone is planned.

Medical Decision-Making: The patient has been under the care of the wound clinic for a previously healed DFU but now has a new diagnosis of osteomyelitis and a Wagner Grade 3 DFU. Amputation of the fourth toe is scheduled within two weeks of presentation to the clinic. The patient has no evidence of wound hypoxia/

ischemia, so the question is whether HBO_2 would be indicated before or after surgery, if at all. Considering all of the VOIDS criteria, the patient has not yet had surgical debridement of the infected tissue, so preoperative HBO_2 would not be recommended, especially in light of normal vascular studies. Once the toe has been amputated, some would consider the question moot because the patient no longer has a DFU, just an amputated toe. This is where a more complete understanding of the original literature educates us that HBO_2 was not used to heal the original DFU, but was used as an adjunctive to surgery to allow the patient's foot to heal from the surgery.[5,15,18-19,46,77-78] At this point, one has to exercise restraint and clinical judgment. While the UHMS CPG does suggest that HBO_2 would decrease the risk of major amputation for this patient, the patient's normal vascular status argues that wound hypoxia/ischemia is not at the root of his ability to heal. Others would argue that the patient, by virtue of his existing DM, the fact that he has already had an amputation of the fifth toe from osteomyelitis, and the fact that there are other physiological effects that HBO_2 provides other than resolution of hypoxia, should receive HBO_2 regardless of what the vascular studies show. The hyperbaric practitioner should have a consistent philosophy to guide medical decision-making at this point for patients with a "qualifying" DFU but without significant PAD. This is precisely the type of patient for which future research should be targeted.

CONCLUSION

There are many reasons for which we would like to use HBO_2, and the treatment of the DFU is one where the literature has more robust evidence than others. With that being said, there are still many controversies and hidden agendas by both advocates and opponents of HBO_2. The literature shows that HBO_2 should be used for the treatment of certain DFUs according to the UHMS CPG,[46] and optimal outcomes in the treatment of DFUs occurs when done as part of a comprehensive limb salvage program.[17]

REFERENCES

1. Abidia A et al. The role of hyperbaric oxygen therapy in ischaemic diabetic lower extremity ulcers: a double-blind randomised-controlled trial. Eur J Vasc Endovasc Surg. 2003;25(6):513-8.
2. Andrews J et al. GRADE guidelines: 14. Going from evidence to recommendations: the significance and presentation of recommendations. J Clin Epidemiol. 2013;66(7):719-25.
3. Andrews JC et al. GRADE guidelines: 15. Going from evidence to recommendation – determinants of a recommendation's direction and strength. J Clin Epidemiol. 2013;66(7):726-35.
4. Balshem H et al. GRADE guidelines: 3. Rating the quality of evidence. J Clin Epidemiol. 2011;64(4):401-6.
5. Baroni G et al. Hyperbaric oxygen in diabetic gangrene treatment. Diabetes Care. 1987;10(1):81-6.
6. Bishop AJ, Mudge E. Diabetic foot ulcers treated with hyperbaric oxygen therapy: a review of the literature. Int Wound J. 2014;11(1):28-34.
7. Bonomo SR et al. Hyperbaric oxygen as a signal transducer: upregulation of platelet derived growth factor-beta receptor in the presence of HBO_2 and PDGF. Undersea Hyperb Med. 1998;25(4):211-6.
8. Boykin JV Jr, Baylis C. Hyperbaric oxygen therapy mediates increased nitric oxide production associated with wound healing: a preliminary study. Adv Skin Wound Care. 2007;20(7):382-8.
9. Brunetti M et al. GRADE guidelines: 10. Considering resource use and rating the quality of economic evidence. J Clin Epidemiol. 2013;66(2):140-50.
10. Camporesi EM, Bosco G. Mechanisms of action. In: Weaver LK, editor. Hyperbaric oxygen therapy committee indications. 2014. p. 241-6.
11. Carter MJ, Fife CE, Bennett M. Comment on: Margolis et al. lack of effectiveness of hyperbaric oxygen therapy for the treatment of diabetic foot ulcer and the prevention of amputation: a cohort study. Diabetes Care. 2013;36:1961-6. Diabetes Care. 2013;36(8):e131.
12. Clarke R. Hyperbaric medicine today: an historically noble discipline challenged by loss of critical access and overutilization – invited commentary. Undersea Hyperb Med. 2017;44(1):5-10.
13. Clinical practice guidelines we can trust. Institute of Medicine of the National Academies; 2011.
14. Davis JC. The use of adjuvant hyperbaric oxygen in treatment of the diabetic foot. Clin Podiatr Med Surg. 1987;4(2):429-37.
15. Doctor N, Pandya S, Supe A. Hyperbaric oxygen therapy in diabetic foot. J Postgrad Med. 1992;38(3):112-4, 111.
16. Duzgun AP et al. Effect of hyperbaric oxygen therapy on healing of diabetic foot ulcers. J Foot Ankle Surg. 2008;47(6):515-9.
17. Eggert JV, Worth ER, Van Gils CC. Cost and mortality data of a regional limb salvage and hyperbaric medicine program for Wagner Grade 3 or 4 diabetic foot ulcers. Undersea Hyperb Med. 2016;43(1):1-8.
18. Faglia E et al. Adjunctive systemic hyperbaric oxygen therapy in treatment of severe prevalently ischemic diabetic foot ulcer. A randomized study. Diabetes Care. 1996;19(12):1338-43.
19. Faglia E et al. Change in major amputation rate in a center dedicated to diabetic foot care during the 1980s: prognostic determinants for major amputation. J Diabetes Complications. 1998;12(2):96-102.

20. Fedorko L et al. Hyperbaric oxygen therapy does not reduce indications for amputation in patients with diabetes with nonhealing ulcers of the lower limb: a prospective, double-blind, randomized controlled clinical trial. Diabetes Care. 2016;39(3):392-9.

21. Fedorko L et al. Response to comments on Fedorko et al. Hyperbaric oxygen therapy does not reduce indications for amputation in patients with diabetes with nonhealing ulcers of the lower limb: a prospective, double-blind, randomized controlled clinical trial. Diabetes Care. 2016;39:392-9. Diabetes Care. 2016;39(8):e136-7.

22. Fedorko study subject #1121 testimonial [video]. 2016. Available from: https://videopress.com/v/MFLcTIBV

23. Fife CE et al. Factors influencing the outcome of lower-extremity diabetic ulcers treated with hyperbaric oxygen therapy. Wound Repair Regen. 2007;15(3):322-31.

24. Fife C. Personal communication about CMS approval of hyperbaric oxygen therapy for diabetic foot ulcers. 2014.

25. Fife CE et al. The predictive value of transcutaneous oxygen tension measurement in diabetic lower extremity ulcers treated with hyperbaric oxygen therapy: a retrospective analysis of 1,144 patients. Wound Repair Regen. 2002;10(4):198-207.

26. Fife CE et al. Transcutaneous oximetry in clinical practice: consensus statements from an expert panel based on evidence. Undersea Hyperb Med. 2009;36(1):43-53.

27. Gallagher KA et al. Diabetic impairments in NO-mediated endothelial progenitor cell mobilization and homing are reversed by hyperoxia and SDF-1 alpha. J Clin Invest. 2007;117(5):1249-59.

28. Game FL et al. A systematic review of interventions to enhance the healing of chronic ulcers of the foot in diabetes. Diabetes Metab Res Rev. 2012;28(Suppl 1):119-41.

29. Game F. Classification of diabetic foot ulcers. Diabetes Metab Res Rev. 2016;32(Suppl 1):186-94.

30. Game FL et al. IWGDF guidance on use of interventions to enhance the healing of chronic ulcers of the foot in diabetes. Diabetes Metab Res Rev. 2016;32(Suppl 1):75-83.

31. Goldman RJ. Hyperbaric oxygen therapy for wound healing and limb salvage: a systematic review. PM R. 2009;1(5):471-89.

32. Goldstein LJ et al. Endothelial progenitor cell release into circulation is triggered by hyperoxia-induced increases in bone marrow nitric oxide. Stem Cells. 2006;24(10):2309-18.

33. Guyatt G et al. GRADE guidelines: 1. Introduction – GRADE evidence profiles and summary of findings tables. J Clin Epidemiol. 2011;64(4):383-94.

34. Guyatt GH et al. GRADE guidelines: 2. Framing the question and deciding on important outcomes. J Clin Epidemiol. 2011;64(4):395-400.

35. Guyatt GH et al. GRADE guidelines: 4. Rating the quality of evidence – study limitations (risk of bias). J Clin Epidemiol. 2011;64(4):407-15.

36. Guyatt GH et al. GRADE guidelines: 5. Rating the quality of evidence – publication bias. J Clin Epidemiol. 2011;64(12):1277-82.

37. Guyatt GH et al. GRADE guidelines: 6. Rating the quality of evidence – imprecision. J Clin Epidemiol. 2011;64(12):1283-93.

38. Guyatt GH et al. GRADE guidelines: 7. Rating the quality of evidence – inconsistency. J Clin Epidemiol. 2011;64(12):1294-302.

39. Guyatt GH et al. GRADE guidelines: 8. Rating the quality of evidence – indirectness. J Clin Epidemiol. 2011;64(12):1303-10.

40. Guyatt GH et al. GRADE guidelines: 9. Rating up the quality of evidence. J Clin Epidemiol. 2011;64(12):1311-6.

41. Guyatt G et al. GRADE guidelines: 11. Making an overall rating of confidence in effect estimates for a single outcome and for all outcomes. J Clin Epidemiol. 2013;66(2):151-7.

42. Guyatt GH et al. GRADE guidelines: 12. Preparing summary of findings tables – binary outcomes. J Clin Epidemiol. 2013;66(2):158-72.

43. Guyatt GH et al. GRADE guidelines: 13. Preparing summary of findings tables and evidence profiles – continuous outcomes. J Clin Epidemiol. 2013;66(2):173-83.

44. Hart G, Strauss M. Responses of ischaemic ulcerative conditions to OHP. In: Proceedings of the 6th International Congress on Hyperbaric Medicine; 1979: p. 312-4.

45. Hingorani A et al. The management of diabetic foot: a clinical practice guideline by the Society for Vascular Surgery in collaboration with the American Podiatric Medical Association and the Society for Vascular Medicine. J Vasc Surg. 2016;63(2 Suppl):3S-21S.

46. Huang ET et al. A clinical practice guideline for the use of hyperbaric oxygen therapy in the treatment of diabetic foot ulcers. Undersea Hyperb Med. 2015;42(3):205-47.

47. Huang ET. Comment on Fedorko et al. Hyperbaric oxygen therapy does not reduce indications for amputation in patients with diabetes with nonhealing ulcers of the lower limb: a prospective, double-blind, randomized controlled clinical trial. Diabetes Care. 2016;39:392-9. Diabetes Care. 2016;39(8):e133-4.

48. Hyperbaric oxygen therapy for the treatment of diabetic foot ulcers: OHTAC Recommendation. 2016. p. 1-3.

49. Internal Clinical Guidelines Team. Diabetic foot problems: prevention and management. London: National Institute for Health and Care Excellence; 2015 Aug.

50. Jeffcoate WJ et al. Reporting standards of studies and papers on the prevention and management of foot ulcers in diabetes: required details and markers of good quality. Lancet Diabetes Endocrinol. 2016;4(9):781-8.

51. Kalani M et al. Hyperbaric oxygen (HBO) therapy in treatment of diabetic foot ulcers. Long-term follow-up. J Diabetes Complications. 2002;16(2):153-8.

52. Kang TS et al. Effect of hyperbaric oxygen on the growth factor profile of fibroblasts. Arch Facial Plast Surg. 2004;6(1):31-5.

53. Kaya A et al. Can major amputation rates be decreased in diabetic foot ulcers with hyperbaric oxygen therapy? Int Orthop. 2009;33(2):441-6.

54. Kessler L et al. Hyperbaric oxygenation accelerates the healing rate of nonischemic chronic diabetic foot ulcers: a prospective randomized study. Diabetes Care. 2003;26(8):2378-82.

55. Kranke P et al. Hyperbaric oxygen therapy for chronic wounds. Cochrane Database Syst Rev. 2012;4:CD004123.

56. LeDez K. Serious concerns about the Toronto Hyperbaric Oxygen for Diabetic Foot Ulcer study. Undersea Hyperb Med. 2016;43(6):737-41.

57. Lipsky BA et al. 2012 Infectious Diseases Society of America clinical practice guideline for the diagnosis and treatment of diabetic foot infections. Clin Infect Dis. 2012;54(12):e132-73.

58. Liu R et al. Systematic review of the effectiveness of hyperbaric oxygenation therapy in the management of chronic diabetic foot ulcers. Mayo Clin Proc. 2013;88(2):166-75.

59. Liu ZJ, Velazquez OC. Hyperoxia, endothelial progenitor cell mobilization, and diabetic wound healing. Antioxid Redox Signal. 2008;10(11):1869-82.

60. Londahl M. Hyperbaric oxygen therapy as adjunctive treatment for diabetic foot ulcers. Int J Low Extrem Wounds. 2013;12(2):152-7.

61. Londahl M. Hyperbaric oxygen therapy as adjunctive treatment of diabetic foot ulcers. Med Clin North Am. 2013;97(5):957-80.

62. Londahl M et al. Hyperbaric oxygen therapy facilitates healing of chronic foot ulcers in patients with diabetes. Diabetes Care. 2010;33(5):998-1003.

63. Londahl M et al. Relationship between ulcer healing after hyperbaric oxygen therapy and transcutaneous oximetry, toe blood pressure and ankle-brachial index in patients with diabetes and chronic foot ulcers. Diabetologia. 2011;54(1):65-8.

64. Londahl M, Fagher K, Katzman P. Comment on Fedorko et al. Hyperbaric oxygen therapy does not reduce indications for amputation in patients with diabetes with nonhealing ulcers of the lower limb: a prospective, double-blind, randomized controlled clinical trial. Diabetes Care. 2016;39:392-9. Diabetes Care. 2016;39(8):131-2.

65. Londahl M, Landin-Olsson M, Katzman P. Hyperbaric oxygen therapy improves health-related quality of life in patients with diabetes and chronic foot ulcer. Diabet Med. 2011;28(2):186-90.

66. Ma L et al. A prospective, randomized, controlled study of hyperbaric oxygen therapy: effects on healing and oxidative stress of ulcer tissue in patients with a diabetic foot ulcer. Ostomy Wound Manage. 2013;59(3):18-24.

67. Margolis D. Discussion on propensity scoring. 2013.

68. Margolis DJ et al. Lack of effectiveness of hyperbaric oxygen therapy for the treatment of diabetic foot ulcer and the prevention of amputation: a cohort study. Diabetes Care. 2013;36(7):1961-6.

69. Margolis DJ et al. Response to comments on: Margolis et al. Lack of effectiveness of hyperbaric oxygen therapy for the treatment of diabetic foot ulcer and the prevention of amputation: a cohort study. Diabetes Care. 2013;36:1961-6. Diabetes Care. 2013;36(8):e132-3.

70. Marx RE. Osteoradionecrosis: a new concept of its pathophysiology. J Oral Maxillofac Surg. 1983;41(5):283-8.

71. Marx RE et al. Relationship of oxygen dose to angiogenesis induction in irradiated tissue. Am J Surg. 1990;160(5):519-24.

72. Moon H et al. The validity of transcutaneous oxygen measurements in predicting healing of diabetic foot ulcers. Undersea Hyperb Med. 2016;43(6).

73. Murad MH. Comment on Fedorko et al. Hyperbaric oxygen therapy does not reduce indications for amputation in patients with diabetes with nonhealing ulcers of the lower limb: a prospective, double-blind, randomized controlled clinical trial. Diabetes Care. 2016;39:392-9. Diabetes Care. 2016;39(8):e135.

74. Murad MH et al. Using GRADE for evaluating the quality of evidence in hyperbaric oxygen therapy clarifies evidence limitations. J Clin Epidemiol. 2014;67(1):65-72.

75. National coverage determination (NCD) for hyperbaric oxygen therapy (20.29). Centers for Medicare and Medicaid Services; 1996.

76. O'Reilly D et al. Hyperbaric oxygen therapy for diabetic ulcers: systematic review and meta-analysis. Int J Technol Assess Health Care. 2013;29(3):269-81.

77. Oriani G et al. Diabetic foot and hyperbaric oxygen therapy: a ten-year experience. J Hyperb Med. 1992;7(4):213-21.

78. Oriani G et al. Hyperbaric oxygen therapy in diabetic gangrene. J Hyperb Med. 1990;5(3):171-5.

79. Roeckl-Wiedmann I, Bennett M, Kranke P. Systematic review of hyperbaric oxygen in the management of chronic wounds. Br J Surg. 2005;92(1):24-32.
80. Sheikh AY et al. Effect of hyperoxia on vascular endothelial growth factor levels in a wound model. Arch Surg. 2000;135(11):1293-7.
81. Stoekenbroek RM et al. Hyperbaric oxygen for the treatment of diabetic foot ulcers: a systematic review. Eur J Vasc Endovasc Surg. 2014;47(6):647-55.
82. Stoekenbroek RM et al. Is additional hyperbaric oxygen therapy cost-effective for treating ischemic diabetic ulcers? Study protocol for the Dutch DAMOCLES multicenter randomized clinical trial? J Diabetes. 2015;7(1):125-32.
83. Strauss MB. The Wagner Wound Grading System. Wound Care Hyperb Med. 2012;3(4):38-45.
84. Strauss MB, Bryant BJ, Hart GB. Transcutaneous oxygen measurements under hyperbaric oxygen conditions as a predictor for healing of problem wounds. Foot Ankle Int. 2002;23(10):933-7.
85. Thom SR. Hyperbaric oxygen: its mechanisms and efficacy. Plast Reconstr Surg. 2011;127(Suppl 1):131S-141S.
86. Thom SR et al. Stem cell mobilization by hyperbaric oxygen. Am J Physiol Heart Circ Physiol. 2006;290(4):H1378-86.
87. Wang Z et al. A systematic review and meta-analysis of tests to predict wound healing in diabetic foot. J Vasc Surg. 2016;63(2 Suppl):29S-36S e1-2.
88. Wang C et al. Hyperbaric oxygen for treating wounds: a systematic review of the literature. Arch Surg. 2003;138(3):272-9; discussion 280.
89. Wattel F et al. Hyperbaric oxygen in the treatment of diabetic foot lesions: search for predictive healing factors. J Hyperb Med. 1991;6(4):263-8.
90. Worth ER, Tettelbach W, Hopf HW. Arterial insufficiences: enhancement of healing in selected problem wounds. In: Weaver LK, editor. Hyperbaric oxygen therapy indications, 13th edition. 2014. p. 25-46.
91. Wunderlich RP, Peters EJ, Lavery LA. Systemic hyperbaric oxygen therapy: lower-extremity wound healing and the diabetic foot. Diabetes Care. 2000;23(10):1551-5.
92. Zamboni WA et al. Evaluation of hyperbaric oxygen for diabetic wounds: a prospective study. Undersea Hyperb Med. 1997;24(3):175-9.

CHAPTER 24 CHAPTER

Fracture Healing and Roles of Hyperbaric Oxygen

CHAPTER TWENTY-FOUR OVERVIEW

Introduction....625
The Physiology of Bone Growth and Fracture Healing....625
Laboratory Studies with Oxygen and Fracture Healing....628
Clinical Review of Hyperbaric Oxygen in Fracture Healing....631
Personal Experiences with Hyperbaric Oxygen in Fracture Healing....632
Discussion....635
Conclusions....638
References....639

Fracture Healing and Roles of Hyperbaric Oxygen

Michael B. Strauss, Anna M. Tan, Lientra Q. Lu

INTRODUCTION

Hyperbaric oxygen (HBO_2) treatments for fracture healing is not an approved indication according to the guidelines formulated in the 13th edition of the *Undersea and Hyperbaric Medical Society Hyperbaric Oxygen Therapy Indications.*[1] Use of HBO_2 for fracture healing is, therefore, considered an "off-label" therapy for this modality. Consequently, the Centers for Medicare and Medicaid Services, as well as most other third-party payers, do not reimburse for using HBO_2 as an adjunct to fracture healing. Since it is estimated that 300,000 (4.7%) of the 6.3 million fractures that occur in the USA yearly are slow to heal or do not heal, other modalities need to be considered to improve these statistics.[2,3] Hyperbaric oxygen is one of them.

Bone is a remarkable tissue. It has multiple functions, including support and protection of the soft tissues of the body, a framework for muscles to act through joints, a fundamental component of calcium homeostasis, a site for generation of hematopoietic elements of the bloodstream and a reservoir for red blood cells. These functions of bone continue to occur while the fracture is healing or even in the presence of delayed or nonhealing of a fracture. Bone can also heal without leaving a scar, a trait it shares with the liver as the only body tissues that have the ability to do such.

Three requirements are essential for fractures to heal: adequate perfusion, appropriate stabilization and an environment for progenitor cells to be induced to form bone. When one or more of these elements is deficient, delayed or nonhealing of the fracture is likely to occur, as in the 4.7% of fractures in the USA that become nonunions. Hyperbaric oxygen has mechanisms to mitigate two of the three reasons fractures become nonunions. These are augmentation of perfusion-oxygenation and enhancement of the environment for fracture healing. This chapter describes the physiology of fracture healing, reports on the laboratory studies that support the use of HBO_2 for bone healing and reviews the limited clinical experiences where HBO_2 was used as an adjunct for fracture healing. From this information, a "new look" is warranted for using HBO_2 in a select complement of fractures.

THE PHYSIOLOGY OF BONE GROWTH AND FRACTURE HEALING

In the developing individual, two types of bone growth occur: enchondral and intramembranous. Enchondral bone formation occurs in the growth plates of long bones.

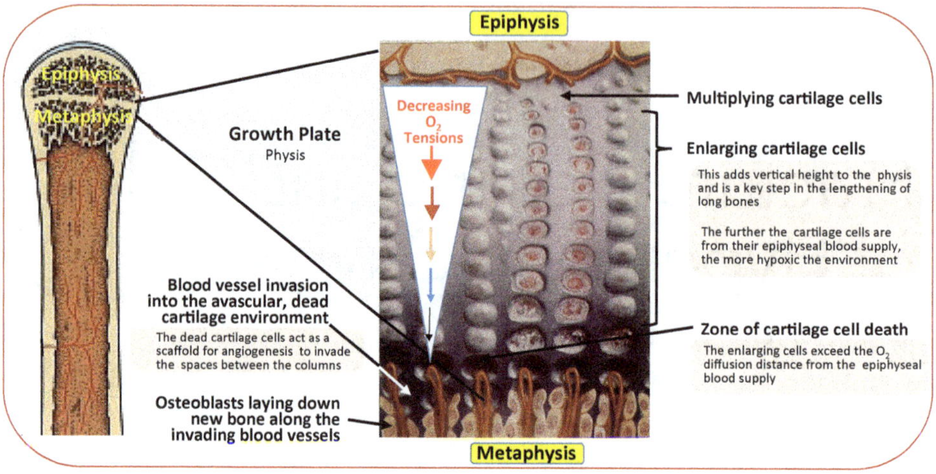

Legend: Oxygen availability is highly regulated in the growth plate. Cartilage multiplies in an oxygenated environment adjacent to epiphyseal blood vessels, but enlarges to lengthen the physis and eventually exceeds the diffusion distance of O_2. The cartilage cells die from hypoxia; this initiates blood vessel invasion between the columns of cartilage. Osteoblasts generate new bone along the blood vessels.

Figure 1. Bone formation at the growth plate.

It starts with a cartilaginous anlage. As the cartilage cells enlarge, they calcify and then outstrip their blood supply (Figure 1). Invasion of blood vessels bring in bone formation cell precursors, which line the calcified cartilage and lay down new bone along the cartilage anlage. The dead cartilage cells are reabsorbed by osteoclasts/chondroclasts. Intramembranous bone formation occurs under the periosteum of flat bones such as the clavicle. Bone formation occurs in situ under the periosteum and is incorporated into the outer surface of the cortical bone.

Fracture healing incorporates features of both types of bone formation with highly regulated oxygen tensions in the healing environment. Intramembranous bone formation is visualized on X-ray as periosteal new bone. Fracture healing has many analogies to soft tissue wound healing (Figure 2). The stages include injury, hematoma formation, inflammatory response, formation of granulation tissue, mitogenesis to soft callus, maturation to hard callus/new bone formation and remodeling. Two factors are essential for each stage to progress to the next. First, there must be adequate perfusion-oxygenation to the fracture site so that the cells in each stage of fracture healing can express themselves with their oxygen-dependent functions. Second, the environment of the bone surrounding the fracture must act as an inducer for the pluripotential cells of the granulation tissue phase to transform to osteogenesis precursors rather than continue to form collagen that would heal the soft tissue wound.

Dr. Bassett in the late 1960s demonstrated fracture cell precursors when compressed in a hypoxic environment formed cartilage and in the hyperoxic environment formed bone (Figure 3).[4] This model conforms to what is observed in nonunions where avascular cartilage and fibrous tissue bridge the bone ends.

Another consideration is that healthy, "raw" bone edges at the fracture site contribute to the induction effect. Death of bone cells immediately adjacent to the fracture is postulated to occur with all but the simplest fracture patterns. This dead bone is removed by the osteoclast, a very oxygen-dependent cell.

Three cell types are associated with bones: osteocytes, osteoblasts and osteoclasts. Osteocytes are the cells embedded in the bone matrix. They are anything but "resting" bone cells, being very metabolically active in directing osteoblastic and osteoclastic activity as well as in the calcium phosphorus regulation in the bone tissue. Osteoclasts are multinucleate giant cells from the macrophage linage that are induced to form alkaline and acid phosphatases to remove calcified tissues. They are very metabolically active and have 100 times the oxygen requirements as the osteoblast.[5] Osteoblasts are the bone-building cells. Their ability to build bone is about one one-hundredth that of the osteoclast's ability to remove bone.[5] Consequently, stabilization (as well as alignment during the remodeling stage), as stated above, is an important component of fracture healing.

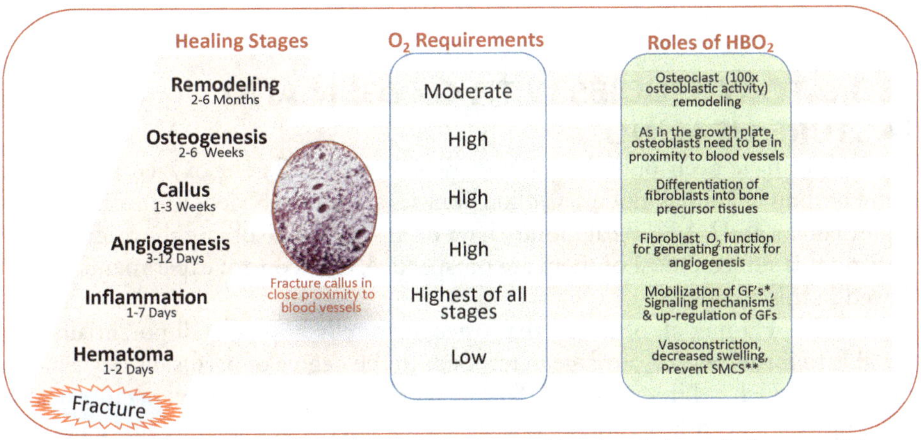

Legend: Oxygen availability and regulation, as in the growth plate, is required throughout the fracture healing process. This occurs without problems in the 95.3% of fractures that heal normally. In the other 300,000 fractures that go onto nonunion in the USA each year, identifiable factors and especially ischemia-hypoxia are the cause. Hyperbaric oxygen can mitigate the ischemia-hypoxia cause.

Key: * = Growth factors, ** = Skeletal muscle-compartment syndrome

Figure 2. Fracture healing, O_2 tensions and roles of hyperbaric oxygen.

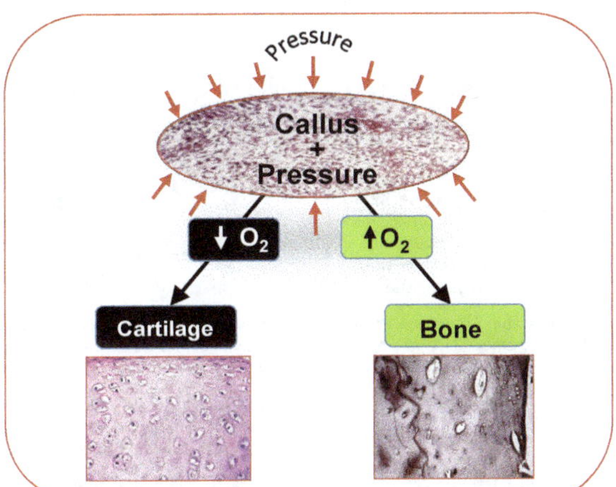

Legend: Dr. Bassett's findings[4] confirmed that undifferentiated pluripotential cells form bone when subjected to compressive forces in an enriched oxygen environment and form cartilage in a hypoxic environment. Cartilage is typically found in the nonunion site.

Figure 3. Effects of pressure and oxygen tensions on undifferentiated mesenchyme

Without it, bone is subject to deformities and, subsequently, pathological fractures, abnormal mechanics leading to arthritis, and wound development at the apex of the deformity.

Bones are in a continual state of remodeling. Structural unsound bone is removed by the osteoclast, while osteoblasts form new bone along lines of stress. When osteoclast function is inhibited by bisphosphonates, an anti-osteoporosis medication, bone remodeling is impaired. Although the bone may appear structurally sound (i.e., thick cortical margins) on X-ray, the failure to remove and rebuild bone along the lines of stress make it subject to pathological fractures, as seen in femurs of longtime bisphosphate drug users.

LABORATORY STUDIES WITH OXYGEN AND FRACTURE HEALING

Many articles have been published about the effects of different oxygen tensions on fracture healing in animal models. Online libraries such as PubMed, Rubicon, Elsevier, Google Scholar, and VA Medical Library have been searched to obtain the most relevant studies on this subject; most of them are prospective, case-control experiments and are reviewed in this section.

In 1932, Ham et al. observed that osteogenic cells have a "dull potentiality" — being able to form bone or cartilage in response to the degree of perfusion-oxygenation in the area in which it differentiates.[(6)] If oxygenation was compromised, fracture healing was disrupted and cartilage formed as is so often observed at a fracture nonunion site. Several earlier fracture-healing animal studies demonstrated that increased vascularity at the fracture site was needed before fracture healing occurred (Table 1).[(7-12)] Degree of perfusion and rate of angiogenesis at the fracture site correlated highly with the speed of callus resorption and bone union. Cavadias and Trueta reported that periosteal and endosteal vessels invaded the undifferentiated mesenchyme at the fracture site.[(12)] This confirmed that perfusion and oxygen delivery is an integral part of bone formation.

TABLE 1. ANIMAL STUDIES WHERE VASCULARITY WAS INVESTIGATED IN FRACTURES

Reference	Animal	Treatment	Results
Kolodny[(7)]	Dog radius	Fracture & disruption of nutrient artery separating bone & soft tissue	Nonunion resulted; decreased to total absence of callus formation vs. control limb
Trueta[(8)]	Rabbit	Kuntscher (clover-leaf) type of intramedullary nailing of fracture model	At 7-10 days, new bone layer appears along the diaphysis → gradually becomes denser. Periosteal callus appears earlier and more robust in rodded side & reflected periosteo perfusion
Gothman[(9)]	Monkey tibia	Intramedullary nailing vs. plating vs. external fixation	In nailed fractures, there was initially an 85.6 % reduction in blood flow, but after 90 days, they had significantly greater blood flow than externally fixed and plate fixed fractures
Wray[10)]	Immature rat	Tibial fracture without immobilization	↑ Fractured femur length (i.e. overgrowth secondary to increased perfusion,; ↑ vascular bed observed at fracture site
Rhinelander[(11)]	Dog	Undisplaced closed fractures vascular pattern vs. normal	Vasodilatation of existing arterial tree, ↑ medullary (predominantly) and periosteal (auxiliary) circulations
Cavadias[(12)]	Rabbit	Permeable barriers implanted in fractures	Periosteal & endosteal blood vessels invade the implant bed

Kolodny's findings also supported the perfusion-oxygenation hypothesis when he created fractures on canine tibia and disrupted the nutrient artery sites to the bone.[7] Nonunions uniformly occurred. Gothman observed that for a fracture to heal in a nonunion fracture model, angiogenesis/revascularization must occur within 14 days after the injury and the blood supply to the site needed to increase by a four- to fivefold factor; otherwise, nonunion would continue.[9] From their study on the vascular pattern of canine's undisplaced closed fractures, Rhinelander and Baragry found that increased blood flow associated with fracture healing stimulated long bone overgrowth.[11]

Reports in animal models demonstrate the harmful effects of hypoxia on bone precursors in fractures (Table 2). When Bassett subjected undifferentiated bone precursors of chick embryonic tissue to a hypoxic environment and pressure, cartilage formed (Figure 3).[4] With induced hypoxia of varying degrees in rats, Vaes and Nichols noted that more lactate accumulated in bones with low oxygen tensions and there was a decrease in synthesis of new bone matrix.[14] In canine tibial fractures exposed to hypoxia, Heppenstall reported that there was a decreased rate of bone union.[24]

With 85% oxygen and 5% carbon-dioxide partial pressures, Sledge and Dingle observed increased rate of cartilage degradation and bone formation in the dog model.[15] With rats subjected to hyperbaric oxygen exposures several hours a day for 14 to 20 days, both Coulson et al. and Wray and Rogers noted an increase in callus formation and decrease in break strength.[16,17] This latter finding was consistent with HBO_2 augmentation of osteoclast activity. This resulted in temporary weakening of bone during the bone remodeling process. Yablon and Cruess demonstrated increased healing of fractures with twice-a-day HBO_2 exposures in rats.[18]

TABLE 2. ANIMAL STUDIES DEMONSTRATING THE EFFECTS OF VARYING OXYGEN TENSIONS ON FRACTURE HEALING

Reference	Animal	Exposure	Results
Bassett[4]	Chick embryo	Compression plus high (35 % O_2) and low O_2 tensions	Bone formation with high O_2 tensions; cartilage formation with low O_2 tensions
Vaes[14]	Rat	Hypoxia of varying degrees	If bone O_2 tensions remained low, lactate accumulated,; ↓ synthesis of new matrix
Sledge[15]	Chick embryo	85 % O_2, 5 % CO_2	Degradation of cartilage septa, conversion of cartilage to bone
Coulson[16]	Rat	3 ATA, 2 hr. daily; 14 days	↑ Breaking strength of fractures
Wray[17]	Rat	2 ATA, 6 hr. daily; 20 days	↑ Callus, decreased strength
Yablon[18]	Rat	3 ATA, 1 hr. BID; 4-40 days	Improved healing with BID HBO_2
Laurnen[19]	Dog	Strontium-85 clearance after 10 minutes in tibiae 12 weeks after fracture	No difference in fx side & control side pO_2, pCO_2, pH. O_2 consumption & CO_2 production increased, reflecting blood flow has stabilized.
Niinikoski[20]	Rat	2.5 ATA, 2 hr. BID; 5-21 days	↑ Callus; ↑ precursors
Penttinen[21]	Rat	2.5 ATA, 2 hr; BID	Callus 19-42 % ↑, nitrogen 15-60 % ↑, minerals (e.g. Ca, Mg, Zn, etc.) 20-63 % ↑; strengths unchanged
Brighton[22]	Rat	Low O_2 initially in the cartilage anlage of the growth plate	Low O_2 → Calcium release; O_2 requirement for proline → OH-proline
Gray[23]	Mice calvaria	2 ATA, 24 hr. continuous exposure	↑ Collagen; ↓ bone formation & bone resorptior
Heppenstall[24]	Dog	Hypoxia (50 %)	Delay fracture healing

Laurnen and Kelly using radioisotopes (strontium-85 washout) showed a sixfold increase in blood flow in dog tibial fractures, while oxygen consumption, carbon-dioxide production and blood calcium and pH changes remained the same as in the opposite control limb.[19] These findings confirm that increased metabolism occurs with the concomitant need for oxygen in fracture healing.

Niinikoski et al. and Penttinen et al. studied biochemical changes in rat tibial fractures.[20,21] They found that increased oxygen tensions stimulated precursors of fracture healing and mineral productions such as Ca, Mg, Zn, etc. This led to increased callus formation at the fracture sites. According to Brighton and Krebs's study on the rat epiphyseal growth plate utilizing mega vitamin A doses and high oxygen tensions, the pretreatment low oxygen tension promoted calcium release from the bloodstream to the growth plate.[22] Subsequently, the high oxygen tensions resulted in hydroxylation of proline, an essential amino acid bone formation precursor generated by the undifferentiated fibroblast. The study also revealed a progressive decrease in oxygen tensions from the epiphysis to the metaphysis of the growth plate (Figure 1). In an experiment on murine calvaria fractures exposed to 2 atmospheres absolute pressures continuously for 24 hours, Gray et al. found an increase in collagen deposition and a decrease in bone formation and resorption.[23]

As the animal review shows, in the 1960s and 1970s there was much interest in studying the roles of oxygen and blood flow in general and HBO_2 in particular on fracture healing in animal studies. Unfortunately, this interest waned after this time probably because of improved orthopaedic fracture fixation techniques, application of callotaxis principles (Ilizarov), new and improved bone grafting alternatives, pulsed electrical stimulation of bone and use of inducers such as bone morphogenetic protein. Consistent findings associated with HBO_2 exposures included increased and speedier callus formation and faster bony union. The fracture strength, however, was initially weaker than compared to the control limbs. These observations substantiate the mechanisms that HBO_2 exhibits in fracture healing. In fracture healing, the oxygenated environment is essential for the pluripotential cells in the precallus to generate bone. In contrast, the physis (growth plate) accounts for the longitudinal growth of long bones in children. In this situation, the cells in the cartilage columns enlarge to the point that they exceed the oxygen diffusion gradient from the epiphyseal arteries and die (Figure 1). This stimulates angiogenesis from the metaphyseal blood vessels, which, in turn, provides a sufficiently oxygenated environment for the osteoblast to lay down new bone along the dead cartilage cell anlage.

In summary, the increased oxygen tensions in the fracture-healing environment accelerate callus formation and osteogenesis. In addition, the activity of the highly oxygen-dependent osteoclast is also stimulated. This results in faster bone resorption for the remodeling and ultimate strengthening process of the fracture. In the interim, because of the speeded-up remodeling process, the bone exposed to HBO_2 is temporarily weaker. By the ends of the observation periods, bone strengths were usually equal in both the HBO_2 and control limbs.

These observations are consistent with the first author's experiences that in about 20% of the cases where HBO_2 was used for fracture healing and/or arrest of refractory osteomyelitis, delayed onset stress fractures occurred after there was X-ray evidence of bone union.

A final observation from the animal studies is that "pulses" of HBO_2, that is intermittent exposures, are sufficient to achieve the bone healing effects. In contrast, the study of a continuous HBO_2 exposure was detrimental to bone healing, which is consistent with oxygen toxicity (probable generation of free radicals) from the single, prolonged HBO_2 exposure.[22]

CLINICAL REVIEW OF HYPERBARIC OXYGEN IN FRACTURE HEALING

While there have been numerous articles exploring the effects of HBO_2 and fracture healing in animal models, little comparative clinical evidence of effectiveness exists. Extensive literature search via Pub Med, Ovid, Cochrane Library, and Google Scholar revealed a dearth of information, with search results consisting primarily of case reports and prospective series. These studies and most recent literature will be summarized in the following section.

Lindstrom et al. reported on 20 subjects requiring intramedullary nailing for closed tibial fractures who received HBO_2 as an adjunct therapy. They measured transcutaneous oxygen tensions in the lower leg, limb temperature and distal arterial flow via Doppler. The trial, however, did not report any clinical outcomes in relation to fracture healing.[25] Porcellini et al. reviewed patients with serious vascular injures in addition to fractures. Hyperbaric oxygen therapy was utilized in 7 out of 34 patients to control bacterial contamination and improve wound healing. Outcomes regarding HBO_2 and its effect on fracture healing, however, were not explicitly reviewed.[26]

Braune et al. detailed the case of a patient with 17-year-old posttraumatic pseudarthrosis of the dens axis following conservative treatment of unstable Anderson's type II odontoid fracture. Following surgical intervention and revisions, X-rays revealed an unstable posttraumatic Blauth's type III odontoid nonunion in association with wound dehiscence, exposed autograft and internal fixation hardware. Hyperbaric oxygen treatments were used as a therapeutic option in conjunction with a surgical salvage procedure. Complete wound healing was observed after 25 days. In addition, radiographs showed bone fusion with incorporation of the autologous bone graft and solid atlantoaxial fusion.[27]

In a 2005 Cochrane review study, the authors were unable to find any articles to meet its inclusion criteria for justifying HBO_2 for fracture healing.[29] Thus, the conclusion was that there was insufficient evidence to support or refute HBO_2 in use for delayed bony healing and nonunion of fractures. There is one randomized, double-blinded controlled trial, however, in which the authors studied fracture healing in crush injuries.[28] Bouachour et al. reported complete healing in 94% of the HBO_2 group versus 33% in the control limb, while need for repeat surgery (after initial debridement and stabilization) was 6% in the HBO_2 group compared to 33% in the patients who did not receive HBO_2. Both observations were statistically significant ($p < 0.05$). All patients had crush injuries (Gustilo grade 2-B open fractures) where vascular compromise and threatened flaps were an integral part of the pathophysiology of the injury.

The most recent studies regarding HBO_2 and fracture healing are from China. Chen observed the effect of intramedullary nail fixation combined with HBO_2 in the treatment of long bone fractures in children. The authors concluded that those in the HBO_2 group had lower levels of pain and swelling with earlier ambulation and shorter healing times.[30] In another study from China, Yu found that HBO_2 significantly improved the formation of callus in 44 patients with delayed union of tibial fractures.[31]

In his randomized controlled study, the 22 patients in the test group who received HBO_2 had a "total effective rate" of 95%. The author concluded that HBO_2 promoted the healing of fractures and reduced the incidence of delayed union and nonunion.

In summary, only meager clinical evidence from the literature supports the use of HBO_2 for fracture healing and especially nonunions. Further studies including prospective series and randomized control trials are needed to advance HBO_2 as an adjunct to fracture healing, prevention of delayed union, and healing of nonunion fractures. Nonetheless, the current knowledge of fracture healing mechanisms and the animal studies reported above are consistent with specialized roles for HBO_2 in fracture management.

PERSONAL EXPERIENCES WITH HYPERBARIC OXYGEN IN FRACTURE HEALING

Through the years, the first author (MBS) has had a number of patients for which hyperbaric oxygen has influenced healing of fractures. This group needs to be differentiated from the multitude of cases where HBO_2 has been used as an adjunct to manage open fractures and crush injuries as described in the Bouachour study previously cited as well as in cases of chronic refractory osteomyelitis.[28,32] The subset of patients in question had delayed or nonunions of their lower-extremity fractures, or fracture healing was likely to be impaired due to the severity of the injury. The first experiences occurred with three active-duty U.S. Navy personnel who had nonunions of their tibia fractures after motorcycle accidents. After nonhealing of the fracture was ascertained, each underwent a segmental (about 5 cm in length) fibula ostectomy and Sarmiento patellar tendon cast bracing. The rationale for the fibular osteotomy was to allow compressive forces to increase across the fracture site with weight bearing. Without subsequent evidence of healing, arrangements were made for the patients to receive three U.S. Navy Treatment Table 5 HBO_2 exposures a week for four weeks at the Naval Special Warfare recompression chamber at the U.S. Naval Amphibious Base in Coronado, California. All three fractures became stable, allowing the discontinuation of cast bracing. X-rays indicated the stability was attributed to periosteal new bone formation.

Subsequently, the first author used HBO_2 for a small number of "last-resort" fracture situations referred to him at Long Beach Memorial Medical Center in Long Beach, California. The following are five anecdotal cases in which HBO_2 appeared to change favorably the patients' outcomes:

One of the earliest cases was a middle-aged male who had bilateral nonunions of his distal femurs after Rush rodding and bone grafting. During the course of 20 hyperbaric treatments, the rods were removed, and then the femoral fractures stabilized with external fixation. The fractures healed after another 10 HBO_2 treatments and subsequent removal of the external fixators 12 weeks after applications.

A second case involved a nonunion of the proximal femoral shaft in a male in his 20s. After cast immobilization failed, an external fixator was applied, but there was hardware failure with breakage of the fixator. With HBO_2 treatments while remaining nonweight bearing on the extremity, the fracture healed.

A third case was that of male smoker in his 40s who after a motorcycle accident sustained a severe proximal tibial fracture that was managed with medial and lateral platings. The proximal 20% of the skin over the anterior aspect of the tibia sloughed, exposing both plates and the necrotic anterior tibial fragment (Figure 4). The patient was referred for HBO_2 treatments as alternative to an above-knee amputation. With staged surgeries while receiving ongoing HBO_2 treatments, the wound was debrided, hardware removed and the fracture stabilized with external fixation spanning from the distal femur to the middle tibia. After granulation tissue covered the cavity, autologous bone grafting was used to fill the defect, and a rotational gastrocnemius muscle flap used to provide soft-tissue coverage. Twenty-five years later, the patient continues to be a community ambulator with moderate loss of knee flexion.

The fourth case was that of a male in his 20s who developed an infected tibial nonunion after plating of a closed shaft fracture and more than 15 subsequent surgeries. Eighteen months after the injury without evidence of healing or control of the infection, he had made the decision to undergo a below-knee amputation (Figure 5). His wife, a nurse at our medical center, convinced him to try HBO_2 as an alternative to an amputation. After two weeks of HBO_2 treatments, the nonunion site was debrided and the fracture site stabilized with an external fixator.

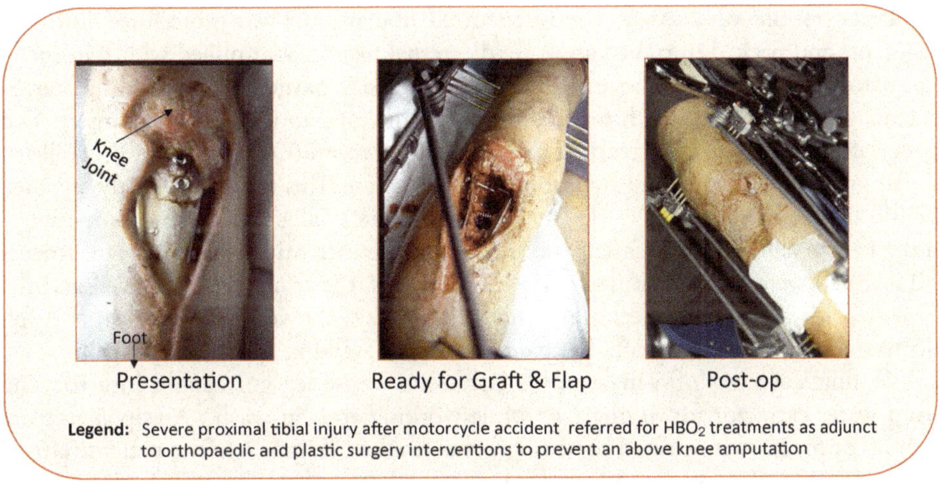

Figure 4. Major skin slough and devitalized proximal tibia bone.

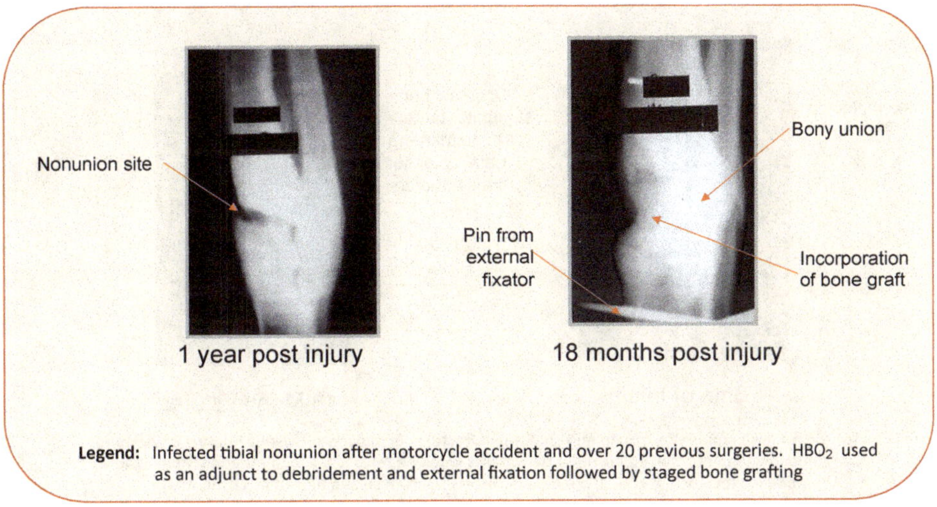

Figure 5. Infected nonunion with multiple surgical attempts to resolve problem.

A week later, when the nonunion site was covered with healthy granulation tissue, autologous bone grafting (Papineau technique) was done. Hyperbaric oxygen treatments were continued for two additional weeks. Blood vessels grew into the open bone graft, and gradually the graft epithelialized over a three-month period. At that time, the fixator was removed, and bony union was confirmed by clinical exam and X-rays.

A fifth case concerned a male also in his 20s who sustained a severely comminuted open distal tibia and fibula fractures with a 5 cm gap due to loss of bone after the initial debridement. A spanning external fixator with single half pins in the calcaneus and proximal to the fracture were used to temporarily maintain alignment until plastic surgeons could perform a microvascular ipsilateral fibular graft to span the defect. Unfortunately, the fixator did not maintain the length, and at the time of the fibular grafting, the gap had shortened 4 cm. The plastic surgeons where stymied as to what to do: Accept the shortening and use 1 cm of the 5 cm fibular graft to span the remaining gap, discard the fibula graft, or seek an immediate second orthopaedic surgeon's opinion. The latter option was chosen. The vascularized fibular graft was morcellized into fine fragments and packed into the gap. A rigid external fixator was applied with transfixing pins placed in the foot and above the fracture. Hyperbaric oxygen treatments were started to manage swelling and the threatened flaps after the four-and-a-half-hour surgery. Two weeks later, the patient was returned to the operating room (OR) where the morcellized fibular graft was stretched out by readjusting the fixator. This maneuver nearly regained the full tibia length. At four weeks, the axial and rotatory alignments were "fine-tuned" in the OR to achieve an essentially normal-appearing extremity, and HBO_2 treatments (40 in total) were stopped at that time. At 12 weeks, the fixator was removed and the leg casted for another six weeks, at which time X-rays showed consolidation and full incorporation of the bone graft. The patient resumed walking with a normal gait.

A final case was of a male in his late teens whose leg got caught in a rotating drum water extractor for drying rags while working at a car wash. An open fracture with 20 or more comminuted bone fragments resulted (Figure 6). The patient refused an amputation and was transferred to our medical center for HBO_2 treatments.

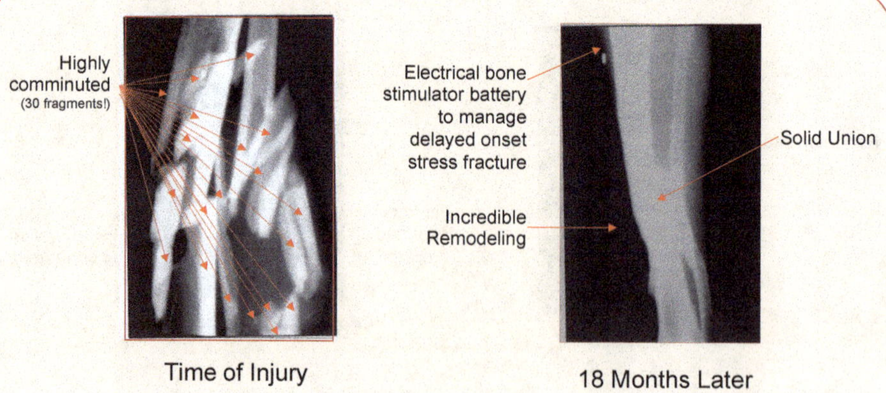

Legend: Extremely comminuted, open mid-shaft tibial fracture secondary to twisting injury. Early wound infection. Patient referred for HBO_2 treatments when he refused a leg amputation. Remarkable remodeling (osteoclast effect), but delayed stress fracture shown healed at 18 months.

Figure 6. Limb-threatening open fracture with recommendation for a below-knee amputation.

Stabilization was achieved with an external fixator. At three months, the fractures had developed callus and the fixator replaced with a walking cast. At six months, bony union was achieved.

Several conclusions can be drawn from these favorable outcomes using HBO_2 as an adjunct for fracture healing. First, HBO_2 was used in conjunction with "state-of-the-art" orthopaedic management. It should always be used as an adjunct to orthopaedic management and not a substitute for it. Hyperbaric oxygen treatments alone would not have achieved the same results. Second, a course of HBO_2 treatments before definitive orthopaedic interventions appeared to help the fracture site respond to the final, definitive orthopaedic intervention. Staged surgeries using HBO_2 before surgery to generate a favorable environment at the nonunion site for bone grafting and after surgery to promote bony union is logical, based on the mechanisms of HBO_2.[33] Third, HBO_2 favored bone formation of the undifferentiated mesenchyme that invaded the fracture site in the fracture milieu. In this capacity, it may have acted as an inducer of osteoblastic and osteoclastic activity as well as providing an oxygen environment sufficient for these cells to function. Fourth, HBO_2 supported angiogenesis (i.e., vascular ingrowth of the avascular bone graft scaffold) in those cases where bone grafting was used in the management. Fifth, early utilization of HBO_2 in the course of healing of fractures that are highly predictable of complications (e.g., the first author's cases 3, 5, and 6 described above) is supported by the above observations. Finally, HBO_2 promotes bone remodeling by the osteoclast, which is the most metabolically active of the three bone cell types. This was apparent in cases 5 and 6 above where extensive remodeling occurred. It is also seen as a minor complication with delayed-onset stress fractures after resuming ambulation. This has been observed in about ⅕ of our patients treated for crush injuries, osteomyelitis and nonunions of long bones.

DISCUSSION

There is much supporting information that perfusion-oxygenation is a key factor in bone formation and growth. This is observed in limb length overgrowth of children's lower-extremity fractures and is attributed to the increased flow associated with fracture healing. For similar reasons, bone overgrowth and hypertrophy are associated with arteriovenous fistulas. The propensity for excessive bone formation is seen after muscle injury (i.e., heterotopic ossification) and after brain and spinal cord injuries. Increased perfusion associates with both the inflammatory reaction in myositis and disruption of sympathetic nervous system vasoconstriction with the neurological conditions. Although acromegaly is attributed to pituitary tumors and increased elaboration of growth hormone, there appear to be concomitant changes in blood flow from the hormone.[34] This may be the reason that increased bone mass is associated with this condition. Finally, the formation of bone spurs is possibly due to an inflammatory response increasing blood flow to bone from repetitive trauma to the site either from traction effects (spurs pointing away from the metaphyses) or over underlying bony deformities.

Additional information showing the importance of blood flow and oxygen availability for bone viability is observed in those situations in which blood supply is lost. Examples include: 1) osteonecrosis of the femoral head associated with fractures, steroids, alcoholism, and dysbarism; 2) osteoradionecrosis of the mandible due to sclerosis of blood vessels from radiation; 3) jaw-bone necrosis from bisphosphonates with failure of bone remodeling (from the osteoclast) to maintain channels for blood vessels to perfuse the mandible; 4) osteonecrosis in conjunction with osteopetrosis for similar mechanisms attributed to jaw-bone necrosis; and 5) bone death in purpura fulminans and frostbite from sludging and obstruction. Bone viability can be confirmed with the technetium nuclear medicine scan.

The approximately one in 25 fractures (4.7 %) in the USA in which healing is delayed is usually predictable. Soft tissue damage, energy exchange, comminution, displacement, contamination, interruption of vascular supply and inadequate management are obvious causes. A multicenter review of more than 300,000 fractures reported that the highest nonunion rates were in the metatarsals (15.5%), scaphoids (15.3%), tibia and fibula (14%) and femur (9%).[3] For all open fractures, the nonunion rate was 10.9% and ranged from 4.4% in those patients with a single fracture to 24% in patients with 7 fractures. Odds ratios were the highest for patients on a combination of nonsteroidal anti-inflammatory drugs and opioids (1.84), management requiring surgery (1.78), open fracture (1.66), concomitant anticoagulation (1.49), high-energy injury (1.38), osteoporosis (1.24), insulin requirement (1.21) and smoking (1.20). Other factors had odds ratios less than 1.20 and included such items as use of antibiotics, use of bisphosphonates for osteoporosis, vitamin D deficiency, use of diuretics and renal insufficiency, in that order. Surprisingly age in 10-year increments from 18 to 63 did not show significant differences in rates of nonunions (range from 4.5 to 5.5%). A surprising omission of the study was absence of information on perfusion to the fracture site. Nonetheless, the five risk factors of multiple fractures, NSAIDs plus opioid use, open fractures, anticoagulation and osteoarthritis plus rheumatoid arthritis increased the risk of nonunion by 50%.[3]

Can information of this sort provide justification for using HBO_2 as an adjunct for prevention of nonunions and achieve fracture healing? The answer is a qualified yes if tools currently available are utilized to justify the decision to use HBO_2. The first step, of course, is the clinical evaluation and assessment of perfusion directly and oxygenation indirectly. Palpation and Doppler detection of pulses provide a direct assessment of perfusion. Skin (and wound base) coloration, skin temperature and

TABLE 3. WELLNESS SCORE

Assessment	2 Points	1 Point	0 Points
ADLs Ability to do activities of daily living	Full	Some	None
Ambulation	Community	Household	None
Comorbidities Except neuro; include obesity	Normal	Impaired	Decompensated
Tobacco/Steroid Use	None	Past	Current
Neuro Function	Normal	Impaired	Decompensated

Note: The "Wellness Score" is a quick-to-obtain evaluation tool to assess how functional a patient is . If scores are 5-points or more, the patient's overall health status as measured by these five easy-to-ascertain assessments justifies limb salvage.

TABLE 4. GOAL SCORE

Assessment	Full 2 Points	Some 1 Point	None 0 Points
	Use half points if mixed or intermediate between 2 grades		
Comprehension			
Motivation			
Compliance			
Support Family, caregiver, institutional			
Insight			

Note: The "Goal Score" is another useful tool to determine how successful and how intent the patient and the family are in avoiding a major amputation. Goal Scores greater than 4 ½ points supports the decision to avoid lower limb amputation and do everything possible for salvage of the nonunion. This score coupled with the Wellness Score (Table 3) provides objectivity for decision-making regarding limb threatening nonunions.

capillary refill provide indirect evidence of perfusion and oxygenation. Finally, juxta-wound transcutaneous oxygen measurements provide objective information as to tissue oxygenation.[35]

Two user-friendly clinical tools can supplement the fracture evaluation information and help justify decision-making regarding salvage or amputation of the lower limb nonunion. These tools are the Wellness and Goal Scores that are also found in Chapter 20: Hyperbaric Oxygen for the Management of Chronic Refractory Osteomyelitis of this textbook (Tables 3 and 4). Each is a 0-to-10 score based on five assessments graded with objective findings from 2 points (best) to 0 points (worst). Scores on these two tools when each is 5 points or greater support the decision to do everything possible to heal the nonunion. If ischemia-hypoxia is associated with the nonunion, and the factors having the highest odds ratios for nonunion (i.e., NSAIDS plus opioid use, operating room treatment, open fracture, anticoagulation and high-energy injury) are present, we feel there is substantial justification for using HBO_2 as an adjunct to other orthopaedic interventions. Even if orthopaedic interventions were used before and failed to resolve the nonunion, repeat bone grafting, callotaxis, use of bone morphogenetic protein, electrical stimulation and/or microvascular bone transplants should be utilized in conjunction with HBO_2 treatments when the indications from the Wellness and Goal Score tools support the decision to heal the nonunion.

Unfortunately, there is minimal clinical information to support the use of HBO_2 for fracture healing (Boauchour et al., Chen, Yu and the first author's anecdotal observations).[28,30,31] Mitigation of hypoxia was the design for most of the animal studies dealing with fracture healing. Impairment of oxygenation on a perfusion basis in tibial nonunions has been documented with transcutaneous oxygen measurements.[36] Information such as this supports the use of HBO_2 since hyperoxygenation of plasma and tissue fluids is a primary mechanism of HBO_2.[33]

TABLE 5. RATIONAL BASED INDICATIONS (RBI) FOR USING HBO_2 WITH NONUNIONS

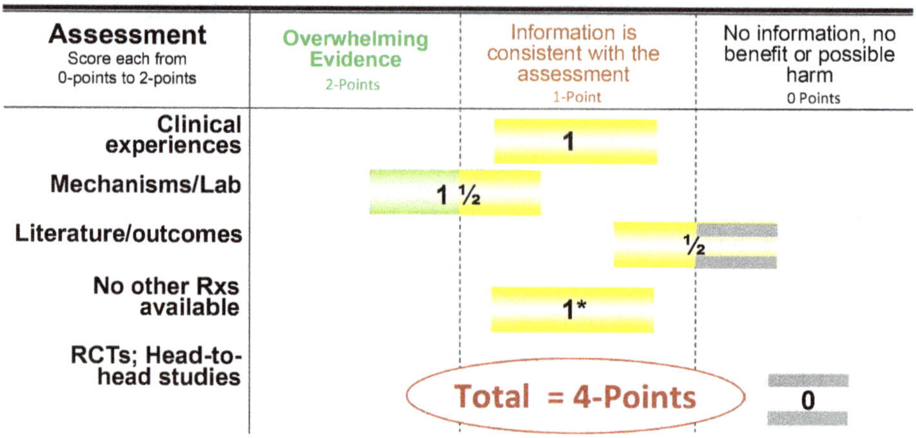

Interpretations: for Using HBO_2 with Nonunions

7 ½ to 10 points Strong RBI for HBO_2 regardless of Wellness & Goal Scores

3 ½ to 7 points Indication for HBO_2 if Wellness & Goal Scores support decision to salvage

0 to 3 points No indication for HBO_2 regardless of Wellness & Goal Scores

When a score we devised titled Rational Indications for Using HBO_2 is applied to fracture healing, only modest justification (i.e., 4 points out of 10 possible points) is summated (Table 5). Obviously, new animal studies using perturbations from the clinical literature associated with nonunions and randomized controlled clinical trials are needed before HBO_2 can be unequivocally recommended for this problem.

CONCLUSIONS

While hyperbaric oxygen is not an approved use for nonunions, its mechanisms support its use when ischemia-hypoxia is contributing to the failure of bone union. Identifiable clinical factors, juxta-wound oxygenation measurements and imaging studies can confirm whether or not perfusion-oxygenation is adequate to the bone at the nonunion site. User-friendly tools such as the Wellness and Goal Scores support decisions to salvage or amputate the nonunion. Although there is only sparse clinical information to support the use of HBO_2 as an adjunct to fracture healing, the laboratory studies consistently validate the need for oxygen in fracture healing in general and the nonunion in particular. Even though only 1 in 25 fractures (300,000) of the 6.3 million fractures that occur in the USA each year go onto nonunions, they present major treatment and financial challenges. When "tried-and-true" orthopaedic interventions such as bone grafting, optimal stabilization, bone morphogenetic protein, callotaxis and pulsatile electrical on sonographic bone stimulation have not resolved the nonunion and there is justification to avoid a lower limb amputation, then HBO_2 should be utilized in the management as an adjunct to one or more of the above orthopaedic techniques. There is no information, study, or observation where bone perfusion-oxygen is not a primary consideration in fracture healing.

REFERENCES

1. Weaver LK. Undersea and Hyperbaric Medical Society Hyperbaric Oxygen Therapy Indications, 13th ed. Best Publishing Company, North Palm Beach, FL; 2014.
2. Physical Fields-OrthoInfo - AAOS. Accessed August 26, 2016 from http://orthoinfo.aaos.org/topic.cfm?topic=A00279
3. Zura R, Ziong Z, Einhorn T, et al. Epidemiology of fracture nonunion in 18 human bones. JAMA Surg. Published online September 07, 2016. Doi: 10.1001/jamasurg.2016.2775.
4. Bassett CA, Herrmann I. Influence of oxygen concentration and mechanical factors on differentiation of connective tissues in vitro. Nature. 1961; 190:460-461.
5. Johnson LC. Kinetics of Osteoarthritis. Lab Invest. 1959; 8:1223-1241.
6. Ham AW. Cartilage and Bone. Special Cytology. 2nd ed. New York, NY; 1932.
7. Kolodny A. The periosteal blood supply and healing of fractures. Experimental Study. J Bone Joint Surg Am. 1923; 5(4):698-711.
8. Trueta J, Cavadias AX. Vascular changes caused by the Kuntscher type of nailing: an experimental study in the rabbit. J Bone Joint Surg Am. 1955; 37-B(3):492-505.
9. Gothman L. Arterial changes in experimental fractures of the monkey's tibia treated with intramedullary nailing. A microangiographic study. Acta Chir Scand. 1961; 121:56-66.
10. Wray JB, Goodman, HO. Post-fracture vascular phenomena and long-bone overgrowth in the immature skeleton of the rat. J Bone Joint Surg Am. 1961; 43-A:1047-1055.
11. Rhinelander FW, Baragry R. Microangiography in bone healing. I. Undisplaced closed fractures. J Bone Joint Surg Am. 1962; 44-A:1273-1298.
12. Cavadias AX, Trueta J. An experimental study of the vascular contribution to the callus of fracture. Surg Gynecol Obstet. 1965; 120:731-747.
13. Gothman L. Vascular reactions in experimental fractures. Microangiographic and radioisotope studies. Acta Chir Scand Suppl. 1961; Suppl 284:1-34.
14. Vaes GM, Nichols G Jr. Oxygen tension and the control of bone cell metabolism. Nature. 1962; 193:379-380.
15. Sledge CB, Dingle JT. Oxygen-induced resorption of cartilage in organ culture. Nature. 1965; 205:140-141.
16. Coulson DB, Ferguson AB Jr, Diehl RC Jr. Effect of hyperbaric oxygen on the healing femur of the rat. Surg Forum. 1966: 17:449-450.
17. Wray JB, Rogers LS. Effect of hyperbaric oxygenation upon fracture healing in the rat. J Surg Res. 1968: 8(8):373-378.
18. Yablon IG, Cruess RL. The effect of hyperbaric oxygen on fracture healing in rats. J Trauma. 1968; 8(2):186-202.
19. Laurnen EL, Kelly PJ. Blood flow, oxygen consumption, carbon-dioxide production, and blood-calcium and pH changes in tibial fractures in dogs. J Bone Joint Surg Am. 1969; 51(2):298-308.
20. Niinikoski J, Penttinen R, Kulonen E. Effect of hyperbaric oxygenation on fracture healing in the rat: a biochemical study. Calcif Tissue Res. 1970; Suppl:115-116.
21. Penttinen R, Niinikoski J, Kulonen E. Hyperbaric oxygenation and fracture healing. A biochemical with rats. Acta Chir Scand. 1972; 138(1):39-44.

22. Brighton CT, Krebs AG. Oxygen tension of healing fractures in the rabbit. J Bone Joint Surg Am. 1972; 54(2):323-332.

23. Gray DH, Hamblen DL. The effects of hyperoxia upon bone in organ culture. Clin Orthop Relat Res. 1976; (119):225-230.

24. Heppenstall RB, Goodwin CW, Brighton CT. Fracture healing in the presence of chronic hypoxia. J Bone Joint Surg Am. 1976; 58(8):1153-1156.

25. Lindstrom T, Gullichsen E, Lertola K, Niinikoski J. Effects of hyperbaric oxygen therapy on perfusion parameters and transcutaneous oxygen measurements in patients with intramedullary nailed tibial shaft fractures. Undersea & Hyperbaric Medicine. 1998; 25(2):87-91.

26. Porcellini M, Bernardo B, Capasso R, Bauleo A, Baldassarre M. Combined vascular injuries and limb fractures. Minerva Cardioangiologica. 1997;45(4):131-8.

27. Braune C, Hamm J, Bohmer D, Scale D, Zichner L. Hyperbaric oxygenation as a successful therapeutic approach in oral wound dehiscence after operative stabilization of an unstable post- traumatic odontoid non-union. Archives of Orthopaedic and Trauma Surgery. 2002; 122(2):115-9.

28. Bouachour G, Cronier P, Gouello JP, et al. Hyperbaric oxygen therapy in the management of crush injuries: A randomized double-blind placebo-controlled clinical trial. J Trauma. 1996; 41:333-339.

29. Bennett MH, Stanford R, Turner R. Hyperbaric oxygen therapy for promoting fracture healing and treating fracture non-union (Cochrane Review). In: The Cochrane Library, Issue 1, 2006. Oxford: Update Software.

30. Chen Guo-ping. Effect of elastic stable intramedullary nail combined with hyperbaric oxygen on children with long bone fractures. Chinese Journal of General Practice. 2012

31. Yu Wenzhong. The effects of hyperbaric oxygen therapy on the treatment of adult patients with delayed union of tibial fracture. China Continuing Medical Education. 2014; 6(8):61-63

32. Strauss MB, Lu LQ, Miller SS, Hart BB. Hyperbaric Oxygen for the Management of Chronic Refractory Osteomyelitis. In: Hyperbaric Medicine Practice, 4th edition, Kindwall (Ed.). In Press.

33. Strauss MB, Hart GB, Lu LQ. Role of Oxygen and Hyperbaric Oxygen Mechanisms. In: Hyperbaric Medicine Practice, 4th edition, Kindwall (Ed.). In Press.

34. Kapitola J, Marek J, Jaboda I, et al. Decreased 133Xe clearance in the proximal femur in acromegaly. Exp Clin Endocrinol. 1986; 87(1):112-115.

35. Moon H, Strauss MB, La S, Miller SS. The validity of transcutaneous oxygen measurements in predicting healing of diabetic foot ulcers. Undersea Hyperb Med. 2016; 43(6):671-678.

36. Kwong LM, Johanson PH, Klein SR. Postocclusive transcutaneous oximetry in followup assessment of tibial nonunion and healed tibia fractures. J Trauma. 1988; 28(7):947-954.

CHAPTER 25 CHAPTER

The Microcirculation and Ischemia-Reperfusion: Basic Mechanisms of Hyperbaric Oxygen

CHAPTER TWENTY-FIVE OVERVIEW

Ischemia-Reperfusion Injury **643**
Pathophysiology **644**
Free Radicals 644
The Microcirculation 644
Hyperbaric Oxygen **647**
Basic Studies 647
Clinical Applications 651
Summary **652**
References **654**

The Microcirculation and Ischemia-Reperfusion: Basic Mechanisms of Hyperbaric Oxygen

Richard C. Baynosa, William A. Zamboni, John Brosious

ISCHEMIA-REPERFUSION INJURY

Patints with high-energy trauma, extremity compartment syndromes, amputated body parts, or failing flaps all experience varying degrees of tissue ischemia. Despite emergent clinical efforts that successfully restore perfusion in these situations, subsequent microcirculatory failure and tissue necrosis may still ensue (Figure 1). Prolonged periods of ischemia followed by reperfusion can actually lead to accelerated microcirculatory injury and ultimate cell death in many tissues.

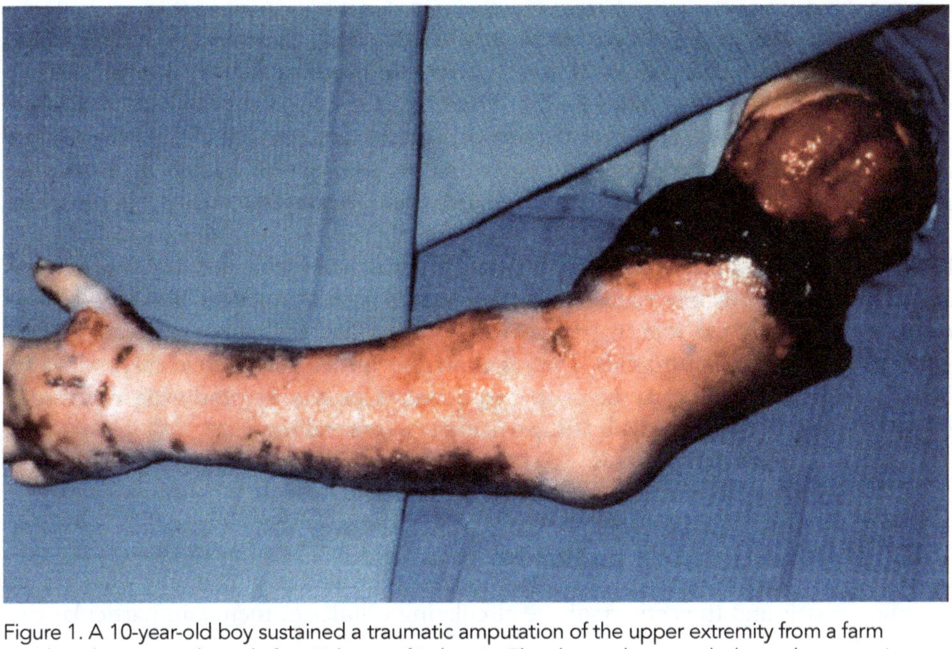

Figure 1. A 10-year-old boy sustained a traumatic amputation of the upper extremity from a farm accident that was replanted after 12 hours of ischemia. The above photograph shows the extremity three days after replantation. Although the arterial and venous anastomosis remained patent and the skin perfused, all of the muscle died as a result of reperfusion injury, necessitating revision amputation.

This phenomenon is known as ischemia-reperfusion (I-R) injury and has been linked to the generation of oxygen-derived free radicals in combination with a dramatic increase in neutrophil adhesion to postcapillary venules during reperfusion. This injury can be severe in extremity traumatic ischemias due to the large muscle mass. Skeletal muscle is very sensitive to ischemia and shows progressive necrosis and loss of function as the ischemic insult is increased. Ischemia-reperfusion injury therefore becomes a significant limiting factor in the successful outcome of the surgical treatment of ischemic skeletal muscle, especially in cases of major limb replantation. Although various tissues have different tolerance levels to ischemia, the final common pathway that results in I-R injury is likely similar. This chapter focuses on the biochemical and microcirculatory mechanisms of I-R injury in addition to the effects of hyperbaric oxygen (HBO_2), particularly in skin and skeletal muscle.

PATHOPHYSIOLOGY

Free Radicals

The biochemistry of I-R injury has been studied extensively and revolves around the production of oxygen-derived free radicals.(1,53) These oxyradicals are highly unstable molecules with an unpaired electron in the outer shell. They are extremely toxic to all biological substances, causing cell death by lipid peroxidation and propagation of more free radicals. Due to the difficulty in isolating oxyradicals, many investigators have turned to the use of free radical scavengers in animal models of ischemia-reperfusion. Several studies have shown that administration of various free-radical scavengers improves survival and function in skin and skeletal muscle subjected to I-R.(22,33,44-45,54) One study showed that edavarone, a synthetic scavenger of free radicals and inhibitor of lipid peroxidation, decreased inflammation and cell infiltration into skeletal muscle following I-R when used as a pretreatment.(32) These studies provide indirect evidence that oxyradicals play a central role in the tissue-destructive events that occur from I-R injury. The oxyradicals most often implicated in I-R (superoxide and hydroxyl free radicals) come from two important sources: xanthine oxidase (XO), from skeletal muscle endothelial cells, and neutrophils.(25,53)

The neutrophil has gained significant attention for its role in I-R injury. Neutrophils are capable of liberating large quantities of extracellular superoxide, which is formed by an enzyme in the cell membrane, NADPH oxidase (Figure 2). Superoxide can then dismutate to hydrogen peroxide, which reacts with ferritin to produce the highly toxic hydroxyl radical. Neutrophilic H_2O_2 can also generate the potent oxidant hypochlorous acid (HOCl) via myeloperoxidase enzymes released from azurophilic granules. HOCl may play an additional role in the activation of proteases (elastase, collagenase, and gelatinase) released by neutrophils. There is growing evidence that free-radical production by activated neutrophils may be more important than XO in producing the tissue-destructive events associated with I-R, particularly in skeletal muscle.(34,49,70)

The Microcirculation

The proliferation of free-radical research has provided a better understanding of the biochemistry of I-R injury. Investigators have more recently begun to study the microcirculatory morphology of reperfusion injury, including dynamic changes in the microvessels and the activity of the circulating cellular elements, in particular the leukocytes.

Zamboni et al.,(70) using an in vivo rat gracilis skeletal muscle preparation, have investigated the effects of I-R on the microcirculation. Quantitative observations of

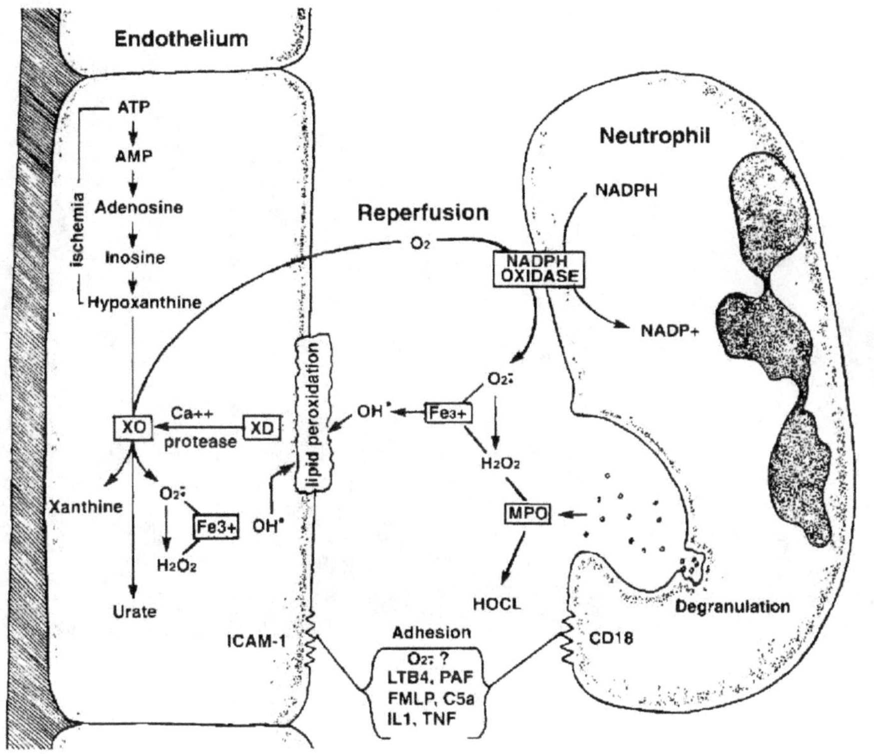

Figure 2. Xanthine oxidase and neutrophil oxygen free radical generating systems associated with I-R injury (adapted from Inauen).[34]

the microcirculation during reperfusion in this study have provided us some insight into the morphology of I-R injury. Following four hours of global ischemia in this model, a significant increase in the number of neutrophils sticking to the endothelium of postcapillary venules was noted, minutes after the initiation of reperfusion, that was not seen in nonischemic control preparations (Figure 3). This increase in neutrophil adhesion was maintained throughout a three-hour reperfusion observation period. As reperfusion progressed, the venule walls became ill defined from adherent marginating and extravasating leukocytes. Disruption of the endothelial basement membrane adjacent to adherent neutrophils was noted on electron microscopy (Figures 4A-4B). These observations suggest that neutrophil adhesion and subsequent release of free radicals is an important early event leading to endothelial damage and microcirculatory failure associated with I-R injury.

Multiple studies have also implicated increased neutrophil-endothelial adhesion as an important pathway in the development of I-R injury.[28,52,59] Additional support of this mechanism is provided by other skeletal muscle microcirculation studies[27,46] as well as several experiments which have demonstrated improved tissue survival by altering the number and adherence properties of neutrophils.[7,41,56,65] The mechanism of I-R-induced neutrophil-endothelial adhesion in skeletal muscle is now known to involve the neutrophil CD18 (beta 2 integrin) adhesion molecule which binds the endothelial ICAM-1 receptor.[40,73] These studies examining this adhesion molecule demonstrated that the neutrophil CD18 adhesion molecule was upregulated by I-R injury and necessary for the initiation of neutrophil-endothelial adhesion.

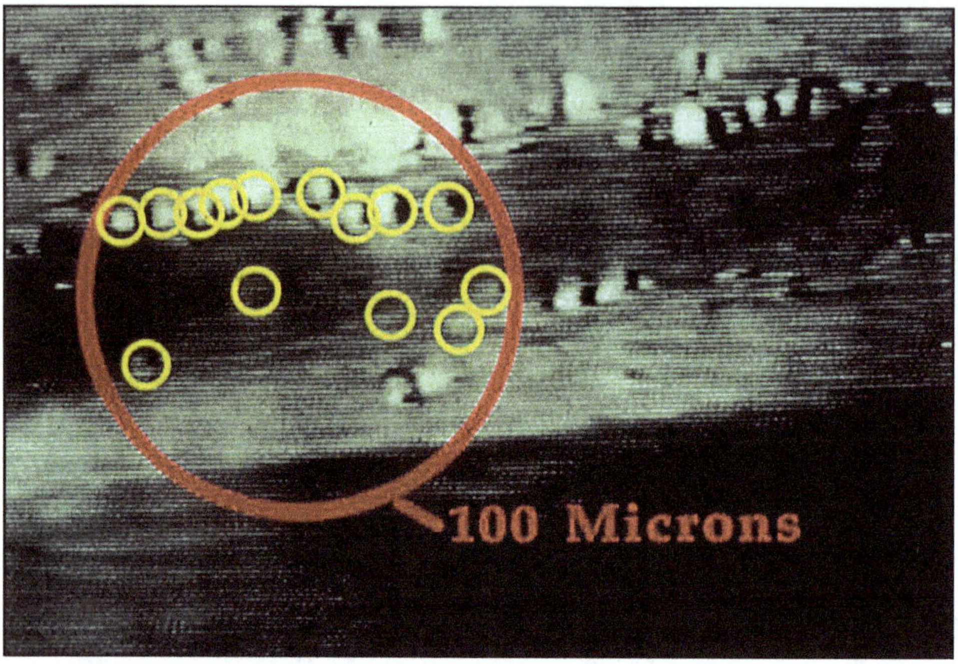

Figure 3. Leukocytes adherent to the endothelium of an ischemic microvenule at 15 minutes reperfusion (700x) were easily identified by their characteristic size and whitish color. [70]

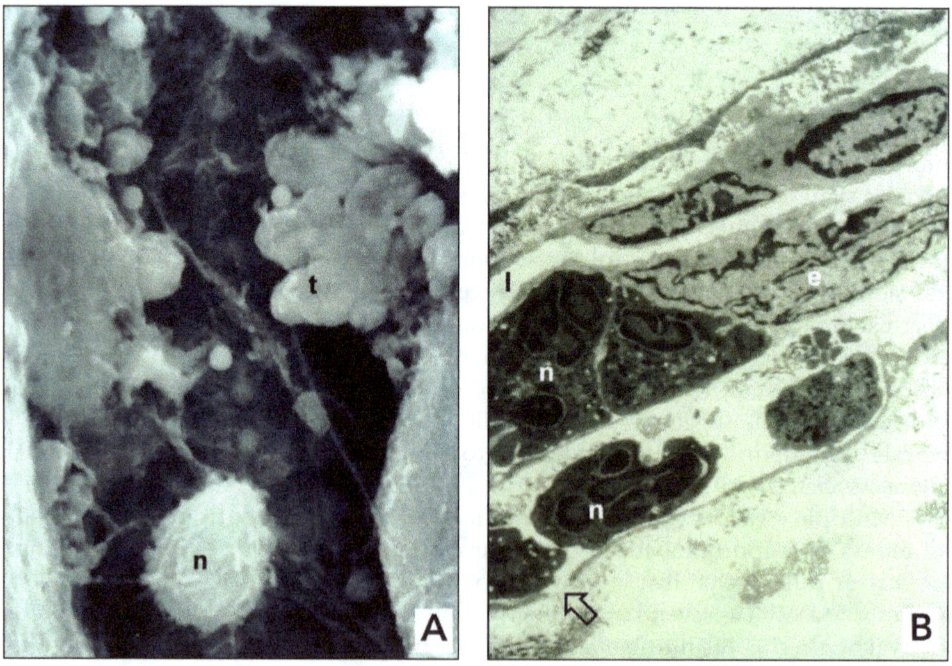

Figures 4A-4B.

A. Scanning EM (4,500K) showing the lumen of an ischemic venule at 2 hours reperfusion. Note the neutrophil (n) and adjacent thrombus-like particulate matter (t) attached to the endothelium.

B. Transmission EM (4,500K) of a similar venule. Note the neutrophils (n) invading the endothelium with disruption of the basement membrane (arrow) e- endothelial cell, l- lumen. [70]

Subsequent confocal microscopy studies have shown that there is not only an upregulation of the CD18 adhesion molecule but also a morphological change leading to polarization of the CD18 adhesion molecules on the neutrophil surface, leading to an increased avidity of neutrophil adhesion to its associated endothelial ICAM-1 receptor.[39] This polarization phenomenon in this study has been termed "capping" of the CD18 adhesion molecules on the neutrophil.

In addition to its role in neutrophil adhesion to vessel walls following I-R, endothelial cells have also been shown to undergo apoptosis and necrosis following I-R.[66] Perhaps endothelial death could be a fundamental cause of endothelial dysfunction, vasoconstriction, and thrombosis seen in skeletal muscle following I-R.

Evaluation of the vasoreactivity and flow characteristics of microarterioles is pertinent to the understanding of I-R injury. Feng et al.[23] measured the venous washout of vasoactive prostaglandins during reperfusion in a rat hind limb ischemia model. He found a significant increase in thromboxane B2 (the stable metabolite of vasoconstricting thromboxane A2) relative to vasodilating prostaglandin E2 in limbs that went on to complete microcirculatory failure. A decrease in venous outflow, in the absence of arteriole thrombosis, was also noted. It was hypothesized from these findings that the impending no-reflow state associated with I-R injury may reflect a global "agonal" vasoconstriction in the microcirculation. Observations of 101 microarterioles in a rat gracilis skeletal muscle preparation have confirmed this hypothesis.[70] Measurement of arteriole diameters during reperfusion after four hours of global ischemia demonstrated an initial reactive vasodilation that was followed at one hour by a progressive and severe vasoconstriction. It was interesting that only arterioles in close proximity to venules showed this vasoconstriction, suggesting that the local environment created by the leukocyte-damaged venule is responsible for the arteriole response. Lew et al.[43] have shown that experimental exposure of the microarteriolar vascular smooth muscle to water-soluble vasoactive substances produces a much greater response than luminal endothelial exposure. It is possible that the neutrophil-damaged venular endothelium results in the release and interstitial diffusion of a vasoactive substance, which causes vasoconstriction in adjacent arterioles. The vasoactive substance causing the I-R-induced vasoconstriction in skeletal muscle microarterioles is unknown at this time. Possibilities include thromboxane, serotonin, leukotrienes, and impaired endothelial-derived relaxing factor, which is now known to be nitric oxide.[11,20,55,67] One study suggests that mast cell degranulation is integral to the arteriolar vasoconstriction seen in skeletal muscle following reperfusion, revealing that many cell lines may be involved in I-R injury.[38]

It is clear from these observations that neutrophil-endothelial adherence and microarteriolar vasoconstriction are important morphological events leading to the microcirculatory failure associated with I-R injury. The fact that vasoconstriction occurs in the subset of arterioles adjacent to leukocyte-damaged venules may explain the "heterogeneity" of I-R injury which results in patchy muscle necrosis. This pattern of injury is seen clinically more often than "global" microcirculatory failure and complete necrosis.

HYPERBARIC OXYGEN

Basic Studies

The controversy surrounding the use of hyperbaric oxygen for I-R injury has been resolved by numerous studies looking at a variety of different tissues and organs. Initial concern was based on the theory that HBO_2 therapy would exacerbate I-R injury by adding extra oxygen to the system and increasing free-radical production.

[8,18] This hypothesis was tested in a rat ischemic axial skin flap experiment in which the authors expected to see decreased flap survival with HBO_2 treatment.[71] Instead, the administration of HBO_2 during reperfusion significantly improved skin flap survival following eight hours of global ischemia. This beneficial effect on I-R injury was also noted in a follow-up study in which laser Doppler analysis during reperfusion showed increased microvascular blood flow in ischemic skin flaps treated with HBO_2.[72] These unexpected findings corroborate the results of Kaelin et al.[37] in which HBO_2 treatment during reperfusion significantly improved free skin flap survival in rats following microvascular reattachment with ischemia times up to 24 hours. Experiments have also shown that hyperbaric oxygen is beneficial after a secondary ischemic insult by significantly reducing necrosis in both skin flaps and skeletal muscle.[57,68] It can be concluded from these animal studies that HBO_2 therapy does not exacerbate, but rather counteracts, the ill effects of I-R injury, resulting in increased microvascular perfusion and improved skin flap survival.

Although the skin flap studies are interesting, the effect of HBO_2 on I-R injury of skeletal muscle has more important clinical significance, especially with regard to limb replantation and the traumatic ischemias. HBO_2 therapy has been shown experimentally to reduce skeletal muscle edema and necrosis in rat hind limb tourniquet ischemia[47] and dog hind limb compartment syndrome models.[58] One hypothesis for this beneficial effect is hyperoxia-induced vasoconstriction, which theoretically decreases edema by reducing capillary pressure. Although hyperoxia-induced vasoconstriction may be marked in cerebral arterioles,[9,19] reducing blood flow 40%, the effect on limb blood flow reduction is minimal (12% to 18.9%),[9,12] making vasoconstriction unlikely as the primary mechanism for reducing skeletal muscle edema. In order to further delineate additional mechanisms, Zamboni et al.[70] studied the effect of HBO_2 on the microcirculatory morphology of I-R in rat gracilis muscle, specifically evaluating leukocyte-endothelial adherence and vasoactivity by measurement of microarteriole diameters. The most striking observation during reperfusion in this study was the significant reduction of leukocytes adherent to venular endothelium in preparations treated with HBO_2 during and immediately following four hours of ischemia (Figure 5). The vein walls in these treatment groups remained clear and well defined throughout the three-hour reperfusion observation period. HBO_2 initiated one hour after reperfusion also significantly reduced leukocyte adherence but not as effectively. The progressive arteriolar vasoconstriction seen in untreated reperfused vessels was also inhibited by HBO_2 therapy administered during and up to one hour following ischemia (Figure 5). HBO_2 administered to nonischemic muscle had no effect on subsequent leukocyte adherence or arteriolar diameters. These results demonstrate that any vasoconstriction in microarterioles occurring during HBO_2 exposure does not persist beyond the treatment. Although HBO_2 therapy initiated one hour after reperfusion prevented ischemic arteriolar vasoconstriction, deterioration of the microcirculation preparation after three hours obviated the addition of delayed-HBO_2-treatment groups. It is likely that the timing of HBO_2 therapy in relation to I-R injury is important in producing a beneficial response.

The beneficial effects of HBO_2 on ischemic tissue are systemic and not local.[71] The systemic mechanism by which HBO_2 decreases neutrophil adherence during reperfusion is not yet known, but ongoing research provides optimism that this mechanism will soon be elucidated. A direct action of HBO_2 at the neutrophil-endothelial interface is one possibility. Kaelin[37] found a significant increase in the activity of the free radical scavenger superoxide dismutase (SOD) in rats with ischemic skin flaps treated by HBO_2.

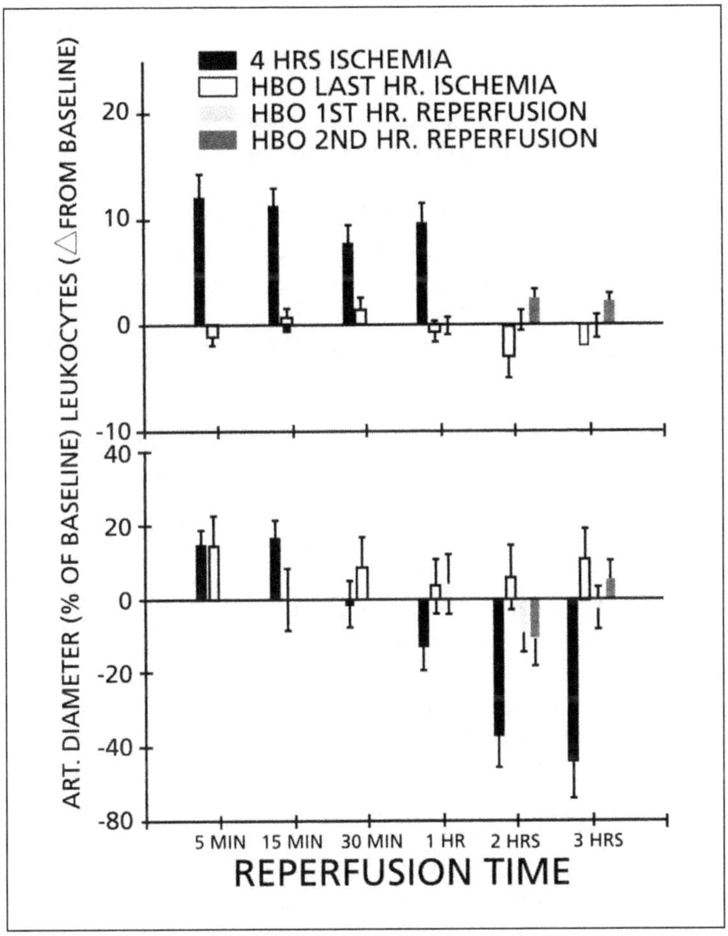

Figure 5. HBO_2 treatment up to one hour reperfusion significantly reduced the number of leukocytes sticking to the endothelium (above) and inhibited the progressive vasoconstriction in arterioles adjacent to venules (below) compared to reperfused, ischemic nontreated vessels. [70]

If superoxide is playing a direct or indirect role in neutrophil-endothelial adhesion, then increased SOD activity may decrease this adherence. Thom[61] studied lipid peroxidation in vitro and demonstrated that hyperoxia alters the free-radical pathway in favor of hydroperoxyl radical formation. These quenching radicals react with lipid radicals to form nonradical products. This termination reaction antagonizes and significantly reduces lipid peroxidation. This stabilizing effect may reduce endothelial activation upon reperfusion, resulting in decreased neutrophil adherence. Although we initially considered the possibility of HBO_2 promoting preferential sequestration of neutrophils in the lungs, it is now known that this does not occur in response to skeletal muscle I-R injury.[74]

Thom[64] studied an animal model of brain reperfusion injury to show that conversion of xanthine dehydrogenase (XD) to the free-radical-forming XO was responsible for lipid peroxidation. More recently, Thom examined the effect of HBO_2 exposure to human neutrophils and noted an inhibition of the CD18 (beta 2 integrin) function that prevented neutrophil adherence while having no effect on the cell-surface expression of the adhesion molecules.[63] This observed HBO_2-mediated inhibition of neutrophil CD18 function would prevent adherence/activation and release of proteases known to stimulate XD-to-XO conversion. It is interesting that the brain biochemical I-R studies by Thom, as well as the skeletal muscle microcirculation morphology studies done in our laboratory, appear to substantiate a final common pathway in which HBO_2 is inhibiting neutrophil adherence and the deleterious cascade of events that follow reperfusion. It is apparent that the endothelial-neutrophil interaction associated with I-R is complex, and multiple studies have recently focused on the effects of HBO_2 on cellular adhesion molecules (CAMs) in attenuating the I-R-induced neutrophil adhesion.

Experiments in a rat skeletal muscle model corroborate the observation that CD18 cell-surface expression is not altered by HBO_2 exposure.[31,40] There is recent evidence that the mechanism by which HBO_2 inhibits neutrophil adhesion involves a qualitative change in the CD18 adhesion molecule through cellular alterations in cyclic GMP.[2,17,40,63] Preliminary work employing harvested neutrophils from an in vivo rat skeletal muscle model using confocal microscopy has suggested that the qualitative change in these CAMs may be secondary to a change in the polarization of the CD18 molecules on the neutrophil surface.[36] This essentially would indicate a reversal of the neutrophil "capping" previously seen using confocal microscopy after I-R injury.[39]

In addition to the scientific work centering on the effect of HBO_2 on the neutrophil, some investigators have focused on the changes encountered by endothelial cells exposed to HBO_2 after I-R injury. Activation of endothelial cells due to ischemia and subsequent reperfusion triggers the expression of CAMs such as E-selectin and ICAM-1 through transcription and translation.[13-14] In vitro studies using both bovine and human endothelial cells by Buras et al. confirmed that mock ischemia with hypoxia and hypoglycemia was capable of inducing increased expression of ICAM-1. These investigators further showed that treatment of the endothelial cells with HBO_2 for 90 minutes at 2.5 ATA decreased the expression of ICAM-1 with a reduction of PMN binding to the endothelial surface.[15] These findings were further corroborated by in vivo studies in a rodent skeletal muscle flap model which also demonstrated that HBO_2 was able to reduce ICAM-1 expression, reduce neutrophil adhesion, and improve overall flap survival.[31] A recent study demonstrated an upregulation in antioxidant gene expression in human endothelial cells following HBO_2 treatment and that these changes lead to increased resistance of these cells to a lethal oxidative stress.[26]

Nitric oxide (NO) has been implicated as an important regulator of several aspects of I-R injury including vascular tone and neutrophil adhesion.[42] Research involving the role of NO in the beneficial effects of HBO_2 has shed further light on the possible basic mechanisms of HBO_2's protective effects. Our laboratory studies have confirmed that HBO_2 reversal of I-R-induced neutrophil CD18 polarization works through a nitric oxide mechanism.[35] We further showed an increase in endothelial-derived nitric oxide synthase (eNOS) mRNA in skeletal muscle suffering I-R injury followed by HBO_2. Not only was this eNOS increase seen in skeletal muscle suffering I-R injury but also in pulmonary tissues not suffering ischemic insult, further suggesting a systemic beneficial response to HBO_2.[5] Using a rat model, other researchers revealed that the decreased neutrophil adhesion provided by HBO_2 treatment was reversed when the experimental rats were treated with the NO-blocker L-NAME.[2] These investigators also suggested that the NO upregulation induced by HBO_2 may inhibit neutrophil CD-18 (beta 2 integrin) function by inhibiting membrane-associated cyclic GMP synthesis.[2] More recent studies have quantitatively documented an increase in nitric oxide in the cerebral cortex and abdominal aorta of rats exposed to HBO_2.[60,62]

While these studies implicate the neuronal-derived form of nitric oxide synthase (NOS) as the source of increased NO, they focus on the cerebral tissue and the periaortic area and not the microcirculation. It is likely that different organs and tissues may be influenced by other forms of NOS, particularly the endothelial-derived form (eNOS) that is associated with the endothelial cells of the microcirculation. Indeed, preliminary work in our laboratory has demonstrated a time-dependent effect of HBO_2 on eNOS activity as well as transcription and translation in examining both the microcirculation as well as the systemic circulation.[3-4,6] These studies suggest that after HBO_2 treatment for I-R injury, there is an early increase in eNOS activity locally followed by a late-phase (24 hours of reperfusion) increase in eNOS transcription and translation in the systemic circulation.[3-4,6] In addition, other preliminary studies have implicated vascular endothelial growth factor (VEGF) as a possible regulating factor by demonstrating an increase in VEGF transcription in the skeletal muscle subjected to I-R injury.[4] Moreover, the decrease in neutrophil adherence seen in our rat muscle flap model with HBO_2 was reversed after pretreatment of the rodents with a functional VEGF monoclonal antibody.[21]

The biochemical and microcirculation studies of HBO_2 and I-R injury are important from a mechanistic point of view and should be continued. Studies evaluating the ultimate function in skeletal muscle subjected to I-R injury may be more important and clinically relevant. Surgical restoration of blood flow following a traumatic crush injury or amputation may result in a viable extremity, but if a significant portion of the muscle dies from I-R injury, then fibrosis will occur and function will be compromised.

Clinical Applications

The primary treatment for traumatic extremity injury with arterial compromise is surgical restoration of blood flow. Fracture fixation, arterial repair, fasciotomy to prevent compartment syndrome, and replantation in selected cases are necessary interventions for limb salvage. Hyperbaric oxygen is an important adjunctive treatment, especially if the tissue is at risk for reperfusion injury. The skeletal muscle is particularly at risk due to its sensitivity to ischemia. The degree of muscle damage from I-R injury is proportional to the ischemic interval, especially in cases of warm ischemia. Some degree of permanent damage to the muscle can be expected when ischemia times exceed four to six hours.

It is important to understand that the majority of microcirculatory damage from ischemia occurs during the first six to seven hours of reperfusion.[48] Therefore, early recognition and treatment become critical. Many centers are using HBO_2 to treat patients with revascularized or replanted extremities, especially with skeletal muscle ischemia times greater than six hours. Another indication would be free-muscle-flap vascular thrombosis requiring re-exploration and anastomotic revision in which a secondary ischemic interval has occurred. These patients can be taken directly from the recovery room, and often from the operating room, to the hyperbaric medical unit for treatment. We have treated patients with ischemia times up to 14 hours (Figure 6A-6B) and have noted excellent muscle survival and a remarkable reduction in soft-tissue edema.

Since most of these patients are still drowsy post anesthesia, they are unable to cooperate with ear-clearing techniques and frequently develop hemotympanum.[50] We are currently placing myringotomy tubes prophylactically in most patients entering the traumatic ischemia protocol, especially in the elderly age group. The HBO_2 treatments are otherwise well tolerated by patients and give us a readily available tool to help ameliorate the ill effects of I-R injury. Although our results have been good,

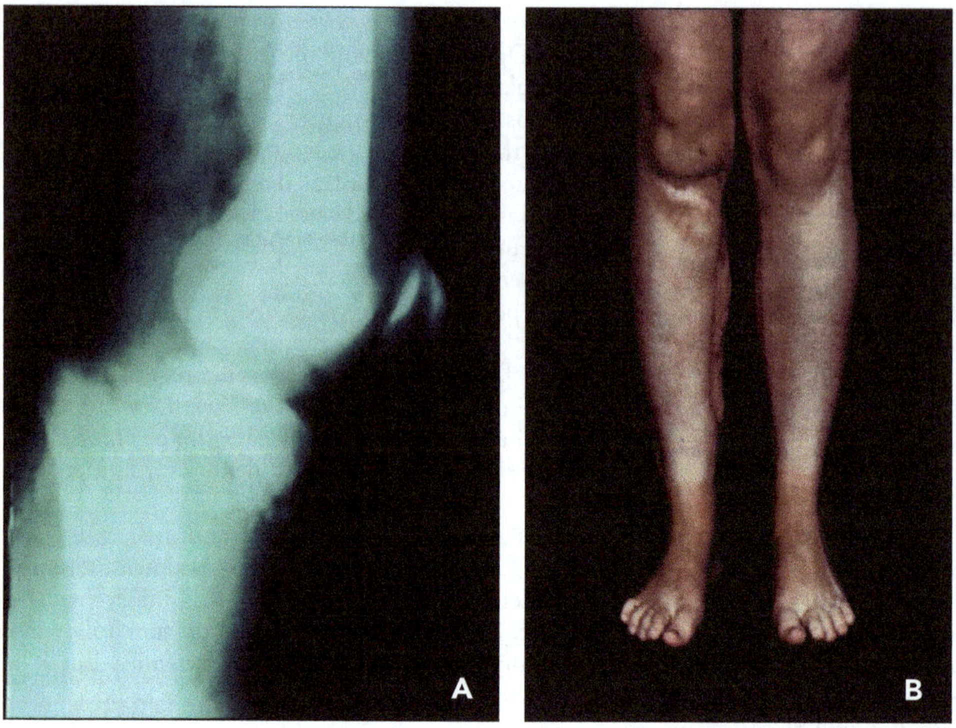

Figure 6A-6B.

A. A teenage cheerleader involved in a three-wheeler accident sustained a severe proximal tibia fracture resulting in popliteal artery disruption. Due to extenuating circumstances, a 14-hour warm ischemia time elapsed before successful revascularization with a vein graft was accomplished. A primary amputation was considered but instead lower-leg fasciotomies were performed and she was treated immediately with HBO_2 using the traumatic ischemia protocol.

B. She obtained 100% survival of the muscle and regained normal function of her leg (photograph taken one year post-op).

we recognize that this information is anecdotal. A recent systematic review by Garcia-Covarrubias et al. regarding the use of HBO_2 in the management of crush injury and traumatic ischemia located eight retrospective uncontrolled studies or case series lacking a standardized methodology and one prospective controlled, randomized trial with some design limitations.(24) Their analysis determined that eight of the nine studies showed a beneficial effect with only one major complication. They concluded that adjunctive HBO_2 is not likely to be harmful and could be beneficial if administered early.(24) Definitive proof of the potential benefit of HBO_2 on I-R injury will require a well-controlled, prospective, randomized clinical trial.

SUMMARY

Acute HBO_2 therapy does not exacerbate I-R injury. Rather, a large body of experimental evidence is accumulating from animal skin flap studies, quantitative skeletal muscle microcirculation observations, and biochemical experiments that demonstrates that HBO_2 treatment antagonizes I-R injury. The microvascular preservation afforded by HBO_2 (Figure 7) appears to play a central role in treating skeletal muscle I-R injury that may accompany extremity crush injury, compartment syndrome, major limb replantation/ revascularization, and acutely failing flaps.

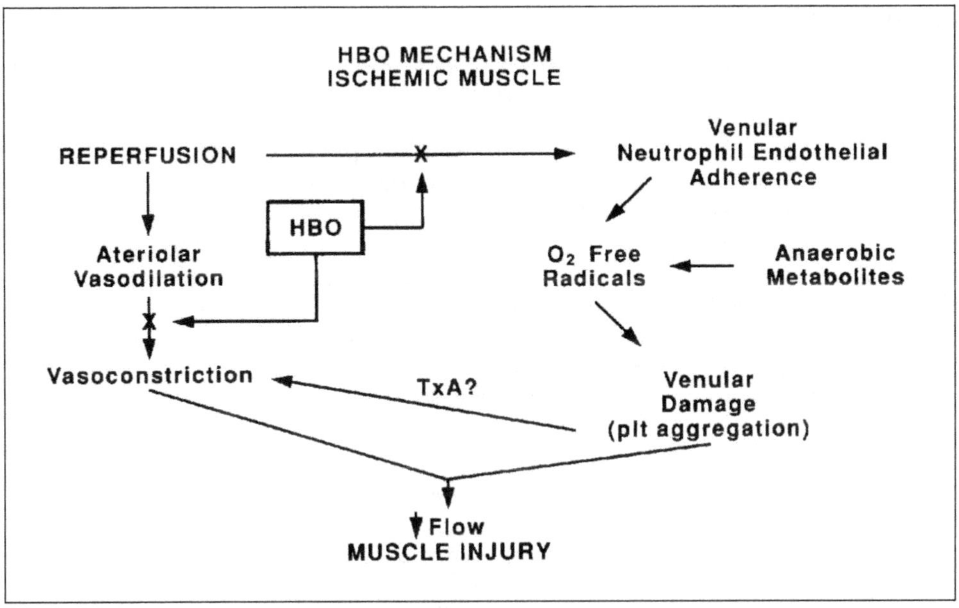

Figure 7. Reperfusion cascade leading to skeletal muscle injury after prolonged ischemia. HBO_2 treatment protects the microcirculation by blocking neutrophil endothelial adherence and inhibiting subsequent arteriolar vasoconstriction.[70]

The application of HBO_2 may eventually extrapolate to other tissues subjected to I-R injury including brain, intestine, kidney, and heart. Indeed, several recent basic science studies in rodents have demonstrated a protective role for HBO_2 in renal, intestinal, and cardiac ischemia reperfusion as well as I-R injury related to hemorrhagic and embolic stroke.[10,16,29-30,51] The progress made in recent years has been significant, but there is still a need for further quality basic-science research, as well as well-controlled prospective clinical studies to fully understand and further define the effectiveness of HBO_2 in the treatment of I-R injury.

REFERENCES

1. Angel MF, Ramasastry SS, Swartz WM, et al. Free radicals: basic concepts concerning their chemistry, pathophysiology, and relevance to plastic surgery. Plast Reconstr Surg. 1987;79:990.
2. Banick PD, Chen Q, Xu YA, Thom SR. Nitric oxide inhibits neutrophil beta 2 integrin function by inhibiting membrane-associated cyclic GMP synthesis. J Cell Physiol. 1997;172:12-24.
3. Baynosa RC, Graves AK, Fang XH, Stephenson LL, Khiabani KT, Wang WZ, Zamboni WA. The effect of hyperbaric oxygen on eNOS protein expression in ischemia reperfusion injury. Plast Reconstr Surg. 2007;120(Suppl):73.
4. Baynosa RC, Khiabani KT, Stephenson LL, Fang XH, Wang WZ, Zamboni WA. The effect of hyperbaric oxygen on nitric oxide synthase and vascular endothelial growth factor expression in ischemia-reperfusion injury. J Amer Coll Surg. 2004;199(Suppl):S65.
5. Baynosa RC, Naig AL, Murphy PS, et al. The effect of hyperbaric oxygen on nitric oxide synthase activity and expression in ischemia-reperfusion injury. J Surg Res. 2013;183(1):355-61.
6. Baynosa RC, Naig AL, Murphy PS, Hansen B, Fang XH, Stephenson LL, Khiabani KT, Wang WZ, Zamboni WA. The effect of hyperbaric oxygen on NOS activity and transcription in ischemia reperfusion injury. J Amer Coll Surg. 2005;200(Suppl):S57-8.
7. Belkin M, LaMorte WL, Wright JG, Hobson RW. The role of leukocytes in the pathophysiology of skeletal muscle ischemic injury. J Vasc Surg. 1989;10:14.
8. Benke PJ. Jessica in the well: ischemia and reperfusion injury. JAMA. 1988;259:1326.
9. Bergofsky EH, Bertun P. Response of regional circulations to hyperoxia. J Appl Physiol. 1966;21:567.
10. Bertoletto PR, Fagundes DJ, De Jesus Simoes M, Oshima CT, De Souza Montero EF, Simoes RS, Fagundes AT. Effects of hyperbaric oxygen therapy on the rat intestinal mucosa apoptosis caused by ischemia-reperfusion injury. Microsurgery. 2007;27:224-7.
11. Billiar TR. Nitric oxide: novel biology with clinical relevance. Ann Surg. 1995;221:339-49.
12. Bird AD, Telfer ABM. Effect of hyperbaric oxygen on limb circulation. Lancet. 1965;1:355.
13. Buras JA. Basic mechanisms of hyperbaric oxygen in the treatment of ischemia-reperfusion injury. Int Anesthesiol Clin. 2000;38:91-109.
14. Buras JA, Reenstra WR. Endothelial-neutrophil interactions during ischemia and reperfusion injury: basic mechanisms of hyperbaric oxygen. Neurol Res. 2007;29:127-31.
15. Buras JA, Stahl GL, Svoboda KK, Reenstra WR. Hyperbaric oxygen downregulates ICAM-1 expression induced by hypoxia and hypoglycemia: the role of NOS. Am J Physiol Cell Physiol. 2000;278:C292-302.
16. Cabigas BP, Su J, Hutchins W, Shi Y, Schaefer RB, Recinos RF, Nilakantan V, Kindwall E, Niezgoda JA, Baker JE. Hyperoxic and hyperbaric-induced cardioprotection: role of nitric oxide synthase 3. Cardiovasc Res. 2006;72:143-51.
17. Chen Q, Banick PD, Thom SR. Functional inhibition of rat polymorphonuclear leukocyte beta2 integrins by hyperbaric oxygen is associated with impaired cGMP synthesis. J Pharmacol Exp Therapeutics. 1996;276:929-33.
18. Davis JC. Jessica in the well. Ischemia and reperfusion injury. JAMA. 1988;259:3558.

19. Dollery CT, Hill DW, Mailer CM, Ramelho PS. High oxygen pressure and the retinal blood vessels. Lancet. 1964;ii:291.

20. Eidt JF, Ashton J, Golino P, et al. Thromboxane A2 and serotonin mediate coronary blood flow reductions in unsedated dogs. Am J Physiol. 1989;257:H873.

21. Ellis CM, Hansen BK, Baynosa RC, Stephenson LL, Khiabani KT, Wang WZ, Zamboni WA. Hyperbaric oxygen decreases neutrophil adherence in ischemia reperfusion by a VEGF-dependent mechanism. J Amer Coll Surg. 2005;200(Suppl):S57.

22. Feller AM, Roth AC, Russell RC, et al. Experimental evaluation of oxygen free radical scavengers in prevention of reperfusion injury to skeletal muscle. Ann Plast Surg. 1989;22:321.

23. Feng LJ, Berger BE, Lysz TW, Shaw WW. Vasoactive prostaglandins in the impending no-reflow state: evidence for a primary disturbance in microvascular tone. Plast Reconstr Surg. 1988;81:755.

24. Garcia-Covarrubias L, McSwain NE, Van Meter K, Bell RM. Adjuvant hyperbaric oxygen therapy in the management of crush injury and traumatic ischemia: and evidence-based approach. Amer Surg. 2005;71:144-50.

25. Gillani S, Cao J, Suzuki T, Hak DJ. The effect of ischemia reperfusion injury on skeletal muscle. Injury. 2012;43(6):670-5.

26. Godman CA, Joshi R, Giardina C, Perdrizet G, Hightower LE. Hyperbaric oxygen treatment induces antioxidant gene expression. Ann N Y Acad Sci. 2010;1197:178-83.

27. Goldberg M, Serafin D, Klitzman B. Quantification of neutrophil adhesion to skeletal muscle venules following ischemia-reperfusion. J Reconstr Micro. 1990;6:267.

28. Granger DN, Benoit JN, Suzuki M, Grisham MB. Leukocyte adherence to venular endothelium during ischemia-reperfusion. Am J Physiol. 1989;257:G683.

29. Gurer A, Ozdogan M, Gomceli I, Demirag A, Gulbahar O, Arikok T, Kulacoglu H, Dundar K, Ozlem N. Hyperbaric oxygenation attenuates renal ischemia-reperfusion injury in rats. Transplant Proc. 2006;38:3337-40.

30. Henninger N, Kuppers-Tiedt L, Sicard KM, Gunther A, Schneider D, Schwab, S. Neuroprotective effect of hyperbaric oxygen therapy monitored by MR-imaging after embolic stroke in rats. Exp Neurol. 2006;201:316-23.

31. Hong JP, Kwon H, Chung YK, et al. The effect of hyperbaric oxygen on ischemia-reperfusion injury: an experimental study in a rat musculocutaneous flap. Ann Plast Surg. 2003;51:478-87.

32. Hori K, Tsujii M, Iino T, et al. Protective effect of edaravone for tourniquet-induced ischemia-reperfusion injury on skeletal muscle in murine hindlimb. BMC Musculoskelet Disord. 2013;14:113.

33. Im JM, Manson PN, Bulkley GB, Hoopes JE. Effects of superoxide dismutase and allopurinol on the survival of acute island skin flaps. Ann Surg. 1985;201:357.

34. Inauen W, Suzuki M, Granger DN. Mechanisms of cellular injury: potential source of oxygen free radicals in ischemia/reperfusion. Microcirc Endothelium Lymphatics. 1989;5:143.

35. Jones SR, Carpin KM, Woodward SM, et al. Hyperbaric oxygen inhibits ischemia-reperfusion-induced neutrophil CD18 polarization by a nitric oxide mechanism. Plast Reconstr Surg. 2010;126(2):403-11.

36. Jones S, Wang WZ, Nataraj C, Stephenson LL, Khiabani KT, Zamboni WA. HBO inhibits IR-induced neutrophil CD18 polarization by a nitric oxide mechanism. Undersea Hyperb Med. 2002;35(Suppl):75.

37. Kaelin CM, Im MJ, Myers RAM, et al. The effects of hyperbaric oxygen on free flaps in rats. Arch Surg. 1990;125:607.

38. Keller MW. Arteriolar constriction in skeletal muscle during vascular stunning: role of mast cells. Am J Physiol. 1997;272(5 Pt 2):H2154-63.

39. Khiabani KT, Stephenson LL, Gabriel A, Nataraj C, Wang WZ, Zamboni WA. A quantitative method for determining polarization of neutrophil adhesion molecules associated with ischemia reperfusion. Plast Reconstr Surg. 2004;114:1846-50.

40. Larson JL, Stephenson LL, Zamboni WA. The effects of HBO treatment on PMN expression of CD18 in a rat model of ischemia reperfusion (IR). Undersea Hyperbar Med. 1998;25.

41. Lee C, Kerrigan CL, Picard-Ami LA. Cyclophosphamide-induced neutropenia: effect on postischemic skin flap survival. Plast Reconstr Surg. 1992;89:1092.

42. Lefer AM, Lefer DJ. The role of nitric oxide and cell adhesion molecules on the microcirculation in ischaemia-reperfusion. Cardiovasc Res. 1996;32:743-51.

43. Lew MJ, Rivers RJ, Duling BR. Arteriolar smooth muscle responses are modulated by an intramural diffusion barrier. Am J Physiol. 1989;257:H10.

44. Manson PN, Anthenelli RM, Im MJ, et al. The role of oxygen-free radicals in ischemic tissue injury in island skin flaps. Ann Surg. 1983;198:87.

45. Marzella L, Jesudass RR, Manson PN, et al. Functional and structural evaluation of the vasculature of skin flaps after ischemia and reperfusion. Plast Reconstr Surg. 1988;81:742.

46. Messina LM. In vivo assessment of acute microvascular injury after reperfusion of ischemic tibialis anterior muscle of the hamster. J Surg Res. 1990;48:615.

47. Nylander G, Lewis D, Nordström H, Larsson J. Reduction of postischemic edema with hyperbaric oxygen. Plast Reconstr Surg. 1985;76:596.

48. Olivas TP, Saylor TF, Wong HP, Stephenson LL, Zamboni WA. The timing of microcirculatory injury from ischemia reperfusion. Plast Reconstr Surg. 2001;107:785-8.

49. Pang CY. Ischemia-induced reperfusion injury in muscle flaps: pathogenesis and major source of free radicals. J Reconstr Micro. 1990;6:77.

50. Presswood G, Zamboni WA, Stephenson LL, Santos PM. Effect of artificial airway on ear complications from hyperbaric oxygen. Laryngoscope. 1994;104:1383-4.

51. Qin Z, Karabiyikoglu M, Hua Y, Silbergleit R, He Y, Keep RF, Xi G. Hyperbaric oxygen-induced attenuation of hemorrhagic transformation after experimental focal transient cerebral ischemia. Stroke. 2007;38:1362-1367.

52. Roth AC, Russell AC, Suchy H, Kalita S. The increased neutrophil adherence seen following ischemia in skeletal muscle is not superoxide dependent. FASEB J. 1990;4:A267.

53. Russell RC, Roth AC, Kucan JO, Zook EG. Reperfusion injury and oxygen free radicals. A review. J Reconstr Micro. 1989;5:79.

54. Sagi A, Ferder M, Levens D, Strauch B. Improved survival of island flaps after prolonged ischemia by perfusion with superoxide dismutase. Plast Reconstr Surg. 1986;77:639.

55. Schumacher WA, Heran CL, Allen GT, Ogletree ML. Leukotrienes cause mesenteric vasoconstriction and hemoconcentration in rats without activating thromboxane receptors. Prostaglandins. 1989;38:335.

56. Simpson PJ, Todd RF, Mickelson JK, et al. Sustained limitation of myocardial reperfusion injury by a monoclonal antibody that inhibits leukocyte adhesion. Circulation. 1990;81:226.

57. Stevens DM, Weiss DD, Koller WA, Bianchi DA. Survival of normothermic microvascular flaps after prolonged secondary ischemia: effects of hyperbaric oxygen. Otolaryngol Head Neck Surg. 1996;115:360-4.

58. Strauss MB, Hargens AR, Gershuni DH, et al. Reduction of skeletal muscle necrosis using intermittent hyperbaric oxygen in a model compartment syndrome. J Bone Joint Surg. 1983;65(5):656-62.

59. Suzuki M, Inauen W, Kvietys PR, et al. Superoxide mediates reperfusion-induced leukocyte-endothelial cell interactions. Am J Physiol. 1989;257:H1740.

60. Thom SR, Bhopale V, Fisher D, Manevich Y, Huang PL, Buerk DG. Stimulation of nitric oxide synthase in cerebral cortex due to elevated partial pressures of oxygen: an oxidative stress response. J Neurobiol. 2002;51:85-100.

61. Thom SR, Elbukin ME. Oxygen-dependent antagonism of lipid peroxidation. Free Radic Biol Med. 1991;10:413.

62. Thom SR, Fisher D, Zhang J, Bhopale VM, Ohnishi ST, Kotake Y, Ohnishi T, Buerk DG. Stimulation of perivascular nitric oxide synthesis by oxygen. Am J Physiol Heart Circ Physiol. 2003;284:H1230-9.

63. Thom SR, Mendiguren I, Hardy K, Bolotin T, Fisher D, Nebolon M, Kilpatrick L. Inhibition of human neutrophil beta2-integrin-dependent adherence by hyperbaric O2. Am J Physiol. 1997;272:C770-7.

64. Thom SR. Xanthine dehydrogenase conversion to oxidase and lipid peroxidation in brain after CO poisoning. J Appl Physiol. 1992;73:1584.

65. Vedder NB, Fouty BW, Winn RK, et al. Role of neutrophils in generalized reperfusion injury associated with resuscitation from shock. Surgery. 1989;106:509.

66. Wang WZ, Fang XH, Stephenson LL, Khiabani KT, Zamboni WA. Ischemia/reperfusion-induced necrosis and apoptosis in the cells isolated from rat skeletal muscle. J Orthop Res. 2008;26(3):351-6.

67. Warren JB, Maltby NH, MacCormack D, Barnes PJ. Pulmonary endothelium-derived relaxing factor is impaired in hypoxia. Clin Sci (Lond). 1989;77:671.

68. Wong HP, Zamboni WA, Stephenson LL. Effect of hyperbaric oxygen on skeletal muscle necrosis following primary and secondary ischemia in a rat model. Surg Forum. 1996;XLVII:705-7.

69. Zamboni WA, Roth AC, Bergman BA, Russell RC, Stephenson LL, Suchy H. Experimental evaluation of oxygen in the treatment of ischemic skeletal muscle [abstract]. Undersea Biomed Res. 1992;19(Suppl):78.

70. Zamboni WA, Roth AC, Russell RC, Graham B, Suchy H, Kucan JO. Morphological analysis of the microcirculation during reperfusion of ischemic skeletal muscle and the effect of hyperbaric oxygen. Plast Reconstr Surg. 1993;91:1110-23.

71. Zamboni WA, Roth AC, Russell RC, Nemiroff PM, Cassas L, Smoot EC. The effect of acute hyperbaric oxygen therapy on axial pattern skin flap survival when administered during and after total ischemia. J Reconstr Micro. 1989;5:343.

72. Zamboni WA, Roth AC, Russell RC, Smoot EC. Effect of hyperbaric oxygen on reperfusion of ischemic axial skin flaps: a laser Doppler analysis. Ann Plast Surg. 1992;28:339.

73. Zamboni WA, Stephenson LL, Roth AC, Suchy H, Russell RC. Ischemia-reperfusion injury in skeletal muscle: CE18 dependent neutrophil-endothelial adhesion and arteriolar vasoconstriction. Plast Reconstr Surg. 1997;99:2002-7.

74. Zamboni WA, Wong HP, Stephenson LL. Effect of hyperbaric oxygen on neutrophil concentration and pulmonary sequestration in ischemia-reperfusion injury. Arch Surg. 1996;131:756-60.

CHAPTER 26 CHAPTER

The Roles of Hyperbaric Oxygen in Crush Injury and Other Acute Traumatic Ischemias

CHAPTER TWENTY-SIX OVERVIEW

Introduction 661
Pathophysiology of Traumatic Ischemias 662
Mechanisms of Hyperbaric Oxygen Applicable to Traumatic Ischemias 668
Clinical Experiences with Hyperbaric Oxygen for Traumatic Ischemias 671
Crush Injuries and Special Considerations for using hyperbaric oxygen 675
Skeletal Muscle-Compartment Syndrome 678
The Role of Hyperbaric Oxygen in Other Traumatic Ischemias 682
Conclusion 683
Summary 685
References 686

The Roles of Hyperbaric Oxygen in Crush Injury and Other Acute Traumatic Ischemias

Michael B. Strauss, Lientra Q. Lu

INTRODUCTION

Hyperbaric oxygen (HBO_2) has been used as adjunct for the management of crush injury and compartment syndrome since its mechanisms and indications were first delineated in 1977.[30-31] Several other conditions including frost bite, thermal burns, threatened flaps/grafts, and compromised re-implantations have similar pathophysiology and hence can be classified along with crush injury and compartment syndrome as acute traumatic peripheral ischemias. In addition to all having trauma (physical, thermal, surgical) as a cause, three unifying factors are present in these conditions, namely (1) tissue ischemia-hypoxia, (2) edema, and (3) a gradient of injury (Figure 1). Tissue hypoxia and edema lead to self-perpetuation, a "vicious cycle" of the injury, and cause tissue damage of and beyond that sustained from the original trauma. The primary role

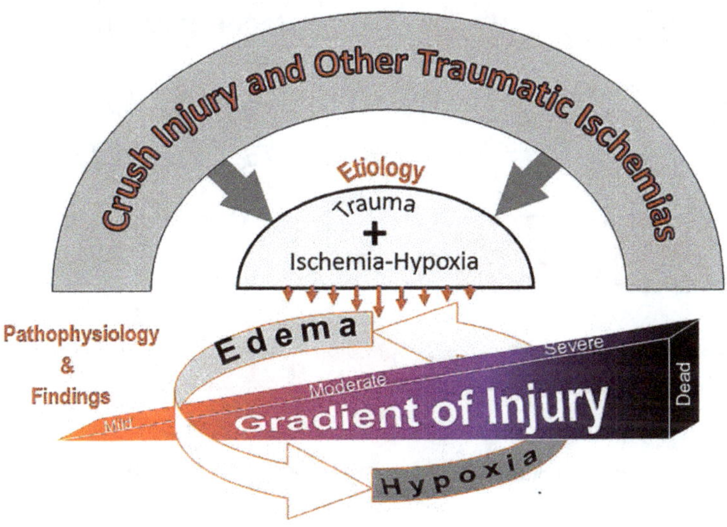

LEGEND: Injury (trauma) leads to a predictable sequence of events. Once into the vicious cycle of edema plus ischemia, the damage to tissues can become self-perpetuating. How the vicious cycle is managed determines outcomes.

FIGURE 1. The sequence of events in crush injuries and other traumatic ischemias.

of HBO_2 for these conditions is to counteract tissue ischemia-hypoxia and edema in order to prevent progression of tissue damage. This chapter will give primary attention to crush injury and compartment syndrome. Information on burns and threatened flaps are presented in other chapters in this text.

PATHOPHYSIOLOGY OF TRAUMATIC ISCHEMIAS

It is essential that an adequate blood supply be maintained to traumatized tissues. Ischemia may arise from injury to large, potentially surgically reparable blood vessels, blood vessels too small to be repaired surgically, or damage to the microcirculation or combinations of these. Local hypoxia occurs because of a direct result of trauma to blood vessels or as an indirect consequence of the injury. In the latter situation, decreased flow in the microcirculation occurs as a consequence of extravasation of intravascular fluid from the damaged blood vessels (with or without vascular collapse from the external pressure of the tissue fluid), stasis, vasoconstriction, thrombosis, or combinations of these mechanisms (Figure 2). Tissue hypoxia is the obvious consequence of the above causes of ischemia. Without the availability of sufficient oxygen, tissues are unable to meet their metabolic needs for maintaining viability, repairing damage, handling the bioburden, and restoring function. During the early phase of healing and infection control, the metabolic needs of tissues increase enormously.[76] Without increased blood flow, these new metabolic demands will not be met. The likelihood of nonhealing wounds, nonfunctional tissues, necrosis, and infections increase in direct proportion to the magnitude of the ischemic insult.

> The essential nature of a blood supply to tissues is mentioned in the Bible. The Bible reads that "the life of all flesh [is] the blood thereof" (Leviticus 17:14) (*King James Bible*).
>
> Perfusion, of course, is fundamental to maintaining the viability of all tissues in the body and is nowhere more important than in understanding the pathophysiology of crush injuries and other traumatic ischemia.

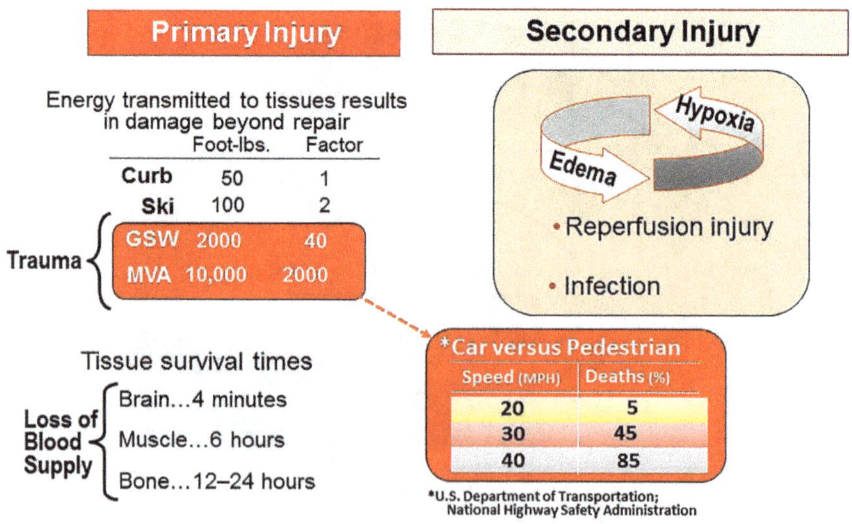

LEGEND: Primary injury leads to immediate death of tissues due to damage as the direct result of trauma to the tissues or damage to the blood supply. The secondary cause of death occurs from manifestations of edema-hypoxia, reperfusion injury, and/or infection.

FIGURE 2. Primary and secondary injury as a cause of tissue death.

We attempted to determine the human body's potential for increasing perfusion to noncritical tissues when needed for repair, bioburden management, and function.[76] Surprisingly, the number derived was in the 20-fold range.

It was determined by the following: 1) blood volume versus potential capacity of the vascular system is 5 liters and 20 liters respectively, so there is a potential for increasing blood flow fivefold to noncritical tissues when the demand for healing and infection control requires redistribution, 2) muscle blood flow can increase up to 50-fold between rest and maximal exercise, 3) oxygen uptake/utilization during the respiratory burst for bacterial killing in the phagocytic vesicle increases a hundredfold or more, and 4) cardiac output has the ability to double by increasing rate and filling. When summated and averaged, these potentials for increasing blood flow exceed the 20-fold range.

If the potential for increased blood flow and oxygen availability to a wound is in the 20-fold range, it is a reasonable assumption that metabolic activity increases a concomitant amount to make healing and infection control possible.

Edema also contributes to tissue hypoxia. It arises from extravasation of intravascular fluid through gap junctions in the endothelium, which appears to lose its integrity for maintaining plasma within its confines when subject to trauma, sepsis, and/or hypoxic insult. Leakage of fluid can also arise after direct trauma to blood and lymphatic vessels, increased tissue-perfusion pressure, decreased venous outflow, and decreased intravascular oncotic pressure, all of which can be associated with trauma. Hypoxia is an important contributor to cytogenic edema since maintenance of intracellular fluid balance is an oxygen-dependent mechanism.[11,42] Edema has detrimental effects on wound healing and infection control. It increases the diffusion distance of oxygen, which is essential for cell metabolic function, through the tissue fluids from capillaries to cells (Figure 3). Oxygen has limited ability to diffuse through tissue flu-

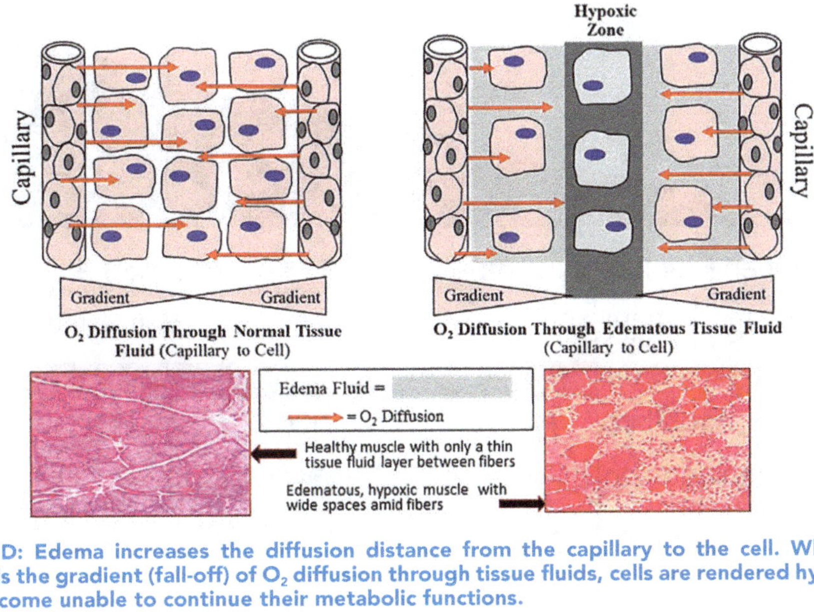

LEGEND: Edema increases the diffusion distance from the capillary to the cell. When it exceeds the gradient (fall-off) of O_2 diffusion through tissue fluids, cells are rendered hypoxic and become unable to continue their metabolic functions.

FIGURE 3. How edema interferes with tissue oxygenation.

> Oxygen diffusability through tissue fluids is 1⁄20 of carbon dioxide and decreases in an exponential fashion as the diffusion distance from the capillary to the cell increases. Edema appreciably interferes with tissue oxygenation. It can be somewhat mitigated by increasing the oxygen tensions in the plasma, for example, with HBO_2.

ids and falls off rapidly as the distance increases. This contrasts sharply to carbon dioxide, a waste product of cellular metabolism, which has 20 times the diffusability through tissue fluids as oxygen does.[86] The diffusion distance of oxygen through tissue fluid is proportional to the square root of the oxygen content in the capillary.[61] Consequently, oxygen diffusion through tissue fluids is decreased by an exponential factor as edema increases the distance from the capillary to the cell.

A second harmful effect of edema is collapse of the microcirculation. This occurs as interstitial fluid pressure around the capillaries increases with accumulation of edema. This is a problem that occurs in closed spaces such as skeletal muscles enclosed in fascia, the intracranial compartment, nerve tunnels, the peritoneum (abdominal compartment syndrome), and perhaps visceral organs that are covered with well-defined serosal membranes. Once the interstitial fluid pressure exceeds the capillary perfusion pressure in the closed space, the capillary bed collapses, flow in the microcirculation ceases, and the oxygen supply to the cell is disrupted. This is the pathophysiology that defines the skeletal muscle-compartment syndrome as well as compartment syndromes in other closed spaces.

A gradient of injury is the third pathophysiological consideration (after ischemia-hypoxia and edema) in traumatic ischemias (Figure 1, Figure 4). A unifying finding of almost all traumatic injuries is a gradient of injury. At the margins of the injury site, minimal or no tissue damage occurs. At the site of maximal injury, tissues may be so severely damaged that they are rendered nonviable. In between these two zones, a continuum of injury occurs from minimal damage, with the tissues still able to carry out their functions, to marginally viable and unable to carry out any healing or

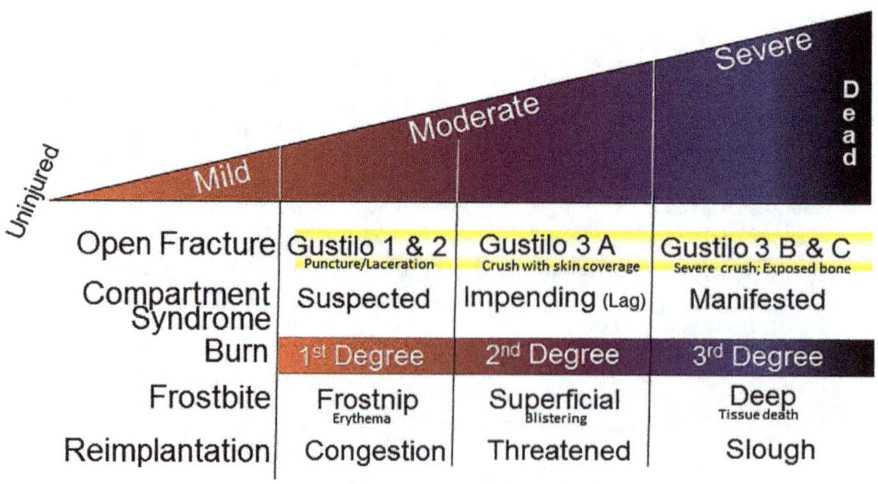

LEGEND: A unifying feature of the traumatic ischemias is the continuum of injury. Somewhat artificial labels have been given to grading the severity. How the injury is managed in the middle section of the continuum determines whether healing is achieved or the traumatic ischemia progresses to tissue loss, infection, and/or amputation.

FIGURE 4. Grading and labeling the continuum of injuries in traumatic ischemias.

infection-mitigating functions. Obviously, the severity of injury and the extent of the continuum of damage vary from injury to injury. This complicates the comparisons of benefits of treatment interventions and outcome measurements. Grading systems are used to measure the severity of injury in traumatic ischemias. They are attempts to establish identifiable but arbitrary points along a gradient of injury (Figure 4). Several of the acute traumatic ischemias have established grading systems; in others, the severity of injury is often described as mild, moderate, or severe, even though other terms may more precisely define the seriousness of the injury. The efficacy of management interventions is based on comparisons of outcomes from injuries that have similar assessments, although the assessment for each injury may only reflects a single point or perhaps a narrow zone on the gradient of injury.

The multitude of presentations of traumatic ischemias essentially makes each one different. Each injury is unique, and no two are exactly alike in terms of cause, severity, extent, location, host responses, etc. Rather than thinking of each as a specific feature in the particular grading system, it is better to consider the injury as a range of injury on a continuum of responses from the damage. Generally, the most severely damaged tissue is used to classify the injury, but size, location, and patient wellness are also important considerations for making management decisions and comparing outcomes.

Another consideration of injury from traumatic ischemias is that they tend to be self-perpetuating due to factors of hypoxia and edema, each contributing to worsening of the other factor (Figure 5).[81,84] As edema worsens, oxygen diffusion distances increase, and cellular hypoxia worsens. Hypoxia interferes with the cell's ability to maintain its intracellular fluid content, which further contributes to edema. In addition, vasodilatation of the intact blood supply proximal to the injury, a reflex response, increases perfusion to the injury site and the intravascular pressure. This potentiates the driving force for extravasation of fluid from the blood vessel to the extracellular fluid compartment and results in increased edema. The increased flow for

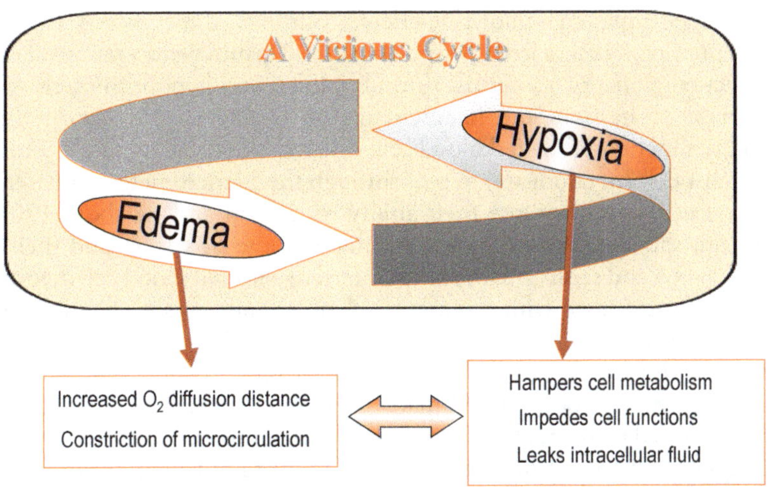

LEGEND: Through the mechanisms described above, edema worsens hypoxia, and hypoxia contributes to edema formation. The result is a self-perpetuating process that can worsen the injury as well as interfere with healing.

FIGURE 5. The self-perpetuating effect of edema coupled with ischemia.

these reasons may be counterproductive, with more bleeding and leakage of fluid into the interstitial spaces, and is something that HBO_2 mitigates as will be discussed later. These self-perpetuating activities may cause further tissue injury after the initial traumatic event has passed. Thus, worsening of the wound can result from continuation of the edema-ischemia vicious cycle. Hence, it may become a cause of secondary tissue loss, delayed healing, and challenges with bioburden management (Figure 2).

The propensity for self-perpetuation (the vicious cycle) is almost a universal finding in the traumatic ischemias. Management interventions are invariably directed at preventing or lessening the amount of injury from self-perpetuation of the injury. Self-perpetuation of the injury is a significant cause of secondary tissue losses and/or amputation (Figure 5).

Primary destruction of tissues arises from the transfer of energy to tissues in amounts that exceed the tissues' ability to absorb the energy and/or from irreversible interruption of blood supply to the tissues. Each tissue has an ischemia interval, which represents the time from the interruption of its blood supply until irreversible injury occurs. For the brain, it may be four minutes or less. The ischemia time for muscle is in the six-hour range. Secondary destruction of tissues is a consequence of the body's attempts to manage the injury, the inability of host reparative and infection-controlling functions to respond adequately, or combinations of the two. The reperfusion injury that occurs after transient periods of ischemia is also a cause of secondary tissue destruction.[49,93] During the time of frank ischemia, the nonperfused tissues remain in a state of suspended animation. During reperfusion, oxygen radicals generated by neutrophils attach to the endothelium, which became hypoxic during the ischemic period, and cause vasoconstriction of the precapillary arterioles. This results in the "no-reflow" phenomenon and the ultimate death of the involved tissues. In addition, toxic oxygen radicals initiate lipid peroxidation of cell membranes and react with endothelial-generated nitric oxide to form peroxynitrite, an extremely destructive radical.[87-88]

Stasis in the microcirculation is another cause of secondary tissue loss in traumatic ischemias (Figure 6). It interferes with the delivery of oxygen and nutrients to tissues. Causes include impaired inflow, restricted outflow, direct vessel injury and/or rheological problems arising from peripheral arterial insufficiency, venous stasis disease, diabetic microangiopathy, vasculitis, thrombophilia, and hypofibrinolysis syndromes. Another cause of stasis in the microcirculation is due to the loss of the normal deformability function of the red blood cell. The red blood cell, with a 7.5-micrometer diameter, must deform (elongate) to pass through the 5-micrometer diameter capillary. As red blood cells age, they lose their ability to deform and, at about 120 days, are removed from the bloodstream by the reticuloendothelial system and their products recycled. Hypoxia and sepsis are known to interfere with red blood cell deformity, both of which can be associated with traumatic ischemias and stasis in the microcirculation and further contribute to tissue injury and destruction.[29,63]

Infection, impaired wound healing, and wound contractures are additional secondary problems that occur in traumatic ischemias (Figure 7). Bacteria grow without restraint in damaged tissues that have impaired blood supplies.[25,91] With the interruption of blood supply, antibiotic delivery to the site of infection is halted. In addition, as tissue oxygen levels decrease, the neutrophil's ability to kill bacteria by oxidative mechanism is impaired. These cells require tissue oxygen tensions in the 30 to 40 mmHg range in order to kill bacteria.[24-26] For similar reasons, wounds will not heal unless there are equally

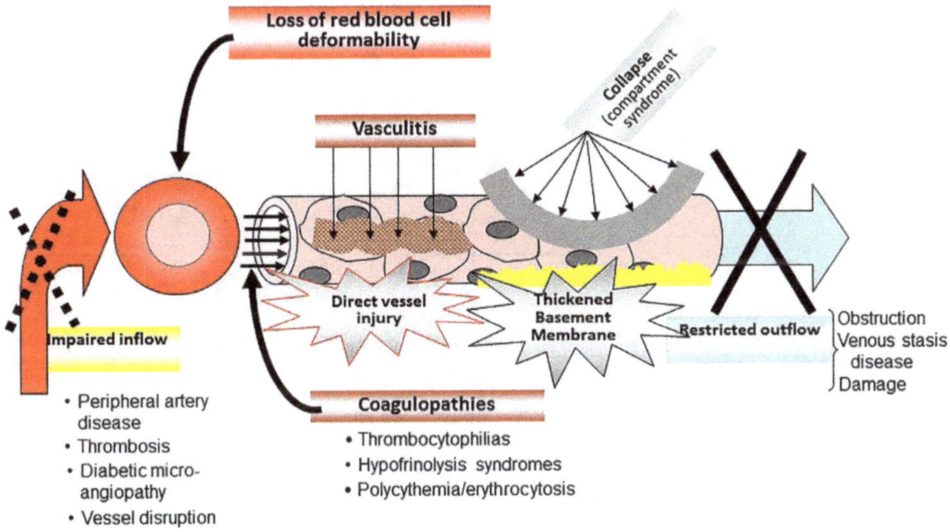

LEGEND: Stasis in the microcirculation has a variety of etiologies. Most act at different sites and have different mechanisms that cause the impaired flow. Several may coexist and have an additive effect on the flow restriction.

FIGURE 6. Causes of stasis in the microcirculation.

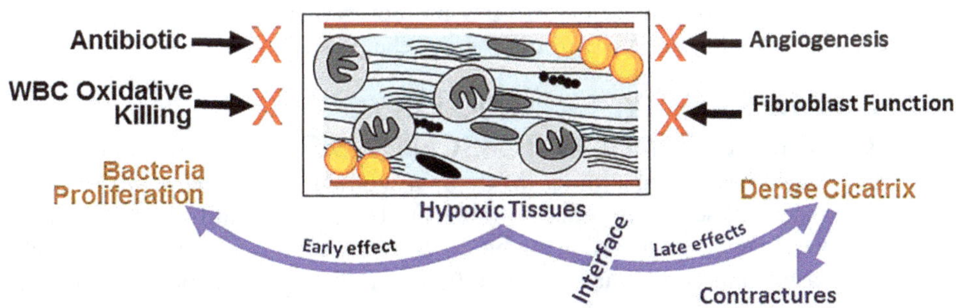

LEGEND: Tissue hypoxia (black letters and arrows and red Xs) impedes wound healing functions. The presence of hypoxia (blue letters and arrows) causes harmful effects with respect to infection control and restoration of function.

FIGURE 7. Hypoxia and its harmful effects on wound healing, bioburden control, and restoration of function.

Adequate oxygen tensions are essential for all aspects of healing from the time of the initial injury, during the control of the bioburden, through the inflammatory, reparative, and remodeling stages of repair and for the rehabilitation and restoration of function (Figure 7.) Although tissues may not die in hypoxic environments, they become nonfunctional. With restoration of adequate oxygen tensions, function returns. This is fundamental to the management of traumatic ischemias.

It is a paradox that at the time of the injury, the oxygen tensions in the wound are likely to be the lowest at any time in the healing process (Figure 8).

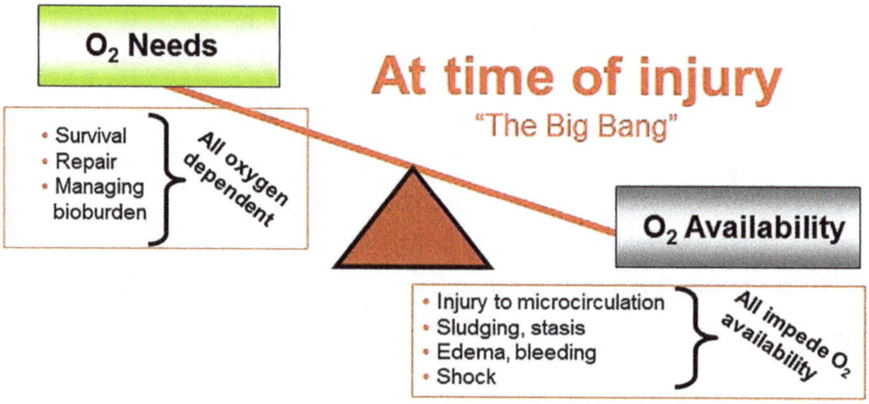

LEGEND: At the time of the injury -"The Big Bang" - oxygen needs are the greatest of any time in the healing process. Ironically, this is the time when they are most likely the lowest due to trauma to the blood vessels, edema, hypotension, bleeding, etc.

FIGURE 8. The paradox of oxygen needs and lack of availability at the time of injury.

high oxygen tensions for fibroblasts to migrate to the injury site, multiply, and produce a collagen matrix that is needed for angiogenesis and wound repair.[27-28]

If tissues die from anoxia and/or infection, they are replaced by scar tissue, a replacement tissue that forms under low oxygen tensions and/or as an attempt by the body to isolate the infection site from the adjacent healthy tissues. As scar tissue matures, it shortens and leads to deformities and contractures, which are sometimes observed as the endpoint responses of traumatic ischemias.

MECHANISMS OF HYPERBARIC OXYGEN APPLICABLE TO TRAUMATIC ISCHEMIAS

Hyperbaric oxygen is a logical adjunct for the management of traumatic ischemias. It has both primary and secondary effects (Table 1). The primary and most important effect of HBO_2 is hyperoxygenation of blood and other tissues. Oxygen physically dissolves in plasma and equilibrates in tissue fluids in direct proportion to the partial pressure of oxygen in the breathing gas. This supplements the oxygen-carrying mechanisms of the red blood cell. The breathing of pure oxygen at 2.0 atmospheres absolute pressure provides sufficient physically dissolved oxygen in plasma to meet tissue oxygen requirements.[3,5] This effect is an important consideration when stasis of cellular elements restricts red blood cell flow through the microcirculation. Plasma will continue to stream through the microcirculation and deliver the physically dissolved oxygen it contains to tissues (Figure 9). With hyperoxygenation of the plasma, dissolved oxygen in the plasma is no more flow limited than any of its other physically dissolved substances. Hyperbaric oxygen may also help improve flow through the microcirculation by enhancement of the red blood cell deformability mechanism.[44] Nemiroff demonstrated the synergistic

> Boerema et al. of the Netherlands published a milestone paper in 1960 reporting survival of piglets under hyperbaric oxygen conditions after removal of their red blood cells. This proved that hyperoxygenated plasma could meet short-term tissue oxygen requirements.[5] For this seminal work, Boerema is regarded as the "father" figure of hyperbaric medicine.

TABLE 1. EFFECTS OF HYPERBARIC OXYGEN USEFUL FOR TRAUMATIC ISCHEMIAS

Type	Mechanism	Effects	Characteristics
Primary (Maintain tissue viability)	Hyperoxygenation	• 10-fold ↑ tissue & plasma O_2 • 25% ↑ blood O_2 content • 3-fold ↑ in O_2 diffusion through tissue fluids	1) Immediate onset 2) Transient effect 3) Proportional to inhaled O_2 partial pressure 4) Dependent on plasma transport
Secondary (To hyperoxygenation) (Facilitate healing & durable effects)	1) Vasoconstriction	20% ↓ in blood flow	Edema reduction
	2) Host Factors • Fibroblast function	Migration, proliferation & secretory activity	Wound healing & matrix for angiogenesis
	• Neutrophil activity	Oxidative killing of bacteria	Formation of superoxides & peroxides
	• Osteoclast and osteoblast effects	Bone remodeling; removal of dead bone	Removal 100 times faster than formation
	3) Microbial actions	Decrease bioburden & its effects	Stasis, killing, ↓ toxin formation & antibiotic synergy
	4) Perturbation of reperfusion injury	Interference with WBC adhesion to endothelium	Interrupts "no reflow" phenomenon after reperfusion
	5) RBC deformability	O_2 exchange through capillary	7.5 μ wide RBC passage through the 5 μ capillary

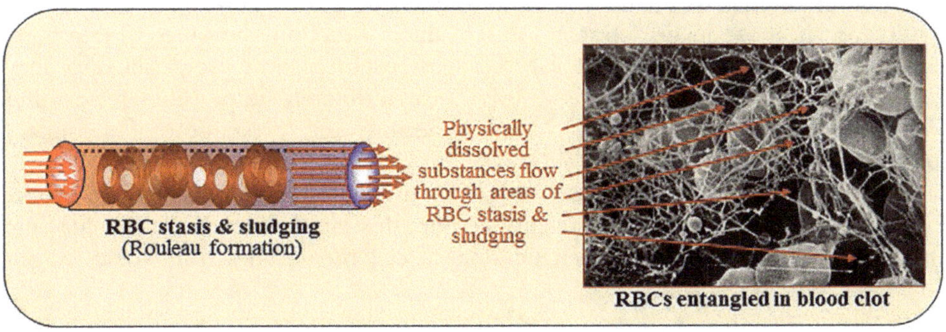

LEGEND: Hemoglobin oxygen transport through the microcirculation is the most flow limited of all the substances carried in the blood due to the mass of the red blood cell.

Plasma will continue to stream by the non-flowing RBCs, and if laden with oxygen - as with HBO_2 - will maintain oxygen delivery to tissues.

FIGURE 9. Augmentation of oxygen transport through the microcirculation with HBO_2.

effects of pentoxifylline, a medication that improves red blood cell deformability, and hyperbaric oxygen on skin flap survival.[55]

Vasoconstriction is a secondary effect of hyperoxygenation, which targets blood vessels. An approximately 20% reduction in blood flow in normal vasculature and corresponding reduction in edema is observed from this effect.[4,51,57,66,72,78-79] Filtration of plasma and/or extravasation of intravascular fluid from blood vessels is reduced secondary to decreased flow (see vasoconstriction role of oxygen in Chapter 13: The Role of Oxygen and Hyperbaric Oxygen Mechanisms). The increased oxygen content of the blood flow secondary to hyperoxygenation of the plasma more than compensates for the decreased flow associated with vasoconstriction.[4] The net effects are edema reduction and maintenance of oxygen delivery in the presence of decreased flow. A secondary effect of

Vasoconstriction of blood vessels in diabetics and patients with other causes of peripheral arterial disease probably does not occur to any significant degree in these conditions. This is due to calcification/atherosclerosis with noncompressibility of blood vessels and autosympathectomy effects.

Consequently, pulses may be palpable or obtainable with Doppler, but perfusion may not be able to increase sufficiently to meet the demands of wound healing and control of infection when needed to do such.

For host factors such as fibroblast, neutrophils, and osteoclasts/osteoblasts to function, 30 to 40 mmHg oxygen tensions are required in the tissue fluids. Transient elevations of oxygen tension as achieved with intermittent HBO_2 (rather than continuous exposures above these levels) appear sufficient for functional activities in these cell types.

edema reduction is improved flow in the microcirculation as edema decreases and results in reduced tissue fluid pressure and less tendency to collapse the thin-walled blood vessels of the microcirculation.

A third mechanism of HBO_2, and another secondary effect of hyperoxygenation for traumatic ischemias, is in its ability to provide a sufficiently oxygenated environment so host factors for wound healing and infection control function adequately. As mentioned earlier, these require oxygen tensions in the 30 to 40 mmHg range.[25-26,28] Pulses of oxygen to achieve or exceed the 30 to 40 mmHg tension as realized with twice- or three-times-a-day HBO_2 treatments are sufficient to meet host-function tissue oxygen requirements. Although these effects may not be important for the survival of tissues immediately after the injury, their function becomes increasingly important as time progresses since they are ultimately responsible for wound healing and prevention of secondary complications, such as infection.

Finally, HBO_2 protects tissues from the harmful effects of reactive oxygen species (Figure 10).[9,17,90,96] Several mechanisms support this effect, including the following: First, HBO_2 antagonizes lipid peroxidation of cell membranes from toxic oxygen

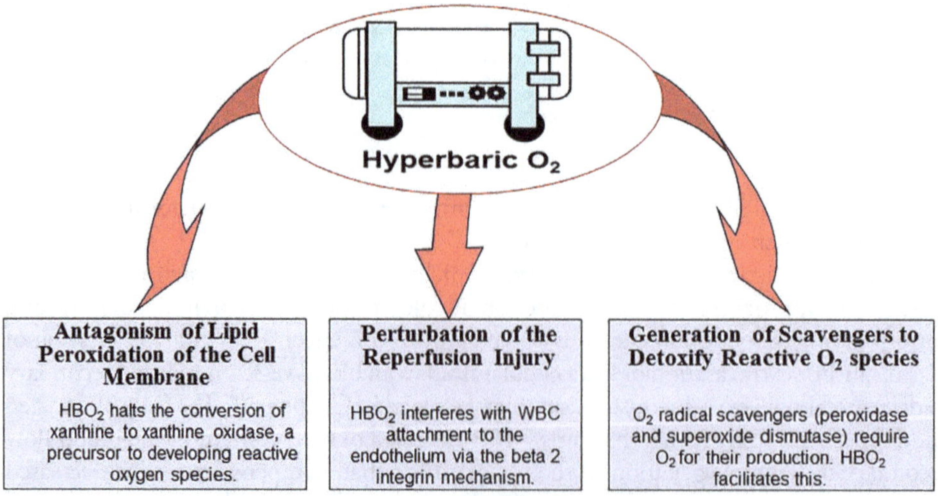

LEGEND: Three mechanisms of HBO_2 interfere with the generation and effects of reactive oxygen species. HBO_2 = hyperbaric oxygen, O_2 = oxygen, WBC = white blood cell

FIGURE 10. Roles of HBO_2 in mitigating the reperfusion injury.

radicals that interact with the lipids in the membrane.[87] Second, HBO_2 interferes with the sequestration of neutrophils on postcapillary venules and consequently perturbs the initiation of the reperfusion injury.[88] This effect results from HBO_2 interfering with the CD-11 beta 2 integrin mechanism which initiates the adherence of neutrophils to the capillary endothelium. There appears to be a window of effectiveness for using HBO_2 for this purpose from one hour before until several hours after the ischemic insult.[68,90,96] Third, HBO_2 provides sufficient oxygen to the reperfused tissues, so they can generate scavengers to detoxify the reactive oxygen species.[13,68]

Although hyperbaric oxygen is a possible source for the generation of reactive oxygen species, this appears to be of no clinical significance as observed in safely treating hundreds of thousands of patients with this modality. More importantly, the mechanisms that protect tissues from the harmful effects of reactive oxygen species are becoming increasingly well defined.

CLINICAL EXPERIENCES WITH HYPERBARIC OXYGEN FOR TRAUMATIC ISCHEMIAS

The complexity and diversity of these injuries makes interpretations of published reports using hyperbaric oxygen difficult. The first successful use of HBO_2 for a traumatic ischemia was reported in 1961, when it helped in the salvage of a foot after a near-avulsion.[74] In 1964, Perrins reported that the survival of threatened flaps was improved by a threefold factor when HBO_2 was used.[62] Subsequently, two literature reviews were published.[15,84] The first review was reported in 1981 and consisted of all the published reports on crush-type injuries and use of HBO_2 to that date.[84] Over 700 case reports were identified.[1,12,16,32-33,37-39,48,67,71,73,85] The cases were separated as to either being published in the English-language literature (63 patients or 13% of the series) or the Soviet literature (634 cases or 87% of the series). The Soviet reports suggested their focus was on using HBO_2 to mitigate injuries resulting from battlefield wounds. Outcomes were almost invariably described in subjective terms such as "useful," "improved," "beneficial," "effective," etc. The most noteworthy observation from this review was that the outcomes for traumatic ischemias improved as the frequency of treatments increased (Figure 11). For example, 59% good responses were

Author	HBO_2 Rxs/Day	Good Outcomes
Schramek[67]	6	100%
Loder[37]	3	80%
Slack[73]	1	59%

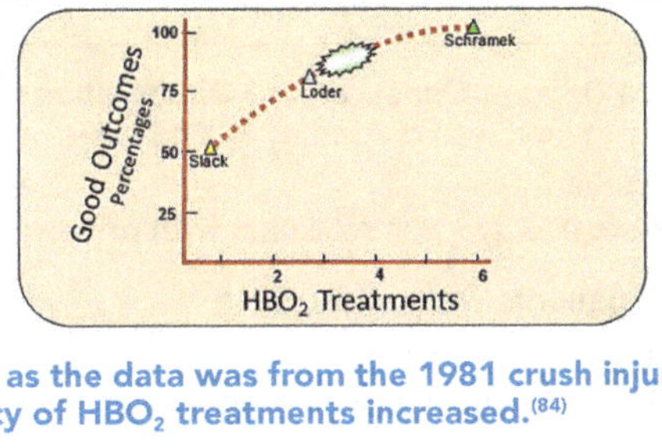

LEGEND: As poor quality as the data was from the 1981 crush injury review, outcomes were improved as the frequency of HBO_2 treatments increased.[84]

FIGURE 11. Observations on outcomes as related to the frequency of HBO_2 treatments.

Perhaps the most important information from the 1981 review was the observation that the more frequent the treatments, the better the outcomes. This assumption is supported by the previously discussed pathophysiology of the crush injury and other traumatic ischemias where the greatest oxygen demands for the injured tissues are highest immediately after the injury and because of the injury are likely to be the lowest of any time in the recovery process. Hyperbaric oxygen helps mitigate this discrepancy.

reported with one HBO_2 treatment a day, 80% complete or partial recovery with three treatments a day, and 100% salvage with six treatments a day.[34,37,94] In the second review, published in 2005, eight reports met the criteria to be included in an evidenced-based approach.[6,15,35,45,52,56,64,69,82,85] Seven of the eight reports were case series, with one of them being a retrospective study and the others prospective series. It is not surprising that only one of the citations in the 1981 review had enough statistical data to be included in the evidentiary review.[85] One randomized controlled trial (discussed next) was included in the review.[6]

In 1996, Bouachour, et al. reported the benefits of HBO_2 for open fracture crush injury (Table 2).[6] Their study was a randomized, double-blinded, placebo-controlled clinical trial. Thirty-six patients were randomized into two groups of 18 each. Standard-of-practice orthopaedic and medical management was provided for one arm of the study and similar management plus adjunctive use of HBO_2 in the other. Complete healing occurred in 94% (17 of 18 patients) of the hyperbaric group as compared to 59% (10 of 18 patients; p = < 0.01) in the control limb. Additional surgical procedures were required in 6% (1 of 18 patients) of the HBO_2 group as compared to 33% (6 of 18 patients; p = < 0.05) of the controls. Finally, healing in patients over 40 years of age was significantly improved in the HBO_2 group, with this occurring in 7 of 8 patients (88%) versus 3 of 10 patients (30%; p = < 0.05) in the control group. The authors also demonstrated the need for adequate oxygenation for healing of open fracture crush

TABLE 2. BOUACHOUR CRUSH INJURY RANDOMIZED CONTROL TRIAL [6]

Observations	HBO_2 Limb	Control Limb	p Value
Patients	**18** (50%)	**18** (50%)	
Primary Healing	**17** (94%)	**10** (56%)	**< 0.01**
Returns to OR	**1** (6%)	**6** (33%)	**< 0.05**
Primary Healing Patients > 40 years old	**7/8** (88%)	**3/10** (30%)	**< 0.05**

Transcutaneous Oxygen Measurement Observations: Ratios (i.e., TCOM value of injured limb divided by TCOM value of HBO_2-treated limb) were recorded.

Ratios of patients (HBO_2 & control limbs**) with primary healing ≥ 0.9**

Ratios in HBO_2 patients were all ≥ 0.9

Conclusions: 1) Limb oxygen tensions predicted healing
2) HBO_2 improved limb oxygen tensions

TABLE 3. OUTCOME COMPARISONS BETWEEN TWO STUDIES WITH & WITHOUT HBO_2

Observations	Matos HBO_2 used as an adjunct to orthopaedic management	Caudle Orthopaedic management without HBO_2
Study Design	Prospective	Prospective
Patients	23	62
Primary Healing	20 (87%)	24 (39%)
Unsatisfactory Outcomes*	3 (13%, all amputations)	38 (61%)

***Unsatisfactory Outcomes:** amputations, infections, nonunions, or combinations

injuries. Transcutaneous oxygen measurements of both the injured and contralateral legs were recorded. This information allowed the authors to generate a ratio (that is, $PtcO_2$(injured leg)/$PtcO_2$(uninjured leg)). In all fractures that healed, the indices were 0.9 or greater, with the differences being statistically significant. All patients who received HBO_2 had ratios greater than 0.9.

In 1999, Matos et al. published an abstract that was not included in the evidentiary review.[45] His study is useful in that it allows comparisons of outcomes in a somewhat head-to-head fashion with those reported in an orthopaedic surgery report where HBO_2 was not used (Table 3). Twenty-three patients with open fracture crush injuries were managed with orthopaedic interventions plus adjunctive HBO_2 treatments. Fractures were subdivided into those where enough soft tissue remained after debridement and stabilization of the fracture to cover all bone tissue (Gustilo type III-A open fracture crush injury) and those where exposed bone remained after the initial orthopaedic management (Gustilo type III-B) and those where there was a concomitant vascular injury (Gustilo type III-C) (Figure 4). Twenty patients (87%) had a successful outcome with preservation of the limb, while three patients (13%) required amputations.

TABLE 4. COUPLING OF THE GUSTILO OPEN FRACTURE CRUSH INJURY CLASSIFICATION WITH THE PATIENT'S HOST STATUS* FOR MAKING DECISIONS TO USE HBO_2

Host Status* / Gustilo Class	Healthy 7 ½ - 10 points	Impaired 3 ½ - 7 points	Decompensated 0 - 3 points
1	No HBO_2	No	No
2	No	Yes HBO_2	Yes HBO_2
3-A	No	Yes	Yes
-B	Yes HBO_2	Yes	No†
-C	Yes	No†	No†

NOTE: *Host status based on a 0-to-10 Wellness Score that summates five assessments each graded from 2 points (best) to 0 points (worst) that includes (1) ability to do activities of daily living, (2) ambulation, (3) comorbidities, (4) smoking/immunosuppressors, and (5) neurological deficits; see Wellness Score details in Chapter 20: Hyperbaric Oxygen for the Management of Chronic Refractory Osteomyelitis.

† Consider a primary amputation

For comparison purposes, an orthopaedic report with analogous fracture crush injuries where HBO_2 was not used had an amputation rate of 25% (13 of 62 patients) and other poor outcomes in 40.3% (25 of 62 patients) giving an overall complication rate of 62.8% (Table 3).[10]

The decision to use HBO_2 treatments for crush injury fractures is determined by two factors. The first is the seriousness of the injury coupled with the patient's wellness status (Table 4). Hyperbaric oxygen treatment protocols for traumatic ischemias vary according to what the pertinent pathophysiological concerns are and what desired effect is being sought from this modality (Table 5). Almost all HBO_2 treatments for traumatic ischemias are done at pressures of 2.0 to 2.4 atmospheres absolute for periods of 90 to 120 minutes of pure-oxygen breathing. Early application of HBO_2, preferably within four to six hours of the injury, is desirable to address the acute wound hypoxia problems, so likely to occur immediately after the injury. Treatment schedules for traumatic ischemias should be tailored to mitigate the suspected pathophysiology. For example, there should be 3 or more treatments in a 24-hour period for critical ischemias, treatments twice a day for threatened flaps and oxygenation of the environment so host factors can function, and daily treatments for infections and/or remodeling/resorption of calcified tissues. For the isolated ischemia-reperfusion injury, for example after a prolonged tourniquet time, revascularization, and/or thrombectomy of an extremity that otherwise has sustained minimal physical trauma, one to two HBO_2 treatments, based on animal studies and limited clinical observations, appears to be adequate.[68,88,90,96] Again, treatments for the ischemia-reperfusion injury should be started as soon as possible after the insult. If the ischemia-reperfusion injury is a component of the surgery, HBO_2 should be started immediately after the surgery is completed.

Recommended HBO_2 treatment guidelines for traumatic ischemias vary with what is the suspected pathophysiology of the underlying condition. Treatment schedules should be altered if justified by clinical findings, such as the need to increase the frequency of treatments for threatened flaps or when additional trailing treatments are indicated. Collaboration is recommended in such situations and provides collective justification for modifying HBO_2 treatment schedules.

When HBO_2 is used as an adjunct for the management of traumatic ischemias, three distinct levels of tissue involvement/injury must be appreciated when considering its benefits and harmful effects (Figure 12).[81] First, normal and noninvolved tissues adjacent to and/or remote from the injury tolerate HBO_2 treatments without apparent

TABLE 5. HBO_2 TREATMENT PROTOCOLS FOR CRUSH INJURIES

Condition	HBO_2 Rxs	Peer Review after # of treatments	Comments
Reperfusion injury	1 or 2	2	**Minimal tissue trauma**; reimplantations, free flaps; transient ischemia, after revascularizations, etc.
Crush injury	TID 1–2 Days BID 2 Days Daily 2 Days	12	If deterioration noted with step-down treatments, resume previous schedule
Crush injury with threatened flaps	BID 10–14 Days	10	Additional treatments after crush injury 5–6-day protocol completed or if HBO_2 not started until the problem arises
Crush injury with bone infection	Daily for 21–40 days	21	(same as above)

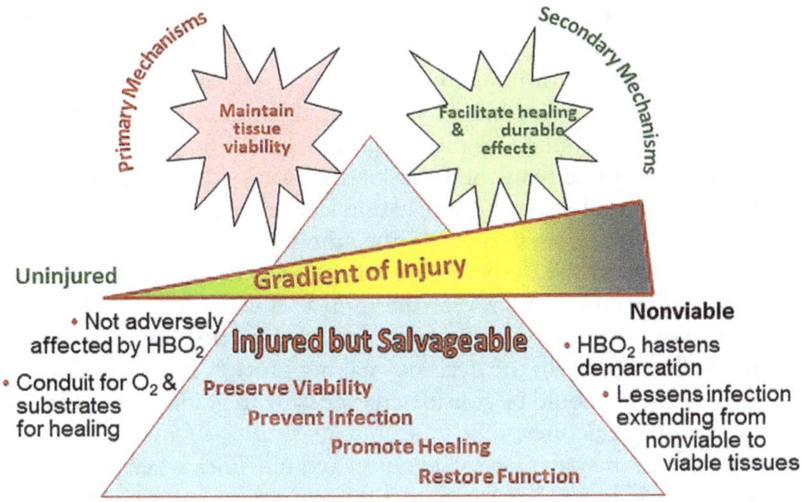

LEGEND: The midportion of the gradient of injury in traumatic ischemias is the zone where HBO_2, acting through its primary and secondary mechanisms, is most beneficial. However, it can also have helpful effects for both uninjured and nonviable tissues.

FIGURE 12. Effects of HBO_2 on the 3 levels of tissue involvement (uninjured, gradient of injury, and nonviable) traumatic ischemias.

untoward effects when accepted treatment protocols as mentioned above are used.[4] Remote and seemingly noninvolved tissues can contribute to the healing process by augmenting perfusion and oxygenation to the injured tissues as well as mobilizing precursors for wound healing and infection control. Systemic vasoconstriction does not adversely affect these activities in the presence of hyperoxia achieved with HBO_2.[4]

Second, the tissues in the gradient of injury are the target area for HBO_2 treatments. Four goals are sought for HBO_2 (as well as all other treatment interventions) for the gradient of injury: 1) preservation of tissue viability, 2) prevention of infection, especially during the critical post-injury hypoxic phase, 3) promotion of healing processes, and 4) restoration of function during the recovery and convalescent phases. The third level of involvement concerns dead, nonviable tissues. Although HBO_2 will not revitalize dead tissue, it hastens demarcation between the nonviable and the adjacent live tissues. As a corollary to this, it helps prevent extension of infection from the very vulnerable margins of the necrotic tissues to the adjacent severely injured tissues.

CRUSH INJURIES AND SPECIAL CONSIDERATIONS FOR USING HYPERBARIC OXYGEN

Crush injuries are traumatic ischemias that cause such severe damage to tissues from the energy transfer that tissue survival is in question.[81] Crush injuries arise primarily from motor vehicle accidents, high-velocity gunshot wounds, falls, and the dropping of heavy objects onto a body part. Invariably, two or more types of tissues are injured severely enough that they are at risk of not surviving. Associated with these findings are the two other components of the traumatic ischemia triad, namely the gradient of injury and the self-perpetuating edema-hypoxia vicious cycle. Gustilo's classification of open fractures is widely used for judging the severity of crush injuries (Figure 4, Table 4). Type III fractures meet the criteria of crush injury.[19-20] In subtype III-B and -C open fracture crush injury, those with insufficient soft tissue to cover bone after debridement is done and concomitant major blood vessel injury respectively, complication rates approach 50%, even with optimal management.[19] Complications include nonunions, infection, amputations, or combinations of these. The Mangled Extremity Severity Score (MESS) provides a guideline to select which injured extremities, after limb-threatening trauma, should undergo primary amputation.[34]

Perhaps a better guide than the Gustilo classification for using HBO_2 in crush injuries is the Tscherne and Oestern classification formulated in 1982.[92] They classified closed fractures into four grades based on the amount of soft-tissue injury and open fractures based on wound size, level of contamination, and fracture pattern (Table 6). The higher the grades, the more severe the injury. This grading system provides an additional source of information for justifying HBO_2 in crush injuries and integrates well with the Wellness Score in the decision-making process. Hyperbaric oxygen as an adjunct or management should be considered especially in grade 3 closed fractures and grades III and IV open fractures.

These classification systems provide objective guidelines when making decisions whether HBO_2 should be used as an adjunct for managing crush injuries. However, it appears that most trauma surgeons classify crush injuries on an analogue scale as mild, moderate, or severe based on their clinical experiences and only intuitively factor in the host status for making decisions regarding management. Hyperbaric oxygen should be considered for the serious injuries whether or not a classification system is used. The wellness and goal statuses of the patient should always be factored into the decision-making process.

Age, while not an absolute criterion, should be considered in the management decisions. While chronological age is important, for decision-making and management

TABLE 6. TSCHERNE AND OESTERN CLASSIFICATION OF FRACTURES & USE OF HBO_2 WITH RESPECT TO WELLNESS SCORE (see Table 4)

Grade	Findings	Comments Use of HBO_2 with respect to Wellness Score		
		Healthy Host	Impaired	Decompensated
Closed Fractures				
0	• Minimal soft-tissue injury • Indirect injury to limb (torsion) • Simple fracture pattern	No	No	No
1	• Superficial abrasion or contusion • Mild fracture pattern	No	No	No
2	• Deep abrasion • Skin or muscle contusion • Severe fracture pattern • Direct trauma to limb	No	No	Yes
3	• Extensive skin contusion or crush injury • Severe damage to underlying muscle • Compartment syndrome • Subcutaneous [tissue] avulsion	Yes	Yes	Yes
Open Fractures				
I	• Open fractures with a small puncture without skin contusion • Negligible bacterial contamination • Low-energy fracture pattern	No	No	Yes
II	• Open fractures with small skin and soft-tissue contusions • Variable fracture patterns	No	Yes	Yes
III	• Open fractures with heavy contamination • Extensive soft-tissue damage • Often, associated arterial or neural injuries	Yes	Yes	Yes
IV	• Open fracture with incomplete or complete amputations	Yes	Yes	Yes

purposes, physiological age is more important. Physiological age reflects what the patient's cognitive function and activity level is compared to someone of a different age. Age, however, has its effects and appears to be mitigated by HBO_2. In the lab, Renstra, et al., showed that the doubling times of fibroblasts from older subjects was reduced by approximately 50% as compared to the doubling times of fibroblasts from newborns.[65] However, when cultured with HBO_2 exposures, these fibroblast doubling times were equivalent to the newborn's.[65] Bouachour, et al., observed that in the subgroup of patients over 40 years of age with open fracture crush injuries, the outcomes were statistically significantly better in the HBO_2 treatment arm.[6] Age over 50 years can account for almost 30% in the decision-making process to amputate a mangled extremity in the MESS system.[92] While HBO_2 is not a "fountain of youth," it does show promise for lessening the detrimental effects aging has in recovery from crush injuries.

Management of crush injuries includes direct interventions that involve surgery, such as debridement, repair of damaged vessels, stabilization of bony elements, and repair of soft tissues. The other component of crush injury care is management of its indirect effects. The mechanisms of HBO, such as hyperoxygenation, increased oxygen delivery in low-flow states, perturbation of the reperfusion injury, and reduction of edema, help to manage the indirect effects of the crush injury. Other considerations for managing the indirect effects of the crush injury include adequate fluid and blood replacement to optimize perfusion, prophylactic antibiotics to prevent infection, venous stasis disease prophylaxis, nutrition management, and measures to improve flow in the microcirculation, such as anti-platelet adhesion, red blood cell deformability, anticoagulation, volume expanders, and/or viscosity-reducing agents. After emergency surgical care is completed, and the patient is stable enough, HBO_2 treatments should commence immediately since the greatest needs for adequate wound oxygenation to ensure primary healing and prevention of infection is during the inflammatory phase of wounds (Figure 8).

It is ironic that in the time immediately after the injury ("The Big Bang"), oxygen requirements are the greatest of any time in the healing and restoration-of-function process. This is because during the first phase of healing, the inflammatory phase, the high oxygen tensions are needed for mobilizing growth factors, white blood cells, fibroblasts, and other mediators to initiate the wound healing process as well as manage the bioburden (Figure 13).

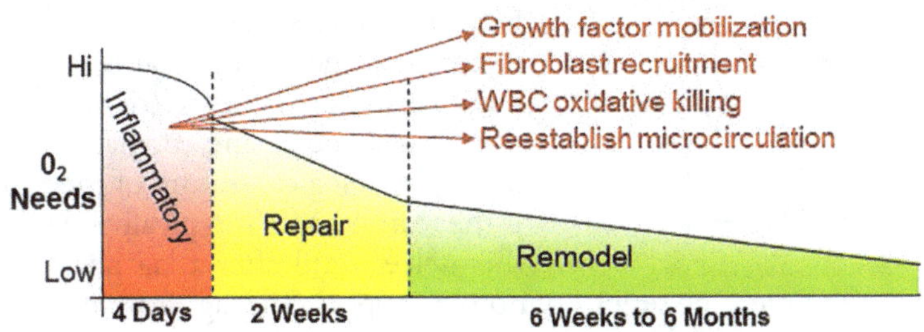

LEGEND: The greatest requirements for oxygen are in the inflammatory (the initial) phase of wound healing. The recruitment of wound-healing and infection-controlling agents is so profound that it takes 20 times as many colony-forming units (CFUs) to initiate an infection in a dog knee model at the end of the inflammatory phase as it does at the beginning of the inflammatory phase (Personal communication TK Hunt ~1980).

FIGURE 13. Oxygen requirements during the three phases of wound healing.

Experiences with HBO_2 as discussed previously show that when this modality is used as an adjunct for managing severe open fracture, crush injury complication rates are in the 20% range.(15,84) This is a sizable improvement from the 50% rates reported when HBO_2 was not used.(19-20,34) The additional expenses associated with HBO_2 treatments would be far less than the costs of managing these high complication rates. In 1977, Brighton estimated that in the United States, $140,000 was the average cost per patient required to resolve the 100,000 open fractures, crush injuries that failed to heal primarily each year.(7) Today, the costs would be many multiples of this. Even with new technologies, the complication rates are predictable for the most severe open fractures, crush injuries.(7,10,18-20) Because of the large number of these injuries that occur in the United States each year, a reduction in complications and the morbidity associated with them could have substantial impact on health-care costs and far outweigh the additional expenses associated with HBO_2 treatments. Mackay, et al., reported in 1986 that lower-limb amputations after failed revascularizations generated medical costs approaching $50,000 when hospitalization, surgery, prosthesis, and rehabilitation costs were considered.(41) Not to be dismissed are the intangible benefits that primary healing and avoidance of amputations have on the patient's mental outlook, ability to function independently, and return to gainful employment.(40) Finally, a lower-limb amputation should not always be considered as a failure in management. When pain, deformity, a functionally useless or unresolved infection in the limb persists, amputation becomes a logical option.

SKELETAL MUSCLE-COMPARTMENT SYNDROME

A skeletal muscle-compartment syndrome (SMCS) occurs when swelling of injured skeletal muscle increases the interstitial fluid within the myofascial compartment above the capillary perfusion pressure. Ischemic injury to the muscle occurs due to blood flow interruption at the microcirculation level. Edema and tissue hypoxia are the important pathophysiological components of the SMCS. While direct trauma to muscle is probably the most frequent cause, other etiologies include (1) prolonged ischemia time from thromboses, (2) arterial injuries, (3) prolonged tourniquet times, (4) venous occlusion or interruption of outflow secondary to injury, (5) external compression from devices such as bandages, casts, or pneumatic compression suits, (6) bleeding into the compartment, (7) intravenous fluid or medication infiltration into the compartment, (8) snake envenomation, (9) crush syndrome (prolonged compression of an extremity secondary to comatose posturing, that is to say, lying on a limb), and (10) overexertion. Self-perpetuation from hypoxia and edema is an important pathophysiological feature of the SMCS. This is the reason SMCSs typically do not manifest themselves until after a lag phase; that is the time from injury to the time serious symptoms appear. The lag phase may range from a few hours, especially with bleeding into the compartment, to several days after the inciting cause.

> Most SMCSs do not manifest themselves until after a lag phase. The exception is frank bleeding into the compartment. The lag phase is the time interval from the injury to the time symptoms and signs of a SMCS occur. The lag phase exemplifies the self-perpetuating hypoxia-edema process.

The SMCS, like the crush injury, represents a continuum of severities that can be divided into *Suspected*, *Impending* (lag), and *Established* stages (Figure 14A, Figure 14B). In the *Suspected* stage, the compartment syndrome is not actually present, but the

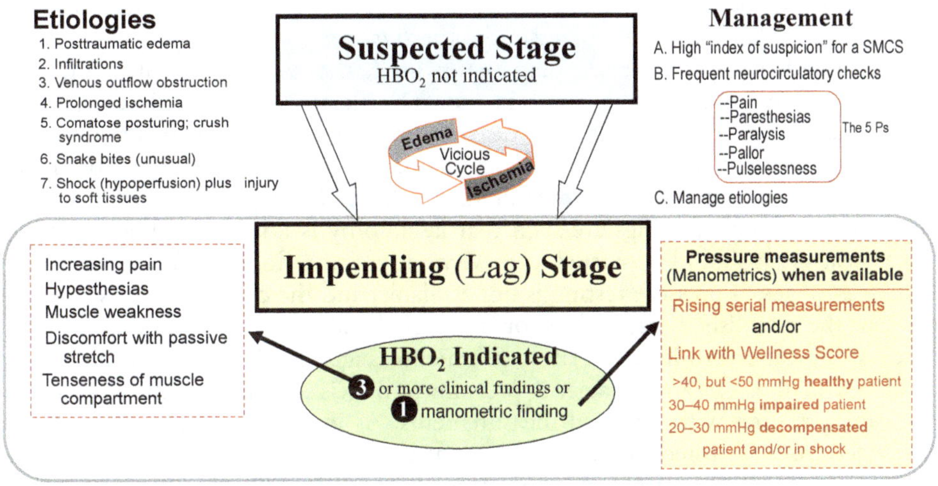

LEGEND: The skeletal muscle-compartment syndrome starts with an injury or an insult (see etiologies) in *Suspected* stage above. If the edema-ischemia vicious cycle progresses, the *Suspected* stage evolves into the *Impending* (Lag) stage. Hyperbaric oxygen is the only known intervention that will mitigate the edema-ischemia vicious cycle progression.

FIGURE 14A. Indications for HBO_2 in the skeletal muscle-compartment syndrome.

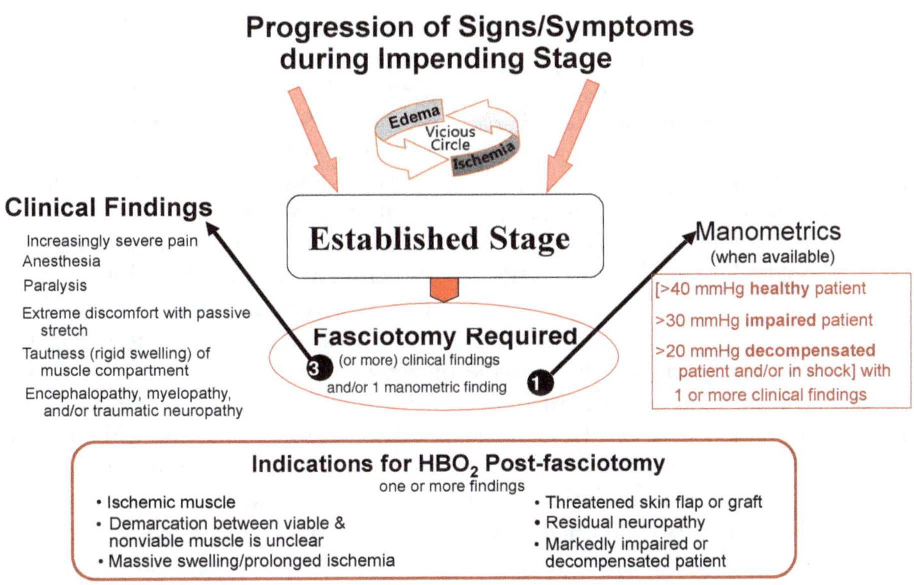

LEGEND: If the *Impending* stage progresses on to the *Established* stage, HBO_2 must not be used as a substitute for fasciotomy. However, HBO_2 should be used post fasciotomy if one or more residual findings are present.

FIGURE 14B. Requirements for fasciotomy in the skeletal muscle-compartment syndrome & indications for HBO_2 post fasciotomy.

severity of the injury or the circumstances (for example, prolonged ischemia time) raise suspicions that a SMCS could develop. In this stage HBO_2 is not recommended, but frequent neurocirculatory checks of the injured extremity are required in order to recognize the earliest possible progression to the *Impending* stage (lag phase).

If the edema-hypoxia cycle perpetuates itself, the condition evolves into the *Impending* stage. In this stage, signs include (1) increasing pain, (2) hypesthesia/paresthesia, (3) muscle weakness, (4) discomfort with passive stretch, (5) tenseness in the compartment, or combinations of these signs. If any of these symptoms or signs exist, compartment pressure measurements should be made. If the compartment pressures and clinical findings are such that fasciotomy is not required at that time, HBO_2 treatments should be started to prevent progression from the *Impending* to the *Established* stages. If pressure testing is not available, and the compartment syndrome is not in the established stage, three or more of the above clinical findings provide sufficient indications to initiate HBO_2 treatments (Figure 14A). A second indication for HBO_2 in the *Impending* stage, if pressure testing is available, is the findings of increasing pressures with repeated measurements. As in crush injuries, the Wellness Score needs to be factored in the compartment pressure measurements when making decisions to use HBO for the *Impending* stage of the SMCS (Figure 14A).

In the *Established* stage of the SMCS, signs and/or pressure measurements confirm the diagnosis and dictate that immediate fasciotomy be done (Figure 14B). Hyperbaric oxygen must not be used as a reason to defer surgery, but if an operating room is not immediately available, a HBO_2 treatment should be given while awaiting fasciotomy surgery. The rationale for this is that HBO_2 will mitigate the vicious cycle of edema and ischemia and help preserve viability and function of the involved tissues.

If the SMCS becomes "full-blown," that is, progresses to the *Established* stage, immediate fasciotomy is required. Hyperbaric oxygen should not be used as a substitute for fasciotomy when surgery is indicated. If significant residual problems remain after the fasciotomy, then HBO_2 should be used as an adjunct to wound, flap, and/or functional recovery management.

After fasciotomy surgery, HBO_2 should be used as an adjunct to wound management if significant residual problems remain such as ischemic muscle, threatened flaps, unclear demarcation between viable and nonviable muscle, residual neuropathy, marked swelling, prolonged (more than 6 hours) ischemia time, and/or significant host impairment as quantified by the Wellness Score (Figure 14B).

Measurements of interstitial fluid pressure within the compartment provide objectivity for assessment of the SMCS. Surgical decompression of the myofascial compartment is recommended when pressure measurements exceed the capillary perfusion pressure. However, there is not uniform agreement as to what pressure criteria justify immediate fasciotomies.[23,43,46-47,53-54,83,94] This is the reason clinical criteria are equally important to compartment measurements in the justification for fasciotomy surgery (Figure 14A). If the initial pressure measurements are in the intermediate range, that is, not elevated enough to justify surgical decompression, three permutations arise: 1) the pressures may decline, 2) the pressures may plateau, or 3) the pressures may rise to a point where surgical decompression is required. Except for the use of HBO_2, no proven interventions are available to interrupt the progression of the SMCS during the *Impending* stage (lag phase). If serial measurements of compartment fluid pressures are done at timed intervals in the patient with a suspected SMCS, the time of critical pressure elevation may be missed. This is due to the fact that initial pressure increases occur gradually until the compliance of the compartment is exceeded (that is, the compartment is filled to capacity with edema fluid without a significant rise in intracompartmental pressures). After that point, additional edema formation in the compartment causes rapid elevations in pressure. This, again, emphasizes the importance of frequent clinical assessments in evaluation and management of the compartment syndrome in its *Impending* stage.

Several problems complicate the evaluation and management of the SMCS. First, when compartment pressure measurements alone are used to provide an objective indication for fasciotomy, there is no agreement in the published reports as to what pressure should be used.(23,43,46-47,53-54,83,94) Furthermore, hypotension is the only host factor considered in the manometric interpretation reports. Hypotension is integrated into four of the above seven reports but without unanimity in opinion as to what degree is considered significant. Hypotension lowers the threshold pressure for the SMCS syndrome because it decreases capillary perfusion pressure, which lowers the threshold for ischemic injury to the muscles within the compartment. Consequently, the criteria for surgical decompression of the compartment based on interstitial fluid pressures alone may not be valid in the presence of shock. Second, if neuropathy develops as a consequence of the SMCS, recovery of function occurs in only a small percentage of cases.(58-59) Finally, once the compartment has been surgically decompressed, it is not always apparent which tissues will survive and how much muscle injury has occurred since a gradient of injury exists as in the other traumatic ischemias.

Hyperbaric oxygen is a logical intervention for the SMCS. The primary pathophysiology problems of this condition, hypoxia and edema, are corrected by the hyperoxygenation and edema-reduction mechanisms of HBO_2. This information was conclusively confirmed by SMCS studies in animal studies.(58-59,78-79) Enhanced recovery of muscle function has been demonstrated in a rabbit SMCS model with HBO_2.(2) Clinical experiences using HBO_2 for the SMCS are consistent with what would have been predicted from knowing the mechanisms of HBO_2, the pathophysiology of SMCS, and the laboratory studies.(14,60,82)

Why is HBO_2 not used more frequently and as a "standard of practice" for the *Impending* (lag) stage of the SMCS? The question is especially pertinent since the mechanisms of HBO_2 have demonstrated conclusively in well-designed laboratory studies to interrupt its pathophysiology.(58-59) Additionally, no other interventions are known to be effective for this stage of the SMCS. Some responses to this dilemma are offered in the conclusion of this chapter.

When HBO_2 was initiated during the *Impending* (lag) stage of the SMCS, no compartment syndromes progressed or required surgical decompression.(82) When HBO_2 was started after surgical decompression had been done because of concerns about wound healing, it sped the reduction of edema and prevented further loss of tissue. This facilitated wound closure, survival of threatened flaps and grafts, and restoration of function. A cost-benefit review showed that when HBO_2 was started during the *Imprending* stage, the total expenses generated (hospitalization, HBO_2 treatments, medicines, and surgeries) were one-quarter of those in patients whose compartment syndromes had progressed to the degree that surgical decompression was required and who then subsequently received HBO_2 treatments to manage the residual problems.(80)

THE ROLE OF HYPERBARIC OXYGEN IN OTHER TRAUMATIC ISCHEMIAS

The mechanisms of HBO_2 useful for crush injury and compartment syndrome also have applications for other traumatic ischemias such as burns, frostbite, threatened flaps and grafts, and compromised reimplantations. Burns demonstrate a gradient of injury: first-, second-, or third-degree severity from the inciting cause being thermal injury (Figure 4). Since hypoxia and edema are also important components of the pathophysiology, they meet the criteria of a traumatic ischemia. Components of a traumatic ischemia are also observed in threatened flaps and grafts. Hypoxia is the predominant finding, but other characteristics of traumatic ischemias, such as edema and a gradient of injury, are important features. In contrast to other traumatic ischemias, there is usually less actual physical injury to the threatened flaps and grafts sites than in crush injuries and burns. The underlying problems are predominantly ischemia and edema from mobilizing the flap during surgery or a wound base with insufficient vascularity to support the flap or skin graft. The exception to this, of course, is the severe open fracture crush injury where physical trauma to the flap is an important consideration in defining the seriousness of the crush injury. As in the other traumatic ischemias, the primary indications for HBO_2 in threatened flaps and grafts are to improve oxygen availability to areas where perfusion is compromised and to reduce edema. Comprehensive discussions of burns and threatened flaps and grafts are found in other chapters of this text. The following discussion supplements information about frostbite and threatened reimplantations.

The pathophysiology of frostbite is similar to that of the other traumatic ischemias, but the etiology is that of cold injury to the tissues. Problems arise in frostbite injuries during rewarming when stasis in the microcirculation, Rouleau formation of red blood cells in the microcirculation, and edema develop as a consequence of reperfusion. During rewarming, oxygen demands are at their greatest point, yet the ability to deliver oxygen to the injured tissues is most compromised. The role of HBO_2 in this condition is obvious, but unfortunately few clinical studies are available.[89] The ideal time to initiate HBO_2 for frostbite is during the rewarming period. After the rewarming is accomplished, HBO_2 treatments should be done twice a day for reducing edema, supporting injured but salvageable tissues, aiding in demarcation between viable and irreversibly damaged tissues, and lessening the chances of infection. Other adjuncts to improve perfusion, such as low-molecular-weight dextran, sympathetic blocks, optimization of intravascular fluid volume, maintenance of cardiac function, and use of antiplatelet, anti-agglutination medications, should be considered. In addition, recombinant tissue plasminogen activator (r-tPA) has shown benefits in reducing injury from frostbite when it was given during the rewarming period.[70]

Due to Rouleau formation and vasospasm, perfusion to the microcirculation can be severely compromised. This additionally qualifies frostbite as an acute peripheral arterial insufficiency condition, which is discussed more extensively in other parts of this text.

Threatened reimplantations demonstrate the same pathophysiology as other traumatic ischemias. Hyperbaric oxygen has been used as an adjunct for managing this problem.[8,36,95] Typically, the pathophysiology of the threatened replantation is a combination of the findings found in crush injury and the threatened flap. Edema reduction appears to be the major benefit of HBO_2 for the threatened replantation.[95] This is because post replantation arterial repairs are usually sufficient to meet the replant's perfusion needs while vein repairs are more tenuous. The consequence is congestion and swelling due to insufficient venous outflow. Medicinal leech therapy supplemented with HBO_2 treatments for its edema-reducing mechanism is an effective combination for dealing with this threatened-replantation problem. If arterial inflow is insufficient and/or the microcirculation has been compromised by the injury causing the amputation, the hyperoxygenation effect of HBO_2 is indicated for this component of the problem. Finally, if the ischemia time is prolonged, as is often the situation with reimplantations, HBO_2 should be used for its perturbation of the reperfusion injury.[88,96]

CONCLUSION

Hyperbaric oxygen is underutilized as an adjunct for the management of traumatic ischemias. The specific mechanisms of HBO_2 mitigate the pathophysiology of these conditions. The laboratory and clinical information demonstrating the benefits of HBO_2 for traumatic ischemias are as substantial as any of the other evidence used to justify adjunctive interventions for other medical or surgical conditions. The relevant question is, why is HBO_2 not included in all traumatologists' algorithms for managing crush injuries and other traumatic ischemia? The answers are several-fold:

- **First**, traumatologists are either unaware or appear to ignore the science of HBO_2 therapy and the research and laboratory-based information that supports its use in traumatic ischemias.
- **Second**, expectations of complications and wound healing failures are the rule with the severest degrees of the traumatic ischemias. Unfortunately, there appears to be a general acceptance of these complications as meeting the "standards of practice," without any consideration for improving the outcomes with the adjunctive use of HBO_2.
- **Third**, HBO_2 is an adjunct to primary surgical and medical management of traumatic ischemias. Because of this role, HBO_2 tends to be considered only after complications arise rather than as a proactive primary intervention to prevent predictable problems.
- **Fourth**, because HBO_2 chambers are not typically available at trauma centers, their lack of immediate availability is used as a reason to defer transfer or not consider HBO_2 treatments at all. However, transfers for other emergencies are done frequently from medical facilities where a higher level of care is unavailable from the referring institution. For example, life- and limb-threatening conditions such as limb reimplantations, neurosurgical emergencies, severe burns, arterial gas embolism, decompression sickness, gas gangrene, and carbon monoxide poisoning are transferred to facilities that can provide the level of care required for these problems. These latter four conditions are typically transferred, regardless of the proximity of the hyperbaric facility, specifically for HBO_2 therapy. Should not the same standards be used to reduce predictable complications with the use of HBO_2 for the most serious types of traumatic ischemias?
- **Finally**, there seems to be reluctance for hyperbaric medicine facilities themselves to encourage the use of HBO_2 for traumatic ischemias. This is a two-part problem. First, the complexity of managing patients with traumatic ischemias, often with associated complex medical problems, is problematic for hyperbaric medical facilities that do not regularly treat critical care

patients. Second, because of implementation of Diagnosis-Related Group (DRG) payments by Medicare, third-party payer contracts, or the patient being uninsured, reimbursements for HBO_2 treatments for traumatic ischemia may be extremely limited or nonexistent.

> Even though there has been a geometric increase in HBO_2 facilities, with over 1400 now operational in the United States, fewer than 40 are willing or equipped to handle the traumatic ischemias and other emergency conditions for which HBO_2 is needed.

Is HBO_2 justified as an evidenced-based indication for crush injury and skeletal muscle-compartment syndrome (SMCS)? Since it is used as an adjunct to surgery and medical management, perhaps HBO_2 therapy needs to be judged differently than how a primary treatment modality is judged. Nonetheless, when the American Heart Association 1999 Guidelines are used, hyperbaric oxygen meets the criteria of a Class I-b indication for crush injury and a Class II indication for compartment syndrome.[21] For crush injury, a favorable randomized controlled trial exists (Class I-b indication), and for the SMCS, it is probably useful and effective with a favorable risk/benefit ratio (Class II indication). The absence of a randomized controlled trial for the SMCS is the reason HBO_2 is not classified at a higher evidence-based indication level for this condition.

> Ian Millar from Melbourne, Australia, coordinated has coordinated an international blinded, randomized control trial study on the use of HBO for crush-injury-related fractures. The study is entitled Hyperbaric Oxygen for Lower Limb Trauma (HOLLT). At the time of this writing, the HOLTT data collection has been completed and according to Dr. Millar is being analyzed for outcomes at one-year-minimum follow-ups. We await Dr. Millar's reports.

It is apparent that factors other than randomized controlled trials need to be considered when making decisions about selecting treatment interventions. This is as valid for using HBO_2 for the traumatic ischemias as it is for selecting interventions for other medical and surgical conditions. We recommend that five assessments be used to make rationally based decisions when using HBO_2 for crush injury and other traumatic ischemias (Table 7).[77] To quantify this approach, each assessment is graded on a 0-to-2-point scale, with two points indicating overwhelming information to support the assessment, one point to indicate that the information is consistent with the assessment, and zero points if there is no information, no benefit, or possible harm for the assessment. By adding up the points of each of the five assessments, a 0-to-10 score (with 10 being best) is determined. If the total is five or greater, we feel a rationally based, evidence-appropriate indication exists for using the treatment. When using this guide, crush injury scores 7 points and SMCS scores 5.5 points, thereby qualifying each as a rationally based, evidence-appropriate indication for using HBO_2 (Table 7).

Since indications for HBO_2 were first formulated by the Undersea and Hyperbaric Medical Society (UHMS), crush injury, SMCS, and other acute traumatic ischemias have been included in the *Hyperbaric Oxygen Therapy Committee Report* as approved indications.[22,30] The U.S. Food and Drug Administration (FDA) uses the *UHMS HBO Committee Report* as a primary source document when inquiries are made regarding the use of HBO_2 therapy. Reimbursement for the use of HBO_2 as an adjunct in the management of acute traumatic peripheral ischemia and crush injuries

TABLE 7. USE OF RATIONALLY BASED INDICATIONS* TO JUSTIFY HBO_2 FOR CRUSH INJURY AND COMPARTMENT SYNDROME

Assessment Score each from 0 to 2 points	Overwhelming Evidence 2 Points	Information is consistent with the assessment 1 Point	No information, no benefit, or possible harm 0 Points
Clinical experiences Observations, case reports		Crush: 1; Compartment: 1	
Mechanisms Supported by laboratory studies	Crush: 2; Compartment: 2		
Literature/outcomes Prospective, retrospective studies		Crush: 1; Compartment: 1	
No other Rxs available After surgical & medical interventions	Crush: 1 1/2	Compartment: 1 1/2	
RCTs; Head-to-head studies	Crush: 1 1/2		Compartment: 0

Crush Injury = 7 Points

Compartment Syndrome = 5 ½ Points

***Note:** 5 points or greater qualifies the intervention as rationally based; **Rxs** = treatments

is authorized by the Department of Health and Human Services (DHHS), Centers for Medicare and Medicaid Services (CMS), and is covered by most third-party insurance carriers.[50] As in all other medical and surgical conditions, appropriate ICD-10-CM (International Classification of Disease, Clinical Modification 10) codes must be used with appropriate documentation to receive reimbursements.

SUMMARY

Hyperbaric oxygen therapy as an adjunct in the management of crush injury, skeletal muscle-compartment syndrome, and other traumatic ischemias has the scientific basis, outcome expectations, and reimbursement justifications for its use. The expectation is that as clinicians become better informed about the use of HBO_2, demands for better outcomes increase, and the availability of HBO_2 treatment facilities expand, this mechanism-sound, under utilized therapy will assume its appropriate role in these conditions.

REFERENCES

1. Barthelemy L, Bellet L, Michaud A, Carbon P. The value of thermography in the appreciation of the effectiveness of hyperbaric oxygen therapy in treatment of acute arteritis of the lower limbs. Bordeux Med. 1976;9:1095-1100.
2. Bartlett RL, Stroman RT, Nickels M, Kalns JE, et al. Rabbit model of the use of fasciotomy and hyperbaric oxygenation in the treatment of compartment syndrome. Undersea Hyperb Med. 1998 Supplement;25:29, #77.
3. Bassett BE, Bennett PB. Introduction to the physical and physiological bases of hyperbaric therapy. In: Davis JC, Hunt TK, editors. Hyperbaric oxygen therapy. Bethesda (MD): Undersea Medical Society Inc.; 1977. p. 11-24.
4. Bird AD, Telfer ABM. Effect of hyperbaric oxygen on limb circulation. Lancet. 1965;1:355-6.
5. Boerema I, Meijne NG, Brummelkamp WK, et al. Life without blood. A study of the influence of high atmospheric pressure and hypothermia on dilution of the blood. J Cardiovasc Surg. 1960;1:133-6.
6. Bouachour G, Cronier P, Gouello JP, et al. Hyperbaric oxygen therapy in the management of crush injuries: a randomized double-blind placebo-controlled clinical trial. J Trauma. 1996;41:333-9.
7. Brighton CT. Quoted in Hospital Tribune. 1988 May 9;4.
8. Buncke HJ, Alpert BS, Johnson-Giebink R. Digital replantation. Surg Clin N Am. 1981;61:383-94.
9. Burt JG, Kapp JP, Smith RR. Effects of HBO on infarcts in gerbils. Surg Neurol. 1987;28:265-8.
10. Caudle RJ, Stern PJ. Severe open fractures of the tibia. J Bone Joint Surg. 1987;69(Am):801-7.
11. Christensen O. Mediation of cell volume regulation by Ca++ influx through stretch-activated channels. Nature. 1987;330:66-8.
12. Davidkin NF. Experience with clinical use of hyperbaric oxygenation in traumas and their compilations. Ortop Travmatol Protez. 1977;9:33-5.
13. Ferrari R, Ceconi C, Curello S, et al. Oxygen-mediated damage during ischaemia and reperfusion: role of the cellular defences against oxygen toxicity. J Mol Cell Cardiol. 1985;17:937-41.
14. Fitzpatrick DT, Murphy PT, Bruce M. Adjunctive treatment of compartment syndrome with hyperbaric oxygen. Mil Med. 1998;163(8):577-9.
15. Garcia-Covarrubias I, McSwain NE, Van Meter K, et al. Adjuvant hyperbaric oxygen therapy in the management of crush injury and traumatic ischemia: an evidence-based approach. Am Surg. 2005;71:141-51.
16. Gismondi AG, Micalella F, Colonna SS. Possible use of hyperbaric oxygen in the treatment of certain vascular disease. Ann Med Nav. 1978;83:547-58.
17. Grief R, Akea, et al. Supplemental perioperative oxygen to reduce incidence of surgical-wound infection. N Engl J Med. 2000;342(3):61-7.
18. Gustilo R. Management of open fractures and their complications. Philadelphia: WB Saunders; 1982. p. 202-8.
19. Gustilo RB, Mendoza RM, Williams DN. Problems in the management of type III (severe) open fractures: a new classification of type III open fractures. J Trauma. 1984;24:742.
20. Gustilo RB, Williams DN. The use of antibiotics in the management of open fractures. Orthopaedics. 1984;7:1617-9.

21. Hazinski ME, Cummins RD, editors. Handbook of emergency cardiovascular care for health care providers. American Heart Association; 1999. p. 3.
22. Hart BB. Refractory osteomyelitis. In: Weaver LK, editor. Hyperbaric oxygen therapy indications. 13th ed. North Palm Beach (FL): Best Publishing Co.; 2014. p. 179-207.
23. Heckman MM, Whitesides TE Jr, Grewe SR, et al. Histologic determination of ischemic threshold of muscle in the canine compartment syndrome model. J Orthop Trauma. 1993;7:199-210.
24. Hohn DC. Oxygen and leukocyte microbial killing. In: Davis JC, Hunt TK, editors. Hyperbaric oxygen therapy. Bethesda (MD): Undersea Medical Society Inc.; 1977. p. 101-10.
25. Howe CW. Experimental studies on determinants of wound infection. Surg Gynecol Obstet. 1966;123:507-14.
26. Hunt TK, Linsey M, Grislis G, et al. The effect of differing ambient oxygen tensions on wound infection. Ann Surg. 1975;181:35-9.
27. Hunt TK, Pai MP. The effect of varying ambient oxygen tensions on wound metabolism and collagen synthesis. Surg Gynecol Obstet. 1972;135:561-7.
28. Hunt TK, Zederfeldt, Goldstick TK. Oxygen and healing. Am J Surg. 1969;118:521-5.
29. Hurd TC, Dasmhapatra KB, Rush BF, Machiedo GW. Red blood cell deformability in human and experimental sepsis. Arch Surg. 1988;123:217-20.
30. Hyperbaric Oxygen Therapy Committee. Kindwall EP, editor. Hyperbaric Oxygen Therapy Committee report. Bethesda (MD): Undersea Medical Society; 1977.
31. Hunt TK, Davis JC, editors. Hyperbaric oxygen therapy. Bethesda (MD): Undersea and Hyperbaric Medical Society; 1977.
32. Illingworth CFW, Smith G, Lawson DD, et al. Surgical and physiological observations in an experimental pressure chamber. Br J Surg. 1961;49:222-7.
33. Isakov YV, Atroschenko ZB, Bailik IF, et al. Hyperbaric oxygenation in the prophylaxis of wound infection in the open trauma of the locomotor system. Bestn Khir. 1979;123:117-21.
34. Johansen K, Daines M, Howey T, Helfet D, et al. Objective criteria accurately predict amputation following lower extremity trauma. J Trauma. 1990;30:568-73.
35. Kiyoshige Y. Effect of hyperbaric oxygen therapy as a monitoring technique for digital replantation survival. J Reconstr Microsurg. 1999;15:327-30.
36. Kiyoshige Y, Tsuchida H, Watanabe Y. Color monitoring after replantations. Plast Reconstr Surg. 1996;97:463-8.
37. Loder RE. Hyperbaric oxygen therapy in acute trauma. Ann R Coll Surg Engl. 1979;(3):39-43.
38. Lukich VL, Filimonova MV, Bazarova VS. Changes of the gaseous exchange in hyperbaric oxygenation in patients with regional ischemia. Vrach Delo. 1979;(3):39-43.
39. Lukich VL, Filimonova MV, Fokina TS, et al. Employment of hyperbaric oxygenation in out-patients. Khirurgiia. 1976;(2):82-6.
40. MacKenzie EJ, Bosse, Pollak AN, et al. Long term persistence of disability following severe lower-limb trauma. Results of a seven-year follow-up. J Bone Joint Surg. 2005;87(A):1801-9.
41. Mackey W, McCullough JL, Conlon TP, et al. The costs of surgery for limb-threatening ischemia. Surgery. 1986;99:26-35.
42. Malinoski DJ, Slater MS, Mullins RJ. Crush injury and rhabdomyolysis. Crit Care Clin. 2004;20:171-92.

43. Matava MF, Whitesides TE Jr, Seiler JG 3rd, Hutton WC. Determination of the compartment threshold pressure of muscle ischemia in the canine model. Orthop Trans. 1993-1994;17(3):667-8.

44. Mathieu D, Goget J, Vinkier L, et al. Red blood cell deformability and hyperbaric oxygen therapy [abstract]. HBO Review. 1985;6-280.

45. Matos LA, Hutson JJ, Bonet H, et al. HBO as an adjunct treatment for limb salvage in crush injuries of the extremities. Undersea Hyperb Med. 1999;26(Suppl):66-7.

46. Matsen FA, Mayo RA, Sheridan GW, Krugmire RB. Monitoring of intramuscular pressure. Surgery. 1976;79:702-9.

47. Matsen FA 3rd, Winquist RA, Krugmire RB Jr. Diagnosis and management of compartment syndrome. J Bone Joint Surg. 1980;62(A):286-91.

48. Maudsley RH, Hopkinson WI, Williams KG. Vascular injury treated with high-pressure oxygen in a mobile chamber. J Bone Joint Surg. 1963;2(B):346-50.

49. McCord JM. Oxygen-derived free radicals in postischemic tissue injury. N Engl J Med. 1985;312:159-63.

50. Medicare Coverage Issues Manual. U.S. Department of Health and Human Services (DHHS), Centers for Medicare and Medicaid Services (CMS). Medicare Coverage Issues Manual. U.S. Department of Health and Human Services (DHHS), Centers for Medicare and Medicaid Services (CMS); CIM 35 2002 Dec 10. Rev. 48 Issued 2006 Mar 17.

51. Meijne NG. Hyperbaric oxygen and its clinical value, with special emphasis on biochemical and cardiovascular aspects. Springfield (IL): Charles C. Thomas; 1970.

52. Monies-Chass I, Hashmonai M, Hoerer D, et al. Hyperbaric oxygen treatment as an adjuvant to reconstructive vascular surgery in trauma. Injury. 1977;8:274-7.

53. Mubarak SJ, Hargens AR. Acute compartment syndromes. Surg Clin North Am. 1983;63:539-65.

54. Mubarak SJ, Owen CA, Hargens AR, Garetto LP, et al. Acute compartment syndromes: diagnosis and treatment with the aid of the wick catheter. J Bone Joint Surg. 1978;60A:1091-5.

55. Nemiroff PM. Synergistic effects of pentoxifylline and hyperbaric oxygen on skin flaps. Arch Otolaryngol Head Neck Surg. 1988;114:977-81.

56. No known authors. Hyperbaric oxygen therapy in replantation of severed limbs. A report of 21 cases. Chin Med J. 1975;1:197-204.

57. Nylander G, Lewis D, Nordstom H, et al. Reduction of post-ischemic edema with hyperbaric oxygen. Plast Reconstr Surg. 1985;76:596-601.

58. Nylander G, Nordstr H, Franzen L, et al. Effects of hyperbaric oxygen in post-ischemic muscle. Scand J Plast Reconstr Surg. 1988;22:31-9.

59. Nylander G, Otamiri DH, Larsson J. Lipid products in post-ischemic skeletal muscle and after treatment with hyperbaric oxygen. Scand J Plast Reconstr Surg. 1989;23:97-103.

60. Oriani G. Acute indications of HBO therapy – final report. G Oriani et al., editors. Handbook of hyperbaric medicine. Springer (NY): 1996. p. 93-103.

61. Peirce EC Jr. Pathophysiology, apparatus, and methods, including the special techniques of hypothermia and hyperbaric oxygen. Extracorporeal circulation for open-heart surgery. Springfield (IL): Charles C. Thomas; 1969. p. 84-8.

62. Perrins DJ. The effect of hyperbaric oxygen on skin flaps. In: Grabb WC, Myers MB, editors. Skin flaps. Boston: Little, Brown and Co.; 1975. p. 53-63.

63. Powell RJ, Machiedo GW, Rush BF. Decreased red blood cell deformability and impaired oxygen utilization during human sepsis. Am Surg. 1993;59:65-8.

64. Radonic V, Baric D, Petricevic A, et al. War injuries of the cural arteries. Br J Surg. 1995;82:777-83.

65. Renstra WR, Buras JA, Svoboda KS. Hyperbaric oxygen increases human dermal fibroblast proliferation, growth factor receptor number and in vitro wound closure. Undersea Hyperb Med. 1998;25(Suppl):53.

66. Schraibman IG, Ledingham IM. Hyperbaric oxygen and local vasodilation in peripheral vascular disease. Br J Surg. 1969;56:295-9.

67. Schramek A, Hashmonai M. Vascular injuries in the extremities in battle casualties. Br J Surg. 1977;64:644-8.

68. Shandling AH, Ellestad MH, Hart GB, et al. Hyperbaric oxygen and thrombolysis in myocardial infarction: the "Hot MI" pilot study. Am Heart J. 1997;134:544-50.

69. Shupak A, Gozal D, Ariel A, et al. Hyperbaric oxygenation in acute peripheral posttraumatic ischemia. J Hyperbaric Med. 1987;2:7-14.

70. Skolnilek AA. Early data suggest clot-dissolving drug may help save frostbitten limbs from amputation. JAMA. 1992;267(15):2008-10.

71. Skurikhina LA. Treatment under altered barometric pressure (barotherapy, vacuum therapy, hyperbaric oxygenation). Vorp Kurortol Fizioter Lech Kult. 1976;3:83-9.

72. Skyhar MJ, Hargens AR, Strauss MB, et al. Hyperbaric oxygen reduces edema and necrosis of skeletal muscle in compartment syndromes associated with hemorrhagic hypotension. J Bone Joint Surg. 1986;68A:1218-24.

73. Slack MD, Thomas DA, DeJode. Hyperbaric oxygen in the treatment of trauma, ischemic disease of limb, and varicose ulceration. In: Brown IW, Cox BG, editors. Proc of the 3rd Int's Conf on Hyperbaric Med. Washington (DC): National Academy of Science, National Research Council, Publish 1404; 1966. p. 621-4.

74. Smith G, Stevens J, Griffiths JC, et al. Near-avulsion of foot treated by replacement and subsequent prolonged exposure of patients to oxygen at two atmospheres pressure. Lancet. 1961;2:1122-3.

75. Strauss MB. Crush injury, compartment syndrome and other acute traumatic peripheral ischemias. In: Kindwall E, Whelan H, editors. Hyperbaric medicine practice. 2nd ed. Flagstaff (AZ): Best Publishing Co.; 1999. p. 753-71.

76. Strauss MB. Diabetic foot and leg wounds. Principles, management and prevention. Primary Care Reports. 2001;7(22):187-97.

77. Strauss MB. Evidence review of HBO for crush injury, compartment syndrome and other traumatic ischemia. Undersea Hyperb Med. 2001;28(Suppl):35-6.

78. Strauss MB, Hargens AR, Gershuni DH, et al. Delayed use of hyperbaric oxygen for treatment of a model anterior compartment syndrome. J Orthop Res. 1986;4:108-11.

79. Strauss MB, Hargens AR, Gershuni DH, et al. Reduction of skeletal muscle necrosis using intermittent hyperbaric oxygen in a model compartment syndrome. J Bone Joint Surg. 1983;65A:656-62.

80. Strauss MB, Hart GB. Cost-effective issues in hyperbaric oxygen therapy: complicated fractures. J Hyperbaric Med. 1988;3:199-205.

81. Strauss MB, Hart GB. Crush injury and the role of hyperbaric oxygen. Top Emerg Med. 1984;6:9-24.

82. Strauss MB, Hart GB. Hyperbaric oxygen and the skeletal muscle-compartment syndrome. Contemp Orthop. 1989;18:167-74.

83. Strauss MB. Hyperbaric oxygen for crush injuries and compartment syndromes: surgical considerations. In: Bakker DJ, Cramer FS, editors. Hyperbaric surgery perioperative care. Flagstaff (AZ): Best Publishing Co.; 2002. p. 341-59.

84. Strauss MB. Role of hyperbaric oxygen therapy in acute ischemia and crush injuries – an orthopedic perspective. HBO Review. 1981;2:87-108.

85. Szekely O, Szanto G, Takats A. Hyperbaric oxygen therapy in injured subjects. Injury. 1973;4:294-300.

86. Textbook of medical physiology. Unit IV, The circulation. Hall JE, editor. Textbook of medical physiology. 13th ed. Unit IV, The circulation. Philadelphia: WB Saunders; 2016.

87. Thom SR. Antagonism of CO-mediated brain lipid peroxidation by hyperbaric oxygen. Toxicol Appl Pharmacol. 1990;105:340-4.

88. Thom SR. Functional inhibition of neutrophil B2 integrins by hyperbaric oxygen in carbon monoxide-mediated brain injury. Toxicol Appl Pharmacol. 1993;123:248-56.

89. Thom SR, Strauss BM. Frostbite: pathophysiology, treatment and role of hyperbaric oxygen. HBO Review. 1985;6:99-113.

90. Thomas MP, Brown LA, Sponseller DR, et al. Myocardial infarct size reduction by synergistic effect of hyperbaric oxygen and recombinant tissue plasminogen activator. Am Heart J. 1991;120:791-800.

91. Tran DT, Miller SH, Buck D, et al. Potentiation of infection by epinephrine. Plast Reconstr Surg. 1985;76:933-4.

92. Tscheme H, Ostern HJ. A new classification of soft-tissue damage in open and closed fractures. Unfallheikunde. 1982;85(3):111-5.

93. Vedder NB, Fouty BW, Winn RK, et al. Role of neutrophils in generalized reperfusion injury associated with resuscitation from shock. Surgery. 1989;106:509-16.

94. Whitesides TE Jr, Haney TC, Morimoto K, Harada H. Tissue pressure measurements as a determinant for the need of fasciotomy. Clin Orthop Rel Res. 1975;113:43-51.

95. Zamboni WA, Roth AC, Russell RC, et al. Morphological analysis of the microcirculation during reperfusion of ischemic skeletal muscle and the effect of hyperbaric oxygen. Plas Reconstr Surg. 1993;91:1110-23.

96. Zamboni WA, Roth AC, Russell RC, et al. The effect of acute hyperbaric oxygen therapy on axial pattern skin flap survival when administered during and after total ischemia. J Reconstr Microsurg. 1989;5:343-7.

CHAPTER 27 CHAPTER

Hyperbaric Oxygen Use in Exceptional Blood Loss Anemia

CHAPTER TWENTY-SEVEN OVERVIEW

Introduction 693
Indications for HBO_2 696
Treatment Routine 697
Treatment Protocol 697
Case Reports 698
Case 1 698
Case 2 698
Costs of Hyperbaric Oxygen 702
Conclusion 702
References 703

Hyperbaric Oxygen Use in Exceptional Blood Loss Anemia

Keith W. Van Meter

INTRODUCTION

Exceptional blood loss anemia in one sense means a severe loss of red blood cells (RBCs) by quantity. This may be through exsanguination, hemolysis, or faulty production. It also may mean the severe loss of oxygen-carrying capacity of RBCs occurs by dysfunctional hemoglobin (Hgb). This loss can happen by Hgb disablement for oxygen transport by toxins (see Chapter 12: Carbon Monoxide).

Hyperbaric oxygen (HBO_2) offers a way to clinically address life support when transfusion of RBCs would not be possible or practical. HBO_2 also provides a solution in instances when RBC transfusion would be contraindicated by religious belief. HBO_2 has offered to all of these clinical transfusion predicaments a short-term therapeutic bridge with little adverse side effect.[18]

In contradistinction, other bridging attempts to address the unavailability or undesirability of RBC transfusion have been multiple. To date, intravascular infusion of stroma-free hemoglobin by hemoglobin polymers,[26,30] fluorocarbons,[8-10,24,27] or lipid oxygen-containing microparticles (LOMs)[20] have resulted in adverse side effects. Erythropoietin, other hematenic drugs, or replacement factors are helpful but too slowly acting for addressing acute hemorrhagic shock. Further, RBC transfusion is not without risk of transmission of infection. Likewise, RBC transfusion has risk of incompatibility or undesirable immunomodulation.[44]

HBO_2 has a respectable track record of patient safety, with a low incidence of adverse side effects, and is a cost-effective, low-technology solution to provide the short-term need to fill a specific clinical gap in the management of exceptional blood loss anemia.[40] To this point, HBO_2 stems the gap in the instance when transfused RBCs cannot be possible by way of immediate availability or by the clinical situation that the patient can ill afford to wait the time to regenerate a sustainable red blood cell mass on his or her own.

At 1 atmosphere, the fraction of inhaled oxygen of 100% (FiO_2 100%) is not enough to support life or health in patients with sudden, severe drops in Hgb by RBC depletion or by Hgb dysfunction. At 1 atmosphere, an FiO_2 100% can provide only 2.3 volumes percent of dissolved oxygen in plasma.

However, most organs in the body require an extraction of 6.6 volumes percent or more of oxygen for maintaining baseline physiologic function. Not enough oxygen can be supplied to tissue at 1 atmosphere of ambient pressure in the absence of RBCs.[41]

At 3 atmospheres of pressurization afforded by HBO_2, a pure-oxygen breathing mix can provide 6.6 volumes percent of dissolved oxygen in plasma. This, in the short term, is enough to provide a bridge for "Life Without Blood" as so well demonstrated by Ite Boerema in the late 1950s.[7] He reported a series of experiments with swine in which the animals could be exsanguinated to very low Hgb levels and could be kept alive by ventilating them with oxygen at 3 atmospheres of pressure in a HBO_2 chamber, with merely intravascular volume replacement by a D5 Ringer's dextran 40 solution. When he took the animals off oxygen but continued their ventilation in the chamber with ambient compressed air still at 3 atmospheres, the ST segments elevated by continuous electrocardiographic monitoring. When he replaced the animals on oxygen at 3 atmospheres in the chamber, the ST segments normalized. He then retransfused the animals with their shed blood before decompressing the chamber back to 1 atmosphere, and the animals walked away without impairment.

We have repeated the exact experiment with swine in our laboratory and have arrived at the same results. More specifically, we have monitored the brain tissue oxygen tension through a cranial burr hole by introduction of a polarographic oxygen-sensing electrode. We have found that an American Surgical Society (ACS) class IV hemorrhage leaves the animal with a brain tissue oxygen tension which is unmeasurable when the animal is resuscitated at 1 atmosphere pressure by FiO_2 100% ventilation with 3:1 intravenous Ringer's lactate to shed-blood intravenous-fluid loading. When the same intervention is done with oxygen ventilation at 3 atmospheres, producing a surface equivalent fraction inhalation of 300% ($SEFiO_2$), the animal developed a brain tissue oxygen tension of 30 mmHg. These animals, when retransfused with shed blood before surfacing of the HBO_2 chamber, walked off post dive with long-term survival (Figure 1, Figure 2).[43]

After the work of Boerema, others in controlled animal trials demonstrated improved survival rates by use of HBO_2 over use of normobaric oxygen (NBO) in

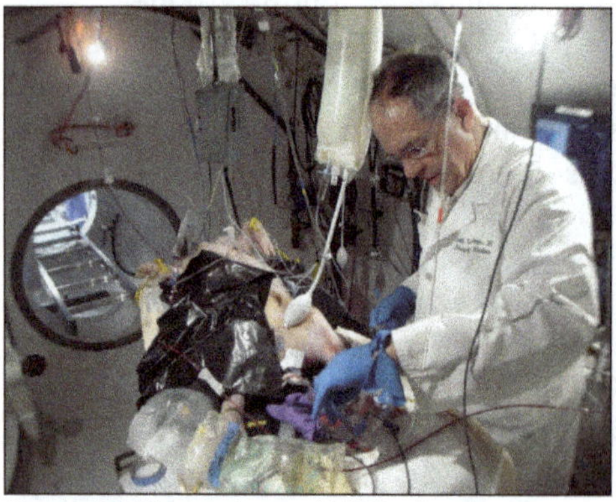

Figure 1. BRI experimental HBO_2 chamber in New Orleans hosting a porcine ACS Class IV exsanguination resuscitation project.

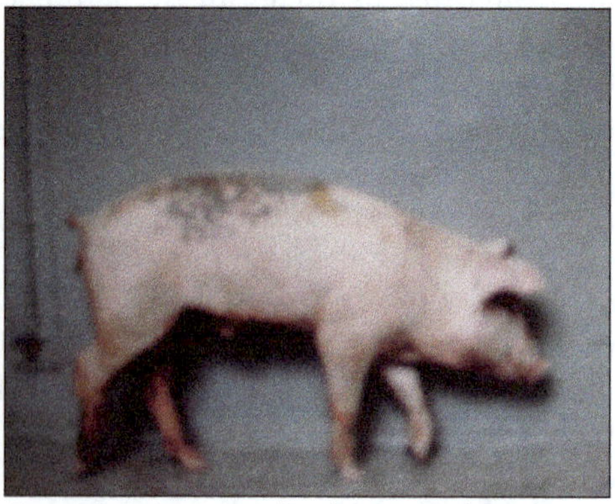

Figure 2. Swine immediately post bridging by a HBO_2 chamber treatment after an ACS Class IV exsanguination with a transfusion of shed blood before returning to 1 atmosphere of pressure.

animals experimentally insulted with hemorrhagic shock.(4) These animal studies have been independently replicated, likewise demonstrating improved survival with use of HBO_2 over that of control animals with use of NBO.(1,6,13,22,28-29,45)

Successful human application of HBO_2 in exceptional blood loss anemia was first reported by Amonic on a patient in chronic hemorrhagic shock.(3) Limited experience on application of HBO_2 in severe hemorrhagic shock in humans followed and was reported in the medical literature.(16) Hart reported on a group of 26 patients treated with HBO_2 to address exceptional blood loss anemia. Remarkably in this case series report, there was a 70% survival in these patients who uniformly had ACS Class IV hemorrhage(11) (or a loss of 40% or more of circulating blood volume) without RBC replacement. If one were to discard those who arrived late, namely patients without cerebral function, there was a mortality rate of one out of nineteen patients or of 5%. Notably, in this case series one patient was treated in a U.S. Navy installation deck decompression chamber where Hart was able to keep a Jehovah's Witness patient with a severe, life-threatening blood loss alive for several days without transfusion of RBCs until the patient, with the aid of administered hematenics, regenerated a RBC count high enough to sustain the patient's life. Isolated reports continue to herald the success of using HBO_2 early and repetitively in similar cases.(25,33)

To explain these encouraging results, subsequent research in controlled animal studies indicate that in exceptional blood loss anemia, HBO_2 protects the synthesis of RNA and DNA.(39) In separate controlled animal research, HBO_2 exerted stimulus for erthropoiesis by causing an increase in circulating erythropoietin.(5) Further, in yet a different controlled animal study, HBO_2 lessened the accumulation of anaerobic by-products in the brains of animals in which hemorrhagic shock was produced.(23)

Acute blood loss anemia imposes an element of a smoldering reperfusion injury in subjects so afflicted. More fundamentally, HBO_2 over and above NBO confers the following therapeutic advantage at ameliorating reperfusion injury:

1. Induction of expression of at least 8,101 genes, half of which oversee reparative function and half of which oversee anti-inflammatory function(14)
2. Lessens impact of intravascular microparticles after ischemic insult(37)
3. Lessens leukocyte-endothelial adherence in reperfusion injury(36)
4. Truncates membrane lipid peroxidation in reperfusion of ischemic tissue(35)
5. Improves leukocyte microbial killing (for both aerobic and anaerobic microbes)(21)
6. Expunges adult modulary stem cells into the central circulation(34)
7. Lessens netosis as an inflammatory event of PMNs in shock states.(14A)

Even more fundamentally, HBO_2 used in resuscitation may confer a way to impart, in extreme ischemic insult imposed by severe blood loss, the necessary 1 mmHg tissue oxygen tension to the mitochondrial intramembrane space to allow the respiratory complexes I–IV and ATP synthase (respiratory complex V) to resupply ATP in quantity enough to sustain salvage and recovery of patients (Figure 3).(42)

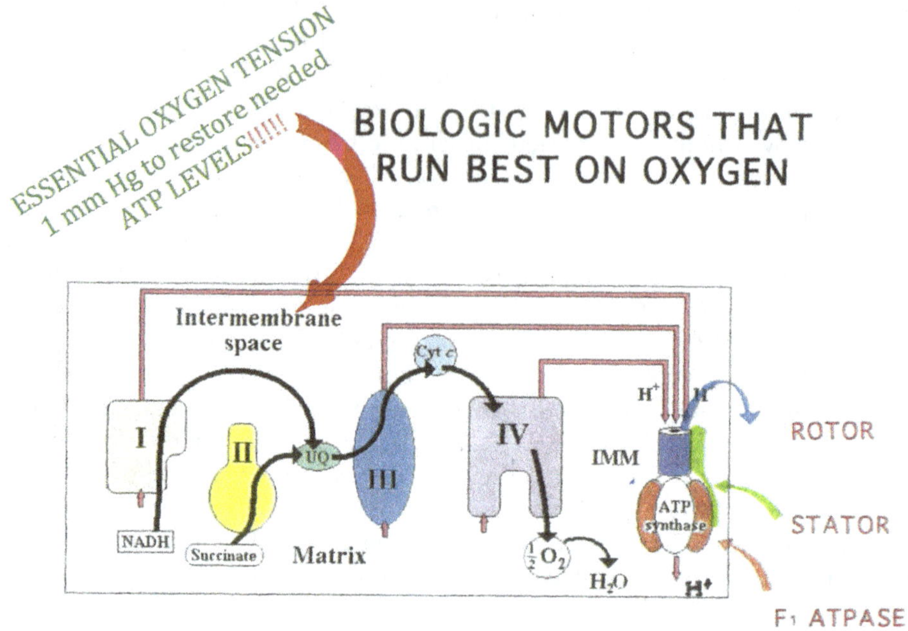

Figure 3. The ETS (respiratory complexes I–IV) fill the intermitochondrial space with H+ to drive the respiratory complex IV (ATP synthase) to churn out ATP. This ETS function is powered by the docking of molecular oxygen on cytochrome aa3 (complex IV) where, in effect, the paramagnetic oxygen atoms draw electrons down the ETC to place H+ in the intramitochondrial membrane space.

INDICATIONS FOR HBO_2

1. HBO_2 may be used for post Class IV Hemorrhage, when the patient cannot accept blood replacement for medical or religious reasons. The following indications dictate the repetitive use of HBO_2:
   a. Shock, systolic blood pressures below 90 mmHg, or vasopressors required to maintain pressures
   b. Disorientation to coma
   c. Ischemic changes of the myocardium as demonstrated on the ECG
   d. Ischemic gut as demonstrated by a sprue-like diarrhea
2. Increased oxygen debt
   a. LD50 oxygen debt in dogs = 113.5 ml/Kg, 12.9 mmol for lactate and -18.8 mmol for base excess (BE)[12]
   b. Oxygen consumption (VO2) – a VO2 deficit of greater than 9.2 L/m2 will result in patient surviving, but with organ death, and, if the deficit attains 33.2 L/m2, all succumb[31]
3. Moderate blood loss

Using HBO_2 for less amount of blood loss to void blood transfusions: HBO_2 accelerates hemoglobin synthesis in an animal model of moderate (30%) blood loss.[45] This is an important observation surgically as in a mass casualty situation where stored blood is unavailable, patients may be supported by using HBO_2!

TREATMENT ROUTINE

1. Replacement of blood volume with crystalloids/plasma expanders for hemorrhage, as recommended by the ACS Committee on Trauma.[11]
2. Medical support for the severe anemia: hematenics, antibiotics, and cardiotonics as needed.
3. HBO_2 to be administered immediately and repetitively. The HBO_2 is repeated as needed, at pressures which are appropriate to relieve the relative hypoxia, and discontinued when the hematocrit and hemoglobin rises to levels which alleviate the preceding symptoms and signs. This (as a rule of thumb) appears to occur at a hematocrit of 22.9% and at a hemoglobin of 7.7 gm% (approximate), based on current experience.

TREATMENT PROTOCOL

1. Multiplace treatment
   a. The first HBO_2 treatment is at 2 to 3 ATA, breathing 100% oxygen, the pressure chosen according to physiological response. Blood pressure should be elevated from shock levels, the pulse rate flowed, while the sensorium clears. In serious cases, we generally proceed to 3 ATA for the first thirty minutes, and then reduce the pressure to 2.5 ATA for an additional hour. We then give an air break on the surface for one hour and re-treat for an hour at 2.5 ATA, if tolerated.

      With improvement over baseline, the duration of the air break is lengthened, and oxygen pressures are reduced with each one-hour HBO_2 exposure. When the air breaks reach two hours, the patient may be removed from the chamber facility for diagnostic or other treatment impossible to perform at pressure. The exposures to HBO_2 remain at one hour per exposure; the pressures are decreased as the patient becomes able to tolerate the ambient air environment. Between HBO_2 treatments, oxygenation may be assisted by oxygen mask or nasal cannula. (Note: Pulmonary oxygen toxicity is avoided by intermittent exposures to air.)

   b. Use volume replacement with Ringer's lactate and the early administration of intravenous hyperalimentation. (Note: We avoid the use of lipids for intravenous hyperalimentation due to the possibility of accelerating pulmonary oxygen toxicity, as demonstrated by Alam and Alam, Hageman and Huna, and Kehrer and Autor.)[2,15,19]
   c. Antibiotics, analgesics and other interventions are prescribed as indicated.
2. Monoplace treatment

Treatment is the same as with the multiplace protocol, with air breaks being given, if an appropriate air supply is available; if not, the patient is removed from the chamber for the ambient-air breaks.

CASE REPORTS

Case 1[(17)]

A previously healthy, twenty-year-old female (110 pounds and 61 inches in height) Jehovah's Witness was brought to Long Beach Memorial Medical Center as a victim of a drive-by shooting in May 1991. She sustained a single penetrating gunshot wound (GSW) to the left chest. The preoperative hematocrit was 24%. She refused any blood transfusions due to her religious convictions.

Operative exploration revealed penetration of the left lung, left hemidiaphragm, spleen, left kidney, and spinal cord. Volume replacement was accomplished with hetastarch solutions and Ringer's solutions.

Postoperatively, the patient was conscious with a complete paraplegia at the level of thoracic cord at T6–T7. Specifically, she had no lower extremity voluntary movement and no response to touch or pain in the lower extremities, and she was areflexic in the lower extremities. Oncotic pressure and blood pressure were maintained with crystalloids and hetastarch. High-dose steroids were given for acute spinal cord injury. The postoperative hematocrit was 18%, and she was started on HBO_2, receiving treatments of 2 ATA for periods of 90 minutes three times a day. The erythropoietin (IPO) levels on the first and second postoperative day were 5.3 and 10.3 MU/ML (normal range is 2.0–19.0 MU/ML).

The EPO level was 86.5 MU/ML on the eighth postoperative day, and EPO 8000 units (8 KU) was started as a daily administration by subcutaneous injection. Nine days following the operation, she had onset of high fever and became confused. Over a two-day period, it was established that she had perforation of an intestine. She was returned to the operating room, and the perforation was repaired on the eleventh day following admission. Following the operation, the erythropoietin was increased to 10 KU and administered intravenously as the reticulocyte count had fallen to 2.7% following repair of the perforation. This dosage was continued for a period of 11 days. HBO_2 was continued postoperatively on an approximately twice-a-day schedule and was discontinued on the 28th day. Iron dextran was given as calculated every other day for ten more days. See Table 1 and Table 2 for a display of the reticulocyte count compared with that of the hematocrit. Exogenous erythropoietin was started on the eighth hospital day, as the patient's endogenous erythropoietin was elevated to only 86.5 MU/ML. Despite the elevated EPO and the administered EPO, there was a remarkable depression of the bone marrow function coinciding with the perforated viscous and the resulting septicemia. It is difficult to assess the value of EPO in this patient due to the administration of the corticosteroids and the septic event; however, it was not the response that was measured in healthy men where a maximum reticulocyte count occurred on the third to fourth day after EPO. She received a total of 138 hours of HBO_2 over 28 days to support the relative ischemia. It was stopped when the hematocrit had climbed to 22%.

The patient remains a complete paraplegic. She has otherwise been rehabilitated to the fullest of her neurologic capabilities.

Case 2 (Reprinted with permission) [(18A)]

Shortly after Hurricane Katrina struck in 2005, a 42-year-old, male commercial diver working in the Gulf of Mexico had a long history of intermittent, gnawing epigastric discomfort. The discomfort sometimes awoke him at night and would not relieve with ingestion of food. He was working in a 300 fsw heliox saturation

TABLE 1. CHARACTERISTICS OF MAJOR OXYGEN THERAPEUTICS

CHARACTERISTIC	BANKED BLOOD	HBOC*	PFC	ALLOSTERICS	HBO
Shelf life	42 days	3 years	2 years	Years	Unlimited
Storage Temp	Refrigeration	Room Temp	Refrigeration	Room Temp	Room Temp
Size	7 micron	0.007 micron	0.2 micron	NA	NA
Cross-matching	Required	Not Required	Not Required	Not Required	Not Required
Risks	Disease transmission, Immune depression, Transfusion reactions, RBC Storage Defects	NO scavenging	Mild decrease in platelet count	None apparent	Oxygen toxicity

*Hemoglobin-Based Oxygen Carrier
**NA Not Applicable

TABLE 2. STATUS OF MAJOR OXYGEN THERAPEUTICS

COMPANY	PRODUCT	TYPE	STATUS
Northfield	Polyheme®	Human	Phase III Elective Surgery / Trauma Resuscitation
Biopure	Hemopure®	Bovine	Phase III:* Approved in S. Africa Elective Surgery
Hemosol	Hemolink®	Human	Phase III Elective Surgery
Alliance	Perflubron (Oxygen)	Perflurocarbon	Phase III Elective Surgery
Allos	RSR 13	Allosteric Modulator	Phase II
NA	Oxygen	Hyperbaric	Approved

*FDA Application filed October 2004. Approved for clinical use in South Africa granted 2001.

chamber system storage depth aboard a diving vessel. He made downward 60 fsw excursions from the storage depth by way of transfer to the Gulf floor by personal transfer chamber (PTC). On one excursion to the floor of the Gulf, he vomited coffee ground emesis, had a melanotic accidental loose stool, and became unconscious. He was fetched by the PTC bellman, who helmeted and dragged him back to the PTC. The PTC was brought to the surface and mated with the saturation deck storage chamber system. He was pushed into the saturation deck chamber and placed in lateral decubitus position on the deck (Figure 4). He was breathing shallowly at a rate of 40 breaths per minute. He was cold, diaphoretic, unconscious, and extremely pale. A diver medic locked-in to place a peripheral intravenous line but was unsuccessful in 32 separate attempts. Interosseous access catheters were not available. Placement of a BIBS mask for enriched oxygen-helium breathing (SEFiO_2 of 300%) improved the diver's initial Glasgow Coma Scale (GCS) score of 3 to a GCS of 10 (eye = 2, verbal = 2, motor = 4). The patient would not comply with ingestion of oral fluids. Slow decompression to surface over three days was started (Figure 5). The medic was instructed to use hypodermoclysis for parenteral administration of crystalloid fluids. Three liters of normal saline was slowly infused in several subdermal intravenous lines attached to subdermal needles placed in his extremities. The chamber SEFiO_2 was kept at 40%, and the mask SEFiO_2 was kept at 250%. His fellow divers noted that his iatrogenically edematous extremities made him look like a Michelin man. He became alert with total return of consciousness (GCS 15) and climbed into an upper bunk under his own power. Without the benefit of a packed red blood cell (PRBC) transfusion, he remained at a GCS of 15 over the three-day decompression to surface. Attempts at getting blood for type and crossmatch as well as for transfusion were unsuccessful. The blood hemolyzed badly on descent and ascent from the heliox storage depths at which the divers resided and could not be used. Type O or patched PRBCs were therefore unavailable to the diver. During decompression to surface, the vessel made its way to port.

An initial HBO_2 treatment was embedded into his saturation decompression profile. Then pulsed, intermittent, tailing breathing HBO_2 treatments of short interval followed and were also embedded into his decompression profile during his slow ascent to surface. He had EKG leads placed on his chest wall shortly after his initial profuse diaphoresis abated and he stabilized. The intervals between HBO_2 treatments were gradually lengthened as long as his ST segments remained unelevated. When the ST segments on the cardiac monitor elevated, he was put back on HBO_2-enriched helium breathing mix (SEFiO_2 300%). His measured hemoglobin (Hgb) on the hemolyzed, locked-out samples of blood was 2 g/dL by this time. Soon peripheral veins could be found and accessed for established intravenous lines. He tolerated oral chicken and beef broth, oral hematenics (folic acid and multivitamins), intramuscular iron injections, and subcutaneous erythropoietin.

When he arrived at surface three days later, he was transfused with type O PRBCs brought by a transport ambulance awaiting the vessel at dockside. He was promptly transferred to the hospital (Figure 6). His pretransfusion Hbg drawn by transport paramedics was 4 g/dL, and his Hbg after six units of PRBC transfusion was 10 g/dL. Endoscopy revealed a mature clot over a duodenal ulcer, which had eroded a duodenal artery. As a precaution, the vessel was endoscopically cauterized without complication. He went on to have an uneventful recovery. He had no

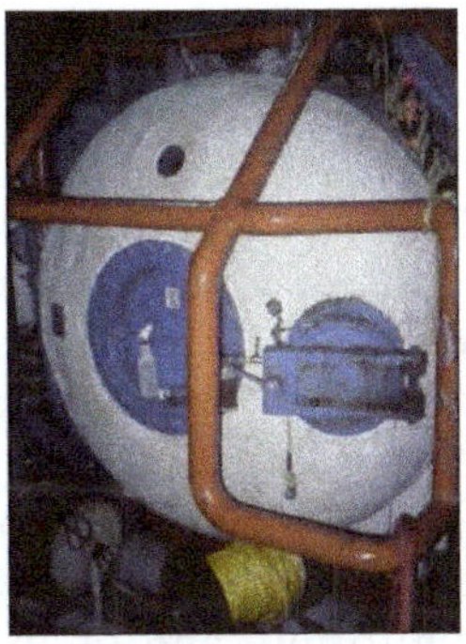

Figure 4. Heliox saturation diving chamber at site of offshore operation where patient sustained a severe blood loss insult when a duodenal ulcer eroded a duodenal artery while he was on a diving work excursion on the Gulf floor. Courtesy of Kewal Jain.[18A]

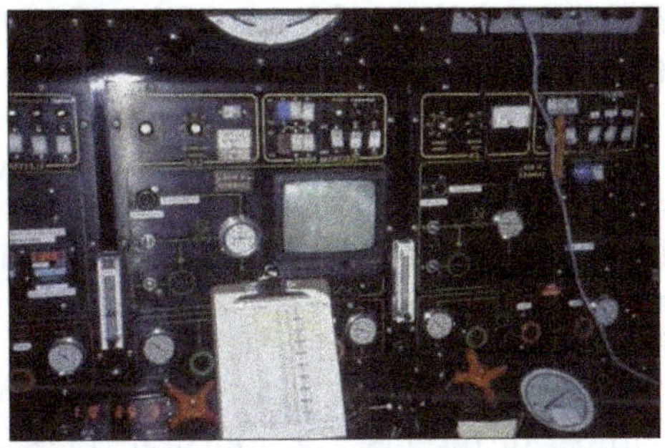

Figure 5. Diver is shown by a topside TV monitor to be in the top bunk in the saturation diving system chamber; the diver is on a $SEFiO_2$ 260% equivalent heliox mix while having a hemoglobin of 2 g/dL. The diver is alert, not short of breath, nondiaphoretic, and normotensive. Courtesy of Kewal Jain.[18A]

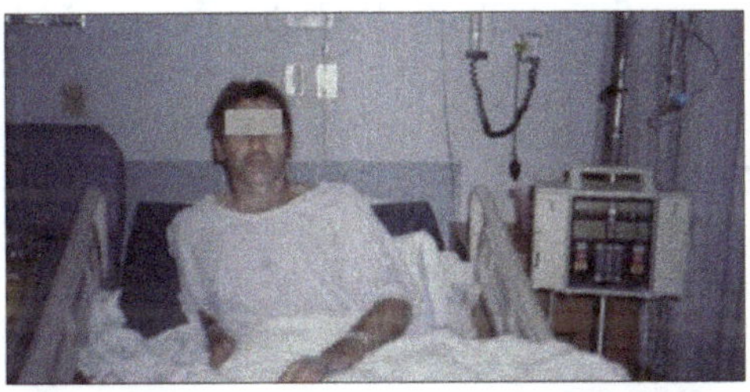

Figure 6. Patient after transfusion of PRBCs and after hospital-based endoscopy – endoscopy which revealed the duodenal ulcer to be hemostatic. Patient was comfortable and was discharged to his home after a two-day hospital stay. Courtesy of Kewal Jain.[18A]

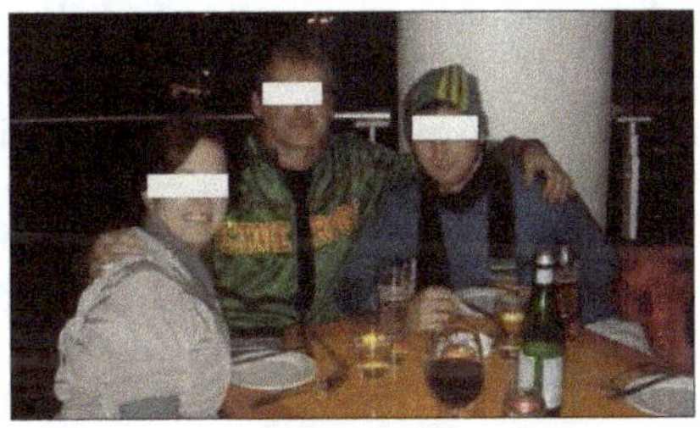

Figure 7. Same diver 10 years later with family, in good health, celebrating the FIFA World Cup as a spectator in South Africa, 2010. Courtesy of Kewal Jain.[18A]

evidence of injury to kidneys (creatinine and BUN and urinalysis were normal), heart (EKG and cardiac enzymes were normal), liver (liver profile was normal), or musculoskeletal system (CPK levels were not elevated). An injury shock state, which may have resulted in multi-organ failure or death in a remote field site three days away from hospital-based intensive care, resolved well (Figure 7).

Shoemaker described accumulated and unresolved oxygen debt after the onset of a shock state as a prognosticator of patient outcome. He contended that if oxygen consumption exceeded oxygen delivery by eight liters during the first four hours of insult, but was afterward promptly resolved, the patient would feel the effects of a bad flu-like syndrome or a mild systemic inflammatory response syndrome. If the accumulated oxygen debt was more than 22 liters over the first four hours before correction, the patient would suffer multiorgan failure. If the uncorrected oxygen debt was in excess of 32 liters in the first four hours, the patient would not survive given conventional attempts at resuscitation to follow.[32] The diver described in this case report suffered an accumulated estimated oxygen debt of 45 liters in the first four hours following his exsanguinations before parenteral fluid and oxygen resuscitation could be fully implemented.

COSTS OF HYPERBARIC OXYGEN

HBO_2 compares favorably with blood transfusions in the following cost analysis using the value of the United States dollar in 2016.

1. The cost of 4 units of PRBCs over the first 24-hour period in a Southern California, private, nonprofit hospital is $1,592.00. This does not include the laboratory costs in typing, crossmatching, and antibody screen that increases the costs to greater than $2,400.00. Fresh frozen plasma, albumin, or other fractions, if needed, would add to this cost.(17)

2. HBO_2 for 5 treatments of 66 minutes each (treatment protocol per the author) in the first 24 hours, at $392.00 per treatment, would cost $1,960.00. There may be additional costs for intensive care, monitoring, and/or use of a respirator, but these are usually facts of life for those receiving transfusions, as well for these seriously ill patients. These costs have recently been evaluated by clinicians in the United Kingdom.(38)

CONCLUSION

HBO_2 is a valuable adjunct when used early in treatment of acute blood loss anemia in those who cannot receive blood replacement for medical or religious or tactical reasons. The low-technology aspect of HBO_2 should make its use appealing in the military far-forward field operations, in prehospital EMS equipped with hyperbaric ambulances, and in trauma centers, emergency departments, and operating rooms as an adjunct to blood bank services. In similar availability, HBO_2 has already has worked in the offshore commercial diving realm as a bridge until transfused units of blood become available.

REFERENCES

1. Adir Y, Bitterman N, et al. Salutary consequences of oxygen therapy on long-term outcome of hemorrhagic shock in awake, unrestrained rats. Undersea Hyperb Med. 1995;22(1):23-30.
2. Alam SQ, Alam BS. Pulmonary lipid peroxides and fatty acids of rats fed different lipids and exposed to oxygen at hyperbaric pressure. Lipids. 1985;20(4):248-51.
3. Amonic RS, Cockett AT, et al. Hyperbaric oxygen therapy in chronic hemorrhagic shock. JAMA. 1969;208(11):2051-4.
4. Attar S, Esmond WH, Cowley RA. Hyperbaric oxygen in vascular collapse. J Thoracic Cardiovasc Surg. 1962;44:759-70.
5. Barkova EN, Petrov AV. The influence of oxygen barotherapy on erythropoiesis in the recuperative period of hemorrhagic collapse. Bull Esp Biol Med. 1976;81(2):156-8.
6. Blair E, Henning G, et al. The effect of hyperbaric oxygenation (OHP) on three forms of shock: traumatic, hemorrhagic and septic. J Trauma. 1964;4:652-63.
7. Boerema I, Meyne NG, et al. Life without blood: a study of the influence of high atmospheric pressure on dilution of blood. J Cardiovasc Surg. 1960;1(2):133-46.
8. Bucala R, Kawakami M, Cerami A. Cytotoxicity of a perfluorocarbon blood substitute to macrophages in vitro. Science. 1983;220(4600):965-7.
9. Castro O, Nesbitt AE, Lyles D. Effect of a perfluorocarbon emulsion (Fluosol-DA) on reticuloendothelial system clearance function. Am J Hematol. 1984;16(1):15-21.
10. Cohn CS, Cushing MM. Oxygen therapeutics: perfluorocarbons and blood substitute safety. Crit Care Clin. 2009;25(2):399-414.
11. Committee on Trauma. American College of Surgeons, Committee on Trauma. ATLS Advanced Life Support for Doctors. 8th ed. 2008.
12. Dunham CM, Siegel HB, et al. Oxygen debt and metabolic acidemia as quantitative predictors of mortality and the severity of the ischemic insult in hemorrhagic shock. Crit Care Med. 1991;19(2):231-43.
13. Elliot DP, Paton BC. Effect of 100% oxygen at 1 and 3 atmospheres on dogs subjected to hemorrhagic hypotension. Surgery. 1965;57:401-8.
14. Godman CA, Chheda KP, et al. Hyperbaric oxygen induces a cytoprotective and angiogenic response in human microvascular endothelial cells. Cell Stress Chaperones. 2010;15(4):431-42.

14A. Grimberg-Peters D, Buren C, et al. Hyperbaric oxygen reduces production of reactive oxygen species in neutrophils from polytraumatized patients yielding in the inhibition of p38 MAP kinase and downstream pathways. PloS One 2016;11(8):e0161343.

15. Hageman JR, Hunt CE. Fat emulsions and lung function. Clinics Chest Med. 1986;7(1):69-77.
16. Hart GB. Exceptional blood loss anemia: treatment with hyperbaric oxygen. JAMA. 1974;228(11):1028-9.
17. Hart GB. HBO and exceptional blood loss anemia. In: Kindwall EP, Whelan HT, editors. Hyperbaric medicine practice. 3rd ed. West Palm Beach (FL): Best Publishing, Co.; 2008. p. 741-52.
18. Hart GB, Lennon PA, Strauss MB. Hyperbaric oxygen in exceptional acute blood-loss anemia. J Hyperbar Med. 1987;2(4):205-10.

18A. Jain, Kewal K. Textbook of hyperbaric medicine, 6th edition. Springer International Publishing; 2017.

19. Kehrer JP, Autor AP. The effect of dietary fatty acids on the composition of the adult rat lung lipids: relationship to oxygen toxicity. Toxicol Appl Pharmacol. 1978;44(2):423-30.

20. Kheir JN, Scharp LA, et al. Oxygen gas-filled microparticles provide intravenous oxygen delivery. Sci Transl Med. 2012;4(140):1-10.

21. Knighton DR, Halliday B, Hunt TK. Oxygen as an antibiotic: the effect of inspired oxygen on infection. Arch Surg. 1984;119(2):199-204.

22. Ledingham IM. Hyperbaric oxygen in shock. Int Anesthesiol Clin. 1969;7(4):819-39.

23. Leonov AN, Yakovlev VN. Role of nitrogen metabolism of the brain in the mechanisms of the therapeutic action of hyperbaric oxygen in hemorrhagic shock. Bull Esp Biol Med. 1977;83(4):418-20.

24. Lutz J, Berthel U, Metzenauer P. Variation in toxicity of Escherichia coli endotoxin after treatment with perfluorated blood substitutes in mice. Circ Shock. 1982;9(2):99-106.

25. McLoughlin PL, Cope TM, Harrison JC. Hyperbaric oxygen therapy in the management of severe acute anaemia in a Jehovah's Witness. Anaesthesia. 1999;54(9):891-5.

26. Moss GS, Gould SA, Sehgal LR, et al. Hemoglobin solution – from tetramer to polymer. Surgery. 1984;95(3):249-55.

27. Nanney L, Fink LM, Virmani R. Perfluorochemicals: morphologic changes in infused liver, spleen, lung and kidney of rabbits. Arch Pathol Lab Med. 1984;108(8):631-7.

28. Navarro RU, Ferguson CC. Treatment of experimental hemorrhagic shock by the combined use of hyperbaric oxygen and low molecular weight dextran. Surgery. 1968;63(5):775-81.

29. Norman JN. Haemodynamic studies in total blood replacement. Bibl Haematol. 1975;41:203-8.

30. Rabiner SF, Helbert JR, et al. Evaluation of a stroma-free hemoglobin solution for use as a plasma expander. J Exp Med. 1967;126(6):1127-42.

31. Sherman DM, Sennik VT, Sidenko VP. The efficacy of hyperbaric oxygenation in experimental hemorrhagic shock. Anestheziol Reanimatol. 1989;2:37-9.

32. Shoemaker WC, Appel PL, Kram HB. Tissue oxygen debt as a determinant of lethal and nonlethal postoperative organ failure. Crit Care Med. 1988;16(11):1117-220.

33. Stark RD, Coatesworth AP, Tucker AG. Management of life-threatening epistaxis in a Jehovah's Witness. Int J Clin Pract. 2003;57(1):60-1.

34. Thom SR, Bhopale VM, et al. Stem cell mobilization by hyperbaric oxygen. Am J Physiol Heart Circ Physiol. 2006;290(4):H1378-86.

35. Thom SR, Elbuken ME. Oxygen-dependent antagonism of lipid peroxidation. Free Radic Biol Med. 1991;10(6):413-26.

36. Thom SR, Mendiguren I, et al. Inhibition of human neutrophil B2-integrin-dependent adherence by hyperbaric oxygen. Am J Physiol. 1997;272(3 Pt 1):C770-7.

37. Thom SR, Yang M, et al. Microparticles initiate decompression-induced neutrophil activation and subsequent vascular injuries. J Appl Physiol. 2011;110(2):340-51.

38. Treweek S, James PB. A cost analysis of monoplace hyperbaric oxygen therapy with and without recirculation. J Wound Care. 2006;15(6):235-8.

39. Tyrtyshnikov IM. Effect of acute massive blood loss during hyperbaric oxygen therapy on nucleic acid metabolism in the albino rat liver. Bull Esp Biol Med. 1974;77(6):611-2.

40. Van Meter KW. A systematic review of the application of hyperbaric oxygen in the treatment of severe anemia: an evidence-based approach. Undersea Hyperb Med. 2005;32(1):61-83.

41. Van Meter KW. Hyperbaric oxygen clinical application in resuscitation from insult of acute severe anemia. Wound Care Hyperbar Med. 2014;5(4):27-32.

42. Van Meter. Hyperbaric oxygen in resuscitation. In: Jain KK, editor. Textbook of hyperbaric medicine. Verlag (NY): Springer; 2016.

43. Van Meter KW. Hyperbaric oxygen therapy as an adjunct to pre-hospital advanced trauma life support. Surg Technol Int. 2012;21:61-73.

44. Van Meter KW. The effect of hyperbaric oxygen on severe anemia. UHM. 2012;39(5):937-42.

45. Wright JK, Ehler W, et al. Facilitation of recovery from acute blood loss with hyperbaric oxygen. Arch Surg. 2002;137(7):850-3.

CHAPTER 28 CHAPTER

Hyperbaric Oxygen in Skin Grafts and Flaps

CHAPTER TWENTY-EIGHT OVERVIEW

Skin Grafts and Flaps **709**
Rationale 709
Animal Studies 710
Clinical Studies 713
General Recommendations 717
Conclusion **718**
References **719**

Hyperbaric Oxygen in Skin Grafts and Flaps

Jenna Cusic, Chelsea Venditto, Hani S. Matloub

SKIN GRAFTS AND FLAPS

Rationale

Hyperbaric oxygen therapy (HBO_2) is unnecessary for the support of normal, uncompromised skin grafts or flaps; however, HBO_2 has been shown to be extremely useful in preservation of tissues following preoperative or postoperative irradiation or in the setting of decreased microcirculation or hypoxia. HBO_2 assists in maximization of the viability of compromised tissue, reducing the need for operative re-intervention.[43A] Similarly, though HBO_2 is not indicated for use in the management of straightforward wounds, HBO_2 can augment healing in complicated acute wounds as well as chronic wounds.[12]

The first description of altering atmospheric pressure to treat medical illness was in 1662 by a British clergyman, Henshaw, who believed that hyperbaric conditions accelerated healing in acute conditions. This led him to construct a sealed chamber called the "Domicillum."[12] In 1772 a Swedish chemist, Carl Scheele, and an English cleric, Joseph Priestley, isolated elemental oxygen; over a century later, incorporating the work of Robert Boyle on physical properties of ideal gases, elemental oxygen was introduced into the barometric chamber to provide hyperbaric oxygen therapy to deep-sea divers. Churchill Davis initiated the modern use of HBO_2 in 1955 for potentiating the effects of radiation therapy in cancer. HBO_2 was introduced into plastic surgery in 1966 when McFarlane and Wermuth described it for use in composite graft salvage in a rat model.[12]

The pathophysiology of tissue ischemia as well as the mechanism by which hyperbaric oxygen therapy counteracts ischemia is multifactorial. Compromised tissues are hypoxic, with oxygen tensions below 15 mmHg.[43A,86] This is much below tissue oxygen tension levels of 30 to 40 mmHg which are necessary for fibroblast synthesis and the subsequent development of collagen matrix for capillary generation in avascular areas.[35,37,43A,45,74,89-90,99] HBO_2 can help deliver this level of oxygen to tissues, thereby stimulating fibroblasts and enhancing collagen synthesis.[43A,85,87] Importantly for this mechanism, the fibroblast is a facultative anaerobe and is postulated to be stimulated by both intermittent hypoxia (via lactate stimulus) and hyperoxia.[36,43A,45,60] Consequentially, through elevating abnormally low tissue oxygen tension values to physiologic levels HBO_2 has been demonstrated to support the otherwise hypoxic tissue until adequate circulation is reestablished.[10,43A]

HBO_2 can elevate arterial oxygen tension to between 400 mmHg and 2000 mmHg in tissues, which creates reactive oxygen species. Depending on their concentration, these reactive oxygen species can have either therapeutic or detrimental effects on wound healing.[(12)] The body's defense mechanisms against these reactive oxygen species are generally adequate; however, hyperbaric treatment protocols must be brief, with periodic "oxygen breaks" during which the patient breathes room air between treatments.[(12)] HBO_2 treatment also improves leukocyte function with increasing oxygen pressure and can reduce surgical-site infections, decrease peripheral edema, and improve skin viability, thus improving skin flap adherence, neovascularization, and penetration of antibiotic therapy.[(12)]

Furthermore, Reinisch[(80-81)] suggested failure of skin flaps may be secondary to development of arteriovenous shunts in the distal aspects of the flap. This would result in a potentially reduced flow to the more critical nutrient capillary network. HBO_2's vasoconstrictive properties may act to help shunt selectively in nonischemic areas, resulting in greater blood flow to the nutrient capillary circulation in ischemic tissue. Thus, HBO_2 contributes to enhanced tissue perfusion via hyperoxygenating tissues, stimulating fibroblasts, encouraging collagen synthesis, promoting neovascularization, and hindering arteriovenous shunts.[(43A)]

Thus, HBO_2 can hyperoxygenate tissues, stimulate fibroblasts, enhance collagen synthesis, promote neovascularization, and close off arteriovenous shunts—all mechanisms contributing to improved tissue perfusion.

A plethora of work as reviewed by Paul Nemiroff in the prior edition has shown the efficacy of HBO_2 on enhancement of flap and graft survival in a variety of experimental and clinical situations. A review of relevant prior animal and human studies as well as more recent literature is presented below.[(43A)]

Animal Studies

In a variety of animal studies, hyperbaric oxygen therapy used on rats has demonstrated favorable results in wound healing, graft take, and flap perfusion. Shulman and Kron reported upon the healing of full- and partial-thickness wounds in rats, concluding that HBO_2 reduced healing time significantly. Furthermore, when HBO_2 was added to skin grafting the healing time of partial-thickness wounds was reduced to one-half that of untreated controls.[(43A)] The study concluded that the combined effect of grafting and HBO_2 has "the startling effect of a reduction in healing time of 50%, thus seemingly improving on nature itself."[(88)] Also noted in the above study was the fact that surgical instruments were not sterilized prior to performing the operations. The assumption was thus made that superficial contamination did occur in all animals, but infection was entirely absent in the groups treated with HBO_2. HBO_2's enhancement of the ability of leukocytes to kill bacteria was demonstrated in a model by Mader in in vivo and in vitro osteomyelitis at tissue oxygen pressures up to 150 mmHg.[(43A, 54,55)] Transplantation has also been improved with HBO_2 via models of rabbit transplantation of epiphyseal growth cartilage where nearly double the success rate occurred with the addition of HBO_2 vs. control in a study by Calderwood.[(9,43A)] Jacobs et al. also found that repeated daily exposure may prolong skin allograft survival.[(40)] Rubin et al. found composite skin grafts in rabbit ears which received 100% O_2 at 2 ATA twice daily for 21 treatments and showed significantly greater survival than grafts in control animals.[(82)]

In non-compromised open wounds where the circulation remains intact, Kivisaari and Niinikoski found HBO_2 at 2 ATA had no effect, yet when compromised open wounds exist as stimulated by devascularizing wound edges, HBO_2 enhanced wound closure rate significantly over control groups by counteracting the delay/disrupted blood supply.[43A,44]

In wound epithelialization in thermal injury, HBO_2 leads to earlier capillary patency and faster epithelialization of second-degree burn wounds in guinea pigs treated with adjunctive HBO_2 at 2 ATA.[43A,47] This was also verified in another study where shallow wounds in pigs treated with HBO_2 at 2 ATA resulted in 80% epithelialization versus 49% in controls.[43A,99]

Hyperbaric oxygen studies in rats have revealed favorable results with regard to flap survival. In a pedicled flap rabbit model, Champion found 100% survival of flaps in rabbits treated with 2 ATA for 2 hours twice daily for 5 days, in comparison to over 40% necrosis of the control flaps. These authors also concluded, as previously suggested, HBO_2 supports hypoxic tissue via increase in oxygen levels until adequate circulation can recur.[10,43A] Similarly, work by McFarlane and Wermuth concluded, "HBO_2 has been of definite value in preventing necrosis in a pedicled flap in the rat and also limited the extent of necrosis in a free composite graft." In addition, the authors noted that their particular design provided a notable result that attests to the value of HBO_2 in preventing necrosis.[52]

Hyperbaric oxygen therapy has been found to improve flap perfusion. Wald et al. found that HBO_2 therapy performed for 2 hours, 4 times daily at 2.4 ATA produced a 22% increase in survival of skin flaps.[96] The timing of HBO_2 treatment has been elucidated. Niinikoski reported a 51% improvement in the length of surviving tubed skin flaps in rats treated with HBO_2 of 2.5 ATA for 2 hours twice daily for 2 days compared to air-breathing controls.[43A,73] Using a cranially-based pedicled flap in rats, Jurell and Kaijser showed that the viable flaps of rats treated with HBO_2 were nearly twice the length than those of controls ($p < 0.001$),[41,43A] of which general benefit remained even if the HBO_2 was delayed for 24 hours after surgery.[41,43A] Yet, if a significant delay in HBO_2 treatment occurs, the beneficial results will be diminished, exemplifying the importance of timing of therapy.[43A,70]

In an experimental study on standard dorsal skin flaps in rats which were designed to present a predictable and constant degree of necrosis, Arturson and Khannan revealed that HBO_2 treatment resulted in significant improvement in flap survival over untreated controls ($p < 0.05$).[1] Other flap-enhancing agents were studied, and in some cases also enhanced flap survival; however, the best results were found in rats treated with hyperbaric oxygen. The authors note that all therapies had a marginal effect on survival of flaps when circulation to the area had ceased completely. This is expected, since no modality will be able to revitalize tissue that is already frankly necrotic.

The effect of varying air pressures on skin flap survival has also been studied, demonstrating hyperbaric air (21% oxygen) and HBO_2 (100% oxygen) showed significant improvement in skin flap survival, whereas HBO_2 at standard room air pressure lended no improvement.[43A,93] Oxygen tension of pedicled flaps is lower than that of uninterrupted skin. Hyperbaric pressure of 100% oxygen, versus 100% oxygen at standard pressure, can help raise tissue oxygen tension. Gruber et al. demonstrated this in his study, where skin flaps in rats treated with HBO_2 at 3 ATA raised mean tissue tensions to 600 mmHg, whereas 100% oxygen at sea level did not raise mean flap pO_2.[30,43A]

HBO_2 furthermore can reduce the extent of ischemic necrosis of skin flaps in previously irradiated flaps. Greenwood and Gilchrist performed a study where rats were given 2,600 rads of radiation, then 6 months postexposure, a pedicled flap was raised. Half the rats were treated with HBO_2 at 2.0 for 14 days and compared to the control of air, showing that treatment significantly ($p < 0.05$) decreased mean flap necrosis.[27,43A]

Nemiroff et al. also concluded that the timing of HBO_2 initiation is also important.[43A,68] In a randomized controlled study, one hundred eighty-five Sprague-Dawley rats were randomly assigned to one of 15 groups after 3 x 9cm cranially based flaps were elevated over the rat's dorsum. The groups included all possible ordering effects of HBO_2, radiation, and flap elevation, as well as controls which included flap elevation only, radiation only, and HBO_2 groups. The length of viable flap was evaluated with fluorescein dye 7 days after the operation. The HBO_2 treatment was given either 24 or 48 hours prior to flap elevation, or within 4 or 48 hours after elevation, and consisted of 4 consecutive 2-hour treatments of 100% oxygen at 2.5 ATA, with half-hour intervals of room air breathing. Radiation consisted of (cobalt 60) and single dose of (cobalt 60) 1000 rads to the rat's dorsum. All groups which received HBO_2 within 4 hours after flap elevation showed significantly longer ($p < 0.05$) viable flaps, with up to a 22% increase in length of flap survival. In comparison to controls, HBO_2 given 48 hours prior to flap elevation significantly improved flap survival ($p < 0.05$), whereas HBO_2 given 24 hours prior to flap elevation resulted in no significant differences. Interestingly, radiation either pre- or post-flap elevation administered with or without HBO_2 had no significant effect on flap survival. Yet, waiting 48 hours prior to initiating HBO_2 did not improve flap survival, which has also been noted in other studies.[7,41,43A,76-79] HBO_2 should be started as soon as a problem or potential problem with a flap's viability is identified.

The assessment of flap perfusion is an important portion of evaluation of effect of HBO_2. Once circulation to the tissue has ceased, HBO_2 will have a marginal effect. For example, if the axial vessel to a flap is violated, rending no significant perfusion to the flap, HBO_2 will not salvage the flap. Viability can be assessed by clinical judgment as well as a variety of other techniques, including intraoperative laser angiography via SPY, fluorescein dye, laser Doppler flow, and measurement of oxygen tension.[43A,53] Of note, using fluorescein dye to assess flap perfusion is not optimal as a prolonged period of flap observation is required.[31,43A]

A number of researchers[34,42,56,62,67] have demonstrated that hyperbaric oxygen enhances wound healing, graft take, and flap perfusion by way of enhancement of capillary proliferation in an animal model. In 1987, Nemiroff and Lungu[67] randomly chose flaps from a previous study[70] and harvested a longitudinal strip of tissue 1x9cm from each flap. The absolute number of blood vessels in the microvasculature and mean surface area of vessels in the flaps (in all but 1 group) was significantly greater for all HBO_2 groups when compared with controls ($p < 0.01$). Manson demonstrated capillaries grew nearly three times further distally in pedicle flaps of guinea pigs that were treated with HBO_2, compared to age-matched controls.[56] Other researchers have shown that HBO_2 can enhance healing and flap survival by affecting angiogenesis.[34,43A56,60,62] Hyperbaric oxygen can significantly enhance flap survival, by increasing and/or maintaining the number and possibly the size of vessels within the microvasculature. To be most effective, HBO2 must be administered as soon after surgery as possible or as soon as tissue malperfusion is suspected.[43A]

In 1988 Nemiroff investigated the effects of HBO2 along with pentoxifylline. This is a rheologic agent that increases red blood cell flexibility, enhancing capillary circulation.[69] Sixty rats were randomly divided into 4 groups: (1) a control group, (2) a pentoxifylline-treated group (20mg/kg intraperitoneally at 24, 12 and 1 hour(s) before flap elevation and every 12 hours after the operation for 7 days), (3) an HBO_2-treated group (14 two-hour treatments of 2.5 absolute atmospheres in divided doses), and (4) a pentoxifylline-plus-HBO_2-treated group. Cranially-based skin flaps were elevated on the dorsum of the rate and the surviving flap length was evaluated with fluorescein dye 7 days after elevation. The viable flap lengths in the pentoxifylline or HBO2-treated groups were significantly greater than those in the control group but were not significantly different from each other. Furthermore, pentoxifylline and HBO2 led to a significantly greater flap survival length than either alone ($p < 0.001$), with 86% improvement over control and 30-39% improvement over either pentoxifylline or HBO2 treatment alone.[43A] Thus, pentoxifylline appears to have a synergistic effect with HBO2 on flap survival.

The effect of HBO_2 on axial pattern flap survival has been studied during flap ischemia and reperfusion.[100] Eighty-one 3 x 6 cm rectangular epigastric skin flaps were elevated and the inferior epigastric pedicle of each flap occluded for 8 hours, then the animals divided into 4 groups. The control group (n = 27) underwent the 8 hours of flap ischemia with no HBO_2. The first experimental group (n = 21) underwent HBO_2 therapy (100% O_2) with three 1.75-hour dives at 2.5 ATA during flap ischemia; the second experimental group (n = 21) underwent HBO_2therapy with two 1.75-hour dives during reperfusion; and the third experimental group (n = 12) underwent HBO_2 treatment during ischemia but with the flap contained in a metal-coated Mylar bag to prevent oxygen diffusion. Flap necrosis was evaluated on post-operative day 6. Mean flap necrosis for controls was 28%; this was reduced with HBO_2 treatment during ischemia or during reperfusion to 9% and 12%, respectively ($p < 0.01$). The percentage of necrosis of the group where the local effect of HBO2 on the flap was blocked by the diffusion barrier, was 5%, also significantly improved from controls ($p < 0.0005$) but not significantly different from the non-impeded HBO_2 groups. HBO2 treatment significantly increased axial-pattern skin flap survival when it is administered during or immediately following total flap ischemia. Additionally, two other controlled animal studies using axial as well as random flap designs have also shown enhanced flap survival with HBO2 treatment.[43A,71,100]

Many varieties of animal model studies have been performed, investigating the clinical effect of HBO_2 treatments on flaps. These have shown efficacy of HBO_2 regarding different types of reconstructions including skin grafts, composite grafts, pedicled flaps, random flaps, axial-pattern flaps, irradiated flaps, and irradiated wounds. Vascular supply does differ between different reconstructive options, yet a central contributor to failure is tissue hypoxia. HBO_2 can assist in reducing the insult of hypoxia on these reconstructions.[43A]

Clinical Studies

Multiple studies have been conducted examining the clinical benefit of hyperbaric oxygen therapy on tissue perfusion. Systematic reviews and randomized, controlled trials support clinical use of hyperbaric oxygen for refractory diabetic wound healing and radiation injuries. HBO_2's role in compromised flaps and grafts and ischemia-reperfusion injury is supported by animal studies and a small number of clinical trials.[94] In their model of a cartilage graft inside an ear lobule graft, Friedman et al. found 1 of 6 patients who did not receive HBO_2 therapy suffered a substantial loss of graft, but when grafts were repeated with HBO_2 therapy, graft take was successful.[21] Therefore, HBO_2 therapy may play a role in supporting the take of larger composite grafts, provided the graft size does not completely overwhelm the recipient site's ability to provide revascularization. HBO_2 may be administered preoperatively in cases of compromised recipient sites with decreased ability to provide revascularization, stimulating vessel proliferation by increasing the oxygen gradient.[21] However, one might routinely expect upwards of 90% take of a typical skin graft in most clinical scenarios; thus, HBO_2 may be beneficial only in areas of poor perfusion.[21]

In 1966 case studies and a prospective, randomized and blinded clinical trial in 1967, Perrin showed the benefit of HBO_2 for skin grafts.[76-79] In this study, 24 patients were assigned to an HBO_2 treatment group and 24 patients were assigned to a control group.[43A] In the HBO_2 group, patients who received postoperative HBO_2 for 2 hours at 2 ATM on postoperative day 0 as well as twice daily for 3 days, compared to a control receiving no HBO_2 therapy, had a 29% improvement in graft take. 64% of grafts were found to survive in the HBO_2-treated group, whereas only 17% survived in the control group ($p < 0.01$).[43A] Perrins also found that random flaps for lip deformities and mucosal flaps had improved success when HBO_2 therapy was initiated after a flap's viability was deemed questionable.[77]

Monies-Chass et al. reported on the utility of hyperbaric oxygen therapy in ischemic limbs. Seven patients sustained acute trauma resulting in limb ischemia and subsequently underwent standard vascular repair. Though technically successful, these repairs failed to restore circulation, and the extremities remained ischemic. Hyperbaric oxygen treatment was initiated and found to be successful, preventing the development of gangrene in all patients.[64]

Mastectomy skin flap necrosis is another clinical area where hyperbaric oxygen therapy may play a favorable role. Mastectomy skin flap necrosis occurs in up to 30% of patients undergoing mastectomy with immediate reconstruction, of which the incidence has increased with nipple-sparing techniques and direct-to-implant reconstruction.[22] Other risk factors for developing necrosis include increasing age (> 65), BMI > 30, large breast size, Wise-pattern skin incision, previous radiation therapy, smoking, tumescent technique, and high intraoperative tissue expander fill volumes (> 65%).[22,63] Treatment options are available for postmastectomy skin flap necrosis such as nitroglycerin paste;[22] however, this modality may not be tolerated by patients with certain medical comorbidities, and HBO_2 may be a viable and important option to consider in high-risk patients. A case report by Copeland-Halperin et al. demonstrated the clinical use of HBO_2 in mastectomy skin flap ischemia. A 71-year-old female with a history of bilateral breast cancer who had undergone left partial mastectomy and radiation therapy, then right partial mastectomy, presented for prophylactic bilateral skin-sparing mastectomies with silicone tissue expander placement. During the reconstruction, the right breast developed signs of ischemia, and the tissue expander was subsequently filled to only 20% volume. By postoperative day 1, ischemic necrosis had developed bilaterally, and HBO_2 was initiated at 2 ATA for 120 minutes, followed by twice-daily 90-minute sessions for 2 days and then 120 minutes daily thereafter. The patient showed substantial improvement after 15 sessions.[11] This allowed her to proceed with future filling of the expanders and eventual implant exchanging, salvaging the reconstruction.[11] This was further supported by another case report by Fredman et al. where a 41-year-old female who developed skin flap ischemia after skin-sparing mastectomy was immediately treated with 5 sessions of HBO_2, achieving resolution of ischemia without complications.[20]

Welsh and Matos[97] as well as Barr et al.[5-6] reported favorable results with HBO_2 improving skin flap survival. In a study of 105 patients with flaps or skin grafts thought to be compromised due to ischemia, Bowersox et al. found that 89% of compromised flaps and 91% of compromised skin grafts survived with adjuvant HBO_2 therapy. Additionally, approximately 90% of these skin graft patients had comorbidities which could further contribute to graft or flap failure. Therefore, this yielded a 10% failure rate which is much lower than the 67% failure or complication rate that several other studies have sited in threatened graft or flap survival.[32,43A]

Hyperbaric oxygen therapy has been studied clinically in the setting of replanted digits, limbs, and even severed ears. In a study by Kim et al. focusing on digital amputations distal to the distal interphalangeal joint, adjuvant HBO_2therapy improved survival rates of the digits to approximately 76%.[43] Bao and colleagues similarly published their research regarding the efficacy of HBO_2therapy contributing to limb survival in limb replantation.[2] Furthermore, in a study reporting on traumatically-severed ears in three males, Neubauer et al. found that HBO_2 therapy was a useful adjunct in survival following reanastomosis.[43A,72]

Hart et al. found benefit of HBO_2 therapy when used in wounds of compromised tissues. Similarly, HBO_2 was found to improve mortality, morbidity and decrease healing time in a randomized, double-blind study of 191 patients with burn wounds. There are several other controlled animal studies which have also shown favorable results of adjuvant HBO_2 therapy on burn wound healing. In a study by Baroni et al., HBO_2 was found to benefit diabetic wounds of the foot as compared to a control group, substantially reducing the risk of limb amputation ($p < 0.0001$).[43A]

Hyperbaric oxygen therapy can be effective in the setting of irradiated tissue as well. A post-radiation surgical complication rate of 67% has been sited by Habel.[32,43A] HBO_2 therapy has been suggested as a treatment to radiation tissue injury in order to improve blood supply. In a Cochrane review, it was found that in osteoradionecrosis, HBO_2 therapy may be more likely to improve mucosal coverage and decrease wound breakdown.[8] It also may reduce the progression to osteoradionecrosis following tooth extraction in an irradiated field.[8] This may be important in head and neck reconstruction, when wound breakdown and infection near a vascular anastomosis could be catastrophic. Furthermore, elective surgery is relatively contraindicated in areas of previous irradiation and impaired wound healing. Lumpectomy with radiation therapy is a breast-conservation treatment modality offered in the cases of certain breast cancers, and these patients often require later recontouring or reconstructive procedures such as oncoplastic reduction. Such secondary procedures are not optimal in irradiated breasts, as the radiated tissue puts these patients at greater risk of having postsurgical complications. In a retrospective review of 5 patients undergoing reduction mammoplasty in previously irradiated breasts who received 20 preoperative HBO_2 therapy sessions at 90 minutes of 2.36 ATM and then 10 postoperative treatments, healing occurred in all patients. Two irradiated and 2 nonirradiated breasts did progress through delayed healing, but the eventual recovery of these patients and the rest of the sample suggests the fact that HBO_2 therapy may be an adjuvant option in previously irradiated breasts undergoing secondary surgeries.[91]

Kveton reported successful treatment of osteoradionecrosis of the temporal bone in a 10-year-old child with rhabdomyosarcoma of the infratemporal fossa. This child had suffered with six years of otorrhea, which was refractory to other forms of therapy, prior to adjunctive HBO_2 treatments.[49]

HBO_2 therapy was found to be helpful in healing radiated laryngectomy wounds in a study by Greenwood and Gilchrist.[28] Additionally, Greenwood and Gilchrist have also found HBO_2 therapy to be beneficial in irradiated flaps in animal models ($p < .05$).[43A] A review by Dauwe et al. found benefit of HBO_2 therapy with level I evidence in late radiation tissue injury, chronic ulcers (diabetic, venous, arterial, and decubitus), acute wounds, migraine headaches, and thermal burns, and level III evidence in osteomyelitis, but found no benefit in necrotizing infections.[12] Also described by Dauwe et al. are studies of hyperbaric oxygen therapy in the setting of burn-wound treatment, in which hyperbaric oxygen was not found to facilitate burn-wound healing in all patients. This may result from hyperoxygenation in the setting of the systemic inflammatory response occurring in burn patients, which may negatively impact wound healing.[12]

Marx et al.[57-60] and other researchers[24,48,95,98] have demonstrated the efficacy of HBO_2 therapy in osteoradionecrosis-associated wounds. Other studies have found benefit of HBO_2 treatment for soft tissue necrosis secondary to radiation injury.[13,18-19,43A,49] Farmer et al. proved the efficacy of HBO_2 in improving radiation injuries of the larynx, nose and floor of mouth.[18] Furthermore, Ferguson reported on HBO_2 in the setting of laryngeal radionecrosis, and found that 7 of 8 patients were successfully treated with adjunctive HBO_2 therapy.[19,43A]

HBO_2 therapy produces sufficient oxygen partial pressures in poorly perfused tissues to allow fibroblastic activity and collagen production, which creates a matrix for capillary budding and neovascularization. The daily elevation of oxygen tension by HBO_2 in hypoxic bone and soft tissue results in the ingrowth of functioning capillaries, fibroblastic proliferation, collagen synthesis, and capillary angiogenesis. By these mechanisms, HBO_2 has been reported to improve reconstructive attempts in the maxillofacial area.[23,60]

HBO_2 has been found useful in other modifications of tissue flaps such as facelifts. In 2010, Stong and Jacono showed that HBO_2 decreased bruising on postoperative day 7 in facelift patients treated for 60 minutes at 2 ATA for 2 days preoperatively and then again on postoperative days 3, 4, and 5 compared to a control group.[92] Hyperbaric oxygen therapy has been found to improve outcomes in periorbital reconstruction, as well as survival of compromised facial flaps.[23,43A]

Additionally, HBO_2 can be used as an adjunct in flaps that may be innervated to improve function or sensation. Although there is no direct evidence, and favorable results may only be extrapolated, Eguiluz-Ordonez et al. found that after nerve transection injury, HBO_2 may have a beneficial effect on nerve regeneration.[17] As shown in their study of 40 rats with nerve transection, the group who underwent HBO_2 therapy showed improved foot-ankle response at 14 weeks as compared with the non-HBO_2 control group.[17]

HBO_2 has been found to improve tissue perfusion, and a substantial amount of animal studies demonstrate the benefit of HBO_2 on improving flap survival.

Despite controversy regarding the value of using animal models in flap studies, Hurn demonstrated that with adequate sample sizes and a protocoled study design, rodent flap studies can be of benefit.[38,43A]

Controversy also exists with regard to the use of double-blind, controlled, randomized studies on human flaps. Due to the variability of the tissues in wounds, grafts, and flaps, it is quite difficult to create double-blind studies in this arena. Furthermore, the fact that HBO_2 therapy proves so effective in wound therapy, flaps and grafts in controlled, randomized, and blinded animal studies, it would be unfortunate to withhold HBO_2 therapy in the control groups of human studies.[43A]

Although numerous alternative methods have been attempted to augment skin flap perfusion, few have been routinely successful in animal or human settings.

Many alternative methods for improving flap perfusion have been reported[15], but a paucity of animal or human studies have shown success. Different mechanisms such as cooling,[46] the use of gravity,[39,66] increasing systemic blood pressure,[66] altering physical characteristics of blood such as with dextran,[25-26] administering vasodilators,[84] and increasing humidity have been attempted to improve flap perfusion. However, other than HBO_2 therapy or use of a delay phenomenon, these attempts have fallen short. Furthermore, the delay phenomenon cannot be employed once a flap has been raised and inset into its recipient bed, and ischemia is less tolerated in delayed flaps than fresh flaps.[65] A study by McFarlane and colleagues[51] found no improved survival in delayed flaps versus fresh flaps.[43A]

The delay phenomenon is employed in specific clinical situations and when used, does require additional surgery, often a longer hospitalization and therefore greater costs. Use of the delay phenomenon in flap reconstruction may not be ideal in scenarios of compromised recipient sites, trauma or previous radiation therapy. However, HBO_2 therapy has been found in both animal and human studies to improve survival of flap reconstructions even in these more complex situations.[43A]

In conclusion, though HBO_2 therapy is not indicated for well-perfused flaps, grafts, or uncomplicated wounds, it has been found to be beneficial in complex wounds or compromised soft tissue reconstructions. Necrosis of soft tissues can have disastrous and sometimes life-threatening consequences, such as in the setting of head and neck reconstruction with complications such as fistula, infection, or carotid blowout. Not only can these complications result in increased morbidity and mortality, but also massive increases in costs due to prolonged hospitalization, readmission, or reoperation. Considering that 20 hyperbaric oxygen therapy treatment sessions at $300/session costs $6,000, and prolonged hospital stay, additional surgeries, or readmission frequently costs upwards of $30,000, HBO_2therapy can help to significantly reduce these costs. Marx and colleagues found that by using HBO_2 to prevent complications associated with radiation therapy such as osteoradionecrosis, there is the potential for substantial economic savings. In a randomized prospective clinical study, patients not treated with HBO_2 therapy had greater post-operative complications resulting in osteoradionecrosis (29%) as compared to the treatment group (5.4%), and the estimated cost savings per patient in the treatment group was $60,000.[43A]

General Recommendations

Recommendation for initial treatment duration is twice daily for 90-120 minutes per session. Once the skin graft, flap or wound appears to be improving, once daily treatment can commence. Treatment pressures are generally administered at 2.0 to

2.5 ATA. Of course, pressures and duration of therapy may change depending on facility or patient specifics.[43A]

CONCLUSION

Hyperbaric oxygen therapy has been found effective in a variety of scenarios involving both animal studies and human clinical studies. Hyperbaric oxygen therapy augments tissue perfusion via multiple mechanisms, including raised tissue oxygen tensions for synthesis of fibroblasts, development of collagen matrix for capillary proliferation, closure of arteriovenous shunts in distal portions of flaps, improvement of leukocyte function (thus decreasing risk of infection,) and increased penetration of antibiotic therapy. Hyperbaric oxygen has been found effective in improving take in composite grafts, cartilage grafts, and straightforward skin grafts. Flap perfusion has been shown to improve in both nonirradiated wounds, irradiated wounds, and delayed wounds. Skin flap perfusion in several clinical scenarios including mastectomy skin flaps, small facial flaps, and even flaps in the setting of facelifts have responded favorably to hyperbaric oxygen therapy. Furthermore, complex wounds involving a variety of different pathologies including osteoradionecrosis, diabetes mellitus, and burn injury have shown improvement with initiation of hyperbaric oxygen therapy. Given the astronomical costs that can be sustained in the case of failed soft-tissue reconstructions due to reoperation and prolonged hospitalization, HBO_2 proves to be a cost-effective means of reconstructive salvage.

REFERENCES

1. Arturson GG, Khanna NN. The effects of hyperbaric dimethyl sulfoxide and complamin on survival of experimental skin flaps. Scan J Plast Reconst Surg. 1970;4:8-10.
2. Bao JYS. HBO_2 therapy in reimplantation of severed limbs: a report of 34 cases. In: Kindwall EP, editor. Proceedings of the 8th International Congress on Hyperbaric Medicine. Flagstaff (AZ): Best Publishing Company; 1984. p.182-6.
3. Barisoni DM, Veall N. Effects of thymoxamine circulation in skin flaps and in denervated skin. Lancet. 1969;1:400-1.
4. Baroni G, Porro T, Faglia E, Pizzi G, et.al. Hyperbaric oxygen in diabetic gangrene treatment. Diabetes Care. 1987;10(1):81-6.
5. Barr PO, Enfors W, Ericksson G. Hyperbaric oxygen therapy in dermatology. Br J Dermatol. 1972;86:631-5.
6. Barr PO, Liljedahl SO, Nylén B. Enfarenheter av hyperbar O2 inom rekonstruktiv kirurgi. Nord Med. 1969;82:1223. Swedish.
7. Bowersox JC, Strauss MB, Hart GB. Clinical experiences with hyperbaric oxygen therapy in the salvage of ischemic skin flaps and grafts. J Hyperbaric Medicine. 1986;1:141-9.
8. Bennett M, Feldmeier J, Hampson N, et al. Hyperbaric oxygen therapy for late radiation tissue injury [review]. Cochrane Database Syst Rev. 2016. doi:10.1002/14651858.CD005005.
9. Calderwood JW. The effect of hyperbaric oxygen in the transplantation of epiphyseal growth cartilage in the rabbit. J Bone Joint Surg. 1974;56B:735-59.
10. Champion WM, McSherry CK, Goulian D Jr. Effect of hyperbaric oxygen on survival of pedicled skin flaps. J Surg Res. 1967;7:583-6.
11. Copeland-Halperin LR, Bruce SB, Mesbahi AN. Hyperbaric oxygen following bilateral skin-sparing mastectomies: a case report. Plast Reconstr Surg Glob Open. 2016;4:680e.
12. Dauwe PB, Pulikkottil BJ, Lavery L, et al. Does hyperbaric oxygen therapy work in facilitating acute wound healing: a systematic review. Plast Reconstr Surg. 2014;133:208e-215e.
13. Davis JC, Dunn JM, Gates GA, et al. Hyperbaric oxygen: a new adjunct in the management of radiation necrosis. Arch Otolaryngol. 1979;105:58-61.
14. DeHaan C, Stark RB. Changes in efferent circulation of tubed pedicles and in the transplantability of large composite grafts produced by histamine ionophoresis. Plast Reconstr Surg. 1961;28:577.
15. Donegan JO. The assessment and enhancement of skin flap viability. Head Neck Surg. 1980;2:470-5.
16. Donovan WE. Experimental models in skin flap removal research. In: Grabb WC, Myers MB, editors. Skin flaps. Boston: Little Brown and Co., Inc.; 1975. p. 11-20.
17. Eguiluz-Ordonez R, Sanchez CE, Venegas A, et al. Effects of hyperbaric oxygen on peripheral nerves. Plast Reconstr Surg. 2006;118:350-7.
18. Farmer JC Jr, Shelton DL, Angelillo JD, et al. Treatment of radiation-induced tissue injury by hyperbaric oxygen. Ann Otol Rhinol Laryngol. 1978;87:707-15.
19. Ferguson BJ, Hudson WR, Farmer JC Jr. Hyperbaric oxygen therapy for laryngeal radionecrosis. Ann Otol Rhinol Laryngol. 1987;96:1-6.
20. Fredman R, Wise I, Friedman T, et al. Spin-sparing mastectomy flap ischemia salvage using urgent hyperbaric chamber oxygen therapy: a case report. Undersea Hyperb Med. 2014;41(2):145-7.

21. Friedman HI, Fitzmaurice M, Lefaivre JF, et al. An evidenced-based appraisal of the use of hyperbaric oxygen on flaps and grafts. Plast Reconstr Surg. 2006;117:175S-190S.

22. Gdalevitch P, Van Laeken N, Bahng S, et al. Effects of nitroglycerin ointment on mastectomy flap necrosis in immediate breast reconstruction: a randomized controlled trial. Plast Reconstr Surg. 2015;135:1530-9.

23. Gonnering RS, Kindwall EP, Goldmann RW. Adjunct hyperbaric oxygen therapy in periorbital reconstruction. Arch Opthalmol. 1986;104:439-43.

24. Goode RL, Linehan JW. The fluorescein test in post-irradiation surgery. Arch Otolaryng. 1970;91:526-8.

25. Goulian D Jr. The use of bromphenol blue in the assay of rheomacrodex effects on flap viability. Plast and Reconstr Surg. 1967;39:227.

26. Grabb WC, O'Neal RM. The effect of low molecular weight dextran on the survival of experimental skin flaps. Plast and Reconstr Surg. 1966;37:406.

27. Greenwood TW, Gilchrist AG. The effect of HBO_2 on wound healing following ionizing radiation. In: Trapp WC et al., editors. Proc of the 5th Int'l Congress on Hyperbaric Med. Vol.1. Burnaby (Canada): Simon Frazier Univ.; 1973. p. 253-63.

28. Greenwood TW, Gilchrist AG. Hyperbaric oxygen and wound healing in post-irradiation head and neck surgery. Br J Surg. 1973;60:394-7.

29. Gruber RP, Brinkley FB, Amato JJ, Mendelson JA. Hyperbaric oxygen and pedicle flaps, skin grafts, and burns. Plast Reconstr Surg. 1970;45:24-30.

30. Gruber RP, Heitkamp DH, Lawrence JB. Skin permeability to oxygen and hyperbaric oxygen. Arch Surg. 1970;101:69-70.

31. Gurtner GC, Jones GE, Neligan PC, et al. Intraoperative laser angiography using the SPY system: review of the literature and recommendations for use. Ann Surg Innov Res. 2013;7:1.

32. Habel DW. Surgical complications in irradiated patients. Arch Oto. 1967;82:382-6.

33. Hart GB, O'Reilly RR, Broussard ND, et al. Treatment of burns with hyperbaric oxygen. Surg Gyn Obst. 1974;139:693-6.

34. Hartwig J, Kohnlein HE, Scherer D. [The influence of hyperbaric oxygen therapy and Dextran 40 on the endangered survival of skin-pedicle flaps.] Chirurg. 1973;44(10):452-6. German.

35. Hunt TK, Pai MP. The effect of varying ambient oxygen tensions on wound metabolism and collagen synthesis. Surg Gyn Obstet. 1972;135:561-7.

36. Hunt TK, Van Winkle W. Fundamentals of wound management in surgery. In: Wound healing normal repair. New York: Appleton-Century-Crofts; 1976.

37. Hunt TK, Zederfeldt BH, Goldstick TK. Oxygen and healing. Am J Surg. 1969;118:521-5.

38. Hurn IL, Fischer JC, Arganese T, et al. Standardization of the dorsal rat flap model. Ann Plast Surg. 1984;2:210-3.

39. Hynes W. The 'blue flap'—a method of treatment. Brit J Plast Surg. 1950;4:166.

40. Jacobs BB, Thuning CA, Sacksteder MR, Warren J. Extended skin allograft survival in mice during prolonged exposure to hyperbaric oxygen. Transplantation. 1979;28:70-2.

41. Jurell G, Kaijser L. The influence of varying pressure and duration of treatment with hyperbaric oxygen on the survival of skin flaps. An experimental study. Scand J Plast Reconstr Surg. 1973;7:25-8.

42. Ketchum SA 3rd, Thomas AN, Hall AD. Angiographic studies of the effects of hyperbaric oxygen on burn wound revascularization. In: Wada J, Iwa T, editors. Proc of the 4th Int'l Congress on Hyperbaric Med. Baltimore: Williams and Wilkins; 1970. p. 388-94.

43. Kim SS, Kim D, Kim W, Baek S. Treatment of amputated digit distal to DIP joint. Plast Surg Forum. 1987;10:241.

43A. Kindwall E, Whelan H, editors. Hyperbaric Medicine Practice. 3rd ed. Flagstaff, AZ: Best Publishing Company; 2008.

44. Kivisaari J, Niinikoski J. Effects of hyperbaric oxygen and prolonged hypoxia on the healing of open wounds. Acta Chir Scand. 1975;141:14-9.

45. Knighton TR, Silver IA, Hunt TK. Regulation of wound healing angiogenesis: effect of oxygen gradient and inspired oxygen concentration. Surgery. 1981;90:262-9.

46. Körlof B, Ugland O. Flaps and flap necrosis. Acta Chir Scand. 1966;131:408-12.

47. Korn HN, Wheeler ES, Miller TA. Effect of hyperbaric oxygen on second degree burn wound healing. Arch Surg. 1977;122:732-37.

48. Kraut RA. Prophylactic hyperbaric oxygen to avoid osteoradionecrosis when extractions follow radiation therapy. Clin Rev Dent. 1985;7:17-20.

49. Kveton JF. Surgical management of osteoradionecrosis of the temporal bone. Otolaryngol Head Neck Surg. 1988;98:231-4.

50. McFarlane RM, DeYoung G, Henry RH. The design of a pedicle flap to study necrosis and its prevention. Plast Reconst Surg. 1965;35:177-82.

51. McFarlane RM, Heazy FC, Rodin A, et al. A study of the delay phenomenon in experimental pedicle flaps. Plast Reconst Surg. 1965;35:245-65.

52. McFarlane RM, Wermuth RE. The use of hyperbaric oxygen to prevent necrosis in experimental pedicle flaps and composite skin grafts. Plast Reconstr Surg. 1966;37:422-30.

53. McGraw JB, Myers B, Skanklin KD. The value of fluorescein in predicting viability of arterialized flaps. Plast Reconst Surg. 1977;60:710-9.

54. Mader JT. Phagocytic killing and hyperbaric oxygen. Antibacterial mechanisms. HBO_2 Review. 1981;2:27-49.

55. Mader JT, Brown GL, Guckian JC, et al. A mechanism for amelioration by HBO_2 of experimental staphylococcal osteomyelitis in rabbits. J Infect Dis. 1980;142:915-22.

56. Manson PN, IM MJ, Myers RA, Hoopes JE. Improved capillaries by hyperbaric oxygen in skin flaps. Surg Forum. 1980;31:564-6.

57. Marx RE. Osteoradionecrosis of the jaws: review update. HBO_2 Review. 1984;5:78-126.

58. Marx RE. Osteoradionecrosis. Part I. A new concept in its pathophysiology. J Oral Maxillofac Surg. 1983;41:283-8.

59. Marx RE. Osteoradionecrosis. Part II. A new concept in its treatment. J Oral Maxillofac Surg. 1983;41:351-7.

60. Marx RE, Ames JR. The use of hyperbaric oxygen therapy in bony reconstruction of the irradiated and tissue deficient patient. J Oral Maxillofac Surg. 1982;40:412-20.

61. Marx RE, Johnson RP, Kline SN. Prevention of osteoradionecrosis: a randomized prospective clinical trial of hyperbaric oxygen versus penicillin. J Am Dent Assoc. 1985;111:49-54.

62. Meltzer T, Myers B. The effect of hyperbaric oxygen on the bursting strength and rate of vascularization of skin wounds in rats. Amer Surgeon. 1986;52:659-62.

63. Mlodinow AS, Fine NA, Khavanin N, Kim JY. Risk factors for mastectomy flap necrosis following immediate tissue expander breast reconstruction. J Plast Hand Surg. 2014;48:322-6.

64. Monies-Chass I, Hashmonai M. Hyperbaric oxygen treatment as an adjunct to reconstructive vascular surgery in trauma. Injury. 1977;8:274-7.

65. Myers MB, Cherry G. Mechanisms of the delay phenomenon. Plast Reconstr Surg. 1969;44:52-7.

66. Myers MB, Cherry G. Enhancement of survival in devascularized pedicles by the use of phenoxybenzamine. Plast Reconst Surg. 1968;41:254-60.

67. Nemiroff PM, Lungu AP. The influence of hyperbaric oxygen and irradiation on vascularity in skin flaps: a controlled study. Surg Forum. 1987;38:565-7.

68. Nemiroff PM, Merwin GE, Brant T, Cassissi NJ. HBO_2 and irradiation on experimental skin flaps in rats. Surg Forum. 1984;35:549-50.

69. Nemiroff PM. Synergistic effects of pentoxifylline and hyperbaric oxygen on skin flaps. Arch Otolaryngol Head Neck Surg. 1988;114:977-81.

70. Nemiroff PM, Merwin GE, Brant T, Cassissi NJ. Effects of hyperbaric oxygen and irradiation on experimental flaps in rats. Otolaryngol Head Neck Surg. 1985;93:485-91.

71. Nemiroff PM, Ryback LP. Applications of hyperbaric oxygen for the otolaryngologist-head and neck surgeon. Am J Otolaryng. 1988;9:52-7.

72. Neubauer RA, Pinella J, Hill K, Bright DE. The use of hyperbaric oxygen in the successful re-anastomosis of the severed ear: three cases. Proc of EUBS Annual Meeting XIV; 1988 Sep 5-9.

73. Niinikoski J. Viability of ischemic skin in hyperbaric oxygen. Acta Chir Scand. 1970;136:567-8.

74. Niinikoski J, Hunt TK. Oxygen tension in human wounds. J Surg Res. 1972;12:77-82.

75. Nylander G, Nordström H, Eriksson E. Effects of hyperbaric oxygen on oedema formation after a scald burn. Burns. 1980;10:193-6.

76. Perrins DJD. Hyperbaric oxygenation of skin flaps. Br J Plast Surg. 1966;19:440.

77. Perrins DJD. Influence of hyperbaric oxygen on the survival of split skin grafts. Lancet. 1967;1:806-71.

78. Perrins DJD. The effect of hyperbaric oxygen on ischemic skin flaps. In: Grabb WC, Myers MB, editors. Skin flaps. Boston: Little Brown and Co., Inc.; 1975. p. 53-63.

79. Perrins DJD, Davis JC. Enhancement of healing in soft tissue wounds. In: Davis JC, Hunt TK, editors. Hyperbaric oxygen therapy. Bethesda (MD): Undersea Medical Society; 1977. p. 229-48.

80. Reinisch JF. Pathophysiology of skin flap circulation. Plast Reconstr Surg. 1974;54:585.

81. Reinisch JF. The role of arteriovenous anastomoses in skin flaps. In: Grabb WC, Myers MB, editors. Skin flaps. Boston: Little Brown and Co.; 1975. p. 81-92.

82. Rubin JS, Marzella L, Myers RA, et al. Effects of hyperbaric oxygen on the take of composite skin grafts in rabbit ears. J Hyperbaric Med. 1988;3(2):79-88.

83. Sasaki A, Fukuda O, Soeda S. Attempts to increase the surviving length in skin flaps by a moist environment. Plast Reconstr Surg. 1979;64:526-31.

84. Sasaki A, Harii K. Lack of effect of isoxsuprine on experimental random flaps in the rat. Plast Reconstr Surg. 1980;66:105-8.

85. Sheffield PJ. Tissue oxygen measurements with respect to soft tissue wound healing with normobaric and hyperbaric oxygen. HBO_2 Rev. 1985;6(1):18-46.

86. Sheffield PJ, Dunn JM. Continuous monitoring of tissue oxygen tension during hyperbaric oxygen therapy. In: Smith G, editor. Proc of the 6th Int'l Congress on Hyperbaric Med. Aberdeen (GB): Aberdeen University Press; 1977. p.125-9.

87. Sheffield PJ, Workman WT. Noninvasive tissue oxygen measurements in patients administered normobaric and hyperbaric oxygen by mask. HBO_2 Rev. 1985;6:47-63.

88. Shulman AG, Kron HL. Influence of hyperbaric oxygen and multiple skin allografts on the healing of skin wounds. Surg. 1967;62:1051-8.

89. Silver IA. The measurement of oxygen tension in healing tissues. In: Herz H, editor. Progress in respiration research. Vol III. Basel (CH): Skarger; 1969. p. 124-5.

90. Silver IA. Oxygenation and epithelialization. In: Maibach HI and Rovee DT, editors. Epidermal wound healing. Chicago: Year Book Medical Publishers; 1972. p. 291-305.

91. Snyder S, Beshlian K, Hampson N. Hyperbaric oxygen and reduction mammaplasty in the previously irradiated breast. Plast Reconstr Surg. 2010;125(6):255e-257e.

92. Stong BC, Jacono AA. Effect of perioperative hyperbaric oxygen on bruising in face-lifts. Arch Facial Plast Surg. 2010;12(5):356-8.

93. Tan CM, Im MJ, Myers RA, Hoopes JE. Effect of hyperbaric oxygen and hyperbaric air on survival of island skin flaps. Plast Reconstr Surg. 1974;73:27-30.

94. Thom SR. Hyperbaric oxygen: its mechanisms and efficacy. Plast Reconstr Surg. 2011;127:131S.

95. Tobey RE, Kelly JF. Osteoradionecrosis of the jaws. Otolaryngol Clin North Am. 1979;12:183-6.

96. Wald HI, Georgiade NG, Angelillo DDS, Saltzman HA. Effect of intensive hyperbaric therapy on survival of experimental skin flaps in rats. Surg Forum. 1968;19:497.

97. Welsh F, Matos L. Medical hyperbaric therapy. Ohio State Med J. 1980;76:582-5.

98. Wilcox JW, Kolodny SC. Acceleration of healing of maxillary and mandibular osteotomies by use of hyperbaric oxygen. Oral Surg. 1976;41:423-9.

99. Winter GD, Perrins DJD. Effects of hyperbaric oxygen treatment on epidermal regeneration. In: Wada J, Iwa T, editors. Proc of the 4th Int'l Congress on Hyperbaric Med. Baltimore: Williams and Wilkins; 1970. p. 363-8.

100. Zamboni WA, Roth AC, Russell RC, et al. Effect of acute hyperbaric oxygen therapy on axial pattern skin flap survival when administered during and after total ischemia. J Reconstr Microsurg. 1989;5:343-7.

CHAPTER 29 CHAPTER

Radiation Injury to Tissue

CHAPTER TWENTY-NINE OVERVIEW

The Unique Character of Radiation Injury 727
Angiogenesis and Fibroplasia in Radiated Tissue 729
Protocols for Hyperbaric Oxygen When Surgery is Performed in Radiated Tissue 733
Mechanisms of Hyperbaric-Oxygen-Induced Angiogenesis and Fibroplasia ... 734
Clinical Applications of Hyperbaric Oxygen 738
- Bony Reconstruction of the Jaws 738
- Soft-Tissue Flaps 739
- Tooth Removal 744
- Osseointegrated Dental Implants 746

Osteoradionecrosis (Orn) 751
Treatment Protocol for Osteoradionecrosis 756
- Stage I 757
- Stage II 758
- Stage III 763

Cost Analysis of Osteoradionecrosis Treatment 769
The Relationship of Hyperbaric Oxygen to Oral Cancer 770
- Animal Studies 771
- Human Studies 773

References 774

Radiation Injury to Tissue

Robert E. Marx

THE UNIQUE CHARACTER OF RADIATION INJURY

The effect of hyperbaric oxygen (HBO_2) on tissues radiated to a dose of more than 5,000 cGy (centigray) is one of capillary angiogenesis and fibroplasia. This effect alone is unique in therapeutics. The mechanism by which hyperbaric oxygen accomplishes this is complex but is related to normal wound revascularization and healing. This mechanism is made possible only because of the unique pattern of tissue injury that radiation creates – a pattern which does not permit the normal revascularization that occurs in other tissue injuries.

When tissue is radiated in the treatment of a malignancy, normal tissue cells are also damaged. In spite of the concerted efforts of radiation therapists to enhance tumor kill and reduce normal nontumor damage such as fractionation, hyperfractionation, supervoltage, beam collimation, charged particles (proton beam), etc., normal tissue is nevertheless damaged.(10,25) The nontumor cells that are in the field of radiation are heterogeneous in their type (fibroblasts, endothelium, muscle, nerve, etc.) and heterogeneous in their sensitivity to radiation. This is partially because of the inherent radiation sensitivity of different cell types. In descending order of sensitivity are tumor cells, endothelium, fibroblasts, muscle cells, and nerve cells. Varying effects may also be seen because radiation may either kill any cell type outright or inflict lethal damage so that it dies later. Radiation may also incapacitate a cell so that it does not produce daughter cells or collagen. The surviving cells may produce defective collagen or defective regulatory enzymes. Individual cells may totally escape damage. The result is a residual tissue which develops a progressive loss of vascularity and cellularity over time as cells live out their life-span and are not replaced or fail to contribute to tissue integrity.

The progressive radiation fibrosis and capillary loss with time have been shown to be almost linear and are an inescapable aftermath of therapeutic radiation (Figure 1).(23,25)

It may even progress to spontaneous radionecrosis of soft tissue or bone if the radiation dose has been sufficiently high. Breakdown may also occur as a complication of surgical wounding when the tissue is required to meet the increased demands of healing.

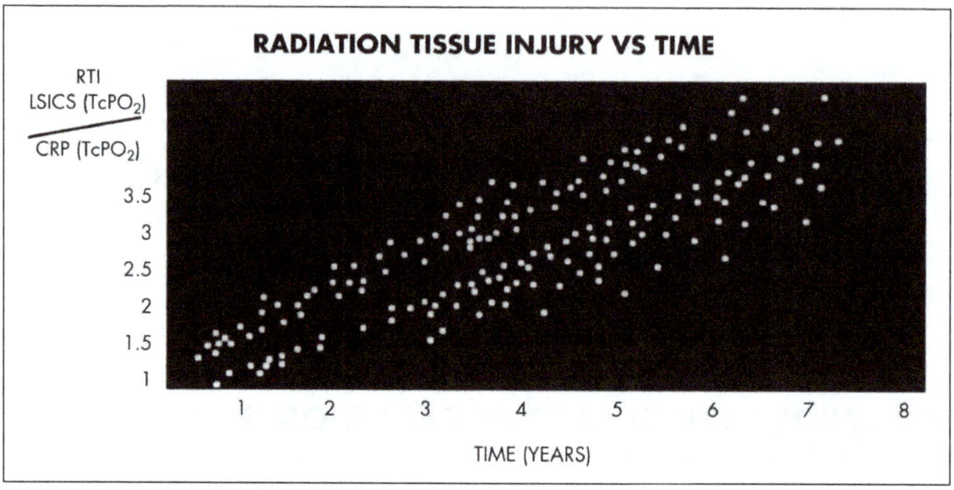

Figure 1. Inverse of capillary density curve shows an increasing radiation tissue hypovascularity with time. It is due to the late cellular effects which stop endothelial cells, and fibroblasts in particular, from replenishing their populations and maintaining sound structures. Therefore they lose their prime function of providing vessels for perfusion and collagen synthesis for tissue repair. The resultant tissue has been termed "three-H" tissue.[23,25-26] It is hypovascular, hypocellular, and hypoxic. Importantly, it will continue to become more so with time (Figures 2 and 3).

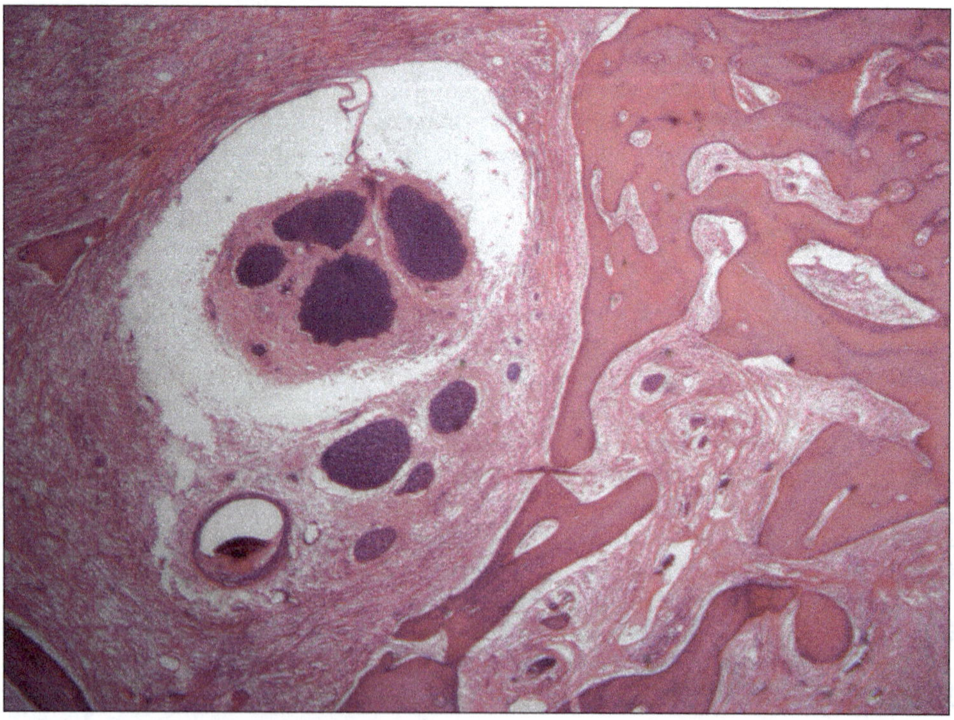

Figure 2. Radiation-induced vascular thrombosis.

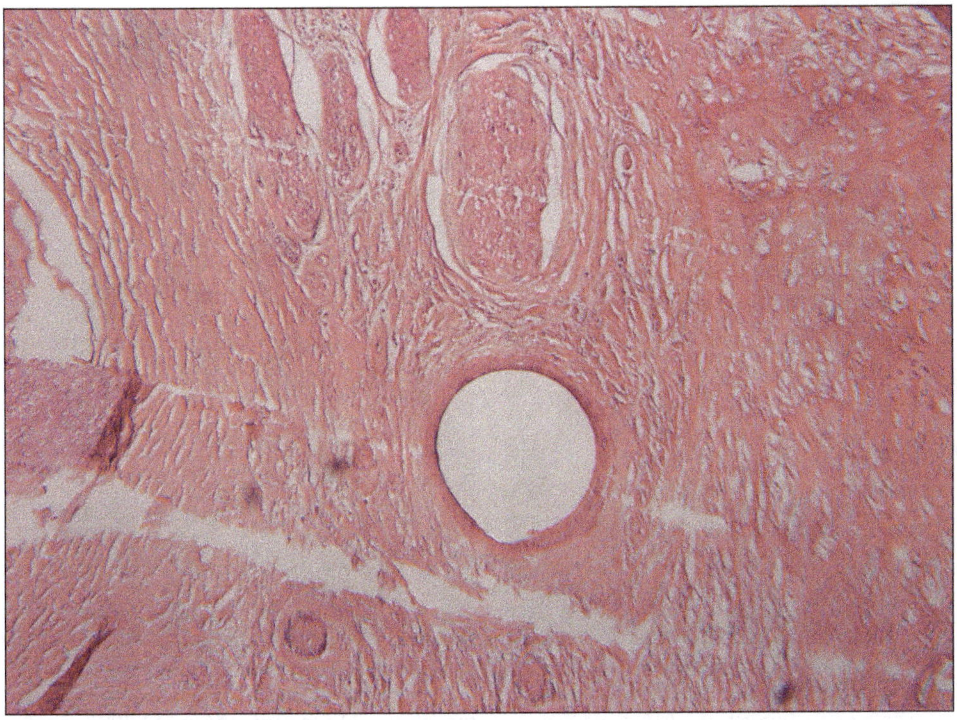

Figure 3. Radiation-induced hypovascular-hypocellular-hypoxic tissue (three-H tissue).

ANGIOGENESIS AND FIBROPLASIA IN RADIATED TISSUE

A hyperbaric chamber, per se, is not the therapeutic agent which produces angiogenesis and fibroplasia in radiated tissue. Oxygen is actually the therapeutic drug, with the chamber serving merely as a dosing device. Oxygen at normobaric (1 ATA) pressure has been shown incapable of producing angiogenesis (Figure 4, Figure 5) or fibroplasia (Figure 6, Figure 7) in animal models.[24]

It seems that increasing pressures to the tested pressure of 2.4 ATA brings the dosage of oxygen into a therapeutic range while avoiding toxicity. Thus, oxygen, like any other medically useful drug, can be applied in insufficient dosage and as such may be subtherapeutic, or it can be given in too high a dose and thus produce toxic symptoms.

The pressures and exposure times necessary to create angiogenesis and fibroplasia in radiated tissue have been elucidated.[23-25] Initially, studies documented both angiogenesis and fibroplasia in radiated head and neck cancer patients through biopsy of human tissues before and after hyperbaric oxygen (Figure 8, Figure 9).[23] Later, human transcutaneous oxygen measurements and animal studies traced the time course of this angiogenesis and fibroplasia (Figure 10).

As seen in Figure 10, angiogenesis and fibroplasia develop in response to HBO_2 of 2.4 ATA, 90 minutes each session, 5 days a week over a 20-session treatment course. Uncomplicated radiated tissue, after the usual dose of 6,000 to 8,000 cGy for malignant tumors, exists with a capillary density only 20% to 40% of that in nonradiated tissue.[24,26] This tissue is hypocellular, hypovascular, and measurably hypoxic and is referred to as "three-H" tissue. The first response of this "three-H" tissue to HBO_2 is known as the "lag phase" because no measurable change is seen with the crudeness of a transcutaneous oxygen monitor.[26]

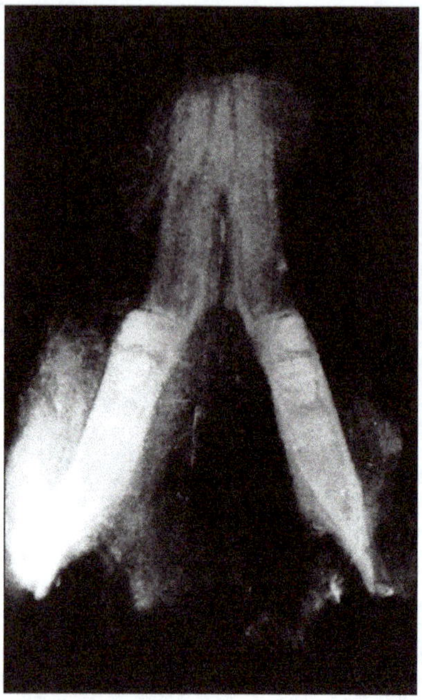

Figure 4. Tissue angiogram of radiation-induced three-H tissue in a rabbit model after 20 exposures to 1 ATA of 100% oxygen. Little angiogenesis is noted.

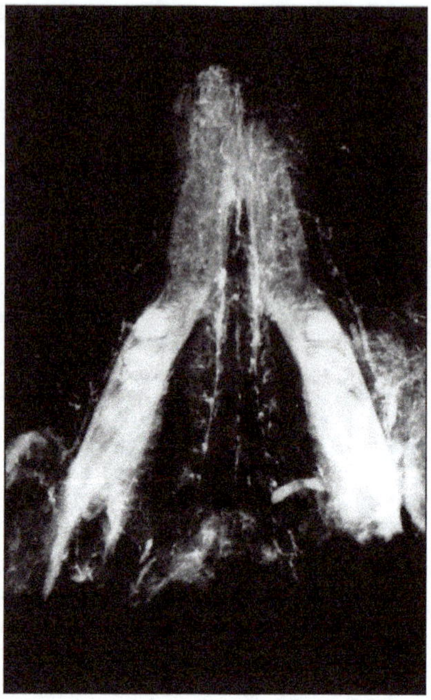

Figure 5. Tissue angiogram of radiation-induced three-H tissue in same rabbit model after 20 exposures to 2.4 ATA 100% oxygen. A measured eightfold increase in vascular density is noted.

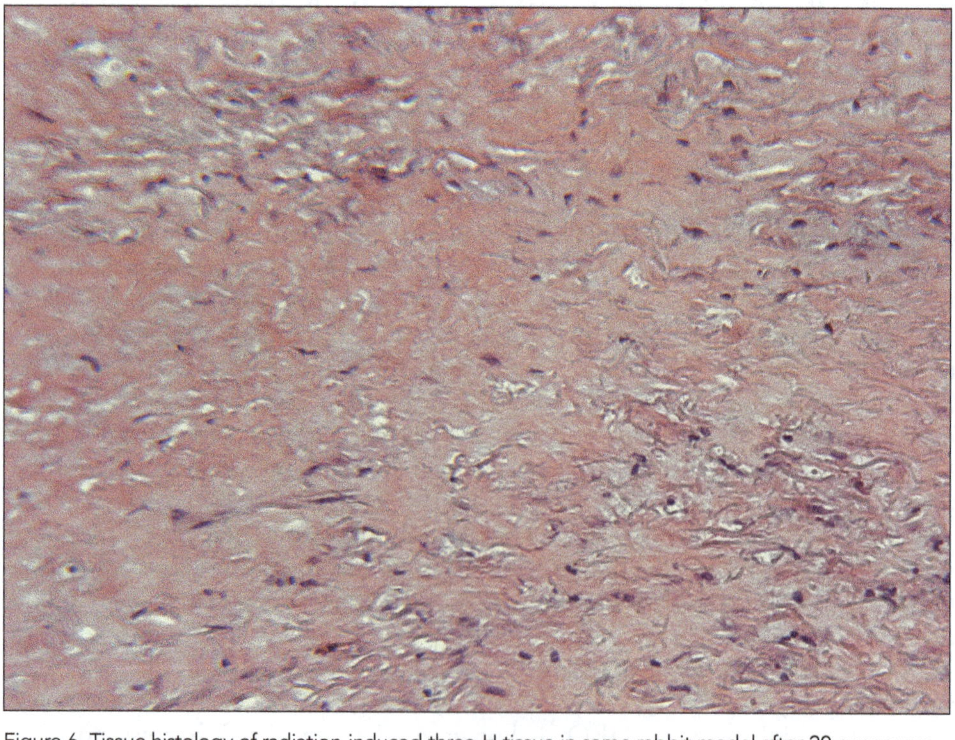

Figure 6. Tissue histology of radiation-induced three-H tissue in same rabbit model after 20 exposures to 1 ATA of 100% oxygen. Marked hypovascularity within a fibrotic stroma.

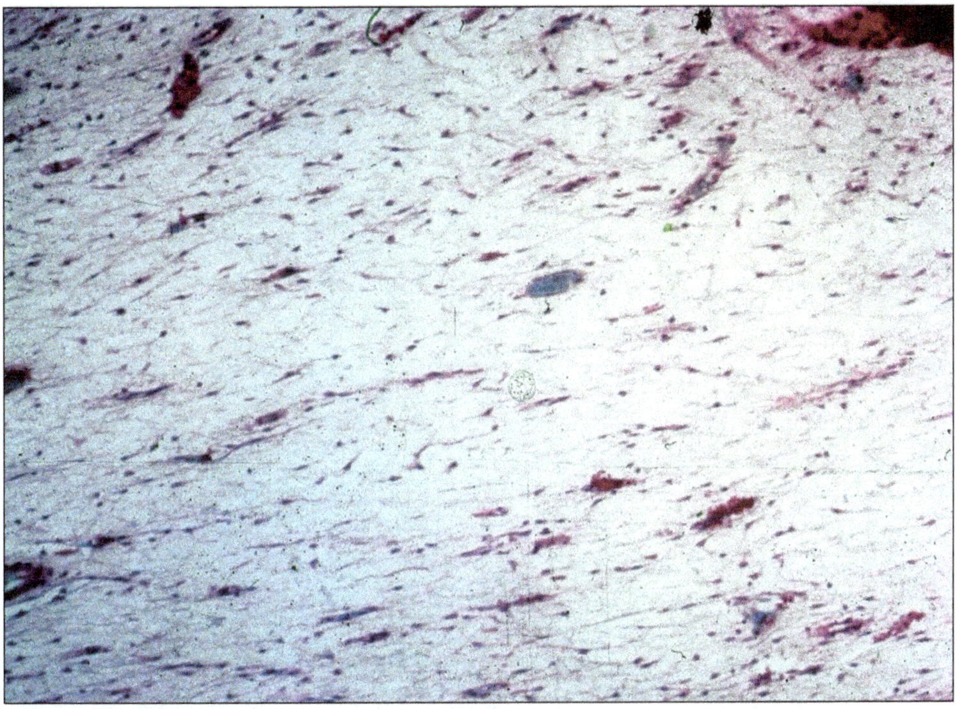

Figure 7. Tissue histology of radiation-induced three-H tissue in same rabbit model after 20 exposures to 2.4 ATA of 100% oxygen. Increased vascular density, reduced fibrosis, and increased cellularity are seen.

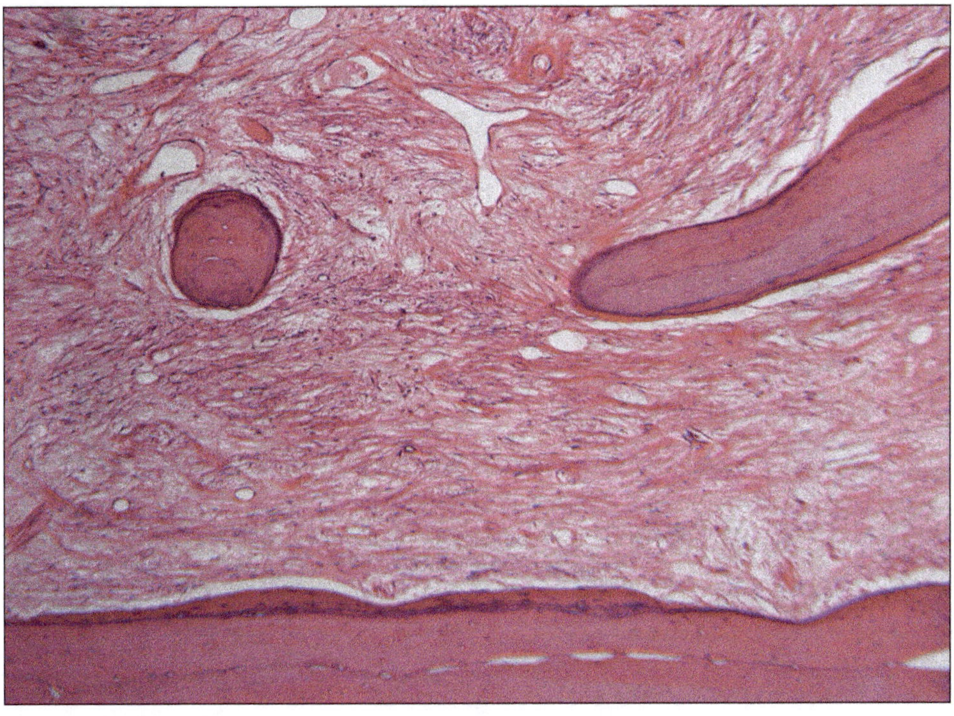

Figure 8. Human tissue histology of radiated tissue prior to hyperbaric oxygen exposures. Three-H picture is evident.

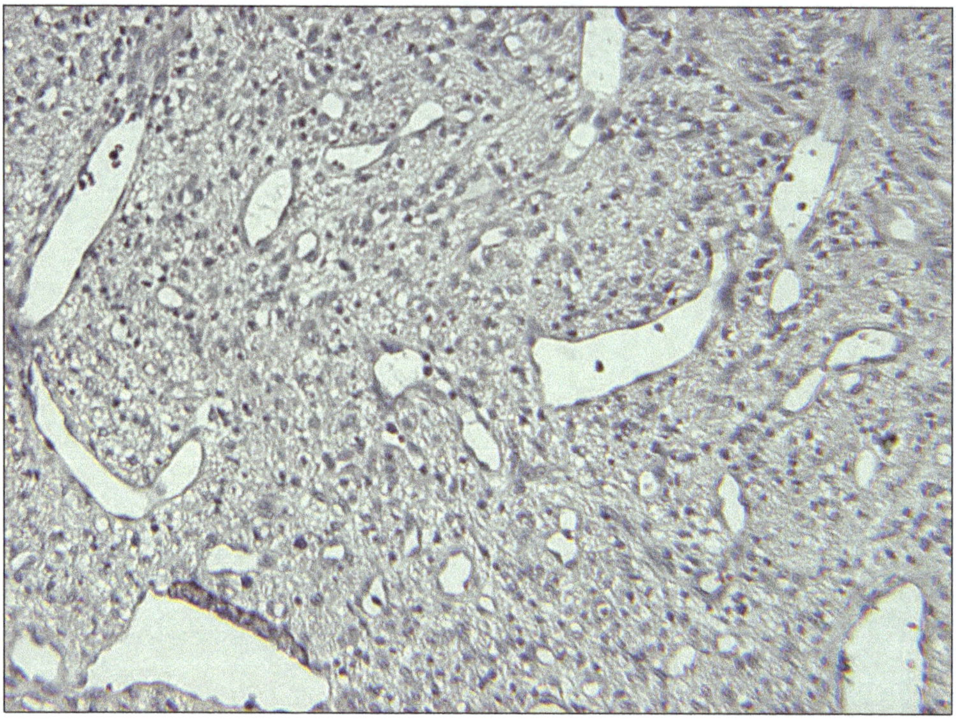

Figure 9. Human tissue histology of radiated tissue after 20 hyperbaric oxygen exposures at 2.4 ATA. Angiogenesis and fibroplasia are apparent.

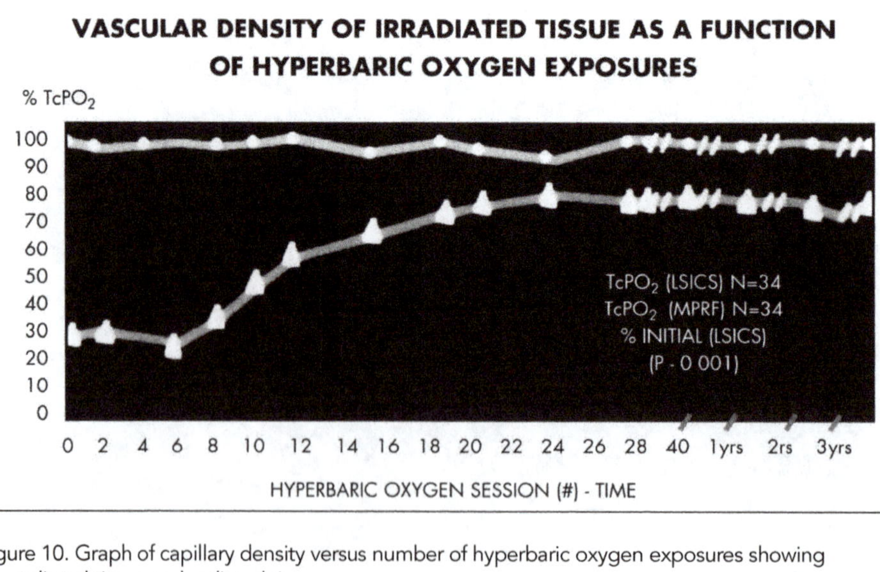

Figure 10. Graph of capillary density versus number of hyperbaric oxygen exposures showing nonradiated tissue and radiated tissue.

However, histologic studies have shown capillary budding and cellular collagen synthesis. The radiated tissue's response begins with macrophage activity, fibroblastic collagen production, and endothelial proliferation, which occur during the first six to eight hyperbaric oxygen exposures.

After eight hyperbaric treatments, the curve in Figure 10 begins a steep upward deflection known as the "rapid rise phase."[26] This rise is caused by the proliferation of lumenized and functional capillaries, which is measured by the transcutaneous monitor as increased perfusion due to an increased capillary density. Histologic evidence shows a geometric development of capillaries from the few preexisting ones. That is, one capillary buds into two, those two into four, and onward at a rate to the exponent of two. This vascular proliferation continues until 20 sessions of hyperbaric oxygen are attained, after which it levels off to between 75% and 85% of that seen in nonradiated tissue. This leveling off of angiogenic response is termed the "plateau phase."

The plateau phase consists of maximum revascularization where the stimulus for further angiogenesis ceases. Histologically, it is associated with an observed reduction in tissue macrophages, capillary budding, and collagen synthesis as compared to the "lag" and "rapid rise" phases. Most importantly, as illustrated in Figure 10, the angiogenic effect is maintained for at least four years. Those patients who were restudied demonstrated the same level of angiogenesis after four years as they had immediately after their hyperbaric oxygen treatment. Apparently, the new vessels induced by hyperbaric oxygen do not involute after cessation of HBO_2 treatment any faster than vessels involute at the normal rate of aging. In fact, surgeries in radiated tissue as much as 25 years after this complete HBO_2 protocol have shown healing equal to a nonradiated tissue, implying a nearly permanent tissue improvement.

Also observed in Figure 10 is the lack of any response in nonradiated tissue. Hyperbaric oxygen does not induce a supervascularization in nonradiated, otherwise normal tissue and therefore cannot be expected to accelerate healing in tissue which does not have a compromised wound healing potential.

PROTOCOLS FOR HYPERBARIC OXYGEN WHEN SURGERY IS PERFORMED IN RADIATED TISSUE

From the research data illustrated in Figure 10, and from a clinical experience of over 30 years, the most effective protocol for the application of HBO_2 as an adjunct to healing in radiated tissue is the following:

1. Twenty sessions prior to surgical wounding
2. Surgical wounding
3. Ten sessions after surgical wounding

A hyperbaric treatment is defined as breathing 100% oxygen for 90 minutes at 2.4 ATA.

Some chamber facilities prefer to use, or can only use, 100% oxygen at 2.0 ATA. This may be less than ideal but is clinically acceptable if, when using the reduced pressure, an increased exposure time of 120 minutes is offered. This protocol has produced clinically similar results to the 2.4 ATA protocol but has been less used. Recent animal studies by the author indicate increasing tissue response up to 3 ATA, but 3 ATA is potentially too toxic to be of clinical use for multiple treatments. The 2.4 ATA protocol has been studied extensively and has been proven effective.

Similarly, some have suggested a twice-daily session of HBO_2 to reduce the time of overall treatment, but this concept is empirical and is untested. A twice-a-day protocol is not recommended because it is both unproven and theoretically may afford insufficient time for the radiated tissue to respond with the angiogenesis and fibroplasia required of tissue healing in radiated tissue.

MECHANISMS OF HYPERBARIC-OXYGEN-INDUCED ANGIOGENESIS AND FIBROPLASIA

The mechanism by which hyperbaric oxygen achieves angiogenesis and fibroplasia in radiated tissue has been studied[26] and found to be stimulated by a similar oxygen-gradient phenomenon that Knighton, Silver, and Hunt have found to be central in the angiogenesis and fibroplasia of normal wound healing.[13,15,38] Radiated tissue does not spontaneously revascularize as do other wounded tissues because of the unique physics and pattern of tumoricidal radiation delivery. Normal wounds have a central area of tissue injury or hematoma surrounded by relatively normal tissue with normal perfusion. Therefore, the oxygen tension in the central area of the wound is extremely low (often 0 to 5 mmHg) and the adjacent tissue is normal (approximately 50 to 60 mmHg). The oxygen gradient is thus naturally steep across a short distance. Such steep oxygen gradients have been shown to be the physio-chemotactic factor attracting wound regulating macrophages to a wound.[14,38] Steep oxygen gradients, along with the lactate, iron, and acid inherent in wounds, stimulate macrophages to secrete vascular endothelial growth factor (VEGF) and basic fibroblast growth factor (bFGF) which in turn promote the capillary budding and collagen synthesis of wound healing.[14]

Radiated tissue does not spontaneously revascularize because the wounding pattern is so diffuse that only shallow oxygen gradients are created (i.e., less than 20 mm Hg). Therefore, the physiochemical response which identifies an injured area as a wound does not develop, and the body, in a sense, does not recognize the radiation injury as a wound. In fact, as the late radiation effect on cells makes the tissue worse with time, the continuation and worsening of the "three-H" pattern make the natural tissue oxygen gradients even less (Figure 1).

The diffuse pattern of radiation injury is created chiefly by the isodose concept of tumoricidal radiotherapy. That is, a tumor is conceptualized as a spheroidal mass with the greatest number of target cells in the diameter of its equator. A greater dose or boost dose is given to the tumor's center. At incremental distances from the equator, the tumor's cellular mass is less, and therefore the delivered radiation dose is less. This progressively diminishing dose from the tumor's center to the periphery of the planned radiated area creates a gradual lessening of tissue injury and therefore a gradual or shallow oxygen gradient. The divergence of the radiation beam from its source further contributes to this shallow oxygen gradient. Even with attempts at higher speed emissions (super- or megavoltage) and collimated beams there is some divergence. This creates greater cellular damage at the center of the radiation port than at the periphery.

The effect of hyperbaric oxygen on the diffuse wounding pattern of radiated tissue is illustrated in Figures 11 through 15.

Studies have identified that the center of an uncomplicated radiation-injured area has oxygen tensions around 5 to 10 mmHg. This value is not far above the 3 mmHg of oxygen tension at which spontaneous wound breakdown is thought to occur. Measurements taken at one-centimeter increments from the center show a gradual improvement in tissue oxygen tensions until one reaches the limits of the radiated field, where the normal 55 to 60 mmHg oxygen tension is found (Figure 11). During exposure of the patient to hyperbaric oxygen at 2.4 ATA, measurements indicate a seven- to tenfold rise at each one-centimeter increment, including the nonradiated tissue outside the radiated field. Since each incremental area shows an increase in oxygen tension, the underlying shallow oxygen gradient is magnified into a steep oxygen gradient (Figure 12). In addition, at every increment, increased oxygen is available at the cellular level. After 10 exposures, when the radiated tissue is in the early portion of the rapid rise phase, the oxygen gradients move centrally, indicating that much of the angiogenesis comes from outside of the radiated field (Figure 13). After 18 exposures, when the radiated tissue is in the later portion of the rapid rise phase (Figure 14), the oxygen gradient is not only seen to move more centrally but is eliminated at the outer areas. This indicates that the bulk of the angiogenesis comes from outside of the radiated field and suggests that angiogenesis in that area eliminates the oxygen gradient altogether. After 20 to 24 exposures, oxygen gradients are either eliminated or are so small that gradients above 20 mmHg cannot be achieved even with hyperbaric oxygen (Figure 15). Thus, hyperbaric oxygen creates steep oxygen gradients in radiated tissues which cannot develop them naturally as do other wounds. These steep oxygen gradients then trigger the recognition of the radiated tissue as a wound and initiate the series of biochemical steps seen in normal tissue angiogenesis. The angiogenesis induced by hyperbaric oxygen remains under the same regulatory control as normal wound angiogenesis so that when sufficient capillary perfusion develops to eliminate oxygen gradients, the biochemical messenger-response sequence shuts off and overangiogenesis is prevented. It is important to emphasize that HBO_2 stimulates angiogenesis to create a vascular architecture of 75% to 85% that of nonradiated tissue. This seems to hinge on the fact that angiogenesis shuts off when oxygen gradients dip below a fixed point (suggested to be 20 mmHg), not necessarily when the gradient is absolutely zero.[34-35]

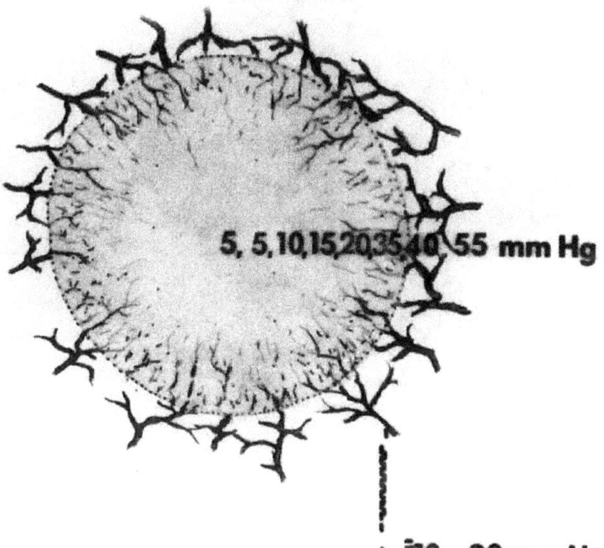

Figure 11. Shallow oxygen tension gradients can be measured within a radiated tissue field. Such shallow oxygen gradients prevent initiation of revascularization.

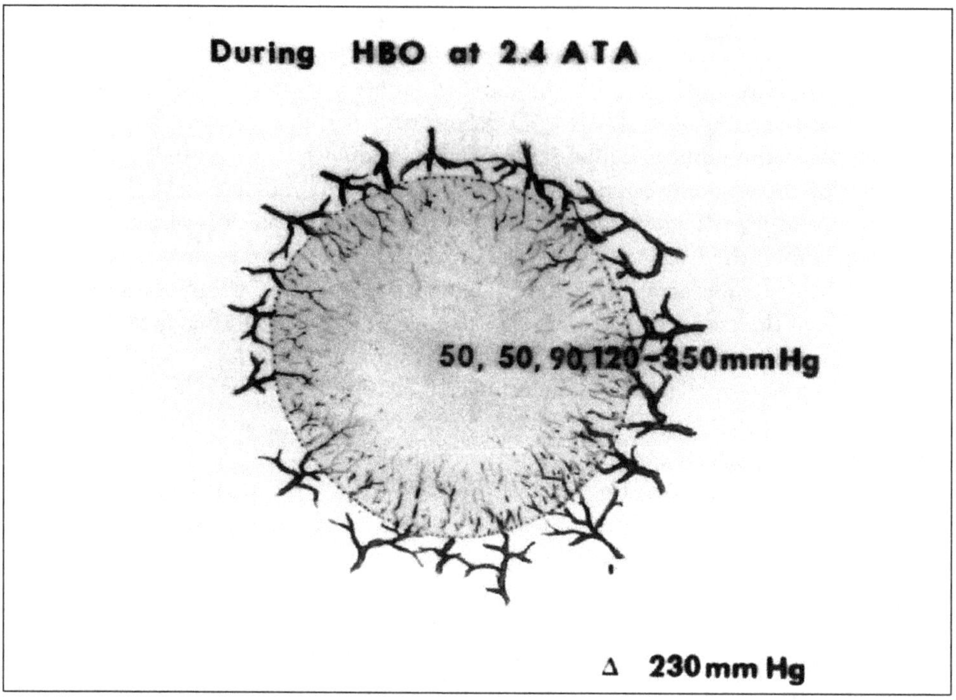

Figure 12. Steep oxygen gradients can be measured within a radiated tissue during hyperbaric oxygen exposures. The creation of oxygen gradients in excess of 20 mmHg is theorized to initiate angiogenesis.

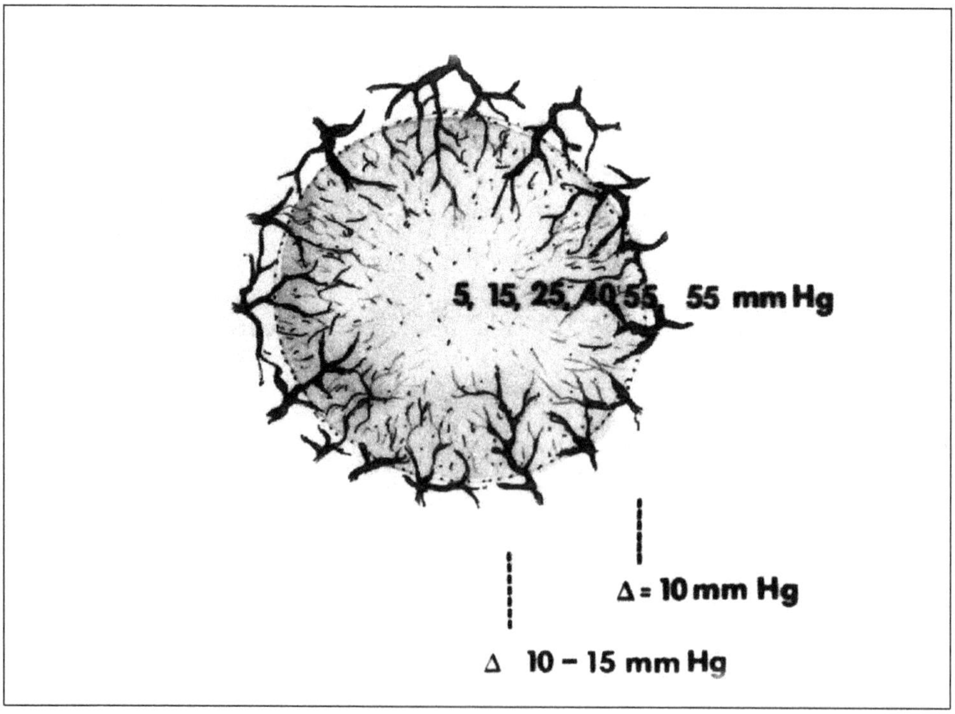

Figure 13. After 10 hyperbaric oxygen exposures, oxygen gradients are observed to move centrally indicating an angiogenesis front from the periphery and the deep wound margin.

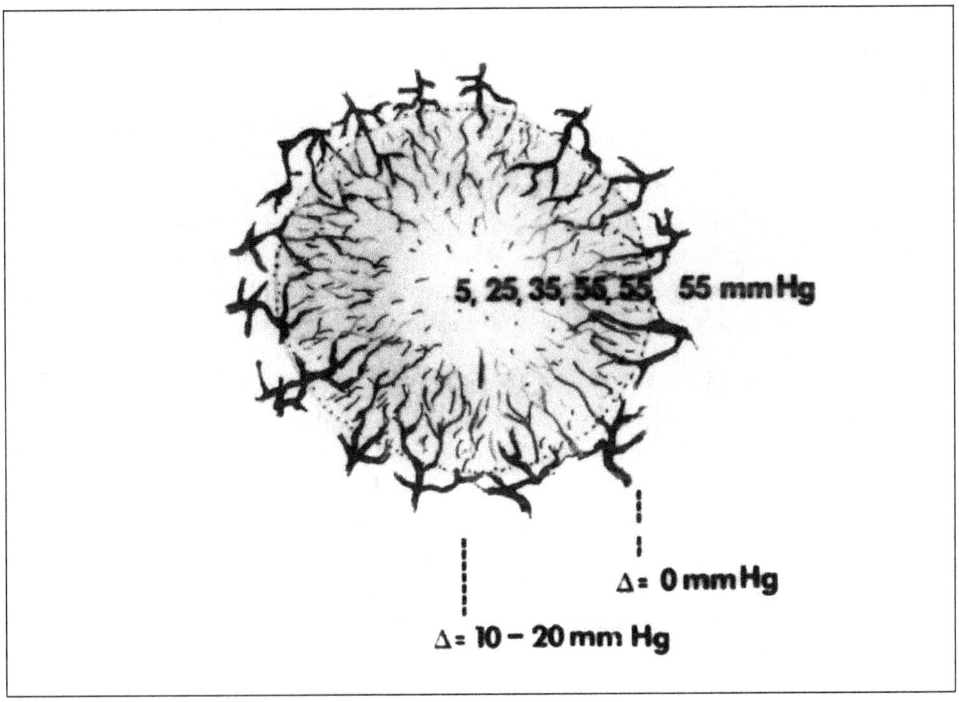

Figure 14. After 18 hyperbaric oxygen exposures, oxygen gradients are observed to continue to move centrally and are actually eliminated at the periphery.

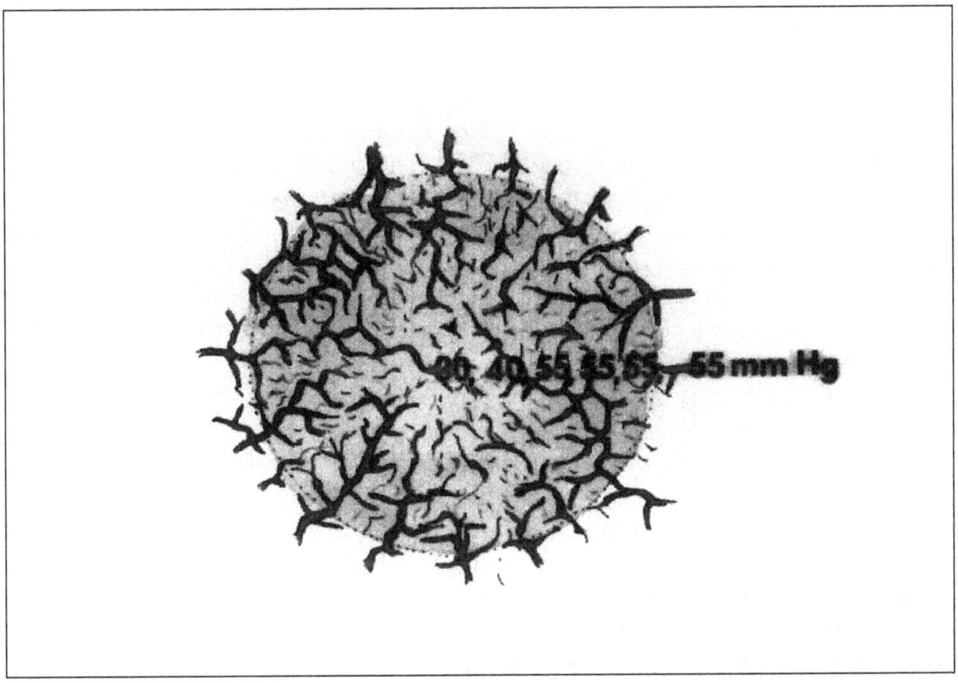

Figure 15. After 24 hyperbaric oxygen exposures, oxygen gradients were either eliminated or reduced to a point where gradients above 20 mmHg can no longer be achieved, even under hyperbaric conditions, and thus further angiogenesis ceases.

This mechanism may also explain why HBO_2 produces angiogenesis in certain other nonradiated wounds such as diabetic ulcers, crush injuries, failing flaps, etc. Compromised wounds have in common a lack of steep oxygen gradients. A notable example is the diabetic ulcer, which has a similarly diffuse, hypoxic vascular pattern due to its microangiopathy.

In nonradiated, noncompromised wounded tissue, there is already a steep oxygen gradient. HBO_2 only adds to the steepness of the gradient which is already producing a maximal stimulus, and the capacity for further response is lost. Since oxygen gradients stimulate angiogenesis, rather than increased oxygen availability, a mere increase in oxygen availability will not enhance wound healing in normal tissue.

CLINICAL APPLICATIONS OF HYPERBARIC OXYGEN

The protocol of 20 sessions of HBO_2 prior to surgery and 10 sessions afterwards (the 20/10 protocol) is the one most commonly used for surgery in uncomplicated radiated tissues. A different and more directed protocol is used in more serious situations where frank soft-tissue necrosis and/or osteoradionecrosis is present. Nevertheless, the 20/10 protocol has now been studied and found effective with randomized, prospective studies in at least three areas of head and neck postradiation surgery: bone graft reconstruction, soft-tissue vascular flaps, and tooth removal. Therefore, it is presently the definitive protocol whenever any elective surgery or wounding is performed within radiated tissues. However, although this protocol prevents wound healing complications, it should be noted that this protocol should not be labeled as a prevention protocol. It is actually a treatment protocol treating a radiation injury.

Bony Reconstruction of the Jaws

Some of the first experiences with hyperbaric oxygen involved jaw surgery and reconstruction.(17) In its early application, hyperbaric oxygen was used only after surgery to oxygenate tissue and enhance healing.(19) Early workers empirically applied hyperbaric oxygen in the postoperative phase because of an insufficient knowledge concerning its mechanism, time course, and the basic tissue angiogenesis response.(11,19) Results were disappointing, as one might anticipate,(11,19) until Marx and Ames focused the attention of hyperbaric oxygen on the preoperative phase.(23) Since then, Marx and Johnson,(25) Marx, Johnson, and Kline,(27) and Marx, Ehler, et al.(24) have elucidated the mechanisms and time course of angiogenesis and fibroplasia as discussed earlier.

The importance of preoperative HBO_2 relates to the basic biology of bone graft healing. Hyperbaric oxygen has literally revolutionized facial bone reconstruction of the radiated patient because it has made outcomes predictable and functional. The patient's healing is less complicated. Prior to the regular use of the 20/10 hyperbaric oxygen protocol, mandibular reconstruction success rates were 40% to 50%.(1,16) With the use of the 20/10 hyperbaric oxygen protocol, success rates meeting 6 rigid criteria have been 90% to 93%(23,26) (Table 1, Table 2). The six criteria are (1) restoration of jaw continuity, (2) restoration of alveolar bone height, (3) alveolar bone width suitable for dental implants, (4) restoration of arch form, (5) maintenance of bone (minimum 18 months), and (6) restoration of facial contours.

Our group conducted a controlled, randomized, prospective study of specific hemimandibular jaw reconstructions in tissue beds radiated to greater than 6,400 cGy. With 485 patients in the hyperbaric group, as compared to 210 patients in the non-HBO_2 group, the complication rate was 8% versus 23% respectively, and the

TABLE 1. HEMI-MANDIBULAR RECONSTRUCTIONS IN RADIATED TISSUE

	N	Complications	Met Criteria	% of Success
Non-HBO_2	210	48 (23%)	1331	(62.3%)
HBO_2	485	30 (8%)	451	(93%)

TABLE 2. SIX CRITERIA TO MEASURE "SUCCESS" IN JAW RECONSTRUCTION

1. Restoration of Jaw Continuity	4. Restoration of Arch Form
2. Restoration of Alveolar Height	5. Maintenance of Bone
3. Restoration of Alveolar Width Suitable for Dental Implants	6. Restoration of Facial Contours

percentage meeting the six rigid success criteria was 93% versus 62.3% respectively (Table 1, Table 2, Figure 16, Figure 17, Figure 18.)

The reason for increased success in the hyperbaric oxygen group relates directly to the induced angiogenesis and fibroplasia. Live bone cell transplantation into HBO_2-treated tissue produces a greater survival of cellular elements and greater bone formation. Such grafts are known to undergo a two-phased regeneration into a functional bone ossicle. The first phase requires a vascular tissue bed to support bone cell survival and the production of osteoid and mineralized early bone. The second phase, which is a bone remodeling/maturation phase, requires a vascular and cellular tissue bed. The vascularity supports the metabolic activity of the bone resorption, bone apposition, bone mineralization sequence inherent in remodeling. Cellularity supplies a cell population of inducible cells which develop into endosteum and periosteum in the grafts (Figure 19, Figure 20).

It is endosteum and periosteum which also make the graft long lasting and capable of withstanding the functional demands of chewing, speech, dentures, and dental implants.

Soft-Tissue Flaps

Extirpative cancer surgery removes significant soft tissue, while radiation more subtly necroses and contracts soft tissue. Therefore, pedicled myocutaneous or free microvascular flaps are often required to reconstruct such defects. Although these flaps will bring with them their own blood supply, they nevertheless must adhere to and heal into the hypovascular-hypocellular-hypoxic radiated tissue. Use of such flaps does not eliminate the need for the hyperbaric oxygen 20/10 protocol. Flaps which bring their own blood supply do not increase the blood supply of the radiated tissue into which they heal. If bone graft placement is required into an area of flap and radiated tissue, the flap tissue will support bone regeneration, but the radiated tissue will not. Use of the 20/10 hyperbaric oxygen protocol, however, will support bone graft healing in all previously radiated tissue and therefore make reconstruction of such patients possible.

Our department at the University of Miami has accomplished a detailed, randomized, prospective study assessing three aspects of wound complications related to soft-tissue flaps and wound healing: wound dehiscence, wound infection, and delayed healing. Two hundred and forty patients were divided into two groups of 120 each.

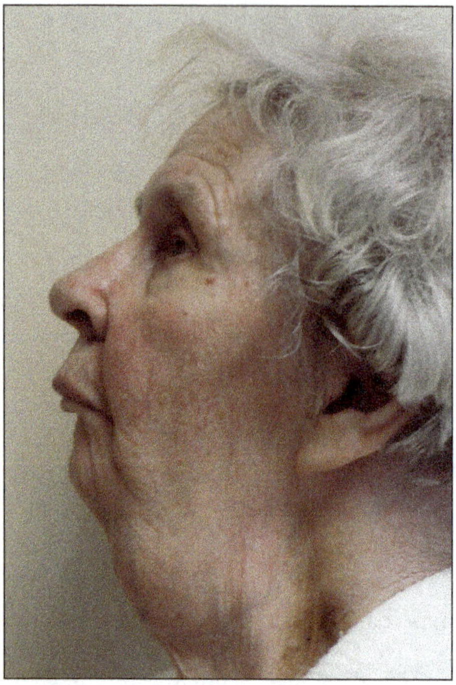

Figure 16. Radiated cancer patient with hemimandibular defect before bone graft reconstruction supported by the 20/10 hyperbaric oxygen protocol.

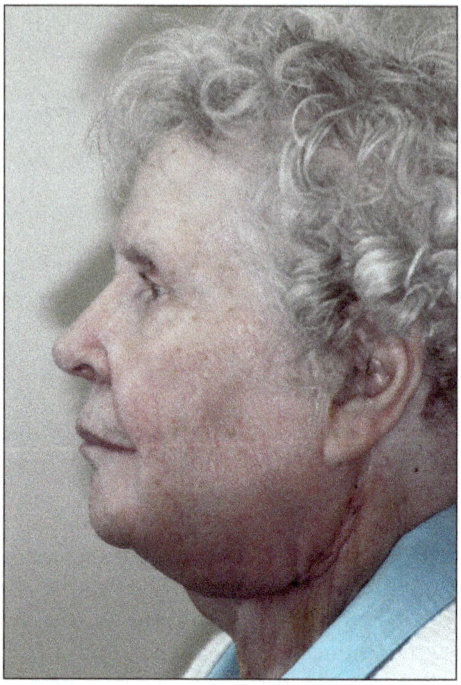

Figure 17. Same radiated cancer patient after bone graft reconstruction supported by the 20/10 hyperbaric oxygen protocol.

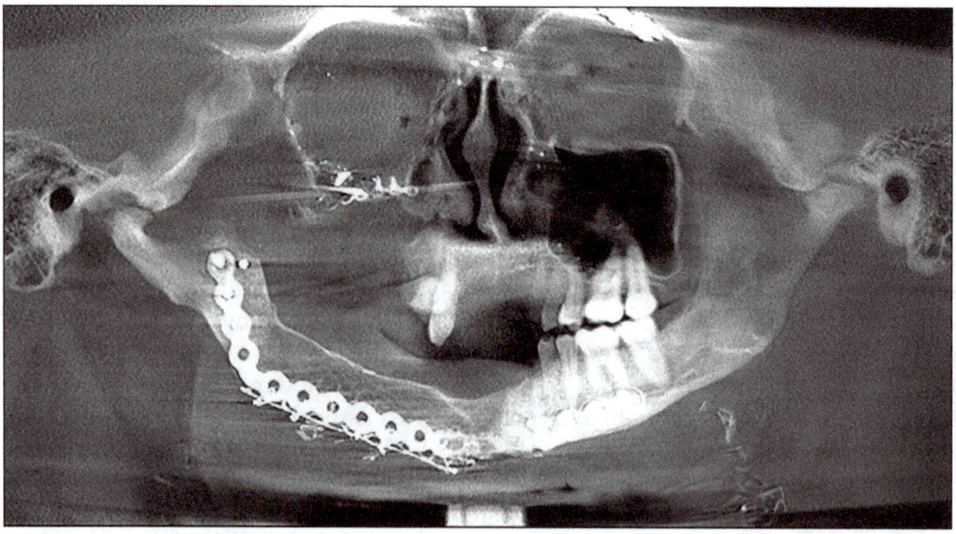

Figure 18. Panoramic radiograph showing seven-year follow-up of same patient's bone grafts, demonstrating a well-consolidated graft, which has withstood functional demands.

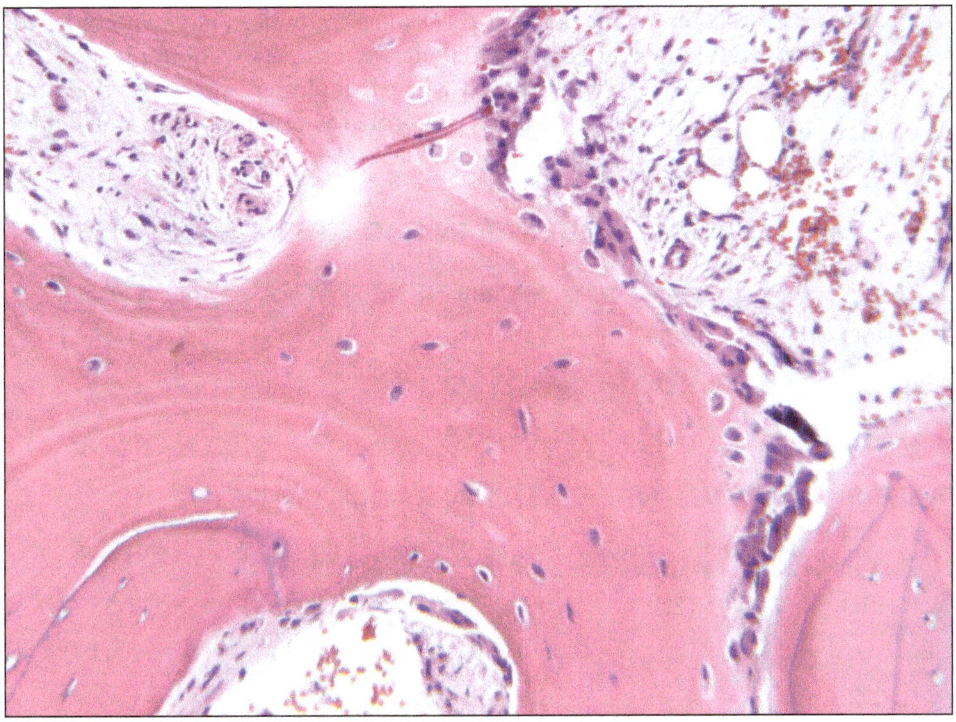

Figure 19. Mature human bone graft in radiated tissue with prominent endosteum derived from hyperbaric-oxygen-induced cellularity in recipient tissue.

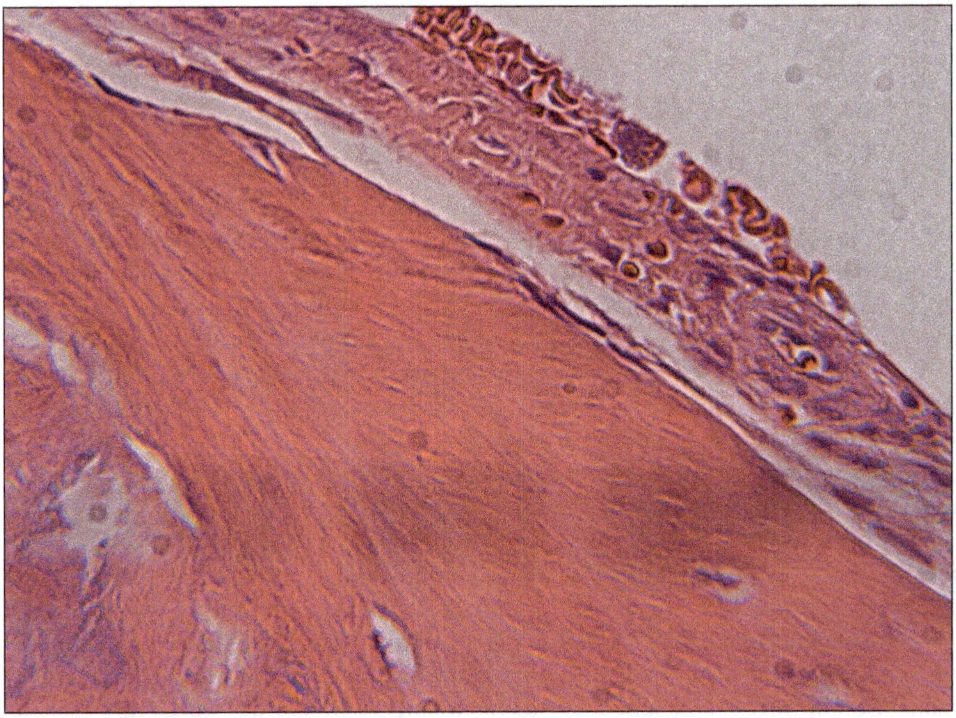

Figure 20. Mature human bone graft in radiated tissue with functioning periosteum derived from hyperbaric-oxygen-induced cellularity in recipient tissue.

Each patient required a major soft-tissue surgery or flap introduced into tissue radiated to a dose greater than 6,400 cGy. One group underwent surgery without preoperative hyperbaric oxygen. The other group underwent their indicated surgery by the same surgeons using the 20/10 hyperbaric oxygen protocol. The results are shown in Tables 3a, 3b, and 3c.

TABLE 3a. WOUND DEHISCENCE IN RADIATED TISSUE

	N	Minor	Major	Total
Non-HBO_2	120	19 (16%)	12 (10%)	31 (26%)
HBO_2	120	4 (3.3%)	2 (1.6%)	6 (5%)
P = 0.005				

TABLE 3b. WOUND INFECTIONS IN RADIATED TISSUE

	N	Minor	Major	Total
Non-HBO_2	120	31 (25.8%)	14 (11.2%)	45 (37%)
HBO_2	120	9 (7.6%)	4 (3.3%)	13 (11%)
P = 0.005				

TABLE 3c. DELAYED WOUND HEALING IN RADIATED TISSUE

	N	Minor	Major	Total
Non-HBO_2	120	26 (22%)	29 (24%)	55 (46%)
HBO_2	120	12 (10%)	5 (4%)	17 (14%)
P = 0.005				

Wound Dehiscence: The control group developed a 25.8% incidence of minor wound dehiscence and a 11.2% incidence of major wound dehiscence, while the 20/10 hyperbaric group developed a 7.6% incidence of minor wound dehiscence and a 3.3% incidence of major wound dehiscence. In this study, a minor wound dehiscence was defined as one which healed within three weeks with wound care and dressings. A major wound dehiscence was defined as one unhealed within three weeks and/or which required secondary surgery or hyperbaric oxygen (Figure 21, Figure 22, Figure 23, Figure 24). The total wound dehiscence difference was 37% to 11% with a p-value of 0.001.

Infection: The control group developed a 16% incidence of minor wound infections and a 10% incidence of major wound infections. The 20/10 hyperbaric group developed a 3.3% incidence of minor wound infections and a 1.6% incidence of major wound infections. In this study, a minor wound infection was defined as one which responded to culture-specific antibiotics and local wound irrigations. A major wound infection required debridement surgery in addition to culture-specific antibiotics and wound irrigations (Figure 25, Figure 26). The total wound infection difference was 26% to 5% with a p-value of 0.005.

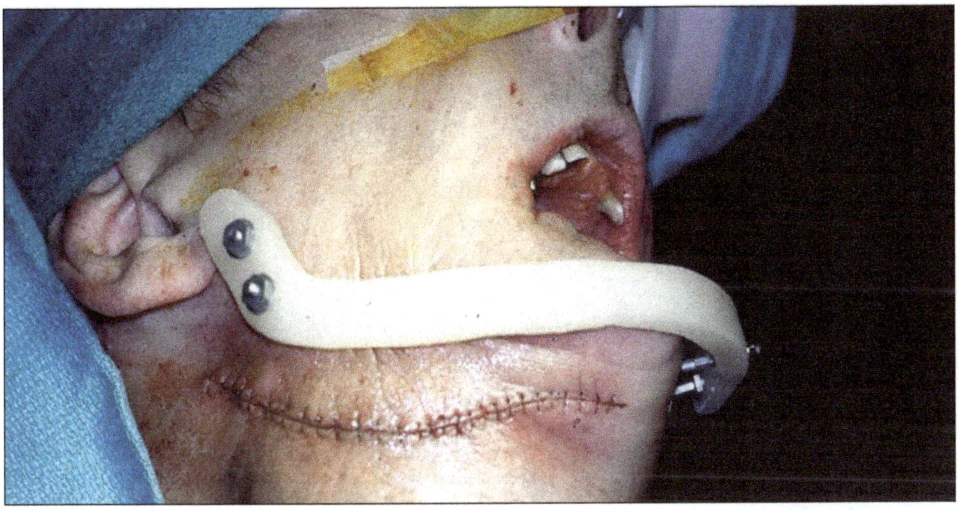

Figure 21. Wound closure of reconstruction patient who did not receive hyperbaric oxygen.

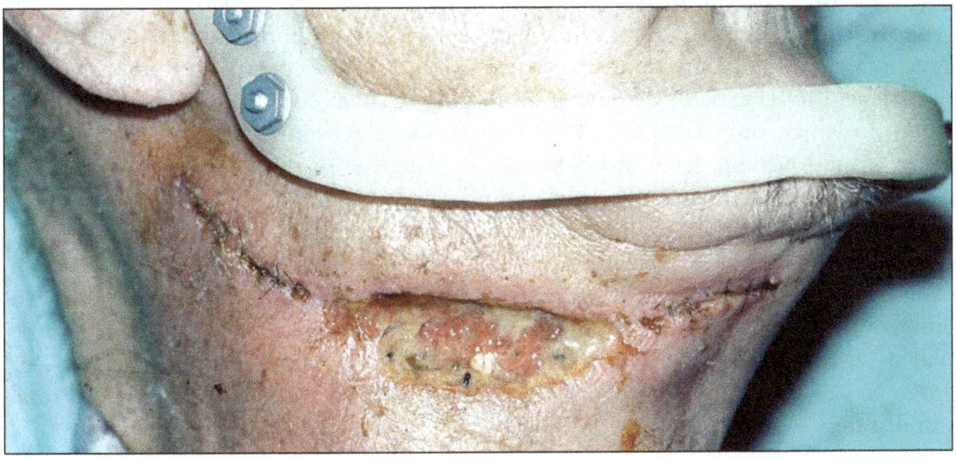

Figure 22. Major wound dehiscence in same patient required hyperbaric oxygen to heal.

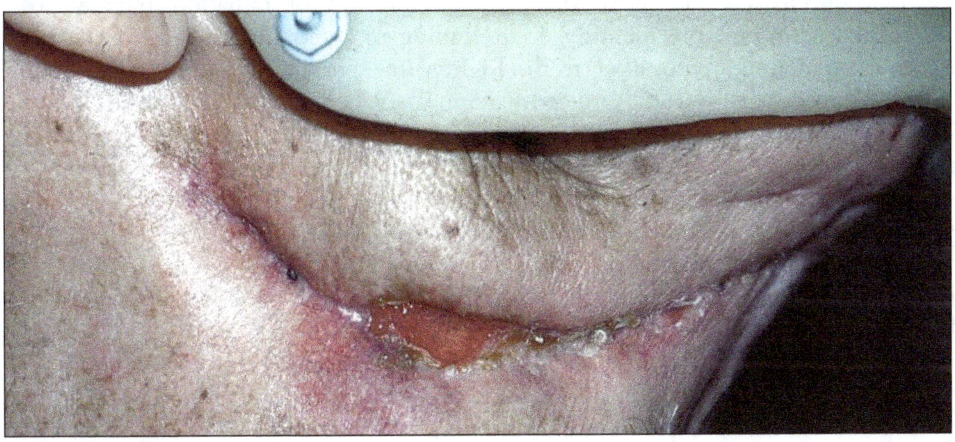

Figure 23. Same patient after 19 hyperbaric oxygen exposures shows granulating tissue base and a periphery-to-central-core direction of healing.

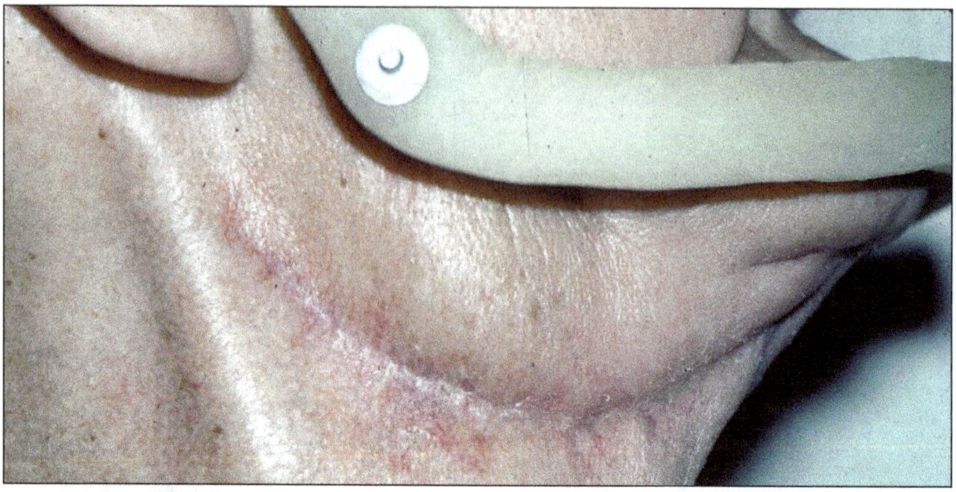

Figure 24. Same patient with completely healed wound after 25 hyperbaric oxygen exposures.

Length of Hospital Stay: Delayed wound healing was evident in many of the patients who developed a dehiscence with or without wound infection or a wound infection alone. The totals of all cases were striking. In the control group, nearly ½ of all patients (46%) experienced a wound healing delay as compared to the hyperbaric group, in which only 14% ($p = 0.005$) experienced a wound healing delay. In this study, wound healing delay was defined as an increase in the inpatient hospital stay specifically to treat the radiated tissue wound (Figure 27, Figure 28).

This study clearly quantitates and confirms the historical observations of many other authors who have reported such complications when surgery is performed in radiated tissues.[9,12,18] It also quantitated the value of the 20/10 hyperbaric oxygen protocol as an adjunct prior to any surgery in radiated tissue. What should also be evident is that use of the 20/10 hyperbaric oxygen protocol reduces the need for prolonged care and additional surgeries. It also reduces deformity, disability, and total cost of care.

Tooth Removal

Osteoradionecrosis is the most dreaded complication of radiation therapy. The single most common precipitating event leading to osteoradionecrosis of the jaws is the postradiation removal of teeth. Eighty-nine percent of all trauma-induced osteoradionecrosis is secondary to tooth removal. When a tooth is removed from a jaw which has previously received 6,000 cGy or more, the bone and surrounding mucosa are wounded. The greater the elapsed time after completion of radiotherapy, the more hypoxic and hypocellular the tissue becomes and the less likely it is to meet the demands of healing. An open tooth socket requires a tertiary type of healing to fill a void and cope with the bacterial contamination of the oral flora. This radiated soft tissue-bone composite, which in the usual case can barely maintain its own physiologic homeostasis, often cannot repair itself postradiation, if a breakdown occurs due to surgical wounding. Hence, it develops into osteoradionecrosis.

In 1985, Marx, Johnson, and Kline published the first randomized, prospective study dealing with the effects of HBO_2 on radionecrosis.[27] The study involved 74 patients who needed teeth removed from high-dose-radiated mandibles. All patients were considered at high risk because of a minimal dose of 6,800 cGy and an average dose of over 7,200 cGy.

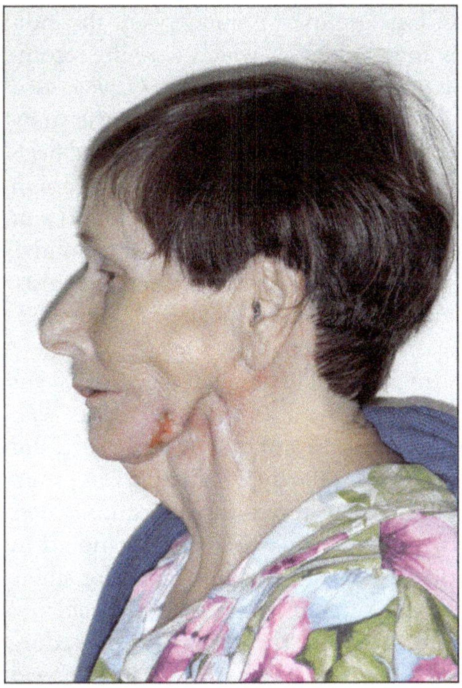

Figure 25. Wound dehiscence and infection in a radiated patient who did not receive hyperbaric oxygen.

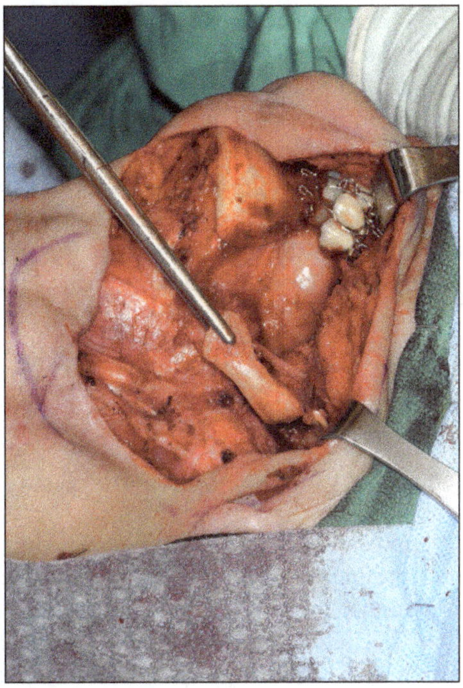

Figure 26. After the standard hyperbaric oxygen protocol, a second wound debridement and bone removal was required.

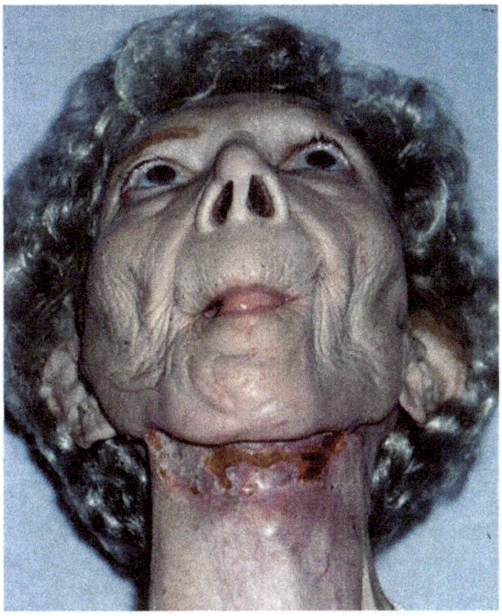

Figure 27. Delayed wound healing due to dehiscence and minor infection extending hospital stay of radiated patient who did not receive hyperbaric oxygen.

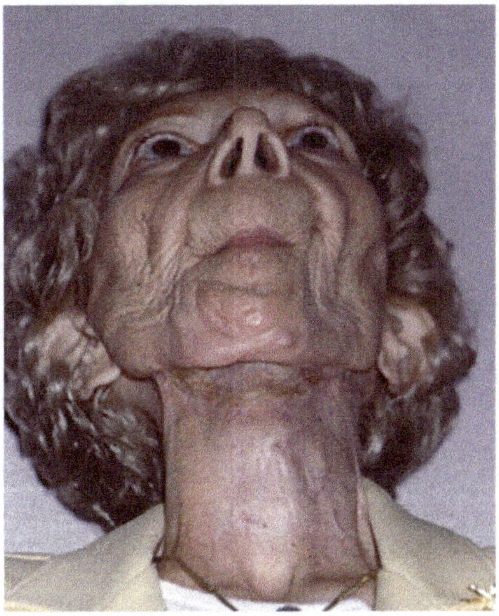

Figure 28. Completed healing of same patient without further surgery or hyperbaric oxygen but delayed by approximately 21 days including an extension of inpatient care for 7 days.

The patients were randomized into two groups. One group of 37 underwent the indicated tooth removals using standard techniques and antibiotics, which were the recommended prophylaxis of the day. In this study, 1 million units of penicillin G were used intraoperatively, followed by 500 mg QID orally for 10 days. Excluded from the study were all penicillin-allergic patients and those with other conditions affecting wound healing. The other group of 37 underwent the 20/10 hyperbaric oxygen protocol. Tooth removal using standard technique was accomplished, and no antibiotics were given at any time. All patients were followed to a single end point to eliminate bias. At six months, those with exposed, nonhealing mandibles were considered to have osteoradionecrosis. The results are shown in Table 4 (Figure 29, Figure 30, Figure 31, Figure 32, Figure 33, Figure 34a, Figure 34b, Figure 34c).

The antibiotic group developed a 29.9% incidence of osteoradionecrosis versus 5.4% in the hyperbaric group ($p = 0.005$). In addition, 8 of the 11 patients who developed osteoradionecrosis in the antibiotic group required jaw resection and hyperbaric oxygen for resolution. Of the two patients in the hyperbaric oxygen group who developed osteoradionecrosis, neither required jaw resection, indicating a less severe form of necrosis. Since 1985, the 20/10 protocol has become the standard in oral and maxillofacial surgery and the dental profession. It is recommended for single and multiple tooth removals alike, as it is for any surgery in a radiated tissue.[25,27] Our unit has continued to collect data on this technically straightforward procedure to remove a tooth/teeth in a radiation field. To date, in 936 patients, we removed 2019 teeth in radiated jaws using the 20/10 hyperbaric oxygen protocol. Seven patients (0.75%) developed osteoradionecrosis.

Osseointegrated Dental Implants

One of the truly great advances that emerged from the orthopedic and dental professions in the 1980s was the biology of osseointegration and its use as anchorage for oral prostheses.[3] Osseointegration is the remodeling of bone about an implanted metal interface without intervening soft tissue. Clinically, root-form metal cylinders become incorporated into bone (osseointegration) and thus may serve to replace individual teeth or several teeth via bridgework. Osteointegrated prostheses offer greater stability and retention over conventional ones.[4]

Head and neck cancer survivors have often undergone removal of all or part of their jaws and many of their teeth. Such missing natural tissues combine with surgical and radiation damage to impair tongue function, palatal function, and the pharyngeal phase of swallowing. The salivary glands are damaged, creating xerostomia which disables these patients greatly. In addition to the soft- and hard-tissue reconstructive surgery which is necessary, osseointegrated implants are needed in these patients, more so than in others. However, implant placement, which is a surgical procedure in itself, as well as the loading forces on these implants when prostheses are constructed, has been a concern and has resulted in osteoradionecrosis (Figure 34b).

TABLE 4. TOOTH REMOVALS IN RADIATED MANDIBLES

	N	# TEETH	ORN	% ORN
Non-HBO_2	37	165	11	(29.9%)
HBO_2	37	156	2	(5.4%)
$P = 0.005$				

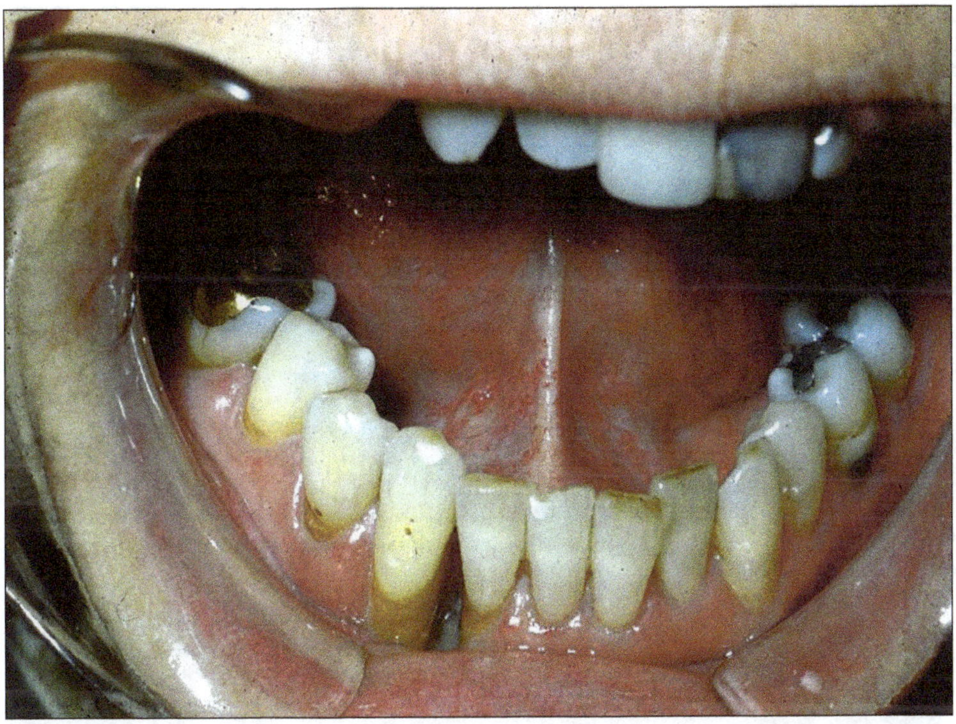

Figure 29. Failing dentition in a patient randomized to the penicillin arm of the study.

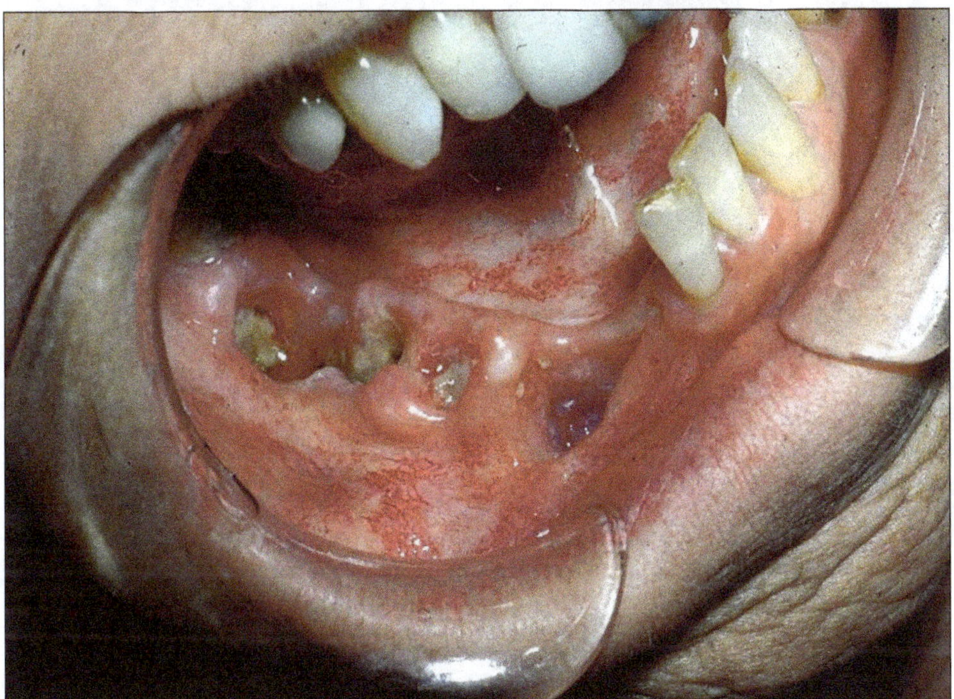

Figure 30. Six months later all tooth removal sockets evidence exposed nonhealing bone indicative of osteoradionecrosis.

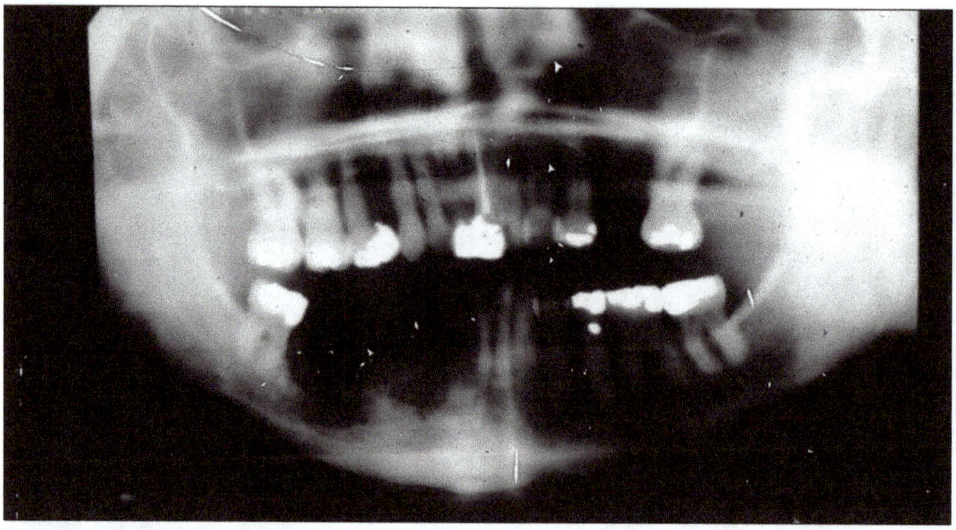

Figure 31. Panoramic radiograph shows extensive bone loss in this patient's osteoradionecrosis that required hemimandibulectomy and hyperbaric oxygen to resolve.

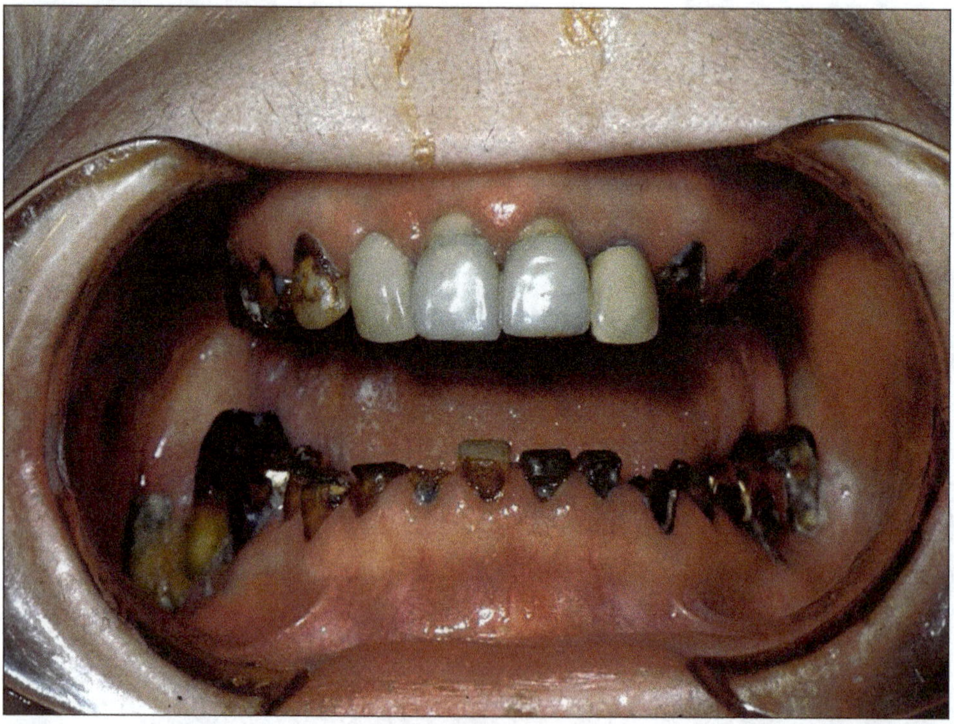

Figure 32. Failing dentition in a patient randomized to the hyperbaric oxygen arm of the study.

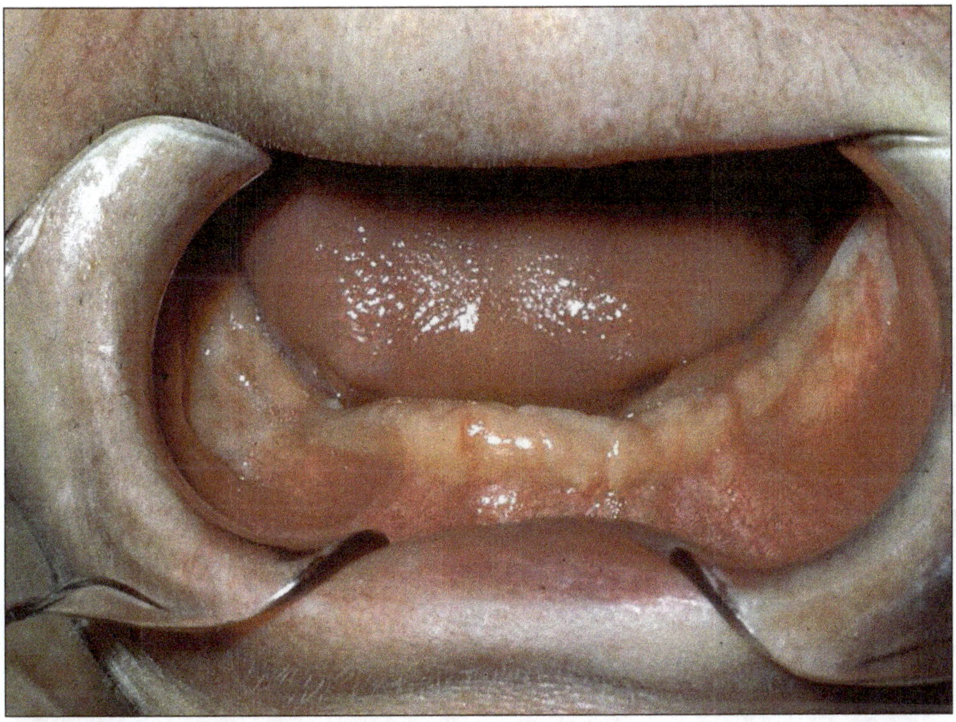

Figure 33. Six months later tooth sockets have healed and bone has remodeled so that a denture prosthesis can be made.

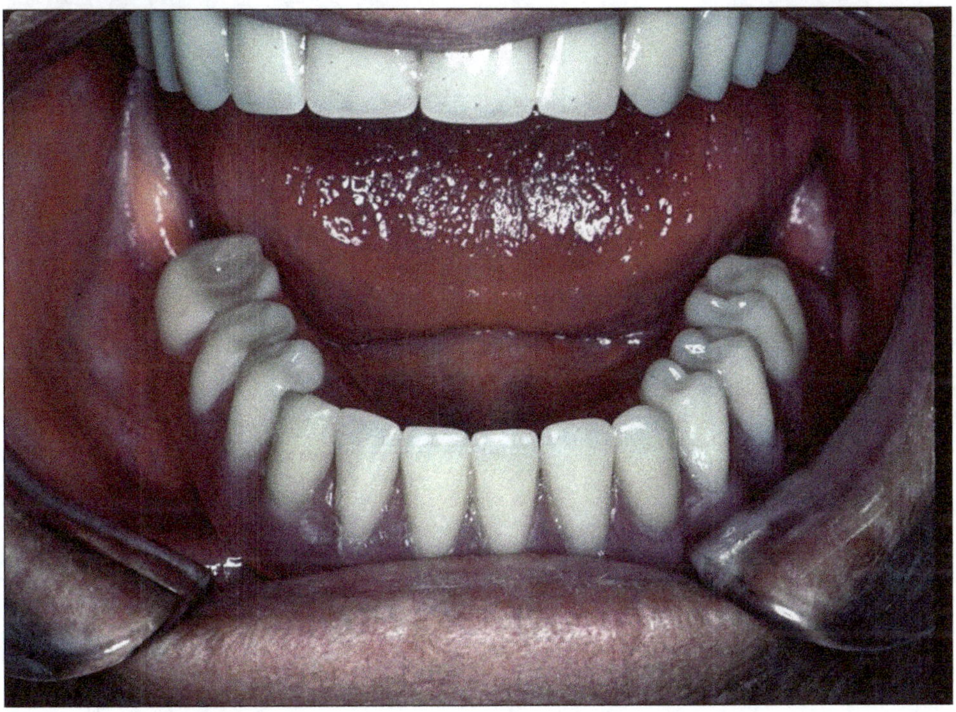

Figure 34a. Same patient functioning with a denture prosthesis on healed radiated tissue without tendency for breakdown.

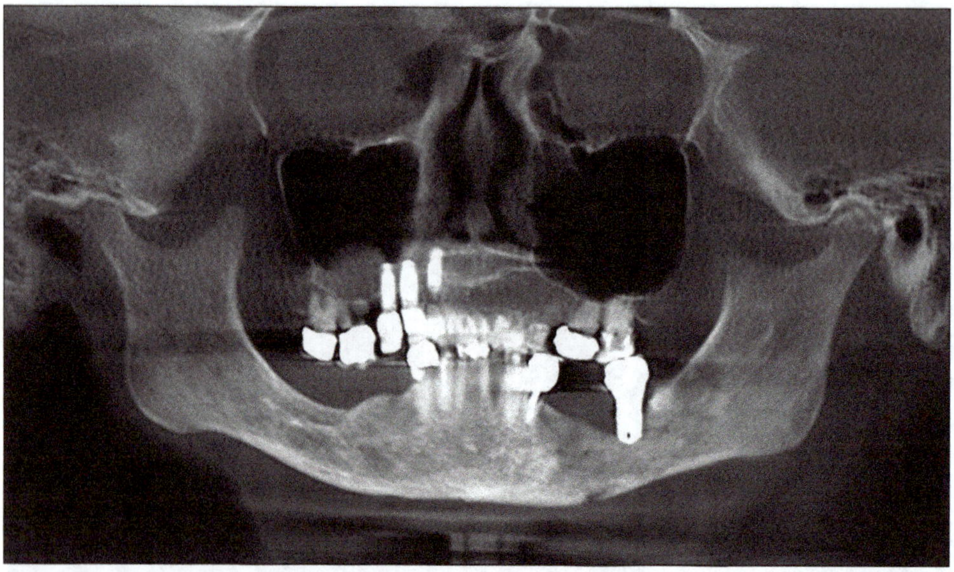

Figure 34b. Osteoradionecrosis developed about this dental implant in traumatic occlusion.

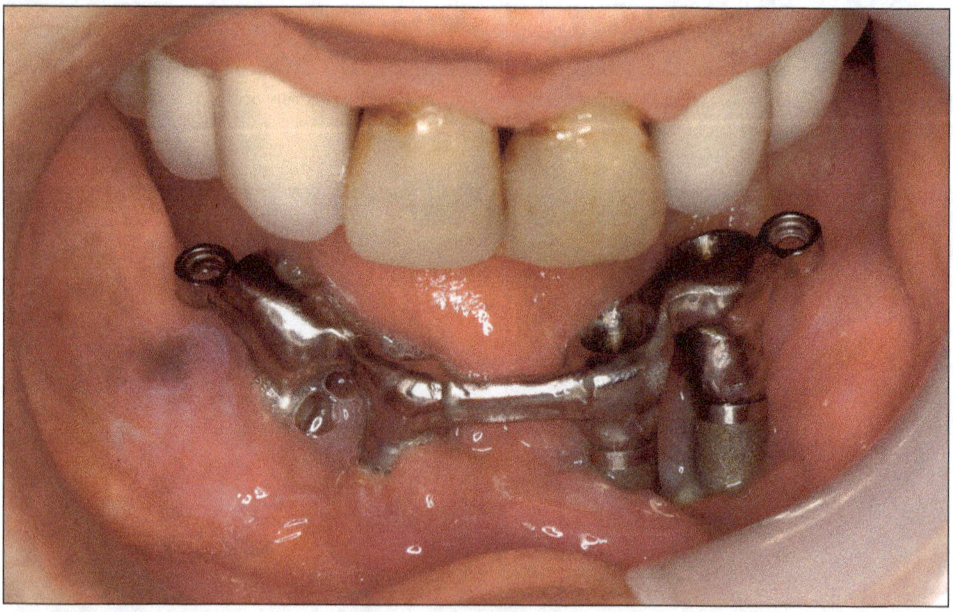

Figure 34c. The placement of these implants resulted in osteoradionecrosis.

Current data indicate that hyperbaric oxygen makes it feasible to afford radiated patients the same advantage of osseointegrated implants as nonradiated patients. To date, our center has placed 2,056 osseointegrated fixtures in bone radiated to greater than 6,400 cGy; of these, 1,727 (84%) have integrated completely and have withstood functional loading by a prosthesis. Three hundred twenty-nine implants (16%) have failed to osseointegrate. Each failed during the initial six months of osseointegration. Each became mobile and was removed. None precipitated an osteoradionecrosis, and all that did integrate are continuing to be functional under loading forces. The lack of development of osteoradionecrosis and the acceptable osseointegration rate of 84% recommends the use of the 20/10 protocol for such implant placement. This is contrasted with our experience with 47 cases where osseointegrated implants precipitated osteoradionecrosis when HBO_2 was not used (Figure 34c). Thus, it appears that HBO_2 has as much value postradiation in osseointegration as it has in bone grafting and soft-tissue repair.

The osseointegration rate of 84% with implants placed into radiated bone using HBO_2 is still less than the 94% published for implants placed into nonradiated bone.[3-4,41] This is probably due to the fact that, although HBO_2 induces an angiogenesis and fibroplasia in all radiated tissues, including bone, it does not seem to increase the osteoblast population. Since osteoblasts are the primary cells in forming and maintaining osseointegration and since radiated bone has a reduced osteoblast population,[2] a lesser success rate is expected. Its greater value is in using HBO_2 for the soft-tissue healing and especially the prevention of osteoradionecrosis (Figure 35, Figure 36, Figure 37, Figure 38, Figure 39a, Figure 39b).

OSTEORADIONECROSIS (ORN)

This disease has been reported in nearly every bone in the skeleton.[5,9,26] However, it is most common in the jaws, particularly the lower jaw due to frequent radiation for oral and oropharyngeal cancers. Serial woundings from periodontal inflammation, pulpal disease, chewing trauma, and the need for oral surgical procedures also contribute to osteoradionecrosis of the jaws. Since 2010, the popular use of intensity modulated radiation therapy (IMRT) has produced a significant rise in the incidence of ORN and its severity. (Figure 25).

The pathophysiology (Figure 35) of osteoradionecrosis was redefined in 1983 as a sequence beginning with (1) radiation, which produces (2) hypovascular-hypocellular-hypoxic tissue, which may undergo (3) tissue breakdown, which is an imbalance where cell death and collagen lysis exceed the homeostatic mechanisms of cell replacement

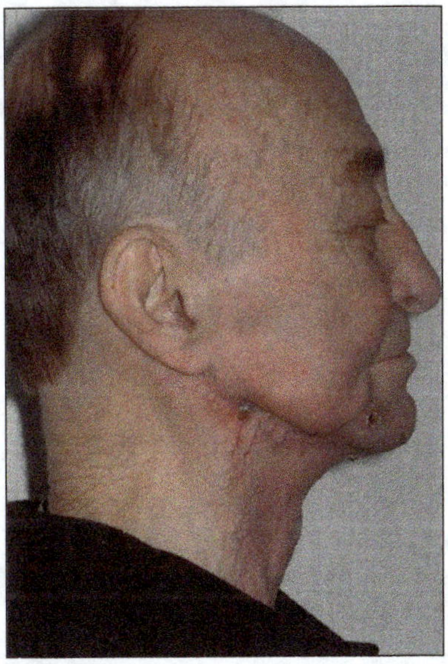

Figure 35. Cancer patient with osteoradionecrosis before hyperbaric oxygen and surgery.

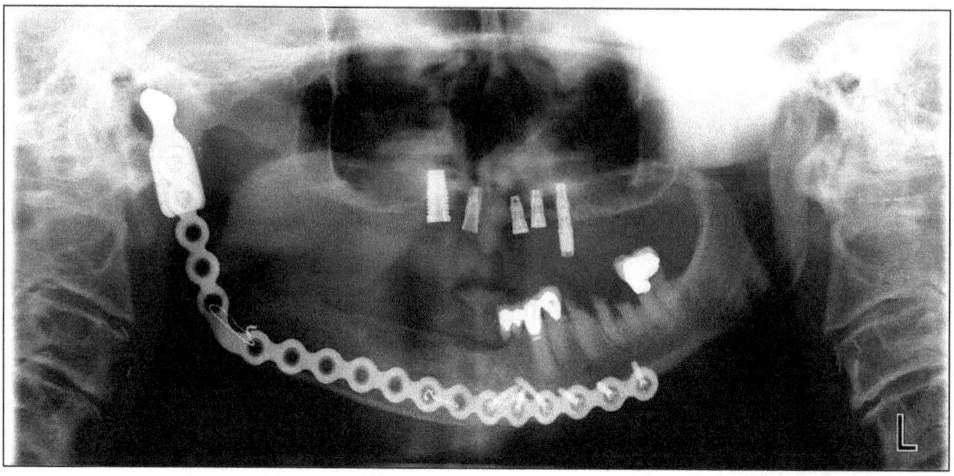

Figure 36. Patient in Figure 35 after standard hyperbaric oxygen protocol, a bone resection, and bone graft reconstruction.

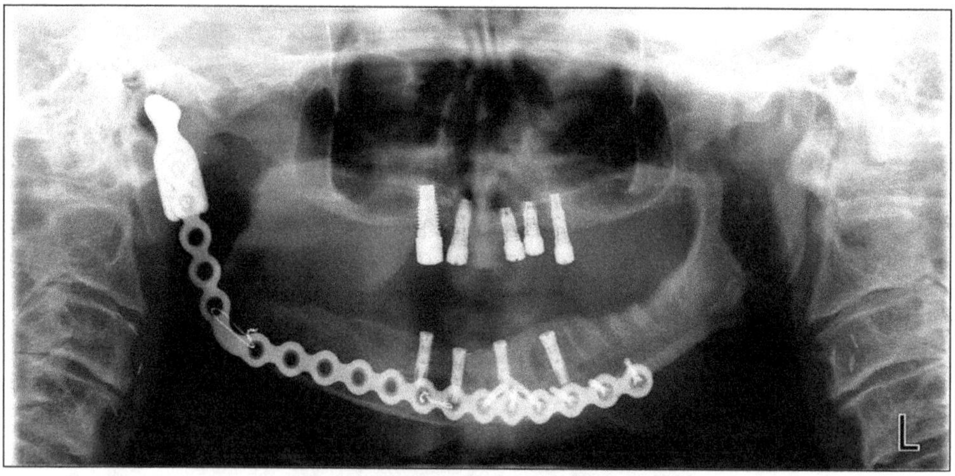

Figure 37. After bone graft maturity, patient requires teeth with radiation caries removed and dental implants placed in bone graft as well as radiated bone.

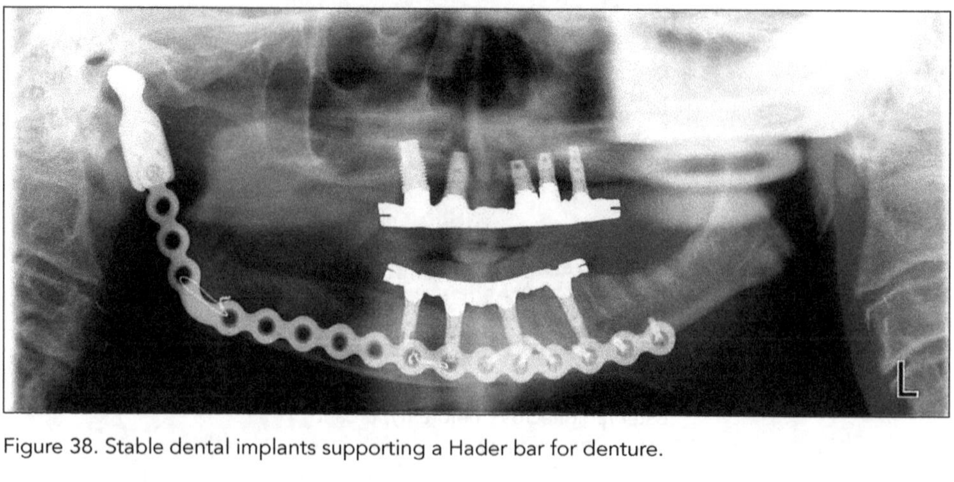

Figure 38. Stable dental implants supporting a Hader bar for denture.

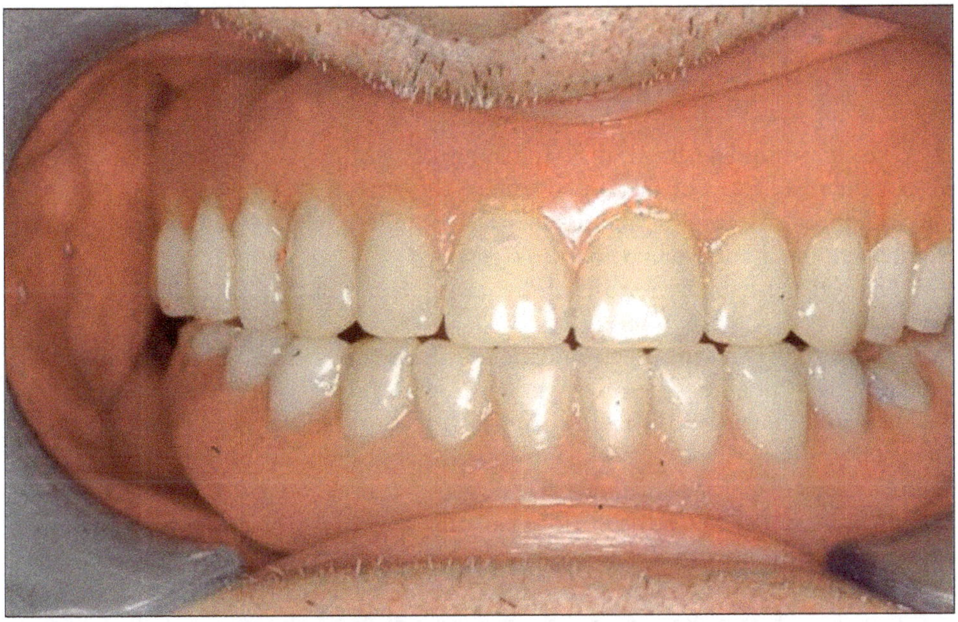

Figure 39a. Fully functional upper and lower denture stabilized on dental implants.

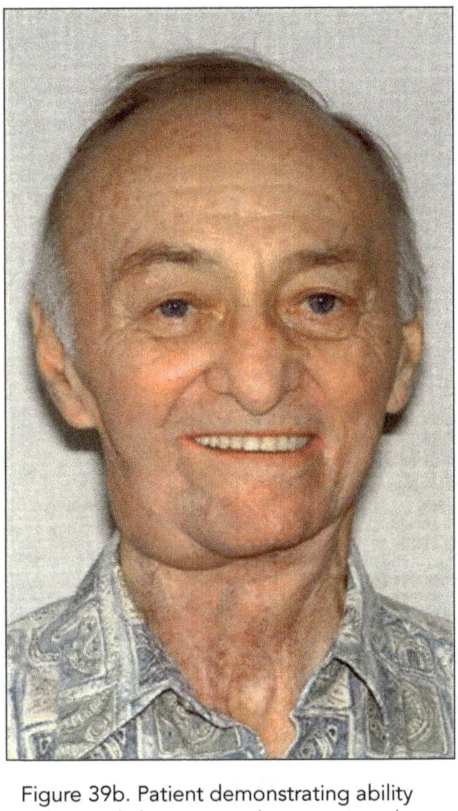

Figure 39b. Patient demonstrating ability to bite with force on implant-supported prosthesis where implants were placed into a highly radiated bone.

and collagen synthesis. This in turn develops into (4) a nonhealing wound, where the metabolic demands exceed the oxygen and vascular supply (Table 5).[21-22]

Prior to 1983, osteoradionecrosis was thought to be an infection of radiated bone.[31,37] However, several good studies have firmly documented osteoradionecrosis as a defect in wound healing.[21,25,27] The importance of this concept is that antibiotics are not the main focus of therapy for osteoradionecrosis.[7] Whenever bone develops osteoradionecrosis, surgical debridement is required, together with the absolute requirement of adjunctive hyperbaric oxygen.

Clinically, osteoradionecrosis of the jaws develops in three situations or as three types (Figure 40).

The first type occurs when radiation and surgical wounding are coupled close together. The woundings become synergistic with hypoxia, and the bone becomes overtly osteoradionecrotic. This happens in three very well-known clinical scenarios. The most common situation is when teeth are removed in a jaw to be radiated and less than 21 days are allowed for tissue recovery and healing. Studies have shown that if 21 days or more can be afforded before radiation begins, osteoradionecrosis will rarely develop, unless the radiation dose becomes extremely high.[25] Fourteen to 21 days have a reduced incidence of osteoradionecrosis, but breakthrough cases do develop in this period of time. Radiation that absolutely must begin within 21 days or even within 14 days to gain better tumor control is in some cases understandable, but this

TABLE 5. PATHOPHYSIOLOGY OF OSTEORADIONECROSIS

1) Radiation
2) Hypovascular-hypocellular-hypoxic tissue
3) Tissue breakdown
4) Nonhealing wound

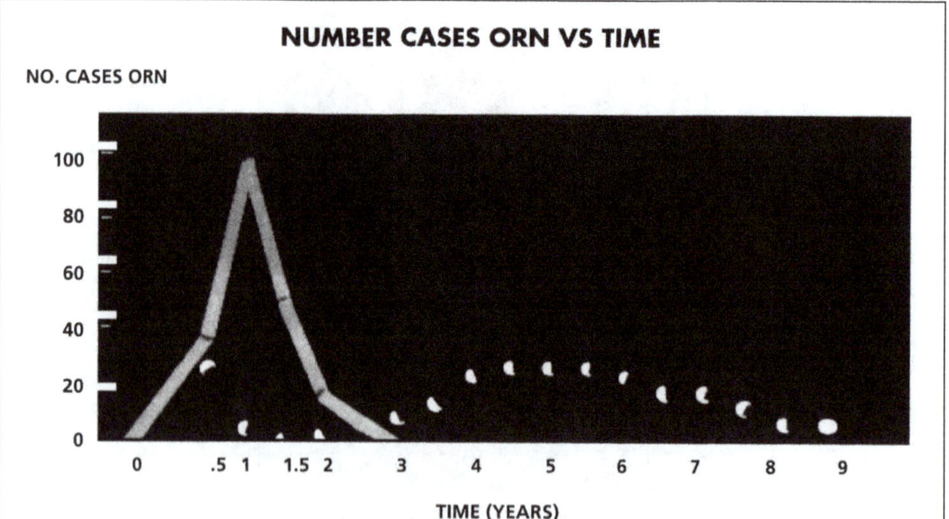

Figure 40. Graph of 536 cases of mandibular osteoradionecrosis showing 3 distinct types and times of occurrence of osteoradionecrosis.

is done with the patient accepting a much greater risk for osteoradionecrosis. The next most common scenario is the mandibulotomy procedure, which is a transection of the mandible to gain access to what is usually a base of tongue or pharyngeal tumor. The reflection of the mandible's vascular periosteum and the fixation methods used in this approach, coupled with the tissue damage of postsurgical radiotherapy, often create an overt osteoradionecrosis. The third scenario is tooth extraction in the middle of a radiotherapy sequence. Teeth that develop symptoms during radiotherapy are best palliated with pulpectomies, drainage, antibiotics, analgesics, etc., rather than treated by removal.[40] The supposedly trivial surgical wounding from even a single tooth removal, if coupled with ongoing radiotherapy, can cause the highest production of osteoradionecrosis. In addition, interrupting a radiotherapy sequence reduces the tumor response through repopulation of tumor cells and requires a greater total dose, thereby worsening the cancer prognosis and increasing the risk of osteoradionecrosis as well. These three causative scenarios of osteoradionecrosis are collectively referred to as "Type I trauma-induced osteoradionecrosis."

The second type of osteoradionecrosis often occurs years after radiotherapy but most commonly within three to six years. Typically, in this scenario, the patient has been functioning well since radiotherapy but may develop dental caries or periodontal disease. The wounding event is most often tooth removal but has also been biopsy, elective dental care, reconstructive surgery, or irritation from dentures.[40] Bone and overlying soft tissues which had been able to maintain homeostasis in the "three-H" state undergo breakdown secondary to the effects of surgical or traumatic wounding. This "Type II trauma-induced osteoradionecrosis" is the one most familiar to both clinicians and laymen.

The third type of osteoradionecrosis is not related to any external trauma or surgery but stems from the effect of radiation alone. It is associated with the higher doses of radiotherapy, IMRT, and interstitial or "brachy therapy." It may also be enhanced or accelerated by concomitant chemotherapy or hyperthermia therapy. This type of breakdown is known as "spontaneous osteoradionecrosis." It usually occurs between six months to two years after completion of radiation treatment.

Figure 41 shows the relationship of the three types of osteoradionecrosis. This graph of radiation pathology also demonstrates the roles of trauma, inflammation, and HBO_2. Clearly defined is subclinical damage or what has been referred to as tissue radiation injury. The graph also defines an arbitrary clinical threshold above which clinical damage occurs. This may present as soft-tissue or bone necrosis.

The first plot shows ascending subclinical damage ending just below the clinical threshold. This point correlates with the cessation of radiotherapy. However, if excessive radiation is given, or, more commonly, surgical wounding occurs, the added damage carries over the clinical threshold into Type I (trauma-induced) osteoradionecrosis (indicated by the **** line). If the first plot peaks just below the clinical threshold, (indicative of very high-dose radiotherapy) but does not cross over the line into overt osteoradionecrosis, there is a recovery period of about four months. In this time period, the histologic inflammation diminishes, and the clinical dermatitis and/or mucositis subsides. However, as the late effects of radiation develop, the progressively more severe "three-H" state in the subclinically damaged area increases. Because the initial radiation dose brought the damage level to just below the clinical threshold with only limited recovery, the late radiation damage may exceed the clinical threshold without an exciting event. This curve describes "spontaneous osteoradionecrosis," which will develop sometime within the patient's lifetime, usually within two years.

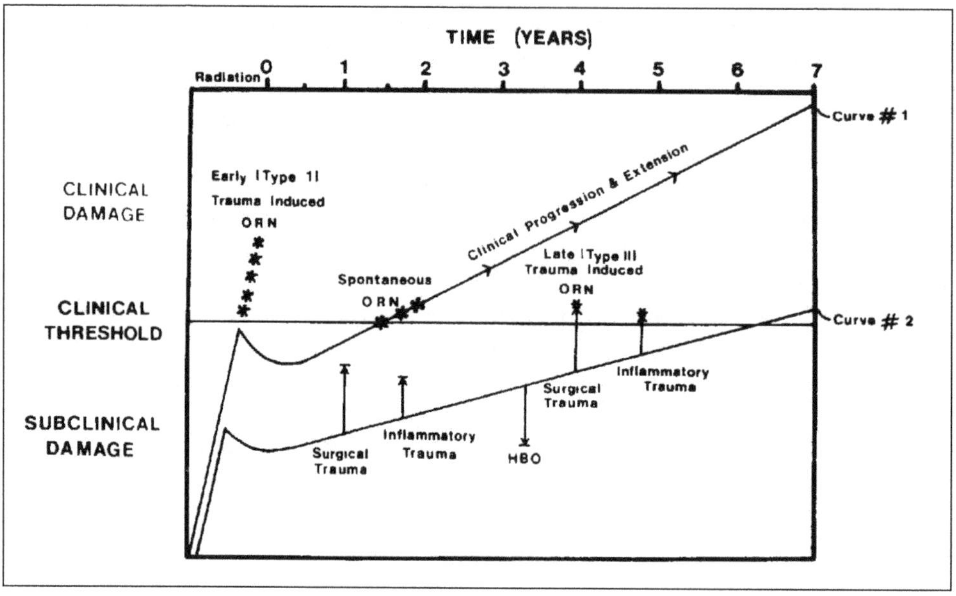

Figure 41. The radiobiology of osteoradionecrosis showing the progress of tissue injury over time.

The usual dosage range of radiotherapy is described by the second plot, which ascends in the subclinical area but ends well below the clinical threshold. After the recovery period, the progressive "three-H" state of late radiation begins. Because the initial dose was less, the slope of the line is less, and the distance it must ascend before it crosses the clinical threshold is greater. In most cases, the time it will take to cross the clinical threshold is longer than the patient's life-span, hence the well-reported low total incidence of osteoradionecrosis, which is estimated to be 8% to 15%. However, if inflammation or surgical trauma occurs, tissue damage vertically accelerates the curve. One sees that trauma inflicted later after completion of radiotherapy has a much greater possibility of exceeding the clinical threshold. By contrast, it is also seen that hyperbaric oxygen deflects the curve vertically downward, reducing the probability of exceeding the clinical threshold. The place of hyperbaric oxygen in the development of osteoradionecrosis is also seen in Figure 42.

The slopes of the lines were derived in a study measuring "before" and "after" vascular densities by histologic examination and transcutaneous oxygen measurements. Not only was hyperbaric oxygen able to reduce the subclinical damage, but it reduced the rate of progression of late radiation effects.

The graph in Figure 41 shows one other noteworthy feature. During the recovery phase after radiotherapy and before the "three-H" state develops, hyperbaric oxygen has no value. This four-month period immediately after radiotherapy has been termed the "golden period" because required surgeries can be accomplished during this time with fewer wound healing complications and without the need for hyperbaric oxygen.

TREATMENT PROTOCOL FOR OSTEORADIONECROSIS

The treatment clinical threat of osteoradionecrosis is different from the 20/10 protocol which is applicable to treat radiation injuries without exposed bone. The osteoradionecrosis treatment is termed the 30/10 protocol because it requires a full 30 sessions prior to any surgical intervention. One reason for the additional 10 treatments is that osteoradionecrosis is an advanced tissue radiation injury which has already

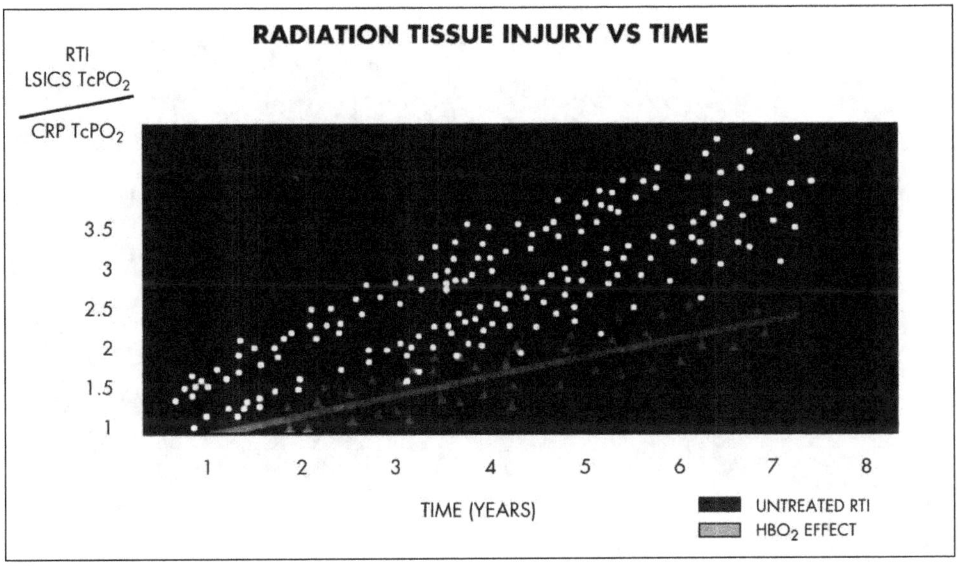

Figure 42. Graph of radiation tissue injury versus time. Two slopes are observed: one without exposure to the 20/10 hyperbaric oxygen protocol, the other after exposure to the 20/10 hyperbaric oxygen protocol.

undergone breakdown resulting in a nonhealing wound. Another reason is that the 30/10 protocol is intended to treat the radiated tissue that is not yet necrotic and which may heal and respond without surgery or with less aggressive surgery. Thus, a full 30 presurgical sessions of HBO_2 are used so that an unequivocal maximum response is obtained. The protocol becomes progressive, beginning with nonsurgical care and advancing to more aggressive debridements. The protocol, initially published in 1983 and developed at the U.S. Air Force Wilford Hall Medical Center and the University of Miami, has stood the test of time and is the standard of care today. It begins by treating all patients who have had at least six months of exposed, nonhealing bone with 30 HBO_2 sessions.[20] These patients begin in what is referred to as Stage I (Figure 43).

However, if the patient initially presents with an orocutaneous fistula (Figure 44), a pathologic fracture (Figure 45), or radiographically evident osteolysis to the inferior mandibular border, he/she is advanced directly to Stage III (Figure 46). Any one of these clinical signs is indicative of advanced disease which requires more aggressive surgery as part of Stage III.

Stage I

In Stage I, all patients undergo an initial trial of 30 sessions of HBO_2. Antibiotics are often discontinued but may need to be used if there is evidence of secondary infection. No surgery or debridement is carried out during this time other than irrigation and removal of sequestered, mobile bone fragments. After 30 sessions, the exposed bone is examined for response. Responding tissue will show a softening of the bone, granulation tissue, and an absence of inflammation (Figure 46). If the tissue is assessed as responding, the softened bone is removed and the patient allowed to undergo an additional 10 sessions of hyperbaric oxygen. If the wound responds with complete healing without further treatment (Figure 47a, Figure 47b), the patient is termed a Stage I responder. If the exposed bone shows no sign of response after 30 sessions of

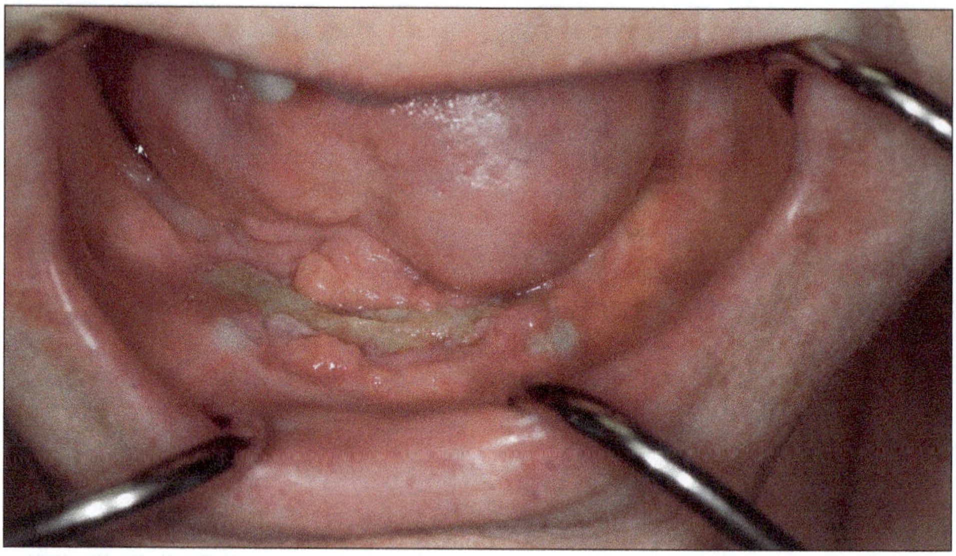

Figure 43. Stage I osteoradionecrosis is an uncomplicated, exposed, radiated bone that has failed to heal over six months.

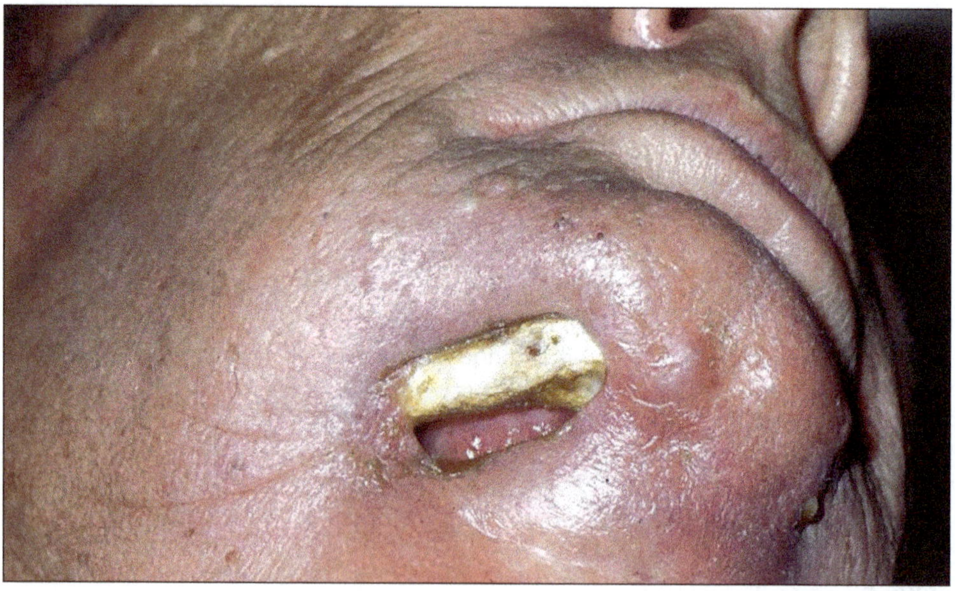

Figure 44. An orocutaneous fistula defines a patient as having Stage III osteoradionecrosis.

hyperbaric oxygen, the patient is termed as a Stage I nonresponder and is advanced to Stage II.

Stage II

In Stage II, the patient has already received 30 sessions of hyperbaric oxygen (Figure 48). Therefore, the patient undergoes a surgical removal of exposed bone. The type of surgery accomplished in Stage II is dependent on the location of the exposed bone but in a general sense is a transoral peripheral resection. If the exposed bone is alveolar,

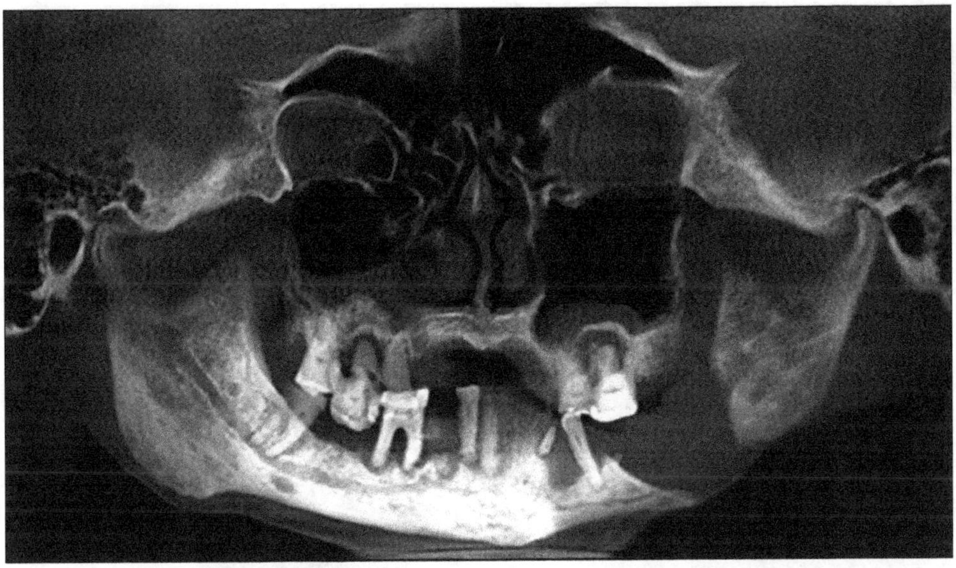

Figure 45. A pathologic fracture also defines a patient as having Stage III osteoradionecrosis.

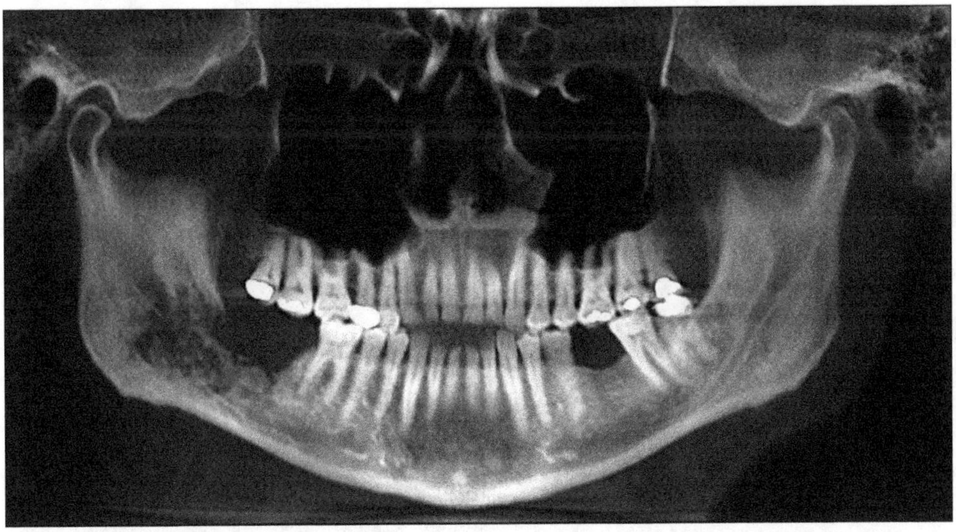

Figure 46. Radiographic evidence of osteolysis to the inferior border of the mandible also defines a patient as having Stage III osteoradionecrosis.

the surgery would be an alveolar sequestrectomy. If the exposed bone were either the lingual or buccal cortex alone, surgery would be a cortical plate removal. All Stage II surgeries retain the inferior border and thus the continuity of the mandible (Figure 49). The bone is removed with a saline-cooled saw rather than a heat-generating burr. The soft tissue is reflected minimally from the bone to preserve the blood supply to the remaining mandible (Figure 50).

Closure is in two or three layers. After surgery, the patient will complete the final 10 hyperbaric oxygen sessions (Figure 51).

If the patient heals without further exposed bone, he or she is termed a Stage II responder (Figure 52).

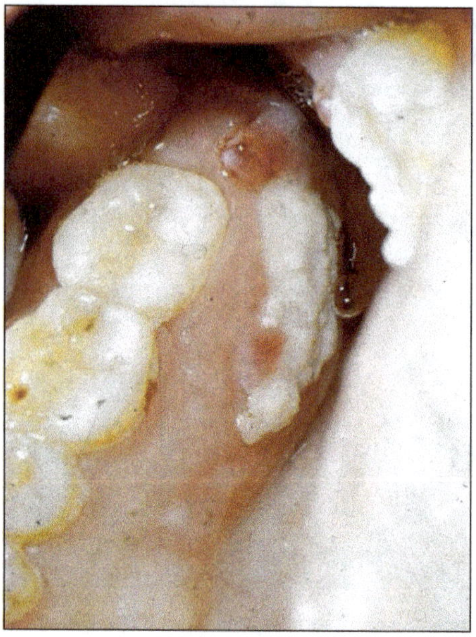

Figure 47a. Osteoradionecrosis after 30 sessions of hyperbaric oxygen showing response by bone softening, absence of inflammation, and granulation tissue.

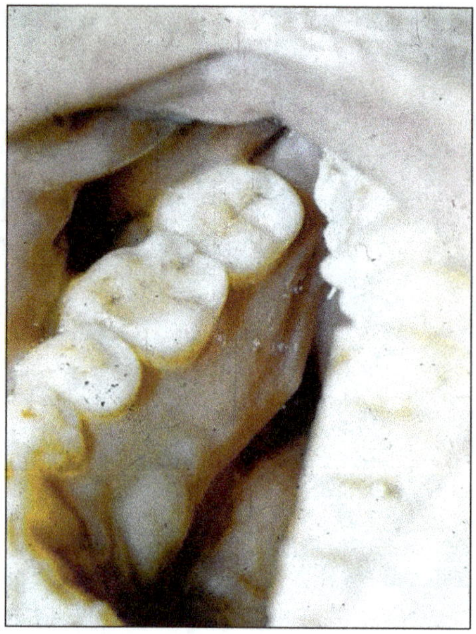

Figure 47b. Stage I responders will sequester nonviable bone and heal over the residual viable bone.

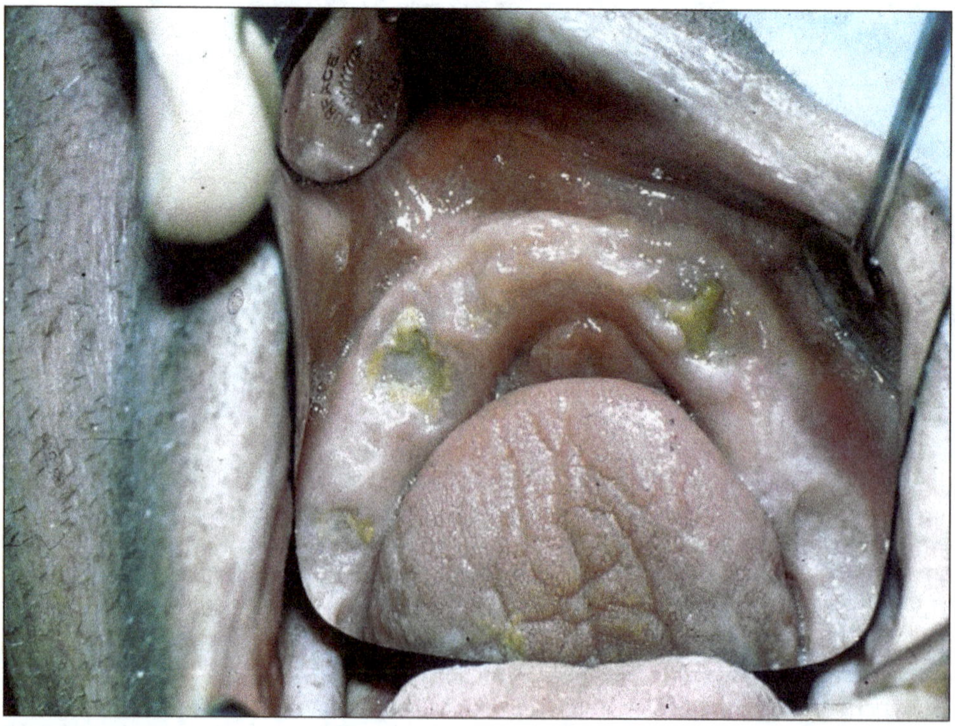

Figure 48. Stage I nonresponder, as evidenced by continued exposure of radiated bone, is advanced to Stage II.

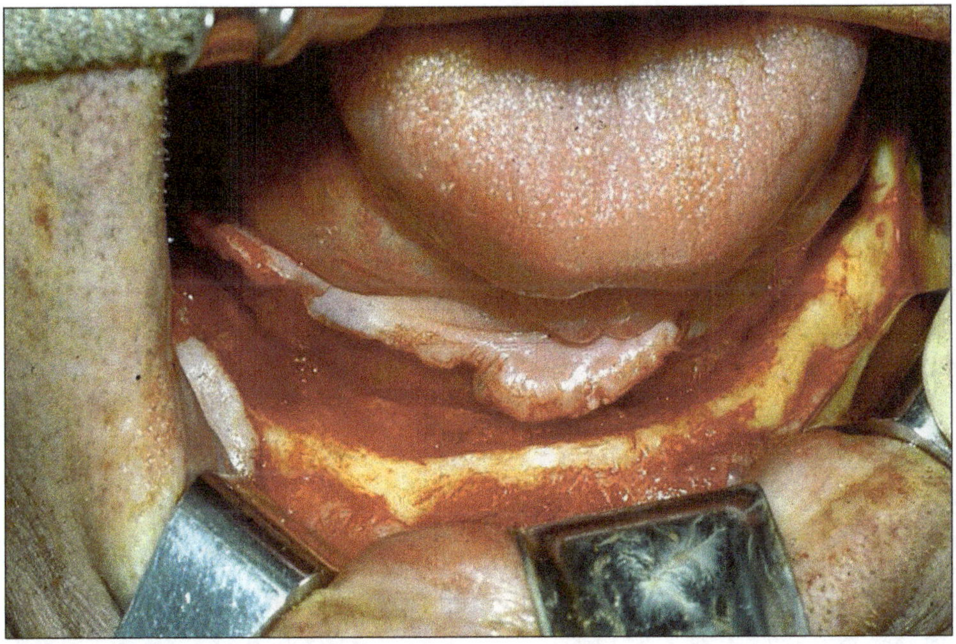

Figure 49. Stage II surgery retains jaw continuity. Here, alveolar resection back to bleeding bone margins retains the mandible's inferior border.

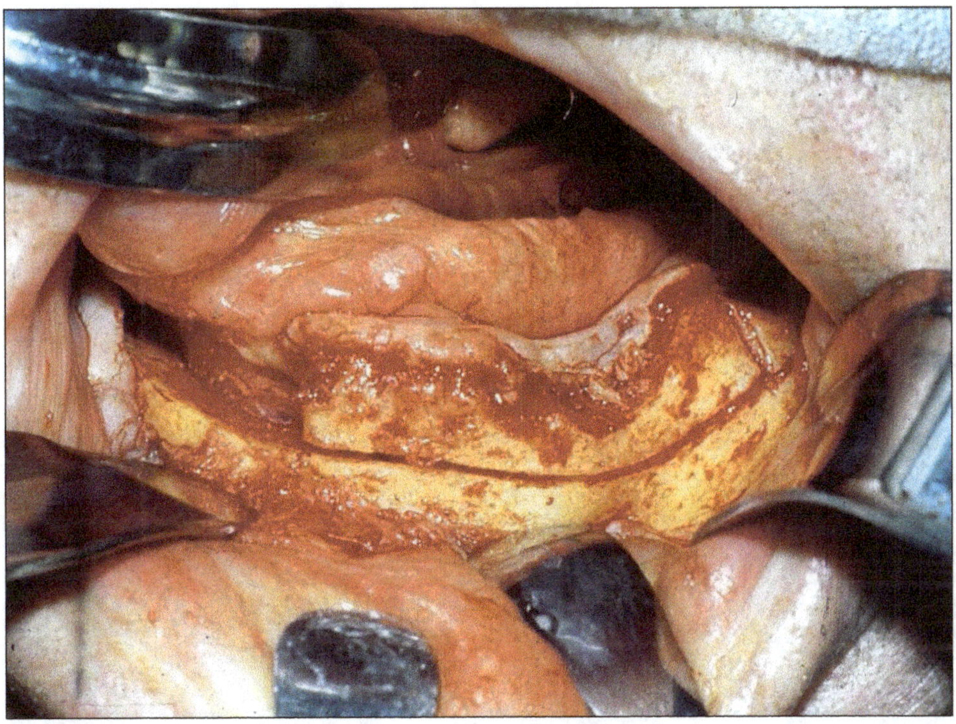

Figure 50. During stage II surgery, it is of paramount importance that the surgeon retain as much vascular tissue attachment to the remaining mandible as possible.

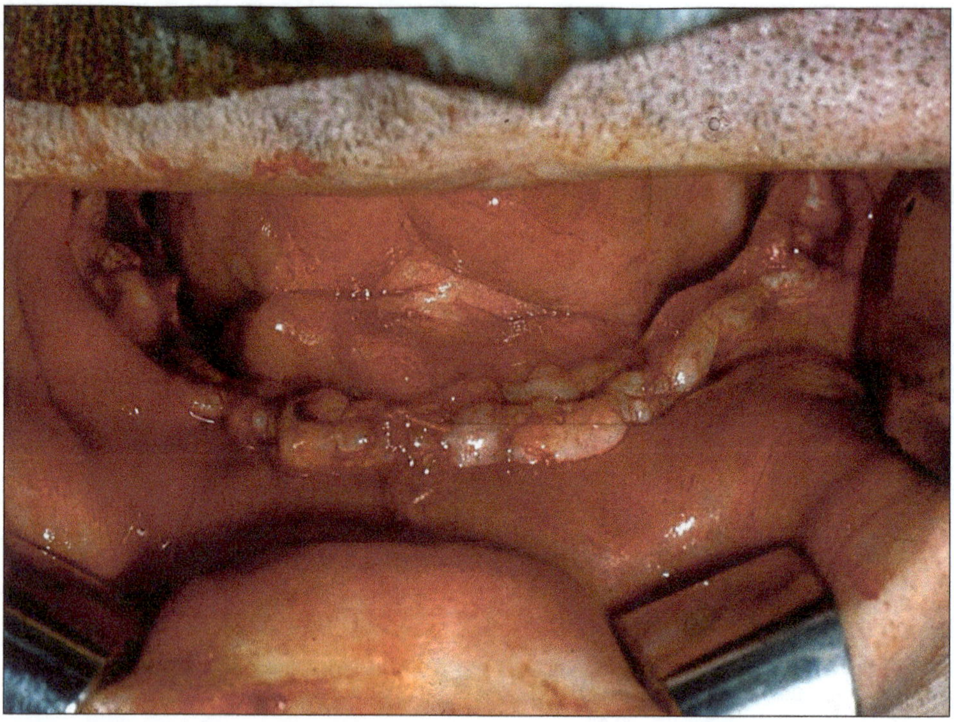

Figure 51. Stage II surgery defines a primary closure over residual viable bone by vascular soft tissue.

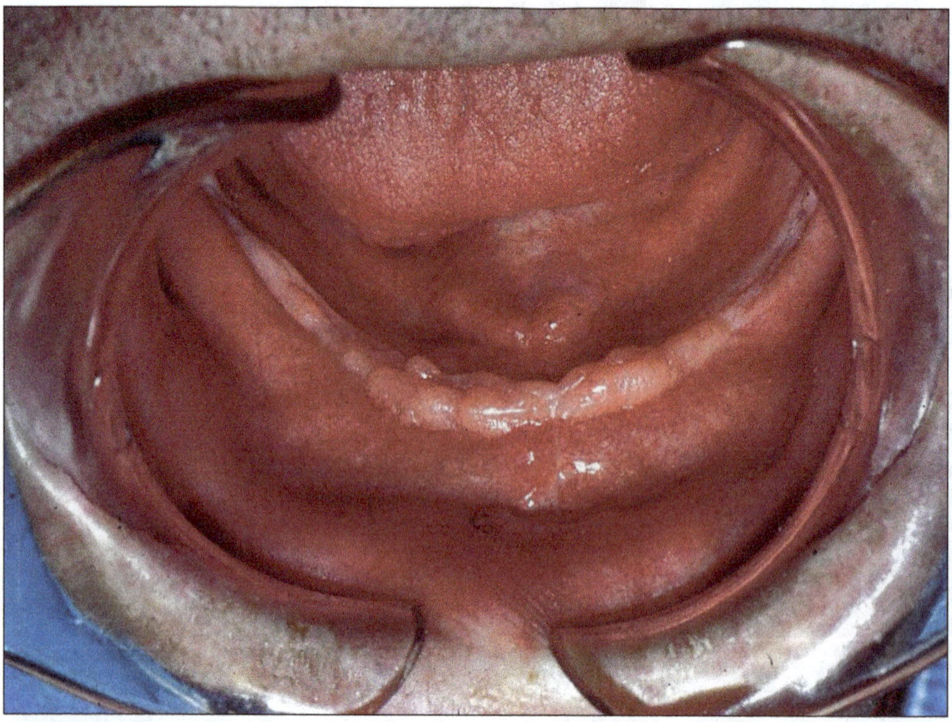

Figure 52. Stage II responders will heal over residual viable bone without further bone exposure.

If the wound dehisces, exposing bone once again, the patient is termed a Stage II nonresponder and is advanced to Stage III.

Stage III

Stage III patients are those who have failed to respond in Stage I and Stage II or have been defined as such on initial presentation. Essentially, this group possesses such a great quantity of nonviable bone that hyperbaric oxygen alone or combined with limited surgical debridement cannot resolve the disease. In Stage III, the patient has already received 30 hyperbaric sessions. The patient will therefore undergo a transcutaneous continuity resection of the involved portion of the mandible and an excision of any necrotic soft tissue (Figure 53, Figure 54, Figure 55).

The resection margins of the mandible are determined by observation at the time of surgery. Bleeding bone margins provide the best guideline as to the viability of the remaining mandibular segments. Similarly, the margins for soft-tissue excision are determined by bleeding observed at the time of surgery. Today, mandibular alignment is gained by rigid internal titanium fixation plates. To reduce the potential for oral or cutaneous dehiscences causing plate exposures, a free vascular or pedicle myocutaneous flap is most often used as well (Figure 56).

At the time of osseous resection, soft-tissue loss must be assessed. If soft tissue has been excised, the soft tissue may be immediately reconstructed with a myocutaneous flap or a free vascular transfer (Figure 57a, Figure 57b, Figure 58). The pectoralis major myocutaneous flap has proven to be one of the most predictable and useful myocutaneous flaps in such defects and the anterior lateral thigh flap the most useful free vascular transfer. Less commonly a free vascular osseocutaneous fibula graft may be used (Figure 59, Figure 60a, Figure 60b).[29]

The patient should then undergo the final 10 hyperbaric oxygen sessions to complete the 30/10 protocol.

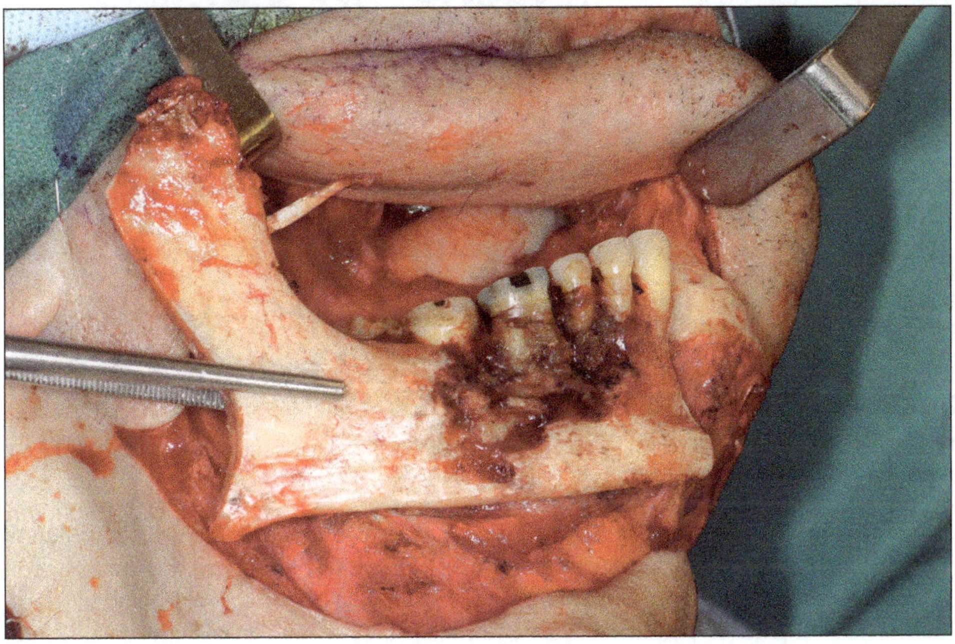

Figure 53. Stage III surgery involves a continuity resection of the mandible and excision of any necrotic soft tissue as well.

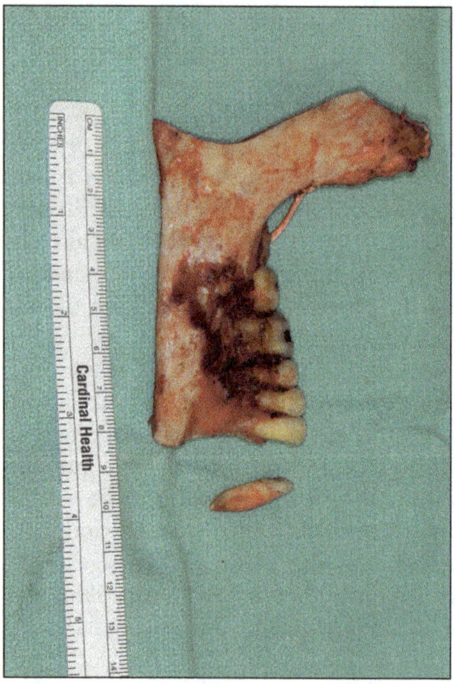

Figure 54. The bony destruction from osteoradionecrosis is readily apparent.

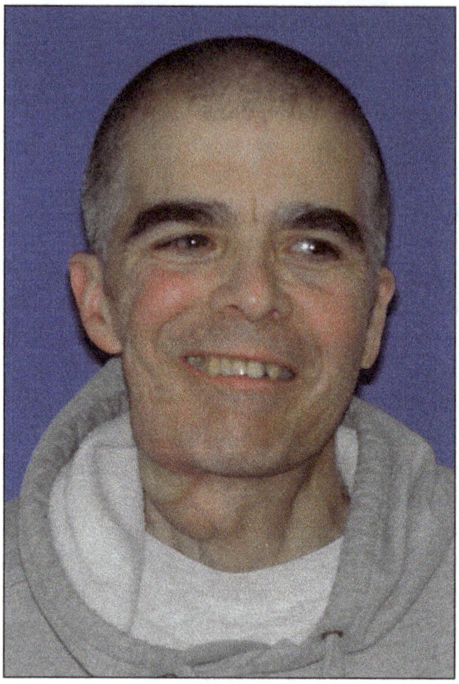

Figure 55. The best jaw fixation is a rigid titanium reconstruction plate hidden beneath the skin and/or a soft-tissue flap.

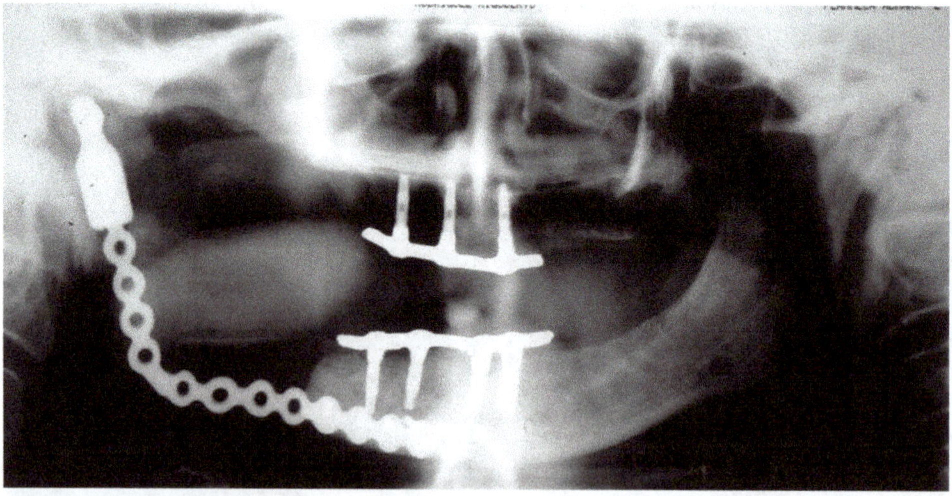

Figure 56. In some cases, the titanium reconstruction plate can be the definitive reconstruction supporting jaw continuity with dental implants providing denture stability.

Patients who require a Stage III approach to resolve their disease usually undergo bony reconstruction of the jaw at three months (Figure 61, Figure 62, Figure 63).

If such bone grafting or other surgery is required, it can be accomplished without the need for further hyperbaric oxygen. Earlier protocols and publications indicated that a retreatment with the 20/10 protocol would be necessary.[20,22,28] However, studies since then[24-26] have shown that the angiogenesis and fibroplasia are long lasting and

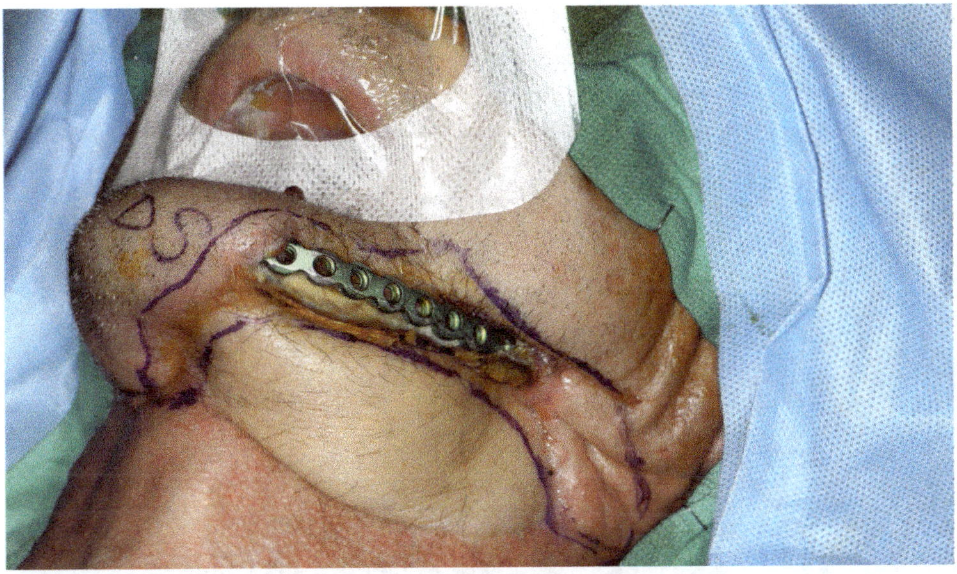

Figure 57a. Soft-tissue radiation necrosis always accompanies osteoradionecrosis and is worsened when surgery is attempted without the standard hyperbaric oxygen protocol.

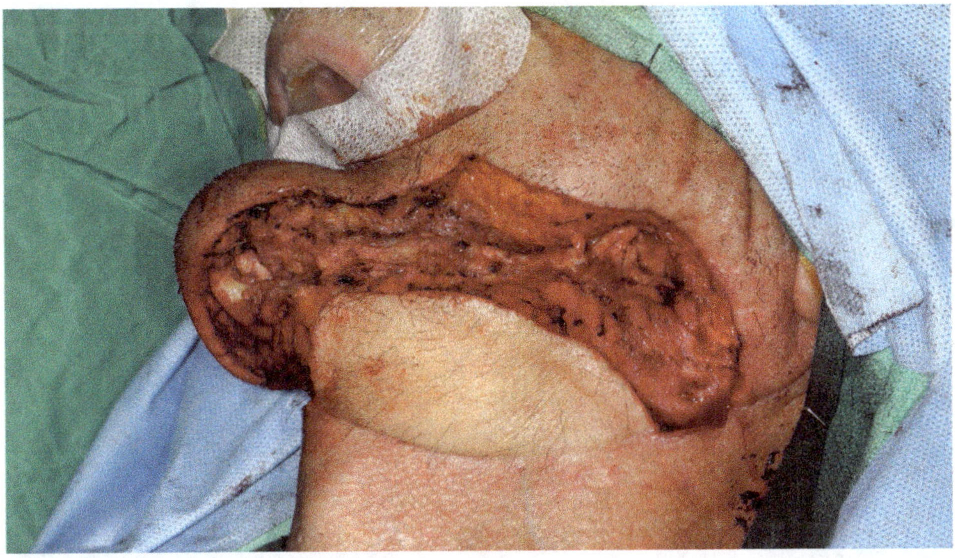

Figure 57b. Excision of soft-tissue radiation necrosis.

need not be reinforced. Indeed, current clinical practice has supported the use of a single but complete protocol of hyperbaric oxygen.

These protocols have been successfully used by most institutions and private practices since 1983. They have generally proven to be effective and predictable, leading to reconstructed patients. Their value resides in the staging of the radionecrotic process, which selects those who can respond to nonsurgical or lesser surgical approaches and expeditiously prepares every patient requiring reconstructive surgery in a minimum of time (three months).

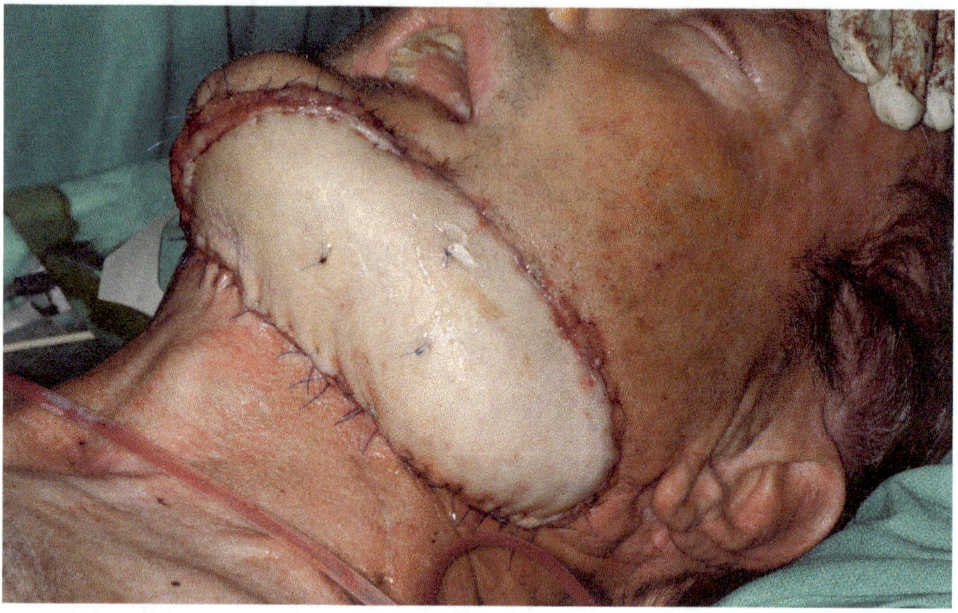

Figure 58. An anterior lateral thigh free vascular flap is commonly used to reconstruct defects from soft-tissue radiation necrosis.

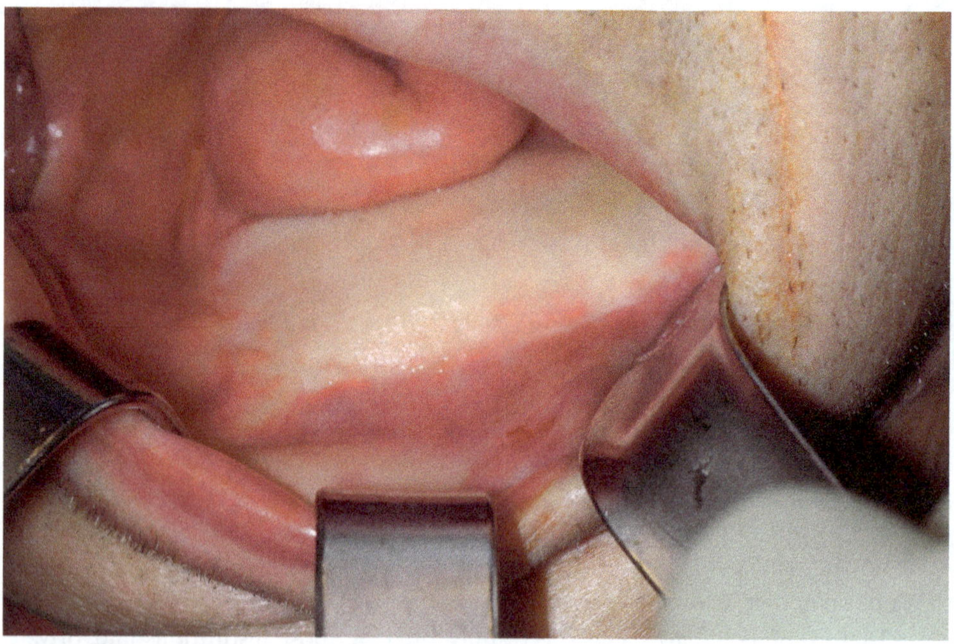

Figure 59. Here the anterior lateral thigh flap was used as a "split paddle" to cover oral lining as well as skin replacement.

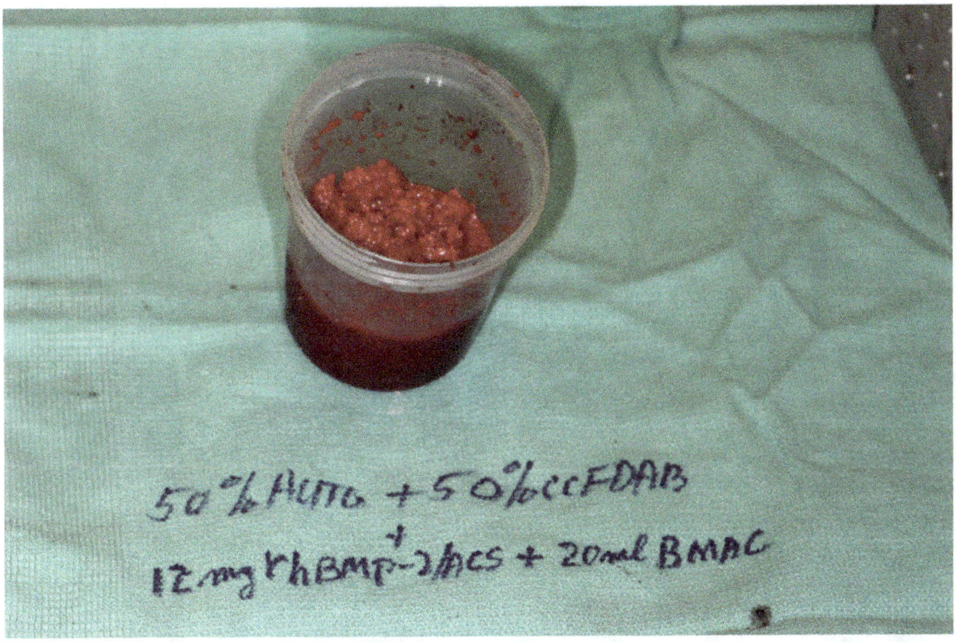

Figure 60a. Today's bone grafts use less autogenous bone by using allogeneic bone, bone-marrow-derived stem cells, and recombinant human bone morphogenetic protein.

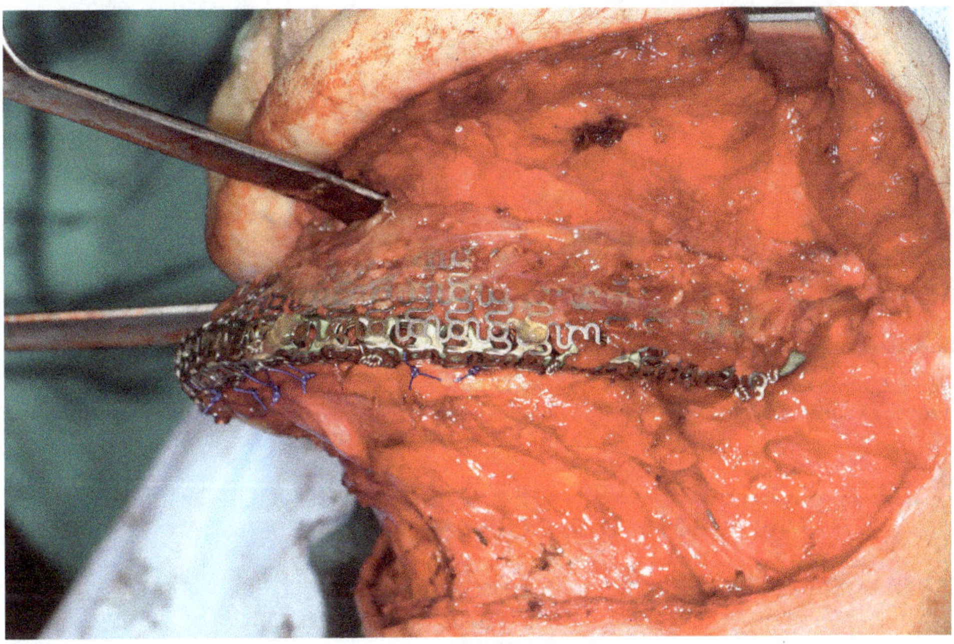

Figure 60b. Composite bone graft as noted in Figure 60a placed.

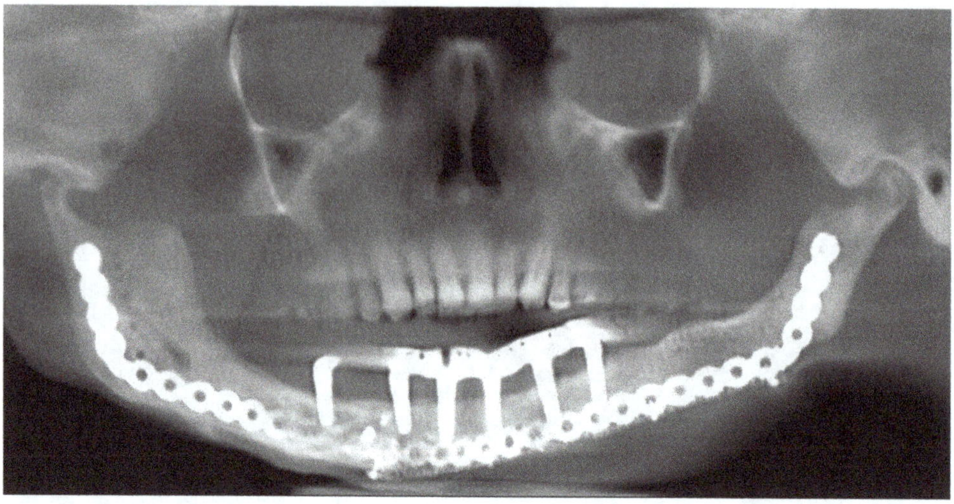

Figure 61. Mature bone graft of 14 cm length with dental implants after the resection for osteoradionecrosis.

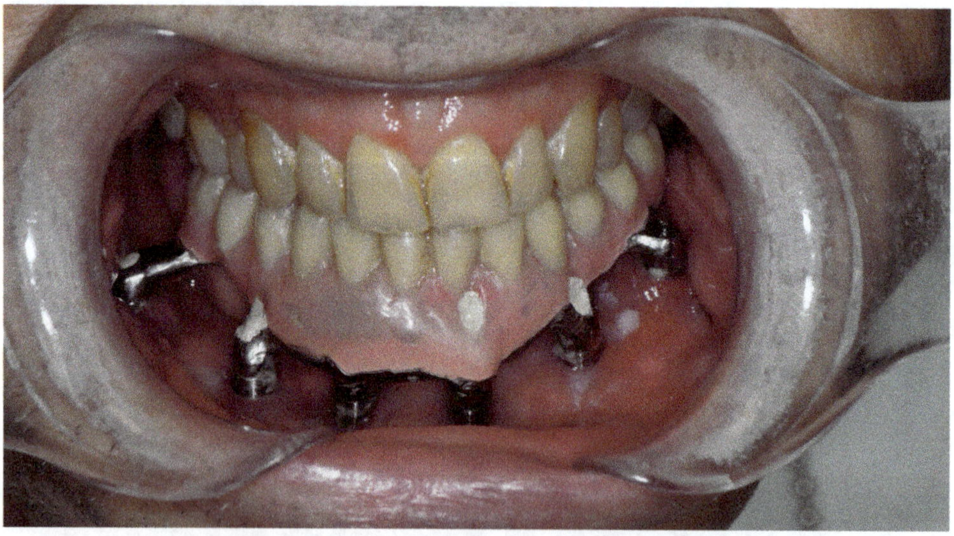

Figure 62. Implant-supported denture after hyperbaric oxygen protocol, osteoradionecrosis resection with anterior lateral thigh flap bone grafting, and dental implants.

TABLE 6. COSTS ANALYSIS OF OSTEORADIONECROSIS PATIENT: JAN 1, 2016, U.S. DOLLARS

TREATMENT	# PATIENTS	AVERAGE ONE-YEAR COST	AVERAGE TOTAL COST	RESOLUTION RATE
Non-HBO_2	197	$65,000	$224,000	10%
HBO_2	108	$60,000	$152,000	16%
Protocol	914	$81,000	$96,000	100%

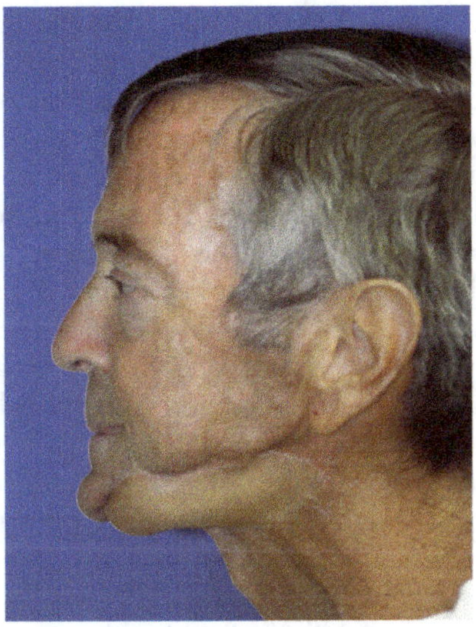

Figure 63. Profile of patient after osteoradionecrosis resection, soft-tissue reconstruction, bone replacement, dental implants, and dentures.

COST ANALYSIS OF OSTEORADIONECROSIS TREATMENT

At the time of the first edition of this book and even more so today this writing, politicians, the press, and the public are voicing concerns about the availability and costs of medical care. No doubt this tug-of-war will continue for even more decades to come. However, where do osteoradionecrosis and hyperbaric oxygen stand in the costliness of today's health care? Table 6 illustrates a complete review of all known cost factors of 1,219 patients who were treated for osteoradionecrosis and has been updated to January 1, 2016, U.S. dollars.

An overall analysis of these findings indicates that osteoradionecrosis is obviously an expensive disease once it develops, no matter how it is treated. Certainly the preventive efforts already known, such as radiotherapy dose fractioning, preradiation dental consultations, fluoride carriers, removing mandibular teeth in the direct radiation path if over 6,000 cGy, and the 20/10 hyperbaric oxygen protocol if surgery is anticipated, are to be encouraged and should continue to be standards.

If one looks carefully at these data, one can see the most costly approach to osteoradionecrosis is one where hyperbaric oxygen is not used. The average yearly costs were USD$65,000, and the total cost was USD$224,000. Worse yet is that USD$224,000 dollars is a low figure because only 10% of cases were resolved. This means that 90% of patients went elsewhere for continued treatment and accrued additional costs not appearing in this table. The high costs were mainly due to hospitalizations and drugs. These patients required serial admissions, serial debridements, many office visits, and great quantities of antibiotics and analgesics. All of this added up to the enormous costs shown in Table 6. What is not shown in Table 6 is the health-care provider's resources which were devoted to these patients' care, the lack of productivity and absence from the workplace, and the degraded quality of family life these patients endured, all of which were significant.

The next most costly approach was when hyperbaric oxygen was used without surgery. This amounted to an average yearly cost of USD$60,000 and an average total cost of USD$152,000. This approach is essentially similar to Stage I cases where HBO_2 by itself was able to resolve the problem in only 16% of the cases. The remaining 84% were treated and retreated with several hyperbaric oxygen courses to build the high total cost of USD$152,000.

The main cost in this approach was the repeated hyperbaric oxygen fees followed by hospitalization and health-care provider fees. This approach to osteoradionecrosis was popular in the late 1960s and 1970s before the pathophysiology of osteoradionecrosis was known and before a definitive protocol to resolve the disease was established,[17,19] yet it is still is use in some areas today. Common approaches during that era called for serial hyperbaric oxygen courses every six months. Such approaches resolved the osteoradionecrosis only on rare occasions because surgical debridement of nonviable bone was not carried out. Such results are a reminder that hyperbaric oxygen cannot resurrect dead bone. Dead bone is best managed by surgical removal. It is also a reminder that the target tissue of hyperbaric oxygen is not the dead tissue but the radiation-damaged tissue which is not yet dead.

The costs for patients treated with the staged protocols discussed in this chapter incurred an average yearly cost of USD$81,000 with a total cost of USD$96,000. The total cost and the yearly cost are nearly the same because the disease is resolved rather than allowed to become chronic with ongoing costs. The USD$96,000 cost in this protocol is indeed expensive, but is an average of Stage I, Stage II, and Stage III responders. The costs include fees for hyperbaric oxygen, surgeons' fees, hospitalization, reconstruction fees, and even prosthetic fees to replace teeth. Stage III patients were the most costly (isolated Stage III costs were USD$118,000) due to a greater requirement for hospitalization and surgery but were still significantly below the costs of any other approach.

Osteoradionecrosis is documented to be an expensive entity. However, HBO_2, if used in a strict protocol along with surgery, has been shown to be the most effective approach. In addition to cost savings, the intangible benefits are immeasurable. By resolving a painful and debilitating disease, patients become productive once again, as they return to their families and to the workplace.

THE RELATIONSHIP OF HYPERBARIC OXYGEN TO ORAL CANCER

The natural concern of many has been the potential effect of increased oxygen levels on cancer which may be residual within patients or within histologically dysplastic mucosa. Patients who have had radiotherapy for head and neck cancers often harbor a treacherous prognosis. They may have residual tumor which surgery or radiation did not fully eradicate. They may also have altered mucous membrane cells from years of tobacco and alcohol use, human papilloma virus, or the spontaneous emergence of oncogenes or loss of tumor suppressor genes that results in premalignant dysplasia. They can also present with tissue breakdown and fistulae which are cancers mimicking osteoradionecrosis. They may even have radiation-induced dysplasias and carcinomas. An entire array of statistics applies to this group. Some of the more important to keep in mind are the following.

Patients who have had one oral cancer and who continue to smoke have a 33% chance of developing a new primary in the foregut within five years.[39] Our statistics indicate that 67% of patients who develop an oral cancer associated with smoking continue to smoke after treatment for their cancer and that, in 46% of oral cancer related to smoking, the patient has stopped smoking for more than ten years. Squamous cell carcinoma of the oral cavity has a 50% overall five-year survival rate. Four percent of patients referred into a major medical center (the University of Miami) with a diagnosis of osteoradionecrosis have residual oral cancer along with their osteoradionecrosis. The point of all these statistics is simply that, even with the best diagnostic techniques, one cannot be sure these patients are tumor free. Because of this, we and several other authors have studied the relationship of cancers, particularly oral cancers, to hyperbaric oxygen.

Animal Studies

The most common and best animal model has been that of the hamster cheek pouch using a 1, 2 9-10 dimethyl Benzanthracene (DMBA) as the carcinogen. Our first study assessed the development of dysplasia and its progression to cancer over 22 weeks as well as the growth rate of the cancers once they emerged. The animals all had the DMBA applied 3 times a week in a 0.5% solution in acetone. One group received daily hyperbaric oxygen at 2.4 ATA for 90 minutes each day; the other group did not receive any hyperbaric oxygen. The results are graphed in Figures 64 and Figure 65. The graph in Figure 64 compares the hyperbaric-oxygen-treated group to the control group, assessing the cheek pouches of serially euthanized animals. The results indicated that, surprisingly, hyperbaric oxygen actually suppressed the dysplasia and delayed the emergence of carcinomas from the dysplasia by one month. Figure 65 shows that the growth rates of tumors induced by the DMBA are equal between the hyperbaric oxygen and nonhyperbaric group.[8,26]

In a similar study, McMillan et al.[30] also found that hyperbaric oxygen suppressed the emergence of oral cancers and suppressed dysplasias. They did observe, however, that tumors in the hyperbaric oxygen group were bigger, but they did not measure growth rates.[30] In related studies, Nemiroff has shown no acceleration of the growth rate of primaries or metastases from lung tumors in mice.[32-33] In a second study, we developed fully mature cheek pouch cancers in the hamsters. One group was exposed

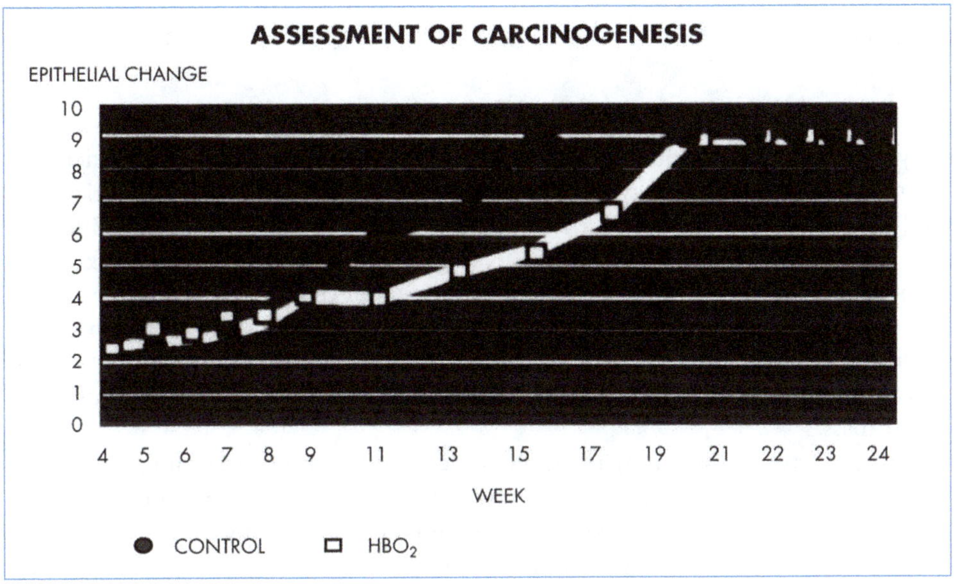

Figure 64. Graph of developing mucosal carcinoma versus time, identifying a suppression of dysplasia and a slowing of overt carcinoma in the hyperbaric oxygen group.

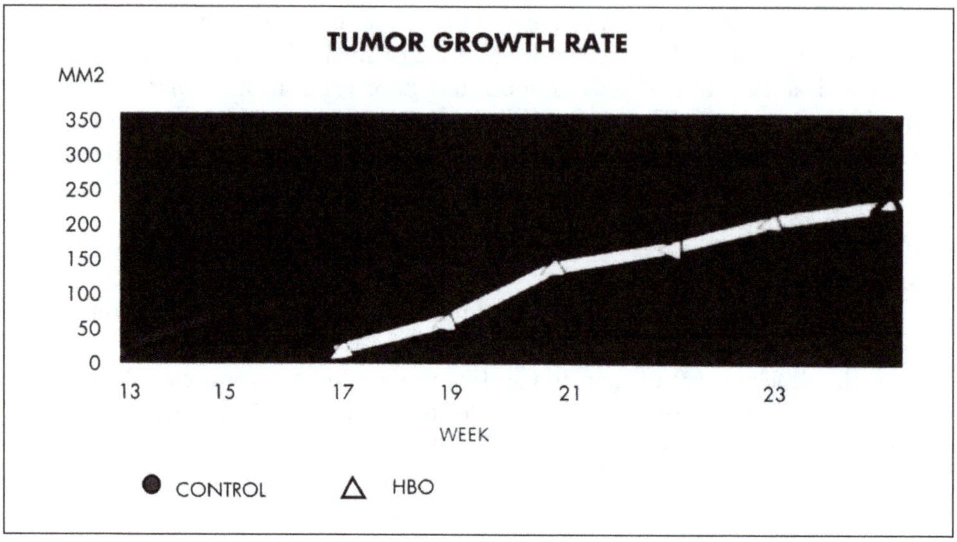

Figure 65. Graph of tumor size versus time, indicating a delayed emergence of carcinoma in the hyperbaric oxygen group and parallel slopes identifying equal growth rates.

TABLE 7. FIVE-YEAR CANCER RECURRENCE: SQUAMOUS CELL CARCINOMA

STAGE	NON-HBO_2	RECURRED	HBO_2	RECURRED
I	55	10 (19%)	31	5 (17%)
II	92	25 (27%)	144	40 (28%)
III	117	44 (38%)	149	39 (26%)
IV	126	52 (41%)	111	40 (36%)
All Stages	390	120 (30.8%)	435	124 (28.5%)
P = 0.82				

to hyperbaric oxygen, another group was injected with an oxygen-radical-generating system of a cross-linked enzyme of glucose oxidase and horseradish peroxidase, a third group received both, and a fourth group served as controls.[6,36] The findings indicated that oxygen radicals (superoxide, singlet oxygen, hydroxyl radical, etc.) have antineoplastic properties based on lipid peroxidation of cell membranes. It seems that tumor cells are somewhat selectively lysed due to their inability to produce superoxide dismutase as a scavenger of oxygen radicals. These studies also indicate that oxygen radicals are more deleterious to smaller tumors and dysplasias than to larger tumors of greater mass.

Animal studies, in summary, imply some suppression of early tumor formation and no acceleration of growth or metastatic potential. However, these animal models, as good as they are, are not the equivalent of human studies. Only human studies can be looked upon as a reliable index of the potential harmful effects of clinical hyperbaric oxygen on a population of patients who have already had one foregut cancer and have been exposed to a variety of carcinogens and other cancer-promoting factors.

Human Studies

From 1995 through 2015, we have followed 825 consecutive patients who were treated for oral squamous cell carcinoma by surgery and radiation therapy or radiation therapy alone. Of these patients, 435 underwent a protocol of hyperbaric oxygen for either reconstructive surgery (the 20/10 protocol) or for the treatment of osteoradionecrosis (the 30/10 protocol). The results of these findings are presented in Table 7, where the results are stratified according to the TNM classification of the Joint Commission on Cancer Staging from Stage I to Stage IV. The higher stages are indicative of more advanced disease and poorer prognosis. Table 7 clearly shows a lesser but nearly equal incidence of recurrence in nearly every stage of squamous cell carcinoma in those who have been exposed to hyperbaric oxygen as those who have not. Therefore, this data shows no ability of hyperbaric oxygen, in humans, to accelerate cancer or cause more to emerge from dysplastic mucosa. It remains a safe and effective modality for radiated head and neck cancer patients despite continued carcinogen exposure and the many forms of their malignancies.

REFERENCES

1. Adamo AR, Szal RL. Timing, results and complications of mandibular reconstructive surgery: report of 32 cases. J Oral Surg. 1979;37:755-62.
2. Boyne PJ. Effect of increased oxygenation on osteogenesis enhancement. In: Davis JC, Hunt TK, editors. Hyperbaric oxygen therapy. Bethesda (MD): Undersea & Hyperbaric Medical Society; 1988. p. 205-16.
3. Brånemark PI, Adell R, Albrektsson T, Lekholm U, Lundkvist S, Röckler B. Osseointegrated titanium fixtures in the treatment of edentulousness. Biomaterials. 1983;4:25-8.
4. Brånemark PI, Lindström J, Hallén O, Breine U, Jeppsson PH, Öhman A. Osseointegrated implants in the treatment of the edentulous jaw. Experience from a ten year period. Scand J Plast Reconstr Surg. 1977;(Suppl 16):1-132.
5. Bump RL, Young JM, Davis JC, et al. Hyperbaric oxygen: treatment of osteoradionecrosis and osteomyelitis. Med Serv Dig. 1971;26:13-8.
6. Ehler WJ, Marx RE, Kiel J, Ravelo JI, Cissik JH. Induced regression of oral carcinoma by oxygen radical generating systems. J Hyperb Med. 1991;6:111-8.
7. Hahn G, Corgill DA. Conservative treatment of radionecrosis of the mandible. Oral Surg. 1967;24:707-11.
8. Harmon FW, Marx RE. The effect of hyperbaric oxygen on carcinogenesis and tumor growth rate. In: Proceedings of the 65th Annual Meeting of the Annual Meeting of the American Association of Oral and Maxillofacial Surgeons; 1983.
9. Hart GB, Mainous EG. The treatment of radiation necrosis with hyperbaric oxygen. Cancer. 1976;37(6):2580-6.
10. Heimbach RD. Radiation effects on tissue. In: Davis JC, Hunt TK, editors. Problem wounds – the role of oxygen. New York: Elsevier; 1988. Chapter 3; p. 53-63.
11. Hong WK, Lippman SM, Itri LM, Karp DD, Lee JS, et al. Prevention of second primary tumors with isotrelinon in a squamous cell carcinoma of the head and neck. N Engl J Med. 1990;323:795-801.
12. Joseph DL, Shumrick DL. Risks of head and neck surgery in previously irradiated patients. Arch Otolaryngol. 1973;97:381-4.
13. Knighton DR, Hunt TK, Schenestuhl H, et al. Oxygen tension regulates the expression of angiogenesis factor by macrophages. Science. 1983;221:1283-9.
14. Knighton DR, Oredsson S, Banda M, et al. Regulation of repair: hypoxic control of macrophage mediated angiogenesis. In: Hunt TK, Heppenstall RB, Pines E, et al., editors. Soft and hard tissue repair. New York: Praeger; 1984. p. 41-9.
15. Knighton DR, Silver IA, Hunt TK. Regulation of wound healing angiogenesis: effect of oxygen gradients and inspired oxygen concentrations. Surgery. 1981;90:262-70.
16. Komisar A. The functional result of mandibular reconstruction. Laryngoscope. 1990;100:364-74.
17. Mainous EG. Hyperbaric oxygen in maxillofacial osteomyelitis, osteoradionecrosis, and osteogenesis enhancement. In: Davis JC, Hunt TK, editors. Hyperbaric oxygen therapy. Bethesda (MD): Undersea & Hyperbaric Medical Society; 1988. p. 191-203.
18. Mainous EG, Boyne PJ. Hyperbaric oxygen in total rehabilitation of patients with mandibular osteoradionecrosis. Int J Oral Surg. 1974;3:297-302.

19. Mainous EG, Boyne PJ, Hart GB, Terry BC. Restoration of resected mandible by grafting with a combination of mandible homograft and autogenous iliac marrow, and post-operative treatment with hyperbaric oxygenation. Oral Surg. 1973;35:13-20.

20. Marx RE. A new concept in the treatment of osteoradionecrosis. J Oral Maxillofacial Surg. 1983;41:351-8.

21. Marx RE. Osteoradionecrosis: a new concept of its pathophysiology. J Oral Maxillofac Surg. 1983;48:283-9.

22. Marx RE. Osteoradionecrosis of the jaws: review and update. HBO Rev. 1984;5:78-128.

23. Marx RE, Ames JR. The use of hyperbaric oxygen therapy in bony reconstruction of the irradiated and tissue deficient patient. J Oral Maxillofac Surg. 1982;40:412-9.

24. Marx RE, Ehler WJ, Tayapongsak PT, Pierce LW. Relationship of oxygen dose to angiogenesis induction in irradiated tissue. Am J Surg. 1990;160:519-24.

25. Marx RE, Johnson RP. Studies in the radiobiology of osteoradionecrosis and their clinical significance. Oral Surg. 1987;64:379-90.

26. Marx RE, Johnson RP. Problem wounds in oral and maxillofacial surgery: the role of hyperbaric oxygen. In: Davis JC, Hunt TK, editors. Problem wounds – the role of oxygen. New York: Elsevier; 1988. Chapter 4; p. 65-123.

27. Marx RE, Johnson RP, Kline SN. Prevention of osteoradionecrosis: a randomized prospective clinical trial of hyperbaric oyxgen versus penicillin. JADA. 1985;111:49-54.

28. Marx RE, Kline SN. Principles and methods of osseous reconstruction. Int Adv Surg Oncol. 1983;61:167-228.

29. Marx RE, Smith BR. An improved technique for development of the pectoralis major myocutaneous flap. Oral Maxillofac Surg. 1990;48:1168-80.

30. McMillan T, Calhoun KH, Nader JT, Stiernberg, Rhaaramans CM. The effect of hyperbaric oxygen therapy on oral mucosal carcinoma. Laryngoscope. 1989;99(3):241-4.

31. Meyer I. Infectious diseases of the jaws. J Oral Surg. 1970;28:27-33.

32. Nemiroff PM. Effects of hyperbaric oxygen on growth and metastases on Lewis lung tumors in mice. J Hyperb Med. 1988;3(2):89-95.

33. Nemiroff PM. Effects of hyperbaric oxygen on tumor metastases in mice. Clin Radiol. 1991;22:538-40.

34. Niinikoski J. Effect of oxygen supply on wound healing and formation of experimental granulation tissue. Acta Physiol Scand Suppl. 1969;334:1-72.

35. Niinikoski J, Hunt TK. Oxygen tensions in healing bone. Surg Gynecol Obstet. 1972;134:746-50.

36. Ravelo JI, Marx RE. The effects of oxygen radicals on tumorigenesis in hamsters. Am Assoc Oral and Maxillofac Surg Scient Abstr Session. 68th Annual Meeting; 1988 Sep 16.

37. Rubin P, Casarett GW. Clinical radiation pathology, Vol. II. Philadelphia: W.B. Saunders; 1968. p. 557-608.

38. Silver IA. Cellular microenvironment in healing and non-healing wounds. In: TK Hunt, Heppenstall RB, Pines E, et al., editors. Soft and hard tissue repair. New York: Praeger; 1984. p. 50-66.

39. Silverman S, Shillitoe EJ. Etiology and predisposing factors. In: Silverman S, editor. Oral cancer. New York: American Cancer Society; 1981. p. 6-35.

40. Strauss SE, Spatz SS. Irradiated dentition: the dentist's responsibilities. J Prosthetic Dent. 1972;27:209-14.

41. Van Steenburghe D, Sullivan DY, et al. A retrospective multicenter evaluation of the survival rate of osseointegrated fixtures supporting bridges in the treatment of partial edentulism. J Prosthet Dent. 1989;61:217-23.

CHAPTER 30 CHAPTER

The Use of Hyperbaric Oxygen for Treating Delayed Radiation Injuries in Gynecologic Malignancies

CHAPTER THIRTY OVERVIEW

Introduction **779**

Methods and Materials **779**

Inclusion Criteria 780

Exclusion Criteria. 780

Results **780**

Radiation Proctitis 780

Radiation Cystitis. 781

Incidence of Radiation Injury in Gynecologic Malignancies 781

Discussion **785**

Level of Evidence 785

Radiation Proctitis 785

Radiation Cystitis. 785

Radiation Necrosis 786

Conclusion **786**

References **787**

The Use of Hyperbaric Oxygen for Treating Delayed Radiation Injuries in Gynecologic Malignancies

Harry T. Whelan, Chris Kilian

INTRODUCTION

Radiation is a well-established therapy for the treatment of many cancers, including those in the female genital tract. Unfortunately, the destruction of cells with radiotherapy is not limited to those with neoplasia, and radiation often has long-term effects on normal, healthy tissue. Histology shows that radiation causes an obliterative endarteritis that leads to the classic "three H" tissue environment: hypovascular, hypoxic, and hypocellular.(12) This is a very difficult tissue environment in which to promote healing. Radiation results in a blurry delineation between normal and damaged tissue, causing a slow, diffuse change in irradiated tissues. This diffuse pattern of damage results in a shallow oxygen gradient between normal and damaged tissue.(9) In normal wounds, a steep oxygen gradient provides a stimulus for macrophages to promote angiogenesis and collagen synthesis.(10) However, in irradiated tissues, this gradient is not present, and thus there is no stimulus for angiogenesis. As a result, necrosis may manifest months to years after initial radiation therapy.

Hyperbaric oxygen (HBO_2) therapy increases the oxygen gradient in damaged and radiated tissues, providing a stimulus for angiogenesis. HBO_2 therapy has been shown to be effective in treating radiation injuries precisely because these tissues have difficulty with angiogenesis.(9) HBO_2 therapy has been used for many years in radiation injuries in head and neck cancers but remains underutilized in many other malignancies.(5) One population of interest is women who have undergone radiation therapy for gynecologic malignancies. The gynecologic cancers most commonly treated with radiation are cervical, uterine, and vaginal. Occasionally it is used in ovarian and vulvar cancer. These patients can develop radiation injuries such as soft-tissue necrosis, cystitis, and proctitis – all of which are U.S. Food and Drug Administration–approved indications for HBO_2 therapy. This paper describes the current evidence for HBO_2 therapy in gynecologic malignancies. We also conducted an analysis of the incidence of radiation injuries in gynecologic cancers at two large medical centers in southeastern Wisconsin.

METHODS AND MATERIALS

We performed a literature search on Google Scholar, PubMed, and Ovid for the search terms "gynecologic malignancies" and "hyperbaric oxygen" paired with "cystitis," "proctitis," and "necrosis." The studies were then reviewed for the highest-quality evidence.

Inclusion Criteria

Articles were included if they reported on the effects of HBO_2 therapy on cystitis, proctitis, and necrosis, particularly with women as the main cohort. Preference was given to prospective and/or randomized studies.

Exclusion Criteria

Articles excluded were case reports, animal studies, editorials, and reviews. Foreign language studies were excluded. To gather incidence data, we accessed cancer databases at Aurora St. Luke's Hospital (ASLH) and Froedtert Memorial Lutheran Hospital (FMLH) in Milwaukee, Wisconsin. The databases were scrubbed of all patient-specific data to maintain confidentiality. We gathered the total number of patients treated at these two institutions for ovarian, uterine, cervical, vaginal, and vulvar malignancies (ICD-9 codes 180–184.9). Those patients were then cross-referenced for necrosis, cystitis, proctitis, and radiation injury NOS (ICD-9 569.49, 623.8, 614.2, 624.8, E926.9, 990).

RESULTS

The efficacy of HBO_2 therapy for radiation injury in head and neck cancers has been well documented. In this paper, we report the results of studies specifically pertaining to gynecologic malignancies. As randomized controlled trials (RCTs) lend the greatest weight toward establishing practice guidelines, we report detailed information on the three randomized controlled trials studying this topic. A summary of articles on this topic is presented in Tables 1 and 2.

Radiation Proctitis

Two RCTs have been published supporting the use of HBO_2 therapy in treating radiation proctitis resulting from pelvic radiation. In 2007, Sidik and colleagues[15] studied 65 women with radiation proctitis after treatment for cervical cancer. Patients were excluded from the study if they had existing pneumothorax, metabolic disease, diabetes mellitus, malnutrition, chronic diseases, or depression. The primary outcomes were improvement on the late effects normal tissue – subjective, objective, management, and analytic (SOMA-LENT) and Karnofsky quality of life scales.

Thirty-two women were randomized to the HBO_2 therapy group, and 33 were controls. Before treatment, the mean SOMA-LENT and Karnofsky scores in the HBO_2 therapy group were 7.7 and 73.8, respectively. In the control group, the scores were 6.8 and 74.6. In the HBO_2 therapy group, most patients underwent at least 18 sessions.

Six months after the intervention, the mean SOMA-LENT and Karnofsky scores improved 33.6% and 15.2% in the HBO_2 therapy group. The control group's mean Karnofsky score improved only 2.4%, and the SOMA-LENT score decreased 19.69% ($p \leq 0.001, 0.008$). This study was limited by the fact that there was no blinding.

In 2008, Clarke and colleagues[4] conducted a randomized, controlled, double-blind trial investigating the use of HBO_2 therapy for radiation necrosis. A total of 226 patients were assessed for eligibility. Of these 226 patients, 76 were excluded and 150 enrolled; 106 were women. Other medical management requirements were discontinued, and advanced interventions were largely avoided.

The HBO_2 therapy group (group 1) was treated with 100% oxygen at 2.0 ATA for 90 minutes, once daily, five times weekly. The control group (group 2) was treated with 21% oxygen (normal air) at 1.1 ATA, once daily, five times weekly. For patient blinding purposes, group 2 patients underwent a brief compression to 1.34 ATA at the beginning of each treatment. The chamber was then slowly decompressed from 1.34 to 1.1 ATA. All patients underwent at least 30 treatments. Sixty-four patients in group 1 and 56 in group 2 completed the intervention. Group 2 was then unblinded and offered treatment. All but three accepted and underwent treatment.

After treatment and before crossover, the mean SOMA-LENT score of group 1 improved from 12.55 to 7.8. Group 2 (sham) improved from 12.85 to 10.23 ($p = 0.0019$). After crossover, the SOMA-LENT score of group 2 approximated that of group 1. After follow-up in years 1–5, there was a trend toward sustained improvement. Based on this, the number needed to treat is 3.

Radiation Cystitis

One randomized controlled study supports the use of HBO_2 therapy in treating radiation cystitis. In 2007, Van Ophoven and associates[13] enrolled 21 women in a randomized, sham-controlled, double-blind study. The primary outcome was marked or moderate improvement on a global response assessment survey (responders). Seven patients were enrolled in the sham group; 14 received HBO_2 therapy. In the HBO_2 therapy group, the women underwent six sessions per week for five weeks. Women in the sham group were placed in hyperbaric chambers and underwent a minimal increase in pressure to simulate HBO_2 therapy but did not receive 100% oxygen. Patients who responded to therapy underwent follow-up for 12 months. Nonresponders were discharged from the study after unblinding.

Two women in the HBO_2 therapy group dropped out of the study. After unblinding, three of the patients in the HBO_2 therapy arm and none of the sham patients were identified as responders. Sham treatment did not result in improvement of any secondary measures. The HBO_2 therapy group had statistically significant improvement in pain scores ($p < 0.05$) and showed a trend toward improved urgency and bladder volume. The authors state a response rate of 21%.

Incidence of Radiation Injury in Gynecologic Malignancies

From 2007 to 2010, the cancer center at FMLH treated an average of 220.5 (range 201–243) patients with gynecologic malignancies, which include ovarian, uterine, cervical, vaginal, and vulvar cancers. Of those patients, an average of 30.5 per year developed delayed radiation injuries, specifically necrosis, proctitis, and radiation injury NOS. There were no cases of cystitis. The average annual incidence of radiation injury in these patients was 13.8%. Results are summarized in Tables 3 and 4. Patients with cervical cancer and vulvar cancer had the highest incidence of radiation complications, at 23% each. Ovarian cancer had the lowest rate of complications, at 6.7%. The most common complication among all malignancies was soft-tissue necrosis.

TABLE 1. SUMMARY OF STUDIES ON HBO_2 THERAPY EFFECTIVENESS IN DELAYED RADIATION INJURIES FROM GYNECOLOGIC MALIGNANCIES

AUTHOR	COMPLICATION	TYPE OF STUDY	NUMBER OF PATIENTS	END POINT	MEAN FOLLOW-UP (MONTHS)	OUTCOME	COMMENT
Warren et al.[16]	Proctitis	Retrospective	14 (12 men, 2 women)	Resolution of symptoms	17	9 out of 14 resolved	3 out of 5 nonresponders improved initially, but then relapsed
Sidik et al.[15]	Proctitis	RCT	65 women (32 HBO_2 therapy, 33 control)	SOMA-LENT score, QOL Karnofsky score	6	Statistically significant improvement in QOL and side effects	
Clarke et al.[4]	Proctitis	RCT	120 (106 women) 64 HBO_2 therapy, 56 control	SOMA-LENT score	24	SOMA-LENT improvement 5.0 versus 2.61	HBO_2 therapy group 6 times more likely to report improvement
Lee et al.[11]	Cystitis	Retrospective	20 women	Resolution of hematuria	14	19 out of 20 patients hematuria free	Only 1 patient required urinary diversion
Bevers et al.[2]	Cystitis	Prospective observational	40 (27 men, 13 women)	Resolution of hematuria	23	37 out of 40 resolved	10 out of 10 gyn cancer patients hematuria free
Del Pizzo et al.[6]	Cystitis	Retrospective	11 (6 women, 5 men)	Resolution of hematuria, urgency, pain	60	3 out of 11 asymptomatic	At 5 years, 5 out of 6 women required urinary diversion

TABLE 1 (CONTINUED)

Chong et al.[3]	Cystitis	Retrospective	60 (55 men, 5 women)	Complete or partial resolution of hematuria	12	80% resolution	If treated within 6 months, 96% patients resolved
Van Ophoven et al.[13]	Cystitis	RCT	21 women	Global symptom improvement	12	21% symptom improvement	No patient in sham group reported improvement
Williams et al.[18]	Necrosis	Prospective observational	14 women	Resolution of necrosis	Not given	13 out of 14 showed complete resolution	One patient died from necrotizing infection
Feldmeir et al.[7]	Necrosis	Retrospective	44 (9 men, 35 women)	Healed versus not healed	Not given	20 out of 23 gyn patients healed	26 out of 41 total patients healed, 31 received adequate amount of HBO$_2$ therapy
Fink et al.[8]	Necrosis	Retrospective	14 women	Complete healing, > 50% improvement, < 50% improvement, no improvement	32	1 out of 8 complete healing, 5 out of 8 showed > 50% improvement, 2 out of 8 showed < 50% improvement	10 out of 14 patients showed > 50% improvement; 8 patients had vaginal or other soft-tissue involvement

TABLE 2. SUMMARY OF STUDIES SCREENED AND REASONS FOR EXCLUSION[7]

	NUMBER OF STUDIES SCREENED	INCLUDED	REASONS FOR EXCLUSION
Cystitis	14	5	Case reports, foreign language
Proctitis	13	3	Case reports, animal study, no gynecologic malignancies, abstract, foreign language
Necrosis	13	3	Case reports, foreign language, no gynecologic malignancies

TABLE 3. TOTAL GYNECOLOGIC CANCER CASES AND RADIATION COMPLICATIONS TREATED AT FMLH FROM 2007 TO 2010

	2007	2008	2009	2010	TOTALS
CERVICAL CANCER					
Total malignancies	38	43	51	52	184
Necrosis	1	6	12	11	30
Proctitis	2	2	3	2	9
NOS	1	2	0	1	4
UTERINE CANCER					
Total malignancies	94	84	105	90	373
Necrosis	10	10	9	12	41
Proctitis	4	7	6	1	18
NOS	1	1	1	0	3
OVARIAN CANCER					
Total malignancies	56	57	71	83	267
Necrosis	1	2	3	5	11
Proctitis	0	5	1	1	7
NOS	0	0	0	0	0
VAGINAL CANCER					
Total malignancies	3	2	2	0	7
Necrosis	1	0	0	0	1
Proctitis	0	0	0	0	0
NOS	0	0	0	0	0
VULVAR CANCER					
Total malignancies	10	15	14	12	51
Necrosis	2	1	4	3	10
Proctitis	0	1	1	0	2
NOS	0	0	0	0	0

TABLE 4. INCIDENCE OF RADIATION COMPLICATIONS IN GYNECOLOGIC MALIGNANCIES AT FMLH

	CERVICAL CANCER	UTERINE CANCER	OVARIAN CANCER	VAGINAL CANCER	VULVAR CANCER
Total incidence	0.234	0.166	0.067	0.143	0.235
Necrosis	0.163	0.11	0.041	0.143	0.196
Proctitis	0.049	0.048	0.026	0.000	0.039
NOS	0.022	0.008	0.000	0.000	0.000

From 2005 to 2010, ASLH treated an average of 839.2 (range 541–1205) patients with gynecologic malignancies. Of those, an average of 46.3 (range 21–60) per year developed complications of radiation therapy. The average annual incidence of radiation complications was 5.5%.

DISCUSSION

Froedtert Hospital, affiliated with the Medical College of Wisconsin, is a tertiary medical center of 433 beds. Aurora St. Luke's Hospital is a 724-bed medical center. Together, the two hospital systems account for nearly 60% of inpatient admissions in the greater Milwaukee area, which has a population of over two million people.[1] FMLH has two monoplace chambers. ASLH has a multiplace chamber that can accommodate 24 patients at once.

The results of our data indicate that if these patients undergo radiation therapy, as many as 23% may develop delayed complications of radiation. The relatively high rate of complications at FMLH may be due to the fact the hospital is a major academic medical center and may treat more complicated or advanced cancers. Certainly, many of these patients may heal with supportive care, but some may be refractory to treatment. It is these refractory cases for which we recommend HBO_2 therapy.

Level of Evidence

Hyperbaric oxygen has been used extensively to treat delayed radiation injuries. In this paper, we presented only studies of HBO_2 therapy and its use in gynecologic malignancies. Using the American Academy of Neurology guidelines on evidence-based medicine, we classified the level of evidence for HBO_2 therapy use in proctitis, cystitis, and necrosis resulting from delayed radiation injuries in gynecologic malignancies.

Radiation Proctitis

The two randomized controlled studies by Clarke[4] and Sidik[15] provide compelling evidence for the effectiveness of HBO_2 therapy for treating radiation proctitis. Based on these two Class I studies, we recommend a Level A rating: HBO_2 therapy should be done for radiation proctitis.

Radiation Cystitis

One randomized controlled study (Van Ophoven et al.[13]) supports the use of HBO_2 therapy in radiation cystitis. However, it was a small pilot study and showed only 21% success rate. The Van Ophoven study showed that in 30 patients, HBO_2 therapy was well tolerated. In the future, more research could be done to identify which patients would benefit most from HBO_2 therapy. The Del Pizzo study[6] could be classified as a negative study, in that only 3 out of 11 patients were asymptomatic after treatment. That study is limited by being a small, retrospective case series. The Bevers[2] study, though large and prospective, was not controlled. That study is significant in the fact that all patients with gynecologic malignancies were hematuria free after HBO_2 therapy. Chong's[3] retrospective review of HBO_2 therapy showed good outcomes, but the results may or may not be generalized to the female population, as the study was mostly of men with prostate cancer. We recommend a Level B rating: HBO_2 therapy should be considered for treating radiation cystitis.

Radiation Necrosis

There is an absence of randomized controlled trials studying the effects of HBO_2 therapy on radiation necrosis in gynecologic cancers. Most of the studies are retrospective; however, they show excellent results, often resolving necrotic wounds and fistulas. Additionally, HBO_2 therapy has been used successfully for years in treating head and neck radionecrosis. Marx et al. reported a controlled, nonrandomized study of soft-tissue radionecrosis of the neck. They showed fewer infections in the HBO_2 therapy group (6% versus 24%), less dehiscence, and improved healing times.[12] Based on this, we recommend a Level B rating: HBO_2 therapy should be considered for radiation necrosis. Despite the lack of RCTs for radiation necrosis, HBO_2 therapy has become standard in many treatment protocols of soft-tissue necrosis in head and neck cancers. Because soft-tissue radionecrosis behaves similarly throughout the body, it is reasonable to apply the same standards used in head and neck cancers to gynecologic malignancies.[17]

The recommendations we have made are limited by the relative paucity of studies on HBO_2 therapy in gynecologic malignancies. This could be a result of the difficulty in performing large studies in hyperbaric chambers. Most treatment protocols require at least 20 daily sessions, as that is the length of time required for angiogenesis. Additionally, a long follow-up is required to establish the lasting effects of HBO_2 therapy, and the treatment is costly. The physiological basis behind HBO_2 therapy has been well studied, and its effects are dramatic, often preventing surgery or other invasive procedures.

Further study on HBO_2 therapy is currently being performed. The Baromedical Research Foundation is completing the Hyperbaric Oxygen Radiation Tissue Injury Study, a multicenter randomized controlled trial evaluating HBO_2 therapy on several different malignancies. The results from this study should provide further insight into the efficacy of HBO_2 therapy.[14]

CONCLUSION

Hyperbaric oxygen has been used for decades with success in treating radiation injuries in head and neck cancers. This paper reviews the best evidence for HBO_2 therapy in treating gynecologic malignancies. The evidence in support of using HBO_2 therapy for radiation proctitis is Level A: it should be used. The evidence for using HBO_2 therapy in radiation cystitis and necrosis is Level B. HBO_2 therapy should be considered in treating women who develop radiation cystitis or necrosis.

Delayed radiation injuries are not theoretical. They may develop in up to 23% of gynecologic cancers treated with radiation. HBO_2 therapy may relieve the significant morbidity these women suffer and save them from invasive surgeries. The side effects of HBO_2 therapy are minimal, limited mostly to mild barotrauma of the middle ear. Some patients may experience visual disturbance, thought to be due to a transient conformational change in the lens. It is a safe, efficacious form of treatment for delayed radiation injuries and should be a routine part of treatment protocols in gynecologic malignancies.

REFERENCES

1. Aurora Health Care FYE 2009 continuing disclosure filing. DAC Bond [Internet]. Digital Assurance Certification, LLC. Aurora Health Care FYE 2009 continuing disclosure filing [cited 2011 Apr 25]. Available from: www.dacbond.com.
2. Bevers RFM, Bakker DJ, Kurth KH. Hyperbaric oxygen treatment for hemorrhagic radiation cystitis. Lancet. 1995;346:803-5.
3. Chong et al. Early hyperbaric oxygen therapy improves outcomes for radiation-induced hemorrhagic cystitis. Urology. 2005;65:649-53.
4. Clarke RE, Tenorio LM, Hussey JR, et al. Hyperbaric oxygen treatment of chronic refractory radiation proctitis: a randomized and controlled double-blind crossover trial with long-term follow-up. Int J Radiat Oncol Biol Phys. 2008;72:134-43.
5. Davis JC et al. Hyperbaric oxygen: a new adjunct in the management of radiation necrosis. Arch Otolaryngol. 1979;105:58-61.
6. Del Pizzo JJ, Chew BH, Jacobs SC, Sklar GN. Treatment of radiation inducted hemorrhagic cystitis with hyperbaric oxygen: long term followup. J Urol. 1998;160:731-3.
7. Feldmeier JJ, Hampson NB. A systematic review of the literature reporting the application of hyperbaric oxygen prevention and treatment of delayed radiation injuries: an evidence based approach. Undersea Hyperb Med. 2002;29:4-30.
8. Fink D, Chetty N, Lehm JP, Marsden DE, Hacker NF. Hyperbaric oxygen therapy for delayed radiation injuries in gynecologic cancers. Int J Gynecol Cancer. 2006;16:638-42.
9. Kindwall EP, Whelan HT. Hyperbaric medicine practice. 3rd ed. Flagstaff (AZ): Best Publishing Co.; 2008.
10. Knighton DR, Silver IA, Hunt TK. Regulation of wound healing angiogenesis: effect of oxygen gradients and inspired oxygen concentrations. Surgery. 1981;90:262-70.
11. Lee HC, Liu CS, Chiao C, Lin SN. Hyperbaric oxygen therapy in hemorrhagic cystitis: a report of 20 cases. Undersea Hyperb Med. 1994;21(3):321-7.
12. Marx RE. Osteoradionecrosis: a new concept of its pathophysiology. J Oral Maxillofac Surg. 1983;41:283-8.
13. Ophoven V et al. Safety and efficacy of hyperbaric oxygen therapy for the treatment of interstitial cystitis: a randomized, sham controlled, double-blind trail. J Urol. 2006;176:1442-6.
14. Radiation tissue injury study. Baromedical Research Foundation [Internet]. Baromedical Research Foundation. Radiation tissue injury study [cited 2011 Apr 28].
15. Sidik et al. Does hyperbaric oxygen administration decrease side effect and improve quality of life after pelvic radiation? Acta Med Indones. 2007;39(4):169-73.
16. Warren DC, Feehan P, Slade JB, Cianci PE. Chronic radiation proctitis treated with hyperbaric oxygen. Undersea Hyperb Med. 1997;24(3):181-4.
17. Weir G. Hyperbaric oxygen therapy for complication of radiotherapy. Wound Healing South Afr. 2009;2:60-2.
18. Williams JA, Clarke D, Dennis WA, Dennis E, Smith ST. The treatment of pelvic soft tissue radiation necrosis with hyperbaric oxygen. Am J Obstet Gynecol. 1992;167:412-6.

CHAPTER 31 CHAPTER

Adjunctive Hyperbaric Oxygen Therapy in the Treatment of Thermal Burns

CHAPTER THIRTY-ONE OVERVIEW

Abstract/Rationale **791**
Background **791**
Pathophysiology **793**
Infection **793**
Experimental Data **794**
Clinical Experience **800**
Recent Perspectives **803**
Pain Management 803
Immunity and Infection 804
Stem Cell Effects 804
Antioxidant Effects 804
Inhalation Injury **804**
2009 Cochrane Review **805**
Patient Selection Criteria **805**
Clinical Management **805**
Surgical Perspectives 806
Hyperbaric Oxygen 808
Utilization Review **809**
Cost Impact **809**
Discussion **809**
Summary **810**
Acknowledgment **811**
Conflict of Interest Statement **811**
References **812**

Adjunctive Hyperbaric Oxygen Therapy in the Treatment of Thermal Burns

Paul Cianci, Ronald M. Sato, Julia Faulkner

ABSTRACT/RATIONALE

A significant and consistently positive body of evidence from animal and human studies of thermal injury supports the use of hyperbaric oxygen as a means of preventing dermal ischemia, reducing edema, modulating the zone of stasis, preventing partial- to full-thickness conversion, preserving cellular metabolism, and promoting healing. The vast majority of clinical reports have shown reduction in mortality, length of hospital stay, number of surgeries, and cost of care. Hyperbaric oxygen has been demonstrated to be safe in the hands of those thoroughly trained in rendering therapy in the critical care setting and with appropriate monitoring precautions. Careful patient selection is mandatory.

BACKGROUND

The National Burn Repository reviewed the combined data of acute burn admissions for the time period between 2006 through 2015. The key findings included data from 96 hospitals, 36 states, and the District of Columbia, totaling 205,033 records. Men outnumber women considerably. The bimodal distribution with the greatest prevalence is the pediatric age range from 1–15, comprising 30% of total burns, and the adult age group from 20–59, making up 54% of burns. Patients age 60 or older represented 14% of burn cases. More than 75% of reported total burn cases were less than 10% total body surface area (TBSA), and these cases had a mortality of 0.6%. The mortality rate for all cases was 3.3% and 5.8% for fire/flame injuries. Seventy-three percent of burn injuries have occurred in the home. Nearly 95% were identified as accidents, with 14% reported as work-related cases. Just over 2% were suspected of abuse, and 1% were self-inflicted. During the 10-year period from 2006–2015, the average length of stay for females declined from 9.3 days to 7.9 days, while that for males declined less significantly, from 9.1 to 8.8 days. The mortality rate for females declined from 4.1% to 2.9%, and in males this decline was 3.9% to 3%. Deaths from burn injury increased with advancing age and burn size as well as presence of inhalation injury. Pneumonia was the most frequently clinically related complication and occurred in 5.4% of fire/flame or flame-injured patients. The frequency of pneumonia and respiratory failure was greater in patients with four days or greater of mechanical ventilation. The rate of complications increases with age. For survivors, the length of stay was slightly greater than one day per percent total body surface area burn. For those who died, the total hospital days were two times that of survivors on the average. However, this trend was reversed in patients with less than 20% total body surface burns. Eighty-seven percent of patients were discharged to home, and 3% were transferred to rehab facilities. Overall, charges for patients who died were three times greater than those who survived. However, this was greatly affected by the large number of patients with less than 10% total body surface area burns. For this group, total charges averaged USD$257,582 for survivors, and nonsurvivors averaged USD$340,474. Age and inhalation injury are major factors in burn mortality. A 20%–39% burn in patients below 60 confers a morality rate of 2.5%. In the presence of inhalation injury, that increases to 14%. The same injury in a 60-year-old shows a mortality of 32%, which increases to 55.8% in the presence of inhalation injury. Thus, age and inhalation injury are important factors in survival.

Burn care is extraordinarily expensive. Charges for a 50%–59% total body surface area averaged USD$1,066,254 in 2015. A 60%–70% burn averaged USD$1,168,006 during the same time frame. Workers compensation or automobile insurance covers approximately 10%, and "no information" or "self-insured" is indicated in 29% of cases.

Significant morbidity attaches to burn injury: pneumonia, cellulitis, respiratory failure, urinary tract infection, wound infection, and sepsis are still the most frequently reported complications and add significantly to mortality. Therapy of burns, therefore, is directed to minimizing edema, preserving marginally viable tissue in the zone of stasis, protecting the microvasculature, enhancing host defenses, and providing the essential substrates necessary to maintain viability. The ultimate goals of burn therapy include survival of the patient, rapid wound healing, minimization of scarring or abnormal pigmentation, prevention of long-term problems such as chronic pain, and cost effectiveness. Optimal outcome, obviously, is restoration as nearly as possible to the preburn quality of life.(5)

A recent report by Wolf et al. summarized problems and research priorities for the coming decade.(118) A major and continuing clinical problem is the innate inflammatory response induced by genetic factors, such as those common in neutrophils and macrophages, which are massively increased while the T-cell adaptive responses are downregulated. The latter are, perhaps, responsible for late effects of severe burns, such as viral and fungal infections. Hyperbaric oxygen therapy has been shown to modulate white cell adherence and to be helpful in the initial stages of inflammation. This could be an area of fruitful investigation.

In fact, the burn injury may be the universal trauma model. Wolf and colleagues point out that control of the hypermetabolic response and the massive inflammation will be important to improvement in burn care.

Despite the advances of early excision in accelerating healing to some degree, we seem to have plateaued in this regard. The authors suggest it may be time to visit the notion of whether healing times can be accelerated. This is another area of potential benefit of hyperbaric oxygen. A continuing problem in burn therapy and one for future investigation, suggested by Wolf et al., is the elimination of pain, both acute and chronic. Neuropathic pain is typically difficult to treat and thought to occur in a large percentage of those suffering severe burns.

PATHOPHYSIOLOGY

Physiologic responses to a major burn include a fall in arterial pressure, tachycardia, and a progressive decrease in cardiac output and stroke volume. Metabolic responses are complex and include metabolic acidosis and hyperventilation. Cellular adenosine triphosphate levels fall, resting cell membrane potential decreases, and an intracellular accumulation of sodium, calcium, and water is paralleled by a loss of cellular potassium.

Immunologic responses include alteration of macrophage function and perturbation of cellular and humoral immunity.(8) The burn wound is a complex and dynamic injury characterized by a zone of coagulation, surrounded by an area of stasis, and bordered by an area of erythema.(6) The zone of coagulation or complete capillary occlusion may progress by a factor of 10 during the first 48 hours after injury. This phenomenon is three-dimensional; thus, the wound can increase in size and depth during this critical period.

Local microcirculation is compromised to the greatest extent during the 12 to 24 hours post burn. Burns are in this dynamic state of flux for up to 72 hours after injury.(8) Ischemic necrosis quickly follows. Hematologic changes include platelet microthrombi and hemoconcentration in the postcapillary venules. Edema formation is rapid in the area of injury secondary to increased capillary permeability, decreased oncotic pressure, increased interstitial oncotic pressure, changes in the interstitial space compliance, and lymphatic damage.(32) Edema is most prominent in directly involved burned tissues but also develops in distant uninjured tissue, including muscle, intestine, and lung. Changes occur in the distant microvasculature, including red cell aggregation, white cell adhesion to venular walls, and platelet thromboemboli.(14)

Inflammatory mediators are elaborated locally, in part from activated platelets, macrophages, and leukocytes, and contribute to the local and systemic hyperpermeability of the microcirculation, appearing histologically as gaps in the venular and capillary endothelium.(73) This progressive process may extend dramatically during the first early days after injury.(7,46)

The ongoing tissue damage in thermal injury is due to multiple factors, including the failure of surrounding tissue to supply borderline cells with oxygen and nutrients necessary to sustain viability.(6) Impediment of the circulation below the injury results in desiccation of the wound, as fluid cannot be supplied via the thrombosed or obstructed capillaries. Topical agents and dressings may reduce but cannot prevent the desiccation of the burn wound and the inexorable progression to deeper layers. Altered permeability is not caused by heat injury alone; oxidants and other mediators (prostaglandins, kinins, and histamine) all contribute to vascular permeability.(70)

Neutrophils are a major source of oxidants and injury in the ischemia/reperfusion mechanism. This complex may be favorably affected by several interventions. Therapy is focused on the reduction of dermal ischemia, reduction of edema, and prevention of infection. During the period of early hemodynamic instability, edema reduction has a markedly beneficial effect as well as modulating later wound conversion from partial- to full-thickness injury.(31)

INFECTION

Infection remains the leading overall cause of death from burns. Susceptibility to infection is greatly increased due to the loss of the integumentary barrier to bacterial invasion, the ideal substrate present in the burn wound, and the compromised or obstructed microvasculature, which prevents humoral and cellular elements from reaching the injured tissue.

Additionally, the immune system is seriously affected, demonstrating decreased levels of immunoglobulins, serious perturbations of polymorphonuclear leukocyte function,[1,2] including disorders of chemotaxis, phagocytosis, and diminished killing ability. These functions greatly increase morbidity and mortality. Certain patients with specific polymorphisms in the tumor necrosis factor and bacterial recognition genes may have a higher incidence of sepsis than the burn injury alone would predict.[10] More recently, fungal infections have become a therapeutic challenge.[20]

Regeneration cannot take place until equilibrium is reached; hence, healing is retarded. Prolongation of the healing process may lead to excessive scarring. Hypertrophic scars are seen in about 4% of cases taking 10 days to heal, 14% of cases taking 14 days or fewer, 28% of cases taking 21 days to heal, and up to 40% of cases taking longer than 21 days to heal.[29]

EXPERIMENTAL DATA

The efficacy of hyperbaric oxygen (HBO_2) in the treatment of thermal injury is supported by animal studies and human clinical data. Edema reduction with HBO_2 therapy has been demonstrated in burned rabbits,[53] rats,[45] mice,[78] and guinea pigs.[55-56] Improvement in healing time has been reported in burned rabbits[58] and rats.[57,74] Decreased infection rates were an additional observation noted in these models.[57-58]

In a seminal study in 1970, Gruber (Figure 1) demonstrated that the area subjacent to a third-degree burn was hypoxic when compared to normal skin and that the tissue oxygen tension could be raised only by oxygen administered at pressure.[42] Ketchum, in 1967, reported an improvement in healing time and reduced infection in an animal model.[58] He later demonstrated dramatic improvement in the microvasculature of burned rats treated with hyperbaric oxygen therapy (Figure 2a, Figure 2b).[57]

In 1974, Hartwig[45] confirmed these findings and additionally noted less inflammatory response and suggested hyperbaric oxygen might be a useful adjunct to the technique of early debridement. Wells and Hilton (Figure 3), in a carefully designed and controlled experiment, reported a marked decrease (35%) in extravasation of fluid

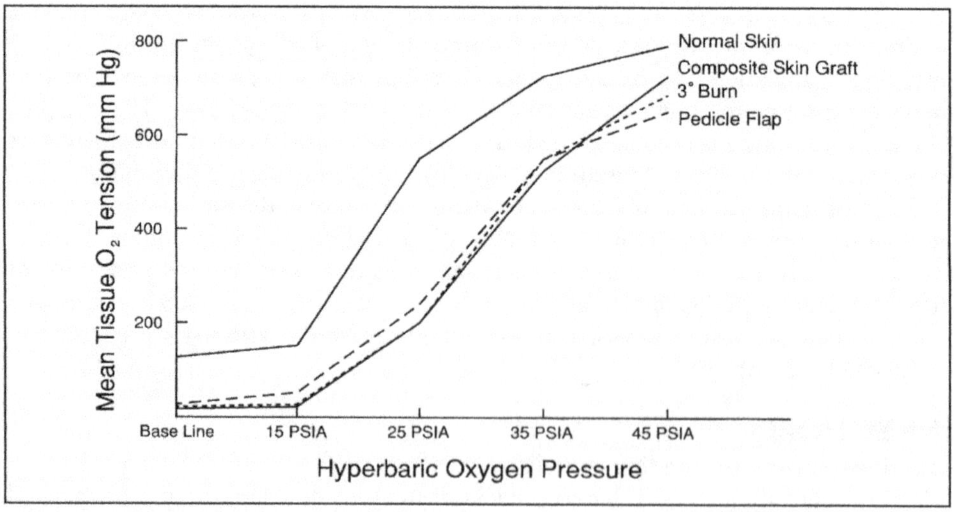

Figure 1. Mean oxygen tension of normal skin and various hypoxic tissues as a function of hyperbaric oxygen pressure. Note: Oxygen tension rises in burned skin only with increasing pressure.[42] (With permission)

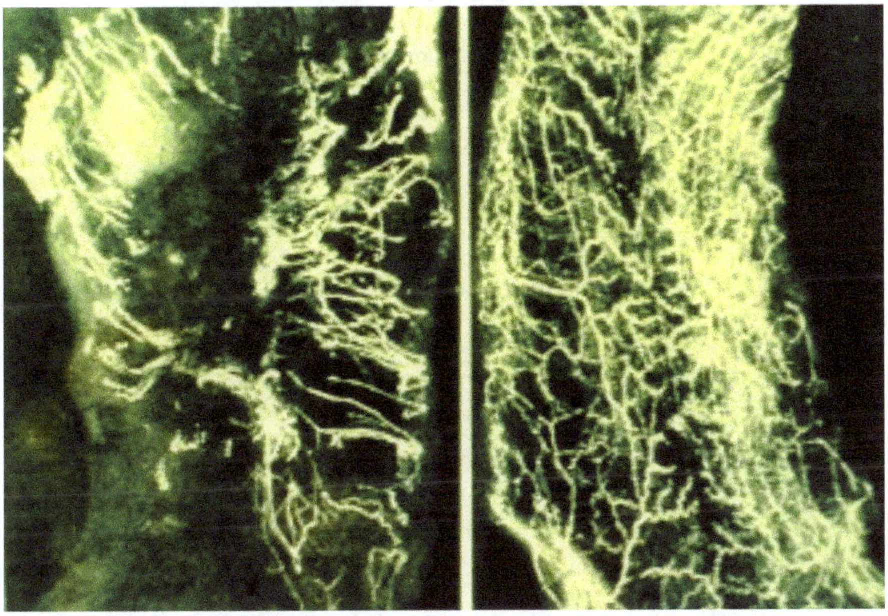

Figure 2a (left panel). Capillary disorganization, inflammation, and leakage of contrast agent in control. Figure 2b (right panel). Restoration of organized capillary arcades and intact circulation in HBO_2-treated animal. From Ketchum.[57]

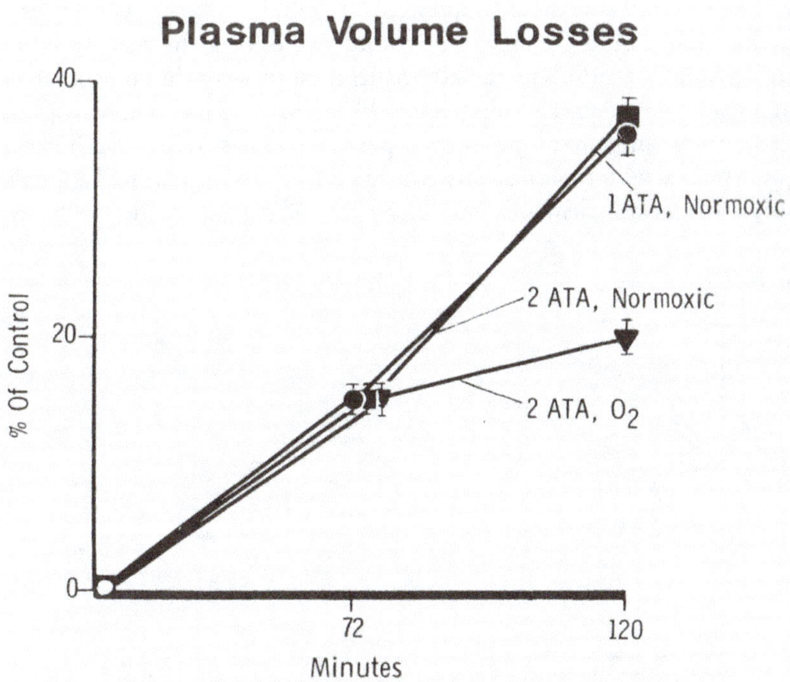

Figure 3. Plasma volume losses after burn in untreated animals (1 ATA, normoxic), animals exposed to hyperbaric oxygen (2 ATA, O_2) and to pressure alone (2 ATA, normoxic).[117] (With permission)

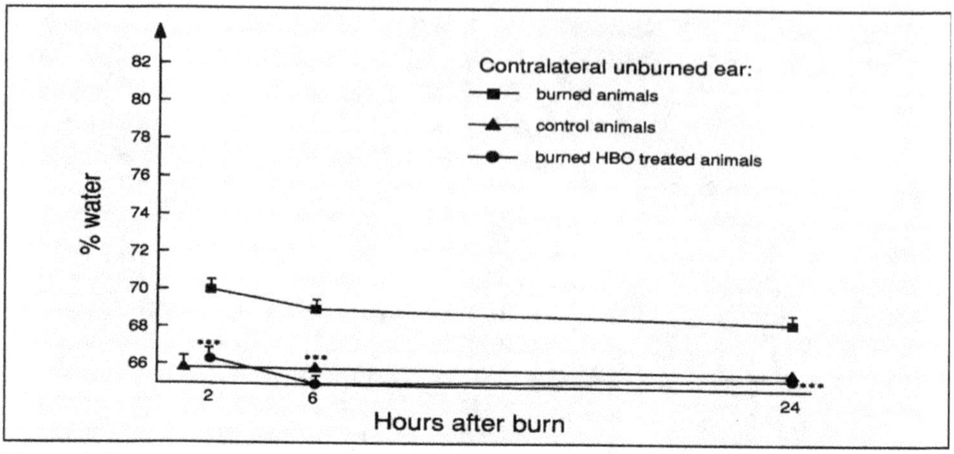

Figure 4. Water content (+) of the contralateral unburned ear in burned animals with and without HBO_2 treatment.[78] (With permission)

in 40% of flame-burned dogs.[117] The effect was clearly related to oxygen and not simply to increased pressure. A reduction in hemoconcentration and improved cardiac output were also noted.

Nylander (Figure 4)[78] in a well-accepted animal model showed that hyperbaric oxygen therapy reduced the generalized edema associated with burn injury.

Kaiser (Figure 5) reported that hyperbaric oxygen treatment resulted in shrinkage of third-degree (full-thickness) injury in a rabbit model. Untreated animals demonstrated the expected increase in wound size during the first 48 hours. At all times, treated animal wounds remained smaller than those of the controls. A reduction in subcutaneous edema was also observed.[55-56] Stewart and colleagues subjected rats to controlled burn wounds resulting in deep partial-thickness injury. Both experimental groups were treated with topical agents. The hyperbaric-oxygen-treated animals showed preservation of dermal elements, no conversion of partial- to full-thickness injury,

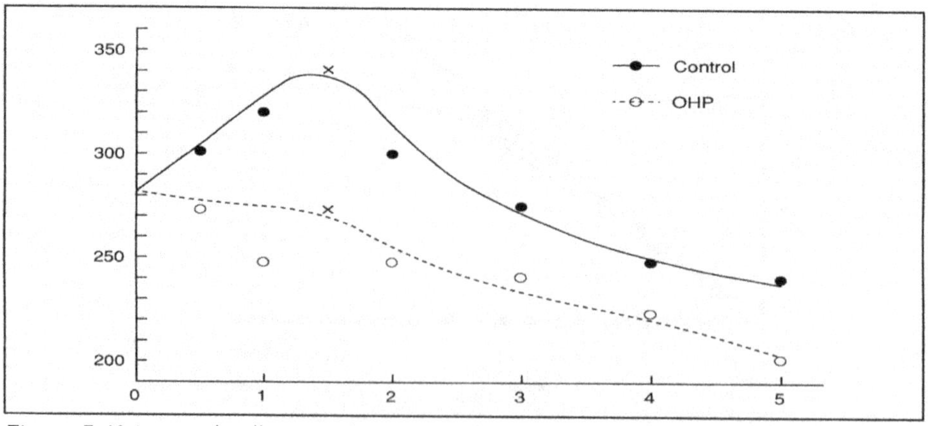

Figure 5. Kaiser and colleagues have recently demonstrated a significant reduction of subcutaneous edema in burned animals treated with HBO_2. He reported progression of the burn wound in controls, while in the hyperbaric-treated animal, wound size decreased.[55-56]

and preservation of adenosine triphosphate (ATP) levels. The untreated animals demonstrated marked diminution in ATP levels and conversion of partial- to full-thickness injury (Figure 6, Figure 7A, Figure 7B).[95-96]

These studies may relate directly to the preservation of energy sources for the sodium pump. Failure of the sodium pump is felt to be a major factor in the ballooning of the endothelial cells, which occurs after burn injury and subsequent massive fluid losses.[7] Germonpré reported decreased extension of burn injury with HBO_2.[37] HBO_2 has also been shown to dramatically improve the microvasculature of burned rats (Hartwig, Ketchum[45,57]). In guinea pigs, earlier return of capillary patency ($p < 0.05$) was demonstrated using an India ink technique.[61]

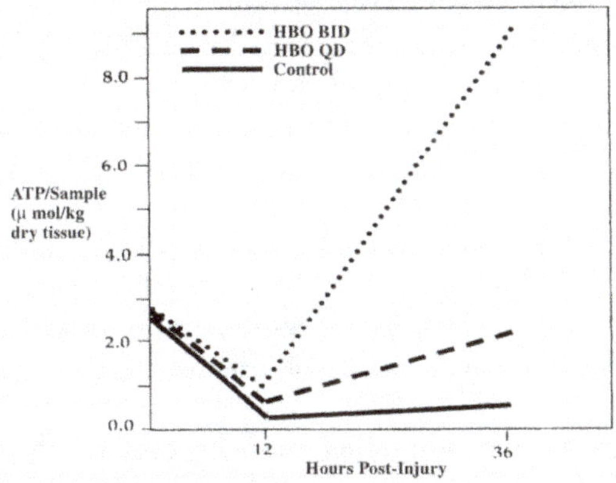

Tissue ATP levels in burn injured skin treated with HBO. Animals treated BID show a ten-fold increase in ATP levels at 36 hours. Biopsies of wounded animals showed progression to full thickness injury in the controls, whereas preservation of the dermal elements and capillary patency was observed in the HBO-treated group.

Figure 6. Rats: burn with Silvadene dressing.[95-96]

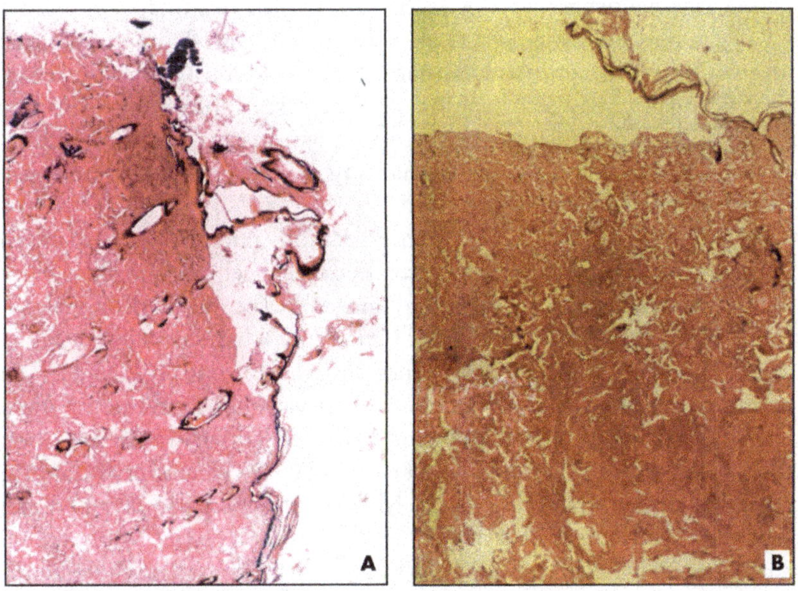

Figure 7A-7B. Biopsy of experimental partial-thickness burns at 5 days.[95-96]

A. HBO_2-treated animals show preservation of the dermal elements.

B. Non-treated animals show coagulation necrosis.

Miller and Korn reported faster re-epithelialization ($p < 0.001$) from these regenerative sites in guinea pigs treated with HBO_2 versus controls. The observed decrease in wound desiccation in the HBO_2-treated group was due to preservation of capillary integrity in the zone of stasis.[70]

Saunders similarly reported improved dermal circulation, preservation of dermal elements, and less collagen denaturation with HBO_2 treatments.[90] Perrins, in a porcine scald model, failed to demonstrate modification of progressive tissue destruction. However, oxygen was administered at 2 ATA for only one hour, and treatment occurred over only a one-day period. No vascular studies were undertaken. It was also noted that the porcine model may not be appropriate given the fact that pigs are resistant to skin infection, do not form a blister following scald wound injury, and do not share many dermal elements with humans, including cutaneous sweat glands.[81]

Niccole reported that HBO_2 provided no advantage in the treatment of full-thickness and partial-thickness burns alone or in combination with topical antibiotic therapy in controlling bacterial counts in a rat model. However, despite a treatment delay of 12 hours, hyperbaric oxygen significantly reduced the time to complete epithelialization in a partial-thickness burn injury.[74]

The pathophysiologic changes within the burn wound show a striking similarity to those noted in the ischemia reperfusion injury, i.e., depletion of ATP, production of xanthine oxidase, lipid peroxidation, activation of polymorphonuclear cells with subsequent endothelial adherence, and generation of reactive oxygen species (ROS).[67,106,114-115]

Recent data regarding HBO_2 cardiac preconditioning (inducing cellular tolerance and protection from ischemia) and adaptive responses resulting in cardioprotection and attenuation of ischemia-reperfusion injury are mediated by HBO_2-induced ROS (e.g., superoxide and hydrogen peroxide) that stimulate the production of nitric oxide. HBO_2-induced reactive oxygen species (ROS) are known to initiate gene expression and reduce neutrophil adhesion (via a decrease in CDl1a/18 function, P-selectin, and downregulation of intracellular adhesion molecule-1). HBO_2 also decreases lipid peroxidation, stimulates neovascularization, and increases antioxidants, thus resulting in cardioprotection.[121] Elucidation of these mechanisms for cardioprotection may provide further understanding of the mechanisms whereby hyperbaric oxygen is of benefit in acute thermal injury.

In a model of reperfusion injury, Zamboni demonstrated that hyperbaric oxygen is a potent blocker of white cell adherence to endothelial cell walls in skeletal muscle, interrupting the cascade that causes vascular damage.[122] The mechanism is felt to be an inhibitory effect on the CD18 locus.[123] As discussed by Wasiak et al.,[116] inhibition of beta 2 integrin activation of intracellular adhesion molecule one (ICAM-1)[17] enables tissues to maintain microvascular flow in areas otherwise subject to the well-described "secondary injury" following a thermal burn.[14] This effect persists for some hours, as demonstrated by both Ueno[108] and Milijkovic-Lolic;[69] Germonpré's data support this observation and may explain the beneficial effect of hyperbaric oxygen therapy on the microcirculation previously observed.[37,45,90,95-96]

Shoshani reported no benefit of HBO_2 in a rat burn model where all animals received standard sulfadiazine treatment.[94] There was no difference in burn wound size, re-epithelialization rate, Doppler blood flow, or healing. In this report, the author erroneously stated that this was the first study utilizing standard burn care (topical agents). These findings contradict the earlier study by Stewart's group, who utilized silver sulfadiazine dressings and confirmed preservation of dermal elements,[95-96] and might be explained by methodological differences.

Bleser and Benichoux, in a very large controlled study in a rat model of 30% body surface area (BSA) burns, reported reduced burn shock and a fourfold increased survival in HBO_2-treated animals versus controls.[13] Tenenhaus and colleagues showed reduction in mesenteric bacterial colonization ($p < 0.005$) in an HBO_2-treated burned mouse model.[101] Bacterial translocation is felt to be a major source of burn wound infection.

In 2005, Magnotti et al. proposed an evolution from bacterial translocation to gut ischemia-reperfusion injury after burn injury as the pathogenesis of multiple organ dysfunction syndrome. Systemic inflammation, acute lung injury, and multiple organ failure after a major thermal injury are common causes of morbidity and mortality. In the normal host, the intestinal mucosa functions as a major local defense barrier, a component of multiple defense mechanisms that helps prevent gut bacteria, as well as their products, from crossing the mucosal barrier. After a major thermal injury, and in other clinical and experimental situations, this intestinal barrier function becomes overwhelmed or impaired, resulting in the movement of bacteria and/or endotoxin to the mesenteric lymph nodes and systemic tissues, defined as bacterial translocation. The importance of this intestinal barrier function becomes clear when considering that the distal small bowel and colon contain 10[10] concentrations of anaerobes and 10[5] to 10[8] each of gram-positive and gram-negative aerobic and facultative microorganisms per gram of tissue and enough endotoxin to kill the host thousands of times over.[65]

Loss of gut barrier function and a resultant gut inflammatory response results in the production of proinflammatory factors; this can cause a septic state, leading to distant organ failure. Splanchnic hypoperfusion causing gut ischemia-reperfusion injury appears to be the dominant hemodynamic event, triggering the release of biologically active factors into the mesenteric lymphatics. The benefits of the early use of hyperbaric oxygen in burn victims may in part be mediated through amelioration of gut reperfusion injury.

The beneficial effects of HBO_2 in ischemic-reperfused tissues have been demonstrated in intestine,[120] skeletal muscle,[79,122] brain[100,102,109] and testicular tissue,[60] and myocardium.[91-92,105,121] In a study of severely burned humans (> 30% TBSA), HBO_2-treated patients compared to controls had increased levels of serum-soluble interleukin-2 receptor ($p < 0.05$) and decreased plasma fibronectin ($p < 0.01$), resulting clinically in a lower incidence of sepsis ($p < 0.05$).[119]

Total enteral nutrition, starting as early as possible after thermal injury, is recommended for burn patients. It results in decreased morbidity and mortality and supports intestinal structure and function. Studies of intestinal barrier function biology, pathophysiology, and consequences of gut barrier failure demonstrate that the ischemic and/or stressed gut can become a proinflammatory organ,[30] and gut-derived factors liberated after periods of splanchnic hypoperfusion can result in acute distant organ, cellular dysfunction and activation of neutrophils and other proinflammatory cells.[28]

Reduction of polymorphonuclear leukocyte (PMNL) killing ability in hypoxic tissue has been well documented.[3,47] The ability of hyperbaric oxygen to elevate tissue oxygen tension and the enhancement of PMNL killing in an oxygen-enriched animal model as demonstrated by Mader[64] suggests that this may be an additional benefit of HBO_2. Hussman and colleagues have shown no evidence of HBO_2-induced immunosuppression in a carefully controlled animal model.[51]

In a 2005 randomized controlled study, Bilic et al. evaluated the effects of HBO_2 on burn wound healing. Standard deep second-degree burns were produced in male Wistar rats treated with silver sulfadiazine and then randomly assigned to either a normoxic, placebo gas or to 2.5 atmospheres absolute (ATA) HBO_2 for 60 minutes for a total of 21 sessions. HBO_2 had a beneficial effect on post-burn edema ($p = 0.022$), neoangiogenesis ($p = 0.009$), numbers of regenerative active follicles ($p = 0.009$), and time to epithelial regeneration ($p = 0.048$). There were no significant differences in necrosis staging or margination of leukocytes. The authors conclude that the data support earlier conclusions that HBO_2 is of benefit in the healing of burn wounds.(11)

Turkaslan et al.(107) reported that hyperbaric oxygen treatment reduced progression of the zone of stasis in the first 24 hours after injury and accelerated the healing process by supporting neoangiogenesis. Prevention of progression in the zone of stasis is a major goal in burn therapy. This report lends further credence to the previously cited work of Miller, Korn, Hartwig, and Ketchum.

HBO_2 has been shown to mobilize stem/progenitor cells in both humans and mice by stimulating bone marrow stromal cell type 3 (endothelial) nitric oxide synthase.(35-36,38,103-104) Findings indicate that some of the mobilized cells will home to peripheral sites where they function as de novo endothelial progenitor cells (EPCs), contributing to wound vasculogenesis, a complement to local angiogenesis. Additionally, at peripheral sites HBO_2 stimulates stem cell growth and differentiation by engaging a physiological autocrine loop responsive to oxidative stress, much the same as lactate.(71-72)

HBO_2 stimulates peripheral site EPCs recruitment and differentiation via a pathway involving thioredoxin-1 and hypoxia-inducible factors-1 (HIF-1) and HIF-2. These findings provide new insight into possible mechanisms for the known clinical benefits of hyperbaric oxygen

Thus, the overwhelming body of evidence in a large number of controlled animal studies demonstrates that hyperbaric oxygen reduces dermal ischemia, reduces edema, prevents conversion of partial- to full-thickness injury, preserves the microcirculation, and preserves ATP and cellular integrity. Additional benefits may be enhancement of PMNL killing and modulation of ischemia reperfusion injury, resulting in improved survival.

CLINICAL EXPERIENCE

In 1965, Wada observed improved healing of burns in coal miners being treated for carbon monoxide poisoning with HBO_2. Later clinical series by Ikeda, Wada, Lamy, Tabor, and Grossman(40,52-53,63,99,111-112) showed improved healing,(112) decreased length of hospital stay,(40) decreased mortality,(40,77) decreased overall cost of care,(22,40,77) improved morbidity,(40) decreased fluid requirements (30%–35%),(77) and decreased number of surgeries ($p < 0.041$).(22) Niu reported a very large clinical outcome series showing a statistically significant reduction in mortality ($p = 0.028$) in 266 seriously burned patients who received HBO_2 when compared to 609 control patients.(77) He also observed a lower incidence of infection and stated that HBO_2 allowed the burn surgeon more time to more accurately define the extent of injury.

Cianci has shown a significant reduction in length of hospital stay in burns up to 39% TBSA.(23) Additionally noted was a reduction in the need for surgery, including grafting, in a series of patients with 40%–80% burns when compared to non-HBO_2-treated controls. HBO_2-treated patients showed an average savings of 36%

(USD$120,000) per case.[22] Adjusted for inflation, this would represent a saving of $227,000 per case in 2016 U.S. dollars.

Hart reported a sham-controlled randomized series showing reduced fluid requirements, mean healing time ($p < 0.005$), mortality, and morbidity in 10%–50% TBSA burn patients treated with HBO_2 when compared to controls and to U.S. National Burn Information Exchange Standards.[44]

In a retrospective paired controlled series of burn patients treated with HBO_2, Waisbren reported increased sepsis, reduced renal function, and decreased circulating white blood cells in HBO_2-treated patients. The author stated he could demonstrate neither a salutary nor deleterious effect on mortality.[113] While frequently cited as a negative study, there was a 75% reduction in the need for grafting ($p < 0.001$) in the hyperbaric group. In a randomized controlled study of 37 partial-thickness burn patients treated with HBO_2 versus 37 controls, Merola reported increased granulation, faster healing, and decreased scarring.[68]

Cianci observed similar results in a series of patients averaging 28% TBSA burns. [26] In a small blinded review, Cianci's group reported a 25% reduction in resuscitative fluid requirements ($p < 0.07$) and maximum (and percent) weight gain ($p < 0.012$) in seriously burned (40%–80% TBSA) patients treated with adjunctive HBO_2 versus controls at a regional burn center[21-22] (Figure 8).[24]

In a controlled pilot series, Maxwell reported reduced surgery, resuscitative weight gain, intensive care days, total hospitalization time, wound sepsis, and cost of hospitalization in the HBO_2 group.[66] Cianci reported reduced surgeries ($p < 0.03$), length of hospital stay (53%), and cost of care (49%) in 40%–80% TBSA burns.[25]

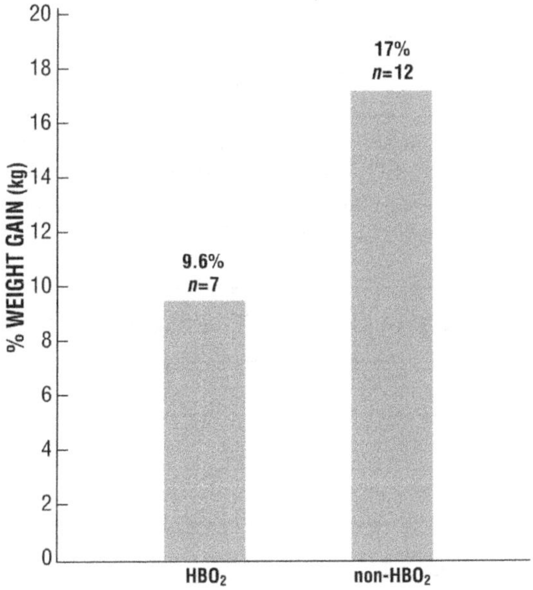

Figure 8. Maximum weight gain at three days expressed as percentage of admission weight. HBO_2-treated patients showed a 45% reduction in weight gain ($p < 0.03$).[24]

2Hammarlund and colleagues showed reduced edema and wound exudation in a controlled series of human volunteers with UV-irradiated blister wounds (Figure 9).[43]

In a subsequent similar study, Niezgoda (Figure 10) demonstrated reduced wound size ($p < 0.03$), laser Doppler-measured hyperemia ($p < 0.05$), and wound exudate ($p < 0.04$) in the HBO_2-treated group. This study was the first prospective randomized, controlled, double-blinded trial comparing HBO_2 with sham controls in a human burn model.[76]

Brannen et al. in 1997[16] reported a randomized prospective trial of hyperbaric oxygen in the treatment of burn injury. Sixty-three patients received hyperbaric oxygen, and 62 served as controls. One-third of the hyperbaric-treated patients received their first treatment within eight hours. However, the average time to treatment was 11.5 hours after the burn injury. The authors noted no difference in the outcome measures of mortality, number of operations, or length of stay and stated they were unable to demonstrate any significant benefit to burn patients from the use of hyperbaric oxygen.

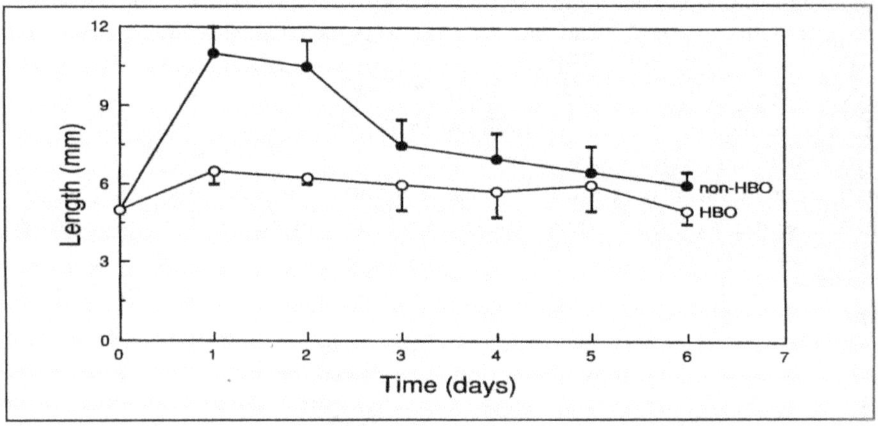

Figure 9. Maximum length (including edema adjacent to the wound) (mean ± s.d.) of UV-irradiated (•) and HBO_2-treated UV-irradiated (°) blister wounds as a function of time. The value on day 0 is approximately the diameter of the suction cup used to create the blister. ($p < 0.05$).[43]

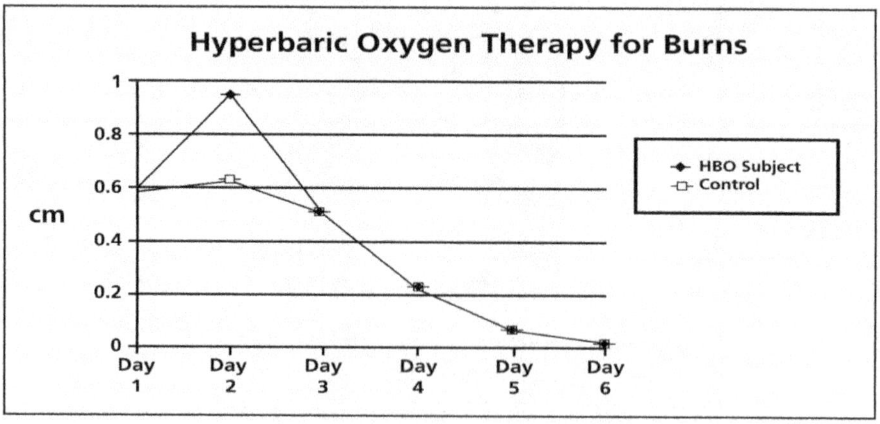

Figure 10. Wound size measurements (cm) of UV-irradiated suction blister wounds in control group (□) and hyperbaric oxygen group (♦).[76]

There were serious limitations in this study. Two-thirds of patients did not receive their first treatment until more than eight hours after burn injury, with a mean of 11.5 hours. Results in the subset of patients receiving earlier treatment were not examined separately. Important outcome measures not studied were functional and cosmetic aspects of facial, hand, and perineal burns. Length of stay, number of surgeries, and extent of grafting are subject to a variety of confounding influences, including economic (e.g., hospital and insurance, utilization management, physician reimbursement) and social considerations (e.g., lack of adequate housing, caregivers, and rehabilitation efforts).

Despite randomization for age, burn size, and inhalation injury, the populations were still heterogeneous. Comorbidity was not examined, and all patients underwent exceedingly early and aggressive excisional therapy with rapid discharge to a lesser level of care. The authors did observe less fluid loss; drier wounds, which necessitated fewer dressing changes; and earlier healing. Further analysis showed a significant reduction in hospital costs in the hyperbaric group.

RECENT PERSPECTIVES

Pain Management

There is a substantial body of evidence reporting the use of hyperbaric oxygen therapy in pain attenuation. In their excellent review of the literature, Sutherland and colleagues concluded that hyperbaric oxygen therapy has been proven to demonstrate a significant antinociceptive effect. They state that early clinical research indicates that hyperbaric oxygen therapy may be useful in modulating human pain; however, further studies are required to determine whether HBO_2 is a safe and efficacious treatment modality.

A particularly difficult problem is that opioid overuse contributes to adaptive immune suppression, and this may be associated with poorer outcomes. Neuropathic pain is typically difficult to treat and thought to occur in a large percentage of those suffering severe burns. Rasmussen and colleagues[84] have reported a series of 17 patients who underwent a controlled first-degree burn. One group was treated at atmospheric pressure $FiO_2 = 0.21$ during hyperbaric treatment. The HBO_2 group was treated at 2.4 ATM breathing 100% O_2. Patients who underwent chamber treatment demonstrated attenuation of secondary hyperalgesia, i.e., an antinociceptive effect. The authors state that hyperbaric oxygen therapy post burns has a potent antinociceptive effect that works at a central desensitization level. The authors suggest this thermal injury model may give impetus to future neurophysiologic studies exploring the central effects of hyperbaric oxygen treatment.

Chong et al.[19] reported a group of 17 burn patients who were treated with hyperbaric oxygen or routine burn care. They noted no difference in inflammatory cytokines or depth of burns, though patients in both groups either increased or reduced estimated depth of injury. There were fewer positive biopsies for bacterial colonization in the hyperbaric group. They also related that this was a preliminary study and of insufficient power to determine any real statistical significance as 40 patients would have been required to achieve this goal. It was unclear as to the average time from injury to the provision of hyperbaric oxygen therapy. However, it was stated that patients were treated during routine hyperbaric treatment sessions and that the HBO_2 patients received two sessions within the first 22 hours. It would be more appropriate to treat as soon as the patient is stable as reported by others.

Jones et al.[54] have reported a series of diabetic patients suffering foot burns. Transcutaneous O_2 studies were performed, and those patients who had low TcO_2s and responded to an oxygen challenge underwent hyperbaric oxygen therapy in addition to standard care. There were 18 patients in the hyperbaric study group. All healed, and there was one amputation. The authors compared this to a group of 68 patients treated with traditional care. Eleven patients in this cohort suffered 31 amputations. The authors reported the observations of their burn surgeons that, with a larger sample size, a definite benefit could be demonstrated. Of note, three of the patients who were scheduled for grafting healed spontaneously with HBO_2 alone.

Immunity and Infection

A major and continuing clinical problem is the innate inflammatory response induced by genetic factors such as those common in neutrophils and macrophages which are massively increased while the T-cell adaptive responses are downregulated. Zhang and colleagues(124) have shown that hyperbaric oxygen attenuates apoptosis and decreases inflammation in an ischemic wound model. The effects of hyperbaric oxygen on modulation of white cell adherence to endothelium has been described. Thom et al. have studied the effect of hyperbaric oxygen and demonstrated that HBO_2 additionally does not alter platelet function but inhibits beta 2 integrin adhesion to endothelium at pressures of 2.8 or more. This would have a beneficial effect on the early stages of burn injury.(34)

Stem Cell Effects

Thom et al. have reported that hyperbaric oxygen increases marrow stem cell populations, and these cells migrate to areas of wounding.(103-104) The previously reported preservation of dermal elements, specifically hair follicles, may represent an additional area for recruitment of native stem cells in the healing of burns. This has been described by Stewart et al.(95-96) and should be an area of fruitful research in burn patients where prolonged healing is a major problem.

Antioxidant Effects

Concern about oxygen toxicity is valid. However, Sureda and colleagues(97) have studied the effect of hyperbaric oxygen therapy in chronic wounds and reported that this modality actually enhanced plasma antioxidant defenses and contributed to the activation of healing resolution, angiogenesis, and vascular tone regulation by increasing the VEGF and IL-6 release and the endothelin-1 decrease, which may be significant factors in simulating wound healing. In clinical practice, acute oxygen toxicity is very rare and usually associated with prolonged treatments utilized in decompression sickness.

INHALATION INJURY

Considerable attention has been given to the use of HBO_2 in inhalation injury due in part to fear that HBO_2 may cause worsening of pulmonary damage, particularly in those patients maintained on high levels of inspired oxygen. The more extensive the burn injury, the higher the incidence of an inhalation injury.(93) Pulmonary injury caused by smoke inhalation is a major cause of fire-related deaths.(9) The airway injury can be worsened by a variety of chemical pyrolysis products, depending on the material burned.(83)

In comparison with a comparable-size burn alone, the combination of a body burn and smoke inhalation injury results in a marked increase in mortality and morbidity, hemodynamic instability, and in burn wound edema, a 30%–50% increase in initial fluid requirements, and an accentuation of lung dysfunction.

Grim studied products of lipid peroxidation in the exhaled gases in HBO_2-treated burn patients and found no indication of oxidative stress.(39)

Ray analyzed a series of severely burned patients being treated for concurrent inhalation injury, thermal injury, and adult respiratory distress syndrome.(85) The author noted no deleterious effect of HBO_2, even in those on continuous high levels of inspired oxygen. More rapid weaning from mechanical ventilation was possible in the HBO_2-treated group (5.3 days versus 26 days, $p < 0.05$). There was a significant reduction in cost of care per case of USD$67,000 in the HBO_2-treated patients ($p < 0.05$). Adjusted to 2016 U.S. dollars, this figure would be $121,000. There is no current evidence to controvert these studies.

2009 COCHRANE REVIEW

In 2009, in the Cochrane Database Systemic Review of the efficacy of HBO_2 for thermal burns, Villanueva et al. identified four randomized controlled studies, of which two satisfied their inclusion criteria.(110)

In the first trial, Hart in 1974,(44) as previously discussed, reported reduced fluid requirements and mean healing time ($p < 0.005$), mortality, and morbidity when compared to controls. There was a reduction in mortality and morbidity when compared to the National Burn Information Exchange standards.

Because of heterogeneity, the studies could not be pooled, though Hart reported mean healing time significantly shorter – 19.7 versus 43.8 days ($p < 0.001$); the authors suggested that the Hart study was particularly constrained by lack of power to detect useful clinical differences. The Brannen study,(16) reporting no difference in mortality, length of stay, or surgeries, was constrained by the previously mentioned limitations. The authors state that while there are promising results from nonrandom clinical reports, there is insufficient evidence to recommend or refute the routine use of hyperbaric oxygen for the treatment of thermal burns and suggest that large, multicenter, randomized study of sufficient power would be needed to address these shortcomings. The Cochrane report did not consider several outcome studies with matched controls showing reduced length of stay, reduction in fluid requirements and edema, reduction of surgery, and cost effectiveness.

While these reports certainly had limitations, they represent valid analysis of the benefits of early treatment in thermal injury and underscore the observations of skilled and experienced physicians which remain an important component of determining therapeutic efficacy. A well-designed, randomized, blinded control study with sham treatment and sufficient power is certainly desirable yet remains to be performed. Most centers see very few large burns; only 4% of burn admissions are for burns > 40% TBSA, certainly necessitating a multicenter format. Attempts at organizing such a study have so far been unsuccessful.

PATIENT SELECTION CRITERIA

Hyperbaric oxygen therapy is recommended to treat serious burns – i.e., greater than 20% total body surface area and/or with involvement of the hands, face, feet, or perineum that are deep partial- or full-thickness injury. Patients with superficial burns or those not expected to survive are not accepted for therapy. Transfer of patients for HBO_2 treatment should be considered carefully and should be sent only to a facility that has experience with burn critical care in the hyperbaric environment

CLINICAL MANAGEMENT

Surgical Perspectives

Over the past 40 years, the pendulum has swung to an aggressive surgical management of the burn wound, i.e., early tangential or sequential excision and grafting of the deep second-degree and probable third-degree burns, especially to functionally important parts of the body.[48,50,87-89] Hyperbaric oxygen, as an adjunctive therapy, has allowed the surgeon yet another modality of treatment for these deep second-degree burns, especially including those to the hands and fingers, face, and ears, and other areas where the surgical technique of excision is often imprecise, and coverage is sometimes difficult.

These wounds, not obvious third-degree, are then best treated with topical antimicrobial agents, bedside and enzymatic debridement, wound care, including biological dressings, and adjunctive hyperbaric oxygen therapy, allowing the surgeon more time for healing to take place and for definition of the extent and depth of injury (Figures 11a-11e, Figures 12a-12c, Figures 13A-13F).

Adjunctive hyperbaric oxygen therapy has drastically reduced the healing time in the major burn injury, especially if the wounds are deep second-degree.[22-23,26,77] There is theoretical benefit of HBO_2 therapy for obviously less well-defined third-degree burns.[56] Fourth-degree burns, most commonly seen in high-voltage electrical injuries,[49] are benefitted by reduction in fascial compartment pressures, as injured muscle swelling is lessened by preservation of aerobic glycolysis and, later, by a reduction of anaerobic infection.

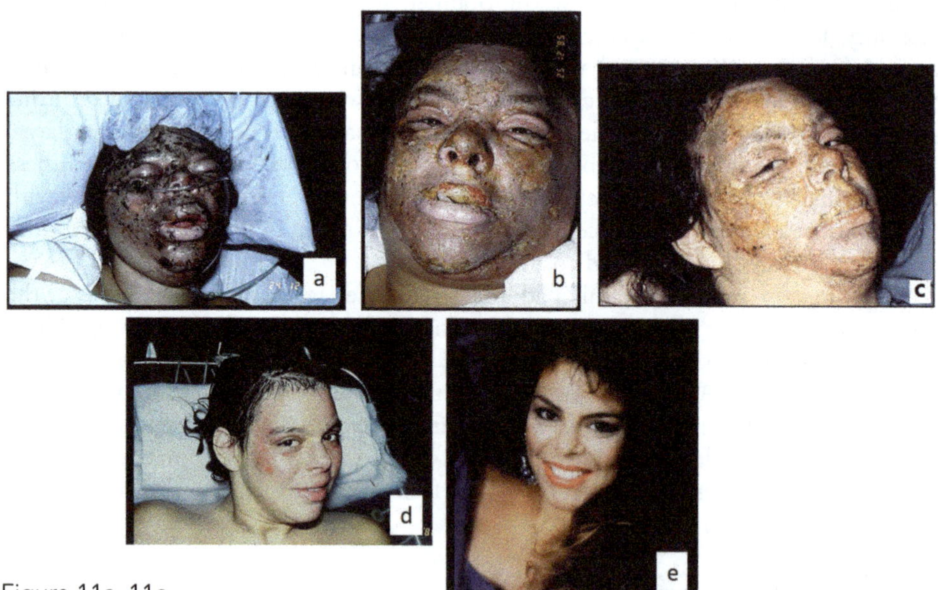

Figure 11a–11e.

a. Twenty-three-year-old female with 50% TBSA burns 12 hours post injury.

b. Twenty-four hours later (36 hours post injury) after 2 hyperbaric oxygen treatments.

c. Seventy-two hours later (post 6 hyperbaric treatments).

d. Shortly before discharge.

e. Long-term follow up at four years (patient now a burn nurse).

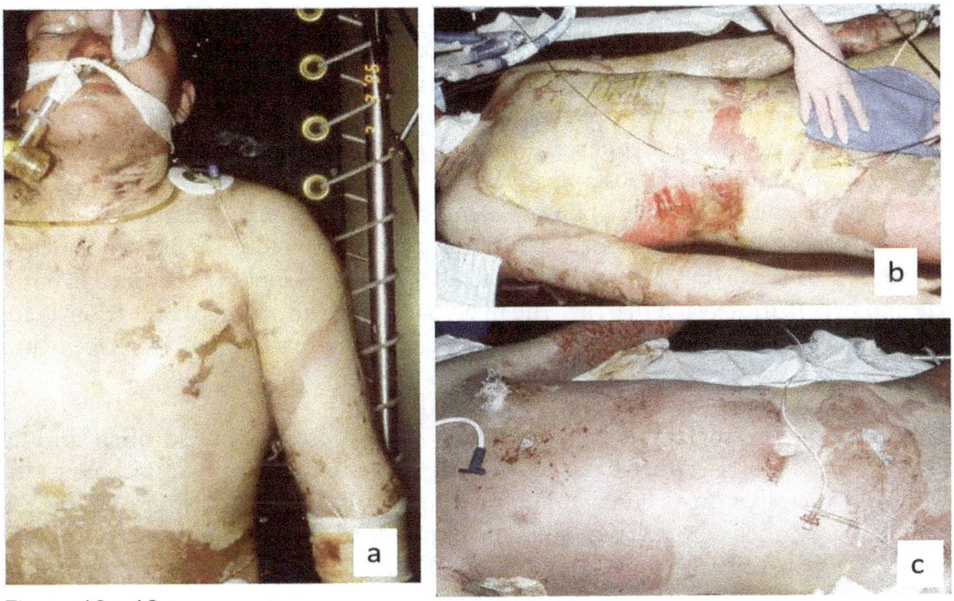

Figure 12a–12c

a. Nineteen-year-old male with inhalation injury and deep partial- to full-thickness flame burn of 70% TBSA. Photo taken pre-HBO_2.

b. Patient six days later after HBO_2 BID.

c. Thirty days later with HBO_2. No skin grafts required on chest and torso.

Figure 13A–13F

A. Deep partial-thickness burn of hand in 30-year-old male with 60% total body surface burn and inhalation injury on admission.

B. Six days later.

C. At surgery, light debridement.

D. Immediately after surgery. Note the preservation of dermal appendages.

E. Two weeks after admission. Note re-epithelialization.

F. Appearance on discharge 25 days post injury. Healed without grafting.

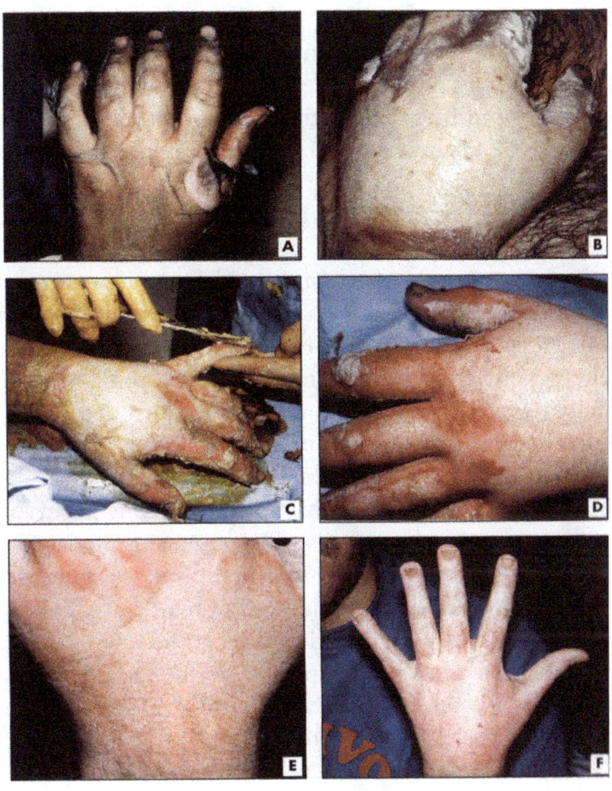

Finally, reconstruction utilizing flaps, full-thickness skin, and composite grafts, i.e., ear-to-nose grafts, has been greatly facilitated using adjunctive HBO_2.[75] Often the decision to use HBO_2 therapy has been made intraoperatively when a surgeon is concerned about a compromised cutaneous or myocutaneous flap. Patients are, in many instances, prepared preoperatively about the possibility of receiving adjunctive HBO_2 therapy immediately postoperatively.

Units planning treatment of burn patients should be experienced in management of critical care patients in the hyperbaric setting and specific problems of burn patients prior to initiation of a therapy program. Preferably, personnel should be certified in burn care and hyperbaric oxygen therapy. The hyperbaric department should function as an extension of the burn unit and participate in the team approach to burn management.

Hyperbaric Oxygen

Hyperbaric oxygen therapy is begun as soon as possible after injury, often during initial resuscitation. Treatments are attempted 3 times within the first 24 hours and twice daily thereafter on a regimen of 90 minutes of 100% oxygen delivery at 2.0–2.4 ATA. Early experience in treating children recommended 45 minutes twice daily,[40] but more recent extensive clinical use of HBO_2 in children demonstrates that adult protocols are safe.

Patients are monitored during initial treatment and as necessary thereafter. Blood pressure can be monitored via transducers or noninvasively using blood pressure cuffs designed for use in monoplace chambers. Patients can be maintained on ventilator support during treatment, which is frequently the case in larger burns with concurrent inhalation injury.

Careful attention to fluid management is mandatory. Initial requirements may be several liters per hour, and pumps capable of this delivery at pressure must be utilized in order to maintain appropriate fluid replacement in the hyperbaric chamber. In larger burn injuries, adequate fluid and electrolyte resuscitation during the first 24 hours can be problematic. Certain patients can develop hypotension shortly after exiting the chamber. Careful volume replacement and assessment of fluid status is mandatory prior to, during, and immediately after HBO_2 treatment. Increasing fluids during ascent may help compensate for any hypovolemia unmasked after hyperbaric oxygen exposure.

Maintenance of a comfortable, ambient temperature must be accomplished. Thermal instability may be a problem within one to two hours of burn wound cleansing and dressing change (depending on the methods used), especially in large TBSA burns. These patients should be carefully assessed prior to an HBO_2 exposure. Febrile patients must be closely monitored and fever controlled, as oxygen toxicity is reported to be more common in this group.

In large burns of 40% TBSA or greater, treatment is rendered for 10–14 days in close consultation with the burn surgeon. Many partial-thickness burns will heal without surgery during this time frame and obviate the need for grafting. Treatment beyond 20–30 sessions is usually utilized to optimize graft take. While there is no absolute limit to the total number of hyperbaric treatments, it is rare to exceed 40–50 sessions, and utilization review is recommended.

Concern has been expressed about the use of the carbonic anhydrase inhibitor mafenide acetate (Sulfamylon) and its removal recommended prior to HBO_2 treatment based on the potential for CO_2 buildup, which can lead to vasodilatation.[59] Sulfamylon is less frequently utilized in burn centers and rarely used at the author's facility except in select cases (small TBSA, severe infection, and/or contraindication to silver sulfadiazine). Its limited use in this setting has not resulted in any observed untoward effects.[82] Silver sulfadiazine is the most widely used topical therapy because of its relatively low toxicity and ease of use.[73]

In larger TBSA burns, especially of the head and neck, otic barotrauma may be a problem, and careful attention should be given to this potential complication. The HBO_2 team should make use of early ENT consultation when indicated.

Patients may be treated in a multiplace or monoplace configuration. Movement over long distances is not recommended, and patients should not be transported to a hyperbaric chamber that is not within the same facility as the burn center.[41]

UTILIZATION REVIEW

Utilization review is recommended after 30 hyperbaric oxygen sessions.

COST IMPACT

Burn care is expensive. During 1997–98, in a Northern California regional burn center (Doctors Medical Center Burn Center), hospital costs for 20 burn patients averaged USD$253,000 ($393,000 in 2016 U.S. dollars).[27] This includes the cost of hyperbaric oxygen that averaged $6,360 ($10,000 in 2016 U.S. dollars) per patient.

Cost data from the 2012 National Burn Repository report indicate that for patients who survive 60% total body surface area burns, charges average $1,297,000,000 (in 2016 U.S. dollars) for the hospital stay alone. This does not include operating room time, surgeon's bills, artificial skin, rehabilitation, and other costs that can reach $637,000 in 2016 U.S. dollars or more for burns over 80% TBSA.[4]

Although not calculated, cost savings as a result of the use of HBO_2 in acute thermal injury are implied in all of the 22 clinical studies in this report by demonstrating reductions in healing time, hospital length of stay, and numbers of surgeries including grafting. In six of the studies, the authors specifically analyzed costs of care in thermal injury with and without adjunctive HBO_2, and estimates of average savings in patients treated with HBO_2 range from USD$76,000 to USD$120,000 per case.

DISCUSSION

Despite the many advances in burn therapy, including early excision, nutritional support, improved ventilation, and infection control, there appears to have been little change in mortality except for patients over 65 with larger burns since the mid-1980s. Early excision seems to have decreased mortality and overall length of stay in smaller burns and those not suffering concurrent inhalation injury.[80] Engrav, in a review of 35 years' experience at the Harborview Burn Center in Seattle, Washington, reported that early excision did not decrease length of stay for larger burns, and there has been little change since 1990.[33] It has also been suggested that burn care may have already achieved a floor of survival.[12] Thus, further improvement in burn care, length of stay, mortality, and cost containment must await future therapeutic developments. Adjunctive hyperbaric oxygen therapy has been shown to reduce length of stay and cost of care in conjunction with early excision and comprehensive burn management. The reader is directed to a comprehensive and recent review on priorities of burn research.[86]

SUMMARY

The beneficial effects of Hyperbaric oxygen in the treatment of burns has been demonstrated in numerous animal studies and human reports over the last 40 years. Observations utilizing hyperbaric oxygen therapy after burns have shown reversal of the zone of stasis, reduction of ischemia and ischemic necrosis, prevention of progression of partial- to full-thickness injury, moderation of inflammation, lessening of the capillary leak, preservation of dermal elements, a reduced need for grafting, shortened hospital stay, and a reduction in cost of care.

The burn community has recognized the need for improvement in our control of pain, speed of healing, and scarring. Wolf and Engrav have both reported the limited progress in burn therapy that has been made in the last 20 years, especially in the control of the inflammatory state, the hypermetabolic syndrome, infection, and scarring. Perhaps the time has come for the burn community to take a serious look at hyperbaric oxygen therapy in the treatment of clinical burns.

As Boykin has observed, "It is clear from review of collected research and clinical data that hyperbaric oxygen therapy provides a unique environment for wound recovery and tissue regeneration for thermal injury that cannot be comparably achieved by our current surgical and medical therapies. Evidence of the reduction in patient morbidity and length of hospital stay are observed in the majority of clinical observations of the use of HBO_2 therapy in burn management and should be expected to be gained from carefully structured programs utilizing these methods. The scientific evidence of the efficacy of HBO_2 therapy as an effective tool for wound healing has made exceptional gains over the past three decades and provides us with a firm biological and physiologic basis for the use of this therapy in patients with complex wounds and burns. The scientific gains made from the observations of HBO_2 therapy-related mechanisms for stem progenitor cell signaling and wound healing have also been significant. Finally, research documenting the vulnerary effects of HBO_2 therapy at the cellular and molecular level also suggest that this therapy has the potential to provide a much-needed elevation of the 'floor of survival' for burn victims and should provide for substantial enhancements in their wound healing and quality of life."[(15)]

Definitive clinical evidence for the efficacy of hyperbaric oxygen therapy in burns awaits a well-designed, multicenter, randomized study of sufficient power. While we await more data,[(86)] we should remember that the observations of seasoned clinicians remain a valid test of efficacy.

Current data show that hyperbaric oxygen therapy, when used as an adjunct in a comprehensive program of burn care, can significantly improve morbidity and mortality, reduce length of hospital stay, lessen the need for surgery, and is cost-effective. It has been demonstrated to be safe in the hands of those thoroughly trained in rendering hyperbaric oxygen therapy in the critical care setting and with appropriate monitoring precautions. Careful patient selection and screening are mandatory.

Given our current understanding of the uniquely beneficial effects of hyperbaric oxygenation on the cellular and molecular mechanisms of wound healing, it is suggested that the formal integration of hyperbaric oxygen therapy in early burn wound management be investigated by the use of well-designed multicenter studies that may provide data for burn wound healing and burn patient outcomes supportive of this role.

ACKNOWLEDGMENT

The authors wish to thank Ms. Helen Doughty, medical librarian at John Muir Medical Center, Walnut Creek, CA, for her invaluable contributions to this manuscript. Also the authors wish to thank the Undersea and Hyperbaric Medicine Society (UHMS) for permission to use content throughout the chapter from the following sources:

Cianci P, Slade JB Jr, Sato RM, Faulkner J. Adjunctive hyperbaric oxygen therapy in the treatment of thermal burns. Undersea Hyperb Med. 2013 Jan-Feb;40(1):89-108.

and

Cianci P, Slade JB Jr, Sato RM, Faulkner J. Thermal burns. In: Lindell K. Weaver, ed. Hyperbaric oxygen therapy indications. 13th ed. UHMS; 2014. p.217-38.

CONFLICT OF INTEREST STATEMENT

The authors have no conflict of interest to declare.

REFERENCES

1. Alexander JW, Meakins JL. A physiological basis for the development of opportunistic infections in man. Ann Surg. 1972;176:273.
2. Alexander JW, Wixson D. Neutrophil dysfunction and sepsis in burn injury. Surg Gynec Obstet. 1970;130:431.
3. Allen DB, Maguire JJ, Mahdavian M, et al. Wound hypoxia and acidosis limit neutrophil bacterial killing mechanisms. Arch Surg. 1997;132:991-6.
4. American Burn Association. National Burn Repository. Version 8.0. 2012.
5. American Burn Association. National Burn Repository. Version 12.0. 2016.
6. Arturson G. Pathophysiology of the burn wound. Ann Chir Gynaecol. 1980;69:178-90.
7. Arturson G. The pathophysiology of severe thermal injury. J Burn Care Rehabil. 1985;6(2):129-46.
8. Atiyeh BS, Gunn SW, Hayek SN. State of the art in burn treatment. World J Surg. 2005;29(2):131-48.
9. Balkissoon R, Shusterman DJ. Occupational upper airway disorders. Semin Respir Crit Care Med. 1999;20:569-80.
10. Barber RC, Aragaki CC, Rivera-Chavez FA. TLR4 and TNF-alpha polymorphisms are associated with an increased risk for severe sepsis following burn injury. J Med Genet. 2004;41:808-13.
11. Bilic I, Petri NM, Bota B. Effects of hyperbaric oxygen therapy on experimental burn wound healing in rats: a randomized controlled study. UHM. 2005;32(1):1-9.
12. Blaisdell LL, Chace R, Hallagan LD, Clark DE. A half century of burn epidemiology and burn care in a rural state. J Burn Care Res. 2011.
13. Bleser F, Benichoux R. Experimental surgery: the treatment of severe burns with hyperbaric oxygen. J Chir (Paris). 1973;106:281-90.
14. Boykin JV, Eriksson E, Pittman RN. In vivo microcirculation of a scald burn and the progression of postburn dermal ischemia. Plast Reconstr Surg. 1980;66:191-8.
15. Boykin JV Jr. Letter to the editor. Undersea Hyperb Med. 2013 Mar-Apr;40(2):212.
16. Brannen AL, Still J, Haynes M, Orlet H, Rosemblum F, Law E, Thompson WO. A randomized prospective trial of hyperbaric oxygen in a referral burn center population. Am Surg. 1997;63:205-8.
17. Buras JA, Stahl GL, Svoboda KK, Weenstra WR. Hyperbaric oxygen down regulates ICAM-1 expression induced by hypoxia and hypoglycemia: the role of NOS. Am J Physiol Cell Physiol. 2000;278:C292-302.
18. Burd F, Chiu T. Allogenic skin in the treatment of burns. Clin Dermatol. 2005;23:376-87.
19. Chong SJ, Kan EM, Song C, Soh CR, Lu J. Work in progress – characterization of early thermal burns and the effects of hyperbaric oxygen treatment: a pilot study. Diving Hyperb Med. 2013;43(3):157-61.
20. Church D, Elsayed S, Reid O, Winston B, Lindsay R. Burn wound infections. Clin Microbiol Rev. 2006;19(2):403-34.
21. Cianci P, Lueders H, Lee H, Shapiro R, Green B, Williams C. Hyperbaric oxygen and burn fluid requirements: observations in 16 patients with 40-80% TBSA burns. Undersea Biomed Res. 1988;15(Suppl):14.

22. Cianci P, Lueders H, Lee H, Shapiro R, Sexton J, Williams C, Green B. Adjunctive hyperbaric oxygen reduces the need for surgery in 40-80% burns. J Hyperbar Med. 1988;3:97.

23. Cianci P, Lueders HW, Lee H, Shapiro RL, Sexton J, Williams C, Sato R. Adjunctive hyperbaric oxygen therapy reduces length of hospitalization in thermal burns. J Burn Care Rehabil. 1989;10:432-5.

24. Cianci P, Sato R. Adjunctive hyperbaric oxygen therapy in the treatment of thermal burns: a review. Burns. 1994 Feb;20(1):5-14.

25. Cianci P, Sato R, Green B. Adjunctive hyperbaric oxygen reduces length of hospital stay, surgery, and the cost of care in severe burns. Undersea Biomed Res. 1991;18:108. Suppl.

26. Cianci P, Williams C, Lueders H, Lee H, Shapiro R, Sexton J, Sato R. Adjunctive hyperbaric oxygen in the treatment of thermal burns – an economic analysis. J Burn Care Rehabil. 1990;11:140-3.

27. Cost statistics (1997-98) from hospital patient accounts, home facility of the authors.

28. Deitch EA. Role of the gut lymphatic system in multiple organ failure. Current Opin Crit Care. 2001;7:92-8.

29. Deitch EA, Wheelahan TM, Rose MP, Clothier J, Cotter J. Hypertrophic burn scars: analysis of variables. J Trauma. 1983;23:895-8.

30. Deitch EA, Xu DZ, Franko L, et al. Evidence favoring the role of the gut as a cytokine generating organ in rats subjected to hemorrhagic shock. Shock. 1994:1:141-6.

31. Demling RH. Burns and other thermal injuries. In: Way LW, Doherty GM, editors. Current surgical diagnosis and treatment. 11th ed. McGraw-Hill Companies; 2003. p. 267.

32. Demling RH. The burn edema process: current concepts. J Burn Care Rehabil. 2005 May-Jun;26:207-227.

33. Engrav LH, Heimbach DM, Rivara FP, et al. Harborview burns – 1974-2009. PlosOne. 2012;7(7):1-23.

34. Fosen KM, Thom SR. Hyperbaric oxygen, vasculogenic stem cells, and wound healing. Antioxid Redox Signal. 2014;21(11):1634-46.

35. Gallagher KA, Goldstein LJ, Thom SR, Velazquez OC. Hyperbaric oxygen and bone marrow-derived endothelial progenitor cells in diabetic wound healing. Vascular. 2006;14(6):328-37.

36. Gallagher KA, Liu ZJ, Xiao M, Chen H, Goldstein LJ, Buerk DG, Nedeau A, Thom SR, Velazquez OC. Diabetic impairments in NO-mediated endothelial progenitor cell mobilization and homing are reversed by hyperoxia and SDF-1 alpha. J Clin Invest. 2007;117:1249-59.

37. Germonpré P, Reper P, Vanderkelen A. Hyperbaric oxygen therapy and piracetam decrease the early extension of deep partial thickness burns. Burns. 1996;22(6):468-73.

38. Goldstein LJ, Gallagher KA, Bauer SM, Bauer RJ, Baireddy V, Liu ZJ, Buerk DG, Thom SR, Velazquez OC. Endothelial progenitor cell release into circulation is triggered by hyperoxia-induced increases in bone marrow nitric oxide. Stem Cells. 2006;24:2309-18.

39. Grim PS, Nahum A, Gottlieb L, Wilbert C, Hawe E, Sznajder J. Lack of measurable oxidative stress during HBO2 therapy in burn patients. Undersea Biomed Res. 1989;16(Suppl):22.

40. Grossman AR, Grossman AJ. Update on hyperbaric oxygen and treatment of burns. Hyperb Oxyg Rev. 1982;3:51.

41. Grube BJ, Marvin JA, Heimbach DM. Therapeutic hyperbaric oxygen: help or hindrance in burn patients with carbon monoxide poisoning? J Burn Care Rehabil. 1988;9(3):249-52.

42. Gruber RP, Brinkley B, Amato JJ, Mendelson JA. Hyperbaric oxygen and pedicle flaps, skin grafts, and burns. Plast Reconstr Surg. 1970;45:24-30.

43. Hammarlund C, Svedman C, Svedman P. Hyperbaric oxygen treatment of healthy volunteers with UV-irradiated blister wounds. Bums. 1991;17:296-301.

44. Hart GB, O'Reilly RR, Broussard ND, Cave RH, Goodman DB, Yanda RL. Treatment of burns with hyperbaric oxygen. Surg Gynecol Obstet. 1974;139:693-6.

45. Hartwig J, Kirste G. Experimentele untersuchungen uber die revaskularisierung von verbrennungswunden unter hyperbarer sauerstofftherapie. Zbl Chir. 1974;99:1112-7. German.

46. Heggers JP, Robson MC, Zachary LS. Thromboxane inhibitor for the prevention of progressive dermal ischemia due to the thermal injury. J Burn Care Rehabil. 1985;6:466-8.

47. Hohn DC, McKay RD, Halliday B, Hunt TK. Effect of oxygen tension on the microbicidal function of leukocytes in wounds and in vitro. Surg Forum. 1976;27:18-20.

48. Hunt JL, Sato RM. Acute electrical burns. In: Greenberg MI, editor. Uncommon problems in emergency medicine. Philadelphia: F. A. Davis Co.; 1982. p. 183-95. CV11.

49. Hunt JL, Sato RM. Early excision of full thickness hand and digit burns: factors affecting morbidity. J Trauma. 1982;22(5):414-9. CV12.

50. Hunt JL, Sato RM, Baxter CR. Early tangential excision and immediate mesh auto-grafting of deep dermal hand burns. Ann Surg. 1979;189(2):147-151.

51. Hussman J, Hebebrand D, Erdmann D, Moticka J. Lymphocyte subpopulations in spleen and blood after early wound debridement and acute/chronic treatment with hyperbaric oxygen. Hanchir Mikrochir Plast Chir. 1996;28(2):103-7.

52. Ikeda K, Ajiki H, Kamiyama T, Wada J. Clinical application of oxygen hyperbaric treatment. Geka (Japan). 1967;29:1279.

53. Ikeda K, Ajiki H, Nagao H, Karino K, Sugii S, Iwa T, Wada J. Experimental and clinical use of hyperbaric oxygen in burns. In: Wada J, Iwa T, editors. Proceedings of the 4th International Congress on Hyperbaric Medicine. Tokyo: Igaku Shoin Ltd.; 1970. p. 370.

54. Jones LM, Rubadue C, Brown NV, Khandelwal S, Coffey RA. Evaluation of TCOM/HBO2T practice guideline for the treatment of foot burns occurring in diabetic patients. Burns. 2015;41:536-41.

55. Kaiser W, Schnaidt U, von der Leith H. Auswirkungen hyperbaren sauerstoffes auf die fresche brandwunde. Handchir Mikrochir Plast Chir. 1989;21:158-63. German.

56. Kaiser W, Voss K. Influence of hyperbaric oxygen on the edema formation in experimental burn injuries. Iugoslaw Physiol Pharmacol Acta. 1992;28(9):87-98.

57. Ketchum SA, Thomas AN, Hall AD. Angiographic studies of the effect of hyperbaric oxygen on burn wound revascularization. In: Wada J, Iwa T, editors. Proceedings of the 4th International Congress on Hyperbaric Medicine. Tokyo: Igaku Shoin Ltd.; 1970. p. 388.

58. Ketchum SA, Zubrin JR, Thomas AN, Hall AD. Effect of hyperbaric oxygen on small first, second and third degree burns. Surg Forum. 1967;18:65-7.

59. Kindwall EP. The use of drugs under pressure. In: Kindwall EP, Whelan HT, editors. Hyperbaric medicine practice. 2nd ed. Flagstaff (AZ): Best Publishing Co.; 1999. p. 326.

60. Kolski JM, Mazolewski PJ, Stephenson LL, Zamboni WA. Effect of hyperbaric oxygen therapy on testicular ischema-reperfusion injury. J Urol. 1998 Aug;160:601-4.

61. Korn HN, Wheeler ES, Miller TA. Effect of hyperbaric oxygen on second-degree burn wound healing. Arch Surg. 1977;112:732-7.

62. Kowalczyk L. A catastrophic cost. The Boston Globe. 2003 Feb 28.

63. Lamy ML, Hanquet MM. Application opportunity for OHP in a general hospital – a two year[s] experience with a monoplace hyperbaric oxygen chamber. In: Wada J, Iwa T, editors. Proceedings of the 4th International Congress on Hyperbaric Medicine. Tokyo: Igaku Shoin, Ltd.; 1970. p. 517.

64. Mader JT, Brown GL, Guckian JC, Reinarz JA. A mechanism for the amelioration of hyperbaric oxygen of experimental staphylococcal osteomyelitis in rabbits. J Inf Disease. 1980;142:915-22.

65. Magnotti LJ, Deitch EA. Burns, bacterial translocation, gut barrier function, and failure. J Burn Care Rehabil. 2005;26(5):383-91.

66. Maxwell G, Meites H, Silverstein P. Cost effectiveness of hyperbaric oxygen therapy in burn care. In: Winter Symposium on Baromedicine; 1991; Aspen, CO.

67. McCord JM. Oxygen-derived free radicals in postischemic tissue injury. N Engl J Med. 1985;312:159-63.

68. Merola L, Piscitelli F. Considerations on the use of HBO2 in the treatment of burns. Ann Med Nav. 1978;83:515.

69. Milijkovic-Lolic M, Silbergleit R, Fiskum G, Rosenthal RE. Neuro-protective effects of hyperbaric oxygen treatment in experimental focal cerebral ischemia are associated with reduced brain leucocyte myeloperoxidase activity. Brain Res. 2003;971(1):90-4.

70. Miller TA, Korn HN. Epithelial burn injury and repair. In: Davis JC, Hunt TK, editors. Hyperbaric oxygen therapy. Bethesda (MD): Undersea Medical Society, Inc.; 1977. p. 251.

71. Milovanova TN, Bhopale VM, Sorokina EM, Moore JS, Hunt TK, Hauer-Jensen M, Velazquez OC, Thom SR. Hyperbaric oxygen stimulates vasculogenic stem cell growth and differentiation in vivo. J Appl Physiol. 2009;106:711-28.

72. Milovanova TN, Bhopale VM, Sorokina EM, Moore JS, Hunt TK, Hauer-Jensen M, Velazquez OC, Thom SR. Lactate stimulates vasculogenic stem cells via the thioredoxin system and engages an autocrine activation loop involving hypoxia-inducible factor 1. Mol Cell Biol. 2008;28:6248-61.

73. Monafo WW. Initial management of burns. NEJM. 1996;335(21):1581-6.

74. Niccole MW, Thornton JW, Danet RT, Bartlett RH, Tavis MJ. Hyperbaric oxygen in burn management: a controlled study. Surgery. 1977;82:727-33.

75. Nichter LS, Morwood DT, Williams GS, Spence RJ. Expanding the limits of composite grafting: a case report of successful nose replantation assisted by hyperbaric oxygen therapy. Plast Reconstr Surg. 1991;87:337-40.

76. Niezgoda JA, Cianci P, Folden BW, Ortega RL, Slade JB, Storrow AB. The effect of hyperbaric oxygen therapy on a burn wound model in human volunteers. Plast Reconstr Surg. 1997;99(6):1620-5.

77. Niu AKC, Yang C, Lee HC, Chen SH, Chang LP. Burns treated with adjunctive hyperbaric oxygen therapy: a comparative study in humans. J Hyperbar Med. 1987;2:75.

78. Nylander G, Nordstrom H, Eriksson E. Effects of hyperbaric oxygen on oedema formation after a scald burn. Burns. 1984;10:193-6.

79. Nylander G, Nordstrom H, Lewis D, Larsson J. Metabolic effects of hyperbaric oxygen in postischemic muscle. Plast Reconstr Surg. 1987;79:91-7.

80. Ong YS, Samual M, Song C. Meta-analysis of early excision of burns. Burns. 2006;32(2):145-50.

81. Perrins DJD. Failed attempt to limit tissue destruction in scalds of pig's skin with hyperbaric oxygen. In: Wada J, Iwa T, editors. Proceedings of the 4th International Congress on Hyperbaric Medicine. Tokyo: Igaku Shoin Ltd.; 1970. p. 381.

82. Personal experience of the authors in a regional burn center.

83. Rabinowitz, PM, Siegel MD. Acute inhalation injury. Clin Chest Med. 2002;23(4):707.

84. Ramussen VM, Borgen AE, Jansen EC, Rotboll Nielsen PH, Werner MU. Hyperbaric oxygen therapy attenuates central sensitization induced by a thermal injury in humans. Acta Anaesthesiologica Scandinavica. 2015;59:749-62.

85. Ray CS, Green G, Cianci P. Hyperbaric oxygen therapy in burn patients: cost effective adjuvant therapy [abstract]. Undersea Biomed Res. 1991;18(Suppl):77.

86. Rowan MP, Cancio LC, Elster EA, Burmeister DM, Rose LF, Natesan S, Chan RK, Christy RJ, Chung KK. Burn wound healing and treatment: review and advancements. Crit Care. 2015. doi: 10.1186/s13054-01509861-2.

87. Sato RM, Baxter CT. Tangential excision of the burn wound. In: Recent advances in emergency and definitive burn wound care. Proceedings of a symposium sponsored by Valley Medical Center; Fresno, CA. 1977 Mar:16-24. CV2.

88. Sato R, Beesinger D, Hunt J, Baxter C. Early excision and closure of the burn wound. CCQ. 1978;1(3):51-62. CV4.

89. Sato RM, Beesinger DE, Hunt JL, Baxter CR. Early excision and closure of the burn wound. In: TL Wachtel et al., editors. Current topics in burn care. Rockville: Aspen Publication; 1983. p. 65-76.

90. Saunders J, Fritz E, Ko F, Bi C, Gottlieb L, Krizek T. The effects of hyperbaric oxygen on dermal ischemia following thermal injury. In: Proceedings of the American Burn Association; 1989; New Orleans. p. 58.

91. Shandling AH, Ellestad MH, Hart GB, Strauss M, Stavitsky Y. Hyperbaric oxygen and thrombolysis in myocardial infarction: the "HOT MI" pilot study. Am Heart J. 1997:134:544-50.

92. Sharifi M, Fares W, Abdel-Karim I, Adler D. Usefulness of hyperbaric oxygen therapy to inhibit restenosis after percutaneous coronary intervention for acute myocardial infarction or unstable angina pectoris. Am J Cardiol. 2004;93:1533-5.

93. Shirani K, Pruitt B, Mason A. The influence of inhalation injury and pneumonia on burn mortality. Ann Surg. 1986;205:82-7.

94. Shoshani O, Shupak A, Barak Y, Ullman Y, Ramon Y, Lindenbaum E, Peled Y. Hyperbaric oxygen therapy for deep second degree burns: an experimental study in the guinea pig. Brit J Plast Surg. 1998;51:67-73.

95. Stewart RJ, Yamaguchi KT, Cianci PE, Knost PM. Surgical Forum. 1988;39:87-90

96. Samadani S, Mason SW, Roshdieh B. Effects of hyperbaric oxygen on adenosine triphosphate in thermally injured skin. Surg Forum. 1988;39:87.

97. Sureda A, Batle JM, Martorell M, Capo X, Tejada S, Tur JA, Pons A. Antioxidant response of chronic wounds to hyperbaric oxygen therapy. PLoS One. 2016;11(9):e0163371.

98. Sutherland AM, Clarke HA, Katz J, Katznelson R. Hyperbaric oxygen therapy: a new treatment for chronic pain? Pain Pract. 2015;2(1):1-9.

99. Tabor CG. Hyperbaric oxygenation in the treatment of burns of less than forty percent. Korean J Int Med. 1967.

100. Takahashi M, Iwatsuki N, Ono K, Koga Y. Hyperbaric oxygen therapy accelerates neurologic recovery after 15-minute complete global cerebral ischemia in dogs. Crit Care Med. 1992 Nov;20(11):1588-94.

101. Tenenhaus M, Hansbrough JF, Zapata-Sirvent R, Neumann T. Treatment of burned mice with hyperbaric oxygen reduces mesenteric bacteria but not pulmonary neutrophil deposition. Arch Surg. 1994;129:1338-42.

102. Thom SR. Functional inhibition of leukocyte B2 integrins by hyperbaric oxygen in carbon monoxide-mediated brain injury in rats. Toxicol Appl Pharmacol. 1993;123:248-56.

103. Thom SR, Bhopale VM, Velazquez OC, Goldstein LJ, Thom LH, Buerk DG. Stem cell mobilization by hyperbaric oxygen. Am J Physiol Heart Circ Physiol. 2006;290:H1378-86.

104. Thom SR, Milovanova TN, Yang M, Bhopale VM, Sorokina EM, Uzun G, Malay DS, Troiano MA, Hardy KR, Lambert DS, Logue CJ, Margolis DJ. Vasculogenic stem cell mobilization and wound recruitment in diabetic patients: increased cell number and intracellular regulatory protein content associated with hyperbaric oxygen therapy. Wound Repair Regen. 2011;19:149-61.

105. Thomas MP, Brown LA, Sponseller DR, Guyton DP. Myocardial infarct size reduction by the synergistic effect of hyperbaric oxygen and recombinant tissue plasminogen activator. Am Heart J. 1990;120:791-800.

106. Traystman RJ, Kirsch JR, Koehler RC. Oxygen radical mechanisms of brain injury following ischemia and reperfusion. J Appl Physiol. 1991;71:1185-95.

107. Turkaslan T, Yogum N, Cimsit M, Solakoglu S, Ozdemir C, Ozsoy Z. Is HBO2T treatment effective in recovering zone of stasis? An experimental immunohistochemical study. Burns. 2010;36(4):539-44.

108. Ueno S, Tanabe G, Kihara K, et al. Early post-operative hyperbaric oxygen therapy modifies neutrophile activation. Hepatogastroenterology. 1999;46:1798-9.

109. Veltkamp R, Siebing DA, Schwab S, Schwaninger M. Hyperbaric oxygen reduces blood-brain barrier damage and edema after transient focal cerebral ischemia. Stroke. 2005;36:1679-83.

110. Villanueva E, Bennett MH, Wasiak J, Lehm JP. Hyperbaric oxygen therapy for thermal burns [review]. Cochrane Database Syst Rev. 2004;(2):CD004727. doi: 10.1002/14651858.CD004727.pub2.

111. Wada J, Ikeda K, Kagaya H, Ajiki H. Oxygen hyperbaric treatment and severe burn. Jap Med J. 1966;13:2203.

112. Wada J, Ikeda T, Kamata K, Ebuoka M. Oxygen hyperbaric treatment for carbon monoxide poisoning and severe burn in coal mine (hokutanyubari) gas explosion. Igakunoaymi (Japan). 1965;5:53.

113. Waisbren BA, Schutz D, Collentine G, Banaszak E. Hyperbaric oxygen in severe burns. Burns. 1982;8:176-9.

114. Ward PA, Mulligan MS. New insights into mechanisms of oxyradical and neutrophil mediated lung injury. Klin Wochenschr. 1991;69:1009-11.

115. Ward PA, Till GO. The autodestructive consequences of thermal injury. J Burn Care Rehabil. 1985;6:251-5.

116. Wasiak J, Bennett M, Cleland H. Hyperbaric oxygen as adjuvant therapy in the management of burns: can evidence guide clinical practice? Burns. 2006;32:650-2.

117. Wells CH, Hilton JG. Effects of hyperbaric oxygen on post-burn plasma extravasation. In: Davis JC, Hunt TK, editors. Hyperbaric oxygen therapy. Bethesda (MD): Undersea Medical Society, Inc.; 1977. p. 259.

118. Wolf SE, Tompkins RG, Herndon DN. On the horizon – research priorities in burns for the next decade. Surg Clin N Am. 2014;94:917-30.

119. Xu N, Li Z, Luo X. Effects of hyperbaric oxygen therapy on the changes in serum sIL-2R and Fn in severe burn patients. Zhonghua Zheng Xing Shao Shang Wai Ke Za Zhi. 1999;15(3):220-3.

120. Yamada T, Taguchi T, Hirata Y, Suita S, Yugi H. The protective effect of hyperbaric oxygenation on the small intestine in ischemia-reperfusion injury. J Pediatr Surg. 1995;30:786-90.

121. Yogaratnam JZ, Laden G, Madden LA, Griffin S, et al. Hyperbaric oxygen: a new drug in myocardial revascularization and protection? Cardiovasc Revasc Med. 2006;7:146-54.

122. Zamboni WA, Roth AC, Russell RC, Graham B, Suchy H, Kucan JO. Morphological analysis of the microcirculation during reperfusion of ischemic skeletal muscle and the effect of hyperbaric oxygen. Plast Reconstr Surg. 1993;91:1110-23.

123. Zamboni WA, Stephenson LL, Roth AC, Suchy H, Russell RC. Ischemia-reperfusion injury in skeletal muscle: CD18 dependent neutrophil-endothelial adhesion. Undersea Hyperb Med. 1994;21(Suppl):53.

124. Zhang Q, Chang Q, Cox RA, Gong X, Gould LJ. Hyperbaric oxygen attenuates apoptosis and decreases inflammation in an ischemic wound model. J Invest Dermatol. 2008;128(8):2102-12.

CHAPTER 32 CHAPTER

Central Retinal Artery Occlusion

CHAPTER THIRTY-TWO OVERVIEW

Introduction 821
Literature Review 821
Patient Selection 821
Physical Exam Findings 821
Differential Diagnoses 821
Patient Management Work-Up 826
Treatment 826
Prognosis 829
Consultations 829
References 830

Central Retinal Artery Occlusion

Heather Murphy-Lavoie, Tracy Leigh LeGros

INTRODUCTION

Central retinal artery occlusion (CRAO) presents as a sudden, unilateral, painless vision loss in the range of counting fingers or less and usually results in permanent, severe, painless vision loss. A wide variety of conventional treatment modalities have been investigated over the years with no success. HBO_2, if instituted prior to retinal necrosis, can improve vision loss. This is accomplished using collateral choroidal circulation and diffusion of oxygen from the choroid to the inner layers of the retina.

LITERATURE REVIEW

There are 39 publications and proceedings over the last 52 years that describe the treatment of 887 patients with CRAO treated with HBO_2. Sixty-four percent of these patients in the literature improved when treated with HBO_2 (Table 1).[43] There are no randomized controlled trials, only retrospective case-controlled series. The best outcomes are achieved when treatment begins within eight hours of symptom onset. HBO_2 should be considered for patients presenting within 24 hours of symptom onset.[23,43]

PATIENT SELECTION

Patients presenting within 24 hours of symptom onset with acute, painless vision loss, a visual acuity < 20/200, and funduscopic findings consistent with CRAO should be considered for emergent HBO_2. While there are a few case reports in the literature showing improvement beyond this time frame, this improvement is rare and even more rarely clinically significant.[2,4,12-13,18,23,40,42,59-60]

PHYSICAL EXAM FINDINGS

Patients with CRAO will have a pale retina on funduscopic exam. They may also have a cherry-red spot on the macula, which portends a poor prognosis.[18] Additional findings often include an afferent pupillary defect and boxcarring of the arterioles of the retina. Patients should be examined for cardiac murmur, stigmata of embolic disease, and signs of giant cell arteritis, such as tenderness over the temporal artery.

DIFFERENTIAL DIAGNOSES

Visual acuity (VA) of light perception only or no light perception may indicate a high-level ophthalmic artery occlusion and lack of choroidal perfusion, portending a poor

TABLE 1. TREATMENT OF RETINAL ARTERY OCCLUSIONS: LITERATURE SUMMARY

REPORT	CRAO/ BRAO	THERAPY	DELAY TO TX
Gool 1965 (17)	BRAO CRAO CRAO BRAO	HBO_2: 3 ATA, anticoagulants, Complamin	5 days, 2 days, Unkn (< 24 hrs) 10 days
Haddad 1965 (19)	CRAO	HBO_2	Unknown
Anderson 1965 (2)	BRAO CRAO BRAO	HBO_2, retrobulbar lidocaine, ocular massage, nicotinic acid	"several hrs" 40+ hrs 6+ days
Takahashi 1977 (54)		HBO_2: 2.5 ATA, ocular massage, paracentesis, vasodilators	1–6 days
Pallota 1978 (46)	CRAO	HBO_2: 2.8 ATA	
Sasaki 1978 (50)	CRAO	HBO_2, stellate ganglion block	
Szuki 1980 (53)	CRAO	HBO_2	
Krasnov 1981 (31)	CRAO	HBO_2	
Zhang 1986 (63)	CRAO	HBO_2	
Desola 1987 (12)	CRAO	HBO_2	
Miyake 1987 (40)	CRAO (53) BRAO (19)	HBO_2: 2 ATA or 3 ATA, vasodilators, stellate ganglion block, 2% carbocaine	18 hrs to 15 days, all but 3 within 12 days
Kindwall 1988 (30)	CRAO	HBO_2	
Cho 1990 (9)	CRAO	HBO_2 x 50 Tx, steroids	15 days
Hirayama 1990 (24)	CRAO	HBO_2, urokinase, steroids, bifemelane	< 1 month
Hertzog 1992 (23)	CRAO	HBO_2: 1.5–2.0 ATA, timolol, acetazolamide, paracentesis, carbogen, vasodilators, steroids, ocular massage, retrobulbar anesthesia	< 24 hours
Beiran 1993 (6)	CRAO	HBO_2: 2.5 ATA, ocular massage, SL nifedipine, oral glycerol	2: < 100 min 1: occluding 1: 6 hrs
Yotsukura 1993 (60)	CRAO	HBO_2, ocular massage, IV urokinase, 2/15 with IV prostaglandin	3 hrs to 6 days

TABLE 1 (CONTINUED)

NOTE: Graph = see full graphs of patient results in original papers, CF = counting fingers, LP = light perception, NLP = no light perception, HM = hand motion, NR = not reported

INITIAL VA	FINAL VA	TOTAL PATIENTS (N)	CASES IMPROVED (N)
1.5% NL P12 5% 1.6%	100% NLP 125% imp VF 1.6%	4	2
NLP CF	NLP CF	2	0
CF 2–3 ft 20/25 20/200	20/20 20/25 impVF Unknown	3	2
Graph	Graph	9	9
NLP	10/10	1	1
		10	7
		6	6
		39	22
		80	49
		20	11
Graph	Graph	72	32
		14	7
HM	0.02	1	1
Graph	Graph	17	12
Graph	Graph	19	14
LP HM CF 2 m HM	6/20 6/6 6/9 CF 60cm	4	4
Graph	Graph	15	8

TABLE 1 (CONTINUED)

REPORT	CRAO/ BRAO	THERAPY	DELAY TO TX
Li 1996 (33)	BRAO OS	HBO_2: 2.32 ATA	< 24 hrs
	BRAO OD (15 mo later)	HBO_2: 2.82 ATA	< 24 hrs
Phillips 1999 (48)	CRAO	100% surface O_2, HBO_2: 2.4 ATA	< 2 hrs
Aisenbrey 2000 (1)	CRAO (8) BRAO (10)	HBO_2 Therapy: 240 kPa, ocular massage, paracentesis, IV acetazolamide	
Matsuo 2001 (38)	BRAO (OU)	HBO_2 Therapy, IV prostaglandin, urokinase	4 days
Beiran 2001 (5)	CRAO (29) BRAO (6)	HBO_2 Therapy: 2.8 ATA; ocular massage, retrobulbar block, timolol, acetazolamide, paracentesis	< 8 hrs
Weinberger 2002 (58)	CRAO	HBO_2, ocular massage, antiglaucoma eye drops	4–12 hrs
Murphy-Lavoie 2004 (42)	CRAO BRAO	HBO_2: 2.0 ATA	6 hrs–4 days
Imai 2004 (27)	BRAO	HBO_2, stellate ganglion block	2 days
Swaby 2005 (52)	CRAO	HBO_2: 2.0 ATA, optic nerve sheath fenestration	3 weeks
Weiss 2009 (59)	CRAO BRAO	HBO_2: 1.5 ATA	Hours–3 weeks
Inoue 2009 (28)	CRAO BRAO	HBO_2: 1.8 ATA	Hours–8 days
Aten 2011 (3)	CRAO	HBO_2: 2.4 ATA	7 hours
Cope 2011 (10)	CRAO	HBO_2: 2.4 ATA	5–144 hours
Telander 2011 (56)	CRAO	HBO_2 x 1, ocular massage, pressure-lowering eye drops	11 hours
Menzel 2012 (39)	CRAO	$HBO_2$2: 2.4 ATA, hemodilution	< 12 hours
Canan 2014 (8)	CRAO	HBO_2: 2.5 ATA, exchange transfusion	< 24 hours

TABLE 1 (CONTINUED)

NOTE: Graph = see full graphs of patient results in original papers, CF = counting fingers, LP = light perception, NLP = no light perception, HM = hand motion, NR = not reported

INITIAL VA	FINAL VA	TOTAL PATIENTS (N)	CASES IMPROVED (N)
20/200 CF 2ft	20/25 20/25	2	2
NLP	20/30	1	1
Graph	Graph	18	12
20/30 20/600	20/15 20/400	2	2
Graph	Graph	35	29
Graph	Graph	21	13
Graph	Graph	16	12
CF	0.08	1	1
20/400	Improved	1	1
Graph	Graph	4	2
Graph	Graph	63	30
NR	20/80	1	1
Graph	Graph	11	8
CF	20/160	1	1
Graph	Graph	51	19
CF	20/30	1	1

TABLE 1 (CONTINUED)

REPORT	CRAO/ BRAO	THERAPY	DELAY TO TX
Hsiao 2014 [25]	CRAO	HBO_2: 2.5 ATA x 6 carbogen, pressure-lowering eyedrops, hemodilution, corticosteroids	4 hours
Masters 2015 [37]	CRAO	HBO_2: 2.8 ATA	< 24 hours
Desola 2015 [13]	CRAO	HBO_2: 2.3 ATA x 15	< 2 months
Lu 2015 [34]	CRAO	HBO_2, ocular massage, anterior paracentsis, aspirin	100 min
Lemos 2015 [32]	CRAO CRVO	HBO_2: 2.4 ATA, ASA	8 hours
Hadanny 2017 [18]	CRAO	HBO_2: 2–2.4 ATA, ocular massage, anterior chamber paracentesis, ASA, acetazolamide, topical beta blocker	< 20 hours
TOTAL			
% Improved			

prognosis. A retinal exam consistent with CRAO associated with a much better VA may indicate the presence of collateral circulation via a cilioretinal artery (14%–32% of the population). The presence of flashes or floaters associated with painless vision loss suggests retinal detachment or vitreous hemorrhage. Ischemic optic neuropathies and posterior circulation strokes may also present with painless vision loss but will not have the classic fundoscopic findings of CRAO. Painful vision loss suggests an alternate diagnosis, such as optic neuritis. Correction of vision loss with pinhole aperture indicates a refractive error and not a retinal pathology.

PATIENT MANAGEMENT WORK-UP

Patients with a diagnosis of CRAO should undergo an evaluation for possible etiologies and risk-factor modifications similar to that of a stroke patient including the following: complete blood count (to screen for platelet disorders or infectious causes), erythrocyte sedimentation rate (for arteritic causes), hypercoagulable panel (fibrinogen, PT/PTT, anti-phospholipid antibody), lipid panel, electrocardiogram, carotid ultrasound, and echocardiography.

TREATMENT

A patient presenting with CRAO should be placed on surface oxygen as soon as possible. Arteritic cases should be treated with concomitant corticosteroids. Oxygen concentration should be titrated up until return of vision. Hyperbaric oxygen can be

TABLE 1 (CONTINUED)

NOTE: Graph = see full graphs of patient results in original papers, CF = counting fingers, LP = light perception, NLP = no light perception, HM = hand motion, NR = not reported

INITIAL VA	FINAL VA	TOTAL PATIENTS (N)	CASES IMPROVED (N)
CF	20/200	1	1
Graph	Graph	29	20
NR	NR	182	138
LP	HM	1	1
20/400	20/40	1	1
Graph	Graph	128	86
		887	568
			64%

Modified from Murphy H, et al., Central retinal artery occlusion treated with oxygen: A literature review and treatment algorithm. Undersea Hyperb Med 2012: 39 (5) Sept - Oct: 943 - 953; and Murphy H, et al. Arterial Insufficiencies: Central Retinal Artery Occlusion (2014). In: Lindell K Weaver (Ed). Hyperbaric oxygen therapy indications: the Hyperbaric Oxygen Therapy Committee Report. North Palm Beach, Florida: Best Publishing Company, with permission.

given at the depth of return of vision for 90 minutes, with a maximum of a USN Treatment Table 6 for the first treatment. In those patients with improvement in vision during initial HBO_2, post-HBO_2 visual acuity should be monitored hourly.

If blindness recurs, oxygen should be retitrated. HBO_2 TID/BID may be necessary until recanalization recurs (usually within 72 hours), or there is no further improvement for 3 treatments.

Fundoscopic findings of CRAO should trigger management as below if symptom onset is within 24 hours or less. Oxygen delivery should be titrated to patient response as follows:

1. Deliver oxygen immediately at 1 atmosphere absolute (ATA) at the highest possible FiO_2.
2. If vision improves significantly with normobaric oxygen within 15 minutes, the patient should be admitted to the hospital and given intermittent normobaric oxygen for 15 minutes every hour alternating with 45 minutes of breathing room air. Visual acuity should be checked at the end of each air-breathing period. This regimen should be continued until angiogram

shows patency, the patient's vision remains stable on room air for 2 hours, or a maximum of 96 hours.

3. Refer for hyperbaric oxygen therapy if no response to normobaric oxygen within the first 15 minutes.
4. Compress to 2 ATA (202 kPa) on 100% oxygen.
5. Other adjunctive therapies to lower intraocular pressure and/or cause retinal vasodilatation may be performed as well but should not delay compression. If vision improves significantly at 2 ATA (202 kPa), remain at this depth for 90 minutes (air-breathing periods at this depth may not be necessary since the incidence of oxygen toxicity seizures is 4 times lower at 2.0 than at 2.4 ATA), and then proceed as outlined in 8 below.
6. If vision fails to improve significantly at 2 ATA (202 kPa) by the first air-breathing period (or 30 minutes), compress to 2.4 ATA (242 kPa). If vision improves significantly at this depth, conduct a USN Treatment Table 9, and then proceed as outlined in 8 below.
7. If vision does not improve significantly at 2.4 ATA (242 kPa), compress to 2.8 ATA (282 kPa). If no improvement occurs after the first 20-minute breathing period, consider conducting a USN Treatment Table 6. If vision improves significantly, proceed as outlined in 8 below. If there is no response to the initial Table 6, options are to discontinue treatment, continue with normobaric oxygen as in 2 above or give 2 additional treatments for 90 minutes at 2.8 ATA (282 kPa) with air-breathing periods on a twice-daily schedule.
8. If the patient has return of vision during hyperbaric treatment, inpatient monitoring and intermittent supplemental oxygen should be considered. Monitoring by a retina specialist should continue. Recovery of vision during the initial treatment of CRAO with HBO_2 indicates retinal viability and the potential for return of vision despite the ischemic period suffered prior to treatment. Patients with such a recovery should have their visual status monitored frequently after completion of HBO_2.

Patients should be monitored at the chamber for two hours post treatment. If vision remains normal, and admission to the hospital is not possible, they can be discharged home with instruction to monitor vision every hour. Should vision loss recur, aggressive use of intermittent normobaric oxygen as described in Section 2 or customized hyperbaric oxygen is indicated to preserve retinal function until CRA recanalization occurs. Ideally, these patients should be admitted to the hospital on a stroke protocol. Twice- or three-times-daily hyperbaric treatments may be necessary until the angiogram normalizes, or the patient has no further improvement for three treatments.

- NOTE: The retina may not tolerate periods of ischemia that persist longer than 90 minutes. Cases of relapse of loss of vision and resultant blindness after discharge home have been reported, and patients should be instructed to return immediately for supplemental oxygen therapy if vision loss recurs after discharge.
- NOTE: One exception to the above regimen is CRAO that results from arterial gas embolism (AGE). In this event, the recommended treatment

regimen for AGE should be followed. Patients with history of DCI, recent hemodialysis, or general anesthesia should always be treated with HBO_2.

- NOTE: All patients who have lost vision in one eye should be directed to present immediately to a hospital or to their ophthalmologist if vision loss occurs in the fellow eye.

PROGNOSIS

The sooner the patient is treated, the higher the likelihood of significant improvement in vision (0.03 logMAR worse for each hour of delay).[18]

Patients with a cherry-red spot on funduscopic exam have a lower likelihood of significant improvement in vision when treated with HBO_2 than those without (49% versus 86%).[18]

CONSULTATIONS

Ophthalmology should be monitoring these patients throughout their treatment course, but oxygen administration should not be delayed pending their arrival. An internal medicine or neurology specialist should be consulted to manage the work-up and risk-factor modification. Best practice is probably to admit these patients to the hospital under the stroke protocol.

REFERENCES

1. Aisenbrey S, Krott R, Heller R, et al. Hyperbaric oxygen therapy in retinal artery occlusion. Ophthalmologe. 2000;97:461-7.
2. Anderson B, Saltzman H, Heyman A. The effects of hyperbaric oxygenation on retinal artery occlusion. Arch Ophthal. 1965;73:315-9.
3. Aten LA, Stone JA, Poli T. Treatment of a patient with acute central retinal artery occlusion with hyperbaric oxygen therapy [abstract]. UHMS Annual Scientific Assembly; 2011; Ft Worth, Texas.
4. Augsburger JJ, Magargal LE. Visual prognosis following treatment of acute central retinal artery obstruction. Br J Ophthalmol. 1980;64:913-7.
5. Beiran I, Goldenberg I, Adir Y, Tamir A, Shupak A, Miller B. Early hyperbaric oxygen therapy for retinal artery occlusion. Eur J Ophthalmol. 2001;11:345-50.
6. Beiran I, Reissman P, Scharf J, Nahum Z et al. Hyperbaric oxygenation combined with nifedipine treatment for recent onset retinal artery occlusion. Eur J Ophthalmol. 1993;3:89-94.
7. Beran DI, Murphy-Lavoie H. Acute, painless vision loss. J La State Med Soc. 2009;161:214-23.
8. Canan H, Ulas B, Altan-Yaycioglu R. Hyperbaric oxygen therapy in combination with systemic treatment of sickle cell disease presenting as central retinal artery occlusion: a case report. J Med Case Rep. 2014;8:370.
9. Cho S, Choi MS, Lee, JY. Effect Of hyperbaric oxygen therapy on central retinal artery occlusion associated with systemic lupus erythematosus (a case report) [abstract]. Abstract of the Undersea and Hyperbaric Medical Society, Inc. Joint Annual Scientific Meeting with the International Congress for Hyperbaric Medicine and the European Undersea Biomedical Society; 1990 Aug; Amsterdam, Netherlands.
10. Cope A, Eggert JV, O'Brien E. Retinal artery occlusion: visual outcome after treatment with hyperbaric oxygen. Diving Hyperb Med. 2011;41(3):135-8.
11. David NJ, Norton EWD, Gass JD, Beauchamp J. Fluorescein angiography in central retinal artery occlusion. Arch Ophthalmol. 1967;77:619-29.
12. Desola J. Hyperbaric oxygen therapy in acute occlusive retinopathies. In: Schmutz J, editor. Proceedings of the 1st Swiss Symposium on Hyperbaric Medicine. Basel, Switzerland: Foundation for Hyperbaric Medicine; 1987. p. 333.
13. Desola J, Papoutsidakis E, Martos P. Hyperbaric oxygenation in the treatment of central retinal artery occlusions: an analysis of 214 cases following a prospective protocol [abstract]. UHMS Annual Scientific Assembly; 2015; Montréal, Quebec.
14. Duker JS, Brown GC. Recovery following acute obstruction of the retinal and choroidal circulations. Retina. 1988;8:257-60.
15. Garcia-Arumi J, Martinez-Castillo V, Boixadera A, Fonollosa A, Corcostgui B. Surgical embolus removal in retinal artery occlusion. Br J Ophthalmol. 2006;90:1252-5.
16. Gaydar V, Ezrachi D, Dratviman-Storobinsky. Reduction in apoptosis in ischemic retinas of two mouse models using hyperbaric oxygen treatment. Invest Ophthalmol Vis Sci. 2011;52:7514-22.
17. Gool J, Jong H. Hyperbaric oxygen treatment in vascular insufficiency of the retina and optic nerve. In: Ledingham IM, editor. Proceedings of the 2nd International Congress on Clinical and Applied Hyperbaric Medicine. Edinburgh, Scotland: Livingstone; 1965. p. 447-60.
18. Hadanny A, Maliar A, Fishlev G, et al. Reversibility of retinal ischemia due to central retinal artery occlusion by hyperbaric oxygen. Clin Ophthalmol. 2016 Dec 29;11:115-25.

19. Haddad HM, Leopold IH. Effect of hyperbaric oxygenation on microcirculation: use in therapy of retinal vascular disorders. Invest Ophthalmol. 1965;4:1141-51.

20. Hayreh SS, Kolder HE, Weingeist TA. Central retinal artery occlusion and retinal tolerance time. Ophthalmology. 1980;87:75-8.

21. Hayreh SS, Podhajsky P. Ocular neovascularization with retinal vascular occlusion: II. Occurrence in central retinal and branch retinal artery occlusion. Arch Ophthalmol. 1982;100:1581-96.

22. Hayreh SS, Zimmerman MB. Central retinal artery occlusion: visual outcome. Am J Ophthalmol. 2005;140:376-91.

23. Hertzog LM, Meyer GW, Carson S, Strauss MB, Hart GB. Central retinal artery occlusion treated with hyperbaric oxygen. J Hyperb Med. 1992;7:33-42.

24. Hirayama Y, Matsunaga N, Tashiro J, Amemlya T, Iwasaki M. Bifemelane in the treatment of central retinal artery or vein obstruction. Clin Ther. 1990;12:230-5.

25. Hsaio S, Huang Y. Partial vision recovery after iatrogenic retinal artery occlusion. Ophthalmology. 2014;14:120.

26. Hwang K. Hyperbaric oxygen therapy to avoid blindness from filler injection. J Craniofac Surg. 2016 Nov;27(8):2154-5.

27. Imai E, Kunikata H, Udono T, Nakagawa Y et al. Branch retinal artery occlusion: a complication of iron-deficiency anemia in a young adult with a rectal carcinoid. Tohuko J Exper Med. 2004;203:141-4.

28. Inoue O, Kajiya S, Yachimori. Treatment of central retinal artery occlusion(CRAO) and branch retinal artery occlusion (BRAO) by hyperbaric oxygen therapy (HBO_2) – 107 eyes over 20 years [abstract]. UHMS Annual Scientific Assembly; 2009; Las Vegas, NV.

29. Karaman S, Ozkan B, Yazir Y, et al. Comparison of hyperbaric oxygen versus iloprost treatment in an experimental rat central retinal artery occlusion model. Graefes Arch Clin Exp Ophthalmol. 2016 Nov;254(11):2209-15. Epub 2016 Aug 2.

30. Kindwall EP, Goldmann RW. Hyperbaric medicine procedures. Milwaukee (WI): St. Luke's Medical Center; 1988.

31. Krasnov MM, Kharlap SI, Pereverzina OK, et al. Hyperbaric oxygenation in the treatment of vascular diseases of retina. In: Yefuny SN, editor. Abstracts of the 7th International Congress on Hyperbaric Medicine. Moscow: USSR Academy of Sciences; 1981. p. 304.

32. Lemos JA, Teixeira C, Carvalho R, et al. Combined central retinal artery and vein occlusion associated with factor V Leiden mutation and treated with hyperbaric oxygen. Case Rep Ophthalmol. 2015 Dec 19;6(3):462-8.

33. Li HK, Dejean BJ, Tang RA. Reversal of visual loss with hyperbaric oxygen treatment in a patient with Susac Syndrome. Ophthalmology. 1996;103(12):2091-8.

34. Lu C, Wang J, Zhou D. Central retinal artery occlusion associated with persistent truncus arteriosus and single atrium: a case report. BMC Ophthalmology. 2015;15:137.

35. Mangat HS. Retinal artery occlusion. Surv Ophthalmol. 1995;40:145-56.

36. Mason JO, Nixon PA, Albert MA. Trans-luminal nd:YAG laser embolysis for branch retinal artery occlusion. Retina. 2007;27:573-7.

37. Masters T, Westgard B, Hendrikson S. Central retinal artery occlusion treated with hyperbaric oxygen: a retrospective review [abstract]. UHMS Annual Scientific Assembly; 2015; Montréal, Quebec.

38. Matsuo T. [Multiple occlusive retinal arteritis in both eyes of a patient with rheumatoid arthritis]. Jpn J Ophthalmol. 2001;45:662-4. Japanese.

39. Menzel-Severing J, Siekmann U, Weinberger A. Early hyperbaric oxygen treatment for nonarteritic central retinal artery occlusion. Am J Ophthalmol. 2012;153:454-9.

40. Miyake Y, Horiguchi M, Matsuura M et al. Hyperbaric oxygen therapy in 72 eyes with retinal arterial occlusion. In: Bove AA, Bachrach AJ, Greenbaum LJ, editors. 9th International Symposium on Underwater and Hyperbaric Physiology. Bethesda: Undersea and Hyperbaric Medical Society; 1987. p. 949-53.

41. Mori K, Ohta K, Nagano S et al. [A case of ophthalmic artery obstruction following autologous fat injection in the glabellar area]. Nippon Ganka Gakkai Zasshi. 2007;111:22-5. Japanese.

42. Murphy-Lavoie H, Harch P, VanMeter K. Effect of hyperbaric oxygen on central retinal artery occlusion. UHMS Scientific Assembly; 2004; Australia.

43. Murphy-Lavoie H, LeGros T, Butler FK, Jain K. Hyperbaric oxygen therapy and ophthalmology. In: Jain, editor. K.K. Jain textbook of hyperbaric medicine. 6th ed. Springer Publishing; 2016.

44. Neubauer AS, Mueller AJ, Schriever S, Gruterich M, Ulbig M, Kampik A. [Minimally invasive therapy for clinically complete central retinal artery occlusion – results and meta-analysis of literature]. Klin Monatsbl Augenheilkd. 2000;217:30-6. German.

45. Olson EA, Lentz K. Central retinal artery occlusion: a literature review and the rationale for hyperbaric oxygen therapy. Mo Med. 2016 Jan-Feb;113(1):53-7.

46. Pallota R, Anceschi S, Costagliola N et al. Recovery from blindness through hyperbaric oxygen in a case of thrombosis on the central retinal artery. Ann Med Nav. 1978;83:591-2.

47. Petterson JA, Hill MD, Demchuk AM et al. Intra-arterial thrombolysis for retinal artery occlusion: the Calgary experience. Can J Neurol Sci. 2005;32:507-11.

48. Phillips D, Diaz C, Atwell G, Chimiak J, Ullman S, et al. Care of sudden blindness: a case report of acute central retinal artery occlusion reversed with hyperbaric oxygen therapy [abstract]. Undersea Hyperb Med. 1999;26(Supp):23-4.

49. Ros MA, Magargal LE, Uram M. Branch retinal artery obstruction: a review of 201 eyes. Ann Ophthalmol. 1989;21:103-7.

50. Sasaki K, Fukuda M, Otani S et al. High pressure oxygen therapy in ocular diseases: with special reference to the effect of concomitantly used stellate ganglion block. Jpn J Anesth. 1978;27:170-6.

51. Stone R, Zink H, Klingele T, Burde R. Visual recovery after central retinal artery occlusion: two cases. Ann Ophthalmol. 1977;9:445-50.

52. Swaby K, Valderrama O, Schiffman J. Treatment Of disc edema and retinal artery occlusion with HBO_2 during the third trimester of pregnancy [abstract]. UHMS Annual Scientific Assembly; 2005; Las Vegas, NV.

53. Szuki H, Inie J, Horiuchi T. Hyperbaric oxygenation therapy in ophthalmology. Part I: incipient insufficiency of the retinal circulation. J Clin Ophthalmol. 1980;34:335-43.

54. Takahashi K, Shima T, Yamamuro M. Hyperbaric oxygenation following stellate ganglion block in patients with retinal occlusion. In: Smith G, editor. Proceedings of the 6th International Congress on Hyperbaric Medicine. Aberdeen: University of Aberdeen Press; 1977. p. 211–5.

55. Tang WM, Han DP. A study of surgical approaches to retinal vascular occlusions. Arch Ophthalmol. 2000;118:138-43.

56. Telander G, Hielweil G, Schwartz S. Diagnostic and therapeutic challenges. Retina. 2011;31(8):1726-31.

57. Weber J, Remonda L, Mattle HP, et al. Selective intra-arterial fibrinolysis of acute central retinal artery occlusion. Stroke. 1998;29:2076-9.

58. Weinberger AWA, Siekmann UPF, Wolf S et al. [Treatment of acute central retinal artery occlusion (CRAO) by hyperbaric oxygenation therapy (HBO_2) – a pilot study with 21 patients]. Klin Monatsbl Augenheilkd. 2002;219:728-34. German.

59. Weiss J. Hyperbaric oxygen treatment of nonacute central retinal artery occlusion. UHM. 2009;36(6):401-5.

60. Yotsukura J, Adachi-Usami E. Correlation of electroretinographic changes with visual prognosis in central retinal artery occlusion. Ophthalmologica. 1993;207:13-8.

61. Yu DY, Cringle SJ, Yu PK, Su EN. Intraretinal oxygen distribution and consumption during retinal artery occlusion and graded hyperoxic ventilation in the rat. Invest Ophthalmol Vis Sci. 2007;48:2290-6.

62. Yuzurihara D, Ijima H. [Visual outcome in central retinal and branch retinal artery occlusion]. Jpn J Ophthalmol. 2004;48:490-2. Japanese.

63. Zhang XZ, Cao JQ. Observations on therapeutic results in 80 cases of central serous retinopathy treated with hyperbaric oxygenation. Presented at: The 5th Chinese Conference on Hyperbaric Medicine; 1986 Sep 26-29; Fuzhow, China.

SECTION 3 SECTION

Hyperbaric Oxygen Used in Off-Label Disorders and Investigational Areas

CHAPTER 33 CHAPTER

Off-Label Indications for Hyperbaric Oxygen Therapy

CHAPTER THIRTY-THREE OVERVIEW

Introduction **839**

What is an Off-Label Indication? **839**

Why is HBO_2 Therapy Vulnerable to Use in Off-Label Indications? 840

Classification of Indications for HBO_2 Therapy 841

What Are the Problems with Treatment of Off-Label Indications for HBO_2 Therapy? 842

Off-Label Indications of Contemporary Interest **843**

Chronic Head Injury and Post-Concussion Syndromes **844**

Ischemic Stroke – Acute Intervention and as an Adjunct to Rehabilitation . . . **848**

Therapy 849

Evidence 849

The Cochrane Review 850

Summary of Data 852

HBO_2 Therapy in Established Ischemic Stroke 852

Acknowledgments **855**

References **856**

Off-Label Indications for Hyperbaric Oxygen Therapy

Michael H. Bennett, Simon J. Mitchell

INTRODUCTION

There are literally hundreds of medical conditions that have been advocated as appropriate for routine treatment with a course of hyperbaric oxygen (HBO_2) therapy. The great majority of these are not endorsed for use by expert medical groups in North America, Europe, or Australia because there is either no reliable evidence to suggest HBO_2 therapy is efficacious or no plausible mechanism of action (or both). Many of these indications are routinely treated at pressures of 1.2 to 1.3 atmospheres absolute (ATA – 122 to 132 kPa) at inspired oxygen proportions well below 100% – often referred to as "mild hyperbaric therapy." Facilities delivering such treatments often operate under the supervision of practitioners unburdened by medical qualifications. The use of such minimal therapy is outside the scope of this chapter, but for any interested readers, an evidence summary was published in 2010.[55] In short, the authors were "not aware of any reliable clinical evidence for therapeutic benefit from mild hyperbaric therapy"[55] and did not recommend the use of this modality for any medical purpose.

This chapter will be confined to a discussion of the meaning of the term "off-label" in the context of HBO_2 therapy – defined for this chapter as the administration of 100% oxygen at pressures of 1.5 ATA (152 kPa) and above. Alternative terms in common use include "unestablished indications," "off-list indications," and "unapproved indications," and we make no distinction between these alternatives. We will propose a subclassification within this broad group of conditions to assist identification of those indications that are worthy of further research. We will then examine 2 specific diagnoses that have received considerable attention over the last 10 years, to illustrate the situation facing the field of hyperbaric medicine in attempting to establish a new indication as broadly accepted by practitioners and health funders.

WHAT IS AN OFF-LABEL INDICATION?

Off-label indications are conditions in which the systematic clinical use of HBO_2 therapy is not supported by adequate proof of benefit.[8] There is a degree of subjectivity in this determination. A body of physicians such as the Undersea and Hyperbaric Medical Society (UHMS) may accept an indication after review of the evidence, often on the existence of credible efficacy and published experience, while the same indication may nevertheless be rejected by a body responsible for funding that treatment, often on the grounds of absent cost-benefit data. It is not the intention of this chapter to explore the reasons for these differences of opinion, and we confine our discussion to conditions not accepted by either type of "labeling" authority.

The great majority of hyperbaric practitioners will be aware of the list of accepted "on-label" indications published by their relevant local craft group. While they will also be aware of a (typically) much shorter list of indications published by the relevant funding authority, this chapter will consider any indication sanctioned by a medical craft group in the Western medical tradition as a legitimate use of HBO_2 therapy. The following discussion will not consider the arguments made by funding bodies that our accepted uses cannot all be supported by clearly established cost-effectiveness data and are therefore "off label" by their own definition. That is an argument for another time and place.

It is argued by some that there is no good reason why we should worry about individuals who promote off-label use of HBO_2 therapy. After all, most legitimate medical practitioners are content to follow the accepted list of indications when defining routine treatment options. In contrast, many off-label users are mavericks, operating in a very distinct way often criticized by their peers – or indeed they are not medically qualified at all – so there should be no confusion with "real" hyperbaric practitioners. We argue, however, that the systematic use of HBO_2 therapy in off-label indications raises ethical concerns about providing misleading information, giving false hope, and taking payment for therapy of doubtful benefit. Any practice perceived as unethical or unscientific has the potential to draw the wider field into disrepute and should be resisted vigorously by legitimate practitioners.

Why is HBO_2 Therapy Vulnerable to Use in Off-Label Indications?

There is a variety of reasons why HBO_2 therapy is frequently advocated in treatment of off-label indications. First, HBO_2 therapy is a physical treatment that strongly lends itself to a placebo or participation effect that may create an impression of efficacy. Treatment involves frequent visits to a dramatic and technical therapeutic environment, where the patient encounters committed and supportive staff as well as a group of fellow patients, all hopeful of success. The delivery of the treatment consists of exposure to an unusual environment that clearly involves some (managed) risk and promotes further collegiality. This has been referred to as "the ritual of hyperbaric oxygen" and is likely to promote a beneficial participation effect.[10,30] This is particularly so for problems where outcomes are subjective or amenable to psychological manipulation or where the results of confirmatory investigations can be easily misinterpreted. Under these circumstances, it is not surprising that well-meaning practitioners may earnestly believe they are achieving good results for their patients through the application of HBO_2. Perhaps not surprisingly, there is a substantial body of emerging evidence that a placebo effect might be responsible for apparent improvement in many off-label indications, and we will return to this issue later in consideration of chronic brain injuries.

Second, the status of oxygen as a drug and the regulations around who may administer it, are uncertain or ambiguous in many countries. It is not uncommon to find so-called "hyperbaric medicine units" owned by members of nonmedical craft groups (like former commercial divers) who see nothing wrong with applying their recompression chamber operational experience to the medical field. Such people may enter relationships of convenience with local doctors for the purposes of billing, but the doctors sometimes know even less about hyperbaric medicine than the chamber operators. Not surprisingly, these scenarios often result in particularly bizarre claims of efficacy. A short visit to the Internet will quickly verify this assertion.

Third, oxygen is easily marketed to the general public as being essential for life. In this paradigm, HBO_2 therapy is portrayed simplistically as "natural," with the underlying assumption that more of a good thing must be better. The mainstream public are vulnerable to such claims, and levels of knowledge about these matters are poor. It takes little effort on the Internet to find apparently qualified scientists prepared to make bizarre claims about oxygen, such as two authors quoted in a recent newspaper article asserting that highly populated and polluted urban locations experience very low levels of oxygen, 15% and possibly even lower at times.[60]

Finally, desperate patients with chronic or progressive problems are frequently willing to "try anything," and it is not difficult to convince such patients to try HBO_2 therapy. This gives rise to several of the ethical concerns we have about the systematic and remunerated treatment of off-label indications.

Three categories of potential indications for HBO_2 therapy. "Unestablished" here is synonymous with "off-label," but an experimental indication is justifiable under some circumstances.[42]

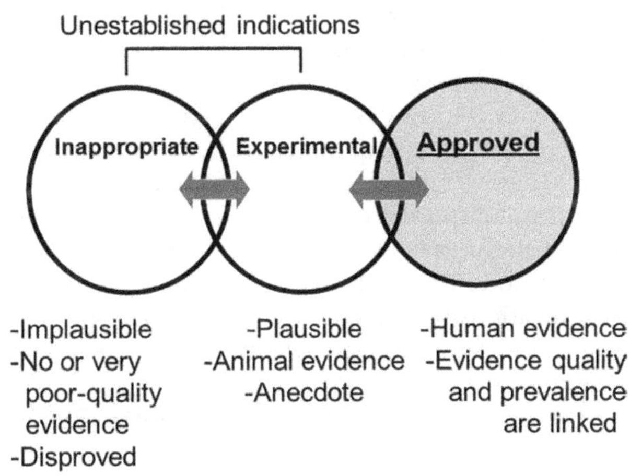

Figure 1. Three categories of potential indications for HBO_2 therapy. "Unestablished" here is synonymous with "off-label," but an experimental indication is justifiable under some circumstances (see text for explanation).[42]

Classification of Indications for HBO_2 Therapy

Figure 1 outlines a simple classification for medical indications for HBO_2 therapy. In this schema, "approved indications" are supported by human evidence of efficacy, subject to clinical expert interpretation. In this regard, it is important to appreciate that the quality of the supporting evidence should reflect the prevalence of the disease in question. Not all approved indications require support by high-quality, large randomized trials. Sporadic, rare, and catastrophic diseases such as necrotizing fasciitis are a good example. Such conditions are difficult to study in randomized trials, and the evidence quality bar may consequently be set lower than would be the case for a prevalent indication like diabetic foot ulcer.

An obvious point of contention in application of this model is who determines whether an appropriate standard of evidence has been met for an indication to be "approved"? The UHMS, an independent and responsible scientific society, has approached the problem by convening a standing committee of experts who periodically review the available evidence and make determinations on the status of new or existing approved indications.[64] This process does not eliminate potential for contentious decisions, but it seems a pragmatic solution to a difficult problem. The double-ended arrows in Figure 1 are intended to indicate that this process of regular review ensures no indication is immutably categorized in the face of emerging evidence. Thus, for example, an "experimental" indication can become "approved" if sufficient evidence emerges to justify this, just as an "approved" indication can move to "inappropriate" in the face of emerging high-quality evidence to suggest HBO_2 therapy is not effective.

We have elsewhere suggested the term "off-label" can be usefully broken down into two distinct subgroups.[42] "Experimental indications" are typically those in which there is a plausible biological rationale for application of HBO_2 therapy and perhaps some supportive animal evidence or human anecdote. However, there is insufficient human evidence to achieve approval. "Inappropriate indications" are typically those with little face validity or biological rationale and little or no supporting evidence. This categorization would also be applied to well-researched indications which may have once seemed plausible but in which the overwhelming weight of available evidence is unsupportive. Some illustrative examples will follow.

As indicated in Figure 1, the "experimental" and "inappropriate" indications collectively constitute what we refer to as "unestablished indications" or "off-label." Such indications may, of course, continue to be studied if it is deemed justified. However, we strongly believe that HBO_2 therapy should not be represented as a proven treatment in these conditions. Medical practitioners should not systematically treat unestablished indications with HBO_2 therapy outside the context of research nor should they (in our opinion) receive payment for such treatment.

What Are the Problems with Treatment of Off-Label Indications for HBO_2 Therapy?

There are two major concerns with the treatment of off-label indications using HBO_2 therapy. The first relates to the ethics of unintentional (or intentional) exploitation of vulnerable patients that we alluded to above. Given the (at best) uncertain benefit from HBO_2 therapy in treatment of such indications, any insinuation of benefit is potentially misleading. Similarly, the acceptance of payment for unproven therapy when the patient has unrealistic or unfounded expectations is widely regarded as unethical. For example, in a standards document, the College of Physicians and Surgeons of Saskatchewan explains that allowing a patient to be administered a treatment not proven to be beneficial over proven care techniques can have dangerous consequences; the patient could be blinded by false hope and his or her condition severely worsen or perhaps become irreversible.[61] The ethics of exposing patients to a therapy with risks when the benefit is unknown or even unlikely are highly questionable.

The second concern relates to the perception the treatment of off-label indications creates among our mainstream medical colleagues. The use of HBO_2 therapy in indications where there is little biological rationale, let alone convincing human evidence, creates the very real risk that hyperbaric physicians will be seen as "alternative medicine" practitioners (or worse). Experienced hyperbaric physicians will remember the 1987 Gabb and Robin article in Chest which labelled HBO_2 therapy a therapy in search of diseases.[21] In support of their thesis, these authors cited a typical long list of indications claimed by enthusiastic advocates and predictably proclaimed that the broad range of conditions speaks for itself.[21]

In 2013, the Food and Drug Administration (FDA) became concerned enough about claims relating to HBO_2 therapy in unestablished indications that it saw fit to issue a communication entitled "Hyperbaric Oxygen Therapy: Don't Be Misled."[20] Although the communication was targeted against claims of efficacy in treating off-label indications like autism, AIDS, cancer, stroke, and depression rather than the approved indications, many readers will have neither grasped the distinction nor advanced beyond the pejorative title.

Over many years, advocates for HBO_2 therapy in off-label indications have attracted ridicule in prominent journals like *JAMA* and *Chest* and provoked admonishment from the FDA. This sort of negative attention from the mainstream medical community is damaging. Few hyperbaric physicians will not have struggled at some time to promote HBO_2 therapy to surgical or medical colleagues, usually based on the latter harboring suspicions of the field as "alternative" or lacking in evidence. Conspicuous promotion of HBO_2 therapy for treatment of off-label indications reinforces such prejudices and almost certainly makes it less likely that patients who would benefit from treatment of approved indications will be referred.

OFF-LABEL INDICATIONS OF CONTEMPORARY INTEREST

While there are many potential indications for inclusion in this chapter, we will confine the discussion to two indications as an illustration of the different types of off-label indication commonly encountered in both the literature and the hyperbaric consulting room. In recent years, the use of HBO_2 therapy for the treatment of various forms of chronic neurological injury has been at the forefront of debate over off-label use of HBO_2 therapy. The evolution of the debate and the related research it has stimulated illuminates many of the issues discussed above, and we provide a summary of it here. These reviews are, of necessity, brief and relatively superficial. Readers are encouraged to appraise the various references themselves and judge their relative merits.

Chronic brain injury states are common areas where HBO_2 therapy has been proposed as a useful therapy. Whether the result of trauma, developmental abnormalities, or immune-related degenerative processes, these conditions have some important characteristics in common. They are in general quite common in the community, are either static or slowly progressive in nature, and have no clearly accepted curative therapy. Most are managed by agents or techniques designed for symptom control or, at best, the slowing of any progressive deterioration. Many are ailments of children or young adults, and for some there are no definitive diagnostic tests available. Importantly, most evaluations of therapeutic effectiveness are based upon symptom relief. Together, these characteristics describe a group of conditions where vulnerable individuals and their caregivers are searching for therapeutic approaches that offer more than the currently available approaches used in "mainstream" medicine.

The "HBO_2 therapy in chronic brain injury debate" first came to prominence in the 1980s in relation to multiple sclerosis (MS) in young adults and later, cerebral palsy (CP) in children. Both are largely historical arguments now, but some practitioners remain active proponents for each.[25,45] Interested readers are referred to published reviews of the evidence.[6-7] The pattern has become familiar. Enthusiastic proponents develop an untested and often novel view of the pathophysiology that allows for a potential mechanistic basis for HBO_2 therapy. Case reports and case series follow that suggest improved outcomes. Convincing animal models are generally unavailable, and so animal evidence is not sought. Unblinded, often historically controlled, comparative studies confirm the potential benefits, and often an early randomized controlled trial (RCT) will similarly support the hypothesis. As other clinicians and researchers become interested, they undertake rigorously designed RCTs that fail to confirm the initial therapeutic effect. Over time, the evidence stacks up against therapeutic benefit, and the practice contracts back to a small number of enthusiasts who remain convinced. The indication slips from "experimental" to "inappropriate" in our schema (Figure 1). Sometimes patient advocates and/or nonmedical practitioners continue to offer treatment as a charity or profit-making venture respectively. To date, no chronic neurological indication has progressed in the opposite direction to become a widely accepted and appropriate routine indication – but this is entirely possible in the future.

In this chapter, we will discuss the treatment of chronic sequelae of mild traumatic brain injury with post-concussion syndromes and ischemic stroke.

CHRONIC HEAD INJURY AND POST-CONCUSSION SYNDROMES

The use of HBO_2 therapy in chronic mild traumatic brain injury (mTBI) has received much attention in the United States, where large numbers of affected servicemen and -women have returned from overseas conflicts. In 2012, Harch and colleagues published a series of 16 returned servicemen with chronic blast-induced mild to moderate traumatic brain injury (TBI)/post-concussion syndrome (PCS) and posttraumatic stress disorder (PTSD) who all received 40 HBO_2 therapy treatments at 1.5 ATA.[23] These patients exhibited improvements in various neurocognitive tests and improvements in regional cerebral blood flow measured by SPECT scan. A second observational study in 63 mTBI patients similarly reported a common subjective perception of benefit but no clinically important changes on more objective neurocognitive testing.[13] A small subset of these patient had SPECT and CT angiographic studies which, as in the Harch series, demonstrated an apparent improvement of regional cerebral blood flow after HBO_2 therapy. The clinical significance of these changes remains a controversial subject.

Several studies under the aegis of the U.S. military were subsequently undertaken in response to strong lobbying for systematic use of HBO_2 therapy in veterans with mTBI. While it is beyond the scope of this paper to describe these studies in detail, some trial characteristics are germane. The methodologies are summarized in an article by Weaver et al.,[69] in great detail in a special issue of *Undersea and Hyperbaric Medicine*,[44] and in the individual papers themselves.[14-15,40,67,71] All three were randomized, double-blinded, sham-controlled trials but with variation between studies in both treatment and sham protocols (Table 1).

The outcome measures in all studies included symptom inventories and neuropsychological testing. Results are reported at one month for the army study; at one and six weeks for the air force study, and immediate post-treatment, one week, and three months for the navy study. The results for all three studies were presented at the Undersea and Hyperbaric Medical Society annual meeting in

2013 and have now been published in full. None of the studies demonstrated any benefit for HBO_2 therapy when compared to the sham protocol. In the army and air force studies, both sham and HBO_2 therapy groups improved more than expected, but there was no difference between the groups. The navy study similarly suggested no difference between groups but failed to confirm the same improvement in either arm. The various authors all considered a placebo effect most likely to account for parallel improvements in both sham (control) and HBO_2 therapy patients.

TABLE 1. KEY CHARACTERISTICS AND OUTCOMES OF THE U.S. MILITARY STUDIES OF HBO_2 THERAPY FOR MILD TRAUMATIC BRAIN INJURY (MTBI).

Note the navy study was designed to factor out any effect of elevated inspired pO_2 in the control group; 1 ATA = 101.3 kPa.
***Rivermead Postconcussion Symptoms Questionnaire**
†Posttraumatic Disorder Check List – Military Version

SERVICE	SUBJECTS	SESSIONS	CONTROL	HBOT	OUTCOMES (NOT AN EXHAUSTIVE LIST)
Army[40]	72	40	Air, 1.2 ATA	100% O_2 1.5 ATA	Mean change in RPQ* 5.4 in HBO_2 and 7.0 with sham P = 0.70
Air Force[71]	50	30	Air, 1.3 ATA	100% O_2 2.4 ATA	PCL-M† between groups P = 0.84
Navy[14,67,15]	60	40	10.5% O_2 2.0 ATA	100% O_2 2.0 ATA 75% O_2 2.0 ATA	Mean change RPQ* and PCL-M† No significant differences after treatment and at 3 months

These outcomes have disappointed enthusiasts.[24] In summary, the proponents of HBO_2 therapy propose an alternative interpretation of these results through postulating a mechanism of action for exposures to air at low pressures. In short, they argue that 1.3 ATA of air is therapeutic in this group and indeed is equally therapeutic as HBO_2 therapy using the outcome measurements used. It is notable the negative results in the military studies contrast sharply with those reported from an Israeli study of HBO_2 therapy (versus standard care) that used an open-label, randomized design with no blinded sham hyperbaric exposures.[11] That study suggested a benefit in the short term when patients randomized to receive HBO_2 therapy were compared to those randomized not to receive it. In this trial, the control group continued their standard treatment regimen and then received delayed HBO_2 therapy after six months (when they too showed similar improvements). Perhaps unsurprisingly, the authors have devoted considerable effort to explaining the different results in comparison to those of the U.S. military mTBI studies.[14-15,40,67,71] They focus particularly on the contention that the U.S. military sham exposures were effective treatments and that this accounted for the equivalent results when sham and HBO_2 therapy groups were compared.

The argument that a low-pressure air sham exposure is an effective treatment (and, therefore, an inappropriate control) is poorly supported. No one has objectively demonstrated that exposure to 1.3 ATA of air is either neuroprotective or capable of resurrecting chronically "idling" neurons in an injured brain. Moreover, there is no body of basic science evidence suggesting that small elevations in inspired pressures of oxygen and nitrogen (or small elevations of pressure itself) would be expected to exert a relevant therapeutic effect. Explanations of the mechanisms underpinning the alleged efficacy of low-pressure air are rarely more sophisticated than the observation that there is a very modest elevation of the arterial pO_2 when breathing air at 1.3 ATA and that this has effects on completely different (usually pulmonary) pathologies in unrelated settings.(11,19) We have seen no cogent arguments to explain why this, of itself, would improve a chronic brain injury. The well-described effects of HBO_2 exposure at pressures above 2.0 ATA, such as stem cell mobilization and effects on nitric oxide synthase, are often cited in the context of these debates, but to our knowledge such effects have never been demonstrated at these minimally elevated oxygen tensions.

One significant problem in relation to the "active air sham" argument is that the same pO_2 achieved breathing air at 1.3 ATA can equally be achieved by breathing 27% oxygen at 1 ATA – without the risks and costs of hyperbaric exposure. This begs an obvious question. If the proponents of 1.3 ATA air treatments truly believe this is an effective regimen because of an oxygen-mediated therapeutic effect, why do they not simply treat their patients with 27% oxygen breathing at 1 ATA – or at least test this intervention, something they have all avoided doing to this point? A cynic might suggest this has much to do with the respective billing potential of the two modalities, but the response from advocates is that the putative neurorehabilitative effect of air at 1.3 ATA depends not only on the elevated arterial pO_2 but also on the small elevation of ambient pressure.(24) To our knowledge, this argument is unsupported by any data demonstrating neuroprotective or neurorehabilitative benefit from exposure to pressure alone, and the notion lacks biological plausibility. Advocates attempt to address this concern by quoting the transduction of small pressure changes by certain cells in marine invertebrates(39) and by citing pressure effects on mammalian neurons(17) revealed in studies whose outcome measures had nothing to do with neurorehabilitation and whose methods involved exposure to far greater pressures than 1.3 ATA.

This seems to be poor science, yet it is tenaciously promoted because the notion that pressure is a key contributor to the apparent benefit accrued from air at 1.3 ATA is crucial to two arguments advanced by those promoting HBO_2 therapy for mTBI. The first, introduced above, is that even if air at 1.3 ATA is as effective as higher doses of HBO_2 therapy, the hyperbaric approach cannot be replaced by breathing the equivalent pO_2 (27% O_2) at room pressure because the patient would not receive the alleged benefit of pressure. The second is that the assumed benefit of pressure alone allows a circular argument which conveniently invalidates the randomized sham-controlled trials that show no benefit from HBO_2 therapy in chronic brain injury, including those designed to exclude any elevation of inspired pO_2 in the sham group.(14) Essentially, this argument holds that while proper blinding of controls cannot be achieved without some pressure exposure, any pressure increase means the controls are receiving an active treatment rather than an inactive sham. If one were to accept this argument, it would make sham-controlled trials virtually impossible to conduct – thus justifying the inferior nonblinded crossover designs employed in recent studies of stroke and mild TBI as "the best we can do."(11,19)

Based on present evidence, we reject the argument that pressure per se is an active treatment in mTBI. We acknowledge the small increase in inspired

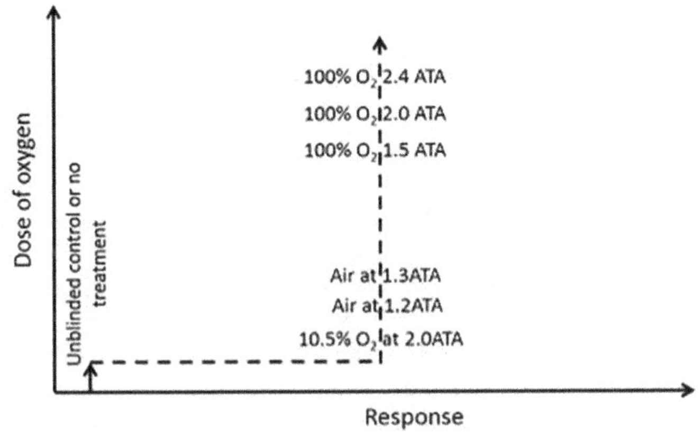

Figure 2. A dose-response curve for oxygen in the treatment of mTBI. There is little or no response for an unblinded control or no-treatment arm in these studies. All other doses of oxygen produce very similar levels of response. There is no sign of a conventional dose-response relationship, suggesting a participation effect is more likely. The same holds for nitrogen dose and pressure. (ATA = atmospheres absolute)

pO_2 to 0.27 ATA that occurs when air is breathed at 1.3 ATA, but we consider there is no convincing evidence for a neurorehabilitative effect of this dose of oxygen. We note that, without exception, every randomized sham-controlled (blinded) study of HBO_2 therapy in chronic brain injury to date has demonstrated equivalent improvement in patients receiving both HBO_2 therapy and a sham exposure. Importantly, these include two studies designed to exclude any elevation of pO_2 in the sham groups.[14,36] This makes for a most unlikely dose-response curve (Figure 2). The corollary is that, unless one believes small increases in ambient pressure or the inspired pN_2 alone can restore function to the chronically injured human brain (notions that are currently unsupported by evidence), the appropriate interpretation of the sham-controlled study results is that there is no true therapeutic effect of HBO_2 therapy in chronic brain injury. We do not accept the assertion that these studies prove that the shams are not inert.

Using the principle of Occam's razor, we believe the most plausible explanation for the results of sham-controlled studies in chronic brain injury is a substantial placebo or participation effect. Given the demonstrated efficacy of cognitive rehabilitation therapy in TBI,[35] it seems very plausible that at least some sequelae of chronic brain injury may improve when highly motivated patients are given a dramatic, prolonged course of treatment in a stimulating, positive, and optimistic clinical environment. It follows that we are not surprised by a 2014 nonblinded, nonrandomized study in cerebral palsy comparing patients treated with conventional methods, air at 1.3 ATA, HBO_2 therapy at 1.5 ATA, and HBO_2 therapy at 1.75 ATA, which found that all "hyperbaric" groups (including air at 1.3 ATA) improved more than conventionally treated controls.[43] It is extraordinary that a peer-reviewed journal allowed this conclusion to be published because it is patently unjustifiable. Indeed, we believe that studies investigating HBO_2 therapy in chronic brain injury that do not include a sham control group are deeply flawed.

Before concluding this discussion, it is appropriate to mention SPECT scan detection of positive changes in regional cerebral blood flow (rCBF) following HBO_2 therapy for mTBI.[11,13,23] These changes are sometimes cited as proof of an HBO_2

therapy effect that cannot be due to placebo. In fact, rCBF as measured by SPECT may be influenced by cognitive therapy for mTBI, and a placebo effect on SPECT results would therefore not be surprising.[35] Indeed, SPECT changes in response to placebo have been demonstrated,[33,47] with one analgesic study concluding that changes in CBF were more linked to the idea of pain or pain relief than to the treatment given.[47] The literature contains many references to placebo-induced changes in rCBF measured by other functional brain imaging techniques, and these are arguably relevant to SPECT. For example, functional magnetic resonance imaging has demonstrated that placebo analgesia causes decreased brain activity in the corresponding brain regions.[66] We acknowledge these findings are related to pain studies rather than brain injury and may therefore prove to be irrelevant at some future date. Equally however, changes in SPECT scans following HBO_2 therapy for mTBI do not constitute a convincing argument against placebo effects.

In the broader context of off label indications, the object lesson arising from the chronic brain injury saga is that there are some prevalent conditions in which HBO_2 therapy may appear to work when observational evidence is considered in isolation. Different conclusions are drawn if sham-controlled studies are undertaken. Uncritical interpretations of observational data or data from trials without blinded sham controls could result in massive expenditure on an expensive, time-consuming "therapy" that may, in fact, only work through a placebo effect. This should be of concern to all hyperbaric physicians who base their practice on evidence and who are striving to build collaborations with skeptical mainstream colleagues.

Conclusion: The treatment of mild TBI/PTSD/post-concussion syndromes has been the subject of several methodologically sound RCTs. While there is an ongoing controversy around what constitutes a true sham treatment in this context, these conditions seem to be moving from the "experimental" to "inappropriate" category of off-label indications.

ISCHEMIC STROKE – ACUTE INTERVENTION AND AS AN ADJUNCT TO REHABILITATION

Stroke may be defined as a sudden neurological deficit that is of presumed vascular origin.[5] It is both a leading cause of mortality worldwide, accounting for an estimated 5.4 million deaths in 2001 (9.6% of all deaths), and a leading cause of disability, accounting for 6% of all disability-adjusted life years in developed countries.[5] About ⅓ of survivors require significant assistance in daily life at one year after an event.[4-5]

Stroke is divided into two broad subgroups: ischemic and hemorrhagic, with the former accounting for 73% to 86% of all cases.[5] On average, ischemic stroke has a lower case fatality rate than hemorrhagic stroke (23% versus 62% at one year). Accepted treatment for ischemic stroke includes anticoagulation, thrombolysis, and endovascular clot retrieval (ECR), while in hemorrhagic stroke such measures are likely to promote further bleeding.[5,58] Therefore, an early and accurate diagnosis is desirable. Because clinical assessment is unreliable in determining the stroke type, neuroimaging (preferably using computerized tomography [CT] scan) is required for optimal management.[68]

During a cerebral ischemic event, neurological tissue suffers hypoxia. When hypoxia is prolonged, neurons lose their ability to maintain ionic homeostasis. Free-oxygen radicals accumulate and degrade the cell membranes,[31,54] leading to irreversible changes resulting in unavoidable cell death. These changes may occur rapidly and before therapy can be instituted, but in some patients the symptoms worsen gradually or in a stepwise fashion over a matter of hours or days.(50) This latter observation suggests that the close management of hemodynamic, respiratory, and metabolic factors designed to maintain oxygenation might be beneficial.

Therapy

Intensive stroke management protocols, thrombolysis, and antiplatelet therapy have been shown to positively influence the outcome following acute events.(12,57,62) Within these protocols, accepted adjunctive measures designed to assist recovery from acute stroke include nutritional supplementation using enteral nutrition via nasogastric tube,(49) tight control of blood glucose,(3) and measures to control arterial blood pressure.(1) The most important therapeutic decisions are whether to administer thrombolysis and/or ECR, and these decisions are based on timing and exclusion of hemorrhagic stroke by brain imaging techniques.

Hyperbaric oxygen therapy (HBO_2 therapy) has been proposed for the adjunctive treatment of ischemic stroke since the 1960s.(26,32) The potential benefits of HBO_2 therapy include the reversal of hypoxia through increased oxygen delivery and the reduction of cerebral edema.(29,59) There are also several specific and potentially beneficial effects of hyperoxia that include decreased lipid peroxidation, inhibition of leukocyte activation, and restoration of the functional blood-brain barrier.(41,63) It has been proposed that HBO_2 therapy protects marginally viable brain (often termed "the ischemic penumbra") from further damage on reperfusion through these mechanisms that act to regulate abnormal cellular metabolites.(2,52) Conversely, oxygen in high doses may increase oxidative stress through the production of oxygen free-radical species and is potentially toxic.(72) Indeed, the brain is particularly at risk.(16) Further, HBO_2 therapy has effects on cerebral blood flow (CBF) that may promote further neuronal damage, including both reductions in CBF secondary to hyperoxic vasospasm and through an inverse steal phenomenon.(48) For these reasons, it is appropriate to postulate that in some stroke patients, HBO_2 therapy may do more harm than good.

Evidence

Most animal studies support the use of HBO_2 therapy, and these have been thoroughly examined by Helms et al. in 2005.(27) The models employed involve the permanent or temporary occlusion of cerebral arteries using ties or intravascular filaments, while the time to institution of HBO_2 therapy in these animals varies from a few minutes to 24 hours. In general, outcomes are improved with HBO_2 therapy in both ischemia/reperfusion models and permanent occlusion models, with infarct size reductions being the most common outcome estimated. While there was a greater variability in results following permanent occlusion, the beneficial effect of HBO_2 therapy following temporary occlusions seemed to hold for delays to treatment of up to several hours in most of these studies. Nevertheless, there was some evidence of reduced benefit with increasing delays to treatment in Weinstein 1987 and Lou 2004(38,70) and (disturbingly) worse outcomes with HBO_2 therapy at 12 hours delay.(38)

Despite this generally encouraging animal evidence and 40 years of interest in the delivery of HBO_2 therapy in stroke patients, little comparative evidence of effectiveness existed before the 1990s. Most reports were of single or multiple cases, with the largest study being a series of 122 cases reported in 1980.(46) A review of these studies calculated that more than half of the patients improved clinically or electrophysiologically with HBO_2 therapy and concluded there was a case for setting up controlled studies.[48] Since 1991, there have been 11 such randomized controlled clinical trials reported in the literature, and these were recently included in a Cochrane Review.[9]

The Cochrane Review

The review included 11 randomized trials enrolling patients with confirmed acute ischemic stroke and using hyperbaric oxygen as an adjunct to standard care. They reported outcomes involving 705 patients, although not all trials contributed to the quantitative meta-analysis.

There was considerable clinical heterogeneity between the included trials, making pooling of data difficult to justify for many outcomes. These trials varied considerably in the time delay from the onset of stroke to the initiation of hyperbaric therapy. Three trials enrolled patients within 24 hours of stroke onset (Sansone 1997, Rusyniak 2003, and Nighoghossian 1995), while Anderson 1991 accepted patients up to two weeks later. Table 2 outlines the trials included in the analysis of major outcomes, the time delay to treatment for each, and the primary outcome measured. There were also wide variations in the dose of HBO_2 therapy used. Rusyniak 2003 delivered a single therapy session at 2.5 ATA for sixty minutes, while both Nighoghossian and Anderson gave multiple treatments at 1.5 ATA.

All trials were small and had low power to detect useful clinical differences between groups. The extent and severity of deficit on enrollment was poorly described and difficult to compare across trials given that most used different neurological and health status scales to establish baseline status.

Four trials did however report death at between three and six months (Figure 3). At that time, there were no significant differences in mortality (six deaths [8.2%] in those receiving HBO_2 therapy versus six [8.5%] with sham therapy), and the relative risk (RR) of dying after receiving HBO_2 therapy was 0.97 (95% CI 0.34 to 2.75). There was no indication of significant statistical heterogeneity between trials (I^2 = 0%), and this analysis suggests HBO_2 therapy has no influence on mortality in this setting. There was some indication of an advantage when the HBO_2 therapy was administered within 24 hours compared to two weeks, but there is no statistical confirmation that such an effect is real.

Many of the three trials employed functional scales scores, and a summary of these outcomes at final follow-up is shown in Table 3. Anderson 1991 also reported that mean infarct volume was smaller in the control group at 4 months (29.0 cm^3 versus 49.2 cm^3) but not significantly so (MD 20.2 cm^3, 95% CI –13.4 to 53.8, p-value 0.24).

Claustrophobia was a significant problem in the monoplace vessels used in all trials for both arms. In the intensive therapy protocol used by Anderson, for example, 39% of participants could not complete scheduled therapy.

TABLE 2. CHARACTERISTICS OF THE INCLUDED STUDIES OF HBO_2 THERAPY FOR ACUTE ISCHEMIC STROKE

STUDY	METHODS	PARTICIPANTS	INTERVENTIONS	OUTCOMES
Anderson 1991	RCT stratified for disease severity and blinded	39 adults with ischemic stroke within two weeks in internal carotid territory.	100% O_2 versus a sham of air, both at 1.5 ATA. 15 treatments over five days.	Neurological examination to one year. Infarct volume at four months.
Nighoghossian 1995	RCT blinded	34 adults with stroke within 24 hours MCA territory.	HBO_2 at 1.5 ATA 40 mins daily for 10 days. Sham at 1.2 ATA.	Three scales of neuro status and disability to one year.
Sansone 1997	RCT abstract only Blinded	17 adults stroke within 24 hours MCA territory	HBO_2 at 1.5 to 1.8 ATA for 60 mins daily for 8–10 days. Unpressurized sham.	Neuro recovery score to one year.
Li 1998	RCT unblinded	86 adults cerebral infarction. Timing not stated.	HBO_2 at 2 ATA for 120 mins daily for 10 days.	No clinical outcomes.
Rusyniak 2003	RCT stratified by time and blinded	33 adults within 24 hours. (0–12/12–24 hours)	HBO_2 at 2.5 ATA for 60 mins once. Sham at 1.14 ATA on air.	Four scales of neuro status and outcome score to 90 days.
Peng 2003	RCT not blinded	60 adults within 1 week of stroke.	HBO_2 at 2.3 ATA for 80 minutes daily for 10 days. No sham.	Chinese clinical neuro score after treatment.
Yang 2003	RCT not blinded	80 adults with CT evidence within 72 hours.	HBO_2 at 2.0 ATA for 80 mins daily for 10 days. No sham.	Neuro recovery scale.
Yang 2004	RCT not blinded	120 adults with CT evidence within 72 hours.	HBO_2 at 2.0 ATA for 60 mins daily for 10 days. No sham.	Neuro deficit and two scales after treatment.
Imai 2006	RCT not blinded	38 adults within 48 hours of stroke in MCA territory.	HBO_2 at 2.0 ATA for 60 minutes daily for 7 days. No sham.	Recovery score and NIHSS.
Hong 2008	RCT not blinded Abstract only	86 adults. No information in timing.	No information on HBO_2 sessions. No sham.	Neuro deficit score.
Zhao 2008	RCT not blinded	112 adults. No information on timing.	HBO_2 unspecified daily for 10 days. No sham.	No clinical outcomes.

Study or Subgroup	HBOT Events	HBOT Total	Control Events	Control Total	Weight	Risk Ratio M-H, Fixed, 95% CI
1.1.1 HBO alone						
Anderson 1991	2	20	2	19	31.0%	0.95 [0.15, 6.08]
Nighoghossian 1995	0	17	1	17	22.7%	0.33 [0.01, 7.65]
Rusyniak 2003	1	17	2	16	31.2%	0.47 [0.05, 4.70]
Subtotal (95% CI)		**54**		**52**	**84.9%**	**0.61 [0.17, 2.20]**
Total events	3		5			
Heterogeneity: Chi² = 0.41, df = 2 (P = 0.81); I² = 0%						
Test for overall effect: Z = 0.76 (P = 0.45)						
1.1.2 HBO and edaravone						
Imai 2006	3	19	1	19	15.1%	3.00 [0.34, 26.33]
Subtotal (95% CI)		**19**		**19**	**15.1%**	**3.00 [0.34, 26.33]**
Total events	3		1			
Heterogeneity: Not applicable						
Test for overall effect: Z = 0.99 (P = 0.32)						
Total (95% CI)		**73**		**71**	**100.0%**	**0.97 [0.34, 2.75]**
Total events	6		6			
Heterogeneity: Chi² = 1.86, df = 3 (P = 0.60); I² = 0%						
Test for overall effect: Z = 0.06 (P = 0.96)						
Test for subgroup differences: Chi² = 1.53, df = 1 (P = 0.22), I² = 34.7%						

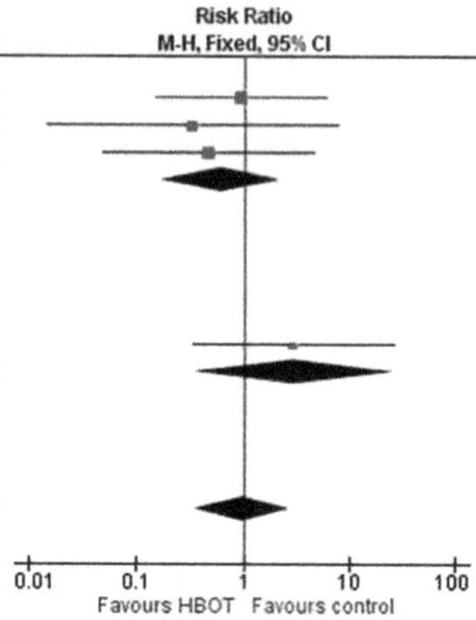

Figure 3. Forest plot for mortality data from randomized trials.[9]

Summary of Data

The ischemic nature of the stroke event, plus the animal evidence when treatment follows soon after the insult, suggests a rational case can be made for the use of HBO_2 therapy for stroke. The animal and uncontrolled human data suggest early treatment is more likely to produce benefit and that late treatment (around 24 hours and beyond) may be ineffective or even deleterious. There is, however, no convincing evidence from randomized controlled trials that HBO_2 therapy improves outcome. Pooled data do not suggest any significant benefit in mortality in the six months following presentation. While there was some indication from one trial (Nighoghossian 1995) for improvement in one disability scale (Trouillas) and one clinical descriptive scale (Orgogozo), these improvements were not reflected in other trials or functional scales and were present at one year but not six months after therapy was completed. There does not appear to be a plausible explanation for this apparent late effect. Further, the analysis of these ordinal scales to produce mean scores for group comparisons may not be appropriate.[65] One review concluded that of nine stroke scales tested, the NIHSS was one of the three most reliable, while the Barthel Index was the most reliable disability scale.[18]

Conclusion: There are few good clinical data on which to base treatment recommendations. Despite a good biological basis and supportive animal research, the routine use of HBO_2 therapy in acute stroke patients cannot be justified from the results of randomized trials at this time. On the other hand, given the small number of participants in the trials included, we cannot be certain that a benefit from HBO_2 therapy has been excluded. This indication may best be classified as "experimental." Future trials will need to be carefully planned to provide information on the effect of disease severity, the appropriate oxygen dose, and the timing of therapy. The use of HBO_2 therapy is now complicated by the increasing availability of emergency clot retrieval services, and any effectiveness for HBO_2 therapy in relation to clot retrieval has not been evaluated.

HBO_2 Therapy in Established Ischemic Stroke

The treatment of ischemic stroke in the acute phase has understandably received a great deal of attention over the last 50 years. More recently, a series of RCTs has established ECR as a life- and function-preserving technique in the acute phase.[22,34,56]

TABLE 3. SUMMARY OF FUNCTIONAL AND ADL SCALES USED AS OUTCOMES IN THESE TRIALS. SIGNIFICANT DIFFERENCES ARE IN BOLD.

*Score designed specifically for Anderson 2001.
#Either National Institute of Health Stroke Scale < 2, Rankin Score < 2, or Glasgow Outcome Score of 5.

FUNCTIONAL SCALE	TRIALS	CONTROL	HBO_2 THERAPY	DIFFERENCE (95% CI) P VALUE
Mean neurological score* [Lower scores = better outcome]	Anderson 1991 One year	25.8	31.4	5.6 (-15.1 to 26.2) P = 0.59
Mean Orgogozo Scale [Higher score = better outcome]	Nighoghossian 1995 One year	78.2	50.3	**27.9 (4.0 to 51.8) P = 0.02**
Mean Trouillas Disability Scale [Lower score = better outcome]	Nighoghossian 1995 One year	4.1	6.3	**2.2 (0.15 to 4.3) P = 0.04**
Mean Modified Rankin Functional Assessment Scale [Lower score = better outcome]	Nighoghossian 1995 One year	2.4	3.0	0.6 (-0.18 to 1.4) P = 0.13
Number of participants to achieve a good outcome	Rusyniak 2003 90 days	10	6	RR 1.8 (0.8 to 3.7) P = 0.13
Barthel Index 95 or 100 [Good outcome]	Rusyniak 2003 90 days	9	8	RR 0.8 (0.43 to 1.6) P = 0.6

The principal of sophisticated and intensive treatment packages are now widely accepted.[49,57] Successful as these strategies have been, there remain many patients with significant neurological impairment that require lengthy periods of rehabilitation. It has been suggested that HBO_2 therapy may allow improvements during or after this rehabilitation phase, based on the principle that some brain regions survive but in a functionally deranged or "stunned" state that may be recoverable – even months or years later.[19,53] These regions may be areas of persistent hypoperfusion following the stroke event and potentially responsive to an angiogenic stimulus such as HBO_2. Enthusiasts for this approach suggest that under such conditions, a course of HBO_2 therapy may evoke neuroplasticity in the late phase of stroke recovery. Indeed, Efrati and his colleagues hypothesize that HBO_2 therapy delivered during the acute phase following a stroke may be deleterious and explain the failure of the studies reviewed above to show a beneficial effect of HBO_2 therapy.[19]

While the postulated mechanism of action in late stroke has developed considerably with our increasing understanding of the effects of HBO_2 therapy, the concept that oxygen may be beneficial is not new. The first reports from the 1960s suggested many patients might benefit, although little detail is available on the time to treatment.[28] The first comparative trial was a randomized crossover study of 16 patients between 3 and 108 months after the stroke event. Patients received a single treatment at 2.0 ATA for 90 minutes breathing either 10.5% or 100% oxygen in random order.[51] There was no evidence of improvement in a range of neurological testing after either the HBO_2 or the sham exposure.

More recently, Efrati et al. published a randomized comparative study of HBO_2 therapy versus no treatment in a group of 74 patients with ischemic or hemorrhagic stroke between 6 and 36 months prior to enrollment.[19] All included subjects needed to have at least one motor dysfunction and to have been stable for a minimum of one month. Twelve individuals were excluded after randomization (seven from the "treatment" group and five from the "cross group"), and three further from the cross group did not return for further evaluation after the initial allocated phase and so did not contribute to the results.

In the light of the discussion above concerning the interpretation of the mTBI trials, the design of this study is of great relevance. Following group allocation, the HBO_2 group received 40 sessions at 2.0 ATA breathing 100% oxygen for 90 minutes daily, while the control group spent the same 2-month period with no specific intervention, following which they returned to the trial site for further evaluation before commencing HBO_2 therapy on the same protocol as the HBO_2 therapy group. Thus, at the point of comparison following completion of the first two months from enrollment, the trial was comparing active HBO_2 therapy versus no-treatment groups. The authors maintain there is no appropriate sham therapy available, given that mild exposures such as to air at 1.3 ATA are also active treatments (see discussion under mTBI above).

Efrati reported several statistically significant differences between the pre-HBO_2 therapy and post-HBO_2 therapy evaluations in both groups. The comparisons between the two groups after the initial allocation period are less clearly presented – in general, the results are presented as showing improvements in both groups after HBO_2 therapy, compared to no evidence of improvement between the initial evaluation and reevaluation after two months of no treatment. We do not believe this to be surprising.

There is some controversy about how the results of this trial are best interpreted. On the one hand, the authors suggest this study provides possible evidence that HBO_2 therapy can promote significant neurological improvement in patients that have suffered a stroke.[19] They also point out that the significance of the improvements in this population is noticeable when compared to the lack of improvement during the control (no-treatment) period of the cross group.

The alternate view, one we share, is that the demonstration of a modest treatment effect immediately after the completion of a course of HBO_2 therapy is not a convincing proof of true benefit where there are no sham-controlled data for comparison. Longer-term follow-up data would be very useful, but the main problem, as with mTBI, is the absence of a convincing, validated, and universally accepted sham procedure. This remains one of the great challenges in the immediate future for hyperbaric medical practice.

Conclusion: There are several observational studies supporting the contention that a course of HBO_2 therapy may be of benefit for stroke patients who have plateaued in their recovery from the precipitating event. The biological basis is contestable, and there is no animal data to support or refute the proposition. The only comparative trial was open label and the results prone to bias. This is a poor basis on which to make treatment recommendations. The routine use of HBO_2 therapy in stroke patients after three months cannot be justified from the results of randomized trials at this time. On the other hand, the observational data is generally supportive, and we cannot be certain that a benefit from HBO_2 therapy has been excluded. This indication is best classified as "experimental." Future trials will need to be carefully planned to include a valid sham therapy for comparison.

ACKNOWLEDGMENTS

This chapter contains some material modified from: Mitchell SJ, Bennett MH. Unestablished indications for hyperbaric oxygen therapy. Diving Hyperb Med. 2014 Dec;44 (4):228-34.

REFERENCES

1. Aslanyan S, Fazekas F, Weir CJ, et al. Effect of blood pressure during the acute period of ischemic stroke on stroke outcome: a tertiary analysis of the GAIN International Trial. Stroke. 2003;34:2420-5.
2. Badr AE, Yin W, Mychaskiw G, et al. Effect of hyperbaric oxygen on striatal metabolites: a microdialysis study in awake freely moving rats after MCA occlusion. Brain Res. 2001;916:85-90.
3. Baird TA, Parsons MW, Phan T, et al. Persistent poststroke hyperglycaemia is independently associated with infarct expansion and worse clinical outcome. Stroke. 2003;34:2208-14.
4. Bamford J, Sandercock P, Dennis M, et al. Classification and natural history of clinically identifiable subtypes of cerebral infarction. Lancet. 1991;337:1521-6.
5. Bath PM, Lees KR. ABC of arterial and venous disease. Acute stroke. BMJ. 2000;320:920-3.
6. Bennett M, Heard R. Hyperbaric oxygen therapy for multiple sclerosis. CNS Neurosci Ther. 2010 Apr 1;16(2):115-24.
7. Bennett M, Newton H. Hyperbaric oxygen therapy and cerebral palsy – where to now? Undersea Hyperb Med. 2007;34(2):69-74.
8. Bennett MH, Mitchell SJ. Hyperbaric and diving medicine. In: Longo DL, Fauci AS, Kasper DL, Hauser SL, Jameson JL, Loscalzo J, editors. Harrison's principles of internal medicine. 18th ed. New York: McGraw-Hill; 2011. e52-1–52-8.
9. Bennett MH, Weibel S, Wasiak J, Schnabel A, French C, Kranke P. Hyperbaric oxygen therapy for acute ischaemic stroke. Cochrane Database Syst Rev. 2014;(11):CD004954. doi: 10.1002/14651858.CD004954.pub3.
10. Bortolami F. The participation effect: is it a question of different expectations and communication? A preliminary investigation. Int J Interdiscip Soc Sci. 2011;5(10):325-54.
11. Boussi-Gross R, Golan H, Fishlev G, Bechor Y, Volkov O, Bergan J, et al. Hyperbaric oxygen therapy can improve postconcussion syndrome years after mild traumatic brain injury – randomized prospective trial. PLoS One. 2013;8(11):e79995. doi: 10.1371/journal.pone.0079995.
12. Chinese Acute Stroke Trial Collaborative Group. CAST: randomised placebo-controlled trial of early aspirin use in 20,000 patients with acute ischaemic stroke. Lancet. 1997;349:1641-9.
13. Churchill S, Weaver LK, Deru K, Russo AA, Handrahan D, Orrison WW Jr, et al. A prospective trial of hyperbaric oxygen for chronic sequelae after brain injury (HYBOBI). Undersea Hyperb Med. 2013;40:165-93.
14. Cifu D, Hart BB, West SL, Walker W, Carne W. The effect of hyperbaric oxygen on persistent postconcussion symptoms. J Head Trauma Rehabil. 2014;29:11-20.
15. Cifu D, Walker W, West SL, Hart BB, Franke LM, Sima A, et al. Hyperbaric oxygen for blast related post-concussion syndrome: 3 month outcomes. Ann Neurol. 2014;75:277-86.
16. Clark JM. Oxygen toxicity. In: The physiology and medicine of diving. 3rd ed. New York: Saunders; 1982. p. 200-38.
17. Dean JB, Mulkey DK, Garcia AJ, Putnam RW, Henderson RA. Neuronal sensitivity to hyperoxia, hypercapnia, and inert gases at hyperbaric pressures. J Appl Physiol. 2003;95:883-909.
18. D'Olhaberriague L, Mitsias P. A reappraisal of reliability and validity studies in stroke. Stroke. 1998;27:2331-6.

19. Efrati S, Fishlev G, Bechor Y, Volkov O, Bergan J, Kliakhandler K, et al. Hyperbaric oxygen induces late neuroplasticity in post stroke patients – randomized, prospective trial. PLoS One. 2013;8(1):e53716. doi:10.1371/journal.pone.0053716.

20. FDA: U.S. Food & Drug Administration [Internet]. U.S. Department of Health and Human Services, U.S. Food & Drug Administration. Hyperbaric oxygen therapy: don't be misled. Consumer health information leaflet [cited 2014 Jun]. Available from: http://www.fda.gov/forconsumers/ consumerupdates/ucm364687.htm

21. Gabb G, Robin ED. Hyperbaric oxygen: a therapy in search of diseases. Chest. 1987;92:1074-82.

22. Gobin YP, Starkman S, Duckwiler G, et al. MERCI 1: a phase 1 study of mechanical embolus removal in cerebral ischemia. Stroke. 2004;35:2848–54.

23. Harch PG, Andrews SR, Fogarty EF, Amen D, Pezzullo JC, Lucarini J, et al. A phase 1 study of low pressure hyperbaric oxygen therapy for blast induced post-concussion syndrome and post-traumatic stress disorder. J Neurotrauma. 2012;29:168-85.

24. Harch PG. Department of Defense trials for hyperbaric oxygen and TBI: issues of study design and questionable conclusions [letter]. Undersea Hyperb Med. 2013;40:469-70.

25. Harch PG. Hyperbaric oxygen therapy for post-concussion syndrome: contradictory conclusions from a study mischaracterized as sham-controlled. J Neurotrauma. 2013 Dec 1;30(23):1995-9.

26. Hart GB, Thompson RE. The treatment of cerebral ischemia with hyperbaric oxygen (OHP). Stroke. 1971;2:247-50.

27. Helms AK, Whelan HT, Torbey MT. Hyperbaric oxygen therapy of cerebral ischemia. Cerebrovasc Dis. 2005;20:417-26.

28. Heyman A, Saltzman HA, Whalen RE. The use of hyperbaric oxygenation in the treatment of cerebral ischemia and infarction. Circulation. 1966 May 1;33(5S2):II-20.

29. Hills BA. A role for oxygen-induced osmosis in hyperbaric oxygen therapy. Med Hypotheses. 1999;52:259-63.

30. Hoge CW, Jonas WB. The ritual of hyperbaric oxygen and lessons for the treatment of persistent postconcussion symptoms in military personnel. JAMA Internal Med. 2015;175(1):53-4.

31. Ikeda Y, Long DM. The molecular basis of brain injury and brain edema: the role of oxygen free radicals. Neurosurgery. 1990;27:1-11.

32. Ingvar DH, Lassen NA. Treatment of focal cerebral ischaemia with hyperbaric oxygen. Report of 4 cases. Acta Neurol Scand. 1965;41:92-5.

33. Joo EY, Tae WS, Jung K-Y, Hong SB. Cerebral blood flow changes in man by wake-promoting drug, modafinil: a randomized double blind study. J Sleep Res. 2008;17:82-8.

34. Kim D, Jahan R, Starkman S, Abolian A, Kidwell CS, Vinuela F, Duckwiler GR, Ovbiagele B, Vespa PM, Selco S, Rajajee V. Endovascular mechanical clot retrieval in a broad ischemic stroke cohort. AJNR Am J Neuroradiol. 2006 Nov 1;27(10):2048-52.

35. Laatch L, Pavel D, Jobe T, Lin Q, Quintana J-C. Incorporation of SPECT imaging in a longitudinal cognitive rehabilitation programme. Brain Injury. 1999;13:555-70.

36. Lacey DJ, Stolfi A, Pilati LE. Effects of hyperbaric oxygen on motor function in children with cerebral palsy. Ann Neurol. 2012 Nov 1;72(5):695-703.

37. Lopez AD, Mathers CD, Ezzati M, et al. Global and regional burden of disease and risk factors, 2001: systematic analysis of population health data. Lancet. 2006;367:1747-57.

38. Lou M, Eschenfelder CC, Herdegen T, et al. Therapeutic window for use of hyperbaric oxygenation in focal transient ischemia in rats. Stroke. 2004;35(2):578-83.

39. MacDonald AG, Fraser PJ. The transduction of very small hydrostatic pressures. Comp Biochem Physiol. 1999;122:13- 36.

40. Miller RS, Weaver LK, Bahraini N, Churchill S, Price RC, Skiba V, et al. Effects of hyperbaric oxygen on symptoms and quality of life among service members with persistent post-concussion symptoms: a randomized trial. JAMA Int Med. 2014 Nov 17. Epub ahead of print. doi: P10.1001/JAMAinternmed.2014.5479.

41. Mink RB, Dutka AJ. Hyperbaric oxygen after global cerebral ischemia in rabbits reduces brain vascular permeability and blood flow. Stroke. 1995;26:2307-12.

42. Mitchell SJ, Bennett MH. Unestablished indications for hyperbaric oxygen therapy. Diving Hyperb Med. 2014 Dec;44(4):228-34.

43. Mukherjee A, Raison M, Sahni T, Arya A, Lambert J, Marois P, et al. Intensive rehabilitation combined with HBO therapy in children with cerebral palsy: a controlled longitudinal study. Undersea Hyperb Med. 2014;41:77-85.

44. Multiple authors. Brain injury and mechanisms of action of hyperbaric oxygen (HBO2) for persistent post-concussive symptoms after mild traumatic brain injury (mTBI) (BIMA) study. Undersea Hyperb Med. 2016;43(5). Special issue.

45. Multiple Sclerosis National Therapy Centres [Internet]. Multiple Sclerosis National Therapy Centres. Oxygen Treatment. Available from: http://www.msntc.org.uk/oxygen_treatment.php

46. Neubauer RA, End E. Hyperbaric oxygenation as an adjunct therapy in strokes due to thrombosis. A review of 122 patients. Stroke. 1980;11:297-300.

47. Newberg AB, Hersh EV, Levin LM, Giannakopoulos H, Secreto SA, Wintering NA, Farrar JT. Double-blind, placebo-controlled, randomized pilot study of cerebral blood flow patterns employing SPECT imaging in dental postsurgical pain patients with and without pain relief. Clin Therapeutics. 2011;33:1894-903.

48. Nighoghossian N, Trouillas P. Hyperbaric oxygen in the treatment of acute ischemic stroke: an unsettled issue. J Neurol Sci 1997;150:27-31.

49. Prosser-Loose EJ, Paterson PG. The FOOD Trial Collaboration: nutritional supplementation strategies and acute stroke outcome. Nutr Rev. 2006;64:289-94.

50. Robertson CS, Narayan RK, Gokaslan ZL, et al. Cerebral arteriovenous oxygen difference as an estimate of cerebral blood flow in comatose patients. J Neurosurg. 1989;70:222-30.

51. Sarno MT, Sarno JE, Diller L. The effect of hyperbaric oxygen on communication function in adults with aphasia secondary to stroke. J Speech Hear Res. 1972;15(1):42-8.

52. Selman WR, Lust WD, Pundik S, et al. Compromised metabolic recovery following spontaneous spreading depression in the penumbra. Brain Res. 2004;999:167-74.

53. Siddique MS, Fernandes HM, Wooldridge TD, Fenwick JD, Slomka P, et al. Reversible ischemia around intracerebral hemorrhage: a single-photon emission computerized tomography study. J Neurosurg. 2002;96:736-41.

54. Siesjo BK, Agardh CD, Bengtsson F. Free radicals and brain damage. Cerebrovasc Brain Metab Rev. 1989;1:165-211.

55. Smart DA, Bennett MH. ANZHMG statement on the administration of mild hyperbaric oxygen therapy. Diving Hyperb Med. 2010;40(2):78-82.

56. Smith WS, Sung G, Starkman S, et al.; MERCI Trial Investigators. Safety and efficacy of mechanical embolectomy in acute ischemic stroke: results of the MERCI trial. Stroke. 2005;36:1432–38

57. Stroke Unit Trialists' Collaboration. Organised inpatient (stroke unit) care for stroke. Cochrane Database Syst Rev. 2013;(9):CD000197. doi: 10.1002/14651858.CD000197.pub3.

58. Sudlow CL, Warlow CP. Comparable studies of the incidence of stroke and its pathological types: results from an international collaboration. International Stroke Incidence Collaboration. Stroke. 1997;28:491-9.

59. Sukoff MH, Ragatz RE. Hyperbaric oxygenation for the treatment of acute cerebral edema. Neurosurgery. 1982;10:29-38.

60. Tatchell P. The oxygen crisis [opinion]. The Guardian [Internet]. 2008 Aug 13. Available from: https://www.theguardian.com/commentisfree/2008/aug/13/carbonemissions.climatechange Quoting Plimer I, Harrison J.

61. The College of Physicians and Surgeons of Saskatchewan [Internet]. College of Physicians and Surgeons of Saskatchewan. Standard: unproven and unconventional treatment [cited 2014 Jul]. Available from: https://admin.cps.sk.ca/CPSS/.

62. The International Stroke Trial Collaborative Group. The International Stroke Trial (IST): a randomised trial of aspirin, subcutaneous heparin, both, or neither among 19435 patients with acute ischaemic stroke. International Stroke Trial Collaborative Group. Lancet. 1997;349:1569-81.

63. Thom SR. Functional inhibition of leukocyte B2 integrins by hyperbaric oxygen in carbon monoxide-mediated brain injury in rats. Toxicol Appl Pharmacol. 1993;123:248-56.

64. Undersea & Hyperbaric Medical Society Committee report. In: Hyperbaric oxygen therapy indications. 13th ed. Flagstaff (AZ): Best Publishing Co.; 2014.

65. Van Gijn J. Measurement of outcome in stroke prevention trials. Cerebrovasc Dis. 1992;2(Suppl 2):23-34.

66. Wager TD, Rilling JK, Smith EE, Sokolik A, Casey KL, Davidson RJ, et al. Placebo-induced changes in fMRI in the anticipation and experience of pain. Science. 2004;303:1162- 7.

67. Walker WC, Franke LM, Cifu DX, Hart BB. Randomized, sham-controlled, feasibility trial of hyperbaric oxygen for service members with postconcussion syndrome: cognitive and psychomotor outcomes 1 week postintervention. Neurorehab Neural Rep. 2013;28:420-32.

68. Wardlaw JM, Keir SL, Seymour J, et al. What is the best imaging strategy for acute stroke? Health Technol Assess. 2004;8:1-180.

69. Weaver LK, Cifu D, Hart B, Wolf G, Miller RS. Hyperbaric oxygen for post-concussion syndrome: design of Department of Defense clinical trials. Undersea Hyperb Med. 2012;39:807-14.

70. Weinstein PR, Anderson GG, Telles DA. Results of hyperbaric oxygen therapy during temporary middle cerebral artery occlusion in unanesthetized cats. Neurosurgery. 1987;20:518-24.

71. Wolf G, Cifu D, Baugh L, Carne W, Profenna L. The effect of hyperbaric oxygen on symptoms after mild traumatic brain injury. J Neurotrauma. 2012;29:2606-12.

72. Yusa T, Beckman JS, Crapo JD, et al. Hyperoxia increases H2O2 production by brain in vivo. J Appl Physiol. 1987;63:353-8.

CHAPTER 34 CHAPTER

Hyperbaric Oxygen Treatment of Avascular Bone Necrosis of the Femoral Head

CHAPTER THIRTY-FOUR OVERVIEW

Introduction 863
AVNFH Pathophysiology 864
Clinical Presentation 865
Standard Management (Summary) and Outcome (HBO_2 Excluded) 866
Rationale for HBO_2 Use 867
Patient Selection for HBO_2 876
Current Protocol 877
Cost Impact 877
Conclusions and Recommendation on the Basis of Previous Studies 877
References 878

Hyperbaric Oxygen Treatment of Avascular Bone Necrosis of the Femoral Head

Giuliano Vezzani, Gerardo Bosco, Enrico M. Camporesi

INTRODUCTION

Femoral head necrosis (FHN), also named avascular necrosis of the femoral head (AVNFH) or osteonecrosis of the femoral head (ONFH), is the frequent presentation of a multifactorial disease that can result in significant clinical morbidity and can affect patients of any age, including young and active patients.

The evolution of femoral head osteonecrosis results in femoral head collapse and subsequent hip joint degenerative lesions.[38]

New technologies have allowed specialist orthopedic surgeons to clearly identify this disease at an earlier stage via radiographic evaluation than was previously possible.[1] Furthermore, it is speculated that a similar pathophysiology might also cause similar avascular syndromes in other sections of the skeleton: compromised blood flow in bony segments with limited vascularity (i.e., femoral condili, the wrist, the head of the humerus, and the distal talus) triggers degenerative processes. The last systematic review of femoral head necrosis and hyperbaric oxygen therapy is masterfully detailed in *Hyperbaric Medicine Practice 2nd edition* with specific tables of patient outcomes and a review of the literature until 1997.[40] That chapter summarized the different pathological outcomes published in multiple papers, rationale for intervention, and a summary of outcome. That chapter also emphasized a scoring classification (scale) to evaluate the presenting grade of bony impairment. Avascular necroses were described in all these regions, and a growing body of literature supports the use of hyperbaric oxygen therapy in all these syndromes.

The current therapeutic choices are well defined for management and care of a hip osteonecrosis but show results that differ from each other according to the specific patient population and the disease stage considered.[5]

AVNFH is essentially the final common pathway of a series of structural derangements, resulting in a sharp decrease in provisional blood flow to the femoral head, leading to cellular death, fractures, and collapse of the articular surface.[20,30]

In the United States, and in the western world at large, the prevalence of AVNFH stands at a mean age of 39 years, and it is considered responsible for at least 10% of hip replacements performed.

From a nosographic point of view, avascular hip osteonecrosis is defined as the usual outcome of an unrelenting course eventually culminating in functional loss of the hip.

It is actually a rare occurrence to have spontaneous regression of AVNFH; most of the untreated diagnoses (67% of asymptomatic patients and 85% of symptomatic hips) proceed towards femoral head collapse.(31)

Although many authors have already suggested and advocated a treatment based on patient's age, symptoms, stage, and/or medical status, the orthopedic community has not yet adopted a univocal algorithm for its treatment.

AVNFH PATHOPHYSIOLOGY

Our understanding of AVNFH risk factors and its pathology is limited by the absence of a bipedal mammalian model and the difficulty of longitudinal studies in humans.

Hallmarks of osteonecrosis (ON) are specific and have a typical pattern of cellular death coupled with a complex process of bone resorption and formation. The first pathologic presentation of AVNFH is necrosis of hematopoietic cells and adipocytes with concomitant edema of interstitial marrow. Though osteocyte necrosis is visible after approximately 2 to 3 hours of anoxia, histological signs of osteocyte death take approximately 24 to 72 hours following oxygen deprivation to appear.(6,41)

Reactive hyperemia and capillary revascularization occur, to some degree, in the periphery of the necrotic zone. The entry of blood vessels propagates a repair process in which both bone resorption and production incompletely replace dead bone with living bone.(1) Dead bone is partially resorbed, and new living bone is laminated onto dead trabeculae. Because bone resorption exceeds formation in the subchondral trabeculae, there is a sequence with net removal of bone, loss of structural integrity of trabeculae, subchondral fracture, and joint incongruity.(11)

The best evidence suggests a common pathophysiological pathway: compromised subchondral microcirculation.(1) A decrease in blood flow by 60% would be expected to reduce the intraosseous pO_2 from 75 mmHg to 50 mmHg, assuming a constant oxygen consumption rate.(25) This reduction will result in marked ischemia. Three pathogenic mechanisms can lead to decreased femoral head blood flow: (1) vascular interruption by fractures or dislocation, (2) intravascular occlusion from thrombi or embolic fat, or (3) intraosseous extravascular compression from lipocyte hypertrophy or Gaucher cells. Though a fourth mechanism, extraosseous venous obstruction, has been experimentally shown to have the same effect, it probably has limited clinical significance. Researchers have focused on elevated intraosseous pressure as a pathogenic mechanism in AVNFH, and literature related to this increase has recently been reviewed. Elevated intraosseous pressures have been measured within osteonecrotic femoral heads associated with venous outflow obstruction and venous stasis.(38)

There are different pathogenic mechanisms which may result in ischemia and osteonecrosis.

1. Intracapsular fractures of the femoral neck can cause direct trauma to vessels that supply the subchondral bone, and relatively high incidences of osteonecrosis of the femoral head (ONFH) have been reported in patients with these fractures.
2. An interruption in the vascular flow to the femoral head may be secondary to endoluminal obstruction. A diverse group of etiologies may cause this obstruction, especially sickle cell aggregations, clots, or lipid thrombi. In these patients, low-oxygen-tension environments are hypothesized to trigger

hemoglobin precipitation which leads to erythrocyte sickling. As the patient's age increased, the rate of AVNFH was noted to increase; presumably, this was a direct result of repeated vascular insults from which these patients suffered over the course of their lives. Also, coagulation factor aberrations have been observed in AVNFH: for example, genetic defects, resulting in hypofibrinolysis or thrombophilia, may lead to increased thrombi formation and a subsequent impaired blood flow in the osseous circulation.

Nevertheless, using a case-control methodology, elevated coagulation factor levels have been reported in patients with osteonecrosis showing absence of known genetic defects.

3. Though it is not a consistently recordable event, the elevations in pressure within the intraosseous extravascular space have already been observed to lead to a decrease in the blood flow in those small vessels passing through it.

   Many times, the increase in extravascular pressure is associated with corticosteroid or alcohol intake, and it has been hypothesized to create an obstruction for arterial inflow or venous outflow; this can lead to ischemia of the marrow elements and osteocytes in the femoral head. Corticosteroids are used to treat a variety of disease conditions including systemic lupus erythematosus, vasculitis, rheumatoid arthritis, asthma, and organ transplantation.(1) Alcohol abuse has also been correlated to AVNFH cases. Also, Gaucher disease has been linked to the development of osteonecrosis of the femoral head, owing to its role in decreasing the capillary blood flow, potentially by increasing the pressures in the intraosseous extravascular space.(36)

Many other dyscrasias and clinical presentations, like hyperlipidemia, hyperuricemia, pancreatitis, leukemia or lymphoma, and hypertriglyceridemia, have been considered as potential causes of osteonecrosis of the femoral head. Osteonecrosis occurrences have also been reported in those undergoing radiation or bone marrow transplantation procedures, in patients suffering from disseminated metastatic malignancies, and in pregnant patients.(1)

Dysbaric osteonecrosis presentation is well characterized by studies of underwater or compressed-air pressure environments with a clear approach outlining diving decompression schedules.(44) A comprehensive summary of the described cases, classification of the radiological presentation, summary of results, and the growing success rate of multiple hyperbaric treatments is presented in the previous edition of this textbook, in the first five tables, summarizing the literature between 1960 and the early 2000s. The present chapter aims to review more recent evidence from 2004 until 2016, presented in Table 1 at the end of this chapter.

CLINICAL PRESENTATION

To ensure optimal treatment of AVNFH, early diagnosis is necessary since treatment success is related to the stage at which the care is initiated.(22)

There are a considerable number of procedures which can be used to detect and stage an AVNFH presentation: histological studies, scintigraphy, bone functional evaluations, radiography and/or magnetic resonance imaging (MRI), or computer-assisted tomography (CT) – most current diagnostic methods available for that aim. AVNFH is usually asymptomatic at early stages; however, some patients may develop knee pain and/or pain radiating from ipsilateral buttock. Patients typically present with a limited range of motion at the hip and stabbing pain, especially during forced internal rotation. A detailed interview may identify associated risk factors in a patient's medical history. AVNFH must be suspected when a patient presents with pain in the hips, shows negative plain radiographs, and no risk factor at anamnesis data; plain radiographs may often appear as normal in the early stages of necrosis. Patients who have had a history of necrosis must be observed for bilateral AVNFH: bilaterality has been reported in up to 70% of observations.[9] Usually the classifications used in the diagnosis of AVNFH include the Ficat, Arlet, and the University of Pennsylvania's Steinberg systems. Ficat classification, based on standard radiograph presentations, consists of the following: Stage I, normal imaging; Stage II indicates a normal contour, but there is evidence of bone remodeling; Stage III is characterized by the evidence of a subchondral collapse, or a flattening of the FH; Stage IV indicates a tight narrowing of the joint space, with secondary degenerative changes in the acetabulum. The Ficat classification system definitely relies on radiographic imaging, and therefore, the lesion size cannot be quantified, making it impossible "de facto" to get a real measure of the disease progression. Steinberg expands the Ficat system into six stages and includes quantification of involvement of the FH, within stage 1–5, with three further subsets each: defining mild (less than 15% radiographic involvement of the head's articular surface), moderate (15%–30% involvement of the head's articular surface), and severe (greater than 30% involvement of the head's articular surface) stages. The Association Research Circulation Osseous (ARCO) recommended shifting towards a new classification system, based on the differences in procedure findings: radiographic, MRI, bone scan, and histologic findings.[5] However, Ficat and ARCO classifications systems, apparently, are still not reliable enough to assess ONFH occurrence.[37]

Currently, ON is diagnosed by a plain AP and frog-leg lateral radiographs of the hip, followed by MRI, but MRI is considered the most accurate benchmark.

Though rarely, other tools for assessing an AVNFH presentation include bone marrow pressure measurements, venography, and core biopsy.

STANDARD MANAGEMENT (SUMMARY) AND OUTCOME (HBO_2 EXCLUDED)

Treatment options are pharmacologic agents and biophysical treatments, as well as joint-preserving and joint-replacing surgeries. An established protocol for the medical management of AVNFH has been increasingly used during the early stages in an attempt to hinder the progression of the disease.

Lipid-lowering agents, anticoagulants, vasoactive substances, and bisphosphonates can all be used to pharmacologically manage AVN. Increases in both the number and size of circulating fat cells have been correlated with the development of AVNFH; therefore, lipid-lowering agents, such as statins, are advantageous due to their capability to reduce the rate of adipogenesis. Statins have been demonstrated to have a protective effect on patients receiving steroids.[33] Anticoagulants such as enoxaparin act via platelet-aggregation inhibition, thus increasing blood flow to ischemic areas of the bone. In those patients with underlying coagulopathy disorders, such as thrombophilia or hypofibrinolysis, these agents are most significantly beneficial. Prostacyclin is a vasoactive agent that improves blood flow, an effect mediated through its vasodilator potential at the level of terminal vessels. Even if prostacyclin has shown significant improvement in both clinical and radiologic outcomes of early-stage AVNFH, possible long-term benefits are still under evaluation.

Bisphosphonates significantly decrease the incidence of collapse of the FH in osteonecrotic hips due to a limitation in the osteoclast activity. Alendronate has been utilized as an adjunctive therapy for some procedures and has been found to reduce pain and the risk of collapse in early stages of AVNFH as well as with hyperbaric oxygen (HBO_2) therapy. Evidence of its utility for the prevention of total hip replacement (THR) and reduction of AVNFH progression remains debated.(12-13,17)

Biophysical treatments for AVNFH under consideration are extracorporeal shockwave therapy (ESWT), pulse electromagnetic therapy, and HBO_2 therapy. ESWT has been demonstrated to restore tissue oxygenation, reduce edema, and induce angiogenesis;(34) ESWT can potentially offer a feasible and good substitute to other more invasive therapeutic modalities targeting AVNFH at different stages. Though not as widely used, pulse electromagnetic therapy is thought to function by stimulating osteogenesis and angiogenesis; however, its role as early-stage AVNFH treatment still needs to be established. A conservative treatment of AVNFH may be effective, especially in the earlier stages of the disease; though medical management can improve pain control, compliance, and functional outcomes, randomized clinical trials (RCT) with long-term follow-up are necessary to determine the effectiveness of therapy.(9) Surgical interventions are not included in this review.

RATIONALE FOR HBO_2 USE

Current literature lacks primary evidence in this area, thus limiting our ability to identify the optimal treatment protocol that must be adhered to in the case management of patients suffering from a precollapse stage of an AVNFH occurrence, or which the early intervention to adopt, so as to avoid bone collapse, getting those desirable outcomes the joint-preserving procedures are aimed to.

Of all possible and feasible therapies that may effectively delay the need for hip arthroplasty, we do believe HBO_2 therapy may show a beneficial effect without the invasiveness of a surgical approach.

HBO_2 increases extracellular oxygen concentration and reduces cellular ischemia and edema by inducing vasoconstriction. Studies have reported radiographic improvement in AVNFH at Stage I according to Steinberg classification, as well as better pain control and compliance, and range of motion (ROM) improvement, in AVNFH at Ficat Stage I–II.(12-13,45)

Effects of HBO_2 include reduced bone-marrow pressure and increased oxygen delivery to ischemic cells, thus relieving compartment syndrome and preventing further necrosis. Moreover, the decrease in bone marrow pressure leads to a significant pain relief.(12-13) Recent works evidence that HBO_2 therapy not only stimulates angiogenesis,(42) but it also influences cells involved in bone remodeling: osteoblasts, responsible for bone deposition, and osteoclasts, responsible for bone resorption.(3-4,19,29) Their activity is finely tuned by osteoprotegerin (OPG)/receptor activator of NF-kB ligand (RANKL)/ receptor activator of NF-kB (RANK) system. Bone remodeling is an important process that continues throughout life and serves to prevent old bone accumulation, adjust bone architecture to meet any possible needs, and repair microdamages. If bone remodeling balance shifts into bone resorption, it may lead to pathological states such as the degradation and collapse of the femoral head. There are studies that report a correlation between severe osteolysis and osteonecrosis with OPG and RANKL expression levels.(18,35,47) Hadi et al., in their published researches, showed that hyperbaric oxygenation accelerates osteoblasts differentiation and suppresses osteoclasts genesis-activation, shifting the balance between bone formation and bone resorption in a direction that promotes regeneration. (3,4,19) The intimate mechanism by which HBO_2 treatment promotes bone formation and repair is still under debate, but, interestingly, a recent published work(46) shows that HBO_2 therapy significantly increases serum OPG concentration but has no significant effect on serum RANKL. These results suggest that hyperbaric oxygenation may exert its action reducing osteoclast activation and formation.

The recent literature is reviewed in Table 1.

TABLE 1. LITERATURE ANALYSIS REPORT OF HBO_2 IN FEMORAL HEAD NECROSIS

LEGEND: ATA stands for Absolute Atmospheres, ARCO for Association Research Circulation Osseus, AVN for Avascular Necrosis, ESWT for Extracorporeal Shock Wave Treatment, FHN for Femur/Femural Head Necrosis, HHS for Harris Hip Score, ONFH for Osteonecrosis Femur Head, SARS for Severe Acute Respiratory Syndrome, SF-12 for Short Form 12, THA for Total Hip Arthroplasty, VAS for Visual Analogue Score, WOMAC for Western Ontario and McMaster Universities Osteoarthritis Index.

STUDY (Authors, Year)	Reis et al., 2003
TYPE	Retrospective cohort study.
NB PATIENTS	12 patients, 16 hips. 10 idiopathic, 13 hips. 1 patient taking steroids (concomitant *systemic lupus erythematosus*), 1 patient taking steroids (concomitant *chronic kidney disease*). **Design of the study:** HBO_2 group 12 patients, 16 hips versus untreated control 47M, 25F; 72 hips
AIM(s)/ EVALUATION CRITERIA	**To evaluate:** Outcomes at MRI, comparing them with an identical size of lesion in an untreated group described earlier (72 FHN lesions at MRI, Vande Berg BC et al. 1999).
INCLUSION/ EXCLUSION CRITERIA	**Inclusion:** Steinberg stage-I cases with lesions ≥ 4 mm thick and/or ≥ 12.5 mm long on MRI. **Exclusion:** All smaller stage-I lesions/bone marrow edema alone and more advanced stages of AVN.
HBO2 PROTOCOL (Pressure, Time, NB of Sessions)	**Study: 100 sessions** Daily Tx, Mon through Sat, 90 minutes $FiO_2 = 1$ at 2.0 ÷ 2.4 ATA Moreover: all patients were asked to use crutches, to minimize weight-bearing during the treatment (as did the comparative, untreated group).
RESULTS	**Outcomes:** 81% complete recovery at MRI after 2 years (mean of 8 [3 ÷ 24] months), in the HBO_2 group, versus 17% in the untreated one. 19% progressed to a higher Steinberg stage.
CONCLUSION/ COMMENT	Retrospective cohort study. Small series. 2 years follow-up, and then a simple yearly clinical control (further MRI only if the imaging was not yet normal). Some difficulties in MRI timing. Favors HBO_2. 1 THA (6.25%) occurrence. Number of HBO_2 sessions need:100 Tx. Moderate level of evidence.

TABLE 1 (CONTINUED)

STUDY (Authors, Year)	Wong et al., 2008
TYPE	Retrospective study. Case series.
NB PATIENTS	4 patients, 8 hips.
AIM(s)/ EVALUATION CRITERIA	**To evaluate:** Outcomes of cocktail therapy in SARS-associated FHN.
INCLUSION/ EXCLUSION CRITERIA	**Inclusion:** ARCO stage 1 (1 out of 8 lesions), ARCO stage 2 (6 out of 8 lesions), ARCO stage 3 (1 out of 8 lesions).
HBO2 PROTOCOL (Pressure, Time, NB of Sessions)	**Study: 100 sessions** Daily Tx, Mon through Fri, 90 minutes FiO_2 = 1 at 2.5 ATA Cocktail therapy Moreover: all patients got oral alendronate sodium 70 mg per week for one year and 6000 impulses of ESWT at 0.62 mJ/mm2 energy flux density (≡28kV) in a single session.
RESULTS	While no progression and no improvement of the lesion compared to baseline (22.4 versus 24.4), HHS improved (86.8 versus 74.2 at 6 months; up to 94.2 at 48 months), VAS pain improved both as per night pain (diminished to 21.3 versus 41.3 at 6 months; reaching 6.3 at 48 months) and on walking as well (36.3 versus 61.3 at 6 months; and 15.0 at 48 months).
CONCLUSION/ COMMENT	Retrospective study. Small case series. 4 years follow-up. Lightly favors HBO_2. No THA occurence. Number of HBO_2 sessions need: 100 Tx. Low level of evidence.

TABLE 1 (CONTINUED)

STUDY (Authors, Year)	Hsu et al., 2009	
TYPE	Randomized controlled trial. Not double blinded.	
NB PATIENTS	Group A (cocktail therapy):28 patients, 50 hips.	Group B (ESWT alone): 35 patients, 48 hips.
AIM(s)/ EVALUATION CRITERIA	**To evaluate versus ESWT alone:** Outcomes in terms of general improvement (as per HHS, Physical & Mental SF-12, VAS pain, and/or WOMAC scores).	Outcomes in terms of specific improvement (as per findings at MRI and/or hip replacement need).
INCLUSION/ EXCLUSION CRITERIA	**Inclusion**: ARCO stage 1 (2 out of 50 lesions), ARCO stage 2 (35 out of 50 lesions), ARCO stage 3 (13 out of 50 lesions).	**Inclusion**: ARCO stage 1 (2 out of 48 lesions), ARCO stage 2 (27 out of 48 lesions), ARCO stage 3 (19 out of 48 lesions).
HBO2 PROTOCOL (Pressure, Time, NB of Sessions)	**Study: 20 HBO_2 sessions** Daily Tx, Mon through Fri, 90 minutes $FiO_2 = 1$ at 2.5 ATA Cocktail therapy Moreover: all patients got oral alendronate 70 mg per week for one year and 6000 impulses of ESWT at 0.62 mJ/mm2 energy flux density (≡ 28kV) in a single session.	**Study: ESWT alone**
RESULTS	**Outcomes:** Neither general improvement as per HHS (74.5 versus 77.2), Physical (31.5 versus 33.7) and Mental (43.2 versus 43.3) SF-12, VAS pain (5.4 versus 5.4), or WOMAC (74.8 versu. 77.2) scores.	No specific improvement as per Hsu findings at MRI (22% cocktail therapy versus 20.8 ESWT) and/or percentages in progression or total hip replacement need (10% versus 10.4% if ESWT alone). Note: Both groups showed significant reduction in bone marrow edema and a trend of decrease in the size of the lesions.
CONCLUSION/ COMMENT	Randomized controlled trial. Follow-up ≥ 2 years; (2.3 ± 0.9 years). Neutral to HBO_2 use, and joint effects of HBO_2 and alendronate over EWST were not observed. ≈ 10% THA occurrences. Number of HBO_2 sessions need: 20 Tx. Low level of evidence.	

TABLE 1 (CONTINUED)

STUDY (Authors, Year)	Camporesi et al., 2010
TYPE	Two phases: a) 0–1.5 months **RCT double blinded.** b) 1.5–84 months **observational study.** Starting as a double-blind randomized controlled trial (for 1.5 months; up to the completion of the 30th Tx). The observational phase starts when, after exposure to 6 weeks of sham to HBA (hyperbaric air, $FiO_2 = 0.21$), the blind was broken, and 6 weeks of HBO_2 (hyperbaric oxygen, $FiO_2 = 1$) were offered to the control group.
NB PATIENTS	17 patients, 17 hips. **Design of the study:** 20 patients, 20 hips (HBO_2 group: 6M 4F; HBA group: 6M 4F). **Drop out:** 1F, HBA group, after first few treatments for personal reasons. **Follow-up:** 17 out of 19 patients.
AIM(s)/ EVALUATION CRITERIA	**To evaluate:** • Pain reduction, if any. • The eventual Improvement in the range of hip motion in flexion, extension, adduction, and abduction. • Stabilometry measurements. • MRI. • Case evolution in hip arthroplasty surgery.
INCLUSION/ EXCLUSION CRITERIA	**Inclusion:** Idiopathic unilateral Ficat II FHN. **Exclusion:** Underlying pathology, pharmacologic treatment, alcohol abuse, trauma to the involved hip, or steroid use.
HBO2 PROTOCOL (Pressure, Time, NB of Sessions)	**Study: 30 sessions** Daily Tx, Mon through Fri, 6 weeks, 60 minutes **$FiO_2 = 1$** at 2.5 ATA. **Control: 30 sessions** Daily Tx, Mon through Fri, 6 weeks, 60 minutes **$FiO_2 = 0.21$** at 2.5 ATA.

TABLE 1 (CONTINUED)

RESULTS	**Pain reduction:** The HBO_2 group showed marked improvement and significance starting after 20 treatment sessions (p = 0.002 versus HBA) through 30 sessions ($p < 0.001$). **Range of hip motion improvement:** • Flexion: clinical evidence of efficacy (nearly doubled at 30 Tx), not any statistical evidence. • Extension, adduction, abduction: statistical evidence starting after 10 Tx and stable at 20 Tx and 30 Tx (p = 0.001 versus HBA). **Stabilometry measurements:** As per the median value difference between the load on the unaffected limb and the load on the affected limb, the HBO_2 group versus HBA: • lower differences, especially at the end of the study, but • no statistical significance. **MRI:** • Most of the improvement registered between the pretreatment MRI and the 12-month MRI. • 7 out of the 9 patients with history of repeated MRI demonstrated continuing radiographic improvement between 12 months and 7 years. **Arthroplasty surgery:** No patient in the study underwent hip arthroplasty surgery.
CONCLUSION/ COMMENT	RCT. Small series. 7 years follow-up Favors HBO_2. No THA occurrence. Number of HBO_2 sessions need: over 30 Tx. High level of evidence.

TABLE 1 (CONTINUED)

STUDY (Authors, Year)	Zhao et al., 2010
TYPE	Prospective study. Case series.
NB PATIENTS	51 patients, 84 hips.
AIM(s)/ EVALUATION CRITERIA	**To evaluate:** The lesion size changes at MRI in ONFH induced by corticosteroid administration in severe acute respiratory syndrome (SARS) patients.
INCLUSION/ EXCLUSION CRITERIA	**Inclusion:** ARCO stage 1 (78 out of 84 lesions), ARCO stage 2 (6 out of 84 lesions).
HBO2 PROTOCOL (Pressure, Time, NB of Sessions)	**Study: 100 HBO_2 sessions** Daily Tx, Mon through Sat, 90 minutes **FiO_2 = 1** at 2.0 ÷ 2.4 ATA. Moreover: all patients received IV injection of prostaglandin E1, ligustrazine and Salvia miltiorrhiza was also used for 10-per-month daily sessions, up to a total of 30 sessions.
RESULTS	**MRI:** Decreased lesion volume, from the baseline of 10.12 ± 8.05 cm^3 to the final value 5.67 ± 6.58 cm^3.
CONCLUSION/ COMMENT	Prospective study. Case series. 5 years follow-up. Lightly favors HBO_2. No THA occurrence. Number of HBO_2 sessions need: 100 Tx. Low level of evidence.

TABLE 1 (CONTINUED)

STUDY (Authors, Year)	Deveci et al., 2013
TYPE	Retrospective study. Case series.
NB PATIENTS	16 patients, 21 hips.
AIM(s)/ EVALUATION CRITERIA	**To evaluate:** Synergistic effect, if any, of a core decompression followed by HBO_2.
INCLUSION/ EXCLUSION CRITERIA	**Inclusion:** Ficat Stage I FHN (9 out of 21 lesions), Ficat Stage II FHN (12 out of 21 lesions).
HBO2 PROTOCOL (Pressure, Time, NB of Sessions)	**Study: 40 HBO_2 sessions** Daily Tx, Mon through Sat, Daily Tx, Mon through Fri, 90 minutes **FiO_2 = 1** at 2.5 ATA.
RESULTS	**Outcomes:** • There are no statistics and/or volume measurements. • A general improvement as per HHS (75.9 versus 55.2), while was registered a worse VAS pain score (8.1 versus. 5.7). • 10% (2 lesions) progression to Ficat Stage III (steroid use in concomitant nephritic syndrome).
CONCLUSION/ COMMENT	Retrospective study. Case series. Average follow-up: ≈ 2 years. Lightly favors HBO_2 as adjuvant therapy. 10% THA occurrence. Number of HBO_2 sessions need: 40 Tx. Low level of evidence.

TABLE 1 (CONTINUED)

STUDY (Authors, Year)	Koren et al., 2015
TYPE	Retrospective study. Case series.
NB PATIENTS	68 patients, 78 hips.
AIM(s)/ EVALUATION CRITERIA	**To evaluate:** The effectiveness of this treatment in a relatively large patient cohort.
INCLUSION/ EXCLUSION CRITERIA	**Inclusion:** Steinberg Stage I (39 out of 78 lesions), Steinberg Stage II (39 out of 78 lesions).
HBO2 PROTOCOL (Pressure, Time, NB of Sessions)	**Study: 78.3 ± 24.2 HBO_2 sessions** Daily Tx, Mon through Sat, 90 minutes **FiO_2 = 1** at 2.0 ÷ 2.4 ATA. All patients followed a protected weight-bearing regimen for the duration of their symptoms.
RESULTS	**Outcomes:** • Mean Harris Hip Score has improved from 21 to 81 ($p < 0.0001$), • the mean physical component of the SF-12 improved from 24 to 46 ($p < 0.0001$), and • the mean mental component of the SF-12 improved from 54 to 59 ($p < 0.0001$). • After the treatment, 88% of hips showed improvement, while at the time of the follow-up 93% of hips survived.
CONCLUSION/ COMMENT	Retrospective study. Case series. Average follow-up: 11.1 ± 5.1 years. Lightly favors HBO_2. 7% THA occurrence. Number of HBO_2 sessions need: ≈ 80 Tx. Good level of evidence.

ANIMAL STUDIES

With regard to the controversy of the opportunity or not of a clinical use of hyperbaric oxygen treatment to stimulate both fracture healing and bone regeneration, animal results (studies on rats) suggest that hyperoxygenation-mediated relief of ischemia enhances fibroblastic, angioblastic, osteoblastic, and osteoclastic activities to realize an accelerated complete recovery of rats' femoral head necrosis.

The Kataoka study(24) in spontaneously hypertensive rats (SHR), was initially oriented to investigate the effects of hyperbaric oxygenation on an ischemic osteonecrosis event and on the ossification disturbance of the femoral head's growth. Authors concluded that HBO_2 prevented both the osteonecrosis and the ossification disturbance of the femoral heads.(24)

In a following Levin study(27) the grade of healing has been measured from vascular deprivation-induced necrosis of the femoral head in rats exposed to hyperbaric oxygen environment, comparing that with the recovery in the untreated ones. The experimental evidence was that newly formed appositional and intramembranous bone was more abundant in the femoral heads of the hyperbaric oxygen-treated rats, and the remodeling phase was more advanced in the rats belonging to the treated group; a smaller amount of necrotic debris in the femoral heads of the treated rats was also noted. There were no observational differences, on the contrary, as per the severity of the degenerative changes in the articular cartilage, and, moreover, the exposure of rats to hyperbaric oxygen does not seem capable of preserving tissue viability after complete exclusion of all those arteries supplying the femoral head. It appears that increased oxygen availability and higher tension in O_2 in tissues created the optimal environment for reparative processes.(27)

Regarding therapeutic options, there are many studies on animals suffering from AVNFH, and each of them tries to reproduce some specific aspect of the wide range of situations that we can find in AVNFH patients (level of lesions, etiologic and pathogenic mechanism). There are also animal studies about the use of medication such as enoxaparin or vascular endothelial factor (to stimulate local revascularization) or zoledronic acid (to decrease osteoclastic activity).

Glucocorticoid-related osteonecrosis shows itself as apoptosis-related, or even depending, therefore differing from the vessel-deprivation-induced tissue coagulation, as usually found in the idiopathic presentation of osteonecrosis. In the glucocorticoid-treated osteoblasts, the quantities of both alpha-TNF and RANK-ligand and osteoprotegerin are upregulated, freezing the osteoclast differentiation.

Nevertheless, it has been observed that a long period under glucocorticoid medication leads to apoptotic behavior in the osteoblasts and osteocytes of the femoral cortex.(8)

Particular mention to the role of the hyperbaric oxygenation in the treatment of vascular deprivation-induced osteonecrosis of the femoral head when HBO_2 is paired to a non-weight-bearing (NWB) approach: in rats, it has been observed to induce the preservation of the femoral heads, and the HBO_2-treated animals demonstrated a well-regenerated hematopoietic tissue. The decrease in the tendency towards FH deformation in the HBO_2-treated group might be a reliable predictor of a general better function of the hip joint.(32)

PATIENT SELECTION FOR HBO_2

The use of HBO_2 therapy when treating osteonecrosis of the femur head has now shifted from clinical evidence and inspirational vision to an evidence-supported treatment option. In fact, HBO_2 therapy has been documented to have a success rate of 81% at seven-year follow-up as compared to only 17% for patients in the control group.[34,45] Interestingly, Vezzani and colleagues, in their retrospective study on AVFNH enrolled from 2004 to 2013 and treated with HBO_2 for one year, showed that upon the therapy about 90% of FICAT I and II patients and half of FICAT III patients had no more need of surgery and remain pain free at four-year follow-up.[45] Another important aspect of HBO_2 is that it is a safe and effective therapy that can be administered in association with several physical treatments to the patients with ANFH.[45] There are numerous physiological and/or pharmacological benefits to HBO_2 therapy: reduction in the edematous component of a lesion, better tissue oxygenation, and the possibility of restoring a venous drainage both recovering the affected bone district (due to a progressive and sharp decrease in the intraosseous pressure) and improving local microcirculation (thanks to an increased angiogenesis).

While there is no significance in the hypothesized joint effect of alendronate and hyperbaric oxygen over ESWT in the literature, there is moderate to strong evidence that HBO_2 therapy is a feasible and efficient treatment modality for Ficat stage I–II FHN and in the earliest stages of hip necrosis, especially when applied with adjunctive fenestration drilling or other intervention of core decompression.

CURRENT PROTOCOL

In Italy, AVNFH is included in the accepted indication with 1Tx/day, 5–6 days/week, ≥ 60 minutes $FiO_2 = 1$, 60 ÷ 90 Tx at an average bathymetry in the range 2.2÷2.5 ATA. Also, the total number of treatments applied to these cases (60 ÷ 90 Tx according to the "Italian Guidelines to HBO_2 Therapy") appears to be very close to Tx gross average in those studies we analyzed: ≈ 70 Tx.

COST IMPACT

Considering the average price/Tx usually applied in Italy as ≈ 100 €/Tx, the average cost per patient appears to be about 8,000 to 9,000 euros. This cost appears reasonable if we compared the amount to the direct and indirect costs related to one or more THA interventional procedures.

CONCLUSIONS AND RECOMMENDATION ON THE BASIS OF PREVIOUS STUDIES

Based on published studies, at the initial stages of FHN we recommend a daily treatment with HBO_2 of ≥ 60 minutes at $FiO_2 = 1$ (5 to 6 days a week, and 4–5 weeks per cycle) at 2.4 ± 2.5 ATA.

The therapy should be applied together with all those adjuvant resources that could accelerate the recovery such as the following: minimize weight bearing (crutch adequate as per height and contralateral to the lesion), ameliorate body mass index (BMI), do physical therapies where applicable, and quit smoking so not to reduce the efficacy of the treatment.

In order to monitor the course of the therapy, we suggest scheduling MRI and orthopaedic clinical evaluation at 3–4 weeks from the end of the HBO_2 cycle.

REFERENCES

1. Aaron RK, Gray R. Osteonecrosis: etiology, natural history, pathophysiology, and diagnosis. In: The adult hip. Philadelphia: Lippincott Williams & Wilkins; 2007. p. 465-76.
2. Agarwala S, Shah SB. Ten-year follow-up of avascular necrosis of femoral head treated with alendronate for 3 years. J Arthroplasty. 2011;26:1128-34.
3. Al Hadi H (sic), Smerdon GR, Fox SW. Hyperbaric oxygen therapy accelerates osteoblast differentiation and promotes bone formation. J Dent. 2015;43(3):382-8.
4. Al Hadi H (sic), Smerdon GR, Fox SW. Hyperbaric oxygen therapy suppresses osteoclast formation and bone resorption. J Orthop Res. 2013;31(11):1839-44.
5. Amanatullah DF, Strauss EJ, Di Cesare PE. Current management options for osteonecrosis of the femoral head: part 1, diagnosis and nonoperative management. Am J Orthop (Belle Mead NJ). 2011;40(9):E186-92.
6. Bauer TW, Stulberg BN. The histology of osteonecrosis and its distinction from histologic artefacts. In: Bone circulation and vascularisation in normal and pathological conditions. New York: Plenum Press; 1993. p. 283-92.
7. Baixe JH et al. Treatment of the osteonecrosis of the femoral head by hyperbaric oxygen. Bull MEDSUBYHP. 1969;1:2.
8. Bejar J, Peled E, Boss JH. Vasculature deprivation-induced osteonecrosis of the rat femoral head as a model for therapeutic trials. Theor Biol Med Model. 2005;5(2):24.
9. Boettcher WG, Bonfiglio M, Hamilton HH, Sheets RF, Smith K. Non-traumatic necrosis of the femoral head – part I. Relation of altered hemostasis to etiology. J Bone Joint Surg Am. 1970;52(2):312-21.
10. Brinker MR, Rosenberg AG, Kull L, Galante JO. Primary hip arthroplasty using non cemented porous-coated femoral components in patients with osteonecrosis of femoral head. J Arthroplasty. 1994;9:457.
11. Brown TD, Baker KJ, Brand RA. Structural consequences of subchondral bone involvement in segmental osteonecrosis of the femoral head. J Orthop Res. 1992;10(1):79-8.
12. Camporesi EM, Bosco G. Mechanisms of action of hyperbaric oxygen therapy. Undersea Hyperb Med. 2014;41(3):247-52.
13. Camporesi EM, Vezzani G, Bosco G, Mangar D, Bernasek TL. Hyperbaric oxygen therapy in femoral head necrosis. J Arthroplasty. 2010;25(6 Suppl).
14. CDC/NCHS National Hospital Discharge Survey, 2000–2010.
15. Chen CH et al. Alendronate in the prevention of collapse of the femoral head in nontraumatic osteonecrosis: a two-year multicenter, prospective, randomized, double-blind, placebo-controlled study. Arthritis Rheum. 2014;64:1572-8.
16. Deveci A, Fırat A, Yılmaz S, Ünal KO, Tecimel O, Bozkurt M, Atabey M. Treatment of femoral head osteonecrosis with core decompression and subsequent hyperbaric oxygen therapy. Cumhuriyet Med J. 2013;35:231-8.
17. Freiberger JJ, Padilla-Burgos R, McGraw T, Suliman HB, Kraft KH, Stolp BW, Moon RE, Piantadosi CA. What is the role of hyperbaric oxygen in the management of bisphosphonate-related osteonecrosis of the jaw: a randomized controlled trial of hyperbaric oxygen as an adjunct to surgery and antibiotics. J Oral Maxillofac Surg. 2012;70(7):1573-83.
18. Grimaud E, Soubigou L, Couillaud S, Coipeau P, Moreau A, Passuti N, et al. Receptor activator of nuclear factor kappaB ligand (RANKL)/osteoprotegerin (OPG) ratio is increased in severe osteolysis. Am J Pathol. 2003;163(5):2021-31.

19. Hadi HA, Smerdon G, Fox SW. Osteoclastic resorptive capacity is suppressed in patients receiving hyperbaric oxygen therapy. Acta Orthop. 2015 Apr;86(2):264–9.

20. Herndon JH, Aufranc OE. Avascular necrosis of the femoral head in the adult: a review of its incidence in a variety of conditions. Clin Orthop Relat Res. 1972;86:43-62.

21. Hsu SL, Wang CJ, Lee MS, Chan YS, Huang CC, Yang KD. Cocktail therapy for femoral head necrosis of the hip. Arch Orthop Trauma Surg. 2010;130(1):23-9.

22. Hungerford DS. Bone marrow pressure, venography and core decompression in ischemic necrosis of the femoral head. In: The hip: proceedings of the 7th Open Scientific Meeting of the Hip Society. St Louis (MO): Mosby; 1979. p. 218-37.

23. Jergesen HE, Khan AS. The natural history of untreated asymptomatic hips in patients who have non-traumatic osteonecrosis. J Bone Joint Surg Am. 1997;79:359-63.

24. Kataoka Y, Hasegawa Y, Iwata H, Matsuda T, Genda E, Miura T, Takahashi H. Effect of hyperbaric oxygenation on femoral head osteonecrosis in spontaneously hypertensive rats. Acta Orthop Scand. 1992;63(5):527-30.

25. Kiaer T, Pedersen NW, Kristensen KD, Starklint H. Intra-osseous pressure and oxygen tension in avascular necrosis and osteoarthritis of the hip. J Bone Joint Surg. 1990;72(6):1023-30.

26. Koren L, Ginesin E, Melamed Y, Norman D, Levin D, Peled E. Hyperbaric oxygen for stage I and II femoral head necrosis. Orthopedics. 2015;38(3):200-5.

27. Levin D, Norman D, Zinman C, Rubinstein L, Sabo E, Misselevich I, Reis D, Boss JH. Treatment of experimental avascular necrosis of the femoral head with hyperbaric oxygen in rats: histological evaluation of the femoral heads during the early phase of the reparative process. Exp Mol Pathol. 1999;67(2):99-108.

28. Lieberman JR, Berry DJ, Mont MA, Aaron RK, Callaghan JJ, Rajadhyaksha AD, Urbaniak JR. Osteonecrosis of the hip: management in the 21st century. Instr Course Lect. 2003;52:337-55.

29. Lin SS, Ueng SW, Niu CC, Yuan LJ, Yang CY, Chen WJ, Lee MS, Chen JK. Effects of hyperbaric oxygen on the osteogenic differentiation of mesenchymal stem cells. BMC Musculoskelet Disord. 2014 Feb 25;15:56

30. Mwale F, Wang H, Johnson AJ, Mont MA, Antoniou J. Abnormal vascular endothelial growth factor expression in mesenchymal stem cells from both osteonecrotic and osteoarthritic hips. Bull NYU Hosp Jt Dis. 2011;69:S56-61.

31. Musso ES, Mitchell SN, Schink-Ascani M, Bassett CA. Results of conservative management of osteonecrosis of the femoral head. A retrospective review. Clin Orthop Relat Res. 1986;207:209-15.

32. Peskin B, Shupak A, Levin D, Norman D, Jacob Z, Boss JF, Misselevich I, Reis DN, Zinman C. Effects of non-weight bearing and hyperbaric oxygen therapy in vascular deprivation-induced osteonecrosis of the rat femoral head. Undersea Hyperb Med. 2001;28(4):187-94.

33. Pritchett JW. Statin therapy decreases the risk of osteonecrosis in patients receiving steroids. Clin Orthop Relat Res. 2001;386:173-8.

34. Reis ND, Schwartz O, Militianu D, Ramon Y, Levin D, Norman D, Melamed Y, Shupak A, Goldsher D, Zinman C. Hyperbaric oxygen therapy as a treatment for stage-I avascular necrosis of the femoral head. J Bone Joint Surg Br. 2003;85(3):371-5.

35. Samara S, Dailiana Z, Chassanidis C, Koromila T, Papatheodorou L, Malizos KN, Kollia P. Expression profile of osteoprotegerin, RANK and RANKL genes in the femoral head of patients with avascular necrosis. Exp Mol Pathol. 2014;96(1):9-14.

36. Schroer WC. Current concepts on the pathogenesis of osteonecrosis of the femoral head. Orthop Rev. 1994;23(6):487-97.

37. Schmitt-Sody M, Kirchoff C, Mayer W, Goebel M, Jansson V. Avascular necrosis of the femoral head: inter and intraobserver variations of Ficat and ARCO classifications. Int Orthop. 2008;32:283-7.

38. Shah KN, Racine J, Jones LC, Aaron RK. Pathophysiology and risk factors for osteonecrosis. Curr Rev Musculoskelet Med. 2015;8:201-9.

39. Solacoff D, Mont MA, Krackow KA. Uncemented total hip arthroplasty in patients less than 45 years with avascular necrosis. Orthop Trans. 1994;17:1085.

40. Strauss MB, Dvorak T, Melamed Y, Reis DN. Femoral head necrosis and hyperbaric oxygen therapy. In: Hyperbaric medicine practice. Flagstaff (AZ): Best Publishing Co.; 2008. p. 943-4.

41. Stulberg BN, Levine M, Bauer TW, Belhobek GH, Pflanze W, Feiglin DH, Roth AI. Multimodality approach to osteonecrosis of the femoral head. Clin Orthop. 1989;240:181.

42. Thom SR. Hyperbaric oxygen: its mechanisms and efficacy. Plast Reconstr Surg. 2011;127(Suppl 1):131S-141S.

43. Tripathy SK, Goyal T, Sen RK. Management of femoral head osteonecrosis: current concepts. Indian J Orthop. 2015;49(1):28-45.

44. Uguen M, Pougnet R, Uguen A, Loddé B, Dewitte JD. Dysbaric osteonecrosis among professional divers: a literature review. Undersea Hyperb Med. 2014;41(6):579-87.

45. Vezzani G, Camporesi E, Mangar D, Bernasek T, Yang Z, Quartesan S, Rizzato A, Bosco G. Beneficial effect of hyperbaric oxygenation in avascular necrosis of the femoral head. Minerva Anestesiol. Forthcoming 2017.

46. Vezzani G, Quartesan S, Cancellara P, Camporesi E, Mangar D, Bernasek T, Dalvi P, Yang Z, Paoli A, Rizzato A, Bosco G. Hyperbaric oxygen therapy modulates serum OPG/RANKL in femoral head necrosis patients. J Enzyme Inhib Med Chem. Forthcoming 2017.

47. Wang J, Wang K, Shi Z, Zhang M. Osteoprotegerin mRNA/receptor activator of NF-kappaB ligand mRNA expressions in bone tissues of glucocorticoid-induced osteonecrosis of the femoral head. Zhongguo Xiu Fu Chong Jian Wai Ke Za Zhi. 2008;22(10):1161-4.

48. Wong T, Wang CJ, Hsu SL, Chou WY, Lin PC, Huang CC. Cocktail therapy for hip necrosis in SARS patients. Chang Gung Med J. 2008;31(6):546-53.

49. Zhao FC, Li ZR, Zhang NF, Wang BL, Sun W, Cheng LM, Liu ZH. Lesion size changes in osteonecrosis of the femoral head: a long-term prospective study using MRI. Int Orthop. 2010;34(6):799-804.

CHAPTER 35 CHAPTER

Use of Adjunctive Hyperbaric Oxygen in the Management of Invasive Fungal Infections

CHAPTER THIRTY-FIVE OVERVIEW

Introduction **883**
Pathophysiology and Rationale for Hyperbaric Oxygen **883**
In Vitro Studies **884**
Animal Studies **884**
Clinical Experience **885**
Mucormycosis 885
Aspergillosis 888
Other 889
Candidiobolus Coronato *889*
Coccidioidmycosis *889*
Pseudosallescheria Boydii *889*
Summary **890**
References **891**

Use of Adjunctive Hyperbaric Oxygen in the Management of Invasive Fungal Infections

Lisardo Garcia-Covarrubias, Diana M. Barratt

INTRODUCTION

Invasive fungal infections (IFIs) are difficult to treat and often fatal in immunocompromised patients, diabetics, and trauma patients. The management of these infections includes antifungal medications, treatment of the underlying or predisposing disease, and surgical debridement. However, in spite of the advancements in new antifungal medications, the morbidity and mortality remain unacceptably high. Hyperbaric oxygen has been advocated as an adjunct to treat IFIs – mainly mucormycosis and aspergillosis. In this chapter, we review the most relevant evidence, including bench and clinical studies on the use of hyperbaric oxygen in IFIs.

PATHOPHYSIOLOGY AND RATIONALE FOR HYPERBARIC OXYGEN

Typically, the fungus enters the body through the respiratory tract. Local proliferation can lead to invasion of the tissues and blood vessels, resulting in hypoxia, hemorrhagic infarction, necrosis, and potential hematogenous extension to distal sites.(28) The hypoxic/acidotic conditions compromise antifungal action and may promote spread of the infection.(7)

Phagocytes, particularly macrophages and neutrophils, play a major role in controlling fungal infections.(42) Their fungicidal activity is mediated by means of different oxygen intermediates; their killing capacity is directly proportional to available oxygen.(33,43)

Sokol-Anderson and colleagues reported that under hypoxic conditions, amphotericin B's (AMB's) fungicidal capacity is reduced as much as 80% compared with normoxic conditions.(39)

Hyperbaric oxygenation elevates oxygen levels in severely hypoxic tissue and has an additive effect when combined with AMB.(23,37) In addition, pulmonary alveolar macrophages' fungicidal activity to *Neurospora crassa* is augmented when exposed to 100% oxygen.(38)

IN VITRO STUDIES

In vitro studies have shown a lag phase in the growth curve of *Candida albicans*, *Aspergillus fumigatus*, and *Mucor.* when exposed to high partial pressures of oxygen.[8,23] Fungicidal activity was achieved using 10 ATA for 28 days.[9] Furthermore, the addition of HBO_2 in presence of AMB exhibited an additive effect on the growth of *Candida albicans.*[23] Sokol-Anderson and colleagues showed that hypoxia severely decreases AMB fungicidal action. Another relevant issue mentioned by these authors was the oxidative antifungal mechanism of AMB. This was elegantly demonstrated by means of combining AMB with catalase and superoxide dismutase, two biological antioxidants, resulting in a significant decrease in the AMB fungicidal activity.[39] Obviously, some of the pressures and lengths of treatment used in the above in vitro studies are incompatible with human life. However, they shed light on the potential application of hyperbaric oxygen in human mycoses.

ANIMAL STUDIES

To our knowledge, there are only two animal studies that have looked at the effect of hyperbaric oxygen in IFIs. The first one, by Barratt and colleagues,[3] was a prospective, randomized, placebo-controlled animal trial designed to determine whether the addition of HBO_2 (2.0 ATA/2 hours BID) to AMB improved survival function in mice with zygomycosis. Infection was induced by injection of *Rhizopus arrhizus* via the tail vein and ethmoid sinus. Prior to the inoculation, mice received intraperitoneal deferoxamine as a predisposing agent for the infection. Next, the animals were randomized as follows: HBO_2/AMB, Air/AMB, and No Treatment. On day 14, survivors were euthanized. Histopathology was performed on 5 brains from the No Treatment animals that died prior to day 14. Survival was as follows: HBO_2/AMB – 42% (21/50), Air/AMB – 46% (22/48), and No Treatment – 31% (15/48). Histopathology revealed branching hyphae in 100% (5/5) of brains. Analysis of survival function (Wilcoxon test) did not demonstrate a significant difference between the HBO_2/AMB and Air/AMB groups ($p = 0.72$). Treatment with either HBO_2/AMB ($p = 0.01$) or Air/AMB ($p = 0.067$) improved survival function over No Treatment by reducing the initial death rate and increasing the survival rate. However, only HBO_2/AMB significantly improved survival function over No Treatment. The authors concluded that the addition of hyperbarics to amphotericin B did not improve survival function over amphotericin B and air.

The second study was by García-Covarrubias and colleagues.[17] In this study, mice were administered intraperitoneal cyclophosphamide to induce immunosuppression before tail-vein injection of *Rhizopus arrhizus.* The animals received AMB in addition to HBO_2. Based on the lack of significant improvement using a pressure of 2 ATA,[3] this study increased the pressure to 2.5 ATA. Each HBO_2 treatment consisted of a 90-minute session. After inoculation, the animals were randomly placed in one of the following groups: AMB plus HBO_2 group (N = 30), AMB group (N = 31), and Control group (N = 22). Three HBO_2 treatments were administered during the first 24 hours after inoculation, followed by twice daily from day 2 to day 6. Thereafter HBO_2 was administered on a daily basis until day 14 post inoculation, for a total of 21 HBO_2 treatments. AMB group (N = 31) received AMB only. Cages of this group were transported to the HBO_2 room along with cages of group number 1 (N = 30) to assure that both groups were exposed to the same stress, temperature, and light intensity. Control group (N = 22) received no treatment. Mice were monitored for 14 days, and time to death was recorded. On day 14, survivors were euthanized, and kidney colony-forming units (CFUs) were assessed. Deaths in all groups began to occur between days four and five post-inoculation. All animals in the control group had died by day nine. Fifteen days after inoculation, survival rate was 40% (12/30) in the HBO_2-AMB group versus 35.4% (11/31) in the AMB group. This difference in favor of the HBO_2-AMB group was not sufficient to achieve statistical significance. Regarding the colony counts, the HBO_2-AMB group showed a slightly lower number (718.5 cfu/gr) compared with the AMB group (799.9 cfu/gr). However, this difference was not significant ($p = 0.92$).

It is important to note that, although neither of the animal studies showed a significant benefit from HBO_2, the models do not replicate the typical clinical scenario. The infection induced in the mice was severely disseminated, and a main component of the standard of care, namely surgical debridement, was lacking. Clearly a better model is needed to further assess the impact of HBO_2 in IFIs. Another limitation of the above studies is that amphotericin B, which was the standard of care at the time, was utilized. Due to less toxicity, the liposomal formulation of amphotericin B is now recommended.

CLINICAL EXPERIENCE

Most of the clinical series on the use of HBO_2 in IFIs deal with its application to mucormycosis. Garcia-Covarrubias et al. reported a small series on aspergillosis, and more recently Segal et al.[36] published a retrospective study from the University of Iowa Hospital and Clinics including two patients with aspergillosis and 12 with mucormycosis. Most of the patients were immunocompromised from hematologic and neoplastic disorders. All patients received standard antifungal medications and HBO_2; surgical debridement was performed in only 13 patients. HBO_2 sessions varied from one to 44; sessions were for 90 minutes at 2 ATA with three 10-minute breaks. The authors reported a 50% survival rate and pointed out the lack of strong evidence to support HBO_2 in the management of IFIs. Reports of treatment on other invasive fungi are so few as to be almost anecdotal. A few of these reports are included in this chapter.

Mucormycosis

The term mucormycosis encompasses a rare group of necrotizing infections caused by fungi belonging to the order of the Mucorales.[40] *Rhizopus* species are responsible for 70% of rhino-orbital-cerebral mucormycosis (ROCM).[44] This infection occurs most commonly in the immunocompromised host. The typical patient profile is that of a poorly controlled diabetic with ketoacidosis. Other common comorbidities include hematologic malignancies, organ and bone marrow transplantation, end-stage renal disease with concurrent deferoxamine administration, major burns, and severe trauma.[10-11]

This order of fungi has the ability to invade blood vessels, with infections localizing at a variety of anatomic sites.[26] In its most common forms, ROCM and pulmonary mucormycosis, inhalation is the natural route of infection. However, traumatic implantation has been described, specifically with the organism *Apophysomyces elegans*.[32]

Apophysomyces elegans is an interesting species as it typically infects previously healthy individuals, and the mechanism of infection is traumatic. García-Covarrubias and colleagues[20] reported a case of a 24-year-old, previously healthy male who sustained severe craniofacial trauma secondary to a motorcycle accident. Initial management was complicated by a right-forehead necrotizing infection requiring right orbital exenteration due to its poor response to antibiotics. *Apophysomyces elegans* was identified as the culprit. The patient was successfully managed with a multidisciplinary approach including liposomal amphotericin B, surgery, hyperbaric oxygenation, and granulocyte colony-stimulating factor (G-CSF). In the same article, the authors reviewed 20 more cases of mucormycosis secondary to *A. elegans,* confirming the fact that the majority of these individuals were previously healthy and infected by a traumatic mechanism.

Prior to 1960, ROCM was almost uniformly fatal.[16] In 1980, Blitzer and colleagues[6] reviewed the English-language literature, analyzing 179 cases. The overall mortality was 50%; a 70% survival was noted in cases reported from 1970 to 1979. This improved survival in later years was, perhaps, related to the increased use of amphotericin B and radical surgery. However, as the authors of this review pointed out, these mortality figures are likely to be inaccurate because of the inclusion of case reports that appear to have been written only because the patient survived. Seventy percent of the survivors had significant residual defects such as blindness, cranial nerve palsies, hemiplegia, ophthalmoplegia, or significant cosmetic defects.

When cerebral extension occurs, a high fatality rate persists, in spite of the use of radical surgery and amphotericin B.[1,29,34] Price and Stevens[35] reported a successful outcome in a case of extensive cerebral mucormycosis.

Ferguson and colleagues[15] reviewed 12 patients with rhinocerebral mucormycosis treated with surgery and amphotericin B from 1969 to 1988. Of the six patients treated with amphotericin B and surgical debridement, without adjunctive HBO_2, prior to 1983, four died as a direct result of fungal infection. Of the six patients treated with surgery, amphotericin B, and adjunctive hyperbaric oxygen therapy, two died, with one of these exhibiting improving mucormycosis, related to a difference in the aggressiveness of the use of amphotericin, medical therapy, or surgery.

Couch and colleagues[13] reported two patients with rhinocerebral mucormycosis with brain mucor abscesses, clinical deterioration, and progression of infection, despite aggressive surgical debridement, amphotericin therapy, and medical control of the underlying diabetic acidosis. Both patients exhibited significant clinical improvement coincident with the addition of adjunctive HBO_2 therapy. Treatments were at 2.5 ATA for 90 minutes, 6 days a week. One patient received a total of 79 HBO_2 treatments; the other received 85 such treatments. No complications of treatment were encountered, and the patients remained free of disease 21 months after hospital discharge. The survival of these patients is particularly noteworthy since both had intracerebral mucor abscesses, with one having total occlusion of an internal carotid artery – complications that had formerly resulted invariably in death. One patient was reported as doing well with only residual blindness, having had to undergo debridement of an orbit. The second patient was reported as being fully alert, ambulatory, and capable of self-care, with only a short-term memory deficit.

Noting that survival is uncommon in bilateral cerebro-rhino-orbital mucormycosis, De La Paz and colleagues[14] achieved eradication of the infection in a 66-year-old diabetic, using HBO_2 combined with bilateral orbital exenteration and amphotericin B. The patient was well one-and-a-half years later.

Melero and colleagues[30] reported a 16-month remission in a diabetic patient with rhino-sinuso-orbital disease who had maintained an active infection despite two debridements and amphotericin B. Further debridement with adjunctive HBO_2 halted the infection.

Okhuysen and colleagues[32] reported a case of a previously healthy man who presented with severe cutaneous and renal mucormycosis due to *A. elegans*. The patient was successfully treated with liposomal amphotericin B, HBO_2, and interferon-gamma, obviating the need for nephrectomy.

Yohai and colleagues[44] reviewed 208 cases in the literature since 1970, 139 of which were presented in sufficient detail to assess factors prognostic for survival. To those were added data from six of their own patients. The histories of those 145 patients were analyzed for the following variables: 1) underlying conditions associated with mucormycotic infections, 2) incidents of ocular and orbital signs and symptoms, 3) incidence of nonocular signs and symptoms, 4) interval from symptom onset to treatment, and 5) the pattern of sinus involvement seen on imaging studies and noted at the time of surgery. Factors related to a lower survival rate include 1) delayed diagnosis and treatment, 2) hemiparesis or hemiplegia, 3) bilateral sinus involvement, 4) leukemia, 5) renal disease, and 6) treatment with deferoxamine. Facial necrosis fell just short of statistical significance but appears clinically important. Hyperbaric oxygen was found to have a favorable effect on prognosis.

García-Covarrubias and colleagues[19] reported a small chart review of mucormycosis patients referred to the HBO_2 service of their institution. Five mucormycosis patients referred for HBO_2 had complete charts available. Four had craniofacial involvement, and one had left upper extremity involvement. The predisposing diseases were leukemia (n = 3), diabetes mellitus plus sarcoidosis (n = 1), and trauma (n = 1). All patients were managed with amphotericin B, surgical debridement, and HBO_2. Survival was 60% (3⁄5) three months after the diagnosis was established. The literature was scarce but favors HBO_2. The authors concluded that, considering the pathophysiology of mucormycosis, adjuvant HBO_2 therapy seems reasonable. However, they acknowledge that the clinical experience is too limited to make HBO_2 part of the standard of care and that prospective, randomized controlled trials will help to define the role of HBO_2 in this devastating infection.

More recently, John BV, Chamilos G, and Kontoyiannis DP[24] reviewed 28 published cases of mucormycosis. Seventeen patients were diabetic, some with ketoacidosis. Five patients had trauma-induced mucormycosis, three had hematological malignancies, two alcoholic liver disease, one was receiving systemic corticosteroids, and three had no known factors for mucormycosis. Most HBO_2 sessions were twice a day lasting 90–120 minutes at a pressure of 2–3 ATA. The median number of sessions was 22 (range 2–85). In most patients, HBO_2 was given after surgical debridement and amphotericin B. Overall survival rate was 86%, with a survival rate among diabetic patients of 94%. Two of the three patients with malignancies died. The authors noted a higher survival rate in patients with correctable predisposing conditions, such as diabetes and trauma, rather than hematological malignancies or bone marrow transplant patients which are associated with a higher mortality rate.

Recommendations for treatment of patients with mucormycosis follow.

All patients should receive standard clinical care including appropriate therapy to control the underlying primary disease, antifungal therapy with either liposomal amphotericin B or amphotericin B lipid complex,[41] and surgical debridement. Recent guidelines from the European Society for Clinical Microbiology and Infectious Diseases and the European Confederation of Medical Mycology support adjunctive HBO_2 in the treatment of mucormycosis with marginal strength only.[12]

Some have suggested that only those patients who exhibit progression of the disease in spite of adequate conventional therapy should be considered for hyperbaric treatment. However, in many cases, the disease is rapidly progressive with extensive intracranial and orbital invasion, despite "adequate" treatment. This, plus the high morbidity and mortality of the disease, indicates that adjunctive HBO_2 could be considered in any patient with invasive mucormycosis.

Based on limited experience reported in the literature, HBO_2 therapy is commonly administered at pressures from 2.0 to 2.5 atmospheres for 90 minutes to 2 hours, with 1 to 2 exposures daily. The optimal duration of treatment with HBO_2 has not been studied prospectively and is generally unknown. Previous reports have suggested 40 treatments to achieve eradication in the usual case; however, up to 80 treatments have been used in the past. Determining the end point may be difficult if the patient becomes asymptomatic, as there is always the fear of stopping too soon and having the patient suffer a recurrence that may be more difficult to eradicate. Nevertheless, fungal cultures obtained from biopsy and the clinical condition of the patient must govern one's judgment.

Aspergillosis

This fungal organism is widespread in nature and usually does not cause disease in healthy individuals; however, it is responsible for opportunistic infections in immunocompromised patients. Invasive aspergillosis is an important cause of morbidity and mortality in hematopoietic stem cell transplant recipients, solid organ transplant recipients, and those with cancer or hematological malignancies. Despite the recent advances in antifungal therapy, morbidity and mortality from invasive aspergillosis in hematopoietic stem cell transplant and solid organ transplant recipients remains unacceptably high. In the Transplant Associated Infection Surveillance Network, the most common clinical presentations were pulmonary, disseminated, and CNS.[(2)]

Oxygen levels are often decreased in the infected tissue of patients with aspergillosis, as this fungus invades blood vessels, causing obstruction, thrombosis, and hypoxia.[(4)] This hypoxic environment results in tissue necrosis, diminishes the oxidative antifungal effect of amphotericin B, and impairs the oxidative killing capacity and phagocytosis of white cells.[(5,33,39)]

There have been few reported cases of invasive aspergillosis treated with hyperbaric oxygen. A case of aspergillosis in the right temporomandibular joint with a history of parotid carcinoma and post-irradiation otitis was reported. Previous treatment attempts with surgery and antibiotics were unsuccessful. Radical debridement of the glenoid fossae, supplemented with amphotericin B and adjunct HBO_2 therapy, successfully resolved the symptoms.[(27)] Price and Stevens[(35)] reported treating invasive aspergillosis with hyperbaric oxygen as a last resort, with success.

The largest experience in this area was reported by García-Covarrubias and colleagues.[(18)] A retrospective study of all the patients with histologic specimens suggestive of invasive aspergillosis referred to a hyperbaric medicine unit located in a large county hospital was conducted. The main assessment of outcome was survival three months after initiation of HBO_2. The study included 10 immunocompromised patients with rhino-sinusinal infection. All patients were managed with AMB, surgery, and HBO_2. In addition, throughout the HBO_2 course four patients received granulocyte colony-stimulating factor (G-CSF), and one patient received granulocyte infusions. The mean time between the onset of symptoms and initiation of AMB was 10.6 days, whereas for HBO_2 initiation, it was 44.1 days. HBO_2 treatments were administered at a pressure of 2 ATA (atmospheres absolute) for 90 minutes. Patients received an average of 19.8 hyperbaric treatments. Complications from HBO_2 included seizures in one patient, mild shortness of breath in two patients, and mild confinement anxiety in one patient. Six patients were alive three months after initiation of HBO_2 therapy. The authors noted that the delay in initiating HBO_2 seemed to indicate that it was utilized as a last resort in most of the patients.

A limitation of the above studies is that they involved the use of amphotericin B, which was the standard of care at the time. Due to toxicity and decreased efficacy, amphotericin B deoxycholate is no longer recommended for use. Voriconazole and isavuconazole are now recommended for first-line treatment of invasive aspergillosis in leukemia and hematopoietic stem cell transplant patients.[41]

The limited experience with HBO_2 and invasive aspergillosis precludes strong recommendations. Nevertheless, on the basis of the pathophysiology of invasive fungal infections and sound physiological principles of HBO_2, prompt initiation of HBO_2 appears reasonable in patients with either overwhelming rhinocerebral fungal infections or host compromise.

The protocol used in García-Covarrubias' report was 10 to 20 initial treatments of 90 minutes at 2.0 to 2.5 ATA, followed by reassessment of the patients' condition. Patients were initially treated every eight hours during the first day and twice a day thereafter. A five minute air break was given every 25 minutes. Once the patient's condition stabilized, once-a-day treatments were given until no further evidence of fungal infection was noted. Higher pressures (2.5 to 3.0 ATA) are used for necrotizing soft-tissue infections such as gas gangrene and necrotizing fasciitis. However, because of the common involvement of the CNS, the treatment benefit of higher pressures for invasive fungal infections must be weighed against the risk of oxygen toxicity seizures.

Other

Candidiobolus Coronato

This extremely rare disorder is caused by another order of Phycomycetes family, the Entomophthorales. But unlike mucormycosis, the lesions caused by these organisms do not cause vascular thrombi or extensive necrosis. Nathan et al. reported the successful eradication of the disease in an otherwise healthy bulldozer operator who had the invasive rhinocerebral form but was very intolerant to amphotericin B.[31] He had been pursuing a downhill course. He received 51 HBO_2 treatments at 2.4 ATA for 90 minutes daily, following a partial maxillectomy and resection of a zygomatic fungoma. This was accompanied by amphotericin B therapy of only 5 to 10 mg per day. He received a total of 1510 mg of the drug. Three weeks after the first surgery, re-exploration revealed no evidence of new necrosis or infection.

Coccidioidmycosis

This disorder, also termed San Joaquin Valley fever, is usually a self-limited respiratory disease, but in the chronic form it can produce cavitation or granuloma ("coin lesion") formation. In endemic areas, people who are exposed for many years may develop the more ominous progressive form with spread to the bones, joints, viscera, skin, brain, and meninges. The fatality rate in the progressive form is 55% to 60%. Therapy is with amphotericin B and ketoconazole. Prolonged intrathecal therapy may be necessary for meningeal involvement. Price and Stevens[35] have reported fulminant coccidioidmycosis to respond to HBO_2 when it has been given as "last resort."

Pseudosallescheria Boydii

Granström and colleagues[21] reported eradication of this organism in a 62-year-old diabetic who suffered from an ear-canal and mastoid infection of the temporal bone for over two years. The CT scan was normal, but the patient developed paralysis of the 5th and 9th cranial nerves. Surgical exploration revealed the mastoid cavity to be filled with granulation tissue containing microabscesses. A scintigram of the external bony part of the auditory canal showed increased uptake. Despite antibacterial antibiotics, the patient's condition deteriorated. Nine months following the initial surgery, a technetium scan revealed increased uptake in the temporal bone, and a CT scan confirmed involvement of the pterygoid apex. Cerebrospinal fluid (CSF) analysis indicated blood-brain barrier damage with leukocytosis. Cultures from the external canal finally yielded *P. boydii*. Oral itraconazole (a congener of ketoconazole) was given for one year. HBO_2 therapy, at 2.4 ATA for 90 minutes, was then conducted daily for 60 days. Following HBO_2, the technetium scan normalized, and repeated cultures were negative. A MRI scan indicated no spread of the infection in the soft tissues of the face. The CSF analysis returned to normal, and the patient remained disease-free one and a half years after diagnosis.

SUMMARY

Invasive fungal infections continue to pose a severe threat to the immunocompromised patient. Current standard of care includes control of the underlying condition, parenteral antifungal medications, and surgical debridement. Nevertheless, morbidity and mortality remain high. Other treatment modalities have been incorporated to the standard of care aiming at improving the poor outcome of these patients. The role of hyperbaric oxygen as an adjuvant therapy has been investigated in the lab and clinically. Results in animal models are somewhat limited because of the poor resemblance with the clinical picture. Case reports and small clinical series, mainly in mucormycosis and aspergillosis, suggest that HBO_2 may be beneficial. From the current evidence, we can also conclude that HBO_2 is not likely to be harmful in this setting. A better animal model and larger clinical studies are needed to better assess the role of HBO_2 in these devastating infections.

REFERENCES

1) Abedi E, Sismanis A, Choi K, et al. Twenty-five years' experience treating cerebro-rhino-orbital mucormycosis. Laryngoscope. 1984;94:1060-2.

2) Baddley JW, Andes DR, Marr KA, Kontoyiannis DP, Alexander BD, Kauffman CA, Oster RA, Anaissie EJ, Walsh TJ, Schuster MG, Wingard JR, Patterson TF, Ito JI, Williams OD, Chiller T, Pappas PG, and the Transplant Associated Infection Surveillance Network. Factors associated with mortality in transplant patients with invasive aspergillosis. Clin Infect Dis. 2010 Jun;50(12):1559-67.

3) Barratt DM, Van Meter K, Asmar P, et al. Hyperbaric oxygen as an adjunct in zygomycosis: randomized controlled trial in a murine model. Antimicrob Agents Chemother. 2001;45;3601-2.

4) Bennett JE. Aspergillus species. In: Mandell GL, Bennett JE, Dolin R, editors. Principles and practice of infectious diseases. 4th ed. New York: Churchill Livingstone; 1995. p. 2306-11.

5) Bjerknes R, Neslein IL, Myhre K, Andersen HT. Impairment of rat polymorphonuclear neutrophilic granulocyte phagocytosis following repeated hypobaric hypoxia. Aviat Space Environ Med. 1990;61:1007-11.

6) Blitzer A et al. Patient survival factors in paranasal sinus mucormycosis. Laryngoscope. 1980;90:635-48.

7) Bullen JJ, Roquers HJ, Spalding PB, et al. Natural resistance, iron and infection: a challenge for clinical medicine. J Med Microbiol. 2006 Mar;55:251-8.

8) Cairney WJ. Developmental effects of hyperbaric oxygen on selected human pathogenic fungi in culture [dissertation]. New York: Cornell University; 1977.

9) Caldwell J. Effects of high partial pressures of oxygen on fungi. Nature. 1963;197:772-4.

10) Cocanour CS, Miller-Crotchett P, Reed RL Jr, Johnson PC, Fischer RP. Mucormycosis in trauma patients. J Trauma. 1992;32:12-5.

11) Cooter RD, Lim IS, Ellis DH, Leitch IOW. Burn wound zygomycosis caused by Apophysomyces elegans. J Clin Microbiol. 1990;28:2151-3.

12) Cornely OA, Arikan-Akdagli S, Dannaoui E, et al. ESCMID and ECMM joint clinical guidelines for the diagnosis and management of mucormycosis 2013. Clin Microbiol Infect. 2014;20(Suppl 3):5-26.

13) Couch L, Theilen F, Mader JT. Rhinocerebral mucormycosis with cerebral extension successfully treated with adjunctive hyperbaric oxygen therapy. Arch Otolaryngol Head Neck Surg. 1988;114:791-4. 14) De La Paz MA, Patrinely JR, Marines HM, et al. Adjunctive hyperbaric oxygen in the treatment of bilateral cerebro-rhino-orbital mucormycosis. Am J Ophthalmol. 1992;114:208-11.

15) Ferguson BJ, Mitchell TG, Moon R, et al. Adjunctive hyperbaric oxygen for treatment of rhinocerebral mucormycosis. Rev Infect Dis. 1988;10:551-9.

16) Ferry AP. Cerebral mucormycosis (phycomycosis). Ocular findings and review of the literature. Surv Ophthalmol. 1961;6:1-24.

17) García-Covarrubias L, Barratt DM, Bartlett R, et al. Hyperbaric oxygen and amphotericin B in the management of mucormycosis: a randomized controlled trial in the murine model. Undersea Hyperb Med. 2002;29:141.

18) García-Covarrubias L, Barratt DM, Bartlett R, et al. Invasive aspergillosis treated with adjunctive hyperbaric oxygenation: a retrospective clinical series at a single institution. South Med J. 2002;95:450-6.

19) García-Covarrubias L, Barratt DM, Bartlett R, et al. Treatment of mucormycosis with adjunctive hyperbaric oxygen: five cases treated at the same institution and review of the literature. Rev Invest Clin. 2004;56:51-5.

20) García-Covarrubias L, Bartlett R, Barratt DM, et al. Rhino-orbitocerebral mucormycosis attributable to Apophysomyces elegans in an immunocompetent individual: case report and review of the literature. J Trauma. 2001;50:353-7.

21) Granström G, Hanner P, et al. Malignant external otitis caused by Pseudoallescheria boydii treated with hyperbaric oxygen [abstract]. Undersea Biomed Res. 1990;17(Suppl):38.

22) Groll AH, Shah PM, Mentzel C, et al. Trends in the postmortem epidemiology of invasive fungal infections at a university hospital. J Infect. 1996;33:23-32.

23) Gudewicz TM, Mader JT, Davis CP. Combined effects of hyperbaric oxygen and antifungal agents on the growth of Candida albicans. Aviat Space Environ Med. 1987;58:673-8.

24) John BV, Chamilos G, Kontoyiannis DP. Hyperbaric oxygen as an adjunctive treatment for zygomycosis. Clin Microbiol Infect. 2005;11:515-7.

25) Latge JP. Aspergillus fumigatus and aspergillosis. Clin Microbiol Rev. 1999;12:310-50.

26) Lehrer RI, Howard DH, Sypherd PS, Edwards JE, Segal GP, Winston DJ. Mucormycosis (UCLA Conference). Ann Int Med. 1980;93:93-108.

27) Lo WL, Chang RC, Yang AH, et al. Aspergillosis of the temporomandibular joint following irradiation of the parotid region: a case report. Int J Oral Maxillofac Surg. 2003;32:560-2.

28) Lopes Bezerra LM, Filler SG. Interactions of Aspergillus fumigatus with endothelial cells: internalization, injury, and stimulation of tissue factor activity. Blood. 2004;103:2143-9.

29) Maniglia AJ, Mintz DH, Novak S. Cephalic phycomycosis: a report of eight cases. Laryngoscope. 1982;92:755-60.

30) Melero M, Kaimen MI, Tiraboschi N, Botargues M, Radisic M. Adjunctive treatment with hyperbaric oxygen in a patient with rhino-sinuso-orbital mucormycosis. Medicina (B Aires). 1991;51:53-5.

31) Nathan MD, Keller AP Jr, Lerner CJ, et al. Entomophthorales infection of the maxillofacial region. Laryngoscope. 1982;92:767-9.

32) Okhuyusen PC, Rex JH, Kapusta M, Fife C. Successful treatment of extensive post-traumatic soft-tissue and renal infections due to Apophysomyces elegans. Clin Infect Dis. 1994;19:329-31.

33) Park MK, Myers RAM, Marzella L. Oxygen tensions and infections: modulation of microbial growth, activity of antimicrobial agents, and immunologic responses. Clin Infect Dis. 1992;14:720-40.

34) Pillsbury HC, Fisher ND. Rhinocerebral mucormycosis. Arch Otolaryngol Head Neck Surg. 1997;103:600-4.

35) Price JC, Stevens SDL. Hyperbaric oxygen in the treatment of rhinocerebral mucormycosis. Laryngoscope. 1980;90:737-47.

36) Segal E, Menhusen MJ, Simmons S. Hyperbaric oxygen in the treatment of fungal infections: a single-center experience. Isr Med Assoc J. 2007;9:355-7.

37) Shefield PJ. Measuring tissue oxygen tension: a review. Undersea Hyper Med. 1998;25:179-88.

38) Smith RM, Mohideen P. One hour in 1 ATA oxygen enhances rat alveolar macrophage chemiluminescence and fungal cytotoxicity. Am J Physiol. 1991;260:L457-63.

39) Sokol-Anderson ML, Brajtburg J, Medoff G. Amphotericin B-induced oxidative damage killing of candida albicans. J Infect Dis. 1986;154:76-83.

40) Sugar AM. Agents of mucormycosis and related species. In: Mandell GL, Bennett JE, Dolin R, editors. Principles and practice of infectious diseases. 4th ed. New York: Churchill Livingstone; 1995. p. 2311-21.

41) Tissot F, Agrawal S, Pagano L, Petrikkos G, Groll A, Skiada A, Lass-Fl⍰rl C, Calandra T, Viscoli C, Herbrecht R. ECIL-6 guidelines for the treatment of invasive candidiasis, aspergillosis and mucormycosis in leukemia and hematopoietic stem cell transplant patients. Haematologica. 2016 Dec. doi: haematol.2016.152900

42) Waldorf AR, Ruderman N, Diamond RD. Specific susceptibility to mucormycosis in murine diabetes and bronchoalveolar macrophage defense against Rhizopus. J Clin Invest. 1984;74:150-60.

43) Washburn RG, Gallin JI, Bennett JE. Oxidative killing of Aspergillus fumigatus proceeds by parallel myeloperoxidase-dependent and -independent pathways. Infect Immun. 1987;55:2088-92.

44) Yohai RA, Bullock JD, Aziz AA, Markert RJ. Survival factors in rhino-orbital-cerebral mucormycosis. Surv Ophthalmol. 1994;39:3-22.

CHAPTER 36 CHAPTER

Treatment of the Brown Recluse Spider Bite with Hyperbaric Oxygen Therapy

CHAPTER THIRTY-SIX OVERVIEW

Background **897**
Distribution **898**
Identification **898**
Venom/Pathogenesis **898**
Diagnosis **899**
Clinical Presentation **900**
Treatment **900**
Hyperbaric Oxygen Clinical Series **902**
Animal Data 902
Human Data 902
Hyperbaric Oxygen Therapy Recommendation 903
Discussion **903**
Conclusion **904**
References **905**

Treatment of the Brown Recluse Spider Bite with Hyperbaric Oxygen Therapy

Matthew Stanton

On May 3, 2007, Dr. Ronald P. Bangasser, who served as California Medical Association president, passed away. Ron, a family practitioner, was always an example of what a doctor should be, operating his wound care clinic and his practice, all the while serving his patients and colleagues through his advocacy for the CMA.

This chapter is dedicated to Ron's contribution to hyperbaric medicine.

BACKGROUND

The *Loxosceles* spider was first mentioned in the literature in 1872 by Caveness.(18) At that time, the envenomation was described to produce fever, hematuria, and jaundice. No further literature was documented until 1929 when Schmaus(70) noted a cutaneous reaction including pain, swelling, and rash from a brown recluse spider. In 1937, Macchiavello(48) reported envenomation caused by a South American relative, *Loxosceles laeta*, and later termed the reaction the "gangrenous spot of Chile" in 1947.(49) MacKinnon and Witkind(50) established "cutaneous arachnoidism" in South America by *L. laeta* in 1953. Shortly after this publication, physicians in the United States, who had diagnosed these necrotic wounds as infectious, began to recognize that wounds in the American Midwest were related to the "gangrenous spot of Chile" and were attributable to the necrotizing properties of the venom. Since then, the term "loxoscelism" has referred to human envenomations from *Loxosceles* spiders which may manifest in a range of symptoms, from mild urticarial rash to dermonecrotic lesion and, rarely, severe life-threatening systemic conditions.(75) While several deaths from loxoscelism have been reported in the literature,(67-68,76,79) none have been definitively proven(75) but are assumed to be from the significant hemolysis that can result.

Over the last five decades, many cases of documented brown recluse spider bites have been reported with varying presentations and treatments.(6,60,69) Advances in science have led to an increased understanding of the venom(20,43) but definitive treatment remains controversial.

DISTRIBUTION

There are approximately 100 species of *Loxosceles* spiders; 80% reside in the Western hemisphere.[78] There are 11 native and 2 nonnative species of *Loxosceles* spiders in North America.[31,63] *Loxosceles reclusa* is the most important species in the United States and responsible for the most American envenomations,[75] with reported occurrences spanning the country from New Jersey to California and Hawaii.[8,17] It is mainly, however, an inhabitant of the South Central United States, primarily western Florida to the eastern third of Texas and as far north as Illinois and southern Iowa.[28] Envenomations outside of the endemic area are rare but suspected to be secondary to travel. However, practitioners should consider other causes of necrotic lesions in areas outside of endemic areas prior to making the diagnosis of loxoscelism.

Loxosceles spiders are usually found in dark, dry, secluded places, e.g., under rocks, wood piles, and debris when outdoors, and in basements, attics, and storage areas indoors.[38] The spider is passive and usually will not bite until provoked or threatened. Due to its nocturnal nature, many envenomations occur at night while the individual sleeps. It is described as rugged as it is capable of surviving up to six months without food or water with a normal life-span of 550 to 625 days. The incidence of bites[36] from the brown recluse spider is highest from April through November.

IDENTIFICATION

The brown recluse spider is unique in many ways, especially in its physical characteristics. It ranges in length from one to five cm leg to leg and is fawn to brown in color, with a distinctive, dark-colored, violin-shaped marking located on its dorsal cephalothorax; thus, it is commonly referred to as "fiddleback" by medical entomologists although lack of expertise causes non-arachnologists to mistake many shaded forms on spider bodies as violin patterns.[78] A more distinctive characteristic is the spider has only three pairs of eyes, in contrast with four pairs in most spiders; however, the eye pattern is not completely exclusive, as genera *Scytodes* and *Sicarius* share similar eye patterns.[14] The legs are long and slender, imparting rapid mobility.

VENOM/PATHOGENESIS

The mechanism of venom toxicity is multifactorial and not completely understood. Most of what is known about the venom of the brown recluse spider was discovered in the 1970s. In the early 1970s, the venom was shown to consist of nine different cytotoxic and inflammatory complex peptides.[23] The venom is a complex mixture of proteins and peptides ranging from 1 to 40 kDa. Several molecules in the crude venom have been identified, including alkaline phosphatase, 5'-ribonucleotide phosphohydrolase, sulfated nucleosides, hyaluronidase, phospholipase-D, metalloproteases, serine proteases, and insecticide toxins.[55] Work by Geren et al. in 1975 and 1976[29-30] revealed that 99.8% of crude venom was composed of a "spreading factor" (hyaluronidases and other enzymes) which allows dissemination of other toxins to surrounding tissues.[55] Only 0.02% of the venom consists of skin-necrotizing factor (SNF). The venom has been shown to significantly disrupt polymorphonuclear (PMN) response by stimulating endothelial cells.[59] Hemolysis may be caused by hemolysin in the venom, a calcium-dependent, heat-labile protein with an optimal activity at pH of 7.1.[27] Phospholipases, which are lipolytic, cause microemboli that occlude capillaries, devitalize tissue, and result in indolent ulcerations in fatty sites.[62]

Phospholipase D is the most studied type of molecule present in the venom from *Loxosceles* species. These toxins are collectively referred to as sphingomyelinase D, due to the first description of enzymes capable of hydrolyzing sphingomyelin substrate.[19] In the late 1970s, Finkle et al.[25] identified the SNF as sphingomyelinase D, the primary constituent of the venom. Sphingomyelinase D activates complement, PMN cells, and platelets.[40] They demonstrated that the direct lytic action of RBCs was secondary to the venom without the aid of complement or the energy systems of the cells.

Both sexes are venomous, but the females may contain twice the concentration of venom than of males.[21] Sphingomyelinase D isolated from *L. laeta* and *L. intermedia* shares similar properties of dermonecrosis, platelet aggregation, and complement-dependent hemolytic activity. Antibodies to the toxin block the dermonecrotic reaction.[24] Rees et al.[64] contributed further scientific findings by producing antivenin raised against brown recluse spider bite venom (crude extract) in New Zealand white rabbits. This study revealed that, if given within 24 hours, the specific antivenin blocked or markedly attenuated the toxic effect of the venom in the rabbit-model system. Humans appear capable of mounting an active humoral immunity to the venom; however, this has not been well studied.[3] Protective immunization of humans is not yet available. Antivenin has been produced, but this too is not readily available for human use in the United States.

DIAGNOSIS

The standard for diagnosing brown recluse spider bites is collection and expert identification of the offending spider.[75] In most cases, the diagnosis of a brown recluse spider bite is purely presumptive, and it is often made in retrospect by obtaining a complete bite history and by the signs and symptoms that later develop. Even pieces of the crushed spider are enough for positive identification by experts. Furbee et al.[28] reported that of the 908 cases of suspected brown recluse envenomation, only 72 (7.9%) had a confirmed spider bite, and 82 (9%) had the spider present for identification. Berger[13] developed an immunologic test that used lymphocytes incorporating thymidine into a nucleoprotein to provide a quantitative response.[5] Pitts et al.[62] developed an ELISA (enzyme-linked immunosorbent assay) directed against circulating venom antigen. More recently, Gomez et al.[34] developed an ELISA which has been used to confirm loxoscelism.[71]

Misdiagnosis frequently occurs since loxoscelism may resemble a wide array of cutaneous diseases. These include staphylococcal or streptococcal infection, herpes simplex, herpes zoster, diabetic ulcer, fungal infection, pyoderma gangrenosum, lymphomatoid papulosis, chemical burn, *Toxicodendron* dermatitis, squamous cell carcinoma, neoplasia, focal vasculitis, syphilis, Stevens-Johnson syndrome, toxic epidermal necrolysis, purpura fulminans, sporotrichosis, Lyme disease, cowpox, and anthrax.[75] The differential diagnosis of necrotic arachnidism must include bites from snakes, ticks, scorpions, and other venomous spiders. Other medical etiologies must be considered, such as foreign body, trauma, injections of drugs, and emboli.

Laboratory studies should include a complete blood count, electrolytes, glucose, blood urea nitrogen, creatinine, protime, partial thromboplastin time, fibrinogen, and urinalysis. Leukocytosis may be present, representing the presence of systemic involvement, but the white count can be normal. A falling hematocrit signifies hemolysis, and severe disseminated intravascular coagulopathy (DIC) may follow. While hemolysis is rare in adults, it is more common in children, likely due to lack of immunity. Hemolysis can be detected by increase in plasma-free hemoglobin, increased haptoglobin, and/or hemoglobinuria, indicating the potential for renal compromise.

CLINICAL PRESENTATION

The clinical presentation ranges from a mild local reaction to death. The severity of clinical response is related to the amount of venom injected, the location of the bite (with areas of high fat content being more severe), and the immune status of the patient. Many bites go unnoticed because they fail to show the characteristic changes or systemic involvement.[13] Less commonly, a stinging sensation will be felt at the same time of the bite, while others will come to recognize the lesion several hours after the skin changes have begun. Mild cases may cause a trivial urticarial reaction. In more severe cases, the bite is initially painless and then followed by a sharp, penetrating, burning sensation over two to eight hours.[75] The pain is theorized to be cytokine-driven.[60]

Pain is accompanied by localized erythema, pruritus, and swelling.[40] Generally within 12 hours, the skin will take on a dusky, mottled appearance, creating concentric rings of erythema and ischemia with a sharply demarcated border around the bite site. A larger area of erythema may evolve as chemical mediators leach into surrounding tissues. Over three to four days, the initial hemorrhagic area will gradually sink below the level of the normal skin and become progressively necrotic. The area of blue necrosis is often surrounded by a ring of pallor which is in turn surrounded by a large area of erythema. This pattern is referred to as the "red, white, and blue sign" and assists in differentiating this bite from nonnecrotic ulcers.[40] The toxic effect of the venom extends beyond the outer border of the lesion. Blisters are frequently present over the involved area. In four to seven days, the ischemic base later results in eschar formation. The area then becomes indurated, and, at 7 to 14 days, the central area becomes mummified, and the eschar falls off, leaving ulceration. The lesion heals slowly over six to eight weeks by secondary intent with minimal scarring if left to heal on its own. In areas of fatty necrosis, some lesions are more extensive and have more severe scar formation.[22,80] Some continue to spread, since some patients can mount only minimal neutralizing effects against the venom. Wounds can extend to 10 cm or more. Most bites are medically insignificant; however, extremely rare ulcers may be 40 cm across and extend deeply into muscles.[75] An estimated 10% of all bites may result in serious dermonecrotic lesions although this number is unreliable as many bites are misdiagnosed or unrecognized.[77]

Some patients, more commonly children, experience systemic involvement, usually with the onset at one to two days post bite. The most common symptoms are fever, chills, headache, nausea/vomiting, malaise, diffuse pruritic morbilliform rash, and arthralgia. Further effects include thrombocytopenia, DIC, and hemolysis leading to hemoglobinemia, hemoglobinuria, renal failure, and, rarely, death.[29,57]

There are two main classification systems for brown recluse spider bites: Wilson-King and Auer-Hershey classifications. Wilson-King evaluates the situation around the bite.[83] This grading allows clinicians to assess the likelihood the bite is from *L. reclusa.* The Auer-Hershey classification analyzes the clinical sequelae of the bite.[8] Grades are 1–4, with grade 4 being severe systemic illness. Patients with any systemic illness will be graded at least a 2b. Even with classification, it is difficult to predict which bites will progress to serious illness. Further, not every patient presents with the classical wound presentation and would be able to be classified using this criteria.

TREATMENT

There are no consensus recommendations for treatment of brown recluse spider bites, and definitive therapy has not been established. Reported therapies include hyperbaric oxygen, dapsone, antihistamines, antibiotics, dextran, glucocorticosteroids, vasodilators, heparin, nitroglycerin, electric shock, curettage, surgical excision, and antivenin.[75] Supportive care is the mainstay of treatment and should include general first aid: elevation, immobilization, local wound care, and tetanus immunization.[75] Ice is not recommended as it may worsen ischemia surrounding the wound. Systemic treatment with opioids may be needed to control pain. Antibiotics should only be used if signs of infection are present and not prophylactically.

Dapsone is a sulfone derivative with a variety of antibacterial and antituberculosis effects, currently used worldwide as a treatment for leprosy.[33] Dapsone has also been found to be effective in skin disorders involving prominent polymorphonuclear (PMN) infiltrates.[9] It is believed that dapsone inhibits PMN myeloperoxidase-hydrogen peroxide-halide generation of oxygen intermediates, as well as inhibiting chemotaxis,[5,9,75] thus decreasing the "innocent bystander" damage to surrounding tissues during acute inflammatory responses. Dapsone causes varying degrees of hemolysis in most patients and can cause severe hemolysis with methemoglobinemia in patients deficient in glucose-6 phosphate dehydrogenase (G6PD).[41,75,82]

Dapsone treatment was first successfully reported in 1983 by King and Rees in a 27-year-old male with documented brown recluse envenomation.[45] This was followed with a prospective study of 31 patients treated with dapsone, with only one patient needing skin grafting.[64] Results of dapsone-treated patients were significantly better than those of a cohort of patients treated with early excision of the lesion. No serious adverse effects were observed with dapsone therapy. Many animal studies have not found definite benefit for dapsone use in loxoscelism.[10,39,61] Likewise, several human studies have not shown conclusive results with dapsone therapy.[1,37,65,81] If utilized, the dosage of dapsone, given orally, is 1–2 mg/kg/24 hours divided into two doses, up to a maximum of 100 mg twice daily, although doses up to 300 mg have been reported.[40] Duration of therapy is two weeks.[35]

Along with ruling out G6PD deficiency, other baseline labs should include complete blood count and liver enzymes. These should be followed weekly while on dapsone therapy. Despite its common use in *Loxosceles* bites, no prospective human trials have proven efficacy, and risks of therapy may outweigh the benefit;[16] thus, this is not a generally recommended treatment in patients with significant envenomations or systemic symptoms.

Glucocorticosteroids have been evaluated in brown recluse spider bites. Although controversy exists based on animal and human studies,[12,51,66] corticosteroids have been used for systemic loxoscelism in Brazil and may help blunt the immune response if given early in acute systemic illness.[40] They can be used for patients to prevent hemolysis and renal injury[4,77] although, even if given early, do not halt skin ulceration. Prednisone was used in three out of five cases of confirmed or probable loxoscelism in pregnancy, all of whom recovered without sequelae and delivered normal infants.[4] No optimal agent or dosing is certain; however, it is reasonable to give prednisone or equivalent in doses of 1–2 mg/kg/day.[83] No clinical trials have assessed the use of steroids in the prevention of hemolysis, but it has been started when hemolysis first presents. The duration of steroids is dependent on symptoms and clinical findings and may start to be weaned when hemolysis has ceased.

Cyproheptadine and nitroglycerin have been studied in animal models but did not show any benefit in preventing skin necrosis or inflammation.[47,61] Studies evaluating electric shock therapy have demonstrated no substantial benefit as well.[10,58] *L. reclusa* antivenom is not available in the United States, but *L. laeta* antivenom is available in South America, though without substantial supporting evidence in humans.[74]

Most bites do not require surgical intervention, and early excision may be both ineffective and unnecessary. Delayed surgical treatment may be best because the lesion may spread for up to two weeks.[56] Early surgical treatment may increase inflammation and venom effects[26,64] and prevents healing. Debridement may be necessary to remove necrotic tissue locally and should be considered over time in wounds that are slow to heal. However, if left alone, many of these wounds will heal by secondary intent without scarring. In some cases, skin grafting later may be required, but this is very rare. Grafting and extensive wound debridement may be preventable with a few sessions of hyperbaric oxygen treatment.

HYPERBARIC OXYGEN CLINICAL SERIES

Hyperbaric oxygen (HBO_2) has been reported for treatment of brown recluse spider bites. HBO_2 is thought to exhibit its effects through enhanced oxygenation to ischemic tissues and possibly direct inactivating effects on *Loxosceles* venom, specifically sphingomyelinase D;[77] however, this was not confirmed in an experimental animal model.[54] It is known that HBO_2 inactivates sulfhydryl groups, which are also thought to play a role in venom toxicity.[52] HBO_2 has been hypothesized to decrease inflammation, stimulate angiogenesis, and decrease envenomation.[2] While the exact mechanism is yet to be elucidated, HBO_2 therapy has been successfully used and can be considered for treatment of brown recluse spider envenomation.

Animal Data

Maynor and Moon et al.[53] demonstrated a significant effect on wound healing in 41 rabbits, 48 hours after envenomation, with reduction in the amount of necrosis and smaller wound sizes; however, other animal models did not conclude these same results.[39,72] The Maynor et al. HBO_2 therapy protocol used 2.5 atmospheres absolute (ATA) for 90 minutes twice daily and found significantly decreased wound size at 10 days. Another study in rabbits, by Strain et al.,[72] demonstrated that twice-daily HBO_2 treatments showed enhanced recovery at the histologic level compared to once-daily treatments and control; however, because no statistical analysis was performed, the magnitude of impact is uncertain. In conflicting reports, Hobbs et al.[39] found no significant differences in necrosis with dapsone, HBO_2, or a combination in a piglet model, and Phillips et al. demonstrated no differences in severity of skin lesions between dapsone, HBO_2, or cyproheptadine.[61] These findings, however, used different HBO_2 treatment protocols from Maynor et al. In a guinea pig model, pretreatment with HBO_2 significantly decreased the lesion size at days three, five, and six compared to dapsone pretreatment or untreated controls.[11]

Human Data

The first mention of HBO_2 therapy in humans for the treatment of brown recluse spider bites was by Svendson in 1986.[73] Six cases of clinically-diagnosed brown recluse bites were treated with hyperbaric oxygen therapy. All lesions healed promptly, without hospitalization, surgery, third-degree skin slough, or significant scarring. Svendson conjectured that the necrosis of tissue in brown recluse spider bites was at least partially caused by tissue hypoxia, secondary to the vasospastic and thrombotic effects of the venom, although no control group was used. The author proposed that if the prolonged ischemia of the wound could be ameliorated, tissue necrosis could be prevented, and speculated that hyperbaric oxygen therapy might actually inactivate the necrotic venom component of the brown recluse spider venom.[73] In the largest nonpublished, non-peer-reviewed human report of clinically diagnosed brown recluse spider envenomation treated with HBO_2, only 1 of 48 patients required grafting.[44] All patients received an average of 5.6 treatments at 2.0 ATA once or twice daily for 90 minutes and were followed for 2 years. No control group was included. Maynor et al.,[52] in 1992, reported on 14 patients, all of whom healed without scarring, disability, or the need for skin grafting. One patient required surgical drainage for a local abscess, and one developed local cellulitis without long-term effects. Broughton documented a case of brown recluse spider bite to the glans penis, which was promptly treated with HBO_2, dapsone, steroids, antihistamines, and antibiotics.[15] HBO_2 was initiated within 24 hours and consisted of 60-minute sessions twice daily at 2.0 ATA for 12 treatments. The patient recovered without sequelae and did not require surgical intervention. More recently, Jarvis et al. described treatment of a periorbital involvement of a brown recluse spider bite in an eight-year-old child. The patient was treated with twice-daily HBO_2 for eight days followed by once-daily treatments for two days, along with steroids and dapsone.[42] Wilson JR et al.[84] reported a 24-year-old female who was treated with 90-minute sessions twice daily HBO_2 at 2.4 ATA for 7 days and then daily for 3 additional days. The patient also received dapsone, steroids, opioids, and required autologous skin grafting. Leach et al. reported successful HBO_2 treatment for two patients that was started four weeks and six months after the initial bite. One patient received a 3-week course, and another patient received 20 sessions, respectively.[46] Other treatment details were not described. Hadanny et al. retrospectively analyzed 3 cases of nonhealing ulcers treated with 2.0 ATA daily for 90 minutes. HBO_2 therapy was started 2–3 months after the initial bite for median 17 treatment sessions. All three ulcers healed without any additional intervention.[34]

Hyperbaric Oxygen Therapy Recommendation

Treatment protocols call for the patient to be seen and diagnosed as soon as possible. With the available literature, if the patient presents in the first 48 hours, and a strong presumptive diagnosis of a brown spider bite is made, treatment with HBO_2 may be considered. The patient can initially be treated twice daily at 2.0 ATA for 90 minutes, for an average of 6 treatments, with a minimum of 2 and a maximum of 20, although more treatments have been used in select cases.[34] A reassessment of the bite site is made after each treatment, and additional treatments and other potential therapies previously discussed can be ordered at the discretion of the clinician. For patients that are not initially treated with HBO_2 for suspected bites, delayed HBO_2 treatments have demonstrated success of nonhealing ulcers.[34] Few patients initially require hospitalization, depending on the severity of the wound and the presence of systemic symptoms. The length of a hospital stay depends on severity of illness. The size of the dermonecrotic lesion and surrounding erythema, along with the continuance and/or disappearance of systemic symptoms, are monitored on a daily basis. After completion of HBO_2 treatment, patients are followed on an outpatient basis.

Other medications used during hyperbaric oxygen treatments are discussed in another chapter.

DISCUSSION

The most difficult aspect of treating brown recluse spider bites is definitively establishing the diagnosis. Most cases are clinically diagnosed based on suspicion and history and without confirmation of the spider bite. The majority of bites result in benign lesions in which treatment with supportive cares is generally sufficient. Severe hemolysis is the most problematic effect and may cause death.

With many potential alternative diagnoses, other etiologies should be ruled out prior to making a presumptive diagnosis of brown recluse spider bite.

Major limitations exist in reported literature due to the anecdotal nature of the evidence and lack of control groups. While HBO_2 has been used for treatment of brown recluse spider bites, conclusive data is absent as no human randomized controlled trials exist. The amount of venom and the time lapse between the bite and the treatment occur under highly variable conditions. In some reported cases, HBO_2 was not started until months after the bite, which implies that the wound may not be related to brown recluse spider bite. A confounding factor in many reported cases is the use of concomitant therapies, making it challenging to decide the magnitude of benefit of HBO_2. While no optimal treatment protocols exist, the most commonly used in human reports were 2.0–2.5 ATA once or twice daily for 60–120 minutes with a varying number of sessions. Initial treatments are generally twice daily.

Although not universally noted, a significant effect reported in the cases of HBO_2 therapy is the healing of the ulcer without significant scarring or need for surgery. A change in the color of the dermonecrotic lesion to normal pink skin color can be noted while in the chamber, but the extent of this effect remains uncertain.

CONCLUSION

Theoretically, treatment of brown recluse spider bites with HBO_2 may reduce scarring and complications. However, there have been no randomized controlled human studies conclusively demonstrating the efficacy of this treatment. Until further research is available, HBO_2 for brown recluse spider envenomation should not be routinely considered. While mortality is not common, future HBO_2 research should focus on limiting morbidity with well-designed trials and optimizing treatment protocols.

REFERENCES

1. Alario A, Price G, Stahl R, et. al. Cutaneous necrosis following a spider bite: a case report and review. Pediatrics. 1987;79:618-21.
2. Andersen RJ, Campoli J, Johar SK, et al. Suspected brown recluse envenomation: a case report and review of different treatment modalities. J Emerg Med. 2011;41(2);e31-7.
3. Anderson PC. Brown recluse spider bites – some immunologic aspects. Illinois Med J. 1978;150-3.
4. Anderson PC. Loxoscelism threatening pregnancy: five cases. 1991;165:1454-6
5. Anderson P. What's new in loxoscelism. Mo Med. 1973;70:711-8.
6. Arnold RE. Brown recluse spider bites: five cases with a review of literature. JACEP. 1976;5(4):262-4.
7. Atkins JA, Wingo CW, Sodemann WA. Probable cause of necrotic spider bite in the Midwest. Science. 1957;126:73.
8. Auer A, Hershey F. Surgery for necrotic bites of the brown spider. Arch Surg. 1974;108:612.
9. Barranco V. Dapsone – other indications. Int J Dermatol. 1982;21(9):513-4.
10. Barrett SM, Romine-Jenkins M, Fisher DE. Dapsone or electric shock therapy of brown recluse spider envenomation? Ann Emerg Med. 1994;24:21-5.
11. Beilman GJ, Winslow CL, Teslow TW. Experimental brown spider bite in the guinea pig: results of treatment with dapsone or hyperbaric oxygen. J Wilderness Med. 1994;5:287-94.
12. Berger RS. A critical look at therapy for the brown recluse spider bite. Arch Dermatol. 1973;107:298.
13. Berger R. The unremarkable brown recluse spider bite. JAMA. 1973;225:1109-11.
14. Brescovit AD, Rheims CA. On the synanthropic species of the genus Scytodes Latreille (Araneae Scytodidae) of Brazil, with synonymies and records of these species in other neotropical countries. Bull Br Arachnol Soc. 2000;11:320-30.
15. Broughton G. Management of the brown recluse spider bite to the glans penis. Mil Med. 1996;161(10):627.
16. Bryant SM, Pittman LM. Dapsone use in Loxosceles reclusa envenomation: is there an indication? Am J Emerg Med. 2003;212:89-90.
17. Butz W. Envenomation by the brown recluse spider and related species. Clin Toxicol. 1971;4:515.
18. Caveness WA. Insect bite complicated by fever. Nashville J Med Surg (2nd series). 1872;10:333.
19. Chaim OM, Trevisan-Silva D, Chaves-Moreira D, et. al. Brown spider (Loxosceles genus) venom toxins: tools for biological purposes. Toxins. 2001;3:309-44.
20. da Silveira RB, dos Santos Filho JF, Mangili OC, et. al. Identification of proteases in the extract of venom glands from brown spiders. Toxicon. 2002;40:815-22.
21. de Oliveira KC, Goncalves de Andrade RM, Piazza RM, et. al. Variations in Loxosceles spider venom composition and toxicity contribute to the severity of the envenomation. Toxicon. 2005;45:421-9.
22. Dos SK et al. Management of brown recluse spider bites. A retrospective study of case impact. Contemp Surg. 1990;35(6).
23. Elgert B, Wright RP, Campbell BJ, Barrett JT. Radiolabeling of polypeptide components of Missouri brown spider venom. Fed Proc Abstract #223. 1973.

24. Fernandes PMF, Junquerira de Azevedo IL, Goncalves de Andrade RM, et al. Molecular cloning and expression of a functional dermonecrotic and haemolytic factor from Loxosceles laeta venom. Biochem Biophys Res Commun. 2002;298:638-45.
25. Finkle J, Campbell BJ, Barrett JT. A diagnostic test for Loxosceles reclusa bites [abstract]. In: Annual meeting of the American Soc. of Microbiology. 1973. p. 97.
26. Forks TP. Brown recluse spider bites. J Am Board Fam Pract. 2000;13:415-23.
27. Forrester LJ, Barrett JT, Campbell BJ. Red blood cells lysis induced by the venom of the brown recluse spider: the role of sphingomyelinase D. Arch Biochem Biophys. 1978;187:355-65.
28. Furbee RB, Kao LW, Ibrahim D. Brown recluse spider envenomation. Clin Lab Med. 2006;26:211-26.
29. Geren CR, Chan TK, Hewell DE, Odell GV. Isolation and characterization of toxins from brown recluse spider venom (Loxosceles reclusa). Arch Biochem Biophys. 1976;174:90-9.
30. Geren CR, Chan TK, Hewell DE, Odell GV. Partial characterization of the low molecular weight fractions of the extract of the venom apparatus of the brown recluse spider and its hemolymph. Toxicon. 1975;13:233-8.
31. Gertsch WJ, Ennik F. The spider genus Loxosceles in North America, Central America and the West Indies (Araneae Loxoscelidae). Bull Am Mus Nat Hist. 1983;175:264-360.
32. Gomez HF, Krywko DM, Stoecker WV. A new assay for the detection of Loxosceles species (brown recluse) spider venom. Ann Emerg Med. 2002;39:469-74.
33. Goodman, Gilman. The pharmacological basis of therapeutics. 7th ed. New York: McMillan Publishing Co.;1985. p. 1212-3.
34. Hadanny A, Fishlev G, Bechor Y, et. al. Nonhealing wounds caused by brown spider bites: application of hyperbaric oxygen therapy. 2016;29:560-6.
35. Hahn I. Arthropods. In: Goldfrank's toxicologic emergencies. 10th ed. New York: McGraw-Hill; 2015. p. 1561-81.
36. Hall RD, Anderson PC. Brown recluse spider bites: can they be prevented? Missouri Med. 1981;78(5):243-7.
37. Herman TE, McAlister WH. Epiglottic enlargement: two unusual cases. Pediatr Radiol. 1991;21:139-40.
38. Hile JM, Gladney WJ, Lancaster JL Jr, Whitcomb WH. Biology of the brown recluse spider. Univ Ark Agr Exp Sta Bull. 1966:711.
39. Hobbs GD, Anderson AR, Greene TJ, et al. Comparison of hyperbaric oxygen and dapsone therapy for loxosceles envenomation. Acad Emerg Med. 1996;3:758-61.
40. Hogan CJ, Barbaro KC, Winkel K. Loxoscelism: old obstacles, new directions. Ann Emerg Med. 2004;44:608-24.
41. Iserson K. Methemoglobinemia from dapsone therapy for a suspected brown spider bite. J Em Med. 1985;3:285-8.
42. Jarvis RM, Neufeld MV, Westfall CT. Brown recluse spider bite to the eyelid. Ophthalmology. 2000;107:1492-6.
43. Jong YS, Norment BR, Heitz JR. Separation and characterization of venom components in Loxosceles recluse-II. Protease enzyme activity. Toxicon. 1979;17:529-37.

44. Kendall TE, Caniglia RJ. Hyperbaric oxygen with treatment of clinically diagnosed brown recluse spider bites: a review of 48 cases. Undersea Biomed Res [Internet]. 1989 Jun [cited 2016 Nov 12];16 Suppl. Available from: http://archive.rubicon-foundation.org/xmlui/handle/123456789/6561

45. King LE, Rees RS. Dapsone treatment of a brown recluse spider bite. JAMA. 1983;250(5):648.

46. Leach J, Bassichis B, Itani K. Brown recluse spider bites to the head: three cases and a review. Ear Nose Throat J. 2004;83(7):465-70.

47. Lowry BP, Bradfield JF, Carroll RG, et al. A controlled trial of topical nitroglycerin in a New Zealand white rabbit model of brown recluse spider envenomation. Ann Emerg Med. 2001;37(2):161-5.

48. Macchiavello A. La Loxoxsceles laeta, causa del arachoidismo cutaneo, a mancha grengrenosa, de Chile. Rev Chil Hist Nat. 1937;41:11.

49. Macchiavello A. Cutaneous arachnidism or gangrenous spot of Chile. Public Health Trop Med. 1947;22:425-466.

50. MacKinnon JE, Witkind J. Arachnidismo necrotico. Ann Fac Med Montevideo. 1953;38:75-100.

51. Mara JE, Myers BS. Brown spider bite: treatment with hydrocortisone. Rocky Mt Med J. 1977;74:257-8.

52. Maynor ML, Abt JL, Osborne PD. Brown recluse spider bite: beneficial effects of hyperbaric oxygen. J Hyperb Med. 1992;7(2):89-101.

53. Maynor ML, Moon RE, Klitzman B, et. al. Brown recluse spider envenomation: a prospective trial of hyperbaric oxygen therapy. Acad Emerg Med. 1997;4(3):184-92.

54. Merchant ML, Hinton JF, Geren CR. Effect of hyperbaric oxygen on sphingomyelinase D activity of brown recluse spider (Loxosceles reclusa) venom as studied by 31P nuclear magnetic resonance spectroscopy. Am J Trop Med Hyg. 1997;56:335-8.

55. Meiri Chaim O, Trevisan-Silva D, Chaves-Moreira D, et. al. Brown spider (Loxosceles genus) venom toxins: tools for biological purposes. Toxins. 2011;3:309-44.

56. Norris K, Misra S. Brown recluse spider bite on the breast. JAAPA. 2014;27(5):32-4.

57. Novak R, Kumar M, Thompson E, Billmeier G. Severe systemic toxicity from a spider bite in a six-year-old boy. J Tenn Med Assoc. 1979;72:110-1.

58. Osborn CD. Treatment of spider bites by high voltage direct current. J Okla State Med Assoc. 1991;84:257-60.

59. Patel KD, Modur V, Zimmerman GA, et. al. The necrotic venom of the brown recluse spider induces dysregulated endothelial cell-dependent neutrophil activation: differential induction of GM-CSF, IL-8, and E-selectin expression. J Clin Invest. 1994;94:631-42.

60. Payne KS, Schilli K, Meier K, Rader RK, Dyer JA, Mold JW, Green JA, Stoecker WV. Extreme pain from brown recluse spider bites: model for cytokine-driven pain. JAMA Dermatol. 2014;150(11):1205-8.

61. Phillips S, Kohn M, Baker D, et. al. Therapy of brown spider envenomation: a controlled trial of hyperbaric oxygen, dapsone, and cyproheptadine. Ann Emerg Med. 1995;25:363-7.

62. Pitts RM, Callahan M, Owings E, King W. Tough spiders: identifying and treating their bites. Emerg Pediatr. 1992;5(4):72-4.

63. Platnick NI. World spider catalogue, version 6.0 [Internet]. 2005. Available from: http://research.amnh.org/entomology/spiders/catalog/INTRO1.html

64. Rees R, Altenbern D, et al. Brown recluse spider bites: a comparison of early surgical excision versus dapsone and delayed surgical excision. Ann Surg. 1985;220(5):659-63.

65. Rees R, Campbell D, Rieger E, et al. The diagnosis and treatment of brown recluse spider bites. Ann Emerg Med. 1987;16:945-9.

66. Rees R, Shack RB, Withers E, Madden J, Franklin J, Lynch JB. Management of the brown recluse spider bite. Plast Reconstr Surg. 1981;68(5):768-73.

67. Rose NJ. Report of fatality: spider bite (Loxosceles). IMJ Ill Med J. 1970;137:339.

68. Rosen JL, Dumitru JK, Langley EW, Meade Olivier CA. Emergency department death from systemic loxoscelism. Ann Emerg Med. 2012;60(4):439-41.

69. Sams HH, Hearth SB, Long LL, Wilson DC, Sanders DH, King LE. Nineteen documented cases of Loxosceles recluse envonmation. J Am Acad Dermatol. 2001;44:603-8.

70. Schmaus LF. Case of arachnoidism (spider bite). JAMA. 1929;92:126-7.

71. Stoecker WV, Green JA, Gomez HF. Diagnosis of loxoscelism in a child confirmed with an enzyme-linked immunosorbent assay and noninvansive tissue sampling. J Am Acad Dermatol. 2006;55(5):888-90.

72. Strain GM, Snider TG. Hyperbaric oxygen effects on brown recluse spider envenomation in rabbits. Toxicon. 1991;29:989-96.

73. Svendson F. Treatment of clinically diagnosed brown recluse spider bites with HBO: a clinical observation. J Ark Med Soc. 1986;83:199-204.

74. Swanson DL, Vetter RS. Bites of brown recluse spiders and suspected necrotic arachnidism. NEJM. 2005;352:700-7.

75. Swanson DL, Vetter RS. Loxoscelism. Clin Dermatol. 2006;24:213-21.

76. Taylor EH, Denny WF. Hemolysis, renal failure and death, presumed secondary to bite of brown recluse spider. South Med J. 1966;59:1209-11

77. Tutrone WD, Green KM, Norris T, et al. Brown recluse spider envenomation: dermatologic application of hyperbaric oxygen therapy. J Drugs Dermatol. 2005;4(4):424-8.

78. Vetter RS. Arachnids submitted as suspected brown recluse spiders (Araneae: Sicariidae): Loxosceles spiders are viturally restricted to their known distributions but are perceived to exist throughout the United States. J Med Entomol. 2005;42(4):512-21

79. Vorse H, Seccareccio P, Woodruff K, et al. Disseminated intravascular coagulopathy following fatal brown spider bite (necrotic arachnidism). J Pediatr. 1972;80:1035-7.

80. Wasserman GS, Siegel CJ. Loxoscelism (brown recluse spider bites): a review of literature. Vet Human Tox. 1977;19:256-8.

81. Wesley RE, Ballinger WH, Close LW, et al. Dapsone in the treatment of presumed brown recluse spider bite of the eyelid. Ophthalmic Surg. 1985;16:116-20.

82. Wille C, Morrow J. Case report: dapsone hypersensitivity syndrome associated with treatment of the bite of a brown recluse spider. Am J Med Sci. 1988;296:270-1.

83. Wilson DC, King LE Jr. Spiders and spider bites. Dermatol Clin. 1990;8:277-86.

84. Wilson JR, Hagood CO, Prather ID. Brown recluse spider bites: a complex problem wound. A brief review and case study. Ostomy Wound Manage. 2005;51(3):59-66.

CHAPTER 37 CHAPTER

Hyperbaric Oxygen in Traumatic Brain Injury

CHAPTER THIRTY-SEVEN OVERVIEW

Introduction 911
Background 911
Preclinical Studies 930
Clinical Trials 933
Availability, Safety, and Oxygen Toxicity Issues 936
Conclusion 938
References 939

Hyperbaric Oxygen in Traumatic Brain Injury

Sarah B. Rockswold, Samuel R. Daly, Gaylan L. Rockswold

INTRODUCTION

The enormous negative social and economic impact of traumatic brain injury (TBI) throughout the world cannot be overemphasized. The major issue is premature death and disability both in civilian and military populations. Nearly four (3.65) million people suffer a TBI each year in the United States, and approximately 2.2 million of them require an emergency room visit; 500,000 are hospitalized, and 50,000 die. This results in direct and indirect costs of 76.5 billion dollars annually to our country. Clinical outcome for severe TBI victims has not improved from 1990 to the present.[73] One major issue is premature death and disability because TBI is a disease of the young. Eighty-four percent of the 3.65 million TBIs are sustained by people age 64 or younger. A successful treatment for severe TBI would result in billions of dollars of savings for the chronically disabled patients, improve the patients' ability to work productively, and relieve a significant amount of human suffering.

Historically, hyperbaric oxygen (HBO_2) was seen as a mechanism to decrease cerebral blood flow (CBF) and intracranial pressure (ICP) while increasing oxygen (O_2) availability to injured brain cells.[45,74-75] As highly technical equipment has become available in both TBI animal and clinical studies, HBO_2 appears to be working at the mitochondrial level to improve cerebral aerobic metabolism after brain injury.[63,77,93] Clinically, HBO_2 has been shown to decrease mortality rates and improve functional outcome in severely brain-injured patients.[1,31,62] As research on HBO_2 continues, the goal is to accomplish a multicenter, prospective, randomized clinical outcome trial by which the efficacy of HBO_2 in the treatment of severely brain-injured patients is evaluated.

BACKGROUND

In examining the HBO_2 clinical literature, it is apparent that the large majority of investigations demonstrated a positive effect (Table 1). However, as our critical appraisal demonstrates, the quality of clinical investigations varied quite widely. The clinical randomized trials for the role of HBO_2 in the treatment of chronic mild TBI with post-concussion are reviewed (Table 2). This review indicates a lack of a positive effect by HBO_2 on this chronic syndrome. This finding is not surprising given a lack of preclinical experimental studies establishing a mechanism and a lack of clinical investigations demonstrating that HBO_2 is physiologically active in these particular

TABLE 1. CLINICAL DATA ON HBO_2 USED FOR ACUTE TBI PHASE 2 DATA:

AUTHOR	TREATMENT GROUPS; N	ELIGIBILITY	NINDS CRITERIA RANKING	FIO_2 AT ATA; WINDOW POST-TBI; DURATION; FREQUENCY
Prakash[58]	(1) HBO_2; 28 (2) Controls; 28	TBI; GCS < 8; No other injuries; Children	2	100% at NM; 10–12 days; NM; Weekly for 3 weeks
Rockswold[64]	(1) HBO_2; 26 (2) Standard of Care; 22	Nonpenetrating TBI; GCS 3–8; 1+ Reactive pupil; Marshall classification > 1; No prior severe brain injury; Mean age 35 years	6	100% at 1.5 ATA; Average = 19 hr; 1 hr; 1 treatment every 24 hrs for 3 treatments
Lin[39]	(1) HBO_2; 22 (2) Control; 22	TBI; GCS 3–12; No multitrauma; Spontaneous respiration; Age > 15	5	100% at 2.0 ATA; 27 days; 1.5 hr; 20 days over the course of 4 weeks

POSITIVE TREATMENT EFFECTS	NEGATIVE TREATMENT EFFECTS	NEUTRAL TREATMENT EFFECTS
• GCS (Elevated after HBO_2 treatment) • Hospital Stay (Shorter stay in HBO_2 group); • Social Behavior (More improvement in HBO_2 group); • Disability (HBO_2 group returned to school earlier)		
• $CMRO_2$ (Increased from pre- to one hour post treatment in Group 1 for those patients with reduced or normal baseline CBF and continued to increase at six hours post treatment*; Elevated Group 1 posttreatment values compared to Group 2*) • CBF (Elevated in Group 1 after treatment compared to pretreatment levels and Group 2 levels*)		
• Dialysate lactate (Decreased after treatment in Group 1 compared to pretreatment and to Group 2*) • PbO_2 (Elevated after treatment in Group 1 compared to pretreatment levels and Group 2*) • Dialysate LPR (Decreased after treatment in Group 1 compared to pretreatment levels and Group 2*) • ICP (Reduced posttreatment values in Group 1 compared to Group 2*) • $AVDO_2$ (Reduced posttreatment values compared to pretreatment*) • CSF F2-isoprostane levels did not change • BAL IL-6 and IL-8 levels did not change		• Dialysate glucose levels did not change • $CMRO_2$ changes between pre- and post treatment did not differ in Group 1 compared to Group 2
• GCS (Elevated compared to controls after HBO_2 treatment*) • GOS (Improvement was better at six months for a subgroup of Group 1 compared to Group 2*)		• GOS at three months was not different between groups

* Significant Finding

TABLE 1 (CONTINUED)

AUTHOR	TREATMENT GROUPS; N	ELIGIBILITY	NINDS CRITERIA RANKING	FIO_2 AT ATA; WINDOW POST-TBI; DURATION; FREQUENCY
Ren[59]	(1) HBO_2; 35 (2) Standard of Care; 20	Closed-head brain injury; GCS 3–8;	4	100% at 2.5 ATA; Acute; 40–60 min; One treatment every four days for three to four treatments
Rockswold[62]	(1) HBO_2; 84 (2) Standard of Care; 84	TBI; GCS 3–9	7	100% at 1.5 ATA; 26 hrs; 1 hr; Every 8 hrs for 2 weeks or until brain death or until they could obey commands
Artru[1]	(1) HBO_2; 31 (2) Standard of Care; 29	Head injuries and in a coma; Age 5–70	3	100% at 2.5 ATA; 4.5 days; 1 hr; Daily for 10 days followed by 4 days of no treatment and another 10 daily sessions
Holbach[31]	(1) HBO_2; 49 (2) Standard of Care; 50	Traumatic mid-brain syndrome; Age Range 3–65 (Mean: 22.6 years old	1	100% at 1.5 ATA; 2–10 days; 20–30 min; Between 1 and 7 times per patient

POSITIVE TREATMENT EFFECTS	NEGATIVE TREATMENT EFFECTS	NEUTRAL TREATMENT EFFECTS
• GCS (Increased significantly after each treatment for Group 1*; Elevated in Group 1 after treatment compared to Group 2*) • BEAM (Reduced abnormality rate after treatments in Group 1 compared to baseline and Group 2*) • GOS at six months (Better outcome in Group 1 compared to Group 2*)		
• ICP (Lower in the subgroup of patients in Group 1 that received a myringotomy compared to those in Group 1 that didn't and Group 2*); • Mortality (Reduced in Group 1 compared to Group 2 at 12 months*); • Mortality (Reduced in Group 1 patients with GCS 4–6 or ICP < 20mmHg compared to same subgroups of Group 2*)		• ICP was not different between Groups 1 and 2 during HBO_2 treatment • GOS at 12 months was not different between groups
• Improvement in coma at 1 month for those patients < 30 years old that had acute nonadapted reaction and were not operated on*		• Mortality at 1 and 12 months was not different between groups • Coma recovery at 1 month was not different between groups
• Mortality (Group 2 had quicker reductions in survival time between day 2 and 7 compared to Group 1; 87% survival rate in Group 1 at day 10 compared to 54% survival rate in Group 2; Largest differences in survival rates between groups is seen in those patients < 30 years old) • Recovery (Complete recovery seen in 33% of Group 1 patients compared to 6% of Group 2 patients; Incomplete recovery seen in 14% of Group 1 patients compared to 20% of Group 2 patients)		
* Significant Finding		

TABLE 1 (CONTINUED)

AUTHOR	TREATMENT GROUPS; N	ELIGIBILITY	NINDS CRITERIA RANKING	FIO_2 AT ATA; WINDOW POST-TBI; DURATION; FREQUENCY
Rockswold[63]	(1) HBO_2; 37	Nonpenetrating TBI; PR GCS 3–8 or deterioration to ≤ 8 within 48 hours of injury; Marshall classification > 2; Age 8–84	1	100% at 1.5 ATA; 9–49 hrs (Average: 23 hours); 1 hr; 2nd treatment was 8 hrs after 1st treatment, and 5 additional treatments were provided at 24-hour intervals
Brown[11]	(1) HBO_2; 2	TBI; Male; Age 5 (MVP; GCS 4–5) and 21 (GSW; GCS 11)	0	100% at 2 ATA; Acute; 1 hour; 4 treatments at 6-hour intervals
Sukoff[75]	(1) HBO_2 with clinically indicated ICP monitor; 10 (2) HBO_2 without ICP monitor; 40	Coma resulting from TBI; Pupillary abnormalities; No operative intracranial lesions	0	100% at 2 ATA; < 6 hrs after ADM; 45 min; every 4–8 hrs for 2–4 days depending on clinical response

POSITIVE TREATMENT EFFECTS	NEGATIVE TREATMENT EFFECTS	NEUTRAL TREATMENT EFFECTS
•CBF (Elevated after treatment in those that began treatment with a low CBF*; Elevated after treatment in those that began with a normal CBF*; Reduced after treatment in those that began with a high CBF*) • CMRO2 (Elevated after treatment for those that began treatment with low and normal levels of CBF*) • CSF lactate (Reduced after treatment, N = 15*) • ICP (Reduced to below baseline levels in those with high pretreatment ICP levels*)	• ICP (Increased linearly during treatment regardless of baseline ICP*; Remained elevated in those with low pretreatment ICP levels*)	• No changes seen between pre- and posttreatment levels of $AVDO_2$, hemoglobin, CPP, and pH
• ICP (decreased during pressurization, increased during treatment and depressurization, and decreased again to below baseline values after treatment) • PaO_2 (Elevated during treatment compared to pre- and posttreatment values)		• No changes seen between pre- and posttreatment levels of $PaCO_2$ and pH
• ICP (decreased during treatment*) (1) • 9/10 patients demonstrated improved awareness and motor activity in the chamber (2) • 22/40 patients demonstrated improved awareness and motor activity in the chamber		
* Significant Finding		

TABLE 1 (CONTINUED)

AUTHOR	TREATMENT GROUPS; N	ELIGIBILITY	NINDS CRITERIA RANKING	FIO_2 AT ATA; WINDOW POST-TBI; DURATION; FREQUENCY
Holbach[32]	(1) HBO_2; 30 (1A) 2.0 ATA (1B) 1.5 ATA	Head Injury (N = 23) or Ischemic brain lesion (N = 7); Age 8–72	2	Progression from air to 100% at 1 ATA to 1.5 ATA to 2 ATA to 1 ATA to air (Only Group A proceeded to 2 ATA – Group B remained at 1.5 ATA); "few days;" NM; 33 treatments in 30 patients
Holbach[30]	(1) HBO_2; 10	Acute cerebral injury	1	Progression from air to 100% at 1 ATA to 1.5 ATA to 2 ATA to 1 ATA to air; Acute; NM; Data from 13 treatments on 10 patients
Hayakawa[29]	HBO_2; 13	Acute cerebral damage (TBI: 9; Brain tumor: 4)	0	100% at 2 ATA; Acute time point; 1 hr; 1 treatment

POSITIVE TREATMENT EFFECTS	NEGATIVE TREATMENT EFFECTS	NEUTRAL TREATMENT EFFECTS
• PaO_2 (Increased as FiO_2 and pressure increased*; Decreased as FiO_2 and pressure decreased*) • AVD glucose (Initial decrease when exposed to 100% at 1 ATA followed by gradual increase throughout treatment*; Elevated after treatment in Group B compared to Group A*) • GOQ (Reduction upon initiation of treatment from abnormally high values*; Group B remained at normal levels throughout treatment) • $AVDO_2$ (Increased upon initiation of 100% FiO2* and again when pressure reached 2 ATA*) • AVD lactate and glucose (Initial decrease upon initiation of 100% FiO_2* and continued to decrease when pressure reached 2 ATA*)	• GOQ (Group A levels increased at 2 ATA above normal values* and decreased to abnormally low values after treatment*)	• No changes seen between pre- and posttreatment levels of PaCO2 and pH
•GOQ (Reduced to normal values at 1.5 ATA*) • Glucose (Elevated at 2 ATA to toxic levels followed by significant reduction when pressure was returned to 1 ATA and when 100% FiO_2 was replaced by air*) • $AVDO_2$ (Increased values upon initiation of breathing 100% FiO_2)	• Glucose (Elevated at 2 ATA to toxic levels)	
• 9/13 patients showed large decrease in CSFP during treatment followed by elevated rebound. These patients tended to show great clinical improvement. • 2/13 patients showed large and maintained decrease in CSFP during and after treatment.*		• 2/13 patients showed little clinical response to treatment.

* Significant Finding

TABLE 1 (CONTINUED)

AUTHOR	TREATMENT GROUPS; N	ELIGIBILITY	NINDS CRITERIA RANKING	FIO_2 AT ATA; WINDOW POST-TBI; DURATION; FREQUENCY
Mogami[48]	HBO_2; 66	Severe brain damage (TBI, tumor, CVD, ischemia)	0	100% at 2 ATA; Acute; 1 hr; 1–2 times per day for as long as indicated

LEGEND: ADM = Admission; ATA = x1 Atmospheric Pressure; AVD = Arterio-cerebral Venous Differences; $AVDO_2$ = Arteriovenous Differences in Oxygen; BAL = Bronchial Alveolar Lavage; BEAM = Brain Electric Activity Mapping; CBF = Cerebral Blood Flow; $CMRO_2$ = Cerebral Metabolic Rate of O_2; CPP = Cerebral Perfusion Pressure; CSF = Cerebral Spinal Fluid; CSFP = Cerebral Spinal Fluid Pressure; CT = Computed Tomography; CVD = Cerebral Vascular Disease; EEG = Electroencephalogram; FiO_2 = inspired oxygen percentage; GCS = Glasgow Coma Scale; GOQ = Glucose Oxidation Quotient; GOS = Glasgow Outcome Scale; GSW = Gun Shot Wound; HBO_2 = Hyperbaric Oxygen Treatment; hr = Hours; ICP = Intracranial Pressure; IL = Interleukin; ICP = Intracranial Pressure; LPR = Lactate/Pyruvate Ratio; min = Minutes; mmHg = millimeters Mercury; MVP = Motor Vehicle vs. Pedestrian; N = sample size; N/A = Not Applicable; NM = Not Mentioned; $PaCO_2$ = Arterial Pressure of CO_2; PaO_2 = Arterial Oxygen Pressure; PbO_2 = Brian Tissue Oxygenation; TBI = Traumatic Brain Injury

patients. Therefore, it is important to differentiate the reported evidence for the effectiveness of HBO in severe acute TBI as opposed to mild chronic TBI.

There are peer-reviewed published animal data from well-established research laboratories which indicate that HBO_2 potentially improves outcome from TBI by multiple mechanisms.[16,40,44,56-57,66,72,80-83,93] These studies have included 8 injury models, 4 different animal species, and at least 12 established laboratories. These mechanisms include improved oxidative metabolism and mitochondrial function, reductions in intracranial hypertension, apoptosis, neural inflammation, and free-radical-mediated damage. These multiple mechanisms may explain why HBO_2 seems to be beneficial in the wide variety of injury models. Cellular energy failure appears to be the initiating event in the complex processes leading to brain cell death.[67,71,76,92] In the first 24 hours after brain injury, ischemia is present, leading to decreased O_2 delivery that is inadequate to maintain efficient oxidative cerebral metabolism.[8-9,79] This abnormal metabolic state appears to trigger a marked increase in the glycolytic metabolism of glucose;[6-7,33] this relatively inefficient anaerobic metabolism results in the depletion of cellular energy. A cascade of biochemical events leads to mitochondrial dysfunction

POSITIVE TREATMENT EFFECTS	NEGATIVE TREATMENT EFFECTS	NEUTRAL TREATMENT EFFECTS
• Neurologic symptoms (Improved during treatment in 50% of patients; Regressed after treatment and when 100% O_2 was replaced with a 98%:2% O_2:CO_2 combination) • EEG (Reduction of abnormalities during treatment) • ICP (Fell during treatment and rose again after treatment; Rose dramatically when 100% O_2 was replaced with a 98%:2% O_2:CO_2 combination) • LPR (Tendency to decrease during treatment)	• ICP (Increased after treatment, during which a decrease was observed)	
* Significant Finding		

and a prolonged period of hypometabolism.(6,38,70-71,78) Diffusion barriers to the cellular delivery of O_2 develop and persist. These barriers appear to reduce the ability of the brain to increase the O_2 extraction fraction (OEF) in response to hypoperfusion.(42) Despite the heterogeneity of TBI, the metabolic derangements related to ischemia and hypometabolism in the brain are seen consistently in the more severely injured TBI patients.(26,35,51,54,60,63-64) Depression of cerebral metabolic rate of oxygen ($CMRO_2$) correlates directly with the overall severity of the brain injury and improvement in $CMRO_2$ with the recovery of the patient. It should be noted that since over 90% of the O_2 delivered to the brain is utilized by mitochondria, $CMRO_2$ is a surrogate maker of mitochondrial function. Hyperbaric oxygen not only improves $CMRO_2$ acutely but continues to do so for at least five days post injury during the time of hypometabolism.(63-64) In both animal and human investigations, HBO_2 markedly increases O_2 delivery to traumatized brain.(16,64-65) Thus, HBO_2 can potentially reverse the ischemia that precipitates cellular energy failure and the subsequent destructive biochemical cascade. Elevated brain tissue oxygen tension favorably influences the binding of O_2 in mitochondrial redox enzyme systems, leading to improved mitochondrial function and adenosine triphosphate (ATP) production.(16,93) In addition, traumatic insult to the brain results in hematomas, contusion, and cerebral edema, all of which lead to intracranial hypertension. Hyperbaric oxygen has been shown in both experimental and clinical studies to reduce ICP(11,29,45,62-66,75) and cerebral edema after severe brain injury.(47,53,56,75) Intracranial hypertension is the major treatable cause of deterioration and death from severe TBI.(36)

TABLE 2. CLINICAL DATA ON HBO_2 USED FOR MILD CHRONIC TBI PHASE 2 DATA:

AUTHOR	TREATMENT GROUPS; N	ELIGIBILITY	NINDS CRITERIA RANKING	FIO_2 AT ATA; WINDOW POST-TBI; DURATION; FREQUENCY
Wolf[91]	(1) HBO_2; 25 (2) Sham HBO_2; 25	TBI resulting in chronic symptoms; Age 20–51	6	(1) 100% at 2.4 ATA; (2) Air at 1.3 ATA; (1–2) 3–71 months; 1.5 hours; Daily for 5 days followed by 1-day break for 30 treatments
Miller[46]	(1) HBO_2; 24 (2) Sham HBO_2; 25 (3) Standard of Care; 23	1+ TBI (GCS 13–15) that resulted in chronic symptoms; No prior moderate or severe TBIs; Mean Age ~30 years	6	(1) 100% at 1.5 ATA (2) air at 1.2 ATA; (1–2) > 4 months with averages ~20 months; 1 hour; weekdays for 40 treatments
Cifu[13]	(1) HBO_2 at 100% FiO_2; 21 (2) HBO_2 at 75% FiO_2; 18 (3) Sham Control; 21	1+ TBI (GCS 13–15) that resulted in 3+ months of PCS symptoms; Military participants; Mean age 23 years	9	(1) 100% at 2 ATA (2) 75% at 2 ATA (3) 10.5% at 2 ATA; (1–3) 8.5 months; 1 hour; 40 treatments over 10 weeks
Cifu[14]	(1) HBO_2 at 100% FiO_2; 21 (2) HBO_2 at 75% FiO_2; 18 (3) Sham Control; 21	1+ TBI (GCS 13–15) that resulted in 3+ months of PCS symptoms; Military participants; Mean age 23 years	8	(1) 100% at 2 ATA (2) 75% at 2 ATA (3) 10.5% at 2 ATA; (1–3) 8.5 months; 1 hour; 40 treatments over 10 weeks

POSITIVE TREATMENT EFFECTS	NEGATIVE TREATMENT EFFECTS	NEUTRAL TREATMENT EFFECTS
		• ImPACT (All groups had similar improvement over time*) • Braincheckers (All groups had similar improvement over time*) • PCL-M (All groups had similar improvement over time*)
		• RPQ (Groups 1 and similarly improved compared to Group 3*) • Neurobehavioral Symptom Inventory (no between group differences) • PTSD Checklist (no between group differences)
		• Neuropsychological outcome (no between group differences) • Psychomotor outcome (no between group differences) • Cognitive functioning measures for attention, memory, and processing speed (no between group differences)
		• Eye tracking abnormalities in fixation, smooth pursuit, and saccades (no between-group differences)

* Significant Finding

TABLE 2 (CONTINUED)

AUTHOR	TREATMENT GROUPS; N	ELIGIBILITY	NINDS CRITERIA RANKING	FIO_2 AT ATA; WINDOW POST-TBI; DURATION; FREQUENCY
Cifu[15]	(1) HBO_2 at 100% FiO_2; 21 (2) HBO_2 at 75% FiO_2; 18 (3) Sham Control; 21	1+ TBI (GCS 13–15) that resulted in 3+ months of PCS symptoms; Military participants; Mean age 23 years	9	(1) 100% at 2 ATA (2) 75% at 2 ATA (3) 10.5% at 2 ATA; (1–3) 8.5 months; 1 hour; 40 treatments over 10 weeks
Boussi-Gross[10]	(1) HBO_2; 36 (2) HBO_2 Crossover; 31	TBI resulting in PCS; < 30 minutes LOC; Negative imaging results at the time of inclusion; Age ~43 years	6	100% at 1.5 ATA; 1–6 years; 1 hour; Daily treatments 5 days a week for 40 treatments
Wolf[89]	(1) HBO_2; 24 (2) Sham exposure to 1.3 ATA; 24	TBI resulting in PCS; Age 20–51; Military participants	7	100% at 2.4 ATA; 3–71 months; 1.5 hours; Daily for 5 days followed by 1-day break for 30 treatments
Barrett[3]	(1) HBO_2 for TBI; 5 (2) TBI; 5 (3) HBO_2 for healthy controls; 5 (4) Healthy controls; 68	Chronic TBI 3–19 years post injury with persistent neuropsychological deficits; Average age 35	3	100% at 1.5 ATA; 3–19 years; 1 hour; 80 treatments followed by 5-month break and another 40 treatments

POSITIVE TREATMENT EFFECTS	NEGATIVE TREATMENT EFFECTS	NEUTRAL TREATMENT EFFECTS
• RPQ (Two symptoms decreased in Group 1 between pre- and posttreatment levels*)		• RPQ (no between-group differences at posttreatment time point) • PCL-M (no between- or within-group differences at posttreatment time point)
• Cognitive functioning (Improvement after treatment in both Group 1 and 2*) • CBF (Global SPECT-measured improvement after treatment in both Group 1 and 2*) • Quality of life (Improvement after treatment in both Group 1 and 2*)		• No improvement in cognitive functioning, quality of life, or SPECT imaging during the control period for Group 2
		• PCL-M (Similar rate of improvement from baseline between groups) • ImPACT (Similar rate of improvement from baseline between groups)
		• PET changes (no between-group differences) • Neuropsychometric testing (no between-group differences) • MRI structural changes (no between-group differences) • rCBF (No consistent patterns of SPECT-measured change over time or compared to patients without HBO_2 treatment)

*Significant Finding

TABLE 2 (CONTINUED)

AUTHOR	TREATMENT GROUPS; N	ELIGIBILITY	NINDS CRITERIA RANKING	FIO_2 AT ATA; WINDOW POST-TBI; DURATION; FREQUENCY
Churchill[12]	(1) HBO_2; 28	TBI 1–29 years prior; GCS 3–13; Age 18–62 (mean age = 37)	1	100% at 1.5 ATA; 6.9 years; 1 hour; 60 daily treatments over 70–105 days
Sahni[68]	(1) Clinically indicated HBO_2; 20 (2) Standard of Care; 20	TBI; GCS 3–15; Age 17–55; Retrospective cohort	3	100% at 1.5 ATA; Months; 1 hour; 1 treatment per day for 30 days
Wolf[90]	(1) HBO_2; 24 (2) Sham exposure; 24	TBI resulting in post-concussive syndrome; Age 20–51; Military participants	7	100% at 2.4 ATA; 3–71 months; 1.5 hours; Daily for 5 days followed by 1-day break for 30 treatments

POSITIVE TREATMENT EFFECTS	NEGATIVE TREATMENT EFFECTS	NEUTRAL TREATMENT EFFECTS
• Feasibility (71% of screened subjects initiated HBO_2 and 64% completed the treatment sessions) • Neuropsychological tests (Improvement seen over time in Logical Memory*) • Self-reported outcomes (Improvements reported in memory function*) • CTA (Normalization in blood flow) • fMRI (Improvement seen in auditory, visual, and motor functioning) • MRS (Improvement seen)	• Safety (6 adverse events related to HBO_2 in 3,403 total treatments)	• Neuropsychological tests (No improvement seen in subscores of Intelligence, Academic Achievement, Memory, Executive Function, Attention, Verbal Fluency, Depression, Anxiety) • Self-reported outcomes (No improvement seen in Depression, Communication, Aggression, Motor Function, Independence, Family Problems, Substance Use)
• Better outcome in Group 1 compared to Group 2 as measured with DRS, Ranchos Los Amigos Scale, and GCS • Best outcome seen in those patients 1–6 months post injury vs. < 1 month and > 6 months post injury		
• No serious adverse events in Group 1 • "Infrequent, mild side effect profile"		

*Significant Finding

TABLE 2 (CONTINUED)

AUTHOR	TREATMENT GROUPS; N	ELIGIBILITY	NINDS CRITERIA RANKING	FIO_2 AT ATA; WINDOW POST-TBI; DURATION; FREQUENCY
Harch[28]	(1) HBO_2; 16	Blast-induced chronic TBI that resulted in LOC and PCS or PTSD; Age 21–45; Military participants	2	100% at 1.5 ATA; Average = 2.8 years; 1 hour; 2 treatments per day, 5 days per week for 40 treatments

POSITIVE TREATMENT EFFECTS	NEGATIVE TREATMENT EFFECTS	NEUTRAL TREATMENT EFFECTS
• rCBF (Global SPECT-measured improvements in blood flow*) • PCS symptoms (Decreased after treatment*) • PTSD symptoms (Decreased after treatment*) • Anxiety and depression (Decreased after treatment*) • General symptoms (80% reported improvement in their symptoms immediately and 92% of those patients maintained improvement at 6-month follow-up) • Physical exam (Improvement seen in 87%–100% of physical exam findings) • Psychometric testing (7 of 13 measures showed improvement after treatment*) • Quality of life (Perception elevated after treatment*)		

*Significant Finding

TABLE 2 (CONTINUED)

AUTHOR	TREATMENT GROUPS; N	ELIGIBILITY	NINDS CRITERIA RANKING	FIO_2 AT ATA; WINDOW POST-TBI; DURATION; FREQUENCY
Neubauer[52]	(1) HBO_2; 1	TBI from MVC, Age 40, 28 days comatose	0	100% at 1.5 ATA twice a day for 28 treatments followed by 100% at 1.75 ATA twice a day for 106 treatments and 100% at 1.5 ATA twice a day for 54 treatments; 6 months
Artru[2]	(1) HBO_2; 6	Coma from head injury	0	100% at 2.5 ATA; ~2 months; 60 min; 1 treatment

LEGEND: ATA = x1 Atmospheric Pressure; CBF = Cerebral Blood Flow; $CMRO_2$ = Cerebral Metabolic Rate of Oxygen; CSF =Cerebrospinal Fluid; CTA = Computed Tomography Angiography; DRS = Disability Rating Scale; FiO_2 = inspired oxygen percentage; fMRI = functional Magnetic Resonance Imaging; GCS = Glasgow Coma Scale; HBO_2 = Hyperbaric Oxygen Treatment; ImPACT = Immediate Post-Concussion Assessment and Cognitive Test; LOC = Loss of Consciousness; MRI = Magnetic Resonance Imaging; MRS = Magnetic Resonance Spectroscopy; N = sample size; N/A = Not Applicable; NM = Not Mentioned; PaO_2 = Arterial Oxygen Pressure; PCL-M = Post-Traumatic Stress Disorder Checklist; PET = Positron Emission Tomography; PCS = Post-Concussive Syndrome; PTSD = Post-Traumatic Stress Disorder; rCBF = regional Cerebral Blood Flow; RPQ = Rivermead Post-Concussion Syndrome Questionnaire; SPECT = Single-Photon Emission Computed Tomography; TBI = Traumatic Brain Injury

PRECLINICAL STUDIES

Daugherty et al. and Zhou et al. from Virginia Commonwealth University have produced experimental mechanistic data that provides strong support for clinical observations of the effect of HBO_2 in TBI reported by Rockswold et al.[16,63-65,93] Both the Daugherty and Zhou studies used a lateral fluid percussion injury (FPI) model in rats to compare sham injured rats, an injured control group, and an injured group treated with 1 hour of HBO_2 (1.5 ATA) followed by 3 hours of normobaric hyperoxia (NBH) (HBO_2/NBH group). The Zhou study also included an injured group treated with NBH only (4 hours of 100% O_2 at 1.0 ATA). Hyperoxia treatments were started 15 minutes following injury. Daugherty et al. found that HBO_2/NBH significantly increased brain tissue pO_2 compared to the control group (247 mmHg versus 37.7 mmHg) and also caused a highly significant increase in global O_2 consumption in both injured and sham injured animals when compared to control animals receiving 30% fraction of inspired oxygen (FiO_2). Mitochondrial redox potential as measured by Alamar blue fluorescence was significantly reduced by the FPI when compared to sham injury which was completely reversed at four hours post injury in animals receiving HBO_2/

POSITIVE TREATMENT EFFECTS	NEGATIVE TREATMENT EFFECTS	NEUTRAL TREATMENT EFFECTS
• Cognitive, motor, linguistic, and speech improvements after 93 treatments • Regional deficits reduced after 160 treatments		
		• No effect of treatment seen in PaO2, $CMRO_2$, arterial lactate, CSF lactate, or CBF

*Significant Finding

NBH therapy. Zhou et al. found that ATP extracted and measured from the cerebral cortex using high-performance liquid chromatography was significantly reduced by the FPI when compared to the sham injury at the completion of the treatment. Both HBO_2/NBH and NBH alone significantly elevated ATP levels one hour post treatment compared to controls. These data indicate that mitochondrial function is depressed after TBI, but there is a potential for mitochondrial functional recovery that HBO_2 can enhance. Injured animals treated with HBO_2/NBH had significant improvement in cognitive recovery as characterized by a shorter latency in the Morris water maze performance (90.5 seconds for controls, 77.4 seconds for NBH, and 60.5 seconds for HBO_2). Significantly decreased neuronal loss in the CA2/3 and hilar regions of the hippocampus was seen in the HBO_2/NBH-treated animals as compared to controls or animals treated with NBH. There was no significant difference in neuronal cell counts between animals that received 30% FiO_2 and those receiving NBH treatment.

A series of elegant experiments conducted by the Tecnion Israel Institute of Technology using a cerebral contusion rat model have provided strong preclinical evidence for the neuroprotective effect of HBO_2.[56-57,72,80-81] A dynamic cortical deformation (DCD) injury model induced by negative pressure applied to the cortex was used. In these studies, DCD-injured rats (control group) were compared to an HBO_2-treated (2.8 ATA) group. Two consecutive 45-minute HBO_2 treatments separated by 5-minute air breaks were given daily for 3 days. The treatment window was three hours after injury. In the first two studies, there were two additional groups: DCD and postoperative hypoxia versus DCD and postoperative hypoxia followed by HBO_2.[56,80] All animals were sacrificed on day four and histological sections taken. Secondary brain damage was assessed by counting the number of terminal deoxynucleotidyl transferase-mediated dUTP nick end labeling (TUNEL) and caspase 3–positive cells in 0.5 mm thick successive increase in the TUNEL-positive cell index for apoptosis in each layer of the cortex. HBO_2 treatment induced a significant decrease in both the radius of the area of the lesion and severity of the brain damage following DCD. The reduction in lesion volume and severity was even more pronounced in HBO_2-treated injured rats compared to controls exposed to posttraumatic hypoxemia.[56] The TUNEL-positive cell index in the first layer in DCD-injured rats treated with HBO_2 was reduced by 53% and by 71.7% in the HBO_2 group exposed to DCD plus hypoxemia. The apoptosis-related proteins of the Bcl-2 family in the traumatic penumbra area were evaluated.[80] The expression of the antiapoptotic protein Bcl-2 was lower in the animals exposed to DCD plus hypoxemia than animals receiving injury from only DCD. A significant increase in Bcl-2 expression was seen in both groups after HBO_2 treatment. The investigators concluded that HBO_2 reduces the area of necrosis, cerebral edema, and secondary brain damage. It was also concluded that apoptotic mechanisms are important in delayed cell death in TBI and that posttraumatic hypoxemia increases the intensity of apoptosis, probably through a decrease in Bcl-2 and Bcl-xL expression that normally represses apoptosis. HBO_2 appears to enhance the expression of Bcl-2 and Bcl-xL, thus suppressing apoptosis.

The effect of HBO_2 on neuroinflammation and on the expression of matrix metalloproteinase (MMP)-9 was studied by Vlodavsky.[81] Neutrophils were revealed by myeloperoxidase staining, and immunohistochemical staining for MMP-9 also was performed. Both HBO_2 and NBH caused a significant decrease in neutrophilic inflammatory infiltration compared to control groups although the effect from HBO_2 was more pronounced and more extended. The expression of MMP-9 also was significantly lower in the HBO_2 group. These results demonstrated that hyperoxia decreased the extent of secondary cell death and reactive neuroinflammation in this TBI model compared to controls. The decline of MMP-9 expression after HBO_2 may also contribute to protection of brain tissue in the perilesional area.

In the final two studies, the investigators hypothesized that HBO_2-mediated enhancement of Bcl-2 expression and increased intracellular O_2 bioavailability may contribute to preserve mitochondrial integrity and reduce the activation of the mitochondrial pathway of apoptosis by involving the 18-kDa translocator protein (TSPO).[57,72] TSPO is mostly associated with the mitochondrial transition pore and its role in mitochondrial respiration. In mitochondria isolated from injured brain tissue, there was a profound loss of mitochondrial transmembrane potential that proved to be substantially reversed (approximately 70%) by HBO_2. This finding correlated with a significant reduction of caspase 3 and 9 activation in HBO_2-treated animals (60%) but not of caspase 8, indicating that the reduction of apoptotic cell death mediated by HBO_2 is achieved by a mitochondrial protective effect. In addition, HBO_2 reduced both the number of TSPO-expressing and TUNEL-positive cells in the perilesional area as compared to control groups (-52.7% of TSPO-positive cells for HBO_2 versus controls, respectively). Hyperoxia resulted in profound decreases in apoptosis in comparison to the control DCD group (-66.5% of TUNEL-positive cells for HBO_2 compared to controls across the perilesional area).

Wang et al. have systematically evaluated the effective treatment window for HBO_2 following TBI in a rat contusion model.[84] This was an exhaustive study utilizing over 300 animals which created a standardized parietal contusion using Feeney's weight-drop model. The neurological scoring systems proposed by Dixon et al. and Hall et al. were adapted, i.e., beam balancing test and prehensile traction test.[21,27] All neurologic evaluations were carried out by a researcher blinded to study group. Gravimetric analysis of brain water content, the incidence of apoptosis, and hippocampal ischemic cell loss also were evaluated. Time windows of HBO_2 effectiveness were evaluated at 3, 6, 12, 24, 48, and 72 hours after TBI. The effectiveness of a single treatment versus three or five treatments on consecutive days was also evaluated. Rats were randomized to either a HBO_2 treatment group receiving 3 ATA for 60 minutes or a sham-operated group. It was found that a single HBO_2 treatment given at 3, 6, or 12 hours post injury significantly reduced the neurology deficit score and brain water content, improved the preservation of neuronal cells in the hippocampus, and reduced apoptosis in the cortex surrounding the primary injury. There was no notable effect when a single treatment of HBO_2 was started at 24, 48, or 72 hours after TBI. However, when the first HBO_2 treatment was started up to 24 hours after TBI, multiple HBO_2 treatments (either 3 or 5 consecutive days) decreased the neurology deficit score and neuronal cell loss significantly more than compared to a single treatment. When the first HBO_2 treatment was carried out at 48 hours after TBI, multiple treatments reduced the neurology deficit score and increased the number of neurons preserved as compared to the control group. However, the improvement was less than that seen with a single HBO_2 treatment administered as early as six hours after TBI. When the first HBO_2 treatment was deferred until 72 hours, there was no improvement in these outcome measures.

CLINICAL TRIALS

Evaluation of the clinical studies utilizing HBO_2 for the treatment of more severe TBI injury indicates a number of weaknesses (Table 1). Most of the protocols were not uniform and the number of subjects relatively small. The severity of brain injury is not well described as the GCS scoring and systematic outcome timing and measures were not utilized. In addition, none of the trials were truly randomized. The clinical trials by Rockswold et al. do not have the same methodologic weaknesses.

The following clinical trial by Holbach et al. represents the trials available in the older literature.[31] A series of 99 patients suffering TBI and what was termed a "mid-brain syndrome" is presented. This study was published in German and was translated. One hundred percent of the patients were described as comatose and 93% with abnormal pupils. Every other patient was treated with HBO_2 at 1.5 ATA for approximately 30 minutes. In most cases, the treatment was performed between the second and tenth day of hospitalization. The patients were followed after discharge and evaluated, although the time post injury is not specified. Seventy-four percent of the control group either died or were left in a vegetative state, and 53% of the HBO_2-treated group were in a similar state. Thirty-three percent of the HBO_2-treated patients made what was termed a complete recovery as opposed to only 6% of the control group. Both of these differences were statistically significant according to our statistician. The trial obviously suffers from a number of deficiencies, including unblended randomization, a variable HBO_2 treatment paradigm, and the outcome not given at a specific time. However, it does suggest a signal of efficacy in these badly injured patients.

The first prospective randomized clinical trial (RCT) by Rockswold et al. randomized 168 patients within 24 hours of injury equally into two groups: a control group and an HBO_2 treatment group (1.5 ATA per 60 minutes).[62] Hyperbaric oxygen treatments were given every 8 hours for 14 days unless the patient began to follow commands or became brain dead. In retrospect, this protocol was chosen very arbitrarily. The dichotomized Glasgow Outcome Scale (GOS) was assessed by a blinded independent examiner. This clinical outcome study demonstrated that HBO_2

can be administered safely and systematically to severe TBI patients and that mortality rates were reduced by a relative 50% (32% for controls and 17% for HBO_2-treated). This effect was especially dramatic in patients with negative outcome predictors, that is intracranial hypertension, evacuated mass lesions, and Glasgow Coma Scale (GCS) scores of 4 to 6. No improvement occurred in clinical outcome using the dichotomized GOS at six months. A reanalysis of the raw data and outcomes was performed by the biostatistical group at the Medical University of South Carolina (unpublished data). Since the favorable impact on mortality rate by HBO_2 occurred in the more severely injured patients, it was hypothesized that patients with GCS scores of 7 or 8 with diffuse injury were "diluting" the treatment effect. This subgroup (49 patients) had a favorable outcome of 71% using the dichotomized GOS. The reanalysis of the remaining patients showed that 19 of 57 (33.3%) in the control group and 27 of 60 (45%) of the HBO_2-treated group had a favorable outcome using the dichotomized GOS. This difference represents an absolute 11.7% improvement in favorable outcome. When the sliding dichotomized GOS was used, 26 of 57 (45.6%) in the control group compared to 35 of 60 (58.3%) in the treatment group achieved a favorable outcome. This difference represents an absolute 12.7% improvement in favorable outcome. Because of the smaller numbers, these differences did not reach statistical significance.

A second prospective, clinical physiologic study to determine the effects of HBO_2 on cerebral metabolism and ICP was performed.[(63)] Thirty-seven patients treated for severe TBI were entered into the study within 24 hours of injury. All patients received HBO_2 at 1.5 ATA for 60 minutes. Treatments were administered once every 24 hours for 5 days. Cerebral blood flow (CBF), arterial venous difference of oxygen (AVDO2), $CMRO_2$, ventricular cerebral spinal fluid (CSF) lactate levels, and ICP measurements were obtained one hour before HBO_2 and one hour and six hours after HBO_2 treatments. CBF and $CMRO_2$ were increased post treatment in patients who began their HBO_2 treatment with a reduced or normal blood flow ($p < 0.05$). Levels of CSF lactate were consistently decreased after HBO_2 sessions ($p = 0.01$). Patients with elevated ICP (> 15 mmHg) prior to HBO_2 showed a consistent and highly significant reduction in their ICP from completion of HBO_2 treatment to 6 hours post treatment ($p = 0.006$). Effects occurred whether their HBO_2 was delivered in the first 24 hours after injury or up to 5 days after injury. The results of this study indicate that HBO_2 may have improved the ability of ischemic or damaged brain tissue to utilize the O_2 received in baseline FiO_2 for at least six hours following the HBO_2. This improved utilization led to improved $CMRO_2$ and decreased CSF lactate levels, which also persisted for at least six hours, indicating a shift toward aerobic metabolism. The authors hypothesized that CBF rises in response to this increased cerebral metabolism. When CBF and $CMRO_2$ are normally metabolically coupled, the ratio between them does not change. In other words, the $AVDO_2$ remains constant. This trend for HBO_2 to normalize metabolic coupling of CBF and cerebral metabolism was most apparent in patients with reduced CBF or with ischemia as documented by high lactate levels.

A third prospective, randomized control trial directly compared the effect of HBO_2 to NBH on surrogate markers of oxidative cerebral metabolism and O_2 toxicity that predict and closely correlate with clinical outcome.[(64)] Sixty-nine patients sustaining severe TBI (mean GCS score 5.8) were prospectively randomized within 24 hours of their injury into 1 of 3 groups: (1) HBO_2: 60 minutes of HBO_2 at 1.5 ATA; (2) NBH: 3 hours of 100% FiO_2 at 1 ATA; and (3) control. Treatments occurred every 24 hours for 3 consecutive days. Brain tissue pO_2 was continuously monitored. Microdialysis lactate, pyruvate, and glycerol as well as ICP were collected hourly. Cerebral blood flow, $AVDO_2$, $CMRO_2$, CSF lactate, F2-isoprostane, and bronchial alveolar lavage (BAL) fluid interleukin (IL)-8 and IL-6 assays were obtained pretreatment and at one and six hours post treatment. Mixed-effect linear modeling was used to statistically test differences between the treatment arms as well as changes from pretreatment to post treatment. Data from the study can be summarized as follows:

1. HBO_2 had a significantly greater positive posttreatment effect than NBH on oxidative cerebral metabolism.
2. Although the treatment effect was not an all-or-nothing phenomenon, a critical brain tissue pO_2 level of 200 mmHg was important in achieving a robust positive effect on cerebral metabolism, especially $CMRO_2$, which reflects mitochondrial function. Brain tissue pO_2 levels of > 200 mmHg were reached in only 51% of the HBO_2 treatment sessions and 5% of the NBH treatments. This finding indicates that higher pressures of HBO_2 may be more effective than 1.5 ATA.
3. HBO_2 had a posttreatment effect lasting between 6 and 24 hours, which suggests that HBO_2 can be delivered intermittently to obtain the treatment effect over many days and reduce potential O_2 toxicity.
4. The treatment effect was as great on day 3 as it was in the first 24 hours, that is, the treatment effect was the same after the first treatment as after the third, which implies that HBO_2 is effective in improving mitochondrial function even when ischemia is not overtly present.
5. ICP was reduced after HBO_2 treatments in comparison with levels following standard care. The NBH group did not demonstrate a reduction in ICP.
6. There was no evidence of cerebral or pulmonary O_2 toxicity in either of the HBO_2 or NBH treatment paradigms administered.

The clinical study described above demonstrated that the positive effect on cerebral oxidative metabolism occurred following, not during, the HBO_2 treatment.(64) The $CMRO_2$ is a surrogate marker of mitochondrial function and was improved significantly at six hours post HBO_2 treatment. The data suggested that the HBO_2 treatment improved the brain's ability to utilize subsequent baseline O_2. This finding strongly supports the concept that O_2 is acting primarily as a signal transducer rather than a respiratory metabolite.(69) This hypothesis was tested in two experimental studies described above.(16,93) Mitochondrial redox potential remained significantly reduced by the FPI at the completion of the HBO_2 treatment. The reduction in mitochondrial redox potential, however, was completely reversed after four hours of NBH following HBO_2. This finding confirmed that HBO_2 improves cerebral metabolism after the treatment rather than during the treatment.

In the final prospective randomized trial by Rockswold et al., 42 patients who sustained severe TBI (mean GCS score 5.7) were prospectively randomized within 24 hours of injury to either (1) combined HBO_2/NBH: 60 minutes of HBO_2 at 1.5 ATA followed by NBH, 3 hours of 100% FiO_2 at 1.0 ATA; or (2) control, standard care.(65) Treatments occurred once every 24 hours for 3 consecutive days. Intracranial pressure, surrogate markers for cerebral metabolism and O_2 toxicity were monitored. Clinical outcome was assessed at six months using the severity-adjusted dichotomized GOS score. Mixed-effects linear modeling was used to statistically test differences between the treatment and control groups. Functional outcome and mortality rates were compared using chi-squared tests. There were no significant differences in demographic characteristics between the two groups.

Data in this study can be summarized by the following key points:

1. The combined HBO_2/NBH treatment significantly improved markers for oxidative cerebral metabolism in relatively uninjured brain tissue, and importantly, also in pericontusional tissue.
2. The combined HBO_2/NBH treatment reduced intracranial hypertension and thereby decreased the therapeutic intensity of treatment of intracranial hypertension.
3. There was no evidence of O_2 toxicity either in the brain or in the lungs, and there was actual demonstrated significant improvement in markers of cerebral toxicity.
4. Combining HBO_2 and NBH into a single treatment potentially has a synergistic therapeutic effect.
5. Although the study was relatively small in terms of numbers, it showed a statistically significant improvement in functional outcome and mortality rate. The mortality rate was 16% for the combined HBO_2/NBH group as compared with 42% for the control group or an absolute percentage reduction of 26% ($p = 0.048$). Thirty-eight percent of the control group and 74% of the HBO_2/NBH group had a favorable outcome based on the sliding dichotomized GOS for an absolute 36% improvement ($p = 0.024$). Based on the dichotomized GOS, 33% of the control group and 58% of the combined HBO_2/NBH group had a favorable outcome for a 25% absolute improvement ($p = 0.077$). This outcome is significantly better than prior experience using HBO_2 as a single treatment or reports from the literature using NBH (Rockswold 1992, Tolias 2004). This improvement in clinical outcome may be secondary to the synergistic effect of combining HBO_2 and NBH treatments.

AVAILABILITY, SAFETY, AND OXYGEN TOXICITY ISSUES

Most neurosurgeons treating severe TBI are familiar with HBO_2 treatment only in a relatively vague way. Even amongst neurosurgeons more familiar with the technique, the idea of placing an intubated, severely brain-injured patient with multiple injuries into an HBO_2 chamber, particularly a monoplace, seems prohibitive.[87] One of the challenges in establishing HBO_2 as an accepted therapy for severe TBI is to establish its safety as well as the efficacy of the treatment.

Several authors have noted that although HBO_2 has shown beneficial effects in animals and humans, this treatment option remains limited because of the expense and very limited availability of HBO_2 chambers.[76-77] Two types of HBO_2 delivery systems exist. One is the traditional multiple-occupancy, large compartment chamber. It is designed to accommodate several patients and attendant medical personnel and has long represented the technology standard. Advantages include the fact that multiple patients can be treated at one time, and there is direct patient attendance during each HBO_2 treatment. There are significant disadvantages, including the greater degree of technology and related support requirements, a larger physical plant footprint, and higher capitalization and operating costs.

An alternate delivery system is the monoplace chamber. It supports a single patient with attendance and support provided from the chamber exterior. The monoplace chamber has been employed across a broad range of patient conditions to an increasing degree over the past two decades. Our institution has found it entirely adequate for the safe care and management of critically ill and ventilator-dependent patients sustaining severe TBI and multiple injuries.[25] The major advantages of the monoplace chamber are (1) minimal physical space footprint, (2) easily incorporate in and adjacent to a critical care support area, (3) minimal technology demands, (4) the delivery system can be effectively and safely operated by existing nursing, respiratory, and standard medical support staff upon appropriate training and preceptorship, (5) lower capitalization and operating costs, and (6) no risk of iatrogenic decompression sickness in support staff. The cost of an HBO_2 monoplace chamber with appropriate adaptations for monitoring critically ill patients and installation is approximately USD$200,000.

Based on our own past clinical trials, as well as that of Weaver et al., placing severe TBI patients in either a monoplace or multiplace HBO_2 chamber is a very low-risk procedure.[61-63,85-87] As above, monoplace chambers are much less expensive than multiplace chambers and can be placed in or near the intensive care unit. In fact, the monoplace chamber becomes an extension of the critical care environment. Continuous monitoring of ICP, mean arterial pressure (MAP), cerebral perfusion pressure (CPP), end tidal carbon dioxide (CO_2), and brain tissue pO_2 can be performed. In addition, central venous pressure or Swan Ganz catheter monitoring are done if needed. Careful evaluation of the patient's pulmonary status prior to HBO_2 treatment is critical. In our work, we have regarded a baseline FiO_2 requirement of greater than 50% and a positive end-expiration pressure (PEEP) of greater than 10 to maintain adequate oxygenation as contraindications to HBO_2. It is essential to maintain adequate ventilation throughout the treatment. In the case of an emergency, an intubated, ventilated patient can be decompressed and out of the chamber in two minutes. We routinely perform myringotomy to reduce patient stimulation during treatment, and thereby, ICP.[62]

The lung is the organ most commonly damaged by hyperoxia since the O_2 tension in the lungs is substantially higher than in other tissues.[37] The mechanism by which pulmonary injury occurs has been termed oxidative stress.[41,88] Central to this process is the release of proinflammatory cytokines by alveolar macrophages, specifically IL-8 and IL-6, and the subsequent influx of activated cells into the alveolar air space.[17-18] Measurement of these proinflammatory cytokines in bronchial alveolar lavage has been shown to be predictive of acute lung injury and pulmonary infection in exposure to superphysiological concentrations of inspired O_2.[50] In two studies by Rockswold et al., there were no increases in these proinflammatory cytokines in HBO_2-treated patients compared to control patients.[64-65] In the clinical trial described previously in which 84 TBI patients received 1688 HBO_2 treatments, no permanent sequelae resulted. [62] Pulmonary complications occasionally occurred (10 of 84 patients), but all were reversible.

Oxygen, especially under increased pressure, also may cause potential cerebral toxicity. Brain tissue is especially vulnerable to lipid peroxidation because of its high rate of O_2 consumption and high content of phospholipids. Additionally, the brain has limited natural protection against free radicals, i.e., it has limited scavenging ability, poor catalase activity, and is rich in iron, which is an initiator of radical generation in brain injury.[19-20,34,55] Brain tissue is especially vulnerable to lipid peroxidation because of its high rate of O_2 consumption and higher content of phospholipids.[19-20,34,55] Cerebrospinal fluid F-2 isoprostanes are a unique series of prostaglandin-like compounds formed in vivo from the free-radical-catalyzed peroxidation of arachidonic acid and have been used to assess peroxidation in patients sustaining severe TBI.[4-5,23,49] Glycerol is an end product of phosolipid degradation and neural tissue cell membranes and is a marker of cell damage whether caused by O_2 toxicity via free-radical formation and lipid peroxidation or secondarily from ischemia.[22,24,43] Levels of both CSF F-2 isoprostanes as well as microdialysate glycerol were significantly decreased following combined HBO_2/NBH treatment in the study performed by Rockswold et al.[65] These findings may not only signify that there were no signs of O_2 toxicity from the combined HBO_2/NBH treatment, but, in fact, that there was a protective effect against neuroinflammation and free-radical-mediated damage.[65]

In conclusion, HBO_2 treatments at a depth of 1.5 ATA can be delivered to the severe TBI patient with or without multiple injuries in either a monoplace or multiplace chamber with relative safety and low risk of O_2 toxicity.

CONCLUSION

The use of HBO_2 in the treatment of TBI has been controversial. Oxygen toxicity and safety concerns have been at the forefront of this controversy. In truth, the complications from HBO_2 have been rare and reversible in the authors' experience. Historically, HBO_2 was seen as a mechanism to decrease CBF and ICP while increasing O_2 availability to injured brain cells.[45,74-75] As highly technical equipment has become available in both TBI animal and clinical studies, however, HBO_2 appears to be working at the mitochondrial level to improve cerebral aerobic metabolism after brain injury.[63,77,93] Clinically, HBO_2 has been shown to decrease mortality rates and improve functional outcome in severely brain-injured patients.[1,31,62] As research on HBO_2 continues, the goal is to accomplish a multicenter, prospective, randomized clinical outcome trial by which the efficacy of HBO_2 in the treatment of severely brain-injured patients is evaluated.

REFERENCES

1. Artru F, Chacornac R, Deleuze R. Hyperbaric oxygenation for severe head injuries: preliminary results of a controlled study. Eur Neurol. 1976;14:310-8.
2. Artru F, Philippon B, Gau F, Berger M, Deleuze R. Cerebral blood flow, cerebral metabolism and cerebrospinal fluid biochemistry in brain-injured patients after exposure to hyperbaric oxygen. Eur Neurol. 1976;14:351-64.
3. Barrett KF, Masel B, Patterson J, Scheibel RS, Corson KP, Mader JT. Regional CBF in chronic stable TBI treated with hyperbaric oxygen. Undersea Hyperb Med. 2004;31:395-406.
4. Bayir H, Kagan VE, Tyurina YY, Tyurin V, Ruppel RA, Adelson PD, et al. Assessment of antioxidant reserves and oxidative stress in cerebrospinal fluid after severe traumatic brain injury in infants and children. Pediatr Res. 2002;51(5):571-8.
5. Bayir H, Marion DW, Puccio AM, Wisniewski R, Janesko KL, Clark RS, et al. Marked gender effect on lipid peroxidation after severe traumatic brain injury in adult patients. J Neurotrauma. 2004;21(1):1-8.
6. Bergsneider M, Hovda DA, Shalmon E, et al. Cerebral hyperglycolysis following severe traumatic brain injury in humans: a positron emission tomography study. J Neurosurg. 1997;86(2):241-51.
7. Bergsneider M, Hovda DA, McArthur DL, et al. Metabolic recovery following human traumatic brain injury based on FDG-PET: time course and relationship to neurological disability. J Head Trauma Rehabil. 2001;16(2):135-48.
8. Bouma GJ, Muizelaar JP, Choi SC, et al. Cerebral circulation and metabolism after severe traumatic brain injury: the elusive role of ischemia. J Neurosurg. 1991;75:685-93.
9. Bouma GJ, Muizelaar JP, Stringer WA, et al. Ultra-early evaluation of regional cerebral blood flow in severely head-injured patients using xenon-enhanced computerized tomography. J Neurosurg. 1992;77:360-8.
10. Boussi-Gross R, Golan H, Fishlev G, Bechor Y, et al. Hyperbaric oxygen therapy can improve post concussion syndrome years after mild traumatic brain injury – randomized prospective trial. PLoS One. 2013;8(11):e79995. doi:10.1371/journal.pone.0079995.
11. Brown JA, Preul MC, Taha A. Hyperbaric oxygen in the treatment of elevated intracranial pressure after head injury. Pediatr Neurosci. 1988;14:286-90.
12. Churchill S, Weaver LK, Deru K, Russo Aa, Handrahan D, et al. A prospective trial of hyperbaric oxygen for chronic sequelae after brain injury (HYBOBI). Undersea Hyperb Med. 2013;40(2):165-93.
13. Cifu DX, Walker WC, West SL, Hart BB, Franke LM, et al. Hyperbaric oxygen for blast-related postconcussion syndrome: three-month outcomes. Ann Neurol. 2014;75(2):277-86.
14. Cifu DX, Hoke KW, Wetzel PA, Wares JR, Gitchel G, Carne W. Effects of hyperbaric oxygen on eye tracking abnormalities in males after mild traumatic brain injury. J Rehabil Res Dev. 2014;51(7):1047-56.
15. Cifu DX, Hart BB, West SL, Walker W, Carne W. The effect of hyperbaric oxygen on persistent postconcussion symptoms. J Head Trauma Rehabil. 2014;29(1):11-20. doi:10.1097/HTR.0b013e3182a6aaf0.
16. Daugherty WP, Levasseur JE, Sun D, et al. Effects of hyperbaric oxygen therapy on cerebral oxygenation and mitochondrial function following moderate lateral fluid-percussion injury in rats. J Neurosurg. 2004;101:499-504.

17. Deaton PR, McKellar CT, Culbreth R, et al. Hyperoxia stimulates interleukin-8 release from alveolar macrophages and U937 cells: attenuation by dexamethasone. Am J Physiol. 1994;267:L187-92.

18. DeForge LE, Preston AM, Takeuchi E, et al. Regulation of interleukin-8 gene expression by oxidant stress. J Biol Chem. 1993;268(34):25568-76.

19. Demopoulos HB, Flamm E, Seligman M, Pietronigro DD. Oxygen free radicals in central nervous system ischemia and trauma. In: Autor AP, editor. Pathology of oxygen. New York: Academic Press; 1982A. p. 127-55.

20. Demopoulos HS, Flamm ES, Seligman ML, Pietronigro DD, Tomasula J, Decrescito V. Further studies on free-radical pathology in the major central nervous system disorders: effect of very high doses of methylprednisolone on the functional outcome, morphology, and chemistry of experimental spinal cord impact injury. Can J Physiol Pharmacol. 1982B;60:1415-24.

21. Dixon CE, Lyeth BG, Povlishock JT, et al. A fluid percussion model of experimental brain injury in the rat. J Neurosurg. 1987;67:110-9.

22. Engstrom M, Polito A, Reinstrup P, Romner B, Ryding E, Ungerstedt U, et al. Intracerebral microdialysis in severe brain trauma: the importance of catheter location. J Neurosurg. 2005;102:460-9.

23. Fam SS, Morrow JD. The isoprostanes: unique products of arachidonic acid oxidation – a review. Current Med Chem. 2003;10:1723-40.

24. Frykholm P, Hillered L, Langstrom B, Persson L, Valtysson J, Watanabe Y, et al. Increase of interstitial glycerol reflects the degree of ischemia brain damage: a PET and microdialysis study in a middle cerebral artery occlusion-reperfusion primate model. J Neurosurg Psychiatry. 2001;71:455-61.

25. Gossett WA, Rockswold GL, Rockswold SB, Adkinson CD, Bergman TA, Quickel RR. The safe treatment, monitoring, and management of severe traumatic brain injury patients in a monoplace chamber. Undersea Hyperb Med. 2010;37(1):35-48.

26. Glenn TC, Kelly DF, Boscardin WJ, et al. Energy dysfunction as a predictor of outcome after moderate or severe head injury: indices of oxygen, glucose, and lactate metabolism. J Cereb Blood Flow Metab. 2003;23(10):1239-50.

27. Hall ED, Yonkers PA, McCall JM, et al. Effects of the 21-aminosteroid U74006F on experimental head injury in mice. J Neurosurg. 1988;68:456-61.

28. Harch PG, Andrews SR, Fogarty EF, Amen D, Pezzullo JC, et al. A phase I study of low-pressure hyperbaric oxygen therapy for blast-induced post-concussion syndrome and post-traumatic stress disorder. J Neurotrauma. 2012;29(1):168-85. doi:10.1089/neu.2011.1895.

29. Hayakawa T, Kanai N, Kuroda R, et al. Response of cerebrospinal fluid pressure to hyperbaric oxygenation. J Neuro Neurosurg Psychiatry. 1971;34:580-6.

30. Holbach KH, Schroder FK, Koster S. Alterations of cerebral metabolism in cases with acute brain injuries during spontaneous respiration of air, oxygen and hyperbaric oxygen. Euro Neurol. 1972;8(1):158-60.

31. Holbach KH, Wassman H, Kolberg T. Verbesserte reversibilitat des traumatischen mittelhirnsyndroms bei anwendung der hyperbaren oxygenierung [Improved reversibility of the traumatic midbrain syndrome using hyperbaric oxygen]. Acta Neurochir. 1974;30:247-56.

32. Holbach KH, Caroli A, Wassmann H. Cerebral energy metabolism in patients with brain lesions of normo- and hyperbaric oxygen pressures. J Neurol. 1977;217(1):17-30.

33. Hovda DA, Yoshino A, Kawamata T, et al. Diffuse prolonged depression of cerebral oxidative metabolism following concussive brain injury in the rat: a cytochrome oxidase histochemistry study. Brain Res. 1991;567(1):1-10.

34. Ikeda Y, Long DM. The molecular basis of brain injury and brain edema: the role of oxygen-free radicals. Neurosurg. 1990;27:1-11.

35. Jaggi JL, Obrist WD, Gennarelli TA. Relationship of early cerebral blood flow and metabolism to outcome in acute head injury. J Neurosurg. 1990;72:176-82.

36. Juul N, Morris GF, Marshall SB, et al. Intracranial hypertension and cerebral perfusion pressure: influence on neurological deterioration and outcome in severe head injury. J Neurosurg. 2000;92:1-6.

37. Klein J. Normobaric pulmonary oxygen toxicity. Anesth Analg. 1990;70:195-207.

38. Lifshitz J, Sullivan PG, Hovda DA, et al. Mitochondrial damage and dysfunction in traumatic brain injury. Mitochondrion. 2004;1-9.

39. Lin JW, Tsai JT, Lee LM, Lin CM, Hung CC, et al. Effect of hyperbaric oxygen on patients with traumatic brain injury. Acta Neurochir Suppl. 2008;101:145-9.

40. Lin K, Niu K, Tsai K, Kuo J, Wang L, Wang L, Chio C, Chang C. Attenuating inflammation but stimulating both angiogenesis and neurogenesis using hyperbaric oxygen in rats with traumatic brain injury. J Trauma. 2012;72(3):650-9.

41. Mantell LL, Horowitz S, Davis JM, et al. Hyperoxia-induced cell death in the lung – the correlation of apoptosis, necrosis, and inflammation. Ann NY Acad Sci. 1999;887:171-80.

42. Menon DK, Coles JP, Gupta AK, et al. Diffusion limited oxygen delivery following head injury. Crit Care Med. 2004;32(6):1384-90.

43. Merenda A, Gugliotta M, Holloway R, Levasseur JE, Alessandri B, Sun D, et al. Validation of brain extracellular glycerol as an indicator of cellular membrane damage due to free radical activity after traumatic brain injury. J Neurotrauma. 2008;25:527-38.

44. Miller JD, Fitch W, Ledingham IM, et al. The effect of hyperbaric oxygen on experimentally increased intracranial pressure. J Neurosurg. 1970;33:287-96.

45. Miller JD, Ledingham IM. Reduction of increased intracranial pressure. Arch Neurol. 1971;24:210-6.

46. Miller RS, Weaver LK, Bahraini N, Churchill S, Price RC, Skiba V, et al. Effects of hyperbaric oxygen on symptoms and quality of life among service members with persistent postconcussion symptoms: a randomized clinical trial. JAMA Intern Med. 2015;175:43-52. doi:10.1001/jamainternmed.2014.5479.

47. Mink RB, Dutka AJ. Hyperbaric oxygen after global cerebral ischemia in rabbits reduces brain vascular permeability and blood flow. Stroke. 1995A;26:2307-12.

48. Mogami H, Hayakawa T, Kanai N, Kuroda R, Yamada R, et al. Clinical application of hyperbaric oxygenation in the treatment of acute cerebral damage. J Neurosurg. 1969;31(6):636-43. doi:10.3171/jns.1969.31.6.0636.

49. Morrow JD. The isoprostanes: their quantification as an index of oxidant stress status in vivo. Drug Metab Rev. 2000;32(3-4):377-85.

50. Muehlstedt SG, Richardson CJ, Lyte M, et al. Cytokines and the pathogenesis of nosocomial pneumonia. Surgery. 2001;130(4):602-9; discussion 609-11.

51. Muizelaar JP, Marmarou A, DeSalles A, et al. Cerebral blood flow and metabolism in severely head-injured children. J Neurosurg. 1989;71:63-71.

52. Neubauer RA, Gottlieb SF, Pevsner NH. Hyperbaric oxygen for treatment of closed head injury. South Med J. 1994;87(9):933-6.

53. Nida TY, Biros MH, Pheley AM, Bergman TA, Rockswold GL. Effect of hypoxia or hyperbaric oxygen on cerebral edema following moderate fluid percussion or cortical impact injury in rats. J Neurotrauma. 1995;12:77-85.

54. Obrist WD, Langfitt TW, Jaggi JL, et al. Cerebral blood flow and metabolism in comatose patients with acute head injury. J Neurosurg. 1984;61:241-53.

55. Ortega BD, Demopoulos HB, Ransohoff J. Effect of antioxidants on experimental cold-induced cerebral edema. In: Reulen HJ, Schurmann K, editors. Steroids and brain edema. New York: Springer-Verlag; 1972. p. 167-75.

56. Palzur E, Vlodavsky E, Mulla H, et al. Hyperbaric oxygen therapy for reduction of secondary brain damage in head injury: an animal model of brain contusion. J Neurotrauma. 2004;21(1):41-8.

57. Palzur E, Zaaroor M, Vlodavsky E, et al. Neuroprotective effect of hyperbaric oxygen therapy in brain injury is mediated by preservation of mitochondrial membrane properties. Brain Res. 2008:126-33.

58. Prakash A, Parelkar SV, Oak SN, Gupta RK, Sanghvi, et al. Role of hyperbaric oxygen therapy in severe head injury in children. J Pediatr Neurosci. 2012;7(1):4-8. doi:10.4103/1817-1745.97610.

59. Ren H, Wang W, Ge Z. Glasgow Coma Scale, brain electric activity mapping and Glasgow Outcome Scale after hyperbaric oxygen treatment of severe brain injury. Chin J Traumatol. 2001;4(4):239-41.

60. Robertson CS, Clifton GL, Grossman RG, et al. Alterations in cerebral availability of metabolic substrates after severe head injury. J Trauma. 1988;28(11):1523-32.

61. Rockswold GL, Ford SE, Anderson BJR. Patient monitoring in the monoplace hyperbaric chamber. Hyperb Oxyg Rev. 1985;6:161-8.

62. Rockswold GL, Ford SE, Anderson DL, et al. Results of a prospective randomized trial for treatment of severely brain-injured patients with hyperbaric oxygen. J Neurosurg. 1992;76:929-34.

63. Rockswold SB, Rockswold GL, Vargo JM, et al. The effects of hyperbaric oxygen on cerebral metabolism and intracranial pressure in severely brain-injured patients. J Neurosurg. 2001;94:403-11.

64. Rockswold SB, Rockswold GL, Zaun DA, Zhang X, Cerra CE, Bergman TA, Liu J. A prospective, randomized clinical trial to compare the effect of hyperbaric to normobaric hyperoxia on cerebral metabolism, intracranial pressure, and oxygen toxicity in severe traumatic brain injury. J Neurosurg. 2010;112(5):1080-94.

65. Rockswold SB, Rockswold GL, Zaun DA, Liu J. A prospective, randomized clinical trial to evaluate the effect of combined hyperbaric and normobaric hyperoxia on cerebral metabolism, intracranial pressure, oxygen toxicity, and clinical outcome in severe traumatic brain injury. J Neurosurg. 2013;118(6):1317-28.

66. Rogatsky GG, Kamenir Y, Mayevsky A. Effect of hyperbaric oxygenation on intracranial pressure elevation rate in rats during the early phase of severe traumatic brain injury. Brain Res. 2005;1047:131-6.

67. Saatman KE, Duhaime AC, Bullock R, et al. Classification of traumatic brain injury for targeted therapies. J Neurotrauma. 2008;25:719-38.

68. Sahni T, Jain M, Prasad R, Sogani SK, Singh VP. Use of hyperbaric oxygen in traumatic brain injury: retrospective analysis of data of 20 patients treated at a tertiary care centre. Br J Neurosurg. 2012;26(2):202-7. doi:10.3109/02688697.2011.626879.

69. Siddiqui A, Davidson JD, Mustoe TA. Ischemic tissue oxygen capacitance after hyperbaric oxygen therapy: a new physiologic concept. Plast Reconstr Surg. 1997;99:148-55.

70. Signoretti S, Marmarou A, Tavazzi B, et al. N-Acetylaspartate reduction as a measure of injury severity and mitochondrial dysfunction following diffuse traumatic brain injury. J Neurotrauma. 2001;18(10):977-91.

71. Signoretti S, Marmarou A, Aygok GA, et al. Assessment of mitochondrial impairment in traumatic brain injury using high-resolution proton magnetic resonance spectroscopy. J Neurosurg. 2008;108:42-52.

72. Soustiel JF, Palzur E, Vlodavsky E, et al. The effect of oxygenation level on cerebral post traumatic apoptosis is modulated by the 18-kDa translocator protein (also known as peripheral-type benzodiazepine receptor) in a rat model of cortical contusion. Neuropath Appl Neurobio. 2008;34:412-23.

73. Stein SC, Georgoff P, Meghan S, Mizra K, Sonnad SS. 150 years of treating severe traumatic brain injury: a systemic review of progress in mortality. J Neurotrauma. 2010;27:1343-53.

74. Sukoff MH, Hollin SA, Espinosa OE, et al. The protective effect of hyperbaric oxygenation in experimental cerebral edema. J Neurosurg. 1968;29:236-41.

75. Sukoff MH, Ragatz RE. Hyperbaric oxygenation for the treatment of acute cerebral edema. Neurosurgery. 1982;10:29-38.

76. Tisdall MM, Tachtsidis I, Leung TS, et al. Increase in cerebral aerobic metabolism by normobaric hyperoxia after traumatic brain injury. J Neurosurg. 2008;109:424-32.

77. Tolias CM, Reinert M, Seiler R, et al. Normobaric hyperoxia-induced improvement in cerebral metabolism and reduction in intracranial pressure in patients with severe head injury: a prospective historical cohort-matched study. J Neurosurg. 2004;101:435-44.

78. Verweij BH, Muizelaar P, Vinas FC, et al. Impaired cerebral mitochondrial function after traumatic brain injury in humans. J Neurosurg. 2000;93(5):815-20.

79. Vigue B, Ract C, Benayed M, et al. Early $SjvO_2$ monitoring in patients with severe brain trauma. Intensive Care Med. 1999;25:445-51.

80. Vlodavsky E, Palzur E, Feinsod M, et al. Evaluation of the apoptosis-related proteins of the BCL-2 family in the traumatic penumbra area of the rat model of cerebral contusion, treated by hyperbaric oxygen therapy: a quantitative immunohistochemical study. Acta Neuropathol. 2005;110:120-6.

81. Vlodavsky E, Palzur E, Soustiel JF. Hyperbaric oxygen therapy reduces neuroinflammation and expression of matrix metalloproteinase-9 in the rat model of traumatic brain injury. Neuropath Appl Neurobio. 2006;32:40-50.

82. Wada K, Ito M, Miyazawa T, et al. Repeated hyperbaric oxygen induces ischemic tolerance in gerbil hippocampus. Brain Res. 1996;740:15-20.

83. Wada K, Miyazawa T, Nomura N, et al. Preferential conditions for and possible mechanisms of induction of ischemic tolerance by repeated hyperbaric oxygenation in gerbil hippocampus. Neurosurgery. 2001;49:160-7.

84. Wang G, Zhang X, Jiang Z, Li X, Peng L, Li Y, Wang Y. Neuroprotective effects of hyperbaric oxygen treatment on traumatic brain injury in the rat. J Neurotrauma. 2010;27:1733-43.

85. Weaver LK, Greenway L, Elliot CG. Performance of the Sechrist 500A hyperbaric ventilator in a monoplace hyperbaric chamber. J Hyperb Med. 1988;3(4):215-25.

86. Weaver LK. Management of critically ill patients in the monoplace hyperbaric chamber. In: Kindwall EP, Whelan HT, editors. Hyperbaric medicine practice. 2nd ed. Flagstaff (AZ): Best Publishing Co.; 1999. p. 245-79.

87. Weaver LK. Operational use and patient monitoring in the monoplace chamber. In: Moon R, McIntrye N, editors. Respiratory care clinics of North America – hyperbaric medicine, Part I. Philadelphia: W.B. Saunders Co.; 1999. p. 51-92.

88. Wispe JR, Roberts RJ. Molecular basis of pulmonary oxygen toxicity. Clin Perinatol. 1987;14(3):651-6.

89. Wolf G, Cifu D, Baugh L, Carne W, Profenna L. The effect of hyperbaric oxygen on symptoms after mild traumatic brain injury. J Neurotrauma. 2012;29(17):2606-12. doi:10.1089/neu.2012.2549.

90. Wolf EG, Prye J, Michaelson R, Brower G, Profenna L, Boneta O. Hyperbaric side effects in a traumatic brain injury randomized clinical trial. Undersea Hyperb Med. 2012;39(6):1075-82.

91. Wolf EG, Baugh LM, Kabban CM, Richards MF, Prye J. Cognitive function in a traumatic brain injury hyperbaric oxygen randomized trial. Undersea Hyperb Med. 2015;42(4):313-32.

92. Zauner A, Doppenberg EMR, Woodward JJ, et al. Continuous monitoring of cerebral substrate delivery and clearance: initial experience in 24 patients with severe acute brain injuries. Neurosurgery. 1997;41:1082-91.

93. Zhou Z, Daugherty WP, Sun D, et al. Protection of mitochondrial function and improvement in cognitive recovery in rats treated with hyperbaric oxygen following lateral fluid-percussion injury. J Neurosurg. 2007;106:687-94.

CHAPTER 38 CHAPTER

Neurological Aspects of Hyperbaric Medicine

CHAPTER THIRTY-EIGHT OVERVIEW

Introduction 947
Stroke 947
Radiation-Induced Cerebral Necrosis 949
Traumatic Brain Injury 950
Cerebral Palsy 951
Multiple Sclerosis 952
Autism 953
Conclusion 954
References 955

Neurological Aspects of Hyperbaric Medicine

Ann K. Helms, Charles C. Falzon, Aliyah Keval, Harry T. Whelan

INTRODUCTION

Since the early days of hyperbaric medicine, there has been interest in using HBO_2 to treat neurologic disease. The exquisite sensitivity of neural tissue to hypoxia makes increased oxygenation attractive as a therapy for disease processes that induce ischemia, edema, and, more recently, apoptosis. This chapter addresses the evidence for using HBO_2 to treat several neurologic diseases, which is an issue that has drawn significant interest and criticism from the press. It is important to note that none of the diseases mentioned in this chapter have received approval from the Food and Drug Administration (FDA) as indications for HBO_2.

STROKE

The largest body of evidence involving the use of hyperbaric oxygen for neurologic illness is found in the field of cerebral ischemia, which was by Helms et al. in 2005.[28] Ischemic stroke occurs when neural tissue receives inadequate vascular supply due to cerebral blood vessel occlusion. At the core, or center, of the infarct, blood flow is completely absent, causing neurons to die within a matter of minutes. The region of the brain that draws the most interest is the penumbra, where evidence has shown that blood flow is diminished but not absent. The cells in this region remain viable for a prolonged period and can be saved if adequate perfusion is restored. The only approved therapy for acute ischemic stroke presently available is Tissue Plasminogen Activator (tPA), which restores blood flow to the ischemic penumbra but must be used within the first few hours of the onset of symptoms to be effective. There is also evidence that a percentage of the cells subjected to prolonged ischemia will inevitably undergo apoptosis, regardless of the efforts made to restore perfusion. As a result, there has been great interest in using HBO_2 to treat ischemic stroke for its ability to improve the delivery of oxygen to deprived tissue and for the added benefit of its anti-inflammatory properties.

There is reasonable evidence from animal studies, involving mice, rats, gerbils, and cats, that focal cerebral ischemia may improve after treatment with HBO_2. Several studies have investigated the efficacy of using HBO_2 therapy that is provided either immediately or delayed minutes to hours after temporary or permanent occlusion of cerebral vessels.[5,12,14,18-19,32,43,56,65,68-69,80] Most studies administer a single, one-hour-long treatment at doses ranging from 2 to 3 ATA, with a few giving similar treatments multiple times. The overwhelming majority of these studies showed a clinical benefit in the treatment group, such as decreased infarct size, improved neurologic function, and increased survival. Only two studies failed to show any benefit from HBO_2 therapy when it was given within the first several hours following the ischemic event.[29,60] Based on these studies, the therapeutic window is limited to the first six hours after restoring perfusion, as treatments given after this window provided no benefit. In addition, the window for observing any improvement from treatment may be even shorter in brains with a permanently occluded vessel.[38,74]

Analyses of brain tissue in HBO_2-treated animals suggest that treatment may provide an indirect benefit to ischemic tissue, in addition to increasing local oxygen levels. In animals treated with HBO_2, there was a significant decrease in neuronal shrinkage, edema, and necrotic tissue, and, more importantly, fewer neurons showed evidence of undergoing apoptosis after ischemia.[13,34,61,74,78-79] These findings indicate that HBO_2 exposure initiates a lasting physiologic change by interrupting the apoptotic cascade that is triggered by the ischemia/reperfusion phenomenon. It also helps to explain studies that show a protective benefit to pretreatment with HBO_2 prior to ischemia.[4,42,70-71]

Several human trials investigating the use of HBO_2 for ischemic stroke have been performed. While most of these lacked controls, uniform standards for inclusion criteria and outcome measurement, or both, there are still three prominent randomized controlled studies that have evaluated HBO_2 in ischemic stroke. Anderson et al. enrolled patients up to 14 days after an ischemic stroke and gave multiple treatments of HBO_2 at 1.5 ATA versus air at 1.5 ATA.[4] After four months of treatments, examiners saw no difference in stroke size on either CT or graded neurologic exam. Nighoghossian et al. also gave HBO_2 at 1.5 ATA, although they limited enrollment to the first 24 hours after onset of symptoms and gave only one 60-minute treatment.[53] Control patients were given a sham treatment of air at a minimal pressure increase. At one year, there was no difference in global function as measured by the modified Rankin scale; however, two other outcome measures, the Orgogozo and Trouillas scores, were significantly higher in the treatment group. The conflicting data from this study suggest that the effect of the regimen was minimal, if at all quantifiable. The most recent study in this field performed by Rusyniak et al. also randomized patients in the first 24 hours after ischemia to receive one 60-minute treatment of either HBO_2 at 2.5 ATA or 100% oxygen at 1.1 ATA.[63] Patients in the "control" group showed a better outcome on two functional scales after three months of treatment, which suggests a potentially harmful effect of HBO_2, but an intention-to-treat analysis showed no statistical difference between the groups.

One might conclude from this that HBO_2 is an ineffective treatment for ischemic stroke; however, it should be noted that these studies enrolled patients well after the therapeutic window of six hours that was suggested by previous animal studies had elapsed. Based on our present understanding of ischemia, one would not expect treatment after two weeks to be effective. Two of the three studies used a very low HBO_2 dose of 1.5 ATA, which is well below the standard dose used for other therapeutic indications. In addition, the control groups in the studies performed by the Anderson and Rusyniak groups received higher doses of oxygen (air at 1.5 ATA and 100% oxygen at 1.1 ATA, respectively) than a patient breathing air, which might be considered intermediate therapy.[2,63] However, with other cardiac situations such as acute coronary syndrome, HBO_2 therapy has been proven to improve oxygen supply to the heart and reduce the volume of cardiac muscle death.[10]

Based on the studies just discussed, HBO_2 cannot currently be recommended for the treatment of ischemic stroke outside of a research protocol. Considering the results that have been produced in animal models, it is imperative that follow-up studies be performed on human subjects to analyze the effects of HBO_2 treatment within the first few hours following an ischemic event using higher doses of oxygen. Potential protocols should also include controls receiving oxygen treatments at percentages closely approximating room air to improve both the rigor of the study and the validity of their results. Until such time as these protocols are thoroughly investigated, there is no definitive answer regarding the role of HBO_2 for the treatment of ischemic stroke.

RADIATION-INDUCED CEREBRAL NECROSIS

Radiation-induced cerebral necrosis (RIN) is a dreaded complication associated with the treatment of brain tumors. The neurologic signs and symptoms that result are often progressive and can be difficult to distinguish from tumor recurrence. The most common presentations involve cognitive changes such as short-term memory loss, poor concentration, personality changes, and focal neurologic abnormalities such as hemiparesis and aphasia.

Radiation injury can develop immediately after treatment, commonly resulting in transient worsening of neurologic symptoms and headaches. This is presumed to be due to both leaky capillaries and edema in the tumor bed, which is frequently reversible with steroid therapy. The symptoms that develop within a few weeks of radiation treatments are usually reversible, often without treatment. Radiation necrosis, however, develops months to years after radiation exposure and is usually irreversible.

MRI scanning following radiation shows signal changes and enhancement that are difficult to distinguish from tumor recurrence. While imaging studies such as MR spectroscopy, PET scanning, SPECT scanning, and MR perfusion studies can be used to distinguish between the two, a biopsy is required for definitive diagnosis. Pathologic examination shows necrosis of white matter and fibrinoid necrosis of blood vessels. This is theorized to be due to endothelial cell damage, which induces a signaling cascade that causes ischemia and necrosis of white matter.[22]

Treatment of radiation necrosis of the brain is difficult. Surgical resection can sometimes stop progression, and some benefit has been seen with antithrombotic medications; unfortunately, these therapies are performed with significant risks and therapeutic limitations.[23] HBO_2 has been very successful in treating soft-tissue radiation injuries that are discussed in other sections of this text. Given that endothelial cell damage and microvascular ischemia are considered to be part of the injury cascade in RIN, hyperbaric oxygen therapy may be a viable treatment alternative.

There has been only 1 small, phase I–II, randomized controlled study investigating the use of HBO_2 in RIN. Hulshof et al. randomized 7 patients with cognitive deficits at least 1.5 years after brain irradiation to receive either 30 HBO_2 treatments at 3.0 ATA for 115 minutes or no treatment.[31] Using a battery of neuropsychological tests as outcome measures, they found a trend towards improved function at three months in the treatment group, but this result was not statistically significant. There have also been numerous anecdotal reports of efficacy and a few short series reporting positive results.[34,36,40,66-67,72] In the largest series, reported only in abstract form, Warnick et al. included 29 patients with RIN of the brain receiving HBO_2 at 2.5 ATA over 90 minutes for 20–60 treatments.[72] All of the patients in the study had focal, progressive neurological deficits with increasing steroid requirements and an MRI showing a ring-enhancing mass with surrounding edema. In this series, 27 of the 29 patients showed improvement or stabilization of symptoms, decreased steroid requirement, and improved MRI appearance. The two patients who worsened were shown to have tumor progression. Interestingly, the greatest benefit was noted in a subset of four patients with benign underlying pathology (meningioma and AVM). Chuba et al. also reported benefit in a group of 10 pediatric patients who underwent HBO_2T after a diagnosis of RIN and failure of traditional steroid therapy.[15] All 10 patients showed clinical improvement or stabilization both initially and at follow-up, while five of the six surviving patients showed continued improvement. The four deaths in this group were attributed to tumor progression.

The evidence suggests that in cases where either the patient is not improving on medical therapies, such as steroids and antithrombotics, or when surgical resection is not possible, HBO_2 should be considered as a treatment option. Due to the lack of studies currently available in this field, there is a definite need for both more and larger randomized trials utilizing HBO_2 for the treatment of RIN.

TRAUMATIC BRAIN INJURY

Traumatic brain injury (TBI) is one of the leading causes of disability in the United States, affecting more than two million people yearly. Although the primary injury to the brain sustained at the time of the trauma is usually not reversible, it is the secondary injury occurring in the hours and days following the initial injury that provides more opportunities for treatment to preserve tissue and function. Unfortunately, the mechanisms by which these secondary injuries occur are not fully understood. In addition to the initial injury, the largest contributor to morbidity and mortality is cerebral ischemia resulting from posttraumatic hypoxia and hypotension. On a microscopic level, abnormalities of calcium and potassium homeostasis, mechanical membrane disruption, excitotoxicity, and altered glucose metabolism also contribute to cellular damage, which in turn cause edema and neuronal cell death. Cell death in the form of both necrosis and apoptosis occurs in the areas surrounding the primary injury but can also occur at more distant areas. Increased intracranial pressure from edema, as well as from contusions and hemorrhages, contributes to secondary injury by increasing the level of ischemia, leading to herniation and death.

Treatment of TBI has traditionally focused on supportive care, but recent studies have changed their focus toward the prevention or reversal of secondary injury cascades. The largest advances in the field have been made regarding early intervention with a focus on minimizing the roles of hypotension and hypoxia, which play a limited role in the development of ischemia.[11] Intracranial hypertension is treated with a combination of ventricular drainage, mannitol, intermittent hyperventilation, hypertonic saline, and barbiturates, although this is not always fully effective.[1] Decompressive craniectomy can be useful, but there are several medical treatments that have been utilized with varying efficacy to limit secondary injury including hypothermia, calcium channel blockers, anticonvulsants, and other neuroprotectants

The interest in using HBO_2 to treat TBI is based upon the premise that hypoxia, edema, and apoptosis play significant roles in the pathophysiology of the disease. HBO_2 has been shown to decrease cerebral edema and to decrease cellular apoptosis after an ischemic event.[13,35,54,64,80,82] There have been several reports showing a benefit from HBO_2 in TBI patients using surrogate markers that were expected to influence the outcome, including the effects of HBO_2 on intracranial pressure which was studied by several teams.[27,59,64] Although intracranial pressure (ICP) sometimes increased during the treatment, some persistent, albeit mild, decreases were seen in several patients. One study was able to correlate this decrease in ICP with clinical improvement; however, analysis of other surrogate markers, such as cerebral blood flow and metabolism, were less reliable as outcome measures.[27,47,59]

Only a few studies have directly compared HBO_2 to standard of care in TBI. In 1976, Artru et al. randomized 60 patients who were in coma after TBI for an average of 4.5 days after their injuries and treated them at 2.5 ATA for 60 minutes daily over 10 days with a 4-day break repeated versus standard of care.[3] At one year, the study showed nonsignificant trends towards shorter coma and higher rate of consciousness in the HBO_2 group, and mortality was not affected. The only significant improvements were in a subgroup of young patients with brain-stem injury who had higher rates of consciousness at 1 month (67% versus control 11%). In 1974, Holbach alternated 99 patients in coma with acute midbrain syndrome to either standard care or HBO_2 at 1.5 ATA and saw significant improvements in mortality (53% versus 74%) and good outcome on the Glasgow Outcome Scale (33% versus 6%).[30] More recently, Rockswold et al. randomized 168 TBI patients between 6 and 24 hours after injury with a Glasgow Coma Score (GCS) of 9 or less to HBO_2 at 1.5 ATA for 60 minutes every 8 hours for 2 weeks versus standard care.[58] At 12 months, blinded examiners saw no change in outcome among survivors, but there was a significant decrease in mortality (17% versus 32%) at 1 year. The smallest and most recent trial randomized patients at day 3 with a GCS of less than 9 to HBO_2 at 2.5 ATA for 400–600 minutes every 4 days for 3 or 4 treatments versus standard care.[57] A markedly larger percentage of patients in the treatment group achieved a good outcome at 6 months (83% versus 30%).

At first glance this data might lead one to question why HBO_2 is not now standard care for TBI. Although the risk for seizures due to the use of HBO_2 therapy is not significant enough for the treatment to be considered unsafe when treating both stroke and traumatic brain injury patients, [24] there are significant points to address regarding the above studies. The problem with them is that none of the studies were blinded, there were no sham controls, and there was extreme variability in criteria of inclusion, time of enrollment, and type of treatment given. In meta-analysis, there does appear to be a positive effect on mortality, but this too is limited by the quality and quantity of studies. More large, well-designed, rigorous studies are needed before HBO_2 can be recommended as a treatment modality for traumatic brain injury.

CEREBRAL PALSY

One of the more controversial uses of hyperbaric oxygen therapy involves the treatment of children with cerebral palsy. The first, and perhaps most difficult, part of any discussion of cerebral palsy (CP) is that it is a poorly defined entity. The term "CP" encompasses many causes and diagnoses that have a common presentation. Recently, an international symposium defined CP as "a group of disorders of the development of movement and posture, causing activity limitations that are attributed to non-progressive disturbances that occurred in the developing fetal or infant brain."[20]

CP presents as spasticity or motor impairment and can be characterized as hemiplegic, diplegic, or quadriplegic, each with a spectrum of symptoms ranging from mild to severe. Motor deficits are often accompanied by other neurologic deficits including visual and other sensory problems, mental retardation, learning disabilities, and epilepsy. The deficits are nonprogressive but can fluctuate over time. There is no cure for CP, and treatment has traditionally consisted of symptomatic therapy aimed at increasing function.

In the 1980s, Dr. Richard Neubauer suggested the theory of "idling neurons" in anoxic brain injury, based on SPECT scan evidence of hypofunctioning cortical neurons that were shown to have increased metabolism after HBO_2 treatment.[(49)] He also reported some improvements in patients with anoxic brain injury, closed head injuries, and stroke with HBO_2 treatments.[(46,48,52)] Despite being either uncontrolled series or case reports done in patients with injuries that would not be characterized as CP, these studies have been used to justify the administration of HBO_2 to treat CP. The same group presented two cases of improvement after HBO_2 in patients with CP; however, the study was not controlled, and the cases were never reported in the literature.[(50)]

There are only a few studies specifically looking at HBO_2 treatment for CP. Montgomery et al. evaluated 25 patients between the ages of 3 and 8 years old with spastic diplegia.[(44)] All patients received 20 treatments of 95% O_2 at 1.75 ATA and served as their own controls. They were evaluated by parental questionnaire as well as several evaluation scales. The patients showed significant improvement in gross and fine motor tasks and much greater improvement in spasticity. The study was the first evidence that HBO_2 might be effective in CP but was criticized for being uncontrolled and unblinded.

The only randomized controlled study was by the same group reported in 2 papers evaluating HBO_2 treatment of 111 children with CP.[(16,25)] In this study, all other therapies were withheld throughout the course of the trial, and patients were randomized to 40 treatments lasting 1 hour at either 1.75 ATA of HBO_2 or sham treatment using air at 1.3 ATA. Investigator assessments of motor function, working memory, and attention, combined with parental evaluations, both immediately and at three months, showed significant improvement in both groups without a trend towards better function in the treatment arm. The benefits experienced by both groups were attributed to the placebo effect, but the study was criticized because the sham group received 1.3 ATA of air, or the equivalent of 28% O_2 by face mask, which some argue might provide a therapeutic benefit.[(51)] A similar study was performed advocating the use of "low pressure hyperbaric oxygen therapy" for other "cerebral hypoperfusion" syndromes, including autism.[(62)] In this small series, 40 one-hour sessions of 1.3 ATA of air were given to 6 autistic children. Analysis of parental evaluations showed a therapeutic benefit in all six cases, but the utility of the results was limited since the study was uncontrolled and unblinded.

At this point, the only randomized study published shows no benefit to treating CP with HBO_2. While there are scattered reports of improvement in uncontrolled small series and case reports, the large placebo effect seen in the randomized study is concerning. Most reviewers agree that more research is needed before HBO_2 therapy is offered to patients with CP and autism.

MULTIPLE SCLEROSIS

Multiple sclerosis (MS) is a disease of the nervous system defined by inflammation and demyelination in the white matter of the brain and spinal cord. In its most common form, relapsing-remitting MS presents with isolated attacks of neurologic symptoms such as visual loss, weakness, or numbness. For the first few years of the disease, patients are normal between attacks, but the cumulative effects of axonal damage in the brain results in permanent deficits. At some point during the disease course, patients experience a steady decline in function, which is termed secondary progressive MS. In another form of the disease, also known as primary progressive MS, patients experience permanent deficits from the onset of symptoms and decline progressively over several years. While the exact cause of MS is not clear, it is known that immune system dysfunction is involved and that both environmental and genetic factors are presumed to contribute. There is no cure for the disease; however, acute attacks often respond well to treatment with intravenous steroids. Over the last 10 years, patients with relapsing-remitting MS have benefited from several recently developed effective immunomodulatory therapies that decrease the attack rate and severity of the disease. Unfortunately, there are few known therapeutic options for primary or secondary progressive MS.

Interest in the use of HBO_2 for MS was particularly high in the 1980s and 1990s when there were few therapies available. Several nonrandomized reports suggested a benefit from HBO_2 for disability in MS.[41,73,81] In response to that, a number of randomized controlled trials of various designs were performed to evaluate the efficacy of HBO_2 in treating MS patients.[6-7,17,21,26,37,45,55,76-77] All of the trials enrolled patients with "definite MS," but many used differing criteria, while others defined a maximum level of disability for enrollment. Most of the studies also required patients to be stable symptomatically with no recent exacerbations. The doses given ranged from 1.75 to 2.5 ATA, but the most common was 2.0 ATA for 90 minutes, and in each trial 20 treatments were given, although a few gave "booster" treatments later on. Outcomes of the various studies included improvement on the expanded disability status scale (EDSS), bowel and bladder function, pyramidal function, number of exacerbations, changes in visual evoked potentials, and MRI appearance. Only 1 small study of 34 patients showed significant differences between the treatment and sham groups, with a decreased mean EDSS seen at the end of treatment and at 6 but not at 12 months after treatment.[41] Two other studies showed small improvements in secondary outcomes of sphincter function and pyramidal function.[6-7,55]

Other outcomes did not exhibit differences between treatment and sham groups in any study. A large registry of 312 MS patients treated at numerous sites did not show any significant improvement in the EDSS.[33] A meta-analysis of these studies did not show any significant effect of HBO_2 on the clinical presentation and progression of MS.[8] Interestingly, it was noted that quite a few patients in the placebo groups in these studies claimed improvement which might explain the presumed benefit seen in uncontrolled studies.

Based on a more modern understanding of MS, the most important distinction to make regarding these studies is assessing both how the disease is defined and at what stage of the disease the patients were treated. In most cases, the patients enrolled at a chronic or advanced stage in the disease and presented with significant disability. The average EDSS for these study groups was approximately 5 or 6, which translates to the inability to work and the requirement of some form of ambulatory assistance, such as a cane, for walking. Although the data available overwhelmingly denies any benefit to MS from HBO_2, it has not been proven that patients with early stages or milder forms of the disease would not benefit from such treatment.

AUTISM

To determine whether hyperbaric oxygen (HBO_2) therapy should be used for the treatment of autism spectrum disorders (ASD), we performed a systematic literature review.[39] A literature search was performed on PubMed, Cochrane Library, and DynaMed for studies evaluating the use of HBO_2 for ASD treatment. The studies were then reviewed for the highest quality evidence. The evidence is weak for the use of HBO_2 in ASD, with only one, likely flawed, randomized control study showing treatment benefit. HBO_2 should not be recommended for ASD treatment until more conclusive favorable results and long-term outcomes are demonstrated from well-designed controlled trials.

Without a doubt, autism spectrum disorder has become part of the public consciousness. News programs and television talk shows frequently feature autism-related topics, and autobiographies by adults who have autism have become best sellers. Popular press and community blogs frequently report and advocate the use of adjuvant treatments, including HBO_2 therapy, for families of children with autism. Some families report using anywhere from 40 to 120 hours of HBO_2 therapy, precious time that might otherwise be spent on other therapies like applied behavior analysis, speech therapy, or occupational therapy.(8) Moreover, the cost of HBO_2 therapy may range up to $150 per hour.

Some families choose to purchase chambers in order to provide therapy at home. Numerous websites focus on renting or selling chambers to families at prices ranging from $5,000 to $28,000. Truly, much remains to be understood regarding the mechanism of autism, and even less has been proven regarding the mechanism of action in how HBO_2 therapy could alleviate autistic behavior. The evidence is very weak for the use of HBO_2 in autism, with only one, likely flawed, randomized control study showing some benefit. Some smaller uncontrolled case reports and series have collected clinical improvements in children's symptom scores after being treated with HBO_2. Given the significant financial and time investment required for families of autistic children and the conflicting study outcomes, HBO_2 should not be recommended as a treatment for ASD until more conclusive favorable results and long-term outcomes are demonstrated from well-designed controlled trials.

CONCLUSION

HBO_2 has been suggested for use in a number of neurological disorders. There are many studies examining the effects of HBO_2 treatment, but none have provided irrefutable evidence supporting any specific neurological disease as an indication for treatment. The case for the use of HBO_2 in ischemic stroke is strong based on animal studies but has yet to be proven in clinical trials. There is data available supporting the use of HBO_2 to treat radiation-induced cerebral necrosis (RIN) on a case-by-case basis; however, larger studies are still warranted. Further study is also necessary to establish the efficacy of HBO_2 in treatment of traumatic brain injury (TBI) because the evidence alleging any benefit is seen in only a small number of low-quality studies. The evidence is also weak for the use of HBO_2 in cerebral palsy (CP), where the only randomized study found no benefit, so its use cannot be supported. The most substantial evidence against HBO_2 is found in studies to treat multiple sclerosis (MS), where it provides no clinical benefit.

REFERENCES

1. Aarabi B, Eisenberg HM, Murphy K, Morrison C, Weinmann M. Traumatic brain injury: management and complications. In: Layton AJ, Gabrielli A, Friedman WA, editors. Textbook of Neurointensive Care. Philadelphia: Saunders Publishing; 2004.
2. Anderson DC, Bottini AG, Jagiella WM, Westphal B, Ford S, Rockswold GL, Loewenson RB. A pilot study of hyperbaric oxygen in the treatment of human stroke. Stroke. 1991;22:1137-42.
3. Artru F, Chacornac R, Deleuze R. Hyperbaric oxygenation for severe head injuries. Preliminary results of a controlled study. Eur Neurol. 1976;14(4):310-8.
4. Atochin DN, Fisher D, Demchenko IT, Thom SR. Neutrophil sequestration and the effect of hyperbaric oxygen in a rat model of temporary middle cerebral artery occlusion. Undersea Hyperb Med. 2000;27:185-90.
5. Badr AE, Yin W, Mychaskiw G, Zhang JH. Effect of hyperbaric oxygen on striatal metabolites: a microdialysis study in awake freely moving rats after MCA occlusion. Brain Res. 2001;916:85-90.,
6. Barnes MP, Bates D, Cartlidge NE, French JM, Shaw DA. Hyperbaric oxygen and multiple sclerosis: final results of a placebo-controlled, double-blind trial. J Neurol Neurosurg Psychiatry. 1987;50(11):1402-6.
7. Barnes MP, Bates D, Cartlidge NE, French JM, Shaw DA. Hyperbaric oxygen and multiple sclerosis: short-term results of a placebo-controlled, double-blind trial. Lancet. 1985;1(8424):297-300.
8. Bennett M, Heard R. Hyperbaric oxygen therapy for multiple sclerosis. Cochrane Database Syst Rev. 2006;3.
9. Bennett MH, Kertesz T, Perleth M, Yeung P, Lehm JP. Hyperbaric oxygen for idiopathic sudden sensorineural hearing loss and tinnitus [review]. Cochrane Database Syst Rev. 2012 Oct 17;10:CD004739.
10. Bennett MH, Lehm JP, Jepson N. Hyperbaric oxygen therapy for acute coronary syndrome [review]. Cochrane Database Syst Rev. 2015 Jul 23;(7):CD004818.
11. Brain Trauma Foundation's guideline for prehospital management of traumatic brain injury [Internet]. Badjatia N et al. Brain Trauma Foundation New York; [cited 2001]. Available from: http://www.braintrauma.org/guidelines/index.php.
12. Burt JT, Kapp JP, Smith RR. Hyperbaric oxygen and cerebral infarction in the gerbil. Surg Neurol. 1987;28:265-8.
13. Calvert JW, Yin W, Patel M, Badr A, Mychaskiw G, Parent AD, Zhang JH. Hyperbaric oxygenation prevented brain injury induced by hypoxia-ischemia in a neonatal rat model. Brain Res. 2002;951:1-8.
14. Chang CF, Niu KC, Hoffer BJ, Wang Y, Borlongan CV. Hyperbaric oxygen therapy for treatment of postischemic stroke in adult rats. Exp Neurol. 2000;166:298-306.
15. Chuba PJ, Aronin P, Bhambhani K, Eichenhorn M, Zamarano L, Cianci PM, et al. Hyperbaric oxygen therapy for radiation-induced brain injury in children. Cancer. 1997;80:2005-12.
16. Collet JP, Vanasse M, Marois P, et al. Hyperbaric oxygen for children with cerebral palsy: a randomised multicentre trial. Lancet. 2001;357:582-6.
17. Confavreux C, Mathieu C, Cacornac R, Aimard G, Devic M. Hyperbaric oxygen in multiple sclerosis. La Presse Medicale. 1986;15(28):1319-22.
18. Corkill G, Van Housen K, Hein L, Reitan J. Videodensitometric estimation of the protective effect of hyperbaric oxygen in the ischemic gerbil brain. Surg Neurol. 1985;24:206-10.

19. Dong H, Xiong L, Zhu Z, Chen S, Hou L, Sakabe T. Preconditioning with hyperbaric oxygen and hyperoxia induces tolerance against spinal cord ischemia in rabbits. Anesthesiology. 2002;96:907-12.

20. Executive Committee for the Definition of Cerebral Palsy. Proposed definition and classification of cerebral palsy, April 2005. Dev Med Child Neurol. 2005 Aug;47(8):571-6.

21. Fischer BH, Marks M, Reich T. Hyperbaric-oxygen treatment of multiple sclerosis. A randomized, placebo-controlled, double-blind study. N Engl J Med. 1983;308(4):181-6.

22. Giglio P, Gilbert MR. Cerebral radiation necrosis. Neurologist. 2003;9:180-8.

23. Glantz MJ, Burger PC, Friedman AH, Radtke RA, Massey EW, Schold SC. Treatment of radiation-induced nervous system injury with heparin and warfarin. Neurology. 1994;44:2020–7.

24. Hadanny A, Meir O, Bechor Y, Fishlev G, Bergan J, Efrati S. Seizures during hyperbaric oxygen therapy: retrospective analysis of 62,614 treatment sessions. Undersea Hyperb Med. 2016 Jan-Feb;43(1):21-8.

25. Hardy P, Collet JP, Goldberg J, et al. Neuropsychological effects of hyperbaric oxygen therapy in cerebral palsy. Dev Med Child Neurol. 2002;44:436-46.

26. Harpur GD, Suke R, Bass BH, Bass MJ, Bull SB, Reese L, Noseworthy JH, Rice GP, Ebers GC. Hyperbaric oxygen therapy in chronic stable multiple sclerosis: double-blind study. Neurology. 1986 Jul;36(7):988-91.

27. Hayakawa T, Kanai N, Kuroda R. Response of cerebrospinal fluid pressure to hyperbaric oxygenation. J Neurol Neurosurg Psychiatry. 1971;34(5):580-6.

28. Helms AK, Torbey MT, Whelan HT. Hyperbaric oxygen therapy of cerebral ischemia. Cerebrovasc Dis. 2005;20:417-26.

29. Hjelde A, Hjelstuen M, Haraldseth O, Martin JD, Thom SR, Brubakk AO. Hyperbaric oxygen and neutrophil accumulation/tissue damage during permanent focal cerebral ischaemia in rats. Eur J Appl Physiol. 2002;86:401-5.

30. Holbach KH, Wassmann H, Kolberg T. Improved reversibility of the traumatic midbrain syndrome using hyperbaric oxygen. Acta Neurochir (Wien). 1974;30(3-4):247-56.

31. Hulshof M, Stark N, Van der Kleij A, Sminia P, Smeding H, Gonzales D. Hyperbaric oxygen therapy for cognitive disorders after irradiation of the brain. Strahlenther Onkol. 2002;178(4):192-8.

32. Kawamura S, Yausi N, Shirasawa M, Fukasawa H. Therapeutic effects of hyperbaric oxygenation on acute focal cerebral ischemia in rats. Surg Neurol. 1990;34:101-6.

33. Kindwall EP, McQuillen MP, Khatri BO, Gruchow HW, Kindwall ML. Treatment of multiple sclerosis with hyperbaric oxygen. Results of a national registry. Arch Neurol. 1991 Feb;48(2):195-9.

34. Kohshi K, Imada H, Nomoto S, Yamaguchi R, Abe H, Yamamoto H. Successful treatment of radiation-induced brain necrosis by hyperbaric oxygen therapy. J Neurol Sci. 2003;209:115-7.

35. Kondo A, Baba S, Iwaki T, Harai H, Koga H, Kimura T, Takmatsu J. Hyperbaric oxygenation prevents delayed neuronal death following transient ischaemia in the gerbil hippocampus. Neuropathol Appl Neurobiol. 1996;22:350-60.

36. Leber KA, Eder HG, Kovac H, Anegg U, Pendl G. Treatment of cerebral radionecrosis by hyperbaric oxygen therapy. Stereotact Funct Neurosurg. 1998;70(Suppl 1):229-36.

37. Lhermitte F, Roullet E, Lyon-Caen O, Metrot J, Villey T, Bach MA, Tournier-Lasserve E, Chabassol E, Rascol A, Clanet M, et al. Double-blind treatment of 49 cases of chronic multiple sclerosis using hyperbaric oxygen. Revue Neurologique. 1986;142(3):201-6.

38. Lou M, Eschenfelder CC, Herdegen T, Brecht S, Deuschl G. Therapuetic window for use of hyperbaric oxygenation in focal transient ischemia in rats. Stroke. 2004;35:578-83.

39. Martin R, Srivastava T, Lee J, Raj N, Koth KA, Whelan HT. Using hyperbaric oxygen for autism treatment: a review and discussion of literature. Undersea Hyperb Med. 2015 Jul-Aug;42(4):353-9.

40. McPherson CM, Warnick RE. Results of contemporary surgical management of radiation necrosis using frameless stereotaxis and intraoperative magnetic resonance imaging. J Neurooncol. 2004;68(1):41-7.

41. Meneghetti G, Sparta S, Rusca F, Facco E, Martini A, Comacchio F, Schiraldi C. Hyperbaric oxygen therapy in the treatment of multiple sclerosis. A clinical and electrophysiological study in a 2 year follow-up. Riv Neurol. 1990 Mar-Apr;60(2):67-71.

42. Miljkovic-Lolic M, Silbergleit R, Fiskum G, Rosenthal RE. Neuroprotective effects of hyperbaric oxygen treatment in experimental focal cerebral ischemia are associated with reduced brain leukocyte myeloperoxidase activity. Brain Res. 2003;971:90-4.

43. Mink RB, Dutka AJ. Hyperbaric oxygen after global cerebral ischemia in rabbits does not promote brain lipid peroxidation. Crit Care Med. 1995;23:1398-404.

44. Montgomery D, Goldberg J, Amar M, et al. Effects of hyperbaric oxygen therapy on children with spastic diplegic cerebral palsy: a pilot project. Undersea Hyperb Med. 1999;26(4):235-42.

45. Neiman J, Nilsson BY, Barr PO, Perrins DJ. Hyperbaric oxygen in chronic progressive multiple sclerosis: visual evoked potentials and clinical effects. J Neurol Neurosurg Psychiatry. 1985;48(6):497-500.

46. Neubauer RA, Gottlieb SF, Pevsner NH. Hyperbaric oxygen for treatment of closed head injury. South Med J. 1994;87:933-5.

47. Neubauer RA, Gottlieb SF, Pevsner NH. Hyperbaric oxygen for treatment of closed head injury. South Med J. 1994;87(9):933-6.

48. Neubauer RA, James P. Cerebral oxygenation and the recoverable brain. Neurol Res. 1998;20(Supp 1):S33-36.

49. Neubauer RA, Kagan RL, Gottlieb SF, James P. Delayed metabolism or reperfusion in brain imaging after exposure to hyperbaric oxygenation—a therapeutic indicator. Proceedings of the XV Annual Meeting of the European Undersea Biomedial Society; 1989 Sep 17-21; Eilat, Israel.

50. Neubauer RA, Uszler J, James P. Hyperbaric oxygen: the recoverable brain in certain pediatric patients. 8th International Child Neurology Congress; 1998 Sep 13-18; Ljubliana, Slovenia.

51. Neubauer RA. Hyperbaric oxygen therapy for cerebral palsy. Lancet. 2001;357:2052.

52. Neubauer RA. The effect of hyperbaric oxygen in prolonged coma: possible identification of marginally functioning brain zones. Med Subacquea ed Iperbarica. 1985;5:75-9.

53. Nighoghossian N, Trouillas P, Adeleine P, Salford F. Hyperbaric oxygen in the treatment of acute ischemic stroke: a double-blind pilot study. Stroke. 1995;26:1369-72.

54. Omae T, Ibayashi S, Kusuda K, Nakamura H, Yagi H, Fujishima M. Effects of high atmospheric pressure and oxygen on middle cerebral blood flow velocity in humans measured by transcranial doppler. Stroke. 1998;29:94-7.

55. Oriani G, Barbieri S, Cislaghi G, Albonico G, Scarlato G, Mariani C, et al. Long-term hyperbaric oxygen in multiple sclerosis: a placebo-controlled, double-blind trial with evoked potentials studies. J Hyperb Med. 1990;5:237-45.

56. Reitan JA, Kien ND, Thorup S, Corkill G. Hyperbaric oxygen increases survival following carotid ligation in gerbils. Stroke. 1990;21:119-23.

57. Ren H, Wang W, Ge Z. Glasgow coma scale, brain electrical activity mapping and Glasgow outcome scale after hyperbaric oxygen treatment of severe brain injury. Chin J Traumatol. 2001;4(4):239-41.

58. Rockswold GL, Ford SE, Anderson DC, Bergman TA, ShermanRE. Results of a prospective randomized trial for treatment of severely brain-injured patients with hyperbaric oxygen. J Neurosurg. 1992;76(6):929-34.

59. Rockswold SB, Rockswold GL, Vargo JM, Erickson CA, Sutton RL, Bergman TA, Biros MH. Effects of hyperbaric oxygenation therapy on cerebral metabolism and intracranial pressure in severely brain injured patients. J Neurosurg. 2001;95:544-6.

60. Roos JA, Jackson-Friedman C, Lyden P. Effects of hyperbaric oxygen on neurologic outcome for cerebral ischemia in rats. Acad Emerg Med. 1998;5:18-24.

61. Rosenthal RE, Silbergleit R, Hof PR, Haywood Y, Fiskum G. Hyperbaric oxygen reduces neuronal death and improves neurological outcome after canine cardiac arrest. Stroke. 2003;34:1311-6.

62. Rossignol DA, Rossignol LW. Hyperbaric oxygen therapy may improve symptoms in autistic children. Med Hypotheses. 2006;67:216-28.

63. Rusyniak DE, Kirk MA, May JD, Kao LW, Brizendine EJ, Welch JL, Cordell WH, Alonso RJ. Hyperbaric oxygen therapy in acute ischemic stroke results of the hyperbaric oxygen in acute ischemic stroke trial pilot study. Stroke. 2003;34:571-4.

64. Sukoff MH, Ragatz RE. Hyperbaric oxygenation for the treatment of acute cerebral edema. Neurosurgery. 1982;10:29-38.

65. Sunami K, Takeda Y, Hashimoto M, Hirakawa M. Hyperbaric oxygen reduces infarct volume in rats by increasing oxygen supply to the ischemic periphery. Crit Care Med. 2000;28:2831-6.

66. Takenaka N, Imanishi T, Sasaki H, Shimazaki K, Sugiura H, Kitagawa Y, Sekiyama S, Yamamoto M, Kazuno T. Delayed radiation necrosis with extensive brain edema after gamma knife radiosurgery for multiple cerebral cavernous malformations. Neurol Med Chir. 2003;43(8):391-5.

67. Tandon N, Vollmer DG, New PZ, Hevezi JM, Herman T, Kagan-Hallet K, et al. Fulminant radiation-induced necrosis after stereotactic radiation therapy to the posterior fossa. Case report and review of the literature. J Neurosurg. 2001;95:507-12.

68. Veltkamp R, Siebing DA, Heiland S, Schoenffeldt-Varas P, Veltkamp C, Schwaninger M, Schwab S. Hyperbaric oxygen induces rapid protection against focal cerebral ischemia. Brain Res. 2005;1037:134-8.

69. Veltkamp R, Warner DS, Domoki R, Brinkhous AD, Toole JF, Busija DW. Hyperbaric oxygen decreases infarct size and behavioral deficit after transient focal cerebral ischemia in rats. Brain Res. 2000;853:68-73.

70. Wada K, Ito M, Miyazawa T, Katoh H, Nawashiro H, Shima K, Chigasaki H. Repeated hyperbaric oxygen induces ischemic tolerance in gerbil hippocampus. Brain Res. 1996;740:15-20.

71. Wada K, Miyazawa T, Nomura N, Nawashiro H, Shima K. Preferential conditions for and possible mechanisms of induction of ischemic tolerance by repeated hyperbaric oxygenation in gerbil hippocampus. Neurosurgery. 2001;49:160-7.

72. Warnick RE, Gessell LB, Breneman JC, Albright RE, Racadio J, Mink S. Hyperbaric oxygen is an effective treatment for radiation necrosis of the brain. Neurosurgery. 2002;51:560.

73. Webster CJ, MacIver C, Allen S, Murray S. The chief scientist reports ... hyperbaric oxygen for multiple sclerosis patients. Health Bull (Edinb). 1989 Nov; 47(6):320-31.

74. Weinstein PR, Anderson GG, Telles DA. Results of hyperbaric oxygen therapy during temporary middle cerebral artery occlusion in unanesthetized cats. Neurosurgery. 1987;20:518-24.

75. Weinstein PR, Hameroff SR, Johnson PC, Anderson GG. Effect of hyperbaric oxygen therapy or dimethyl sulfoxide on cerebral ischemia in unanesthetized gerbils. Neurosurgery. 1986;18:528-32.

76. Wiles CM, Clarke CR, Irwin HP, Edgar EF, Swan AV. Hyperbaric oxygen in multiple sclerosis: a double blind trial. Br Med J (Clin Res Ed). 1986;292(6517):367-71.

77. Wood J, Stell R, Unsworth I, Lance JW, Skuse N. A double-blind trial of hyperbaric oxygen in the treatment of multiple sclerosis. Med J Aust. 1985;143(6):238-40.

78. Yang Z, Camporesi C, Yang X, Wang J, Bosco G, Lok J, Gorji R, Schelper RL, Camporesi EM. Hyperbaric oxygenation mitigates focal cerebral injury and reduces striatal dopamine release in a rat model of transient middle cerebral artery occlusion. Eur J Appl Physiol. 2002;87:101-7.

79. Yin D, Zhou C, Kusaka I, Calvert JW, Parent AD, Nanda A, Zhang JH. Inhibition of apoptosis by hyperbaric oxygen in a rat focal cerebral ischemic model. J Cereb Blood Flow Metab. 2003;23:855-64.

80. Yin W, Badr AE, Myechaskiw G, Zhang JH. Down regulation of COX-2 is involved in hyperbaric oxygen treatment in a rat transient focal cerebral ischemia model. Brain Res. 2002;926:165-71.

81. Zannini D, Formai C, Bogetti B, Sereni G. 40 cases of multiple sclerosis treated with hyperbaric oxygen therapy. Minerva Med. 1982 Nov 3;73(42):2939-45.

82. Zhilyaev SY, Moskvin AN, Platonova TF, Gutsaeva DR, Churilina IV, Demchenko IT. Hyperoxic vasoconstriction in the brain is mediated by inactivation of nitric oxide by superoxide anions. Neurosci Behav Physiol. 2003;33:783-7.

CHAPTER 39 CHAPTER

Hyperbaric Oxygen in the Treatment of Hansen's Disease

CHAPTER THIRTY-NINE OVERVIEW

Introduction 963
Background 964
Discussion 968
Conclusion 968
References 969

Hyperbaric Oxygen in the Treatment of Hansen's Disease

David A. Youngblood, Tomaz A.P. Brito

INTRODUCTION

Hansen's disease is a chronic infection caused by *Mycobacterium leprae*, affecting the peripheral nerves and skin. Internal organs, the spinal cord, and the brain are not affected. The disease spectrum ranges from the paucibacillary forms (indeterminate, polar tuberculoid, and tuberculoid) to multibacillary forms (borderline, borderline lepromatous, and lepromatous). The latter group is characterized by greater infectivity, cellular immunodeficiency in the host, and a tendency to relapse despite prolonged drug therapy. The clinical attack rate among close family contacts exposed to the multibacillary form of the disease is less than 10%, and the paucibacillary form is essentially noninfective.[9]

The prevalence of Hansen's disease in the world today as estimated by reports to the World Health Organization (WHO) is about 11 million,[3] but this takes no account of the number of countries where Hansen's disease is endemic but reliable health statistics are lacking. The Leprosy Study Center of London estimates that the total number exceeds 15–16 million. Fewer than 20% of these cases are considered to be under treatment.[3]

According to the World Health Organization *Weekly Epidemiological Record*, the prevalence of leprosy in the world in the first quarter of 2012 was 181,941, while the total incidence of new cases in 2011 was 219,075 and in 2013 was 215,557. [18] These numbers show that Hansen´s disease will be a social and economic challenge for the years ahead.

Effective drug therapy in Hansen's disease began in the 1950s with the introduction of dapsone (DDS: 4, 4-Diaminodiphenyl sulphone). This remains the primary drug for the control of Hansen's disease in most of the world since it is relatively inexpensive and side effects are minimal. Secondary resistance to dapsone was first reported in 1964,[9] and primary dapsone resistance in previously untreated patients appeared in the 1970s.[17] Resistance rates of up to 40% have been reported.

Rifampin (rifampicin), clofazimine, and ethionamide have been recommended in a combined regimen with dapsone to retard the development of resistance. These drugs, unfortunately, have some undesirable side effects, and they are expensive, requiring foreign exchange credits, which may be limited in developing countries where Hansen's disease is endemic. Despite the use of a combined regimen, the emergence of drug resistance so far seems inevitable, and the predicted development of a vaccine probably remains decades away. Hyperbaric oxygen therapy has yet to prove its potential as an effective adjunct in the treatment of Hansen's disease.

BACKGROUND

"Yet, they themselves, by only employing the power of understanding, have not adopted a fixed rule, but have laid their whole stress upon intense meditation and continual exercise and perpetual agitation of mind." - F. Bacon, *Novum Organum*

The third decade of the twentieth century brought a new era for hyperbaric medicine. In those days, the time of compressed-air therapy had just ended, and the AMA (American Medical Association) had recently forced the closure of Dr. Cunningham`s steel ball "hyperbaric" hospital in Cleveland, OH.[(8)] There were some researchers, like Hugel and Muller, who were trying to improve tissue oxygen tension by means of local injections around phlegmons, but this method, obviously, would never be as efficient as necessary to achieve enough oxygen tension and diffusion for therapeutic effect.[(2)]

Actually, genuine hyperbaric oxygen (HBO_2) therapy was not in practice until 1937 when two Brazilian researchers – Alvaro Ozório de Almeida, who had been a disciple of Paul Bert in Paris, and Eduardo Rabello – begun their studies on the treatment of Lepromatous leprosy with hyperbaric oxygen.[(11)] They presented their first formal report of the favorable effect of HBO_2 therapy on Lepromatous leprosy before the Brazilian National Academy of Medicine on November 25, 1937. The same paper was read by invitation before the Brazilian Dermatological Society on December 6, 1937. The following year, a paper by E. Rabello and A. Ozorio de Almeida entitled "Essai de Traitement de Lepre Par L'Oxygène Sous Pression"[(14)] appeared in the journal of the *Société Francaise de Dermatologie and Syphiligraphie.* This is believed to be the first published report on the use of HBO_2 in the treatment of Hansen's disease. It was followed in the same year by Ozorio de Almeida and Enrique Moura Costa's paper, "Treatment of Leprosy by Oxygen under High Pressure Associated with Methylene Blue" in the *Revista Brasileira de Leprologia,*[(9)] and also, the same paper in the *International Journal of Leprosy.*[(10)]

These studies brought a new light over a hopeless social and sanitary problem, when there was no other medication or treatment for Hansen´s disease, and isolation of the patients was a general rule.

Ozorio de Almeida and his associates had noted clinical improvement in Hansen's disease patients participating in an experimental HBO_2 anticancer therapy. During these studies the two investigators noted that methylene blue intensified the toxic effect of oxygen upon various organisms. Finding that *Mycobacterium leprae* fixes methylene blue, they predicted that the effect of HBO_2 on the bacillus could be intensified without adversely affecting the human host.

The treatment of Hansen's disease patients with the combination of HBO_2 and methylene blue commenced in August of 1937 at the recently inaugurated Hospital Gaffrée & Guinle in Rio de Janeiro, in a brand-new chamber specifically manufactured for their researches (Figure 1). By November, 9 patients had been treated on a variety of oxygen regimens at pressures between 3.0 and 3.5 ATA for durations of 70–80 minutes per treatment and a cumulative average of 10 chamber hours per patient. Posttreatment clinical changes consisted of a marked decrease in skin infiltration,

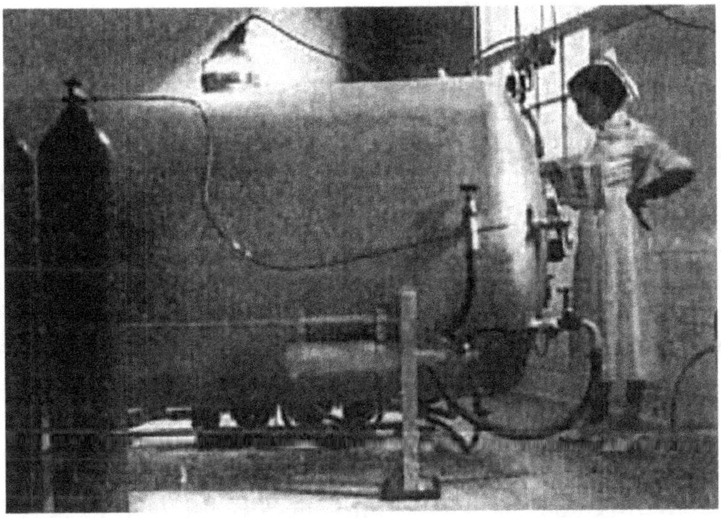

Figure 1.

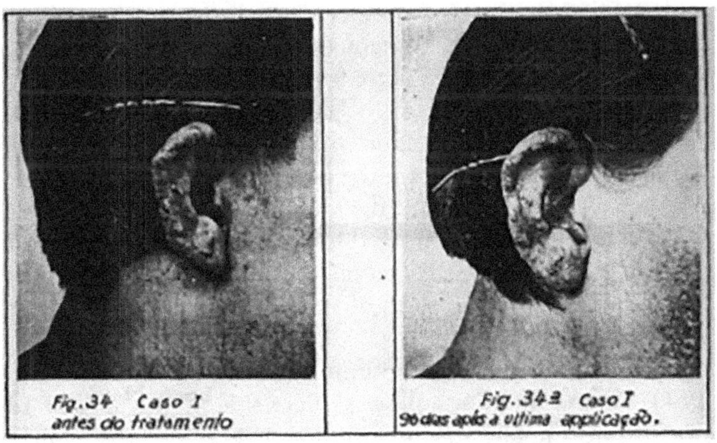

Figure 2. Case 1 before treatment – 96 days after last HBO$_2$.

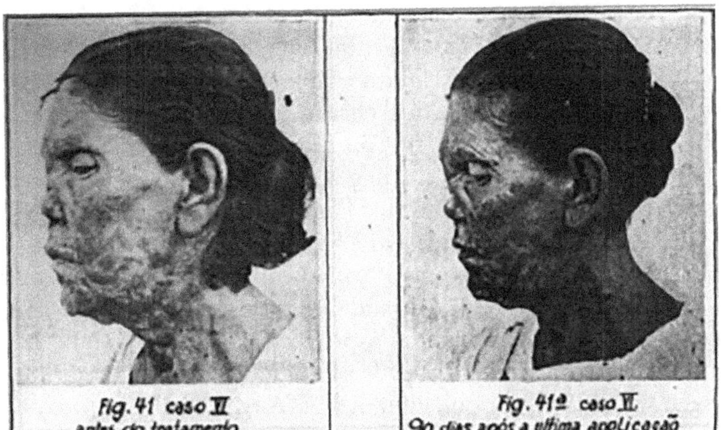

Figure 3. Case VI before treatment – 90 days after the last HBO$_2$.

a disappearance of tubercles, a gain in weight, and general improvement (Figure 2, Figure 3). The bacteria decreased in number, and their morphology was altered. In six cases the bacilli disappeared completely. A. Ozorio de Almeida and his colleague, Henrique Moura Costa, claimed that oxygen under pressure plus methylene blue was the most effective treatment regimen of their era for Hansen's disease.[9]

More than 30 years elapsed before reports on the use of HBO_2 in Hansen's disease reappeared. On August 15, 1969, at the Second National Reunion of the Argentine Society of Leprology in Formosa, Argentina, Doctor Felix F. Wilkinson[20] and his colleagues presented a report on their results using HBO_2 in the leprotomous form of Hansen's disease. They were unaware of the previous Brazilian studies at the time of their presentation, but the published version, "Conclusiones Preliminares Sobre el Uso del Oxígeno Hiperbarico en Lepra Lepromatosa" from the *Revista de Leprologia* included a preface which acknowledged the pioneering work of Ozorio de Almeida and his colleagues in Brazil.

Interest in the application of HBO_2 in the treatment of Hansen's disease apparently was confined to Argentina until the Fifth International Hyperbaric Conference in Vancouver, BC, in 1973, where Dr. Sebastian A. Rosasco,[15] representing his colleagues, reported on 200 patients with the leprotamous form of the disease who had been treated with 3 ATA of oxygen for 1 hour twice daily for 3 consecutive days. Drug therapy was stopped at the time of treatment and not resumed. Ten patients available for five-year follow-up showed no signs of recurrence. Dr. Rosasco's presentation stirred international interest.

In the United States, Dr. Sheldon Gottlieb recognized their findings as confirmation of his earlier predictions on the possible use of HBO_2 in the treatment of Hansen's disease.[4] With the advent of the mouse footpad as an animal model[16] to evaluate the efficacy of drug therapy in the disease, Drs. Hart and Levy conducted an unpublished trial on the effect of HBO_2 on the growth of *Mycobacterium leprae*. Their experiment did not demonstrate any effect of HBO_2 on the growth of the organism in the mouse footpad model.[5]

Repeated attempts were made to communicate with the researchers in Argentina during the 1970s, but only Kindwall was successful. Dr. Kindwall received an impressive set of before-and-after-treatment photographs. Then all contact was lost during the long period of civil strife in Argentina during the late 1970s.

Fortunately, the author found Drs. Wilkinson and Rosasco in Buenos Aires, Argentina, in July of 1981. Frustrated by the continual skepticism and occasional ridicule from their leprologist colleagues, the Argentine investigators had all but abandoned efforts to find support for a formal clinical trial complete with long-term follow-up, although they continued to treat occasional charity patients. Armed with their published and unpublished data on the use of HBO_2 in Hansen's disease, the author returned to Washington, DC, where Dr. Charles Shilling and Ms. Nancy Riegle-Hussey obtained funding from the Max and Victoria Dreyfuss Foundation for a pilot study which would attempt to replicate and refine the work of the South American researchers.

The pilot study protocol required patients with a recent diagnosis of the leprotamous form of Hansen's disease and no previous or current drug therapy. After an appropriate medical evaluation, a pretreatment biopsy would be obtained, analyzed, and inoculated into the footpads of a control group of mice. The patient would be treated with HBO_2 for one hour at 3 ATA twice daily for 5 days. Following the completion of this HBO_2 regimen, a second biopsy from the same site would be implanted in the footpads of a posttreatment mouse group. After an incubation period of approximately 10 months, tissue specimens from the footpads of both groups of mice would be harvested and analyzed to compare the viability, morphology, and relative number of bacteria between the control and treatment groups.

Due to administrative changes at the National Hansen's Disease Center in Carrville, Louisiana, the study was never implemented as planned. The author[22] treated only 1 patient under the protocol, a 30-year-old native of South Texas who had never been out of the United States. He presented with moderate facial edema and reddish macular lesions over the trunk. By the third day of treatment there was a centripetal blanching of the truncal lesions, and the facial edema had disappeared. The skin biopsies were shipped to the laboratory at the National Hansen's Disease Center and inoculated into the footpads of 10 mice for each group for studies of viability and bacterial propagation. Eight months later, mice from each group were studied. There was no significant difference in the bacterial density in the footpads of mice from either the pretreatment or the posttreatment samples. (The patient had been placed on a conventional drug regimen following the completion of his experimental HBO_2 therapy, and he made a rapid clinical recovery.)

Interest had also been stimulated in other parts of the world: during the Fifth International Conference on Hyperbaric Medicine in Aberdeen, Scotland, in 1977, Dr. Sheldon Gottlieb exchanged ideas with Dr. R.R. Pai of Bombay, India, on the possibility of conducting clinical trials in that country. These plans were interrupted, however, by Dr. Pai's unfortunate illness, but he did communicate in 1980 that preliminary studies in Bombay had included 33 patients treated with HBO_2 supplemented with rifampicin (rifampin) and dapsone, relaying in a letter to Dr. Gottlieb that while HBO_2 has been proven to be effective treatment in some leprosy cases, there are other cases that it has not been. More patients will need to be studied before formally reporting any particular way on the subject.[12]

Meanwhile, Dr. Mokashi from Bombay reported in a personal communication to Dr. K.K. Jain on the results of a controlled study in a group of 20 drug-resistant Hansen's disease patients, half of which received HBO_2 at 2.5 ATA twice daily for 3 days after drug therapy had been halted. On follow-up at eight months, the biopsy specimens from the HBO_2-treated patients were all negative, whereas no changes were present in the non-HBO_2 control group.[7]

In Argentina, Dr. Wilkinson[19,21] and his colleagues continued to follow a few of their original patients as well as treat occasional new cases, including 2 patients with the paucibacillary tuberculoid form, 1 of which demonstrated a disappearance of the lesions within 15 days following the second HBO_2 series, but no reports appeared in the literature until Wilkinson et al. (1987) presented their findings from a double-blind study in which 10 patients with the leprotamous form of Hansen's disease receiving DDS, clofazimine, and rifampicin were randomly allocated to a 3-ATA-HBO_2 group or an air control group. They reported a statistically significant reduction in the bacillary population in the HBO_2-treated group.[20]

There are rumors of clinical studies elsewhere in the world – Brazil, India, and Latvia – but none have appeared in the literature except for the report by M. Bertholds et al.,[1] from Riga, Latvia, regarding the failure of HBO_2 to induce or enhance free-radical activity in one patient with the leprotamous form of Hansen's disease.[1]

DISCUSSION

HBO_2 is not a "magic bullet" that kills *Mycobacterium leprae*. In the few mouse footpad experiments it has shown no tendency to inhibit the growth of the bacteria. The beneficial effect of HBO_2 on the multibacillary forms of Hansen's disease in the human host could be a combination of factors: a mild alteration in immune response, interference in some fashion with the oxygen metabolism of this obligate intracellular parasite, or perhaps some improvement in leukocyte function. Although the clinical effect may have been spectacular in some cases, much of the benefit could have been secondary. In looking at the larger series, the overall effect of HBO_2 is less impressive.

But perhaps we have been sidetracked to some extent by our enthusiasm for the discoveries reported from Argentina. In attempting to continue in the direction of their investigations, we apparently overlooked the important details of Ozorio de Almeida's[9] work which preceded the independent discoveries in Argentina.

By 1937, Ozorio de Almeida had already observed the beneficial effects of HBO_2 alone on Hansen's disease among subjects participating in an entirely separate study of the effects of HBO_2 on cancer. The observation intrigued him, but he apparently did not feel that the beneficial effects of HBO_2 were likely to be of clinical significance unless they could be amplified by some synergistic drug. He chose methylene blue because it was known to increase the toxic effect of oxygen on living organisms, and it is firmly fixed by the *Mycobactium leprae* bacillus and held fast while the remainder of the drug is rapidly eliminated from the human host. At that point, he reasoned, high-dose HBO_2 could be administered with devastating effect to the bacillus and little or no harm to the human host.

Methylene blue is a dye, and so is clofazimine. Perhaps the elegant strategy employed by Ozorio de Almeida could be utilized in a similar fashion using clofazimine or a related chemical. Furthermore, we know now that the generation time for *Mycobacterium leprae* is very long – around 12 days in the mouse footpad and perhaps even longer in the human. If the combined or synergistic effects of HBO_2 and the experimental drug happen to be limited to a particular phase in the lifespan of the bacillus, it could be that all previous treatment protocols have halted the HBO_2 prematurely. It would seem that we might need to apply our treatment protocol for at least two weeks in order to measure the effects of the HBO_2 and experimental drug combination on all of the maturation phases of *Mycobacterium leprae*. These approaches merit further study.

CONCLUSION

Despite the decades of frustration and false promises, the role of HBO_2 in Hansen's disease remains to be determined. A new research based on Ozorio de Almeida´s protocol should be funded, not only in the name of science but also in the name of thousands of patients who are condemned to a long, expensive course of therapy.

REFERENCES

1. Bertholds M, Andreyev G, Goldstein N. Effect of hyperbaric oxygen on free radical activity in a patient with leprotamous leprosy. J Hyperb Med. 1989;4(3):131-4.
2. Boerema I, Brummelkamp WH, Meijne NG. Clinical application of hyperbaric oxygen. Best Publishing Co. Treatment of infections with clostridium welchii by oxygen therapy at 3 atmospheres. A report on 37 cases; p. 20-1.
3. Browne SG. Leprosy control: – chimeras and possibilities. Bull Acad Med Belg. 1980;135:208-18.
4. Gottlieb SF. The possible use of high pressure oxygen in the treatment of leprosy and tuberculosis. Dis Chest. 1963;44(2):215-7.
5. Gottlieb SF. Oxygen under pressure and microorganisms. In: Davis JC, Hunt TK, editors. Hyperbaric oxygen therapy. Bethesda (MD): Undersea Medical Society;1977. p. 79-99.
6. Harboe M. Tropical and geographical medicine. New York: McGraw-Hill; 1984. p. 799-808.
7. Jain KK. Textbook of hyperbaric medicine. Toronto (ON): Hogrefe and Huber; 1990. p. 184-6.
8. Kindwall EP, Whelan HT. Hyperbaric medicine practice. 2nd ed. Best Publishing Co. p. 2-5.
9. Ozorio de Almeida A, De Moura Costa H. Treatment of leprosy by oxygen under high pressure associated with methylene blue. Rev Bras Leprol. 1938;6:237-65.
10. Ozorio de Almeida A, De Moura Costa H. Treatment of leprosy by oxygen under pressure associated with methylene blue. Int J Lepr. 1938;6:456.
11. Ozorio de Almeida A, Rabello E. Ensaio de tratamento da lepra pelo oxygenio sob pressão. Comm To Acad Nac de Med. Jornal do Commercio. 1937 Nov 26. Portuguese. 12. Pai RR. Personal communication to: SF Gottlieb. 1980 Jun 4.
12. Pettit JH, Rees RJ. Sulphone resistance in leprosy: an experimental and clinical study. Lancet. 1964;2:673-4.
13. Rabello E, Ozorio de Almeida A. Essai de traitement de la lepre par l'oxygène sous pression. Bull Soc Fr Dermatol Syphiligr. 1938;5:810-23. French.
14. Rosasco SA, Wilkinson FW, Calori B. Hyperbaric oxygen and mycobacterium leprae: preliminary report on 200 cases. In: 5th International Conf Proc. Vancouver (BC): Simon Fraser University; 1974.
15. Shepard CC. The experimental disease that follows the injection of human leprosy bacilli into footpads of mice. J Exp Med. 1960;112:445-54.
16. Shepard CC. Leprosy today. New Eng J Med. 1982;307(26):1640-1.
17. Weekly epidemiological record [internet]. World Health Organization; 2012 [Cited 2016 September]. Report No.: 34. Available from http://www.who.int/wer/2012/wer8734.pdf?ua=1.
18. Wilkinson FF. Respuesta de la forma clinica tuberculoide al oxígeno hiperbarico. Leprologia. 1970;15(2):69-70. Spanish.
19. Wilkinson FF, Rosasco Palau SA, Besuschio S, Calori BA, Bertholds M. Hyperbaric oxygen (HBO_2) as a complementary treatment of patients with multibacillary leprotamous leprosy. Nihon Rai Gakkai Zasshi. . 1987;56:159-65.
20. Wilkinson FF, Rosasco SA, Calori BA, Equia OF, Rubio RA. Conclusiones preliminares sobre el uso del oxígeno hiperbarico en lepra lepromatosa. Revista de Leprologia. 1970;7(5):459-71. Spanish.
21. Youngblood DA. Hyperbaric oxygen in the treatment of Hansen's disease. HBO_2 Rev. 1984;5(4):244-50.

SECTION 4 SECTION

Diving, Submarine Rescue, and Life in the Sea

CHAPTER 40 CHAPTER

Emergency Management of Stricken Divers in Remote Areas

CHAPTER FORTY OVERVIEW

Background 975

Consensus Statements 979

Contraindications to IWR 981

Absolute Contraindications 981

Relative Contraindications 983

Logistical Considerations for Performing IWR 983

Case Study 986

Opposition and Risk Analysis 987

IWR Using Air 988

Role of Rebreathers in Oxygen Administration 988

Management of Neurologic Oxygen Toxicity in Water 989

Follow-Up Care for a Stricken Diver 990

Conclusion 990

References 992

Emergency Management of Stricken Divers in Remote Areas

Joseph Dituri, Carla Renaldo

BACKGROUND

The definitive care for decompression sickness (DCS) has always been 100% oxygen combined with pressure. The majority of oxygen is carried on the hemoglobin molecule. At sea level, the alveolar gas equation predicts that during air breathing,

$$paO_2 = \{(P_{atm} - P_{H20}) \text{ x } FiO_2) - (PaCO_2 \ / \ R)\}$$
$$paO_2 = \{((760 \text{ mm} - 47) \text{ x } .21) - (40 \ / \ 0.8)\}$$
$$paO_2 = \{(713 \text{ x } .21) - 50\}$$
$$paO_2 = \sim 100 \text{ mmHg (driving force)}$$

However, under pressure breathing 100% O_2 at 60 fsw and without significant CO_2 retention, the paO_2 is

$$paO_2 = \{((2128 - 47) \text{ x } 1.0) - 50\}$$
$$paO_2 = \{2081 - 50\}$$
$$paO_2 = 2031 \text{ mmHg (driving force)}$$

Key:
paO_2 = Alveolar partial pressure of oxygen
P_{atm} = Atmospheric pressure at sea level
P_{H20} = Water vapor pressure at 37 degrees C
$PaCO_2$ = Arterial partial pressure of carbon dioxide
FiO_2 = Fractional concentration of inspired oxygen in breathing gas mixture
R = respiratory quotient

The above equations demonstrate that the partial pressure of oxygen in the alveoli and blood is significantly increased using 100% oxygen at elevated ambient pressure. This driving force of oxygen allows enhanced diffusion into the body's tissues even in the face of microvascular obstruction and reduced perfusion.

The purpose of this chapter is to introduce physicians to the history of in-water recompression (IWR) and the details of various methods for treating victims of DCS in the water. We also describe the capabilities and limitations of IWR and ensure the reader understands there are multiple logistical issues that need to be considered prior to attempting IWR. Finally, we describe current best practices as recommended by an industry consensus.

The goal of recompression therapy, in any form, is to reduce the size and number of bubbles by pressure and to facilitate the off-gassing of inert gases (e.g., nitrogen, helium). The treatment for DCS works in two ways. First, the absolute size of the bubble(s) is decreased by the direct mechanical effects of compression. Second, the maximization of oxygen within the surrounding tissues and the minimization of inert gases displaced by the oxygen create a gradient which enhances inert gas diffusion out of the bubble(s), eventually leading to bubble dissolution. Gases extracted from bubbles are dissolved in solution, transported to the lungs, and eventually off-loaded in the alveoli and removed during exhalation.

Immediate controlling actions for DCS are significant and can aide in resolution of symptoms. If recompression can be made almost immediately available at or near the diving site, the chances of a full recovery are more likely to be maximized.(7) The choice of management depends upon a great many factors such as weather, time of onset of symptoms, time until treatment can be accomplished in a recompression chamber, water temperature, and severity of the symptoms. Time as an independent variable is dependent upon severity of symptoms and can range from the need to treat almost immediately (< 30 min in the case of profuse intravascular bubbling) or up to 2 hours after (in the case of other emergent symptoms). An analysis of this situation produces only three viable options if a traditional (hospital-based) recompression chamber is unavailable in adequate time:

1. Treat the affected diver with oxygen at the surface
2. Treat the affected diver with oxygen in a portable recompression chamber
3. Treat the affected diver with oxygen in the water

IWR is not a new consideration. IWR predates the recompression chamber itself. In the nineteenth century when a diver was in pain on the surface post-dive, the diver would reenter the water and "redo" decompression stops. The main benefit of IWR is that it can be initiated rapidly, which provides immediacy of care. Similar to a recompression chamber, IWR increases the pressure, which may resolve the symptomatic bubbles before more serious problems occur.

Myriad tables/profiles exist currently because their potential risks are thought to be outweighed by the potential benefit. Control of the victim once in the water is considerably less than in a recompression chamber. Finally, the logistics for many of these methods is considerable and requires significant practice to conduct properly.

The Australian IWR Table (Figure 1)(14) was developed by the Royal Australian Navy in the 1960s in response to their need for treatment in remote locations far away from recompression chambers. The treatment was similar to the shallow portion of the table developed for recompression chamber use. Oxygen is breathed for the entire duration of the treatment without any air breaks and is followed by alternating periods of oxygen and air breathing on the surface. The maximum operating depth is 30 feet seawater (fsw) or 9.1 meters of seawater (msw) for between 30–90 minutes with an ascent rate of 1 fsw every 4 minutes.

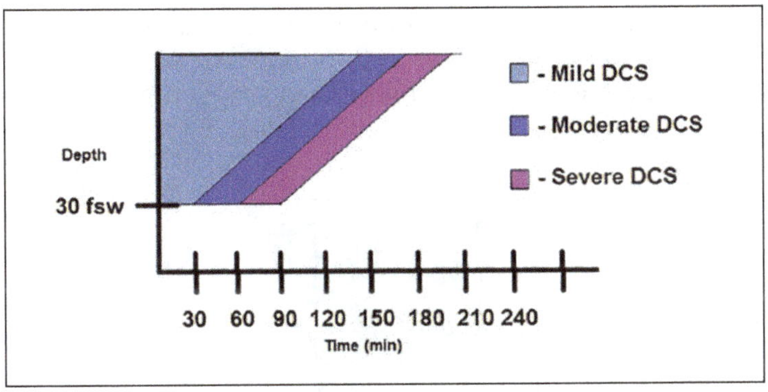

Figure 1. Australian IWR Table.

The Clipperton IWR Tables (2 variants – depending upon equipment availability) [2] were developed for use on a scientific mission to Clipperton Atoll, which is 1,300 km from the Mexican southwest coast. On the first variant, oxygen is breathed the entire portion of the treatment at 30 fsw without any air breaks for 70 minutes. Ascent rate is ~3 fsw/min. For the second table (Figure 2) used in Clipperton, initial descent is to 100 fsw using a rebreather and ascends gradually (~3 fsw/min) to 30 fsw maintaining 1.4 pO_2 on the deeper portion (~20 min). The rebreather is then purged, and pure oxygen (as close to possible) is then breathed at 30 fsw without any air breaks for 70 minutes. Ascent rate is ~3 fsw/min. Substantial oxygen prebreathe and postbreathe is required.

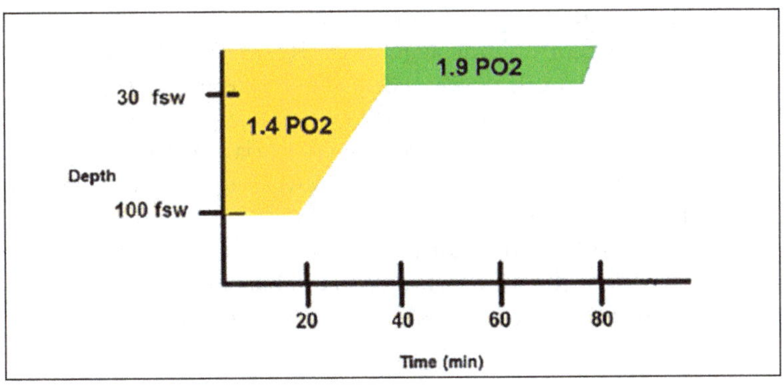

Figure 2. Clipperton (a) IWR Table.

The Hawaiian IWR table was first described by Farm et al.[9] while studying the diving of Hawaii's diving fishermen. These individuals were commonly known to have horrible DCS.[1] The initial portion of the treatment involves descent on air to the depth of relief plus 30 fsw or a maximum of 165 fsw for 10 minutes. The ascent from initial treatment depth to 30 fsw occurs over the course of 10 minutes. The diver then completes a long-duration treatment breathing oxygen at 30 fsw. The Hawaiian IWR Table with Pyle modifications (Figure 3)[16] is the shortest version of the Pyle Hawaiian Table. Longer versions include allowing for a 10-minute decision point to descend to different depths of relief but still starts at and spends a majority of time at 25 fsw. For unresolved symptoms at decision point, divers switch to air or nitrox and descend 25 feet and self-evaluate after 2 minutes. For further unresolved symptoms divers can descend to up to 125 fsw maximum depth of relief with varying ascent times from deeper depths back to 25 fsw in 25 fsw depth increments. Air or nitrox breaks are performed every 20 min for 5 minutes. Following the oxygen time the diver ascends at 3 fsw/min.

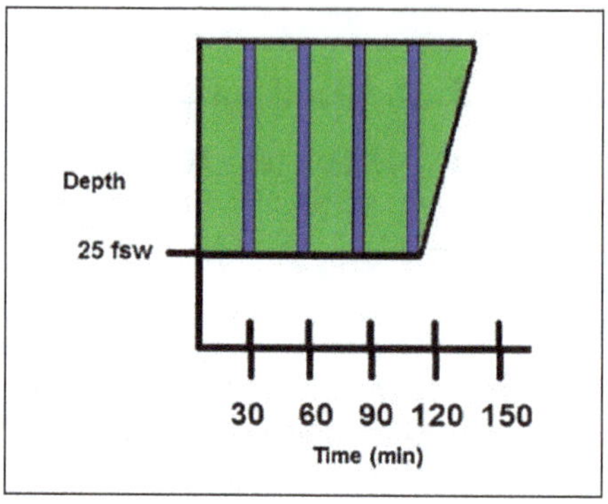

Figure 3. Pyle IWR Table (shortest).

The U.S. Navy developed 2 IWR treatment tables (Figure 4). The table used depends on the symptoms diagnosed by a diving medical officer. The first table is 60 minutes at 30 fsw, and the second table is 90 minutes at 30 fsw. Upon completion of time at 30 fsw, both tables have a stepped ascent to 20 fsw and 10 fsw all while breathing oxygen. No air breaks are considered for this table. The ascent rate is 2 fsw/min. Surface oxygen is required upon completion.

Finally, in 2013, a major training agency, the International Association of Nitrox and Technical Divers (IANTD), developed the first international program to teach IWR. They have certified almost 200 practitioners in the use of IWR as of May 2016. The recommended table (Figure 5) focused on an initial treatment depth of 30 fsw for 10 minutes using pure oxygen followed by an ascent to 25 fsw. It incorporated air breaks and had a 1 fsw/min ascent rate.

IWR has been a viable method of treating affected divers for over a century in one form or another. All of the previous suggested tables exposed the victim to partial pressures of oxygen in excess of 1.6 ATA pO_2 for long durations with complexity

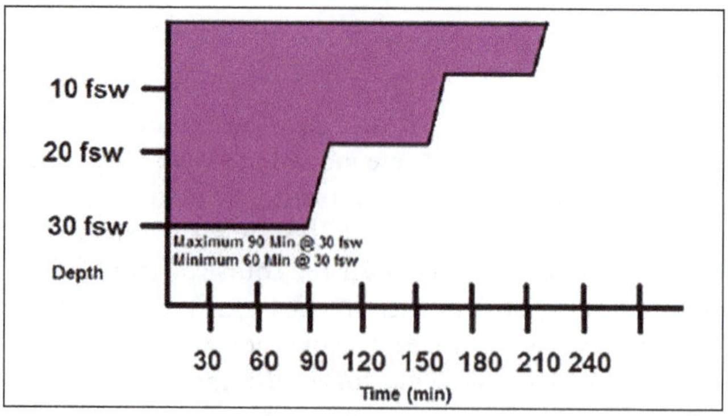

Figure 4. U.S. Navy IWR Table.

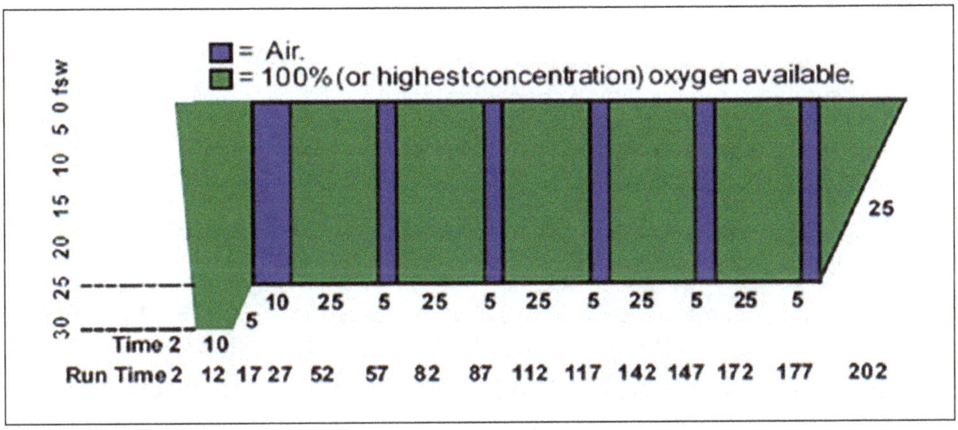

Figure 5. IANTD IWR Table.

and other logistical concerns. Excessively high pO_2 represents a significant risk. Some compromise was needed because IWR has been shown anecdotally to help divers overcome decompression sickness (DCS). In-water management of DCS may significantly reduce the severity of symptoms and improve the likelihood of permanent resolution of symptoms in follow-up professional medical care.

CONSENSUS STATEMENTS

On April 28–29, 2014, in San Diego, California, Richard Sadler, MD, FACS, CDR; Joseph Dituri USN (ret), MS; Simon Mitchell, MB, ChB, DipOccMed, PhD, FANZCA; Craig Jenni, JD; Richard Moon, MD, CM, MSc, FRCP(C), FACP, FCCP; and Richard Pyle, PhD, met to discuss the topic of IWR with the intent of polling industry-leading physicians and divers in the use and practice of IWR. The following is a consensus statement and list of guidelines that came from the invited speakers and input of dive industry professionals.[17]

This consensus statement is a set of recommendations and general guidelines developed using available evidence and expert opinion in areas where high-quality clinical data is limited or does not exist. These guidelines were developed systematically and resulted in specific recommendations that assist the practitioner and diver in making decisions. These recommendations may be adopted, modified, or rejected according to needs and constraints and are not intended to replace local institutional policies. They are not to be considered a standard or "best practice" for emergency response of DCS. Their use cannot guarantee any specific outcome. These guidelines are subject to revision as warranted by the evolution of medical knowledge, technology, and practice. They represent basic recommendations that are supported by a synthesis and analysis of the current literature, expert opinion, and open forum commentary combined with any existing data.

These statements represent the opinion, beliefs, and best judgments of the aforementioned subject-matter experts. As such, they have not been subjected to the same level of formal scientific review as some medical standards. Each person, institution, or practice should decide individually whether to implement the principles in this statement based on a careful evaluation of risk versus benefit and on the sound judgment of the participants involved in the situation at that time.

1. The definitive emergency response of DCS continues to be a combination of pressure and oxygen in high concentrations.
2. Oxygen and pressure are preferred over surface oxygen alone in the emergency response of DCS.
3. It is determined that IWR is a viable methodology for first aid (an intermediate step) prior to definitive emergency response of DCS.
4. Immediacy of emergency response with oxygen and pressure may be fundamental to affect optimal outcomes in selected symptomatic divers.(13)
5. The intrinsic advantage of immediacy in IWR surpasses the potential risks for appropriately selected symptomatic divers.
6. IWR has potential for improving outcomes in those divers with symptoms that have rapid onset and a poor prognosis.
7. IWR is rarely a complete and sole emergency response for DCS. All symptomatic divers of DCS shall, if they opt for IWR, be evaluated by a physician knowledgeable in diving and hyperbaric medicine as soon as possible following IWR.

New consensus recommendations for implementation of IWR:

1. During IWR the diver must be accompanied by a tender.
2. The effectiveness of IWR will be lessened if the diver becomes cold. Maintenance of optimal thermal comfort is therefore important.
3. Indications: While acknowledging the potential benefits of IWR, the potential risks of IWR limit its applications to those divers with symptoms associated with poor outcomes.
4. The breathing mixture should be as close as possible to 100% oxygen (with the goal of achieving a pO_2 of 1.6 atm/bar); mixtures containing less than a minimum FiO_2 of 0.80 (80% inspired oxygen concentration) should not be used for IWR.
5. Emergency response depth should not exceed 20 ft (6 m), even if the breathing mixture contains less than 100% oxygen.
6. Emergency response time should extend 60 minutes after the resolution of symptoms; the total emergency response time must NOT exceed 120 minutes at depth. Figure 6 (pictured at the end of this chapter) is a visual depiction of the treatment table.
7. Periods of breathing air ("air breaks") are not required due to additional complexity.
8. The planned ascent rate should be 1 fsw (0.3 msw)/min if possible.
9. The emergency response protocol should be terminated at any time if deemed necessary by either the tender or diver/symptomatic diver.

10. In the event of an emergency (such as loss of consciousness in the treated diver), a rapid ascent should be made to the surface. If the diver is convulsing and the mouthpiece is retained, (e.g., during use of a retaining strap or if a full-face mask is used) ascent should be delayed until the seizure has stopped. If the mouthpiece is not retained, an ascent should be made immediately, even if the convulsion continues.
11. If symptoms return during ascent from the planned IWR, the diver may return to 20 fsw (6 msw) if the total time at 20 fsw (6 msw) has not yet exceeded 120 minutes.
12. After exiting the water following IWR, the symptomatic diver must not reenter the water even if symptoms recur.
13. Mild activity (i.e., gentle finning movement) is acceptable and encouraged during IWR.
14. For severe DCS (e.g., paralysis), judgment will be required to weigh the benefits of quicker IWR with short delay to evacuation versus immediate evacuation to a hyperbaric facility that may be many hours away. Consultation with an offsite diving medical expert is recommended.

Note: Consideration should be given to combining the last 5 fsw 1-minute stops due to logistics and wave action if needed.

CONTRAINDICATIONS TO IWR

The following is a list of noted absolute contraindications to IWR. All of these conditions have in common a condition that poses a potential uncontrollable risk to the diver.

Absolute Contraindications

1. Isolated hearing loss and vertigo (a sense of spinning) are both potential symptoms of DCS that can lead to permanent injury and technically belong in the most serious category of decompression sickness. However, when they occur in isolation – that is, with no other symptoms of DCS – it is possible that they have been caused by ear barotrauma rather than DCS. If this is the case, then IWR is contraindicated. Isolated hearing loss and vertigo must be differentially diagnosed to ensure no ear barotrauma is present.
2. Airway compromise: Inability to perceive and clear secretions (stupor), active coughing of blood (hemoptysis) or frothy sputum of any sort, collapsed lung (pneumothorax), and "chokes" with paroxysmal coughing all represent risks to a clear airway, which is critical to safe diving. Similarly, emesis represents a potentially unsecure airway, and a victim should not be replaced in the water if such conditions exist.
3. Cardiac arrest: Resuscitation and stabilization always take priority. Successful resuscitation in no way reverses this contraindication, since relapse and instability are common.
4. Extreme anxiety: The risk of barotrauma from an underwater panic attack is prohibitive. The idea of "sedation" or other pharmacologic aid in this

setting is never appropriate and should never be considered. Only a trained Diving Medicine Physician is allowed to medicate a patient/diver.

5. Moderate or severe hypothermia: By definition, moderate hypothermia (core temperature 83°F–90°F)[18] produces uncoordinated muscle movement. This would make it impossible for the diver to safely manage his or her dive gear underwater. Additionally, it is unlikely that the body temperature can be raised while in water. Any potential benefit from IWR would be offset at the point of hypothermia due to the reduction in circulation to the extremities. Finally, at the onset of hypothermia the chattering of teeth would decrease the ability of a tender to accurately detect CNS oxygen toxicity.
6. Altered mental status or altered consciousness: A mental state which would prevent autonomous or volitional control of diving equipment. This could also include weakness or any other symptom of such severity that it would prevent safe diving practices (e.g., equipment use).
7. Severe tachypnea: A respiratory rate of > 24/minute.
8. Loss of consciousness (LOC): Occurring within 15 minutes of surfacing. LOC in this setting strongly implies AGE/CAGE ([cerebral] arterial gas embolism).

   Many dive sites do not have adequate facilities to check for shock or hemodynamic instability. Because these are clear contraindications, a physician must ensure these are checked or obvious to the casual observer not to be present prior to IWR.

9. Shock: A rare presentation of severe DCS where there is a massive capillary leak with loss of intravascular volume. This can be quickly fatal, and the diver is too unstable to consider IWR. Inadequate organ perfusion and low blood pressure will only get worse with the inability to give fluids while doing IWR. Intravenous fluid resuscitation is obligatory.
10. Hemodynamic instability or CPR: A victim with hemodynamic instability is a potential liability for management in water as well as any victim who has had CPR.

Relative Contraindications

1. Vertigo: Even when caused by DCS, vertigo is a potentially debilitating symptom which is usually accompanied by nausea and vomiting and may make IWR hazardous. Differential diagnosis must be performed to ensure the dizziness is not caused by middle-ear barotrauma.
2. Logistical issues: Myriad logistical issues are relative contraindications to IWR such as water temperature, wave action, insufficient oxygen, lack of trained individuals, hazardous marine life, adequate distance to a chamber, and correct equipment, to name a few.
3. Mild symptoms or more serious symptoms and signs that resolve or nearly resolve and remain improved on surface oxygen: An evaluation of benefit-to-risk ratio may not support IWR. These cases should still be monitored for deterioration and discussed urgently with an appropriate expert

authority. It is likely they will require evacuation to a hyperbaric medicine unit for evaluation and treatment.

The diver may only be recompressed in water if there are no overt signs of pulmonary compromise such as pneumothorax or hemoptysis, and he or she is fully conscious and cooperative.

Logistical Considerations for Performing IWR

The following is a group of practical and logistical considerations for equipment. Preemergency response informed consent of all potential IWR participants should ideally be obtained. In order to facilitate this, a webinar or video online should be used where IWR is explained and a standard waiver is signed. Trained IWR divers should practice IWR regularly in order to maintain proficiency.

Absolute control of a symptomatic diver must be ensured, and the diver should be tethered. The symptomatic diver's depth should be controlled by the use of a stable reference line. Some form of positive contact with the symptomatic diver is mandatory. Some examples of positive control include the symptomatic diver being connected to the down line with a separate line, the symptomatic diver being tethered to the accompanying diver with a line, or the use of a quick release (snap) shackle in either of those first two examples is reasonable. Additionally, the surface support team and tender should be prepared for a sudden deterioration of the diver/symptomatic diver. Finally, if reasonably foreseeable adverse conditions cannot be mitigated, the IWR protocol should be terminated.

Some form of device to ensure the diver's airway breathing source remains in place should be used. A regulator retention (gag) strap (RRS) is strongly recommended to hold the regulator in place in the unlikely event of an oxygen seizure. The use of a full-face mask (FFM) is recommended for trained users. Significant caution is advised for the untrained user. The consensus recommendation of a maximum oxygen partial pressure of 1.6 ATA minimizes but does not remove the risk of seizure. The consequences of aspiration underwater are potentially life-threatening.

FFM is the traditional "best practice" for IWR. Advantages include the airway being maximally protected from ambient water in the event of a seizure, allowance for communication, and additional thermal protection. Disadvantages of a FFM include lack of training in most cases, imperfect fit or discomfort, difficulty in clearing water or vomitus (creating an additional risk of aspiration), the necessity in most cases to remove the full mask to change gas supplies (unless a gas switching block is used), and being costly (approximately USD$500–USD$750).

RRS consists of a strap around the head/neck attached to the second stage regulator and a rubberized flexible flange around the mouth, preventing loss of regulator and creating a barrier to water in the event of seizure. Advantages of RRS include lesser costs than a FFM (< USD$100) and requirement of minimal training. Disadvantages of an RRS include it is not as protective of the airway as a FFM, and properly designed devices are not widely available.

All previous IWR protocols require or strongly advocate the use of a FFM, primarily to mitigate the consequences of a hyperoxia-induced seizure underwater. These previous protocols also incorporate breathing 100% (or close to it) oxygen at depths in excess of 6 msw (20 fsw), where the inspired oxygen partial pressure is in excess of 1.6 ATA. As advantageous as a FFM may be in the event of a seizure underwater (for reducing the probability of drowning), as discussed earlier, the use of a FFM also imposes some difficulty (and risk) for divers who are not trained in their use.[4]

In the context of these recommendations, a maximum depth of 20 fsw (6 msw) is advocated for IWR (a depth at which near-100% oxygen is commonly breathed by technical divers for decompression). At 20 fsw (6 msw) the incidence of hyperoxia-induced seizure is extremely low, and the potential net benefits of using a FFM depend on the degree of training and familiarity the afflicted diver already has with this equipment prior to attempting IWR. Therefore, a RRS is recommended in cases where the symptomatic diver is not already trained in the proper use of a FFM or when a FFM is not available.

Although more controversial than a FFM for this purpose, the RRS is arguably supported by data. Gempp et al. reported[10] 54 underwater loss-of-consciousness events in military divers leading to only 3 fatal drownings. In this series there were 26 cases of CNS oxygen toxicity with seizures, with an 11.5% major complication rate: 2 deaths (caught under a barge) and 1 nonfatal moderate water aspiration. The use of the Drager-style gag strap with strap and lip-sealing flange was used in all cases. Although this is an uncontrolled series, and notwithstanding the potential for other factors to influence outcome in the military setting, the unexpectedly high survival following these events suggests that gag straps are effective in most cases. Improvisation of gag straps by divers is not encouraged.

In the event sufficient oxygen is not available and all the other factors are met for selecting IWR, EMS should be activated and the victim prepared for evacuation. The affected diver can be immersed in water (head out of water) using the table and schedule discussed, breathing the highest percentage of oxygen available until 15 minutes prior to the arrival of reliable transportation or the end of the protocol. This idea, while not clinically proven, assists in redistribution of the fluid throughout the body[8] and has the potential to be a low-risk method to "increase" the volume of blood and improve the overall prognosis of a diver with DCS who has a delay in treatment.

As mentioned earlier, there are several IWR protocols, but there are no statistically valid trials favoring one over another. The answer to which one is better is "nobody knows." However, exceeding a maximum pO_2 of 1.6 ATA is strongly discouraged because it can lead to CNS oxygen toxicity in the water. The mechanism of CNS oxygen toxicity is not well understood. On a normal dive, the best protection against CNS oxygen toxicity is to keep below 1.6 ATA pO_2. Exceeding 1.6 ATA pO_2 is dangerous during normal sport diving activity. Be mindful the normal diver does not have a depth-limiting device which prevents accidental descent as well as a buddy whose express function is to monitor and assist in the event of a symptom of CNS oxygen toxicity. Contrary to a sport diver, the stricken diver is to do nothing during IWR except breathing and light motion to improve circulation. Exercise in excess of light motion may hasten the onset of CNS oxygen toxicity. Light movement to increase circulation is not recommended below 20 fsw. Light movement may assist in off-gassing 20 fsw and shallower. The stricken diver is also to be kept as warm as possible and well hydrated.

Prior to administration of oxygen, a safe oxygen environment must be established, removing possible sources of ignition as well as sources of fuel such as petroleum products, paper, or highly flammable objects. All oxygen tanks and sources should be secured, and only equipment designated "oxygen safe" should be used. Oxygen should be provided with either a demand valve/regulator or another means of providing 100% oxygen. If the victim is conscious, the rescuer should obtain permission before administering oxygen. If the victim is unsure or doesn't want oxygen, the rescuer may advise the victim of the benefits of oxygen and that it could help. If the victim is unconscious, the rescuer should activate the EMS, administer oxygen, and perform an exam to determine possible causes.

As discussed, there should be some means of ensuring the stricken diver is not able to descend deeper than 20 fsw (6 msw) as well as a means of retrieval such as a line tied or clipped. A flat ocean floor would be best for this purpose; however, surge may be a factor if swells are high enough. Avoid excessive movement of the stricken diver (in the surge) as to cause any symptoms which could be confused with CNS oxygen toxicity. Alternatively, a line could be affixed to a boat with 20 feet of slack and a weighted bottom. The diver could then clip into the line and have a fixed position not affording the possibility of descending below 20 fsw (6 msw). Specific consideration should be given to slightly overweighing the stricken diver, provided the recommendations about tethering the diver to the line are adhered to. This will reduce the motion of the diver and, in the event of an oxygen seizure, assist the buddy diver in holding the victim at depth. If operating from a boat in a strong current, consideration should be given to drifting rather than having the boat anchored. Drifting eliminates any effect of the current which can complicate depth control and cause fatigue in the divers trying to maintain position.

The tethering or down line should be fixed to the boat so that there is an immediate connection that divers can follow between the surface support and treated diver. Avoid using an anchor line because it tends to move with wave action, which becomes fatiguing for divers trying to stay attached.

A community database of IWR incidents and outcomes is being maintained at http://www.ibum.org/iwr.html. The group of experts from the GAVI IWR symposium determined the most important information required during assessment of an injured diver and IWR is a timeline or chronology of events, along with key relevant data describing the symptomatic diver and circumstances of the incident. The following information should be captured:

1. Was victim referred for evaluation, hyperbaric emergency response, etc. (give details)
2. Outcome/degree of recovery
3. Type of thermal protection (mm of wet suit or dry suit/type)
4. Temperature of water (°F)
5. Did you have any complications with the IWR (detail them)
6. IWR protocol followed (percentage oxygen/depth/time at depth)
7. Surface oxygen use (yes/no) and duration
8. Time of symptom resolution (minutes after surfacing)
9. Order of symptom progression (list all Sx and when they started as well as pain level on a scale of 1–10
10. Time of onset of symptoms (how many minutes after surfacing was first Sx)
11. Dive profile
12. Gender
13. Race

This information will be added to a community database of IWR incidents; outcomes will be maintained by IBUM and available to the general public. This information will be shared freely with all interested parties.

CASE STUDY

IWR has been of benefit to some DCS victims in numerous circumstances. Only three recorded attempts at IWR clearly led to deterioration of the condition of a DCS victim. It is necessary to stipulate there is likely to be a bias against reporting any IWR study results because if successful the diver feels no need to report, and if a failure, divers may become embarrassed. There are hundreds of additional cases where IWR was of benefit that was, in some cases, significant.[19] While myriad anecdotal evidence/ case studies exist for using IWR, perhaps none is more powerful or convincing as this case. Following the Gallant Aquatic Ventures International IWR Symposium where the above consensus statement was formed by industry-leading experts in hyperbarics, there was an apparent need to gather objective quality evidence concerning IWR. A group of concerned researchers worked through IRB and received approval to conduct a study.[5] The team wanted to ensure accurate depths for the in-water study, so they were working to place a platform at the exact depth in the water. The divers planned their dive and dove their plan. They planned for workload and wore computers to ensure the plan was matched. The dive team consisted of a physician who was UHMS trained and board certified in hyperbarics, a retired Navy Saturation Diving Officer and partial owner of IANTD who was also the principle investigator on the In-Water Recompression study and protocol and coauthored the IWR course and manual, as well as a local dive store owner and experienced cave instructor for IANTD who was also a trained IWR Instructor through IANTD.

The dive itself was unremarkable, except for a few "sawtooth" ascents (short cyclical ascents and descents), which were part of the dive plan. All decompression requirements as advised by the Sherwood dive computer were completed without incident. The team exited the water together. Approximately 15 minutes following final ascent to the surface, 1 of the divers experienced difficulty removing his drysuit and started rubbing his back and complained of back pain. Surface oxygen was administered, and a gross neurological assessment was performed including mental status, cranial nerves, strength, coordination and sensory. The victim seemed lucid, and there was no obvious loss of sensation nor any noticeable decrease in strength or coordination. The only symptom was radicular back pain which peaked at an 8 on a scale of 1 to 10. It was readily apparent that this back pain was not attributable to strain or mechanical injury, as it was worsening rapidly. During this time the local dive store owner/IWR Instructor geared up and set up logistics.

The dive site was approximately two hours from the nearest hyperbaric chamber. The rapid tempo of the pain was concerning. There were minimal logistical concerns for using IWR in the dive site. No sea state existed, nor was there an issue with hazardous marine life. Twenty-two minutes post dive, the victim reentered the water and descended to 10 feet with an experienced tender for in-water oxygen. An additional tender entered the water for full IWR using the IWR symposium recommendations as a guide. Twenty-seven minutes post dive, the 3-person team descended to 20 fsw (6 msw).

After less than 2 minutes at 20 fsw (6 msw) breathing oxygen, the pain had been completely relieved and there was complete resolution of all symptoms 31 minutes after surfacing. The remaining protocol was performed per the IWR consensus statement including an ascent rate of 1 foot per minute to the surface. There were no residual symptoms, and the physician had a neurological assessment post dive as well as followed up with several other physicians knowledgeable in hyperbaric medicine. No additional treatment was required. The affected diver was administered a Doppler echocardiogram approximately 24 hours post dive and was noted as still having 1 bubble per 4 cardiac cycles. No abnormal heart defect such as a patent foramen ovale (PFO) was noted. Never before had such a well-informed group been faced with a situation such as this and reported this positive result.

OPPOSITION AND RISK ANALYSIS

As reported by Pyle and Youngblood (1995), some opponents to IWR declare that certain DCS symptoms can be relieved at the surface when the victim breathes pure oxygen.[16] As discussed earlier, this has limitations but is presently an accepted and recommended response to DCS. If symptoms do resolve with surface oxygen, and recompression treatment facilities are relatively close, then the additional risks incurred with reimmersion may not be warranted. However, in cases where chamber facilities are not available, or when symptoms persist in spite of surface oxygen, recompression may be necessary to relieve symptoms and prevent permanent damage, and IWR should be considered.[16]

There is no magic formula that will ensure safety or resolution of symptoms. The overriding theme of IWR is to pressurize the stricken diver, use oxygen to reduce or eliminate the size of the problematic bubbles, and improve the stricken diver's likelihood of full recovery. The placement of a person stricken with a very poorly understood and potentially debilitating malady into a relatively hostile and uncontrolled environment[15] may seem ill-advised. However, this emergent effort has prevented long-term injury and probably saved lives. As pointed out by Pyle and Youngblood, at the root of the controversy surrounding the practice of IWR is a basic conflict between theory and practice. The list of theoretical reasons why IWR has historically been discouraged is long and includes the following:

1. The risks of additional nitrogen loading (with air or enriched air nitrox)
2. The risk of oxygen-induced convulsions (with pure oxygen)
3. The risk of drowning
4. The need for and risk to tending divers
5. Thermal considerations
6. Adverse environmental conditions (e.g., rough seas, marine life, etc).
7. Reduced capacity for the afflicted diver and treatment supervisor to assess the nature of symptom progression during treatment

Many more risks exist and should be discussed prior to IWR.

There are two theoretical considerations supporting IWR. First, there is the obvious advantage of the effect of immediate recompression on bubble growth. A recent human study[3] showed that following a dive to 100 feet for 30 minutes, compression back to 1.6 ATA breathing oxygen reduced venous bubble formation substantially more than breathing oxygen at 1 ATA. Second, there is the advantage of increased inspired oxygen partial pressure (when pure oxygen is breathed), which can have a variety of positive effects on the pathophysiology of DCS (including amelioration of inflammatory events and correction of tissue hypoxia).

A more recent pilot study[5] investigated the efficacy of an IWR treatment on decompression stress measured by semiquantitative counts of venous gas emboli in the central venous circulation. This pilot study had promising results; however, further study is warranted to obtain conclusive results. There is a substantial body of anecdotal evidence of benefit when IWR has been used by divers in the field.

IWR USING AIR

IWR using air is considered less preferable than in-water recompression using oxygen. It must be remembered that the crucial drug used in the treatment of DCS is oxygen. However, it must also be remembered that the vast majority of documented successful IWR cases used air. The authors recommend not using the USN Diving Manual IWR Protocol (20.4.4).[20] The use of air at approximately 5 ATA (pO_2 = 1.0, same as surface O_2 at 100%) incurs inert gas loading with nitrogen at dangerous levels, negating any benefit. USN Air Treatment Table 1A should be avoided for IWR without oxygen for those reasons as well as the fact that the logistical needs are formidable, and it is unlikely that it could be done with the expectation of benefit, at the cost of great risk. At one time, divers were treated in recompression chambers using the U.S. Navy protocols breathing air instead of oxygen. The failure rate was high. It is unlikely that in-water recompression using air is more effective than those treatment tables. While these air tables still remain in the navy dive manual, they are not commonly used due to the lack of effectiveness of air treatments.

ROLE OF REBREATHERS IN OXYGEN ADMINISTRATION

Always consider the potential role of the rebreather for the administration of first aid following a DCS incident. A rebreather allows prolonged administration of 100% oxygen to the conscious victim. Rebreathers can increase duration of an AL 80 cylinder (2,265 liters) from 150 minutes in open circuit to as much as 2,900 minutes. This increase of more than 19 times can help with storage concerns for adequate oxygen reducing the overall footprint of emergency transport gas by approximately 90%. The stricken diver need not be certified or trained in rebreather operation as long as the victim is merely using it on the surface to extend the amount of surface oxygen provided. The rebreather must be set up by a qualified individual and closely monitored by a competent person on the surface. While rebreathers are recognized as a potential tool for administration of oxygen during IWR, their use in IWR by divers untrained in their use should only be attempted under expert supervision.

The volume of oxygen required to complete this management in water is about 6,000 liters. For those who choose this option, using a rebreathing apparatus would reduce consumption to about 300 liters, but the victim must be trained in the use of a rebreather prior to going in the water, and the rebreather must have sufficient carbon dioxide–scrubbing capacity remaining. This savings of 5,700 liters means the in-water management could be accomplished on a single rebreather cylinder as opposed to having another diver shuttle three or four bottles filled with oxygen to the stricken diver. If a rebreather is chosen, this amount will be decreased, but the carbon dioxide scrubber duration and the diver's ability to use the device must be considered.

MANAGEMENT OF NEUROLOGIC OXYGEN TOXICITY IN WATER

The stricken diver should be observed closely as the statistical probability of CNS oxygen toxicity increases when hyperoxic (< 1.6 bar pO_2) mixtures are used in the water. The symptoms of CNS oxygen toxicity are located in Chapter 3: Oxygen Toxicity and will not be mentioned herein for brevity.

The following suggestions can be used by a diver if oxygen toxicity symptoms (other than seizures) arise:

1. The diver being treated should report the symptoms to the accompanying safety diver immediately.
2. If possible, the victim's breathing gas should be changed to air.
3. The safety diver must watch the victim constantly and be ready to intervene (see below) immediately if a seizure occurs.
4. The relationship of premonitory symptoms to the onset of a seizure is variable and unpredictable, as is the efficacy of lowering the inspired pO_2 in preventing progression to a seizure. Given that a seizure in the water is a very dangerous event, the safest course of action when premonitory symptoms occur is to abandon IWR.
5. The safety diver and victim should surface over one to two minutes. The safety diver must be ready to intervene immediately should a convulsion occur.
6. Retrieve the diver from the water, place on oxygen, and consider evacuation for recompression in a hyperbaric chamber.

What to do when a seizure occurs follows:

7. If the diver is wearing a full-face mask or the regulator is retained in the mouth, the safety diver must make every attempt to hold the mask or regulator in place, and the diver should be kept at depth until the seizure is resolved.
8. The moment the seizure appears to abate, the diver should be brought directly to the surface and removed from the water as quickly as possible and an ABC (airway breathing, circulation) protocol instituted.
9. If the regulator is lost from the mouth, and the airway is obviously unprotected, the safety diver should not attempt to replace the regulator. Instead, the victim should be brought to the surface immediately, even if the seizure appears to be continuing. Remove from the water and initiate an ABC protocol.
10. Continue the administration of oxygen on the surface after ABC is complete, and the diver has been conscious for 15 minutes.[11]

Pulmonary oxygen toxicity is highly unlikely with this protocol, as the absolute exposures are too low. The previous dive profile may have a bearing on this, but in general the risk of neurologic toxicity limits the exposure. Some of the earliest symptoms is pain behind the breast bone and cough. Should paroxysmal coughing occur and become uncontrolled, the diver must surface.

There is a small but definite chance of pulmonary oxygen toxicity, especially if a long high exposure dive was the proximate cause. In this case, symptoms of chest discomfort or coughing would be present. Should this occur, 5-minute "air breaks" every 20 minutes may lessen or alleviate the symptoms. However, continuation of oxygen therapy is strongly encouraged, and air breaks should not be instituted without prior discussion with a diving medicine expert.

FOLLOW-UP CARE FOR A STRICKEN DIVER

Upon completion of the IWR protocol and safe return to the boat or remote shore, the stricken diver must be hydrated, be kept warm, and lay supine. Transport to the nearest hyperbaric facility for evaluation by a physician knowledgeable in hyperbaric medicine is required. The use of supplemental oxygen en route, if practical, is advisable. After three hours of surface oxygen, alternating one-hour periods with air is acceptable if symptoms have resolved. Cessation of diving activities is obligatory until evaluation by a physician trained in diving medicine.(6)

The stricken diver should be carefully monitored. The diver and all supporting documentation including dive profile, treatment profile and assessments, diver response, and any medical history as well as any interventions including first aid should be brought to the professional medical staff at the hyperbaric facility. Additionally, it is recommended that copies of all of the material stated above should be sent to the central database repository for IWR to gather data.

CONCLUSION

Divers who have DCS can present in many ways and may have a variable course. Caring for that diver entails diligence in the primary and subsequent evaluations, with awareness of the natural history of the disease. A well-executed plan for accurate diagnosis, aggressive hydration in the situational context, environmental management, and immediate use of oxygen will optimize the chances for better outcomes. Consider using IWR if the situation is warranted but know the contraindications. The placement of a person stricken with a poorly understood and potentially debilitating malady into a relatively hostile and uncontrolled environment(15) just may be the best thing you can do for him or her.

The decision to place a diver back in the water should be very carefully considered. The benefits of IWR should not be equated with recompression in a chamber at a medical treatment facility, and the risks may be substantially higher. With a chamber, additional resources are available to treat complications of DCS, and oxygen toxicity can be safely managed. In the case of IWR, the inherent isolation of the diver from other support requires serious consideration of risk versus benefit.

Though there are no data that would support definitive statements or guidelines, it is probably true to say that the milder forms of DCS do not justify exposure of the diver to the extra risk of IWR in order to achieve early recompression. At a workshop(12) convened to consider management of mild or marginal DCS in remote locations, it was agreed that such milder symptoms could be managed adequately without recompression. This is not to say that you would not recompress such a diver if a chamber was readily available, but the extra risks of IWR may not justified in such cases. Most importantly, the poorer prognosis of more severe symptoms recompressed after substantial delays would suggest that the benefits of immediacy of care offered by IWR may justify the risk in suitable divers. The injured diver must be able to participate in the recompression plan. This includes mental clarity to properly evaluate his or her status, progress, and needs as well as communication with the tender and topside support. The diver must also be able to easily manage his or her airway and secretions.

It is the opinion of the authors and contributors that IWR has an extensive empirical evidence to justify its use in some circumstances. Properly equipped and trained teams caring for a diver with serious DCS should consider the victim's suitability for IWR. The recommendations herein are tools a physician can use to optimize the outcome of a diver with DCS when no chamber is readily available. Above all physicians should analyze the secondary consequences of all decisions. Finally they should know the risks the diver and person dealing with the DCS have assumed and try to do no more harm than good.

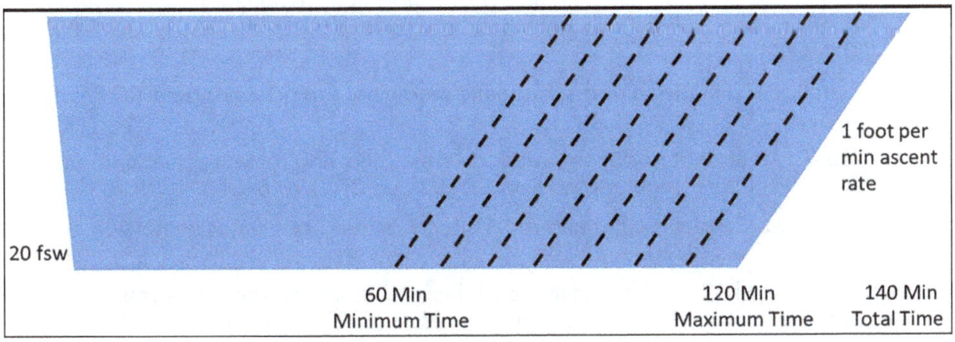

Figure 6. Graphical representation of consensus IWR table timeline that the authors feel is the newest and safer option for IWR.

REFERENCES

1. Black coral [motion picture]. Winn B, Winn J, Winn T, producers. Maui (HI): 2016.
2. Blatteau JE, Jean F, Pontier JM, Blanche E, Bompar JM, Meaudre E, Etienne JL. Decompression sickness accident management in remote areas. Use of immediate in-water recompression therapy. Review and elaboration of a new protocol targeted for a mission at Clipperton atoll. Ann Fr Anesth Reanim. 2006 Aug;25(8):874-83.
3. Blatteau J, Pontier J. Effect of in-water recompression with oxygen to 6 msw versus normobaric oxygen breathing on bubble formation in divers. Eur J Appl Physiol. 2009;106:691-5.
4. Dituri J, Sadler R. In-water recompression (manual). IANTD Press; 2013. p. 1-37.
5. Dituri J, Sadler R, Siddiqi F, et al. Echocardiographic evaluation of intracardiac venous gas emboli following in-water recompression. Undersea Hyperbar Med. 2016;43(2):103-12.
6. Edmonds C. In: Diving and subaquatic medicine. 5th ed. London: CRC Press; 2015. p. 500.
7. Elliot D. Treatment of decompression illness following mixed gas recreational dives. South Pac Underw Med Soc J. 1997 Jun;27(2):90-5.
8. Epstein M. Cardiovascular and renal effects of head-out water immersion in man. Circ Res. 1976 Nov;39(5).
9. Farm, Hayashi, Beckman. Diving and decompression sickness treatment practices among Hawaii's diving fishermen. Honolulu: Sea Grant; 1986. Sea Grant Technical Report UNIHI-TP-86-01. Located at: Sea Grant Library.
10. Gempp E, Louge P, Blatteau J-E, Hugon M. Descriptive epidemiology of 153 diving injuries with rebreathers among French military divers 1979-2009. Mil Med. 2011;176:446-50.
11. Mitchell S, Bennett M, Bird N, et al. Recommendations for rescue of a submerged unresponsive compressed-gas diver. Undersea Hyperb Med. 2012;39:1099-108.
12. Mitchell S, Doolette D, Wacholz C, Vann R, editors. Management of mild or marginal decompression illness in remote locations – workshop proceedings. Washington (DC): Undersea and Hyperbaric Medical Society; 2005. 240 p. ISBN: 0 9673066 6 3.
13. Moon R; editor. In: Bove and Davis' diving medicine. Philadelphia: Elsevier; 2004. p. 202-4.
14. Pyle RL. In-water recompression [letter]. South Pac Underw Med Soc J. 1997;27(3).
15. Pyle R. Keeping up with the times: application of technical diving practices for in-water recompression. In: Kay E, Spencer MP, editors. In-water recompression: the forty eighth workshop of the undersea and hyperbaric medical society. Undersea and Hyperbaric Medical Society; 1999. p.74-88. Co-published by the Diver's Alert Network.
16. Pyle RL, Youngblood DA. In-water recompression. AquaCorps J. 1995 Oct/Nov 11:35-46
17. Sadler R, Dituri J, Mitchell S, et al. GAVI consensus statement regarding in-water recompression. 2014 Apr. p. 1-7.
18. Sterba JA. Field management of accidental hypothermia during diving. U.S. Naval Experimental Diving Unit technical report. 1990. NEDU-1-90. Retrieved 2017 Jan 1. http://www.dtic.mil/dtic/tr/fulltext/u2/a219560.pdf

19. UHMS Workshop #48. In: Kay E, Spencer M, editors. Water recompression. Kensington (MD): Undersea Hyperbaric Medical Society; 1999.

20. U.S. Navy diving manual. 6th rev. Vol. 5, Diving medicine and recompression chamber operations. Washington (DC): Aqua Press; 2008.

CHAPTER 41 CHAPTER

Ketogenic Diet and Ketogenic Supplementation for Central Nervous System Oxygen Toxicity

CHAPTER FORTY-ONE OVERVIEW

Mechanisms and Manifestations of Central Nervous System Oxygen Toxicity . . . 997

Fasting Ketosis and Nutritional Ketosis as an Anticonvulsant Therapy . . . 999

Anticonvulsant Mechanisms of Ketosis . . . 1000

Evidence Supporting Nutritional Ketosis for CNS-OT . . . 1002

Is Ketosis Safe and Feasible for the Diver? . . . 1003

Feasibility of Living in Ketosis . . . 1004

Exogenous Ketone Supplements . . . 1005

Additional Advantages to the State of Ketosis for the Diver . . . 1005

Enhanced Oxygen Efficiency . . . 1005

Reduction in Anxiety-Related Behavior . . . 1006

Neuroprotection from Environmental Harm . . . 1007

Enhancement of Physical and Neurological Performance . . . 1008

Conclusion . . . 1009

References . . . 1010

Ketogenic Diet and Ketogenic Supplementation for Central Nervous System Oxygen Toxicity

Angela M. Poff, Heather Annis, Harry T. Whelan, Csilla Ari, Joseph Dituri, Dominic P. D'Agostino

MECHANISMS AND MANIFESTATIONS OF CENTRAL NERVOUS SYSTEM OXYGEN TOXICITY

Oxygen was independently discovered in the late eighteenth century by two preeminent chemists, Wilhelm Scheele of Sweden and Joseph Priestley of Great Britain. It is now one of the most commonly utilized medical treatments worldwide, but its therapeutic use is limited by a significant potential for toxicity. The French physiologist Paul Bert was the first to report on the toxic effects of oxygen on the central nervous system (CNS) in the late nineteenth century. These effects were termed "central nervous system oxygen toxicity" (CNS-OT) and are a result of pathological effects induced by elevated partial pressures of oxygen. While other organ systems are affected by oxygen toxicity (OT), namely the lungs (pulmonary oxygen toxicity, P-OT) and the eye, this article will focus on CNS-OT which manifests largely as seizures.

Oxygen toxicity is a potential risk for any person encountering an elevated partial pressure of oxygen (pO_2), such as patients receiving hyperbaric oxygen (HBO_2) therapy and professional or recreational divers breathing oxygen or mixed gases at depth. HBO_2 therapy is a treatment in which patients breathe 100% oxygen in a pressurized chamber, thus increasing both the percent of oxygen being breathed and the barometric pressure at which it is being breathed. This condition is similar to the environment experienced in the scuba diving scenario, where individuals breathe air or oxygen-containing mixed gases in a hyperbaric environment. Both scenarios increase the percent of oxygen dissolved in the plasma, aiding oxygen delivery to the tissues by increasing its diffusion distance and delivery to the tissues independent of hemoglobin. HBO_2 therapy is an approved therapy by the Undersea and Hyperbaric Medical Society (UHMS) for a variety of disorders, including decompression sickness, chronic wounds, and radionecrosis, among others.[29,85] The risk and severity of CNS-OT rises with increasing inspired pO_2 and duration of exposure; therefore, the potential of OT limits the depth and time of hyperbaric exposure, serving as the basis for the diving tables and HBO_2 treatment protocols. Thus, HBO_2 therapy is typically administered at pressures of 2 to 3 atmospheres absolute (ATA) for 1.5 to 2 hours at a time, and divers are limited in their depth and time at depth.[76]

At 50 feet of seawater, a diver breathing 100% O_2 could encounter CNS-OT within just 10 minutes.[13] In this article, we will focus primarily on mitigating CNS-OT in divers.

In order to effectively assess CNS-OT in the diver, it is crucial to gain an understanding of the potential symptoms and measures of the onset of CNS-OT in individuals when diving. Signs such as facial pallor, inspiratory predominance, sweating, hiccups (diaphragmatic spasms), bradycardia, nausea, palpitations, spasmodic vomiting, depression, fibrillation of lips, apprehension, lip twitching, visual field constriction, twitching of cheek, nose, and/or eyelids, tinnitus, syncope, auditory hallucinations, convulsions, vertigo, headaches, faintness, retching, anxiety, and seizures are underlined as common symptoms[5,25,39,69] and can conceivably be used as an early predictor or measure. There is a limitation to the use of some of these signs in the underwater environment; however, some signs demonstrated a specific relationship to seizures underwater, such as tinnitus, hyperventilation, hearing disturbances, disorientation, amnesia, and facial twitching. In dives where the event led to unconsciousness, divers reported between three and nine precipitating events,[4] suggesting that the documented signs can be used as predictors of CNS-OT. The linking of OT to illness and incidents including death underwater is supported by Alcaraz-García et al.[1] This work highlighted that using a closed-circuit breathing apparatus with high pO_2 increased the chances of suffering oxidative hyperoxia-induced stress. The divers recovered from an impacted total antioxidant status during the process, suggesting that they are able to adapt to the experience of hyperoxia. Arieli et al.[6] and Kindwall and Whelan[39] have also found no residual effects of CNS-OT and seizure to date. This suggests that by decreasing the incidence of CNS-OT, we are unlikely to be negatively impacting neurologic outcomes.

The literature also suggests that, to date, there has been limited study of CNS-OT accidents, and it is important to assess the possible risk of seizure, death, and other complications when diving at deep depths using closed-circuit rebreathers (CCRs). A study by Arieli, Yalov, and Goldenshluger[7] aimed to assess the impact of diving at different depths and for different amounts of time, confirming that symptoms of CNS-OT increased when diving at deeper depths and for longer periods of time.[4] The incidence of CNS-OT-related events at high pressure has been evaluated in two studies of note. Arieli et al.[5] researched the occurrence of CNS-OT in Israeli navy divers. They found an incidence of 2.5% CNS events at oxygen pressures of 1.1 ATA–1.4 ATA amongst actively diving subjects. Smerz et al.[69] found an incidence of 2% CNS events at pO_2 2.6–2.9 ATA in sedentary divers within a hyperbaric dive chamber. This data allows us to estimate that there is approximately a 2.5% incidence of CNS-OT at 1.2 ATA with a potentially increasing incidence with increases in pressure and depth. Both of these studies found incidence of actual seizures at $< 1\%$. In all and from all causes, CCR diving has a mortality rate ten times that of open-circuit diving.[26] There appears to be ample evidence to suggest that specific symptoms can be used as measures of oxygen toxicity in CCR divers. These include inspiratory predominance, (feeling of choking), hiccups (diaphragmatic spasms), bradycardia, nausea, retching, spasmodic vomiting, palpitations, depression, fibrillation of lips, apprehension, lip twitching, visual field constriction, twitching of cheek, nose and/or eyelids, tinnitus, syncope, auditory hallucinations, convulsions, headaches, faintness, retching, anxiety, and seizures.

Breathing an inspired pO_2 greater than is experienced during normobaric normoxia will increase tissue production of reactive oxygen and nitrogen species (RONS).[61,77] RONS are highly reactive molecules capable of oxidizing cellular biomolecules such as proteins, lipids, and nucleic acids.[9] Oxidative stress (OxS) occurs when the rate of RONS production exceeds the antioxidant capacity to protect against them, resulting in biomolecule oxidation and damage. It is widely thought that CNS-OT is due in part to RONS-mediated OxS and thus may be amenable to mitigation strategies that target this underlying pathology. However, dietary antioxidants have not proven effective against CNS-OT, highlighting the complexity of this mechanism. Studies have demonstrated that a variety of antiepileptic drugs (AEDs) are effective to variable degrees against CNS-OT, but often the side effects of these medications make them less than ideal for use by divers. Such side effects include drowsiness, fatigue, poor coordination, unsteadiness, behavior changes, headache, vomiting, irritability, and depression, among others.[2] Any of these effects could significantly enhance the risks of the underwater environment and make it difficult for professional divers to safely and efficiently complete a task or mission. Thus, in an attempt to identify safe and effective alternative mitigation strategies for CNS-OT, researchers have begun investigating an approach that has been successfully used clinically for pediatric refractory seizures for nearly 100 years – dietary-induced nutritional ketosis.

FASTING KETOSIS AND NUTRITIONAL KETOSIS AS AN ANTICONVULSANT THERAPY

Ketosis is a physiological state characterized by an elevation in blood ketones, namely beta-hydroxybutyrate (βHB), acetoacetate (AcAc), and acetone (ACE). When the hormone insulin is suppressed, such as during fasting, calorie restriction, starvation, a carbohydrate-restricted diet, or prolonged exercise, the liver metabolizes fatty acids to acetyl CoA, and a portion of this is shunted towards ketogenesis rather than the Kreb's cycle. Excluding diabetic ketoacidosis (specific to type 1 diabetics), the physiologic state of fasting ketosis or nutritional ketosis has long been accepted as a powerful metabolic therapy that confers remarkable seizure control, even independent of etiology. The earliest links reported appear in texts from antiquity, in which fasting was known to be an effective treatment for seizures. Hippocrates and Erasistratus wrote of treating epileptic patients with fasting in the third and fourth centuries BC, and a similar recommendation was provided by Jesus in the Biblical New Testament.[8] In the 1920s, clinicians at the Mayo Clinic sought to develop a diet that mimics the physiological state of fasting in hopes of designing a more sustainable method of maintaining seizure control than fasting. Since the body subsists on the mobilization of stored fat reserves during fasting, the clinicians at the Mayo Clinic designed a diet which was composed primarily of fat, with the remaining calories primarily coming from protein and only trace amounts of digestible carbohydrate. This diet was called the ketogenic diet (KD) for its propensity to induce an elevation of blood and urine ketones (βHB, AcAc), and it indeed proved to be a very effective method for reducing seizures. The KD is still used clinically today for both pediatric and adult patients who do not respond to antiepileptic drugs (AEDs) or who become refractory. Since its inception, studies have confirmed its remarkable anticonvulsant efficacy.

On average, > 50% of patients experience > 50% reduction in seizures, another ⅓ of patients experience > 90% seizure control, and approximately 10%–15% of so-called "super responders" experience rapid, total, and permanent seizure control, even after multiple AEDs have failed.[41]

Anticonvulsant Mechanisms of Ketosis

The exact mechanisms that underlie the anticonvulsant properties of ketosis are not well understood but likely include a number of related yet distinct variables.[65] It is also likely that for any specific seizure disorder, a particular mechanism may be the most important, and this may differ between disorders of varied etiologies. Some of the most well-supported theories include 1) reduction of oxidative stress, 2) glucose and insulin stabilization, 3) enhanced brain energy reserves and anapleurosis, and 4) alteration in neurotransmitter signaling.

Reduction in Oxidative Stress

OxS is characteristic of epileptogenesis, and the KD has been demonstrated to reduce oxidative stress in a number of preclinical and clinical reports, including in seizure disorders.[31,65] Veech and colleagues elucidated one mechanism by which this occurs.[34] They demonstrated that ketone metabolism increases oxidation of ubiquinol (Q) in the electron transport chain (ETC). This reduces the abundance of the semiquinone radical (Q·) which is sensitive to oxidation by oxygen and produces the major precursor ROS superoxide anion ($O_2^{-}\cdot$). Simultaneously, ketone metabolism also increases reduction of the mitochondrial NAD and cytoplasmic NADP couples, which aids in regeneration of reduced glutathione (GSH), an important endogenous antioxidant enzyme depleted in epileptic brain tissue. Indeed, the KD increases the ratio of reduced to oxidized glutathione (GSH:GSSG) in rat brains,[31] and ketone treatment reduces neuronal ROS production following glutamate exposure[48] and inhibits cell death in neurons exposed to hydrogen peroxide (H_2O_2)–induced OxS.[38] Ketones reduce basal levels of ROS production, as well as following administration of the mitochondrial inhibitor oligomycin.[38] The KD was also shown to increase reduced glutathione levels[66] through an Nrf2-dependent pathway.[74] Interestingly, Nrf2 overexpression and the resulting endogenous antioxidant capacity has been shown to decrease seizures in a rat model of temporal lobe epilepsy,[55] which has been posited to be the locus of seizure generation in CNS-OT. One key study by D'Agostino et al. found that "ketones may prevent synaptic dysfunction by preserving brain metabolism during metabolic stress or ROS- induced oxidative stress."[20] Furthermore, Verdin and colleagues demonstrated that βHB functions as an endogenous histone deacetylase inhibitor (HDACI) to increase expression of multiple oxidative stress resistance factors,[67] which could conceivably have an effect of suppressing OxS-induced seizures.

Glucose Reduction

The KD induces a slight reduction in blood glucose and subsequent decrease in oxidative glucose metabolism which may contribute to its anticonvulsant effects.[53,57,89] Powerful homeostatic mechanisms prevent a significant lowering of baseline glucose on the KD (unless calorie restricted), but the postprandial rise in glucose and insulin is significantly attenuated with a ketogenic meal compared to a standard mixed diet. Carbohydrate ingestion can rapidly reverse seizure control in keto-adapted patients, supporting the idea that glucose restriction and insulin suppression are key components of KD efficacy.[30]

Further confirming this hypothesis is the success of glycolytic inhibitors for seizure control. 2-deoxyglucose (2-DG) is a glucose mimetic structurally identical to glucose, but lacking the 2' hydroxyl group, thus preventing its glycolytic metabolism past the point of phophoglucoisomerase. 2-DG suppresses seizures in multiple preclinical models, including audiogenic and chemical-induced seizure rodent models[71] and is currently being using in human clinical trials. Toxicity of 2-DG becomes an issue at higher doses (> 25 mg/kg), so its use for prevention of CNS-OT may be limited.

Enhanced Brain Energy Reserves and Anaplerosis

It is known that seizure activity can cause energy depletion in the brain, and, interestingly, evidence suggests that energy failure may also contribute to epileptogenesis.[42] Brain ATP levels fall prior to seizure onset, and ATP can become depleted during its manifestation.[42] This is thought to exacerbate neuronal damage and cognitive sequelae. Proper maintenance of ion balance and preservation of resting membrane potential are ATP-dependent processes; therefore, energy depletion will undoubtedly affect neuronal firing and may contribute to seizure pathology, especially in areas of the brain that are under high metabolic demands and selectively vulnerable to energy crisis. Anaplerosis is the replenishing of the Kreb's cycle (a.k.a. TCA cycle), thus increasing available metabolic intermediates which can be utilized for energy production, neurotransmitters, and membrane biosynthesis. The KD has been shown to increase anaplerosis, Kreb's cycle enzyme expression, and energy availability in the brains of animals with seizure disorders, and therefore it may work in part through this mechanism.[42] Furthermore, mitochondrial metabolic defects are common in epileptogenesis, and the KD has been shown to support mitochondrial function through a variety of mechanisms involving oxidative metabolism, bypassing rate-limiting enzymes (e.g., PHD), shifting redox homeostasis, and gene regulation.[65] For example, the KD upregulates the gene expression of numerous mitochondrial proteins and mitochondrial biogenesis in the hippocampus of rats.[11]

Alteration in Neurotransmitter Signaling

Ketosis has been shown to alter the signaling of neurotransmitters involved in epileptogenesis, including the primary excitatory neurotransmitter glutamate and the primary inhibitory neurotransmitter γ-aminobutyric acid (GABA). GABA is known to counteract excess glutamate hyperexcitability, which is a known consequence of CNS-OT.[22] In general, nutritional ketosis appears to increase the GABA-to-glutamate signaling ratio through a variety of mechanisms, including an increased activity of glutamic acid decarboxylase (GAD).[18,21,24,84] During ketosis, astrocytes increase conversion of glutamate to glutamine, which is then converted to GABA, resulting in increased neuronal inhibition.[88] Glutamate signaling in the ketotic brain may be directly inhibited by affecting vesicular glutamate transporters (VGLUTs), which function to fill presynaptic vesicles with glutamate. AcAc, and to a lesser degree βHB, directly competes with Cl- as an allosteric activator of VGLUT activity, thus lessening glutamate release from presynaptic terminals.[32] These findings are further supported by evidence that AcAc inhibits glutamate release from rat and mouse neurons and suppresses glutamate release and seizure activity in vivo.[32] The relationship between ketosis and these two neurotransmitters remains unclear, as studies in children on the KD have revealed increased GABA but unchanged glutamate levels in the cerebrospinal fluid,[21] while studies in rats on the KD have revealed reduced brain glutamate and no change in GABA.[57]

Another potential neurochemical mediator of the KD is adenosine, a purine ribonucleoside neurotransmitter produced from ATP that inhibits neuronal excitability and elicits potent neuroprotective and anticonvulsant effects.[51] Recently, studies have revealed that the anticonvulsant effects of the KD may be due in part to stimulation of adenosine receptor signaling, as the KD reduces seizures in wild-type mice but not in those with targeted deletion of the A_1R adenosine receptor subtype.[52]

Effect on Neuronal Membrane Potential

Neuronal excitability and epileptogenesis are significantly affected by energy metabolism, which is almost certainly one link between the KD and its antiseizure effects. The neuronal ATP-sensitive potassium channel (K_{ATP}) is an inwardly rectifying K^+ channel inhibited by ATP which tightly links cellular energy status to neuronal membrane potential and excitability. Thus, when cellular energy (ATP) is low, K_{ATP} channels are activated and hyperpolarize the membrane, suppressing seizure activity. Ketones affect both the expression and activity of these channels. Tanner and colleagues demonstrated that βHB increases both basal K_{ATP} channel levels and the amount of stimulus required to evoke K_{ATP} channel opening.[75] The specific relationship between ketosis and K_{ATP} channel–mediated alterations in neuronal membrane potential is unclear, but it has been hypothesized that the KD decreases glycolytic ATP production, resulting in a compartmentalization of intracellular ATP that subsequently enhances K_{ATP} channel activity.[86]

Evidence Supporting Nutritional Ketosis for CNS-OT

As described, there has been ample research into the effects of a ketogenic diet on refractory epilepsy, and the utilization of this diet is now mainstream for children and adults.[27] However, research into the particular area of the ketogenic diet and CNS-OT, as related to humans and diving, is sparse – hence the importance of the current research efforts in this arena. The little data which exists in this field is encouraging, however, including the demonstration that fasting ketosis attenuates CNS-OT.[16] To further investigate the effects of acute administration of ketogenic agents on CNS-OT, a study of juvenile Sprague-Dawley (SPD) rats (2–4 months) was used to assess the neuroprotective effect of acute nutritional ketosis with 1,3-butanediol acetoacetate diester (10 g/kg; ketone diester) on animals subjected to a pO_2 of 5 atmospheres absolute (5 ATA O_2). The ketone diester is a calorically dense (6 kcal/g) and highly stable ketogenic compound that hydrolyzes to produce a 1:1 ratio of βHB to AcAc in the blood. Oral gavage administration of ketone diester resulted in a 575% increase in the latency to seizure.[20] This dosage of ketone diester caused rapid (15–30 minutes) and sustained (> 4 hours) nutritional ketosis above what can be achieved with fasting alone or a strict (4:1 ratio) KD. The ketone diester produces a dose-dependent elevation of βHB and AcAc. AcAc spontaneously decarboxylates to acetone which was also elevated in the blood and known to have potent antiseizure effects at subnarcotic levels. Elevating βHB alone with 1,3-butanediol did not confer protection against CNS-OT from 5 ATA $O_{2,}$ suggesting that the specific elevation of AcAc or ACE may be important for this effect. Ongoing dose-response studies (unpublished) have demonstrated that the use of lower doses of ketone diester (5 g/kg) combined with ketogenic fats in the form of medium-chain triglycerides (MCTs, 5g/kg) increased time to latency by ~200% compared to control treatment (water) in older rats (18 months).

The antiseizure doses of ketogenic supplementation administered (5–10 g/kg) supply a significant source of energy-dense calories (single dose = 25% of daily needs) and thus can serve as a food that can be used alone or as a means to further augment the antiseizure efficacy of the KD. MCTs have the added benefit of delaying gastric absorption and thus can extend the pharmacokinetic curve of the ketone diester while also stimulating de novo hepatic ketogenesis. Formulating ketone esters with MCTs significantly reduces the required dose of ketone esters needed for prevention of CNS-OT and can improve palatability Treatment with βHB in the form of a mineral salt (5g/kg NaCa βHB) with 5g/kg MCT did not significantly delay latency to CNS-OT seizure[3A], which supports previous studies that an elevation of both βHB and AcAc are essential for suppressing CNS-OT seizures. These observations suggest that therapeutic ketosis with ketone supplementation may need to mimic the physiological ratios that are achieved with fasting ketosis or the ketogenic diet. These findings strongly support further investigation into the hypothesis that nutritional ketosis achieved with ketone supplementation or the KD may be an effective mitigation strategy for CNS-OT.

IS KETOSIS SAFE AND FEASIBLE FOR THE DIVER?

Early humans experienced regular periods of limited food availability and episodic starvation; thus, ketosis is a natural physiologic state that influenced the evolution of our species. Evolutionary pressures favored the preservation and even enhancement of physical and cognitive performance during starvation ketosis as a means of food provision. The CNS has the highest demand for ketones during starvation, and humans are particularly adept at experiencing ketosis due to our high brain-to-body weight ratio. Thus, at its most basic function, ketosis evolved as a mechanism to provide fuel to the brain during starvation. Since there is relatively little energy stored in the human body in the form of carbohydrate (glucose as glycogen), these reserves are depleted within two to three days of starvation. If the human brain were entirely reliant on glucose, the body would begin to break down muscle to liberate gluconeogenic amino acids to supply glucose to the starving brain within days of cessation of eating. This would result in death by cardiorespiratory failure within two to three weeks. However, an average human can live for two to three months or more without eating or even up to one year depending on the individual's amount of stored body fat.[73] Unlike glucose, fat is the primary storage form of energy in the body, with a typical adult human holding approximately 70,000 kcal of energy in adipose tissue. While some fatty acids can indeed cross the blood-brain barrier (BBB), studies have suggested that they are incapable of supporting the significant cerebral energy requirements during starvation. Rather, ketones are the only other primary fuel for the brain aside from glucose and, under certain conditions, lactate. During starvation, stored body fat is metabolized, and beta-oxidation of fatty acids in the liver generates excess acetyl-CoA, which stimulates hepatic ketogenesis. Ketones readily cross the BBB and provide up to ⅔ of the brain's energy requirements in this condition.[14] Thus, ketosis was a key component in our evolution, and it is likely a significant contributing factor to the development of the large human brain and success of our species. Furthermore, because of the high medium-chain triglyceride (MCT) content of human breast milk, breastfed babies are in ketosis during perhaps the most rapid and critical period of neurological development. During this time, ketones provide approximately 25% of the infant's brain energy requirement.[12]

Although the physiologic state of ketosis is a natural one, there are known side effects of prolonged use of the classical KD – all of which are generally considered mild and treatable with minor adjustments in food selection and supplementation. If not properly planned, the foods consumed on the KD can be deficient in certain vitamins and minerals, such as calcium, selenium, zinc, copper, and vitamin D.[41] Vitamin and mineral supplementation can be used to prevent or reverse these deficiencies. Due to the slight increase in urine acidity caused by ketosis, those on the classical KD (4:1 ratio) have a mild increased risk of developing kidney stones. Urine alkalinization with potassium citrate can mitigate this risk. While studies suggest that the blood lipid profile of individuals on the KD typically improves,[83] some individuals may experience lipid abnormalities or high cholesterol, but the chance of higher risk of cardiovascular problems caused by these transient changes is debated. Regardless, monitoring of routine blood work (CBC, CMP) and overall lipid profile (NMR) is suggested. Loss of bone mineral content and growth retardation are also potential side effects but are most often seen in children rather than adults. Bone metabolism can be supported with vitamin D supplementation. There are certain individuals who should not implement a KD. Known absolute contraindications include primary carnitine deficiency, carnitine palmitoyltransferase I or II deficiency, carnitine translocase deficiency, β-oxidation defects, pyruvate carboxylase deficiency, and porphyria. Relative contraindications include liver disorders, pancreatitis, gall bladder disease, and kidney disorders.

Feasibility of Living in Ketosis

Living in ketosis can be difficult but is certainly feasible for a dedicated individual. In fact, it is the preferred lifestyle of many people, including high-level athletes, prominent academics, celebrities, and laypeople alike. Public interest in the ketogenic lifestyle has surged over the past decade, and there are now numerous online resources and lifestyle groups dedicated to ketogenic living. These new resources are helping to make the ketogenic lifestyle significantly more mainstream and feasible than it was even a few years ago. Companies are beginning to produce and sell premade ketogenic meals and snacks, and low-carbohydrate food alternatives are readily available in nearly all grocery stores and restaurants, which all make implementation far easier now than in years past. We now realize that a less restrictive modified version of the diet (e.g., modified Atkins diet, MAD) improves compliance and has similar antiseizure efficacy in adults.

Despite these advances, the classical KD is undoubtedly a strict diet which can be difficult to follow. A 4:1 ratio of fat:carbohydrate+protein results in nearly 90% of calories coming from fat. However, more recent evidence suggests that this strict of a macronutrient ratio is not absolutely necessary for acceptable levels of seizure control. Over the past decade, practitioners in the epilepsy community have developed and tested a number of modified ketogenic diets in order to improve patient compliance. The MAD allows for more protein and slightly more carbohydrate (~60% kcal fat, ~30% kcal protein, ~10% kcal carbohydrate). The Low Glycemic Index Treatment (LGIT) is another such diet, which limits intake to foods with a glycemic index of less than 50. The MCT ketogenic diet also allows for increased protein and carbohydrate intake (10%–15% kcal/each), but the fat intake is primarily composed of MCTs which are highly ketogenic. Studies have demonstrated that these alternative diets also elicit significant seizure control, often to similar levels as the cKD.

Although they have not been tested in CNS-OT, it is likely that these modified KDs would elicit some level of benefit, and their pleasing palatability may improve feasibility.

Exogenous Ketone Supplements

Achieving and sustaining therapeutic levels of ketonemia (> 1 mM blood ketones) or ketonuria (> 40 mg/dL) is generally considered necessary for the antiseizure efficacy of the KD. Despite its proven efficacy, the strict dietary restrictions of the KD can result in cessation of treatment.[40,44] In attempts to circumvent this problem, researchers are developing a variety of exogenous ketone supplements which are metabolized to release or endogenously produce the ketone bodies, namely βHB and AcAc, following ingestion.[19-20,37,64] Recently, researchers are reporting that, although it conventionally takes about 24 to 48 hours to achieve nutritional ketosis, the induction of therapeutic ketosis can be achieved in as little as 10 to 15 minutes under laboratory conditions using ketone supplementation.[36,81] Exogenous ketone supplements elevate blood ketone levels in a dose-dependent fashion and therefore allow for a rapid and controlled induction of ketosis without requiring severe dietary carbohydrate or calorie restriction. Exogenous ketone supplements have been shown to mimic many of the metabolic and physiologic effects of the KD which are suggested to contribute to its anticonvulsant properties, including a suppression of blood glucose, glycolysis, oxidative stress, and inflammation, and an enhancement of anaplerosis, mitochondrial biogenesis, and ATP and adenosine production.[35,37,42,50,70-72]

As previously described, one of the earliest reports of the antiseizure efficacy of exogenous ketone supplementation occurred in a rat model CNS-OT.[20] In this study, a single oral dose of the BD-$AcAc_2$ ketone ester induced rapid and sustained ketosis (> 3mM βHB and > 3mM AcAc) and prolonged the latency to seizure nearly sixfold.[20] Importantly, this study also evaluated the efficacy of another exogenous ketone supplement, 1,3-butanediol, which elevated blood βHB to greater than 5 mM but did not elevate AcAc or acetone, nor did it affect latency to seizure. Thus, it appears that an elevation in AcAc or ACE is necessary for delaying or preventing seizures in this model. The ketone ester which was effective in CNS-OT has been demonstrated to be effective against other seizure conditions, including both transgenic rodent and chemical-induced models, such as pentylenetetrazole (PTZ)–induced seizures, the WAG/Rij rat model of absent epilepsy (unpublished), the Ube3a m-/p+ mouse model of Angelman syndrome, and the kainic acid-induced mouse seizure model.[18,81] Valadao et al. showed that diving in ketosis is safe and that ketosis can be induced through diet in less than 48 hours.[78] Ongoing research by Viggiani et al. using nutritional ketosis in rebreather divers has not evidenced any negative effects to date, and phase two is likely to utilize supplemental ketosis.

ADDITIONAL ADVANTAGES TO THE STATE OF KETOSIS FOR THE DIVER

Enhanced Oxygen Efficiency

Henry Lardy first described the superior metabolic efficiency of ketones in the 1940s, when he demonstrated that βHB and AcAc were unique amongst a panel of 16 major carbohydrate, lipid, and intermediary metabolites in their ability to increase bull sperm mobility while simultaneously decreasing oxygen consumption.[43] In the 1990s, Veech and colleagues reported similar findings in working perfused rat heart, demonstrating that ketone supplementation to glucose-containing perfusate increased cardiac hydraulic work by 25%, also while decreasing oxygen consumption.[34] They went on further to describe a mechanism by which ketone metabolism reduces the mitochondrial NAD couple and oxidizes the coenzyme Q couple, thus increasing the energy of the redox span between those two sites. This phenomenon causes increased energy to be released by electrons in the ETC, allowing more protons to be pumped into the inner mitochondrial space and thereby enhancing the electrochemical gradient across the inner mitochondrial membrane and increasing the energy of ATP hydrolysis. Bomb calorimeter experiments have confirmed that ketones produce more energy per two-carbon moiety than glucose.[15] Studies in fasted obese subjects in ketosis support these molecular findings, revealing a reduction in cerebral blood flow and oxygen consumption in this condition.[56] Ketones therefore appear to be superior to glucose for ATP production per unit oxygen and are likely among the most metabolically efficient energy metabolites. This enhanced oxygen efficiency could provide benefits to divers who are exposed to extreme environments and could potentially attenuate the neurological effects of pressure, such as nitrogen narcosis. As the increase in the partial pressure of nitrogen produces an altered mental state similar to alcohol intoxication, it can compromise the diver`s ability in decision-making and can lead to fatal accidents. No studies have been conducted so far on how nutritional ketosis or ketone supplementation would affect nitrogen narcosis, but increased ATP production and enhanced oxygen efficacy in the brain may be beneficial in such circumstances.

Reduction in Anxiety-Related Behavior

The most prevalent type of mental disorders today is anxiety disorders.[45] Generalized anxiety and panic disorders can also affect warfighters and divers and may be masked or aggravated by other mental or physical illnesses. The symptoms that are present in anxiety-related behaviors, such as fear and worry, can interfere with a person`s quality of life or can compromise the success of a warfighter`s mission.

Based on our current knowledge, the amygdala and the hippocampus play a key role in the neurobiology of anxiety, while, interestingly, the same brain regions are involved in a significant proportion of patients with focal epilepsy.[23,45] It is also believed that serotonergic, glutamatergic, and GABAergic systems play a role in the regulation of anxiety,[23,33,45,60] and ketosis is believed to balance brain neurotransmitter homeostasis.

According to anecdotal reports, nutritional ketosis can promote a reduction in anxiety, while current studies show convincing evidence to indicate that ketone supplementation reduces anxiety in rodent models.[3] Rapid and sustained increase in blood ketone levels can be induced by ketone supplementation, which might induce an anxiolytic effect by increasing the GABAergic effects[18,45,87] or through other neuropharmacological pathways.[65] The effect of ketone supplementation on anxiety was assessed by using the elevated plus maze (EPM) behavioral assay in SPD rats, as well as in WAG/Rij rats which have reduced activity of the GABAergic system.[46] Both SPD and WAG/Rjj rats were fed exogenous ketone supplements subchronically (7 days daily via intragastric gavage bolus), while chronic (15 weeks ketone supplements in food) effects were also tested in the SPD line. The effects of ketone supplements were different on the anxiety-related behavior in the rat strains with and without pathology. In this study, chronic and subchronic feeding of ketone supplements (ketone esters and βHB mineral salts) not only elevated blood ketone levels similar to fasting and KD, but also reduced anxiety-related behavior. The anxiolytic effect of nutritional ketone supplementation may provide a desirable effect for patients undergoing HBO_2 therapy and for warfighters achieving nutritional ketosis without dietary restrictions.

Neuroprotection from Environmental Harm

Ketosis is broadly neuroprotective, an effect that has been consistently observed and reported across neurological diseases linked to metabolic dysregulation and oxidative stress such as epilepsy, neurodegenerative conditions such as Alzheimer's and Parkinson's diseases, and acute neurological insults such as stroke and traumatic brain injury.[28] Neuroprotective effects of ketosis are not fully understood but likely include preservation of brain energy reserves and reductions in glutamate excitotoxicity, oxidative stress, and inflammation. Deficits in cerebral energy metabolism are a hallmark characteristic of most brain pathologies, and it is thought that the enhanced energy reserves provided by ketosis contributes to its neuroprotective effects. As mentioned, ketones are the only other primary fuel for the brain. βHB is a more efficient fuel than glucose per unit of oxygen,[79] an attribute that would certainly be beneficial during an energetic crisis. Also, ketosis stimulates mitochondrial biogenesis, further supporting energy reserve capacity. These effects allow for preservation of cellular function during stress and the survival of neurons that would otherwise succumb to such insult.[28] Glutamate excitotoxicity is another major mechanism underlying neuronal injury and death which may be affected by ketosis as AcAc has been shown to protect neurons against this specific insult in vitro.[63] Oxidative stress is also a common characteristic of neuronal pathology, and, as previously mentioned, ketosis reduces oxidative stress by decreasing the production of free radicals and enhancing endogenous antioxidant defenses. Thus, ketosis may offer neurological resilience against the stressors and potential damage caused by CNS-OT seizures.

There is an increased risk of toxicity at deeper depths, as well as increased risk of death after a seizure because of the length of time it takes to get the diver to the surface. A diver rendered incapacitated at depth can be resuscitated only at the surface, necessitating a rapid ascent (unless a submarine or underwater facility/platform is available, and this is not likely with the vast majority of dives). Underwater events at depth therefore increase the risk of decompression illness (DCI) in the affected diver as well as the rescue diver during ascent.[80] From the research presented above, it is now safe to say that OT can cause seizures at partial pressures of oxygen in CCR divers and that divers who seize underwater are at extreme risk of drowning, placing them and the rescuers at risk for DCI through rapid-ascent rescue attempts. DCI, unlike oxygen toxicity CNS events, can cause permanent CNS damage. Ketosis likely reduces seizures from OT by increasing latency, and ketogenic diets are neuroprotective. From this we can hypothesize that diving on a ketogenic diet should decrease incidence of oxygen-toxicity-induced seizures, thereby decreasing risk of DCI, while also protecting the CNS from potential damage from increased high pO_2 exposure and other neurological insults related to DCI. Future studies would expect to find more of these positive signs among those on the ketogenic diet.

When the nervous tissue is damaged, along with the underlying neurons, glia, axons, myelin, and synapses, the availability of glucose is limited for fueling brain function. As such, nervous tissue must undergo regrowth or repair in order to restore proper functionality. The capacity for CNS regeneration and repair is limited, even compared to the peripheral nervous system (PNS), but recent studies have revealed mechanisms which may support this function.[68] In preliminary studies (unpublished), the effects of a βHB on cell regeneration of primary neuron cell cultures were tested by utilizing a scratch assay that was followed for 24 hours by taking 100 serial photographs. Significantly more cells were found to migrate into the damaged area when the cell culture was treated with βHB, and the cell coverage was higher than in control cell cultures. This resulted in cell migration and regeneration of the damaged area in response to ketone treatment and thus may lead to promising applications for treating traumatic brain injury or other injury to the central nervous system, such as caused by DCS or CNS-OT seizures.

Enhancement of Physical and Neurological Performance

Ketosis provides positive effects in a number of neurological disorders.[27] While underresearched, the impact of ketosis on the individual's ability to prevent or delay illness is apparent, but, interestingly, ketosis is also associated with enhanced functioning in the absence of known pathology. A recent paper by Veech and colleagues demonstrated that exogenous ketone supplementation increased performance on tasks of learning and memory by 38% and increased physical performance by 32% compared to isocaloric, starch, or fat-supplemented standard diet.[59]

Conditions that induce a bioenergetic challenge, such as exercise or intermittent fasting, have consistently been shown to elicit neuroprotective effects, and it is thought this effect is mediated at least in part by the release of signaling molecules from the peripheral tissues.[49] Increased fatty-acid oxidation and ketone synthesis are hallmark characteristics of these conditions, and the recently described signaling properties of ketones make them likely candidates that may mediate these effects.[62] Ketones serve as alternative fuel during reduced glucose availability or metabolism, which is often associated with bioenergetic challenges as well as brain injury and neurodegenerative diseases. Mattson and colleagues recently described an intriguing new mechanism by which βHB stimulates neurological function through the brain-derived neurotrophic factor (BDNF).[49] BDNF is a neurotrophic factor that elicits numerous survival and growth-promoting effects in a variety of neurons.[10] It enhances neurogenesis and is involved in synaptic plasticity which is critical for learning and memory, and, unsurprisingly, decreased BDNF activity is associated with numerous neurological diseases.[58] Mattson and others have proposed that the cognitive-enhancing effects of ketones have ties to our evolutionary history – in times of a food deficit, it was most critical that an organism perform at its optimal cognitive and physical capacity in order to acquire food and avoid starvation. Indeed, all normal physiologic conditions that stimulate ketogenesis are associated with enhanced neurological function, including fasting, intermittent fasting, the ketogenic diet, exogenous ketone supplementation, and vigorous exercise.[17,47,54,90]

It is also thought that some aspects of physical performance, such as endurance, could be enhanced during ketosis, but this is not well studied. The aforementioned increased oxygen efficiency of ketone metabolism provides a clear potential benefit which could allow more work output for less oxygen requirement. Ketosis is also known to be anticatabolic in a catabolic state, which is consistent with its evolutionary role of minimizing protein degradation during starvation. And more recently, studies have revealed novel mechanisms by which ketones promote protein synthesis. Zhu and colleagues reported that AcAc accelerates muscle regeneration and mitigates muscular dystrophy by activating the MEK/ERK pathway.[91] Volek and colleagues are studying the potential benefits of fat adaptation in high-level athletes.[82] There is an obvious benefit of efficiently accessing and utilizing fat stores during prolonged physical tasks, which is that the body has on average 10–20 times more fat kcals stored in it than carbohydrate. Cognitive and physical performance can therefore deteriorate in a carbohydrate-fueled athlete when readily available fuels (approximately 2,000 kcal in glycogen) are utilized, forcing the athlete to consistently refuel throughout the task. Paradoxically, this occurs while typically > 40,000 fat kcals are available in the adipose tissue but are inefficiently accessed in those individuals that are not fat adapted. There are a number of other effects of ketosis which may benefit the warfighter, including improved cerebral blood flow, reduced oxidative stress, improved insulin sensitivity, protein-sparing effects, reduced lactate production, improved body composition, and reduced inflammation chronically and in response to high intensity exercise, among others.[82]

CONCLUSION

The data described in this paper can be taken collectively to hypothesize that diving in ketosis should decrease incidence of oxygen-toxicity-induced seizures and may provide further benefits and protection for divers, such as enhanced neurological and physical performance and protection against various environmental stressors. We propose that being in the state of nutritional ketosis will be beneficial to recreational divers diving deep with regular air, to divers diving on hyperbaric (high partial pressure) oxygen using closed-circuit rebreather (CCR) apparatuses, or to those shallow diving on 100% O_2.

REFERENCES

1. Alcaraz-Garcia MJ, Albaladejo MD, Acevedo C, Olea A, Zamora S, Martinez P, Parra S. Effects of hyperoxia on biomarkers of oxidative stress in closed-circuit oxygen military divers. J Physiol Biochem. 2008;64(2):135-41.
2. Anti-seizure medication and their side effects. Epilepsy Foundation Western/Central Pennsylvania [Internet]. Epilepsy Foundation Western/Central Pennsylvania. Anti-seizure medication and their side effects. Available from: http://www.efwp.org/programs/ProgramsSideEffects.xml
3. Ari C, Kovacs Z, Juhasz G, Murdun C, Goldhagen CR, Koutnik AM, Poff AM, Kesl SL, D'Agostino DP. Exogenous ketone supplements reduce anxiety-related behavior in Sprague-Dawley and Wistar Albino Glaxo/Rijswijk rats. Front Mol Neurosci. 2016;9:137.

3A. Ari C, Koutnik AP, DeBlasi J, Landon C, Dean JB, D`Agostino DP. Comparison of exogenous ketone supplements on delayed latency to cns oxygen toxicity (cnsot) seizures. ONR-NAVSEA Undersea Medicine Program Review. 2017.

4. Arieli R, Arieli Y, Daskalovic Y, Eynan M, Abramovich A. CNS oxygen toxicity in closed-circuit diving: signs and symptoms before loss of consciousness. Aviat Space Environ Med. 2006;77(11):1153-7.
5. Arieli R, Shochat T, Adir Y. CNS toxicity in closed-circuit oxygen diving: symptoms reported from 2527 dives. Aviat Space Environ Med. 2006;77(5):526-32.
6. Arieli R, Truman M, Abramovich A. Recovery from central nervous system oxygen toxicity in the rat at oxygen pressures between 100 and 300 kPa. Eur J Appl Physiol. 2008;104(5):867-71.
7. Arieli R, Yalov A, Goldenshluger A. Modeling pulmonary and CNS O(2) toxicity and estimation of parameters for humans. J Appl Physiol (1985). 2002;92(1):248-56.
8. Bailey EE, Pfeifer HH, Thiele EA. The use of diet in the treatment of epilepsy. Epilepsy Behav. 2005;6(1):4-8.
9. Bellance N, Lestienne P, Rossignol R. Mitochondria: from bioenergetics to the metabolic regulation of carcinogenesis. Front Biosci (Landmark Ed). 2009;14:4015-34.
10. Binder DK, Scharfman HE. Brain-derived neurotrophic factor. Growth Factors. 2004;22(3):123-31.
11. Bough KJ, Wetherington J, Hassel B, Pare JF, Gawryluk JW, Greene JG, Shaw R, Smith Y, Geiger JD, Dingledine RJ. Mitochondrial biogenesis in the anticonvulsant mechanism of the ketogenic diet. Ann Neurol. 2006;60(2):223-35.
12. Bougneres PF, Lemmel C, Ferre P, Bier DM. Ketone body transport in the human neonate and infant. J Clin Invest. 1986;77(1):42-8.
13. Butler FK Jr, Thalmann ED. Central nervous system oxygen toxicity in closed circuit scuba divers II. Undersea Biomed Res. 1986;13(2):193-223.
14. Cahill G. Fuel metabolism in starvation. Ann Rev Nutr. 2006;26:1-22.
15. Cahill GF Jr, Veech RL. Ketoacids? Good medicine? Trans Am Clin Climatol Assoc. 2003;114:149-61; discussion 162-3.
16. Chavko M, Braisted JC, Harabin AL. Attenuation of brain hyperbaric oxygen toxicity by fasting is not related to ketosis. Undersea Hyperb Med. 1999;26(2):99-103.
17. Cherif A, Roelands B, Meeusen R, Chamari K. Effects of Intermittent fasting, caloric restriction, and Ramadan intermittent fasting on cognitive performance at rest and during exercise in adults. Sports Med. 2016;46(1):35-47.

18. Ciarlone SL, Grieco JC, D'Agostino DP, Weeber EJ. Ketone ester supplementation attenuates seizure activity, and improves behavior and hippocampal synaptic plasticity in an Angelman syndrome mouse model. Neurobiol Dis. 2016;96:38-46.
19. Clarke K, Tchabanenko K, Pawlosky R, Carter E, Todd King M, Musa-Veloso K, Ho M, Roberts A, Robertson J, Vanitallie T, et al. Kinetics, safety and tolerability of (R)-3-hydroxybutyl (R)-3-hydroxybutyrate in healthy adult subjects. Regul Toxicol Pharmacol. 2012;63(3):401-8.
20. D'Agostino D, Pilla R, Held H, Landon C, Puchowicz M, Brunengraber H, Ari C, Arnold P, Dean J. Therapeutic ketosis with ketone ester delays central nervous system oxygen toxicity seizures in rats. Am J Physiol Regul Integr Comp Physiol. 2013;304(10):R829-36.
21. Dahlin M, Elfving A, Ungerstedt U, Amark P. The ketogenic diet influences the levels of excitatory and inhibitory amino acids in the CSF in children with refractory epilepsy. Epilepsy Res. 2005;64(3):115-25.
22. Demchenko IT, Piantadosi CA. Nitric oxide amplifies the excitatory to inhibitory neurotransmitter imbalance accelerating oxygen seizures. Undersea Hyperb Med. 2006;33(3):169-74.
23. Dias BG, Banerjee SB, Goodman JV, Ressler KJ. Towards new approaches to disorders of fear and anxiety. Curr Opin Neurobiol. 2013;23(3):346-52.
24. Erecinska M, Silver IA. Tissue oxygen tension and brain sensitivity to hypoxia. Respir Physiol. 2001;128(3):263-76.
25. Farmery S, Sykes O. Neurological oxygen toxicity. Emerg Med J. 2012;29(10):851-2.
26. Fock AW. Analysis of recreational closed-circuit rebreather deaths 1998-2010. Diving Hyperb Med. 2013;43(2):78-85.
27. Freeman JM, Kossoff EH. Ketosis and the ketogenic diet, 2010: advances in treating epilepsy and other disorders. Adv Pediatr. 2010;57(1):315-29.
28. Gasior M, Rogawski MA, Hartman AL. Neuroprotective and disease-modifying effects of the ketogenic diet. Behav Pharmacol. 2006;17(5-6):431-9.
29. Gill AL, Bell CNA. Hyperbaric oxygen: its uses, mechanisms of action and outcomes. QJM. 2004:97.
30. Huttenlocher PR. Ketonemia and seizures: metabolic and anticonvulsant effects of two ketogenic diets in childhood epilepsy. Pediatr Res. 1976;10(5):536-40.
31. Jarrett SG, Milder JB, Liang LP, Patel M. The ketogenic diet increases mitochondrial glutathione levels. J Neurochem. 2008;106(3):1044-51.
32. Juge N, Gray JA, Omote H, Miyaji T, Inoue T, Hara C, Uneyama H, Edwards RH, Nicoll RA, Moriyama Y. Metabolic control of vesicular glutamate transport and release. Neuron. 2010;68(1):99-112.
33. Kakui N, Yokoyama F, Yamauchi M, Kitamura K, Imanishi T, Inoue T, Koyama T. Anxiolytic-like profile of mirtazapine in rat conditioned fear stress model: functional significance of 5-hydroxytryptamine 1A receptor and alpha1-adrenergic receptor. Pharmacol Biochem Behav. 2009;92(3):393-8.
34. Kashiwaya Y, Sato K, Tsuchiya N, Thomas S, Fell DA, Veech RL, Passonneau JV. Control of glucose utilization in working perfused rat heart. J Biol Chem. 1994;269(41):25502-14.
35. Kesl S, Poff A, Ward N, Fiorelli T, Ari C, D'Agostino D. Methods of sustaining dietary ketosis in Sprague-Dawley rats. In: Federation of the American Societies for Experimental Biology; 2014; San Diego, CA.

36. Kesl SL, Poff AM, Ward NP, Fiorelli TN, Ari C, Van Putten AJ, Sherwood JW, Arnold P, D'Agostino DP. Effects of exogenous ketone supplementation on blood ketone, glucose, triglyceride, and lipoprotein levels in Sprague-Dawley rats. Nutr Metab (Lond). 2016;13:9.

37. Poff AM, Kesl S, D'Agostino DP. Ketogenic diet and metabolic therapies: mechanisms and applications. Oxford University Press; 2016. Chapter 32; Ketone supplementation for health and disease; p. 310-27. ISBN: 9780190497996.

38. Kim do Y, Davis LM, Sullivan PG, Maalouf M, Simeone TA, van Brederode J, Rho JM. Ketone bodies are protective against oxidative stress in neocortical neurons. J Neurochem. 2007;101(5):1316-26.

39. Kindwall EP, Whelan HT. Hyperbaric medicine practice, 3rd edition. Flagstaff: Best Publishing Co.; 2008.

40. Klein P, Tyrlikova I, Mathews GC. Dietary treatment in adults with refractory epilepsy: a review. Neurology. 2014;83(21):1978-85.

41. Kossoff E, Turner Z, Doerrer S, Cervenka M, Henry B. The ketogenic and modified atkins diets: treatments for epilepsy and other disorders. Springer Publishing Co.; 2016.

42. Kovac S, Abramov AY, Walker MC. Energy depletion in seizures: anaplerosis as a strategy for future therapies. Neuropharmacology. 2013;69:96-104.

43. Lardy HA, Phillips PH. Studies of fat and carbohydrate oxidation in mammalian spermatozoa. Arch Biochem. 1945;6:53-61.

44. Levy RG, Cooper PN, Giri P. Ketogenic diet and other dietary treatments for epilepsy. Cochrane Database Syst Rev. 2011;(3).

45. Li X. Using the conditioned fear stress (CFS) animal model to understand the neurobiological mechanisms and pharmacological treatment of anxiety. Shanghai Arch Psychiatry. 2012;24(5):241-9.

46. Luhmann HJ, Mittmann T, van Luijtelaar G, Heinemann U. Impairment of intracortical GABAergic inhibition in a rat model of absence epilepsy. Epilepsy Res. 1995;22(1):43-51.

47. Maalouf M, Rho J, Mattson M. The neuroprotective properties of calorie restriction, the ketogenic diet, and ketone bodies. Brain Res Rev. 2009;59(2):293-315.

48. Maalouf M, Sullivan PG, Davis L, Kim DY, Rho JM. Ketones inhibit mitochondrial production of reactive oxygen species production following glutamate excitotoxicity by increasing NADH oxidation. Neuroscience. 2007;145(1):256-64.

49. Marosi K, Kim SW, Moehl K, Scheibye-Knudsen M, Cheng A, Cutler R, Camandola S, Mattson MP. 3-Hydroxybutyrate regulates energy metabolism and induces BDNF expression in cerebral cortical neurons. J Neurochem. 2016;139(5):769-81.

50. Masino SA, Geiger JD. The ketogenic diet and epilepsy: is adenosine the missing link? Epilepsia. 2009;50(2):332-3.

51. Masino SA, Kawamura M Jr, Ruskin DN, Geiger JD, Boison D. Purines and neuronal excitability: links to the ketogenic diet. Epilepsy Res. 2012;100(3):229-38.

52. Masino SA, Li T, Theofilas P, Sandau US, Ruskin DN, Fredholm BB, Geiger JD, Aronica E, Boison D. A ketogenic diet suppresses seizures in mice through adenosine A(1) receptors. J Clin Invest. 2011;121(7):2679-83.

53. Masino SA, Rho JM. Mechanisms of ketogenic diet action. In: Noebels JL, Avoli M, Rogawski MA, Olsen RW, Delgado-Escueta AV. Jasper's basic mechanisms of the epilepsies. 4th ed. Bethesda (MD); 2012.

54. Mattson MP, Longo VD, Harvie M. Impact of intermittent fasting on health and disease processes. Ageing Res Rev. 2016.

55. Mazzuferi M, Kumar G, van Eyll J, Danis B, Foerch P, Kaminski RM. Nrf2 defense pathway: experimental evidence for its protective role in epilepsy. Ann Neurol. 2013;74(4):560-8.

56. McHenry LC Jr. Cerebral blood flow. N Engl J Med. 1966;274(2):82-91.

57. Melo TM, Nehlig A, Sonnewald U. Neuronal-glial interactions in rats fed a ketogenic diet. Neurochem Int. 2006;48(6-7):498-507.

58. Murer MG, Yan Q, Raisman-Vozari R. Brain-derived neurotrophic factor in the control human brain, and in Alzheimer's disease and Parkinson's disease. Prog Neurobiol. 2001;63(1):71-124.

59. Murray AJ, Knight NS, Cole MA, Cochlin LE, Carter E, Tchabanenko K, Pichulik T, Gulston MK, Atherton HJ, Schroeder MA, et al. Novel ketone diet enhances physical and cognitive performance. FASEB J. 2016;30(12):4021-32.

60. Nagy J, Zambo K, Decsi L. Anti-anxiety action of diazepam after intra-amygdaloid application in the rat. Neuropharmacology. 1979;18(6):573-6.

61. Narkowicz CK, Vial JH, Mccartney PW. Hyperbaric oxygen therapy increases free-radical levels in the blood of humans. Free Radic Res Commun. 1993;19(2):71-80.

62. Newman JC, Verdin E. Ketone bodies as signaling metabolites. Trends Endocrinol Metab. 2014;25(1):42-52.

63. Noh HS, Hah YS, Nilufar R, Han J, Bong JH, Kang SS, Cho GJ, Choi WS. Acetoacetate protects neuronal cells from oxidative glutamate toxicity. J Neurosci Res. 2006;83(4):702-9.

64. Puchowicz MA, Smith CL, Bomont C, Koshy J, David F, Brunengraber H. Dog model of therapeutic ketosis induced by oral administration of R,S-1,3-butanediol diacetoacetate. J Nutr Biochem. 2000;11(5):281-7.

65. Rho JM. How does the ketogenic diet induce anti-seizure effects? Neurosci Lett. 2015.

66. Rowley S, Patel M. Mitochondrial involvement and oxidative stress in temporal lobe epilepsy. Free Radic Biol Med. 2013;62:121-31.

67. Shimazu T, Hirschey MD, Newman J, He W, Shirakawa K, Le Moan N, Grueter CA, Lim H, Saunders LR, Stevens RD, et al. Suppression of oxidative stress by beta-hydroxybutyrate, an endogenous histone deacetylase inhibitor. Science. 2013;339(6116):211-4.

68. Shoichet MS, Tate CC, Baumann MD, LaPlaca MC. Strategies for regeneration and repair in the injured central nervous system. In: Reichert WM, editor. Indwelling neural implants: strategies for contending with the in vivo environment. Boca Raton (FL); 2008.

69. Smerz RW. Incidence of oxygen toxicity during the treatment of dysbarism. Undersea Hyperb Med. 2004;31(2):199-202.

70. Srivastava S, Kashiwaya Y, King M, Baxa U, Tam J, Niu G, Chen X, Clarke K, Veech R. Mitochondrial biogenesis and increased uncoupling protein 1 in brown adipose tissue of mice fed a ketone ester diet. FASEB J. 2012;26(6):2351-62.

71. Stafstrom CE, Ockuly JC, Murphree L, Valley MT, Roopra A, Sutula TP. Anticonvulsant and antiepileptic actions of 2-deoxy-D-glucose in epilepsy models. Ann Neurol. 2009;65(4):435-47.

72. Stafstrom CE, Roopra A, Sutula TP. Seizure suppression via glycolysis inhibition with 2-deoxy-D-glucose (2DG). Epilepsia. 2008;49 Suppl 8:97-100.

73. Stewart WK, Fleming LW. Features of a successful therapeutic fast of 382 days' duration. Postgrad Med J. 1973;49(569):203-9.

74. Suzuki T, Motohashi H, Yamamoto M. Toward clinical application of the Keap1-Nrf2 pathway. Trends Pharmacol Sci. 2013;34(6):340-6.

75. Tanner GR, Lutas A, Martinez-Francois JR, Yellen G. Single K ATP channel opening in response to action potential firing in mouse dentate granule neurons. J Neurosci. 2011;31(23):8689-96.

76. Thom S. Hyperbaric oxygen – its mechanisms and efficacy. Plast Reconstr Surg. 2011;127(Suppl 1).

77. Thom S. Hyperbaric oxygen therapy. J Intensive Care Med. 1989;4:58-74.

78. Valadao JM, Vigilante JA, DiGeorge NW, O'Connor SE, Bear A, Kenyon J, Annis H, Dituri J, Dituri AE, Whelan HT. Ketogenic diet for high partial pressure oxygen diving. Undersea Hyperb Med. 2014;41(4):331-5.

79. Veech RL, Chance B, Kashiwaya Y, Lardy HA, Cahill GF Jr. Ketone bodies, potential therapeutic uses. IUBMB Life. 2001;51(4):241-7.

80. Verdier C, Lee DR, Scoff H. Unconscious recreational rebreather diver and rescue techniques [Internet]. DIRrebreather; 2008. Available from: http://archive.rubicon-foundation.org/xmlui/bitstream/handle/123456789/7826/DIRrebreather_Rescue_Procedures.pdf?sequence=1

81. Viggiano A, Pilla R, Arnold P, Monda M, D DA, Coppola G. Anticonvulsant properties of an oral ketone ester in a pentylenetetrazole-model of seizure. Brain Res. 2015;1618:50-4.

82. Volek JS, Aragon A. Low carbohydrate diets for athletes. In: Personal Trainers Conference: Application in Motion; 2013; Las Vegas, NV.

83. Volek J, Phinney S, Forsythe C, Quann E, Wood R, Puglisi M, Kraemer W, Bibus D, Fernandez M, Feinman R. Carbohydrate restriction has a more favorable impact on the metabolic syndrome than a low fat diet. Lipids. 2009;44(4):297-309.

84. Wang ZJ, Bergqvist C, Hunter JV, Jin D, Wang DJ, Wehrli S, Zimmerman RA. In vivo measurement of brain metabolites using two-dimensional double-quantum MR spectroscopy – exploration of GABA levels in a ketogenic diet. Magn Reson Med. 2003;49(4):615-9.

85. Weaver LK. Hyperbaric oxygen therapy indications. 13th ed. Undersea and Hyperbaric Medical Society; 2014.

86. Yellen G. Ketone bodies, glycolysis, and K_{ATP} channels in the mechanism of the ketogenic diet. Epilepsia. 2008;49(Suppl 8):80-2.

87. Yudkoff M, Daikhin Y, Melo TM, Nissim I, Sonnewald U, Nissim I. The ketogenic diet and brain metabolism of amino acids: relationship to the anticonvulsant effect. Annu Rev Nutr. 2007;27:415-30.

88. Yudkoff M, Daikhin Y, Nissim I, Grunstein R, Nissim I. Effects of ketone bodies on astrocyte amino acid metabolism. J Neurochem. 1997;69(2):682-92.

89. Yudkoff M, Daikhin Y, Nissim I, Horyn O, Lazarow A, Luhovyy B, Wehrli S, Nissim I. Response of brain amino acid metabolism to ketosis. Neurochem Int. 2005;47(1-2):119-28.

90. Zheng HQ, Zhang LY, Luo J, Li LL, Li M, Zhang Q, Hu XQ. Physical exercise promotes recovery of neurological function after ischemic stroke in rats. Int J Mol Sci. 2014;15(6):10974-88.

91. Zou X, Meng J, Li L, Han W, Li C, Zhong R, Miao X, Cai J, Zhang Y, Zhu D. Acetoacetate accelerates muscle regeneration and ameliorates muscular dystrophy in mice. J Biol Chem. 2016;291(5):2181-95.

CHAPTER 42 CHAPTER

Submarine Rescue Diving and Hyperbaric Medicine

CHAPTER FORTY-TWO OVERVIEW

Introduction....1017
Pressurized Rescue Likelihood....1021
History of Pressurization....1021
Problem with Pressure....1022
Decompression of Occupants....1023
Undersea Rescue Command....1024
The Future of Submarine Rescue....1029
Appendix....1031
References....1048

Submarine Rescue Diving and Hyperbaric Medicine

Joseph Dituri, Harry T. Whelan

INTRODUCTION

The unfortunate reality is that submarines sink purposefully. They often operate in shallow portions of depths that exceed their design depth. In the unlikely event of a submarine "issue," the crew has few escape methods. The U.S. Navy's Undersea Rescue Command (URC) hosts America's submarine rescue assets. The Navy's newest submarine rescue asset, the pressurized rescue module (PRM), has been certified and has retired the deep-submergence research vehicles. The PRM is a tethered, manned remotely operated vehicle (ROV) that can hold two internal attendants (IAs) and 16 rescuees from a downed submarine up to 2,000 fsw deep (Figure 1, Figure 2a, Figure 2b). The IAs need to be divers because the disabled submarine may be pressurized.

Naval Sea Systems Command has plans for a transfer under pressure (TUP) system that will consist of two 32-man chambers and a deck transfer lock along with flexible manways to allow saturated rescuees to be evacuated and decompressed from a submarine (Figure 3). TUP is scheduled for initial testing in February 2017 in San Diego, California. Meanwhile, the PRM continues to descend to the submarine's watery vault to retrieve another load from Davy Jones' Locker. The transport of the PRM requires at least two C-5 type aircraft to get it to the scene of the incident, illustrating its enormity. The entire PRM and TUP system as well as other parts are

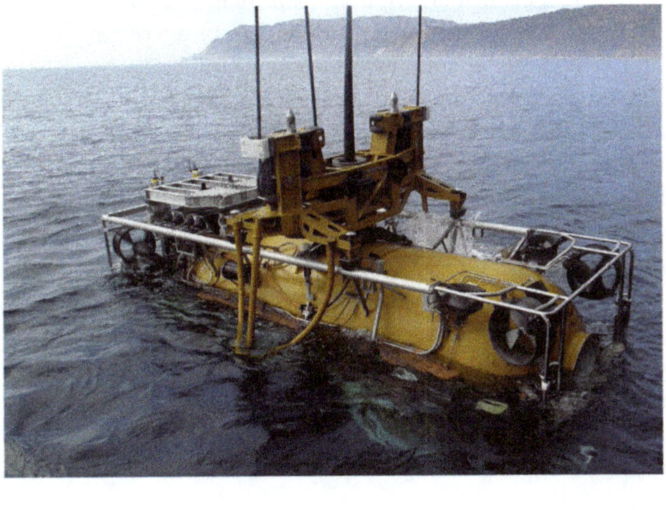

Figure 1. Launch of the U.S. Navy's pressurized rescue module (PRM-1) *Falcon* into the water for the PRM's first dive of the operational readiness evaluation (ORE) on July 19, 2015. (Photo courtesy of the U.S. Navy)

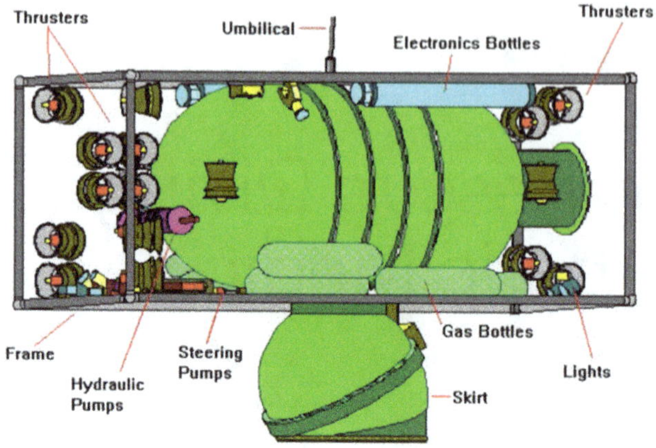

Figure 2a. Animated diagram of pressurized rescue module (PRM). (Image courtesy of the U.S. Navy)

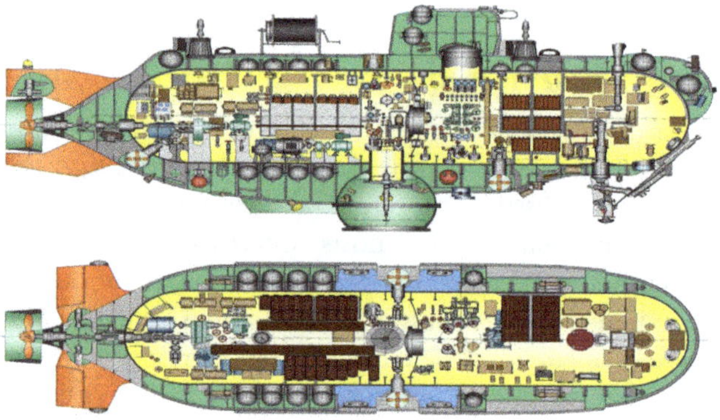

Figure 2b. Russian modernized saving and rescue deep-water vehicle (project 18551). (Image courtesy of the U.S. Navy)

encompassed in the Submarine Rescue Diving and Recompression System (SRDRS) (Figures 4a, Figure 4b, Figure 4c, Figure 4d). This entire SRDRS system will take five C-5s to transport it to a rescue site.

A historical review of disabled submarine (DISSUB) events demonstrates a wide spectrum of anticipated medical conditions, ranging from no or minimal injuries to death. It is anticipated that any event significant to the extent of a distressed submarine on the seabed unable to surface is likely to result in injuries to at least a portion of the crew. These immediate injuries are anticipated to fall into one or a combination of the following categories: (a) trauma, either blunt or penetrating; (b) thermal injury; (c) submersion related; and (d) pulmonary injury.

Surface abandonment is an event that results in a surfaced submarine requiring assistance that necessitates crew members to abandon the vessel; it is almost identical to any other maritime surface abandonment event. Due to either a low freeboard or a high sea state, however, crew members who must abandon a submarine on the surface will be forced to exit through the sail and therefore may be potentially subjected to blunt traumatic injuries from impact with the hull or the sail.

Prolonged survival aboard a DISSUB will be a physiologically stressful period and will be compounded by any comorbid condition incurred during the submarine disabling event. Survivors within a DISSUB will be threatened by progressively worsening environmental and atmospheric conditions, hypothermia, hyperthermia, prolonged exposure to elevated pressure, exhaustion, and possible injury or contamination such as those which purportedly occurred on the Russian submarine *Kursk*.

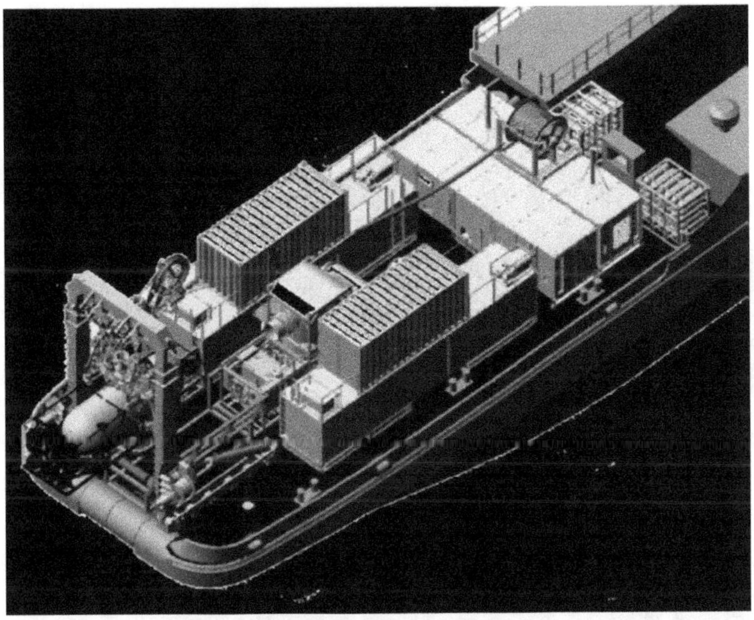

Figure 3. Transfer under pressure (TUP) system. Once the transfer of rescued submariners is complete, the PRM will detach from the submarine and ascend to the submerged cursor frame suspended from the launch and recovery system (LARS). The PRM is then recovered from the sea and landed on a deck cradle installed onboard the vessel of opportunity (VOO). Upon recovery, the PRM docks with the submarine decompression system (SDS) to allow transfer and decompression of personnel. The attendants and those rescued are then transferred under pressure to the SDS from the PRM via a pressurized flexible manway. (Image courtesy of the U.S. Navy)

The primary risk of escape is related to physiologic responses to significant changes in atmospheric pressure. Assuming that conditions aboard the DISSUB have deteriorated to the point that they are no longer compatible with survival, the decision to escape will be made by the DISSUB senior survivor. Escaping from the progressively deteriorating atmosphere presents another set of risks that must be given equal consideration. The escape process requires the escapee to experience a rapid pressurization while in the escape trunk to a pressure equal to the ambient water depth. The escapee will then experience a rapid decrease in pressure as he or she ascends to the surface. Although every effort has been made through training, escape-trunk engineering, and escape-suit design to make this process as safe as possible, risks still remain. Barotrauma and decompression injuries of any type and severity are possible. The proper treatment for many of these injuries requires the use of hyperbaric chambers. If hyperbaric chambers are unavailable, the minimal standard of care would be to administer high concentrations of oxygen.

Other than potentially minor traumatic injuries, relatively few additional risks are incurred to the survivor if a rescue vehicle is able to mate to the DISSUB and maintain the same atmospheric pressure that was experienced on the DISSUB. Although escape is the more likely resulting scenario, rescue is normally the preferred method of evacuation. Decompression injuries are likely if the survivor experiences a sudden decrease in pressure either within the rescue vehicle or on a vessel of opportunity (VOO). Additionally, hyperthermia is a potential risk to the rescue vehicle passengers as the ambient temperature increases. Monitoring and cooling measures should be implemented if operating for prolonged periods in warm waters.

Submarine Rescue Diving and Recompression System (SRDRS). (Images courtesy of the U.S. Navy)

From top:

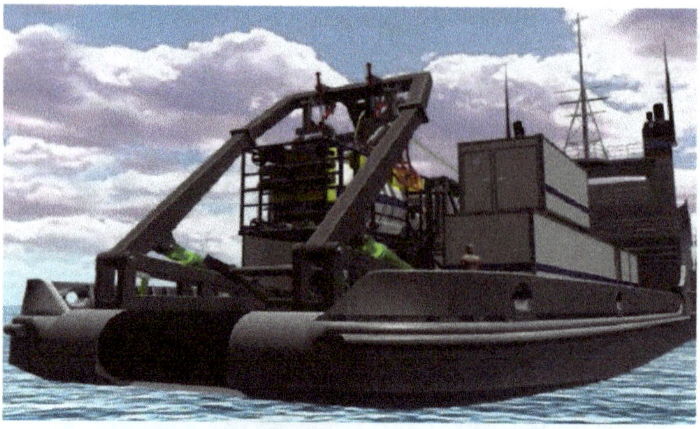

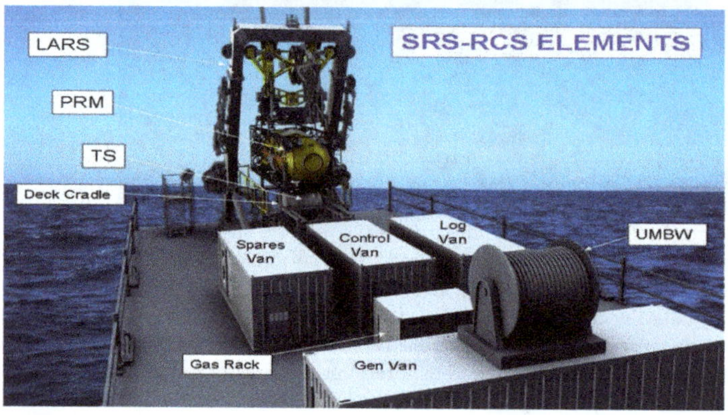

Figures 4a–4b. SRDRS mission requirements:

- Rescue 155 personnel from pressurized DISSUB
- Five-hour round trip with PRM (second sortie and on)
- 16 rescues per trip
- Two PRM inside operators
- Requires 10 trips to rescue crew
- SDCs hold 36 rescues each (takes two PRM sorties to fill)

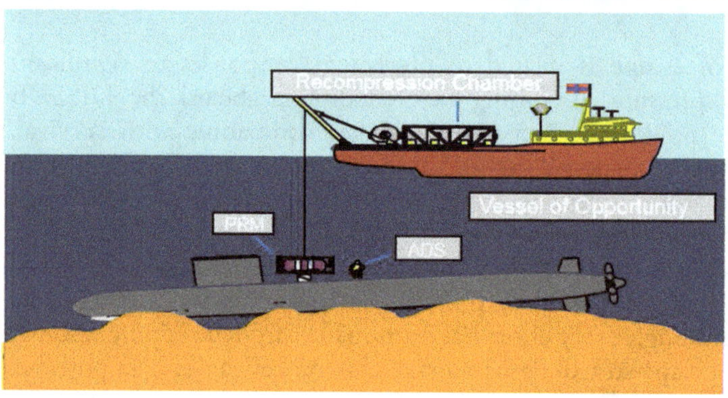

Figure 4c. Mission profile: PRM operators/SDC tenders will not be available for repetitive mission due to decompression requirement.

- There should be a surface interval of 24 hours before PRM operators/SDC tenders are available for next sortie.
- A minimum of 20 PRM operators/SDC tenders are required for 10 PRM sorties.
- PRM operator/SDC tender should be a Second Class Diver (qualified as inside chamber tender)/Diving Medical Technician (DMT).

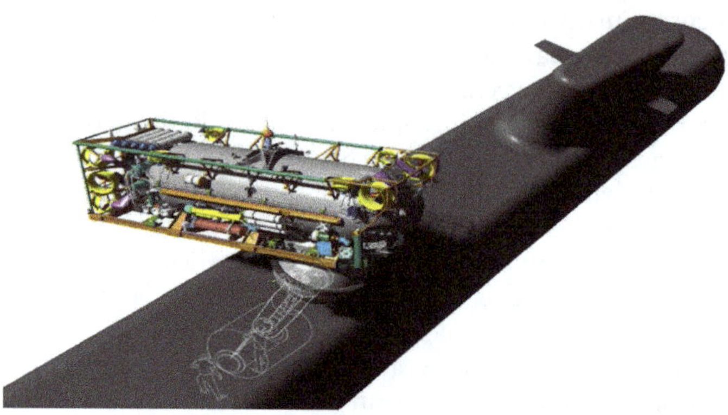

Figure 4d. Once the PRM is mated with the submarine, two onboard attendants will assist with the transfer of submariners into the PRM. The attendants also control and monitor life-support functions.

The potential for decompression injuries and death increases significantly as the atmospheric pressure within the DISSUB increases and the length of time the survivor is exposed to that pressure increases. Decompression injuries can certainly be expected if the survivor is exposed for more than 12 hours to a pressure of more than 1.7 ATA (23 feet of seawater) and then is rapidly decompressed to the surface pressure either by escape or rescue. DISSUB atmospheric pressure will increase due to either a reduction in air space volume, such as flooding, or an increase in gas in the air space, such as emergency air breathing (EAB), gas/airline ruptures and leaks, and escape-trunk cycling.

PRESSURIZED RESCUE LIKELIHOOD

The PRM is capable of rescue but not pressurized rescue beyond 1.6 ATA (20 fsw). In the unlikely event of a DISSUB, the submarine would likely become pressurized. The crew of the DISSUB would remain pressurized until saved and decompressed. The minimal time to first rescue is 72 hours. After 72 hours at any depth deeper than 20 fsw, there would be a required offgas or decompression time to allow the extra nitrogen absorbed at depth to slowly come out of solution. A DISSUB can become pressurized by several means. The most likely scenario for pressurization probably would be a combination of the following events rather than a single one:

1. A leak in an air/O_2 system could cause pressurization of the DISSUB. As seems evident, flooding will increase air pressure by displacing part of and consequently compressing the remaining volume. Another method is intentional pressurization (IP) by the crew to keep water out. This is a less likely situation for discussion because at the depths in which submarines operate, open communication to the sea could be thwarted by IP, but rescue would be beyond the capabilities of any system in existence. A hybrid of this might be when IP becomes a contributing factor to pressure — i.e., the crew may need to pressurize the submarine a slight amount to keep a system from flooding, which can be secured in short order.
2. The use of a breathing gas mask that is external to the DISSUB environment, such as an emergency breathing system (EBS) or emergency air breathing system (EABS), allows the exhaled (CO_2-rich) air to exhaust into the DISSUB. While this will cause a minute increase in pressure, if 155 people over a four-day period must be on EBS and/or EABS, the internal pressure of the DISSUB could increase significantly. This scenario is more unlikely.
3. Another method of pressurization is using air to provide oxygen that is metabolized. This is unlikely as modern submarines contain O_2 generation equipment. There is, however, a scenario in which O_2 generation may not be functioning and/or O_2 in storage could be depleted, thus requiring the need for supplemental metabolic makeup. There are myriad sources of pressurization in a DISSUB, and the submarine rescue experts agree that the probability of a pressurized rescue is likely.

HISTORY OF PRESSURIZATION

B.A.P. *Pacocha* of the Peruvian Navy experienced a pressurization of a DISSUB in August 1988, and the results were catastrophic. Twenty-three souls immediately escaped at night, prior to sinking. The DISSUB sank to a depth of 140 fsw in five minutes.

Four souls died during sinking. Twenty-two souls were trapped for 20–24 hours in the forward torpedo room, which had been pressurized to 54 fsw from flooding and air bank use. The decision was made to escape, and 20 sailors developed decompression sickness (DCS). All of these sailors were treated with recompression. There was one death and one severe central nervous system (CNS) injury along with many permanent injuries from DCS.[4]

In May 1939, the USS *Squalus* sank off Portsmouth, New Hampshire, with all hands. Within five minutes of the order to submerge the submarine, she rested on the bottom in 242 feet of water with her three after-compartments flooded and 26 crew dead. The forward two compartments were not flooded, but they were pressurized. The pressure in the DISSUB prior to the first McCann bell run was about 28 fsw. The forward torpedo room was ventilated from the rescue bell for about five minutes on the first sortie. This may have lowered the pressure in the DISSUB somewhat, but five minutes is a fairly short period of time given the size of the exhaust line from the bell to the surface. Thirty-two men were rescued and decompressed over a 40-hour period.[6]

PROBLEM WITH PRESSURE

The problem is not with the pressurization itself. Mammalian tolerance is pressurization in excess of 2,000 fsw. While there are ramifications involved with this level of pressurization, the fact remains that humans can withstand the pressure. The problem comes with the rapid (case-pendant) depressurization of those individuals saturated with inert gas. As the external pressure is reduced at a decreased depth, tissues begin the process of off-gassing. The tissues are attempting to return to equilibrium equivalent with external pressure by releasing the previously absorbed gas into the bloodstream, where it is carried to the lungs for filtering.

The amount of blood filling the capillary bed at any one time is about 5% of the entire body's blood volume. The capillary bed is the area where the exchange of O_2 and other nutrients with CO_2 and wastes takes place. The exchange can take place only at the capillary bed because it is lined with one thin layer of porous endothelial cells capable of allowing solutes smaller than proteins to diffuse between blood and tissue.

When the inert gas solubility capability is exceeded such that the gas is forced out of solution, a bubble is formed to transport the gas out of the system. Upon realizing the presence of the gas bubble, the body immediately sends antibodies to inspect this new foreign body. When it is discovered to be a foreign element to the body, the immune system dispatches phagocytes and leukocytes to attack and remove the bubble by attaching themselves onto the bubble. Another problem associated with the gas bubble trapped in the bloodstream is that the surface of the gas bubble tends to attract other particles found in the bloodstream, such as fat. The result is a large mass consisting of the gas bubble, fat, and phagocytes/leukocytes making its way through the bloodstream.[3]

Additionally, as internal pressure rises, the increased partial pressure of O_2 in the DISSUB can cause respiratory and nervous system effects, such as respiratory failure and seizures. The risk of these conditions increases rapidly when atmospheric pressure in the DISSUB exceeds five atmospheres. A pressurized rescue of a DISSUB beyond five ATA is beyond the capability of TUP design.

Given the above, there is a need to "bridge the gap" between PRM capability and TUP capability with a contingency plan. The purpose of this chapter is to illuminate the potential barriers to a decompression contingency plan as well as promulgate the steps required to develop a plan that could be used. It is recognized that any plan would be an emergent response to a recognized hole in capability, and the need for the TUP system still exists.

DECOMPRESSION OF OCCUPANTS

There are several methods for decompressing the occupants of a DISSUB given the pre-TUP constraints. Recompression chambers to hold 18 people are not readily available and abundant. These recompression chambers do not mate with the PRM allowing a transfer under pressure. The exact protocols have been vetted, and their discussion is beyond the scope of this text, but the logistics behind each different protocol will be considered.

1. **Decompression inside DISSUB:** The rescue team, once on site, could connect hoses (using the 1-atmosphere suits described below) to the salvage air fittings on a DISSUB and slowly vent the pressure out of the DISSUB. This is dependent upon the reason for pressurization and may not work in all cases. It would require an ability to "throttle" the valves such that decompression rates would be manageable. If the DISSUB could be depressurized to the first decompression stop of the protocol, the decompression of all occupants could begin on the submarine, hastening the completion for any of the scenarios below. This concept would be limited in depth to about 1,000 fsw due to the length of hoses available and logistic requirement. Portsmouth Naval Shipyard had an engineering study done on this topic that is worthy of further discussion.[5]
2. **Decompression inside the PRM:** After the sortie, the occupants of the PRM could decompress within the PRM, allowing them to remain pressurized for the entire time. There are a few ways the occupants could breathe O_2, decreasing the decompression requirement. For specific times, see the Director of Ocean Engineering and Supervisor of Diving and Salvage letter dated 17 February 2006.[1]

   While decompression inside the PRM has merit, it is not practical in most instances. The PRM contains no pressure lock to remove the waste generated by these occupants during the 5- to 58-hour decompression. Because there is no pressure lock, there is no way of getting required medicines or hydration supplies into the PRM. Since dehydration is one of the contributing factors to DCS, and rescuees would likely already be partially dehydrated from their time on board the DISSUB, hydration is important. All supplies would have to be prestaged inside the PRM for use during decompression. Prestaging would affect the amount of personnel (weight) that could be recovered from a DISSUB. The PRM was not designed as a decompression chamber, so quarters are cramped, and flow rates between the makeshift cross-ventilation systems may not be adequate to control the atmosphere or for climate control. PRM would be occupied during the decompression, extending the sortie time and lengthening the time to rescue the full crew from DISSUB. Generally speaking, decompression inside the PRM would work for rescues involving less than four hours duration.
3. **Surface decompression:** One idea that has been loosely explored is to prebreathe oxygen inside the PRM, which decreases the probability of DCS during surface decompression.[2] The occupants could prebreathe 85% O_2 on the way up to the surface inside the PRM. Upon arrival of the PRM on

the deck of the ship, the occupants could be rapidly decompressed to the surface and transported to available chambers. This would allow the PRM to resupply in short order and continue lifesaving sorties (Figures 5a-5q).

There is significant risk of DCS when omitting required decompression to come to the surface and transfer occupants to decompression chambers. The ascent rate of the PRM is an important consideration for this scenario, as the transition from pressure to surface and back to pressure should be less than 15 minutes total.

The use of additional chambers adds a logistic burden that will need to be planned. Additionally, a method is required to transfer personnel from the PRM to the chambers in less than 10 minutes. Evacuating a fully loaded PRM in 10 minutes seems plausible unless occupants are nonambulatory. Additional chambers are isolated systems that have climate control and have a medical lock to get hydration and medicine into the occupants. They also come with their own O_2 supply. Standard Navy fly-away recompression chambers (FARCs) hold up to eight people. Two FARCs could hold all occupants of the PRM, thus allowing the PRM to be resupplied and return to the mission of saving the occupants of the submarine.

Consideration must be given to the backlog and ratio of decompression time to sortie time. Sortie times (from one specific point in the mission until the PRM is at the specific point for the next run) were five hours at Operation Bold Monarch in 2008. Minimum decompression time using accelerated oxygen is 70 minutes given 25-foot saturation, and the times increase almost exponentially from there. As seems evident, almost any treatment would be longer than PRM sortie times forcing a backlog. This same scenario could be used sans the O_2 prebreathe, but that scenario should be considered only in the absence of the ability to prebreathe.

UNDERSEA RESCUE COMMAND

In addition to the PRM, the URC hosts the only two remaining submarine rescue chambers (SRCs) in active service for the U.S. Navy. Navy divers and submariners operate and maintain these systems. Some of the old salts remember these from the old submarine rescue ships, which used to have one SRC on board each ship. The SRC is capable of rescues to a depth of 850 fsw with a capacity of six rescuees (Figure 6). A large set of air racks and a valve console make this reminiscent of hyperbaric chamber operations but on a larger scale (Figure 7). This system offers a lightweight and highly portable alternative to other systems because it can fit on a single plane.

The last deep submergence rescue vehicle (DSRV), called *Mystic*, was located at URC and was relieved by the PRM in 2008 (Figure 8). Divers were required to support the launch and recovery; this type of diving was purportedly the most perilous scuba diving evolution that the U.S. Navy performed. Divers have also been used for evacuation of DSRV personnel in the unlikely event of a problem.

URC also hosts four of the world's 2,000 fsw 1-atmosphere diving suits (ADS). This ADS is not a typical off-the-shelf commercial suit. They were custom designed for the U.S. Navy, and each piece of the suit is made from a solid block of aluminum that is milled out to fit a diver inside (Figure 9). The multiple pieces allow a diver to move with much more dexterity than would normally be afforded by an ROV. The ADS suit also allows topside personnel to have "live eyes" on the project with a person in the suit. The diver enters the suit and is sealed inside at one atmosphere. Oxygen is trickled in for metabolic makeup, and a large scrubber and fan remove the natural byproduct of oxygen metabolism, maintaining the pressure at one atmosphere inside the suit. Life support is monitored, and the dive is supervised from the surface. The "pilot" flies the

Submarine Rescue Diving Recompression System (SRDRS) Concept of Operation Brief. Step-by-step process of surface decompression of 155 personnel aboard pressurized DISSUB. (Images courtesy of the U.S. Navy)

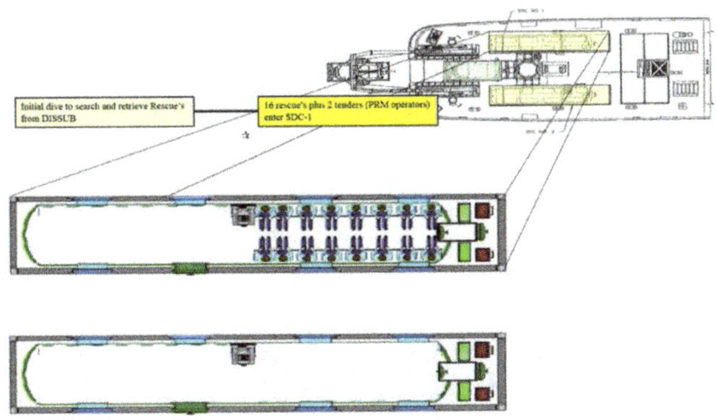

Figure 5a.

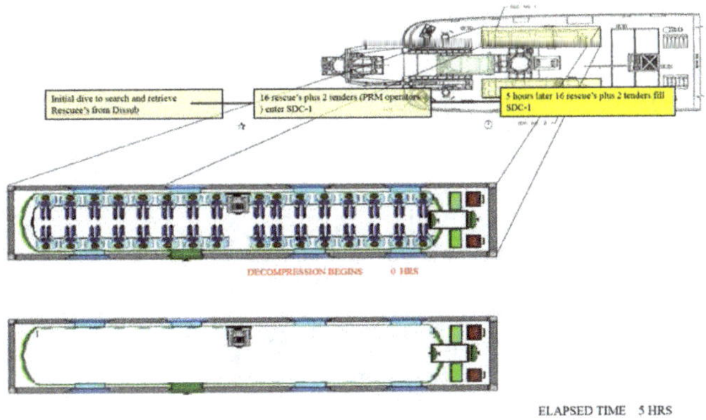

Figure 5b.
Elapsed time: 5 hours

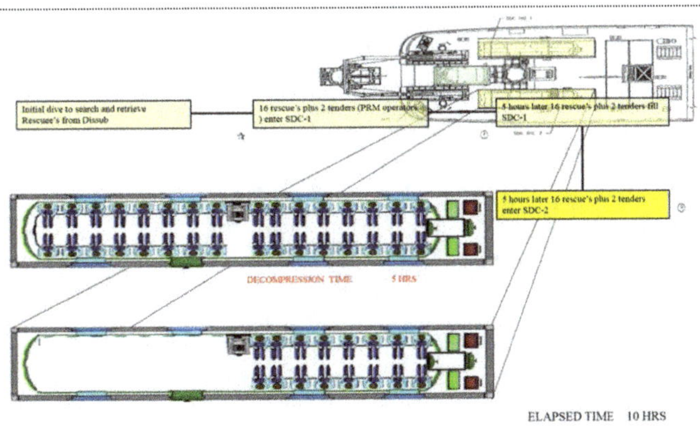

Figure 5c.
Elapsed time: 10 hours

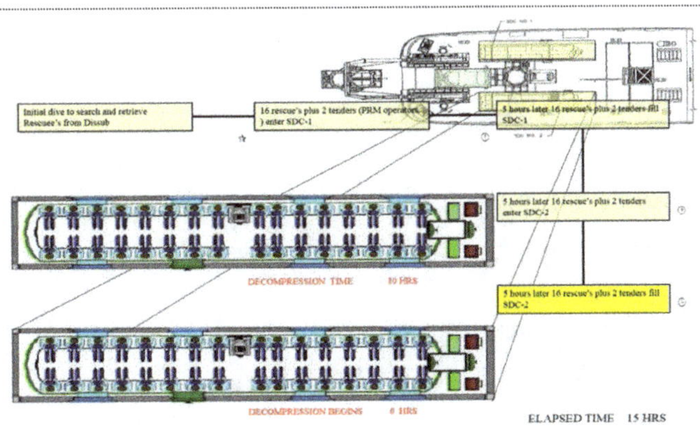

Figure 5d.
Elapsed time: 15 hours

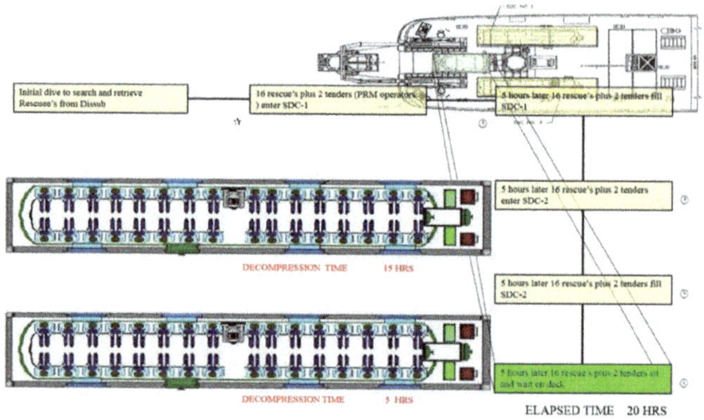

Figure 5e.
Elapsed time: 20 hours

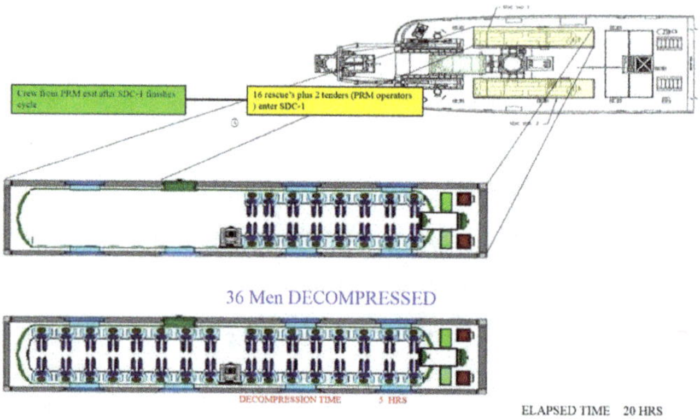

Figure 5f.
Elapsed time: 20 hours

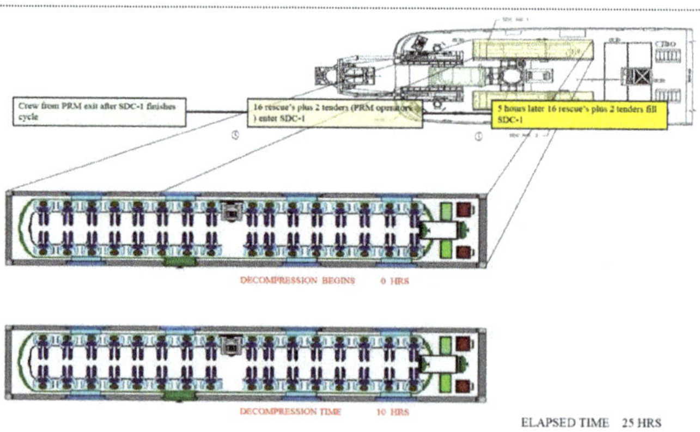

Figure 5g.
Elapsed time: 25 hours

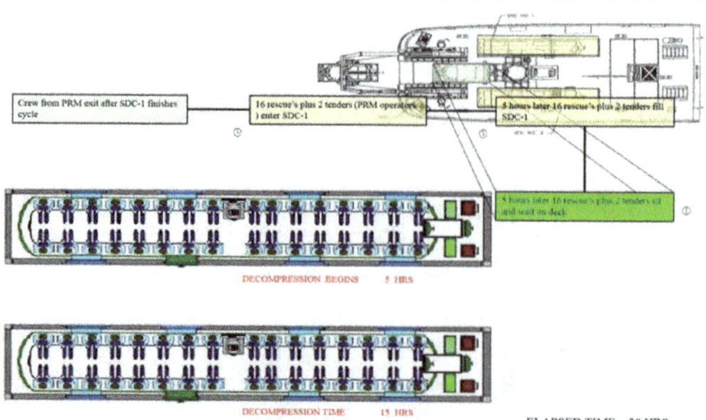

Figure 5h.
Elapsed time: 30 hours

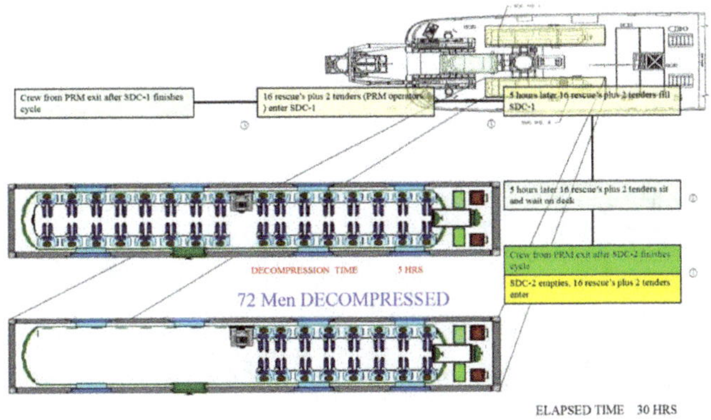

Figure 5i.
Elapsed time: 30 hours

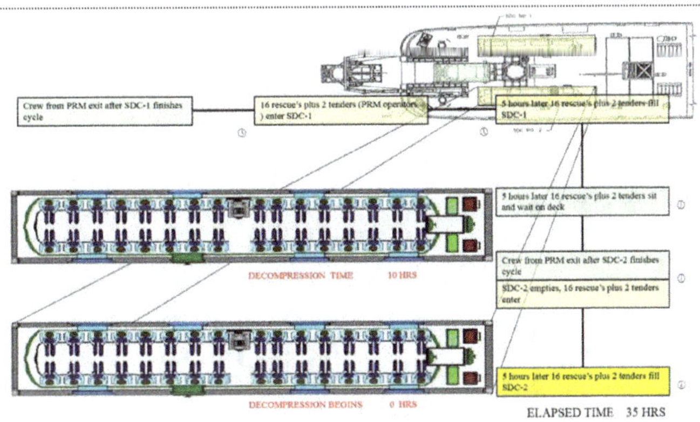

Figure 5j.
Elapsed time: 35 hours

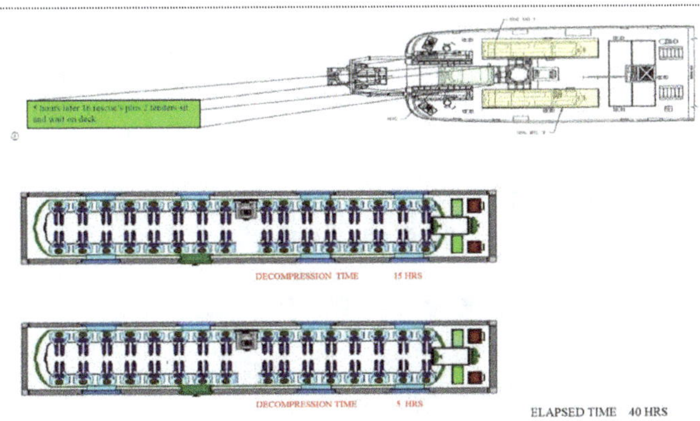

Figure 5k.
Elapsed time: 40 hours

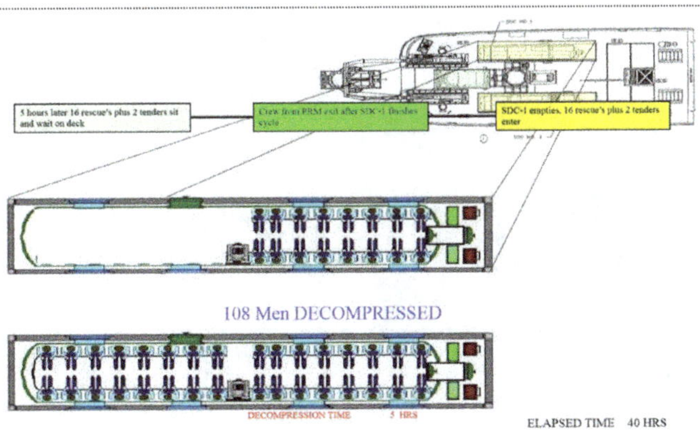

Figure 5l.
Elapsed time: 40 hours

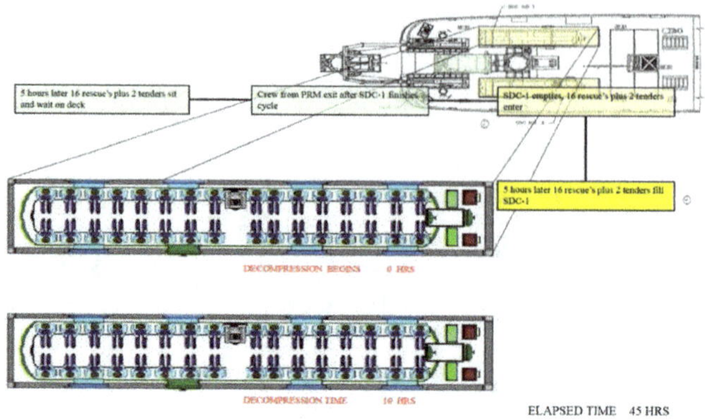

Figure 5m.
Elapsed time: 45 hours

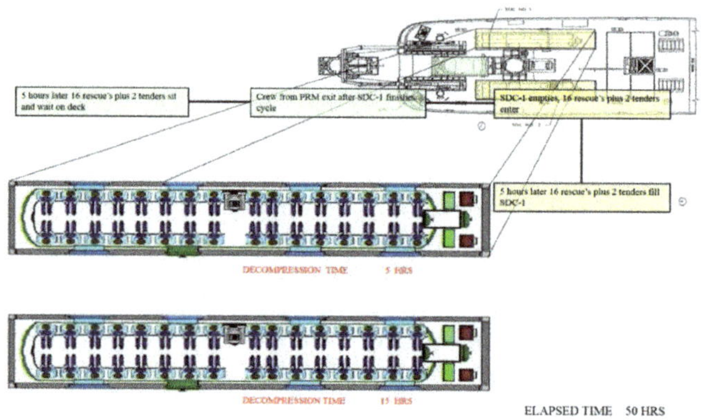

Figure 5n.
Elapsed time: 50 hours

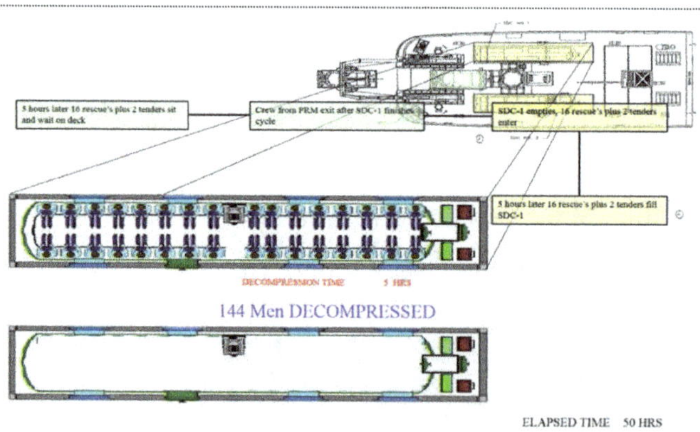

Figure 5o.
Elapsed time: 50 hours

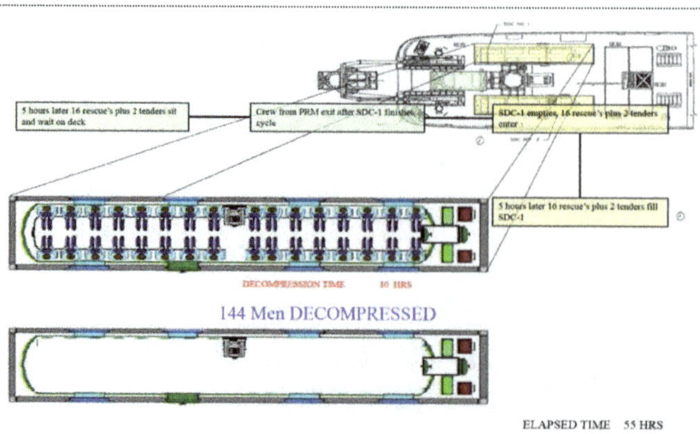

Figure 5p.
Elapsed time: 55 hours

Figure 5q.
Elapsed time: 60 hours

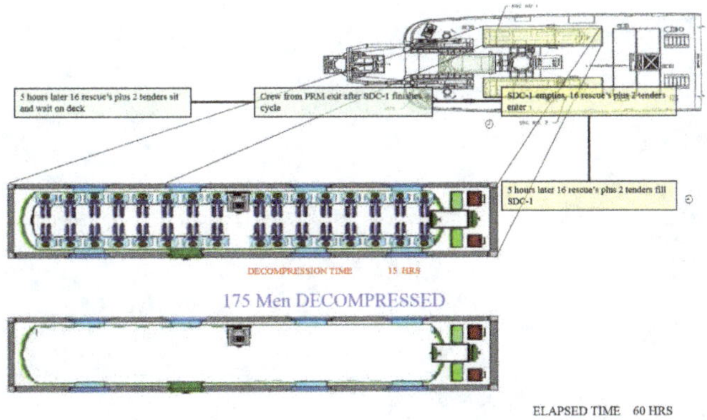

suit up, down, left, and right with the use of foot controls, while the hands remain free to work on projects through the use of manipulators. Because of the innovative design, the suit affords no-decompression diving to 2,000 fsw for up to six hours. This asset is used for intervention, defined as surveying the disabled sub, clearing the escape hatch, and connecting a downhaul cable for the SRC.

If the aforementioned "toys" were not enough, URC also has a hard hat and full-face-mask-capable surface-supplied MK-3 system with the 600-foot umbilicals and the extra air rack to attain depths of up to 190 fsw. This asset is used for intervention in shallower depths and for training and proficiency of the navy divers who come to the command. URC also has a transportable recompression chamber system (TRCS) for treatment and practice and to serve as a mobile transfer lock for the new TUP system. Lifting and rigging evolutions are aplenty, and they regularly lay legs of lightweight mooring systems. The side-scan sonar system and small ROVs are also used in many operations.

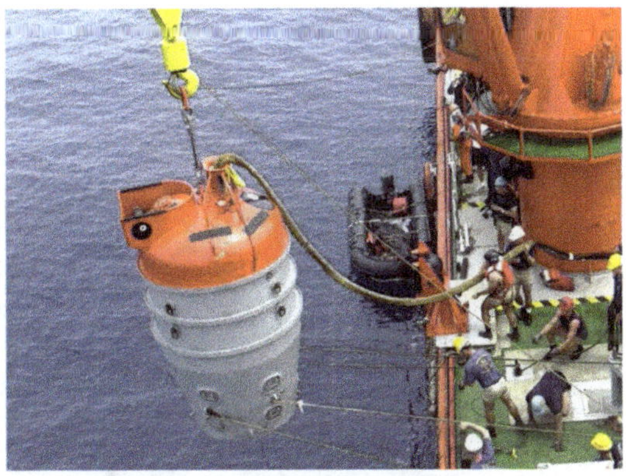

Figure 6. The outside of a submarine rescue chamber (SRC) The U.S. Navy's SRC deploys from MV *Kendrick* to dive to the Republic of Singapore submarine *Conqueror*. (Photo courtesy of the U.S. Navy)

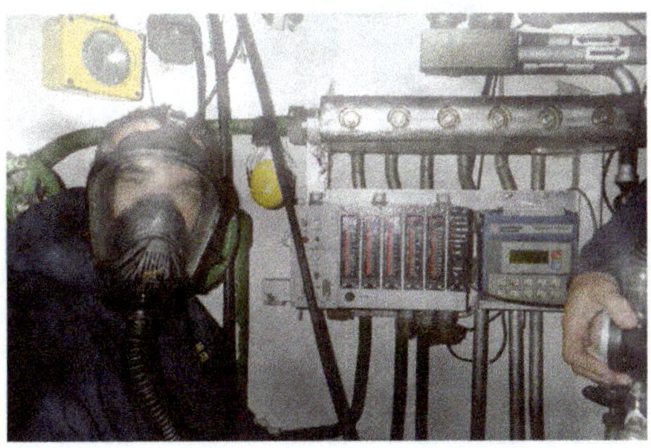

Figure 7. Inside submarine rescue chamber (SRC). Emergency air supply donned in the SRC during operational primary air system failure. The oxygen and carbon dioxide monitoring system is shown to the right of the diver. (Photo courtesy of the U.S. Navy)

THE FUTURE OF SUBMARINE RESCUE

Since its concept more than 90 years ago, the idea of submarine rescue has grown into a capability that provides those nations with undersea vessels a solution to catastrophes beneath the sea. Admittedly most of the areas of the ocean are considered "unrescuable"

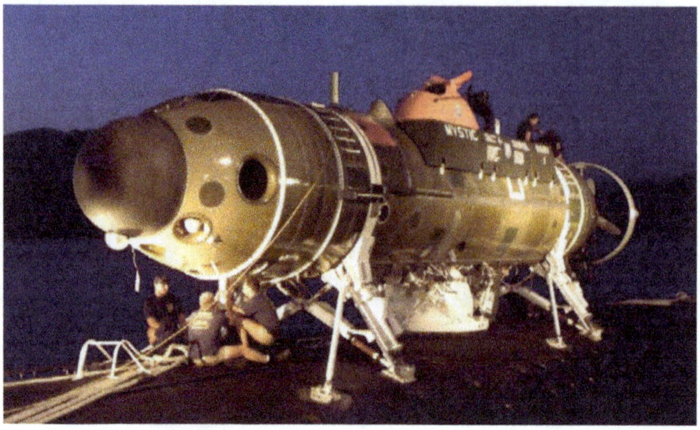

Figure 8. The last deep submergence rescue vehicle (DSRV) is called *Mystic*. (Photo courtesy of the U.S. Navy)

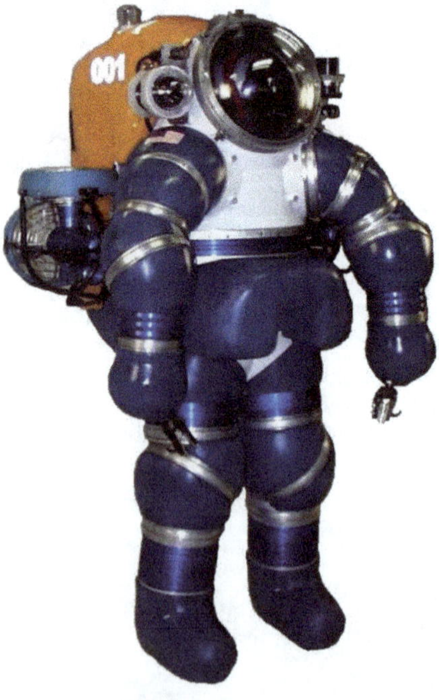

Figure 9. A 2,000 fsw one-atmosphere diving suit (ADS). (Photo courtesy of the U.S. Navy)

waters because they exceed 2,000 fsw, but the concept of rescuing submariners from a watery grave is held in the highest regard. URC is currently conducting testing, evaluations, and training for TUP, the U.S. Navy's newest addition to undersea rescue. The safe decompression of about 155 personnel from a DISSUB may take more than 100 hours and require 95 personnel for rescue, decompression operations, medical treatment, and command and control. The TUP system uses accelerated decompression treatment profiles designed specifically for submarine rescue. Significant work was done at the Naval Submarine Medical Research Laboratory in the early 1990s to reduce the decompression times required, and a plan to achieve it was budgeted and planned for many years ago. The future of submarine rescue is upon us. Due to the complexity of submarine operations and the unforgiving deep ocean environments, any submarine-hosting navy will require capabilities such as TUP. Submarine rescue is an international concern, and, regardless of country of origin, nearly all submarine-capable countries are networked for submarine rescue support to save their greatest assets: their sailors.

APPENDIX

(Adapted material from COMSUBDEVRON FIVE: U.S. Navy Submarine Development Squadron FIVE, *written by Dr. Harry T. Whelan as Senior Undersea Medical Officer at Deep Submergence Unit in 2008. It has been further adapted for use in this chapter on submarine rescue.)*

Submarine Medical Services

1. General

   a. *Purpose.* This ANNEX will provide a concept of operations, assign tasks and responsibilities, and provide guidance for use during a distressed submarine (DISSUB) incident to ensure optimal delivery of all aspects of health care for the purpose of saving lives, minimizing the effects of wounds and injuries, and preserving the force.

   b. *Applicability.* This plan may be applicable to any supporting health-care personnel tasked to assist in submarine escape and rescue operations.

2. Situation

   a. *General.* The optimal outcome of survivors from a DISSUB is dependent on many variables, one of which is a rapid and appropriate medical response with assets capable of providing various levels of medical care in a complex and remote mass casualty situation. The medical team and the consideration of medical issues, personnel, and equipment must be carefully integrated into the crew rendezvous phase during either rescue or escape scenarios.

   b. *Anticipated Medical Conditions.* A historical review of DISSUB events demonstrates a wide spectrum of anticipated medical conditions ranging from no or minimal injuries to death. The following are listed as an overview of potential injury patterns:

      (1) *DISSUB.* It is anticipated that any event significant to the extent of a distressed submarine on the seabed unable to surface is likely to result in injuries to at least a portion of the crew. These immediate injuries are anticipated to be categorized into one or a combination of the following: (a) trauma, either blunt or penetrating; (b) thermal injury; (c) submersion related; and (d) pulmonary injury.

      (2) *Surface Abandonment.* An event that results in a surfaced submarine requiring assistance that necessitates crew members to abandon the vessel is virtually identical to any other maritime surface abandonment event. However, due to either a low freeboard or a high sea state, crew members who must abandon a submarine on the surface will be forced to exit through the sail and therefore potentially be subjected to blunt traumatic injuries from impact with the hull or the sail.

      (3) *Onboard Survival.* Prolonged survival onboard a DISSUB will be a physiologically stressful period and will be compounded by any comorbid condition incurred during the submarine disabling event. Survivors within a DISSUB will be threatened by progressively worsening environmental and atmospheric conditions, hypothermia, hyperthermia, prolonged exposure to elevated pressure, exhaustion, and possible injury or contamination.

(4) *Escape.* The primary risk of escape is related to physiologic responses to significant changes in atmospheric pressure. Assuming that conditions aboard the DISSUB have deteriorated to the point that they are no longer compatible with survival, the decision to escape will be made by the DISSUB Senior Survivor. Escaping from the progressively deteriorating atmosphere presents another set of risks that must be given equal consideration. The escape process requires the escapee to experience a rapid pressurization while in the escape trunk to a pressure equal to the ambient water depth. The escapee will then experience a rapid decrease in pressure as he or she ascends to the surface. Although every effort has been made through training, escape-trunk engineering, and escape-suit design to make this process as safe as possible, risks still remain. Barotrauma and decompression injuries of any type and severity are possible. The proper treatment for many of these injuries requires the use of hyperbaric chambers. If hyperbaric chambers are unavailable, the minimal standard of care would be to administer high concentrations of oxygen.

(5) *Rescue.* Other than potentially minor traumatic injuries, relatively few additional risks are incurred to the survivor if a rescue vehicle is able to mate to the DISSUB and maintain the same atmospheric pressure that was experienced on the DISSUB. Although escape is the more likely resulting scenario, rescue is normally the preferred method of evacuation. Decompression injuries are likely if the survivor experiences a sudden decrease in pressure either within the rescue vehicle or on the VOO (see note below). Additionally, hyperthermia is a potential risk to the rescue vehicle passengers as the ambient temperature increases. Monitoring and cooling measures should be implemented if operating for prolonged periods in warm waters.

NOTE: The potential for decompression injuries and death increases significantly as the atmospheric pressure within the DISSUB increases and the length of time the survivor is exposed to that pressure increases. Decompression injuries can certainly be expected if the survivor is exposed for more than 12 hours to a pressure of more than 1.7 ATA (23 feet of seawater) and then is rapidly decompressed to the surface pressure either by escape or rescue. DISSUB atmospheric pressure will increase due to either a reduction in air space volume, such as flooding, or an increase in gas in the air space, such as EAB use, gas/airline ruptures and leaks, and escape-trunk cycling.

3. Definitions and Concepts

a. *Health Service Support (HSS).* HSS refers to all aspects of health care during the response phase. Medical care provided to the DISSUB survivors is a major aspect. However, HSS also incorporates medical, dental, and psychiatric care of the responding forces. HSS will also extend to force health protection measures and considerations that may be encountered when operations require non-U.S. military resources such as vessels of opportunity (VOOs) or medical treatment facilities (MTFs).

b. *DISSUB Medical Response Team (DMRT).* Various medical staff and assets are intrinsic to Commander, International Submarine Escape and Rescue Liaison Organization (ISMERLO) Participating Navies, and its subordinate commands and detachments, including the reserve component. In most DISSUB scenarios, all of these medical assets will be notified and mobilized to either Deep Submergence Unit (DSU) or other common points of embarkation. This responding ISMERLO Participating Navies intrinsic medical team is referred to as DMRT. The DMRT is mobilized to the scene of any DISSUB event regardless of whether an escape or rescue scenario is expected. Although it is anticipated that all medical assets will be mobilized to form the DMRT, some DISSUB scenarios, such as a small submersible with a small crew size, may necessitate that only a portion of the medical assets mobilize. The COMSUBDEVRON FIVE Senior Medical Officer (SMO) in coordination with the Rescue Element Commander (REC) and Undersea Medical Officer (UMO) will make recommendations to the REC and ISMERLO Participating Navies as to the exact composition of medical personnel and assets that should be mobilized. The DMRT may arrive at locations and VOOs that have organic medical assets. However, the DMRT will have training and experience specific to the unique medical considerations of the DISSUB event. Typically, the ISMERLO Participating Navies SMO will serve as the SMO of the DMRT.

c. *DISSUB Medical Treatment Team (DMTT).* The DMTT is a subcomponent of the DISSUB Entry Team (DET), those individuals in the rescue vehicle who will rendezvous with the survivors in the DISSUB. The necessity for and composition of the DET and DMTT members will vary greatly depending on the circumstances of each event. The DMTT may not be needed, or it may include a single or multiple individuals. The composition and disposition of the DMTT will ultimately be determined by the Coordinator Rescue Forces (CRF) based on recommendations from the REC and SMO DMRT.

d. *DISSUB Advisory Panels.* Two advisory panels will be activated and made available for technical advice and recommendations during any DISSUB event.

   (1) *ISMERLO Participating Navies.* This advisory panel will provide technical advice pertaining to conditions on the DISSUB to include such areas as onboard survivability equipment, onboard atmospheric considerations, and prediction of onboard survival times.

   (2) *The Decompression Advisory Panel* is headed by ISMERLO Participating Navies Senior Medical Officer or Duty Diving Medical Officer. This panel will provide technical advice pertaining to DISSUB survivors who have been or are currently exposed to hyperbaric conditions. Recommendations and advice addressing such areas as decompression treatment options and decompression injury mitigation options will be provided.

e. S*urge Medical Assets.* The DMRT will be the most prepared and equipped medical team to provide care of the DISSUB survivors. The DMRT can be mobilized to the scene of a DISSUB with relative ease and expediency. The DMRT may not be adequate to optimally manage all medical aspects of certain DISSUB events. Circumstances such as extended medical operations and the extent and number of survivor injuries may necessitate that additional medical personnel and equipment is mobilized to the DISSUB scene. The SMO DMRT is responsible for assessing and recommending what, if any, additional medical assets are required. Additional medical assets beyond the DMRT are referred to as extrinsic surge medical assets.

(1) *Extrinsic Surge Medical Assets.* Any medical asset or personnel not assigned to ISMERLO Participating Navies detachment or subordinate command, including the reserve component, may be called upon and mobilized to provide assistance to the DMRT. Activation and utilization of these assets will be coordinated through the appropriate force medical officer and fleet surgeon as required.

4. Assumptions and Considerations

a. Survivors within a DISSUB will have been gradually exposed to deteriorating atmospheric conditions and therefore will have developed some compensatory physiologic reactions. Members of the DET who have not developed these compensatory physiologic reactions will be at a greater risk of impairment once suddenly placed in a DISSUB environment. Therefore, appropriate protective measures should be considered for DET members.

b. Survivors from a DISSUB are anticipated to be in severely weakened physical condition. Considerations should be made to incorporate optimal transfer assistance equipment and procedures to and from rescue vehicles, recovery craft, VOOs, and hyperbaric chambers.

c. Survivors from a DISSUB are anticipated to have some degree of respiratory compromise due to inhaled atmospheric toxins, fumes, and contaminants and thermal injury. This condition may reduce their ability to tolerate hyperbaric oxygen therapy.

d. Survivors may escape to the surface at any time, even before the arrival of the first Submarine Search, Escape and Rescue (SUBSAR) forces. In this situation, SUBSAR units first on the scene may be required to provide basic first aid and/or oxygen as needed for potential decompression injuries.

e. Sufficient medical personnel or units will be available through service component augmentation and mobilization to provide medical support to submarine rescue operations.

f. Surge medical assets can be made available as needed.

g. Adequate aeromedical evacuation (AE) assets and supporting communications equipment will be available throughout the DISSUB operations area. Lines of communications (LOCs) will remain open and are available for AE. Necessary overflight rights will be granted. DISSUB survivors may require transportable decompression chambers and one atmospheres absolute (ATA) AE assets during transit to definitive care locations.

h. Logistical medical support will vary with DISSUB location. Although potentially challenging, adequate Class VIII A supplies will be available and methods of resupply sufficient to perform rescue- and/or escape-scenario medical operations.

i. Deployed response and support personnel will rely on intrinsic HSS of local platforms during DISSUB operations.

j. Each friendly force nation will establish to the best of its ability sufficient health service support and evacuation support for its own forces.

5. Limitations
   a. DISSUB location in relation to proximity and capabilities of rescue vessels and medical treatment facilities may vary considerably.
   b. Medical responders will need to act before having complete information and adapt plans to the developing situation, as it becomes known.
   c. Local weather conditions may affect rescue efforts, including patient transport, relief personnel, or supplies.
   d. As currently configured, survivors must be decontaminated prior to transport from the DISSUB.
   e. The VOO will not have sufficient space and resources to medically manage injured survivors for a prolonged period of time. Stabilization and transfer to another location will be a priority. This limitation may necessitate periodic transfer of injured survivors along with a medical attendant.
   f. U.S. Navy rescue assets do not currently possess the capability to rescue survivors under pressure and directly transfer under pressure (TUP) into a decompression chamber. Some surface interval will occur, which may lead to varying clinical manifestations of decompression illness if the DISSUB is pressurized in excess of 23 feet of seawater.
   g. Hyperbaric chambers may not be available for use during a rescue mission due to operational limitations. In this case, morbidity and mortality rates will be directly related to the degree of DISSUB pressurization.
6. Responsibilities
   a. Fleet Surgeon shall:
      (1) Act as fleet medical advisor to SAR Coordinator.
      (2) Coordinate fleet medical assets.
      (3) Ensure AE assets are in place.
      (4) Coordinate bed status and inpatient admissions on afloat, fixed, and nonfixed MTF.
   b. ISMERLO Participating Navies Fleet Medical Officer (FMO) shall:
      (1) Act as medical advisor to the Submarine Search Rescue Authority (SSRA).
      (2) Serve as shore-based central medical coordination point of contact responsible for coordination and liaison with:
         (a) Fleet Surgeon for:
            1. Identification and resourcing of appropriate surge medical assets, equipment, and personnel.
            2. Coordination of inpatient bed utilization at various MTFs.
            3. Assistance with the identification and utilization of appropriate medical evacuation vessels.
         (b) SMO DMRT for determination of requirements and situational reports.
         (c) DISSUB Advisory Panel for technical advice.
         (d) Area medical personnel and units as potential extrinsic surge medical assets.

(3) Ensure regional UMOs and independent duty corpsmen (IDCs) maintain proficiencies and credentials to serve as potential extrinsic surge medical assets.

(4) Provide direction and guidance for HSS activities and initiatives that are not otherwise provided in this operation plan (OPLAN).

(5) Ensure appropriate HSS resources and infrastructure are deployed to support forces deploying into the DISSUB rescue area of operations (AO).

c. SMO DMRT shall:

(1) Planning, preexecution phase

(a) Advise CRF on medical readiness and status.

(b) Establish communications with:

1. FMO

2. DISSUB Advisory Panels

3. Rescue element UMO

(2) Execution phase of response

(a) Proceed as directed to the scene of any DISSUB incident regardless of escape or rescue scenario.

(b) Act as principal medical advisor to the Chief Operations Specialist (OSC)/CRF.

(c) Exercise technical authority over all medical resources allocated for rescue operations, to include medical staffing, medical logistics, and optimal delivery of HSS to DISSUB survivors and response forces.

(d) Establish appropriate watch bill for all DMRT personnel.

(e) Advise CRF or appropriate DMTT members regarding equipment to be included with the DISSUB Entry Team.

(f) Provide policy and guidance for HSS in the rescue area; develop HSS plans and review of subordinate plans and operations.

(g) Monitor and maintain the status of medical supplies.

(h) Liaison with component medical elements, DISSUB advisory panels, FMO, and HN and coalition medical elements as needed.

(i) Supervise patient evacuation to ensure safe and effective evacuation to an appropriate medical facility. Maintain effective tracking of all patient movement.

(j) Coordinate HSS planning and execution, including international medical support if available.

(k) Ensure timely medical situation reports (MEDSITREP) are provided to the AO FMO during rescue/escape operations.

(l) Brief arriving medical units/personnel on operating procedures and AO medical regulating system.

d. UMO for Rescue Element Commander shall:

(1) Planning, preexecution phase

(a) Communicate with ISMERLO Participating Navies medical personnel during preparation phase prior to mobilization to ensure communication link and provide situational report.

(b) Ensure all rescue element medical equipment is properly maintained, accounted for, and in a state of continuous readiness.

(c) Maintain all appropriate credential and training requirements.

(2) Execution phase of response

(a) As directed, deploy with the medical equipment to the DISSUB scene.

(b) Assume all duties of the SMO DMRT if so designated.

(c) Establish appropriate medical treatment and triage area on the VOO.

(d) Report to SMO DMRT status of medical equipment and personnel.

e. Senior member of DMTT shall:

(1) Be either a UMO or IDC designated by the SMO DMRT.

(2) Deploy to the DISSUB as a component of the DET with appropriate medical equipment to perform initial triage, assist crew transfer, and perform environmental assessment.

(3) Communicate, as best as possible, with the DMRT regarding atmospheric conditions on the DISSUB, medical conditions of the DISSUB crew, and needed supplies.

(4) Coordinate and assist DISSUB medical personnel in stabilization and triage any injured survivors for treatment and transport to the VOO.

(5) Provide medical/environmental SITREP (Commander's Situation Report) updates from the DISSUB to the SMO DMRT.

f. UMO overseeing hyperbaric operations shall:

(1) Maintain and possess expertise in diving/hyperbaric medicine.

(2) Recommend appropriate decompression tables to the Master Diver responsible for chamber operations. Consult with Decompression Advisory Panel as needed.

(3) Provide patient data to SMO DMRT, and alert early if potential for emergent AE needs exist.

(4) Integrate with divers manning the chamber. Identify operational limitations/safety issues for chamber operations, and report status periodically per SMO DMRT.

7. Execution

a. *Concept of Operations.* Commanders and medical unit leaders will establish conditions to deploy a healthy and fit force, achieve situational awareness, mobilize appropriate medical equipment and personnel, expeditiously triage and transfer DISSUB survivors, stabilize patients using forward resuscitative methods, and move patients to definitive afloat, fixed, or nonfixed MTFs with hyperbaric facilities as indicated. Initial focus of medical operations will be limited to stabilization of patients prior to evacuation and accelerated decompression as needed and as hyperbaric chambers are available. Patients requiring medical treatment beyond the capabilities onboard the VOO will be evacuated to an appropriate treatment facility. Treatment of casualties in the area of operations (AO) will be at one of three levels, with the fourth level occurring outside the AO. Level 1 is that immediate treatment performed by medical or nonmedical personnel. Level 2 provides for medical treatment including stabilization and basic resuscitative care and limited dental and psychiatric care. Levels 1 and 2 will be provided by the DMRT. Level 3 provides medical care to include resuscitative surgery and further stabilization, hospitalization with capabilities of more definitive nursing, and surgical, dental, and psychiatric care along with more robust laboratory and radiological diagnostic capabilities. Level 4 includes definitive and restorative care. Levels 3 and 4 are beyond the authority of this OPLAN. Concept by phase follows:

(1) *Transition to DISSUB Response Phase Operations.* As rescue forces prepare for mobilization, the U.S. submarine medical force structure is sized to provide HSS only to U.S. forces unless otherwise directed. U.S. submarine medical forces may not be the sole specialist or lead nation for area/regional medical support. Activation of DMRT andintrinsic and extrinsic medical assets calls for early augmentation and activation of these units as determined by early planning and coordination between the FMO and SMO DMRT. HSS will be conducted in the following phases:

(a) Phase 1 – Notification

1. Notification of the ISMERLO Participating Navies FMO is made immediately upon initiation of SUBLOOK. No recall is initiated, and no resources are diverted. The COMSUBFOR/COMSUBPAC FMO is notified of any subsequent change in the status, including initiation of SUBMISS or SUBSUNK. This information is relayed to the fleet surgeon to begin communication and coordination of potential augmentation of extrinsic medical assets.
2. The COMSUBFOR/COMSUBPAC FMO makes positive notification to the medical department head, COMSUBDEVRON FIVE, upon the initiation of SUBLOOK. No recall is initiated, and no resources are diverted. Positive communication will be made of any subsequent changes, including initiation of SUBMISS or SUBSUNK. These procedures do not replace any recall procedures; they promote direct and timely communication between principles.
3. The cognizant FMO informs ISMERLO Participating Navies Undersea Medicine Command Authority.
4. SMO DMRT and UMO for the Rescue Element establish positive communications and commence preliminary medical mobilization plan.
5. SMO DMRT establishes contact with both the DISSUB Advisory Panel and DISSUB Survivability Advisory Panel.

(b) Phase 2 – Preparation. The objectives for this phase are to assess operational conditions affecting medical needs, plan integration with assets as indicated with HN or international medical response, review berthing for staff and potential patients, assess AE availability and routes, anticipate hyperbaric chamber requirements and mobilization, and plan HSS for responding personnel.

(c) Phase 3 – Deployment. Staged allocation of assets can be made in an expeditious manner accounting for potentially limiting operational factors such as berthing, adverse weather, and VOO deck space availability. This phase begins with the early-deployed DMRT, to stage medical response areas, set up equipment, and familiarize medical personnel. Care will be given to minimize injury to responding personnel during the deployment phase that could impact staffing at the DISSUB site. The HSS focus will be on rapid and forward intervention to stabilize critically ill or injured members and transport stabilized patients from the rescue site. There will likely be limited operational U.S. MTFs/platforms in the AO. Early in the deployment, HSS will be provided by the DMRT and any organic medical personnel already on the DISSUB scene. HSS in this phase requires the rapid buildup of HSS capability through coordination with the AO Fleet Surgeon, FMO, and SMO DMRT. The desired end state of this phase is the successful deployment of adequate HSS to support DISSUB operations.

(d) Phase 4 – Rendezvous Operations (either escape or rescue scenarios). This phase begins upon notification of SUBSUNK and continues until operations are complete. The SMO DMRT will be in regular communication to support the OSC/CRF. The HSS focus will be to preserve the health of rescue forces, to save lives, and to minimize the effects of wounds, injuries, and disease on DISSUB survivors. Hyperbaric chambers may be used for accelerated decompression of pressurized DISSUB survivors. The desired end state of this phase is the successful retrieval and treatment of all DISSUB survivors.

1. The initial actions of the survivor rendezvous phase will be to effectively and safely recover all survivors to the VOO or other support ship where initial Level 2 care can be provided, including any potential hyperbaric treatments.
2. The later actions of the rendezvous phase include survivor transfer to Level 3 care if required and any follow on hyperbaric treatments. These later actions of the rendezvous phase are anticipated to require significant logistical, transportation, and communication support as survivors are transferred to various platforms to receive a higher level of care.

(e) Phase 5 – Redeployment. This phase begins on order, when DISSUB operations are complete. The HSS focus for this phase is the methodical return of HSS assets to designated areas while continuing to provide support to submarine rescue forces. The desired end state of phase 5 is maintenance of force health protection in the AO during rescue system retrieval.

b. *Hospitalization*

(1) All attempts will be made to utilize U.S. fixed and nonfixed MTFs. Organic medical capabilities of the rescue platform aboard the VOO are considered Level 1 and 2, providing basic resuscitative care and stabilization of casualties before evacuation to Level 3, inpatient facilities.

(a) U.S. standards of clinical treatment will be planned for in all instances.

(b) Allied forces personnel will be provided HSS by ISMERLO Participating Navies forces on an emergency basis or in accordance with existing agreements. Foreign DISSUB survivors will be repatriated to national medical authorities as soon as medically indicated.

c. *Patient Movement and Evacuation*

(1) Any appropriate means of conveyance may be utilized to transport patients to the optimal treatment location. The SMO DMRT is responsible to identify transport requests to the OSC. Tracking of all patient movements until the patient enters the Global Patient Medical Regulating Center (GPMRC) will be the responsibility of the SMO DMRT (to include medical regulating, patient evacuation, and theater evacuation policy).

(2) Survivors from both escape and rescue may require pressurized transportation. DISSUB survivors may have been subjected to a hyperbaric environment prior to rescue or escape, placing them at risk for developing decompression illness. In this situation, the receiving afloat, fixed, or nonfixed medical facility should have hyperbaric treatment capability onsite.

(3) The potential exists for evacuation of up to 155 patients, some of whom may be critically injured, utilizing pressurized transportation as indicated, to a facility prepared for handling many casualties, some or all of whom would require surgical and/or hyperbaric capabilities.

(4) Referral to host nation hospitals will be limited to only those situations where there is a risk of loss of life, limb, or eyesight. Such referrals will be coordinated through and approved by the FMO.

d. *Adjunct Medical Support*

(1) Coordination and synchronization of efforts with coalition medical assets. In the event of an international submarine rescue effort, a diverse medical personnel response will occur. Preference for use of English to relay information will be made known. If the foreign medical personnel are not able to communicate, then translators should be made available to facilitate HSS delivery.

(2) Eligibility of Care

(a) HSS will be provided to members of host nation military, coalition forces, and/or multinational forces deployed in support as applicable during DISSUB operations.

(b) Civilians/foreign military that are injured during the DISSUB operations will be treated by U.S. forces.

(c) ISMERLO Participating Navies civilians and contractors who are deployed with ISMERLO Participating Navies forces during DISSUB operations are eligible for treatment.

e. *Submarine Search, Escape and Rescue (SUBSAR).* Component commanders will ensure SUBSAR operations are supported medically. DISSUB survivors who escape from a submerged submarine will potentially add a layer of complexity to the typical SUBSAR operations as these individuals may require treatment in hyperbaric chambers. Therefore, members of the DMRT will deploy and advise the OSC/SSRA even in DISSUB events that appear to be completely an escape scenario.

f. *Host Nation Support (HNS).* Should HNS agreements be negotiated upon ISMERLO Participating Navies OPLAN execution, specific guidance will be followed regarding their use in DISSUB operations.

g. *Joint Blood Program.* No blood products will be stored or maintained on the VOO. If blood products are required, survivors will be transferred to higher levels of care after stabilization. Blood programs will vary with the type of support ships responding to the AO.

h. *Elements of Force Health Protection*

(1) The ISMERLO Participating Navies FMOs are responsible for developing liaisons with the regional fleet surgeons to ensure adequate staffing of HSS and effective AE in submarine rescue operations.

(2) Deploying rescue personnel will be healthy, fit, in a Class 1 or 2 dental status, and will have received appropriate prophylaxis.

(3) Organic force health protection capabilities will be utilized.

(4) All water obtained from non-navy VOOs will be considered nonpotable and will be treated prior to use.

i. *Ancillary Support*

(1) Dental Services. Not applicable.

(2) Veterinary Service. Not applicable.

(3) Radiological Services. The DMRT may deploy with a portable ultrasound device. This device will be used as a screening tool and not as a definitive diagnostic device.

(4) Electronic Medical Equipment. Any electronic devices used in a hyperbaric chamber will have been previously certified for hyperbaric use. Electric generators used for medical devices should be of such quality to ensure proper functioning of the devices.

(5) Mortuary Service. Decedent affairs for submarine rescue operations are coordinated with Logistics. Any medical officer present may be utilized to pronounce time of death as required.

(6) Mass Casualties. The DMRT will be prepared to treat mass casualties, to include those possibly exposed to petrochemical and radiological substances. The principles of triage will be applied. If personnel augmentation is required, the SMO DMRT will request assistance from the designated ISMERLO Participating Navies FMO.

j. *Coordinating Instructions*

(1) Direct liaison and coordination among subordinate activities and supporting commands is authorized and required during planning and execution. Subordinate activities and supporting commands will avoid unilateral actions, which may significantly and adversely impact medical support provided to DISSUB rescue operations.

(2) All dedicated undersea medical assets from ISMERLO Participating Navies and detachments and subordinate commands that are not accompanying the initial transit will rendezvous at a predetermined location or be transferred to the DISSUB site. Parent commands of medical personnel will be responsible for arranging transportation. Any mode of available travel, military or commercial, may be utilized to transfer personnel. Maintenance of communication channels between DISSUB operations and staff en route is essential to ensure integrated planning. Estimated time of arrival (ETA) of medical personnel and situational updates if delays occur should be provided to the CRF.

(3) The DMRT must accompany the rescue force and establish operating capabilities before rescue forces begin operations. All attempts must be made to avoid having the DMRT arrive later than the rescue forces they support. Employment of those rescue forces prior to reception, staging, onward movement, and integration (RSOI) and activation of the associated HSS resources/infrastructure increases morbidity and mortality and is a force health protection issue.

k. *Administration and Logistics.* Medical supply/resupply support is a service component responsibility. Forces will deploy with accompanying supplies in accordance with service guidelines. Supporting HSS supply units will identify the locations and procedures for requisition and issue of HSS supplies/materiel to supported units.

(1) Reports. All medical reports will be submitted in accordance with U.S. message text formatting system and the specific formats. Commands should submit medical regulating reports IAW.

(2) Medical Material

(a) DMRT will deploy with an initial supply sustainability of 48–72 hours for stabilization of a small number of critical patients and general care of minor medical conditions. Limited DMRT personnel will necessitate treatment based on triage management and allocation of resources accordingly.

(b) Resupply will be needed if extended operations or increased numbers of critical patients are encountered during operations.

l. *Command, Control, Communications, and Computers.* Refer to Basic Operation Plan. Ensure medical communication requirements are identified and are fully coordinated.

(1) Medical information will be transmitted via electronic media, satellite, telephone, fax, or courier. Medical information will not be classified unless locations or other operational security or classified information is divulged

but will be handled in compliance with all relevant instructions regarding patient confidentiality.

(2) Organic medical units shall receive communications support from their parent commands.

(3) U.S. medical units will be under operational control to the deploying OSC/CRF, with technical control and HSS policy enforcement provided through the deploying SMO DMRT.

Medical Team Clinical Considerations, Response, and References

1. Principles of Triage
   a. The principles of triage should be used whenever the number and severity of casualties exceeds the resources available.
   b. Since triage is a dynamic process, it is important that the rescue plan allow for the redesignation of patients to appropriate triage categories depending upon their response to treatment over time.
2. Senior Member of DMTT/Triage Medical Officer (TMO)
   a. Responsible for the rapid assessment of survivors and their placement into relevant triage categories, which determines the patient's designated treatment station.
   b. Identify survivors with a casualty identification number written clearly on both their bodies and on casualty report forms.
   c. Maintain and update a triage casualty log.

Triage/Decompression Treatment Categories

1. Introduction. Clinicians involved in DISSUB scenarios require knowledge of both clinical conditions and treatment modalities that are considered beyond the scope of those provided by current clinical assessment systems that are used in traditional land- or surface-based mass casualty scenarios.

When assessing traditional mass casualty injuries, the standard clinical categories (red, yellow, green, and black) should be used to designate patients for appropriate medical treatment.

In addition, survivors must be categorized according to their need for hyperbaric therapy (C1, C2, C3) to treat any conditions that may result from inadequate decompression under the various rescue/escape scenarios.

2. Triage Categories
   a. Red
      (1) Applied to casualties who require IMMEDIATE lifesaving medical and/or surgical treatment which is not overly time-consuming, and who have a high probability of survival.
      (2) Examples include hemorrhagic shock, tension pneumothorax and other respiratory emergencies, and acute surgical abdomen.
   b. Yellow

(1) Applied to casualties requiring time-consuming, major medical and/or surgical treatment, and whose general condition permits delay in such treatment without endangering the patient's potential for survival.

(2) Examples include second-degree burns (< 20%), open fractures, inhalation pulmonary injuries, major lacerations, and moderate hypothermia.

c. Green

(1) Applied to casualties with relatively minor injuries that may be managed by first-aid trained personnel, or who have no outward evidence of injury.

(2) Examples include closed bony fractures without vascular compromise, minor lacerations, first-degree burns, mild hypothermia, and survivors who require observation for DCS.

d. Black

(1) Applies to patients with such severe injuries that they would have an extremely low probability of survival, even under optimal medical and logistical circumstances.

(2) This scenario involves patients who would possibly require medical/surgical management, recompressive treatment, or any combination of those modalities.

(3) These patients should receive simple palliative treatment and available comfort measures, including analgesics.

3. Decompression Treatment Categories

a. Category C1

(1) Applies to patients with symptoms of severe or life-threatening DCI, and who require IMMEDIATE treatment in an onboard recompression chamber.

(2) Delaying treatment to these patients would entail a significant risk to their survival and substantially increase their risk for permanent injury.

b. Category C2

(1) Applies to patients with minor and life-threatening DCI symptoms at the time of assessment.

c. Category C3

(1) No indication that recompression is required.

4. Triage Considerations for Radiation Casualties

a. These patients should be designated no lower than yellow.

b. Survivors who are known or suspected to have received a radiation dose in excess of 2 Gy will require hospitalization within 24 hours.

c. If they are either asymptomatic despite having a life-threatening decompression obligation or show immediate signs of significant DCI, these patients should not be transferred to another medical treatment facility for management of their ionizing radiation exposure until completion of the required hyperbaric treatment.

APPENDIX TABLE 1. TRIAGE/DECOMPRESSION TREATMENT CATEGORY IMMEDIATE MANAGEMENT (BOLD), TREATMENT AREA BY CATEGORY (ITALICS)

	C1	C2	C3
RED	• **Immediate life-saving medical** • **Immediate recompression** • *PRIMARY/DECO chamber*	• **Immediate life-saving medical** • Non-urgent recompression • *PRIMARY*	• **Immediate life-saving medical** • Recompression not required • *PRIMARY*
YELLOW	• Non-lifesaving, major medical • **Immediate recompression** • *DECO chamber*	• Non-lifesaving, major medical • Non-urgent recompression • *Secondary*	• Non-lifesaving, major medical • Recompression not required • *Secondary*
GREEN	• Minor medical care/observation • **Immediate recompression** • *DECO chamber*	• Minor medical care/observation • Non-urgent recompression • *Tertiary*	• Minor medical care/observation • Recompression not required • *Tertiary*
BLACK	• Supportive care	• Supportive care	• Supportive care

Management of Recompression Therapy for DISSUB Survivors

1. Initial Considerations

    a. All diving-related casualties should be attended by a UMO. If a UMO is not available to manage these issues, then ISMERLO Participating Navies should be consulted immediately.

    b. The senior member of DMTT and UMO overseeing hyperbaric operations may have to cope with either multiple cases of DCI or multiple survivors with decompression obligations.

    c. In the event of DISSUB escape instead of rescue, the medical officer may need to treat multiple exposure injuries including, but not limited to, heat or cold injury, hypothermia, dehydration, and sources of contamination.

    d. When in doubt regarding serious DCI, the DISSUB survivor should undergo recompression.

2. Decompression Illness (DCI)

    a. Recompression to provide hyperbaric oxygen therapy is the standard of care for DCI and omitted decompression.

b. Treat DCI or omitted decompression early before symptoms develop to decrease the likelihood of potential recompression emergencies.

c. Treatment with oxygen at the highest concentration possible should be given to all cases of suspected DCI or omitted decompression where chamber treatment is not on site, but adequate oxygen supplies are immediately available.

d. If assets are overwhelmed by the number of casualties:

(1) Oxygen supplies from the initial response will likely be inadequate.

(2) If resupply is not possible prior to exhausting the available oxygen, it may be necessary to conserve the supply by initially treating only the most severe cases of DCI.

(3) Recompression on air is a viable alternative to treat less severe cases of DCI.

(4) Backup chambers and evacuation support must be requested as early as possible.

e. If transport to a treatment center is necessary and available, care should be taken to avoid exacerbating or accelerating the course of DCI.

(1) Use of pressurized aircraft.

(2) Maintaining altitudes less than 1,000 ft.

(3) Hyperlite stretchers to provide recompression, or, if possible, to initiate hyperbaric treatment.

3. Pressurization of Survivors Aboard DISSUB

a. If it is known that the DISSUB survivors experienced pressure changes at depth for a significant amount of time prior to escape or rescue, they may require specialized hyperbaric care using either saturation or accelerated decompression protocols.

b. In the event of this scenario, the Decompression Advisory Panel can be activated by calling the ISMERLO Participating Navies quarterdeck and asking for the Senior Medical Officer or Duty Diving Medical Officer.

Management of Contamination for DISSUB Survivors

1. Treatment of Contaminated Casualties

a. In the event of known chemical, biological, or radiological (CBR) contamination of survivors, the spread of contamination should be minimized by implementing standard decontamination and containment procedures.

b. The urgent stabilization and treatment of casualties must not be delayed because of known or potential contamination.

c. Clean areas may only be accessed once casualties and treatment personnel from designated “dirty” areas have been decontaminated.

d. Contaminated casualties should not pose a significant hazard to the treatment teams.

e. Prior to exposure, all members of the treatment team should be briefed regarding:

(1) The nature of the potential contaminants.

(2) Strict adherence to a policy of no drinking, eating, or smoking in designated treatment areas.

(3) Implementation of appropriate personal protective equipment (PPI), including, but not limited to, coveralls, gloves, masks, and eye protection.

f. Most contamination can be eliminated by having the survivors and treatment team members:

(1) Remove contaminated clothing.

(2) Wash with soap and water.

(3) Tag their contaminated clothing and place them into polyethylene bags.

(4) Store bags in an isolated part of the ship.

2. Treatment of Irradiated Casualties

a. Treatment personnel should follow the decontamination protocol, as outlined above, for contamination casualties.

b. The availability of radiation monitoring equipment can assist in the management of survivors by confirming and identifying areas of contamination, but are not essential to the decontamination of either survivors or casualties.

c. External radiation contamination

(1) Survivors pose no radiation hazard to the crew of a rescue vessel, unless the radioactive fission products are allowed to spread.

d. Internal radiation contamination

(1) Not a hazard to treatment teams.

(2) If a survivor did not receive iodine aboard the DISSUB, then treatment should be initiated and documented by the attending UMO.

e. Acute Radiation Syndrome (ARS)

(1) Suspect if survivors report a dose of ionizing radiation above 1 Gy.

These conditions should not interfere with the provision of emergency medical services, including airway management, obtaining vascular access, or recompression in a chamber.

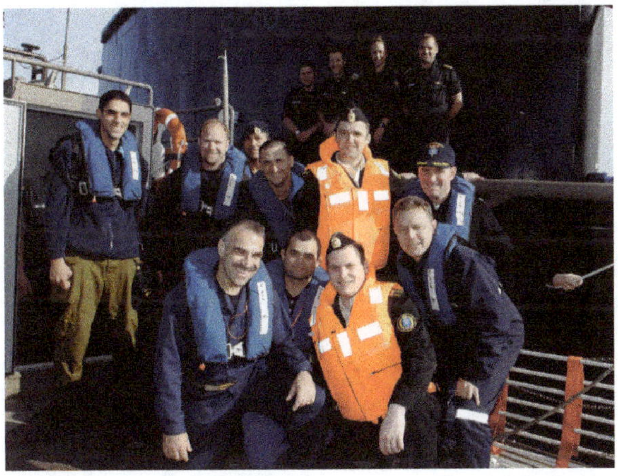

Figure 10. Ismerlo Operation Bold Monarch off the coast of Norway in the North Sea, 2008. The Russian rescue system AS34 has opened the hatch on the Norwegian submarine *Uthaug* and conducted the first transfer between a Russian escape system and a foreign submarine. Shown are multinational NATO and Russian sailor participants after successful mission accomplishment.

REFERENCES

1. Director of Ocean Engineering and Supervisor of Diving and Salvage letter. 2006 Feb 17. 06 Ser 00CM/0011.
2. Director of Ocean Engineering and Supervisor of Diving and Salvage letter. 2006 Feb 17. 06 Ser 00CM/0011.
3. Dituri J. Leading Navy diving into the 22nd century, NAVSEA Engineering Duty Officer technical paper. 2002. p. 15-6.
4. Harvey C, Carson J. The B.A.P. Pacocha (SS-48) collision: the escape and medical recompression treatment of survivors. The Naval Submarine Medical Research Laboratory: Naval Medical Research and Development Command; 1989 Mar 30. NSMRL Special Report SP89-1.
5. Higgins J. Use of the submarine rescue chamber and its umbilical to decompress a pressurized disabled submarine. 2000. p. 1-9. Ser 205/097.
6. USS *Squalus* (SS-192): the sinking, rescue of survivors, and subsequent salvage, 1939 [Internet]. Naval Historical Center; 2008 Sep. 9. Available from: http://www.history.navy.mil/faqs/faq99-1.htm

CHAPTER 43 CHAPTER

Dive Medicine

CHAPTER FORTY-THREE OVERVIEW

Introduction to Diving Medicine **1051**

Diving Physics **1051**

Boyle's Law 1052

Dalton's Law 1052

Henry's Law 1052

Diving Apparatus **1052**

Self-Contained Underwater Breathing Apparatus 1053

Surface-Supplied Underwater Breathing Apparatus 1053

Abnormal Gases **1054**

Hypoxia 1054

Hypercapnia (CO_2 Toxicity) 1054

Nitrogen Narcosis 1055

Carbon Monoxide Poisoning 1055

Hyperventilation 1056

Oxygen Toxicity 1056

High-Pressure Neurological Syndrome 1057

Breath-Hold Diving **1058**

Drowning **1060**

Decompression Sickness and Arterial Gas Embolism **1062**

Decompression Sickness 1062

Arterial Gas Embolism 1062

Barotrauma **1063**

Pulmonary Barotrauma 1063

Pneumothorax 1064

Mediastinal Emphysema 1064

Subcutaneous Emphysema 1064

Arterial Gas Embolism 1064

Nonpulmonary Barotrauma **1065**

External-Ear Barotrauma 1065

Middle-Ear Barotrauma 1065

Facial Baroparesis 1066

Middle-Ear Oxygen Absorption Syndrome 1066
Inner-Ear Barotrauma 1067
Sinus Barotrauma 1068
Barodontalgia 1068
Mask Barotrauma 1068
Skin Barotrauma 1068
Thoracic Barotrauma 1068
Gastrointestinal Barotrauma 1068
Pregnancy and Diving 1069
Diving in the Elderly 1070
Long-Term Physiological Effects 1071
Medications 1073
Antihistamines 1073
Decongestants 1073
Anti-Motion Sickness 1074
Analgesics/Anti-Inflammatories 1074
Diving Hazards 1074
Human Factors 1075
Altitude 1076
Flying after Diving 1078
Saturation Diving 1079
Conclusion 1081
Disclaimer 1081
References 1082

Dive Medicine

Terrance L. Leighton III, Jonathan E. Strain

INTRODUCTION TO DIVING MEDICINE

Humans have been exploring the sea for thousands of years, and, although the undersea environment is generally inhospitable to humans, it has not deterred humanity from exploring the mysteries of the deep. In ancient times, free diving was the only means by which the hidden treasures of the sea were explored. Simple mechanical devices to aid in exploring underwater were described as far back as Aristotle, but the first modern diving bell was invented in the seventeenth century. As new techniques and equipment were developed, dives became deeper and longer. These dives to greater depths increased the stresses on the body and brought to light unique pathologies associated with diving, which led to the development of the field known as diving medicine.

Hyperbaric medicine and diving medicine are intimately associated with each other, and the hyperbaric medical practitioner should have an understanding of diving medicine and diving-related injuries. The environment of the hyperbaric chamber and the undersea environment place similar physiologic challenges on the body. In addition, the most significant diving-related injuries are treated with hyperbaric chambers.

Diving is performed in military, commercial, and recreational settings. Recreational sport diving has become increasingly popular, and with the demand for pushing the limits, the complex systems in use by military and commercial divers have become increasingly available for recreational use. The distinctions between professional and recreational diving are disappearing and will likely continue to do so. Understanding the unique pathologies associated with diving requires an understanding of the kinds of underwater breathing apparatus (UBA) in use, the undersea environment, the physiologic challenges associated with changes in ambient pressure, the challenges associated with breathing air at increased pressure, and the challenges of breathing gas mediums of different compositions than atmospheric air.

DIVING PHYSICS

To understand diving medicine and diving-related injuries, one must have a basic knowledge and appreciation of the physics involved with diving. While there are many important laws that govern the way the human body interacts with the undersea environment, there are a few that are of particular importance in understanding the development of diving pathologies; these explain the reasons that most diving injuries occur. The physical laws that govern chamber operations also apply to diving. These laws are discussed at length elsewhere but are briefly explained as follows.

Boyle's Law

Sir Robert Boyle is credited with defining the relationship between the pressure and volume of a gas at a constant temperature. Boyle's law states that at a constant temperature, the volume of a gas is inversely proportional to the pressure. In other words, as pressure increases volume decreases and vice versa. Gas volume is reduced to 1/2 of the original volume when the absolute pressure is doubled. The changing pressures exerted on the gas-filled spaces of the body while diving lead to changes in the volume of the gas within those spaces. If these spaces are not equalized with the surrounding environment through proper venting, damage to the tissue will occur. Based on Boyle's law, a relative volume change from 2 to 3 atmospheres absolute (ATA) (33–66 feet seawater [fsw]) is less than the change from 1 to 2 ATA (surface to 33 fsw); thus, for a given change in depth, the gas volume change is greater when closer to the surface.[7] This means that the risk of injury to the body from changes in gas volume (barotrauma) is greatest with changes in depth closer to the surface. Boyle's law is applicable to diving medicine in the following: pulmonary overinflation syndromes, squeeze injuries, air consumption, and the minimum manifold pressure required to overcome the pressure of water on air hoses in surface-supplied diving.

Dalton's Law

An English chemist named John Dalton described the relationship of the pressures of various gases in mixtures. Dalton's law of partial pressures states that, in a mixture of nonreacting gases, the total pressure exerted by the gas is equal to the sum of the partial pressures of the individual gases. The partial pressure of a gas equals the product of ATA and percentage of the gas being used (PP = ATA x % gas). In other words, as the depth of a dive increases (and the ATA is also increasing), the partial pressure of each gas in the breathing medium is increased as well. This can become problematic, as some gases are not toxic at 1 ATA where we normally live but can become toxic at increased partial pressures. Therefore, the application of Dalton's law to diving medicine is primarily related to gas toxicities at depth.

Henry's Law

William Henry was an English chemist and contemporary of John Dalton. He described the relationship between the partial pressure of a gas and the amount of that gas that dissolves in a liquid. His law states that at a constant temperature, the amount of a given gas dissolved in a given type and volume of liquid is directly proportional to the partial pressure of that gas in equilibrium with that liquid. In other words, as a gas comes in contact with a solution, the amount that will dissolve into that solution is dependent on the partial pressure of the gas (if the temperature remains constant). As dives increase in depth, the partial pressure of the gases in the breathing medium increases as well. This escalation of partial pressures increases the gas load that each tissue must bear. The converse is also true: as the depth decreases on ascent (and thus the partial pressure of each gas decreases), it will come out of solution. If this is done too quickly, the tissues are not able to handle the gas load, and injury occurs. The applicability of Henry's law to diving medicine is primarily related to understanding inert gas absorption, decompression sickness (DCS), and the development of dive tables.

DIVING APPARATUS

There are many different diving systems in use, and they all follow a few basic principles. The two overarching types of diving systems are (1) self-contained underwater breathing apparatus (SCUBA), where the diver's air supply is carried on his or her person, and (2) surface-supplied underwater breathing apparatus, where the diver's breathing medium comes from the surface to the diver via a hose attached to the diver. The former is used in recreational, commercial, and military diving, while the latter is most often seen with commercial and military diving.

Self-Contained Underwater Breathing Apparatus

The most common type of underwater breathing apparatus in use is the self-contained underwater breathing apparatus, or SCUBA, systems. There are two types of SCUBA systems: open-circuit and closed-circuit.

Open-circuit SCUBA systems consist of demand regulator assembly, air cylinders, cylinder valve, manifold assembly, and backpack or harness. The demand regulator assembly is a dual-stage system that allows air to flow from the air tank through a hose to the diver. The first stage of the regulator serves as a pressure reducer to decrease the highly compressed air in the air tank (usually around 3,000 PSI [pounds per square inch]) to a predetermined level over ambient pressure. Upon inhalation from the mouthpiece of the second-stage regulator, a diaphragm opens, and the pressure of the air is further reduced to the pressure of the surrounding environment and the diver's lungs. Exhaled air is transmitted through an exhaust system on the second-stage regulator and is discharged into the surrounding water. There are a variety of tank systems, manifold assemblies, and harnesses in use.

Closed-circuit SCUBA systems, or oxygen rebreathers, use a tank with 100% oxygen. The oxygen is supplied to a breathing bag that supplies oxygen to the diver. The exhaled gas is cycled through a "scrubbing system" that removes carbon dioxide, and the oxygen is recycled to the diver. The carbon dioxide reacts with the calcium hydroxide in the scrubber and forms calcium carbonate, which is retained in the absorber unit. Closed-circuit systems significantly reduce the volume of gas required for a dive. Another key benefit for military special operations is that they do not produce bubbles. This allows special operators to work underwater covertly and unbeknownst to enemy forces on the surface.

Surface-Supplied Underwater Breathing Apparatus

All SCUBA dives are limited by the amount of breathing medium available to the diver. Surface-supplied underwater breathing systems provide an almost unlimited supply of breathing gas. In addition, they allow for communication between the diver and the surface. This direct line from the topside to the diver also allows for potential removal of a diver if underwater catastrophe develops.

There are different surface-supplied UBA in use. Regardless of the equipment in use, the diver's air supply comes from an air compressor, a bank of high-pressure air flasks, or a combination of both. The gas must be supplied at sufficient pressure to overcome the hydrostatic pressure at the depth of the diver and the decline in pressure as the air flows through the hoses and valves of the system. In addition to the breathing hose, a communication cable is available for voice communications from diver to diver or diver to topside. Line-pull signals have also been developed in the event that voice communication is lost. While the direct connection with the surface provides many advantages, special care must be taken with surface-supplied diving as this also means that the danger of a fouled or entangled line is always present.

ABNORMAL GASES

Human life is uniquely suited to be supported by atmospheric air. Being underwater requires one to breathe atmospheric air at higher partial pressures or breathe gas mixtures different from air. Both expose the body to unique stressors and provide an opportunity for uncommon pathology. The symptom complexes that arise from the breathing or accumulation of nonphysiologic gases may have similar presentation. The dive profile, the UBA being used, and the timing of presentation all help elucidate the underlying pathophysiology.

Hypoxia

Oxygen is essential to sustain life. It is the means by which cellular aerobic metabolism is sustained due to its role as the final electron acceptor in the electron transport system. Without this, efficient production of the cellular energy currency, adenosine triphosphate (ATP), cannot be maintained. Hypoxia is defined as oxygen deficiency, and the diving environment places the diver at risk of this for many reasons. Oxygen debt may occur due to an interruption in gas supply, loss of gas, or contamination of gas. Symptoms of hypoxia usually begin when the pO_2 is less than 0.16 ATA. Symptom onset is often sudden, and the first sign that a diver's oxygen supply has been compromised may be an unresponsive diver. Other symptoms include lack of concentration, lack of muscle control, drowsiness, weakness, agitation, and/or euphoria. If such symptoms occur, the cornerstone of treatment is to reestablish sufficient oxygen to the diver. If the diver is in the water, then shifting to an alternate gas source is required. Once the diver is on the surface, 100% oxygen should be administered.

Hypercapnia (CO_2 Toxicity)

Hypercapnia may be encountered in the diving environment. Like hypoxia, the first indication of hypercapnia may be an unconscious diver. Other symptoms include headache, dizziness, shortness of breath, decreased work tolerance, rapid pulse, burning eyes, and confusion. Treatment involves lowering the inspired CO_2 or increasing alveolar ventilation. This is done by increasing helmet ventilation, decreasing exertion, shifting to an alternate breathing source, or aborting the dive if faulty equipment is suspected.

Buildup of carbon dioxide can be encountered for many reasons, but each instance can be broken down into two primary mechanisms: 1) excess carbon dioxide in inspired gas and 2) decreased alveolar ventilation. These can be present individually or simultaneously.

The most likely reason for excess CO_2 in inspired gas is contamination or inadequate ventilation of the UBA. The rebreathing apparatus in use by military special forces (and increasingly by recreational divers) relies on a CO_2 absorbent to remove exhaled CO_2. Equipment failure or exhaustion of the absorbent leads to reinhalation of expired CO_2 and subsequent CO_2 toxicity.

Decreased alveolar ventilation is often the result of increased resistance to breathing at depth. There are several causes of increased resistance, as the dense gas must flow through an extensive pathway where resistance is potentially increased including valves, hoses, regulators, and the diver's own airway.

There are other factors that lead to increased total body CO_2 while diving. The increased partial pressure of inspired oxygen suppresses respiratory drive, further increasing the body's CO_2 load. The increased work associated with diving leads to increased production of CO_2, and novice divers may be tempted to "skip breaths" in order to conserve air supply, which also leads to buildup of CO_2.

Hypercapnia, although potentially fatal by itself, also increases the risks of nitrogen narcosis, DCS, and O_2 toxicity.

Nitrogen Narcosis

Breathing inert gases at increased partial pressures can lead to a state of stupor or "narcosis." The most common form of this is due to nitrogen gas and is known as nitrogen narcosis. While at the time the etiology was not known, the effects of what is now known as inert gas narcosis were described as early as 1826 by a French physician named Colladon.[16] After descending in a diving bell to 20 meters, he described "a state of excitement as if I had drunk some alcoholic liquor."

Typically, symptoms of nitrogen narcosis are first noticed at around 100 fsw. The severity increases with depth and rate of descent. Symptoms include loss of judgment, a false sense of well-being, lack of concern for safety, apparent stupidity, or inappropriate laughter. In addition, numbness or tingling of the lips, gums, and legs may be noticed. The symptom complex is associated with decreased intellectual abilities more than psychomotor or manual abilities.

The treatment of nitrogen narcosis is aimed at lowering nitrogen partial pressure, which is done by ascending in the water column. Divers may also be able to develop tolerance to the affects through repetition and "self-control." Fatigue, hypercapnia, hypothermia, and rapid descent increase one's risk of developing nitrogen narcosis. Gas mixtures using other inert gases such as helium have been developed to combat the difficulties associated with breathing nitrogen at depth.

The mechanism of nitrogen narcosis is likely multifactorial and includes the hypothesis of both physical changes in lipid-rich membranes of neurons and also biochemical mechanisms. The Meyer-Overton hypothesis suggests that the more lipid soluble an inhaled substance is, the more narcotic effects it will have.[16] This may be due to swelling of the lipid-rich membranes of neurons as gas is solubilized within them. The swelling of the membrane leads to alterations in cell surface proteins and affects ion channel function.

There is also evidence to suggest that inert gases may bind to hydrophobic pockets within proteins, changing their activity, which may also play a role in nitrogen narcosis. Protein kinase C, guanine nucleotide-binding proteins, GABA alpha, and ligand-gated ion channels on sensory and motor neurons have all been suggested as targets for narcotic agents, which will lead to narcosis symptoms.[16]

Carbon Monoxide Poisoning

Carbon monoxide comes from the incomplete combustion of hydrocarbons, often from internal combustion engines, fire, or tobacco smoke. The gas supply to a diver may become contaminated with carbon monoxide (CO) leading to CO poisoning. The symptoms of CO poisoning can be mild with headache, nausea, or vomiting. Severe symptoms may also develop including mental status changes, neurologic symptoms, and loss of consciousness.

Carbon monoxide displaces oxygen from hemoglobin, creating carboxyhemoglobin, and shifts the oxygen dissociation curve to the left. This becomes problematic as oxygen delivery to tissue fails leading to hypoxia.

The onset of symptoms associated with CO buildup in the body is different in the diving environment due to the increased pressures of both oxygen and carbon monoxide. The partial pressures of both oxygen and carbon monoxide increase linearly with depth and would be expected to offset the effects of each other in a way that would lead to similar effects as those seen on the surface.

However, the increased partial pressure of oxygen at depth allows for continued delivery of oxygen to tissue at a rate sufficient to overcome the effects of reduced usable hemoglobin, delaying the onset of hypoxia. Depending on the level of CO contamination, symptoms may appear at depth. However, more commonly, symptoms manifest during ascent or on the surface as the protective effect of increased oxygen partial pressure is lost.[10]

The initial treatment is to remove the source of the carbon monoxide. If symptoms are mild, they can be treated with 100% oxygen on the surface. If severe, they may require hyperbaric treatment.

Hyperventilation

Hyperventilation is defined as rapid breathing in excess of metabolic requirements. This may be seen more commonly in novice divers who are more prone to anxiety and who are still gaining familiarity with the undersea environment. Its physical manifestations are due to the lowering of carbon dioxide in the blood. Symptoms include dizziness, twitching or tingling of the extremities, and spasm of the small muscles of the hands and feet. The symptoms can be mistaken for oxygen toxicity. A thorough history and exam will usually distinguish the two entities. The spasms of the small muscles of the hands and feet also point to a diagnosis of hyperventilation, as these are not seen in oxygen toxicity. The treatment is to slow down the breathing rate. With direction and reassurance, the condition corrects itself.

Oxygen Toxicity

Oxygen (O_2) is a requirement to sustain human life as it acts as the final electron acceptor in the electron transport chain creating energy in the form of ATP. If oxygen is supplied in excess of the body's need, buildup of reactive oxygen species (ROS) can overcome the body's antioxidant mechanisms. This becomes toxic to the organism as the increased generation of oxygen free radicals leads to a breakdown in normal cellular function and, ultimately, cell death. The potential for oxygen toxicity in diving is due to prolonged exposure of the body to oxygen at higher pressure than is experienced on the surface. The primary toxicities associated with diving are central nervous system toxicity, pulmonary toxicity, and ocular toxicity. The cornerstone of treatment is to decrease the diver's exposure to high-pressure oxygen to prevent further insult and treat the pathology that has developed.

Central nervous system O_2 toxicity has the greatest potential to lead to catastrophe in the water due to the possibility of developing seizures, which may lead to drowning. The primary risk factor for central nervous system (CNS) O_2 toxicity is prolonged exposure to high pO_2. Other risk factors include presence of inert gas in the breathing medium, hypercapnia, immersion (more likely in the water than in a chamber), and darkness. Increased metabolic rate, often due to exercise, cold water immersion, and increased sympathetic nervous system activity are also risk factors. The symptoms of CNS O_2 toxicity are often remembered with a pneumonic: VENTIDC (**V**ision, **E**ars, **N**ausea, **T**witching, **I**rritability, **D**izziness, and **C**onvulsions). Decreased peripheral vision or blurry vision may be an indication of CNS O_2 toxicity. The diver may also experience tinnitus and nausea and vomiting. Twitching or tingling of the face, lips, eyes, and extremities may develop and are fairly specific to oxygen toxicity. The diver may become irritable, confused, agitated, or anxious. Dizziness may develop, leading to loss of coordination and fatigue. Convulsions are the most serious manifestation and may be the first sign that reactive oxygen species have overwhelmed the body's antioxidant defense mechanisms.

There is current research and early development of a watch designed to detect changes of oxygen toxicity that would alert a diver of the impending overload of antioxidant mechanisms and prevent development of life-threatening convulsions.

Pulmonary oxygen toxicity is divided into two distinct entities: moderate pO_2 toxicity and high pO_2 toxicity. Histopathological analysis of lung tissue in both cases shows two distinct patterns.[17] Moderate pO_2 injury is a diffuse injury mediated primarily by an inflammatory response. Edema and destruction of the alveolar-capillary barrier are seen. It is typically seen with pO_2 of less than 1.5 ATA. High pO_2 injury seems to be a CNS-mediated injury potentiated by nitric oxide derived from neuronal nitric oxide synthase. It is characterized by epithelial damage of cells in the alveolar spaces.[17]

Regardless of the type of pressures leading to pulmonary O_2 toxicity, the symptoms are similar. Divers may experience a sensation of a "tickle" in their throats, hoarseness, inspiratory burning, cough, chest tightness, and dyspnea. The clinical manifestations may or may not be accompanied by decreases in pulmonary function indices (FEV1, FVC, FEF25-75, peak flow, and DLCO). As might be expected, the higher the pO_2 and the longer the exposure time, the greater the chance of developing symptoms. There is a wide degree of variation among divers in regard to propensity for pulmonary O_2 toxicity and the degree of symptom development. Symptoms may manifest quickly or may not become apparent for up to three days. The symptoms may resolve within hours, or they may take several days. Most signs and symptoms are self-limiting; however, permanent damage may occur.

The eye is another known target of hyperbaric oxygen. There are four primary ocular pathologies that may develop from nonphysiologic exposure to oxygen: neuritis, cataracts, hyperoxic myopia, and retinopathy of prematurity. Neuritis is associated with high pO_2 and is characterized by temporary loss of peripheral vision. Cataracts development is seen in prolonged treatments with hyperbaric therapy and is usually not associated with diving. The incidence of hyperoxic myopia increases with increasing exposure to hyperbaric oxygen. It is characterized by changes in the refractive index of the lens and is usually self-reversing. It may be more common in divers with preexisting presbyopia. Retinopathy of prematurity (formerly known as retrolental fibroplasia) is not typically associated with diving and diving injury. As the name suggests, it is seen in premature infants who are receiving supplemental oxygen. The retinal vasculature is constricted, leading to endothelial cell destruction, loss of retinal circulation, and disorganized cell proliferation and fibrous growth.[5,66] This can ultimately lead to retinal detachment and permanent blindness.[5]

It is important to note that not all changes in vision after diving are due to oxygen toxicity. While it is important to consider oxygen toxicity and more sinister etiologies, some symptoms may be due to accommodative fatigue or dry eyes. These may be due to the sustained visual effort required in the undersea environment or from air flowing through a full-face mask, respectively.

High-Pressure Neurological Syndrome

Due to the depth-limiting effects of nitrogen narcosis, breathing mixtures were developed using other inert gases whose narcotics effects were much less due to their lower lipid solubility. Helium was first used, and this allowed divers to explore depths not previously attained. However, this development led to another problem associated with breathing nonphysiologic gases at high pressures, a syndrome that came to be known as high-pressure neurological syndrome (HPNS).

This is usually encountered in long saturation dives at pressures exceeding 15 atm.[40] The signs and symptoms of HPNS are due to a state of hyperexcitability and consist of tremor, severe myoclonic jerks, fatigue, imbalance, nausea, dizziness, somnolence, and potentially convulsions.[40] The tremor of the extremities is at a frequency of 8–12 Hz, which is sometimes referred to as a "helium tremor."[60] The development of HPNS is directly related to the rate of compression and the depths attained. Faster compression to greater depth leads to more severe signs and symptoms of HPNS. The treatment for such is decreasing the compression rate. Prevention of symptoms is obtained by extremely slow compression rates. In addition, some prolonged stages at a constant pressure allow for adaptation and reduction/prevention of HPNS symptoms. Due to some similarities in symptomatology with the serotonin syndrome, some have suggested a role of 5-HT1A receptor antagonists in the future.[40] This requires further investigation.

The pathophysiology of HPNS is complex, but it is generally felt that it is a direct compression effect of high ambient pressures on the lipid components of the neurons. The high pressure causes compression and alterations in cellular function and signaling. This is in contrast to the effects of nitrogen, which causes swelling of the lipid membranes due to its solubility. This theory has led to the development of alternative breathing mixtures to minimize these effects. These mixtures (trimix, etc.) minimize HPNS by "swelling the membranes" with nitrogen to counteract the compression of the lipid membranes. High pressure has also been shown to increase neuronal excitability and augment the synaptic responses of some subtypes of the N-methyl-D-aspartate receptor (NMDAR).[50]

There does seem to be some inter-diver variability in susceptibility to HPNS. In addition to selecting the least susceptible divers, other means of minimizing HPNS are prolonged rates of compression, stages of constant pressure for adaptation, and allowing time for adaptation once the desired depth is reached before starting work.[40]

BREATH-HOLD DIVING

The closing of our foramen ovale results in humans always having to hold their breath when submersing themselves. The breath hold is the limiting factor when under water as one has a limited space to store oxygen in each breath. As we breathe in and fill our lungs, the oxygen-carbon dioxide (CO_2) exchange begins. The rate at which oxygen is consumed varies, and, as a result, due to the limited oxygen supply, time submersed is also a variable. Breath holding leads to oxygen consumption and CO_2 buildup. CO_2 first accumulates in the lungs and the blood, and then after approximately a minute the gas starts to be stored in the muscles and viscera. This accumulation is what all breath-hold divers battle as it is what triggers the hypercapnic respiratory drive. As the point of hypoxia is reached, the risk of unconsciousness is increased, exponentially increasing the risk of drowning and death.

Hyperventilation effectively decreases the body's CO_2 levels, which leads to an increased time required to reach the point triggering the hypercapnic respiratory drive. This allows for longer breath-hold times but also is quite dangerous because the subsequent decrease in CO_2 from hyperventilation is not accompanied by an increase in O_2. As a result, the delayed response for the urge to breathe is met with potential hypoxia and unconsciousness.

During descent, water pressure increases, and the lung capacity responds inversely. As a result, the alveolar partial pressure of oxygen dissolved in the blood (PaO_2) is increased, which allows for the diver to use more of the stored oxygen in the lungs and prolong breath-hold dives. Unfortunately, there is a debt to be paid; as a diver ascends, the ambient pressure decreases and with it so does the lungs' PaO_2. This leads to a risk of hypoxia and potential unconsciousness.[31]

Any time divers immerse themselves, the body begins to react in a manner of increased metabolic activity. This primarily is the result of cooler water temperature and the increased hydrostatic pressure. The pressure changes affect the lungs' capacity and diffusion rates; meanwhile, the increased metabolic activity increases the oxygen consumption, leading to a shorter time period before the body reaches its hypoxic breaking point.

Immersion, pressure change, and breath holding are all factors that the body can adapt to, but there is a breaking point, and with that the danger arises. Air trapping in combination with pressure change on ascent can lead to pulmonary overdistension and possible rupture, which can result in a pneumothorax, pneumomediastinum, and/or arterial gas embolism.

In addition to the pulmonary aspects, it is essential to evaluate and discuss the cardiovascular effects of breath-hold diving, as there is no other way to get the oxygen to the body and the CO_2 out. Paul Bert, a French physiologist, first documented the heart's natural response to breath-hold diving in 1870. He noted "diving bradycardia" in ducks, which is a vagal-mediated reflex that is also accompanied by peripheral vasoconstriction, a reduction in cardiac output, and maintenance of arterial blood pressure. This response was then expanded on by Irving and colleagues in 1935 who suggested that this reflex/response is to conserve the limited oxygen supply for the vital organs that are more sensitive to ischemia, i.e., the brain and the heart. As a result of this conservation, the peripheral vasoconstriction greatly reduces the blood flow to the ischemia-resistant organs (muscles, skin, and viscera). This in turn leads to an anaerobic metabolism and the accumulation of lactic acid.[9]

Arrhythmias are a very common side effect of the human diving response. Per Bove and Davis, factors that contribute to the development of arrhythmias are high vagal tone, heart distension from blood redistribution into the chest secondary to immersion and the drop in intrathoracic pressure, apneic face immersion in cold water, and subendocardial ischemia from the large increase in blood pressure. Diving bradycardia is seen with long, deep dives, while tachycardia is often noted in divers just prior to diving. This tachycardia is thought to be driven by the pulmonary stretch receptors, which are stimulated with deep inspiration. Pre-dive hyperventilation and anxiety may also have roles in the tachycardia. During cold-water dives, arrhythmias have been found to be more prevalent and are not limited to vagal tone inhibition but have also been documented to be premature in character.[8]

Elevated blood pressure is a natural human diving response with recorded systolic pressures reaching up to 345 mmHg in elite breath-holds divers per Ferrigno and colleagues. This is likely due to the baroreceptor stimulation and the natural vasoconstriction in the human diving response.[25] As a result, it is essential to advise individuals with hypertension of the risks that are associated with their condition and diving.

In 2005, Divers Alert Network (DAN) fatality surveillance data reveals that cardiac conditions are the number two cause of death, second only to drowning in the United States and Canadian recreational diving. Approximately 80% of fatalities were in people 40 years or older, and, for those whose medical history was available, hypertension and heart disease were the most common conditions reported.[20] The Recreational Scuba Training Council, Undersea and Hyperbaric Medical Society (UHMS), and DAN recommend that divers over the age of 40 undergo risk assessment for coronary artery disease. Exercise stress testing may be recommended for asymptomatic divers with multiple cardiac risk factors.[20,30,45] Routine screening would not be advised for young, low-risk divers because of the low positive predictive value of exercise stress testing in these individuals.[45]

As the lungs and heart are affected by breath-hold diving, the consequences of such have neurological ramifications. Consciousness is essential at all times while under water. When the brain becomes deprived of oxygen or overwhelmed by CO_2, the natural response is unconsciousness, which exponentially increases the risk of death.

The ears and sinuses are highly susceptible to barotrauma in breath-hold dives, particularly due to repeat exposure to rapid pressure changes. In modern, record-breaking, assisted breath-hold dives, individuals can descend rapidly. Because all humans must come back to the surface for air, ascent at rapid rates is also essential. While deep dives have a large pressure differential, it's actually the shallower breath-hold dives with multiple changes in direction and pressure variability that greatly put the middle ear and sinuses at risk of barotrauma.

DROWNING

Drowning is responsible for approximately 7,000 deaths in the United States alone every year.[2,61] There are a multitude of causes found throughout all ages, races, and in both sexes. In the United States, males are five times more likely than females to die by drowning and blacks twice as often as whites.[19] An unfortunate reality is that drowning is often directly associated with alcohol. This can be the result of boating accidents, overconfidence, decreased motor function, or sheer incoherence putting individuals in harm's way and increasing the likelihood of fatality.

Another common cause of drowning is with individuals who are attempting to rescue others who are/appear to be drowning. The panic that ensues in an individual who is struggling and fighting for his or her life in the water becomes overwhelming to the rescuer. This survival instinct will often lead to the death of the victim and the rescuer.

Drowning while diving is uncommon; however, it is a concern that must be considered before every dive. Scuba-related drownings are most commonly associated with entanglement, running out of air, toxic gas mixes, or cave diving.[12]

There is strong evidence that intentional hyperventilation before breath-hold diving greatly increases an individual's risk of death via drowning. This is due to the reduced partial pressure of arterial CO_2 ($PaCO_2$) to the point where an individual's breath-hold breaking point is prolonged beyond an individual's hypoxia breaking point. When the breath-hold breaking point surpasses the hypoxia breaking point, unconsciousness and best-case-scenario near-drowning are the result with death via drowning looming as a more probable outcome.

A common misconception is that drowning is secondary to immersion and fluid-filled lungs and that death results from aspiration. Instead, drowning is the result of hypoxemia, and aspiration is irrelevant. It's the hypoxemia that leads to unconsciousness, and unconsciousness in combination with immersion results in death.

Now with the underlying cause of drowning being hypoxemia, aspiration does play a large role in the event of near-drowning. After removal from the water, the presence of fluid in the lungs plays a large role in the rates of morbidity and mortality. The fluid medium also matters. The fluid medium compounds not in matter of increased complications but in the manner that those complications occur. Saltwater aspiration leads to fluid transudation across the alveolar membrane secondary to the hyperosmotic nature of saltwater. The excess fluid leads to less ventilation and a prolonged hypoxemia, even after one is pulled out of the water. On the other hand, freshwater is hypothesized to rinse the alveoli, which results in surfactant removal and alveolar collapse. Collapsed alveoli are unable to appropriately ventilate, leading to a low ventilation/perfusion ratio and hypoxemia.(12)

When a near-drowning victim is recovered and presents to the emergency department, a range of respiratory complications can occur, including severe pulmonary edema and acute respiratory distress syndrome (ARDS) requiring positive end-expiratory pressure (PEEP). In regards to PEEP, only modest amounts are necessary to achieve and maintain adequate oxygenation. Although PEEP does not alter the course of the underlying pulmonary injury, it allows for adequate oxygenation while the lungs are recovering. This usually takes approximately 48 to 72 hours post immersion injury.(13)

In addition, pneumonia is common with aspiration. Chest X-ray in these individuals is likely to show patchy infiltrates, most commonly in the periphery.(27,34,52,59)

The role of antibiotics in the treatment of near-drowning victims has been a point of debate. Per KW. Kizer,(38) near-drowning victims who aspirate ocean water or swimming pool water generally do not need antibiotics, except in the setting of fever, new pulmonary infiltrates, or purulent secretions. In fact, it has been determined that most pulmonary infections in near-drowning victims are hospital acquired.(48)

Near-drowning victims may suffer a myriad of complications resulting from hypoxemia and hypercapnia. The hypercapnia is a result of decreased ventilation and increased CO_2 production. Concurrently, an increased level of lactic acid is produced from inadequate oxygen supplies, which leads to a decrease in pH. The severity of acidity has been found to be a predictor of renal insufficiency and subsequent renal failure. Additional complications found in near-drowning victims are pneumonia, hemoglobinuria, diffuse intravascular coagulation, acute tubular necrosis, albuminuria, and rhabdomyolysis.(11)

It has been found that the greatest cause of death in male SCUBA divers over the age of 45 is cardiac related. Cardiac risk factors that increase the likelihood of a cardiac event on land can be exacerbated underwater, and, as a result, when a cardiac arrest occurs underwater, resuscitative measures by bystanders, like CPR, respond moderately well. Sinus tachycardia is the most common rhythm seen in victims and is secondary to hypoxemia and acidosis.(37,56)

Per Hoff, Putman, and Causey, et al.,(15,33,58) the patient's clinical status should be the basis for the decision to admit a near-drowning victim to a hospital. Criteria for admission include significant respiratory symptoms, an abnormal-appearing chest X-ray, significant abnormal arterial blood gas (ABG), or the need for supplemental oxygen or ventilator support. It has been determined that pulmonary damage is usually evident within a few hours of the initial event, and therefore a patient who remains asymptomatic can safely be sent home.

At the end of all evaluations, the prognosis remains speculative. Certain factors increase likelihood of full recovery, but inevitably a response to a near-drowning event will be based on an array of factors. Recovery prognosis greatly relies on the length of anoxic period and the duration of immersion. As the time period of hypoxemia lengthens, secondary damage neurologically is increased exponentially. Per J. Orlowski(54) a poor outcome is anticipated after immersion reaches and exceeds five minutes. If an individual arrives to the emergency department neurologically intact, a very positive outcome is to be expected, as it has been mentioned previously that the lungs can recover within 48 to 72 hrs.

Cardiac arrest, on the other hand, can go in one of two ways. If an individual suffers from cardiac arrest while diving and positively responds to initial CPR dive side, the prognosis is great, but if the individual does not respond well to CPR initially, a poor prognosis can be anticipated as is the case in most cardiac cases, diving or otherwise.

DECOMPRESSION SICKNESS AND ARTERIAL GAS EMBOLISM

Decompression sickness (DCS) and arterial gas embolism (AGE) are two of the most deadly forms of diving-related injuries.

Decompression Sickness

DCS is an injury related to bubble formation from excess dissolved gas when ambient pressure is reduced (decompression). Based on Henry's law, inert gas in breathing mediums is dissolved in tissues as divers spend time under pressure. The amount of inert gas dissolved is based on the depth and length of the dive. Longer, deeper dives result in increasing whole-body inert gas load until saturation occurs. On ascent, decompression occurs, and, based on Henry's law, the dissolved inert gas comes out of tissues.(29) This can lead to the formation of intravascular and extravascular bubbles. During the decompression phase of a dive, the rate must be controlled and done in a fashion that allows the body to "off-gas" or "decompress." If done appropriately, the gas bubbles are filtered by the lungs, and the gas is exhaled. If done incorrectly, the gas load becomes too great, and decompression sickness develops. These bubbles can lead to mechanical compression of tissue, causing damage to the endothelium. This results in capillary leak, extravasation of plasma, and impairment of endothelial function. In addition, the bubbles can act as a foreign body and evoke a strong inflammatory response.

DCS classification was developed by Golding et al. in 1960(28) and is categorized into type 1 and type 2 based on the organ systems involved. Type 1 DCS is bubble formation that affects the musculoskeletal, cutaneous, and lymphatic system. Type 2 DCS affects the pulmonary, neurologic, and vestibular system. The mainstay of treatment is recompression in a hyperbaric chamber with controlled decompression. Type 1 DCS rarely becomes life threatening, and treatment may not even be pursued. Type 2 DCS is of greater concern due to the organ systems involved. It may become life threatening, and urgent recognition and treatment with recompression is necessary to prevent development of long-term sequelae. Type 2 DCS may manifest with paresthesia, cranial nerve deficits, hemiparesis, mental status changes, and/or respiratory symptoms that may rapidly progress to cardiopulmonary collapse, vertigo, and hearing loss.

Arterial Gas Embolism

AGE is a potentially deadly complication, usually from the development of a pulmonary overinflation syndrome (POIS) injury. In contrast to DCS, AGE is neither time nor depth dependent and may occur early in a dive and from very shallow depths.(29) POIS injuries are the result of rapid expansion of gas in the lungs, usually from rapid, uncontrolled ascents. This is based on Boyle's law and can lead to rupture of the alveoli and introduction of air into the pulmonary vasculature. This gas may proceed to the left side of the heart and subsequently be delivered to the systemic arterial vasculature. The symptom complex has wide variability and is dependent on the location these gas bubbles settle and prevent delivery of oxygen to the distal tissue. The most deadly scenario is if the gas bubbles lodge in the brain or cardiac vasculature, presenting as a stroke or myocardial infarction respectively. The treatment is recompression in a hyperbaric chamber while on supplemental oyygen as soon as possible.

Of note, the symptoms of neurologic DCS and AGE may at times be identical. While the treatment for both is recompression, an attempt to distinguish between the two should be made, as it may help elucidate concurrent underlying pathology or predilection to injury. The key feature to distinguish between AGE and neurologic DCS is timing of symptom onset relative to surfacing from a dive. Neurologic symptoms that appear within 10 minutes are considered to be from AGE, while those that appear after 10 minutes are considered to be neurologic DCS. In 1 study of 116 cases of AGE, 10 occurred during ascent, 97 occurred within 5 minutes of surfacing, and 9 occurred between 5 and 10 minutes.[43] There are at least 2 case reports of delayed-onset AGE occurring well after the 10-minute window;[32,40] therefore, neurological deficits, no matter the time frame, should be appropriately monitored and managed.

BAROTRAUMA

The U.S. Navy Diving Manual defines barotrauma as "damage to body tissues from the mechanical effects of pressure that result when the pressure differentials between body cavities and the hydrostatic pressure surrounding the body, or between the body and the diving equipment, are not equalized properly." Boyle's law states that for any gas at a constant temperature, the volume of the gas will vary inversely with the pressure. Diving exposes the body to pressures greater than the atmospheric pressures commonly encountered. The human body has many gas-filled spaces, and the increased hydrostatic pressure of the diving environment causes changes within these spaces in accordance with Boyle's law. If the pressure within these air-filled cavities is not equalized with the ambient pressure, barotrauma will occur. There are five requirements for barotrauma to occur. They are commonly remembered with the pneumonic GRAVE (**G**as-filled space, **R**igid walls, **A**mbient pressure change, **V**ascular-lined space, **E**nclosed space).

Pulmonary Barotrauma

Pulmonary barotrauma is an important subset of barotraumas and is the result of the inability of expanding gas to exit the lungs, which leads to increased alveolar pressure causing alveolar damage. In diving, this is usually the result of rapid or uncontrolled ascent. The rapid ascent leads to overinflation of the lungs, resulting in a type of diving injury known as pulmonary overinflation syndrome, or POIS. POIS is an umbrella term for four distinct manifestations with the same underlying etiology, pulmonary overinflation. The four comorbidities of POIS are pneumothorax, mediastinal emphysema, subcutaneous emphysema, and AGE.

As hydrostatic pressure is decreasing during ascent, the pressure of the gas within the body cavities is increasing in accordance with Boyle's law. If the rate of ascent is appropriately controlled, the air within the body cavities has time to "off-gas." However, if the rate is too rapid, appropriate equalization of spaces is not achieved, leading to a POIS injury. The alveoli rupture, and air enters the pulmonary interstitial spaces. This air can then move into the pleural space, mediastinum, subcutaneous space, or the pulmonary vasculature, leading to the myriad of symptoms associated with POIS.

Pneumothorax

As alveoli rupture, air contained within the lungs may extravasate and enter the pleural space, causing a pneumothorax. Symptoms associated with pneumothorax include chest pain (often pleuritic) and shortness of breath. Decreased breath sounds and hyperresonance to percussion are seen on exam. In patients who are clinically stable, observation may be appropriate. In some cases, needle decompression may be needed. If this fails, or if the patient is clinically unstable, then chest tube insertion may be required. It is important to note that if the patient is also suffering from arterial gas embolism and requires recompression, decompression of the pneumothorax with thoracostomy must be done prior to recompression. The reason for this is to prevent the potential development of a tension pneumothorax from a simple pneumothorax, which is possible during the ascent phase of recompression.

If a tension pneumothorax does occur, then subjectively the patient may complain of symptoms like chest pain, cough, and shortness of breath. Tachypnea, tachycardia, narrowed pulse pressure, asymmetric chest wall movement, tracheal deviation, and neck vein distension may be seen on exam. Immediate medical attention is needed, as patients are more clinically unstable due to the increased cardiovascular compromise. Treatment principles are similar to those of a simple pneumothorax; however, these are likely to require more emergent treatment and chest tube insertion.

Mediastinal Emphysema

Gas from alveolar rupture can dissect along the perivascular sheaths and enter the mediastinum, which is known as mediastinal emphysema. Symptoms may include substernal chest pain or burning and likely will be worsened by inspiration. On exam, a crunching sound that is synchronous with the heartbeat may be heard and is known as Hamman's sign. This distinct crunching is produced from the heart beating against air-filled tissue. Treatment is rarely required, as the air will over time be reabsorbed. If treatment is pursued, some recommend 100% surface oxygen or, for more severe symptoms, shallow recompression.

Subcutaneous Emphysema

As air from ruptured alveoli travels superiorly within the mediastinum, it may dissect into the subcutaneous space of the neck and supraclavicular area. Symptoms may be similar to those of mediastinal emphysema (chest pain, substernal burning) but may also include notable crepitus of the skin, sore throat, hoarseness, and dysphagia. Patients will often note a change in their voice as air impinges on the nerves supplying the larynx. Treatment is rarely required but may be pursued in the same fashion as treatment for mediastinal emphysema.

Arterial Gas Embolism

Arguably the most deadly sequelae from pulmonary barotrauma, arterial gas embolism occurs as air enters the pulmonary vasculature and is transported to the left atria via the pulmonary vein. It then travels through the systemic arterial circulation and becomes lodged in tissues, leading to ischemia, infarction, and the ensuing inflammatory cascade. This is discussed more extensively in Chapter 15: Gas Embolism. The presentation of an AGE is quick and dramatic. The central nervous system and the heart are the most commonly affected organs, and the symptoms are similar to what would be expected from stroke and myocardial infarction depending on location. Treatment is immediate recompression with oxygen supplementation. When treatment is initiated quickly, most victims achieve full recovery with no sequelae. However, few people may have residual neurologic signs or symptoms.

NONPULMONARY BAROTRAUMA

While pulmonary barotrauma is typically of greater concern due to its risk of more severe morbidity and mortality, there are many other forms of barotrauma that both divers and medical personnel should be aware of. The principles and underlying physics are the same as pulmonary barotrauma; if a vascular lined, enclosed, gas-filled space is subject to pressure change without proper venting, barotrauma will occur.

External-Ear Barotrauma

The external auditory canal serves as the conduit through which sound reaches the tympanic membrane. If obstructed, the requirements for barotrauma can be met as divers descend in the water column. Potential anatomic obstructions include cerumen impaction, otitis, and exostosis. Exostosis is common in divers due to the extensive history of aquatic activities, especially in cold water. This ear-canal exostosis is also known colloquially as "surfer's ear." While most lead to only a small narrowing of the canal, some can cause near complete occlusion and may require complete cessation of diving activity until surgically corrected.

There are also nonanatomic obstructions that prevent the air in the external ear canal from properly venting. These include things like earplugs and wet suit hoods.

The symptoms of external ear barotrauma include ear pain on descent, hearing loss, and hemorrhage in the ear canal. The primary means of treatment is to stop the descent and relieve the obstruction if it is amenable. An ascent in the water column may aid in one's effort as well. If otitis externa is present, it should be treated in accordance with treatment guidelines. Some divers prophylactically use a 2% acetic acid and aluminum acetate solution after diving in squalid conditions for the prevention of otitis externa.

Middle-Ear Barotrauma

The most common type of barotrauma experienced by divers is middle-ear barotrauma (MEB).[3,39] Normally the middle ear is a closed, vascular lined space and thus subject to pressure change. The normal means by which the middle ear remains at an equal pressure with the surrounding environment is through the opening of the eustachian tube. During descent in the water column, the increasing pressure of the surrounding water leads to a "middle-ear squeeze." The diver can prevent this squeeze and resultant trauma with an effective Valsalva maneuver, which is a manual, intentional opening of the eustachian tube allowing for equalization of pressure. If a diver is suffering from eustachian tube dysfunction, he or she likely will be unable to equalize and will subsequently develop middle-ear barotrauma.

There are numerous etiologies for eustachian tube dysfunction including otitis media, mastoiditis, seasonal allergies, upper respiratory infections, large adenoids/tonsils, and nasal septum deviation.

The most notable initial symptom of middle-ear barotrauma is ear pain during descent. If descent is stopped immediately, the diver may ascend a few feet and perform an effective Valsalva. If descent is not stopped, and MEB occurs, divers may experience transient conductive hearing loss, vertigo, and tinnitus. In severe cases, tympanic membrane (TM) perforation may occur and is often described as severe pain followed by instant relief upon rupture. An additional sign may be blood in the face mask as a diver surfaces. This is because bleeding from tissue disruption travels through the nasopharyngeal passages and is trapped in the mask.

Treatment of MEB consists of cessation of diving activity until all signs and symptoms have resolved. The clinician must also monitor for signs of infection and treat appropriately. If the tympanic membrane has perforated, complete healing prior to continuation of diving is a must and usually occurs spontaneously within a couple of weeks.

A U.S. Navy submarine medical officer in World War II named Wallace Teed developed a classification system for MEB, known as the TEED scale. The degree of trauma is classified on a scale of 0–5 by the appearance of the tympanic membrane.

MEB is usually easily avoided with some simple preventive measures. If a descent is well controlled, and Valsalva is achieved every one to two fsw, then MEB is uncommon. One should always attempt a Valsalva on the surface prior to a dive. If a diver is unable to "clear the ears" on the surface, then diving should be avoided until a cause is identified and corrected. Frequently this only requires the use of nasal or oral decongestants.

The phenomenon known as "reverse middle-ear barotrauma" occurs on ascent. The underlying physics is the same, except that the trauma occurs due to expansion of the middle ear space during ascent. The risk factors are the same as those of MEB, and the underlying pathology is eustachian tube dysfunction leading to ineffective opening of the eustachian tubes. Symptoms are usually just ear pain on ascent. However, TM rupture, alternobaric vertigo, and facial baroparesis may also occur.

Facial Baroparesis

Facial baroparesis is a cranial nerve VII palsy associated with ipsilateral MEB. The underlying pathophysiology is based on the anatomy of the middle ear. The horizontal branch and chorda tympani of cranial nerve VII pass through the middle ear and are thus subject to the effects of increased pressure. The symptoms usually resolve within one hour of depressurization of the middle ear. This condition, however, must be distinguished from AGE, which may have a similar presentation. AGE will likely be accompanied by other signs and symptoms (e.g., other neurological deficits, altered consciousness, dive profile/history consistent with AGE) and will usually worsen with time. In contrast, facial baroparesis will typically improve with time and will likely be associated with other signs and symptoms of MEB.

Middle-Ear Oxygen Absorption Syndrome

Middle-ear oxygen absorption syndrome is a form of barotrauma that can occur after a dive when a dive using a diving apparatus containing a gas mixture with higher partial pressures of oxygen (O_2) occurs. As the gas with increased oxygen content is breathed during the dive, the middle-ear cavity fills with O_2. Once the dive has been completed, negative pressure in the middle-ear space can be created as the increased O_2 is absorbed and metabolized. This is known as "Draeger ear" after the most common rebreather diving system in use (the Draeger or MK 25). Middle-ear oxygen absorption syndrome can also occur after treatment tables using O_2.

The signs and symptoms are similar to those seen with middle-ear barotrauma. The treatment is equalization with Valsalva, which may need to be performed multiple times until all of the O_2 has been absorbed and metabolized. Prevention is also possible with periodic Valsalva after O_2 dives.

Inner-Ear Barotrauma

The inner ear is a neuroanatomically complex organ and is subject to the effects of inappropriate pressure change. Sound is propagated through the middle ear and is converted to waves that travel through the perilymph to the organ of Corti for sound detection. There are several membranes at work in the inner ear, and rapid changes in pressure may lead to their loss of integrity and subsequent development of inner-ear barotrauma (IEBT). The membranes separating the middle and inner ear consist of the oval window and the round window. There are also membranes within the cochlea separating the regions of the perilymphatic space.

The primary forms of inner-ear barotrauma are perilymph fistula, intralabyrinthine membrane tear, and inner-ear hemorrhage, but other, rarer pathologies exist.[24] Pressure differentials in the middle ear from the inability to equalize are transmitted to the membranes associated with the inner ear. In addition to the pressure change in the middle ear, increased intracranial pressure (usually from a forceful Valsalva) is transmitted to the round window membrane via the cochlear aquaduct.[39] Risk factors for IEBT are similar to the risk factors for middle-ear barotrauma, and the two often occur simultaneously due to their similar genesis.

There are anatomic anomalies and malformations of the cochlea that may also predispose a diver to IEBT. Membrane loss of integrity may lead to perilymph leakage into the middle ear, introduction of gas into the perilymph, or mixing of the perilymph and endolymph.[24] There may also be damage to the blood supply to the inner ear leading to inner-ear hemorrhage.

Regardless of the underlying injury, the symptom complex is similar and includes a combination of sensorineural hearing loss, tinnitus, and vestibular dysfunction (e.g., dizziness, vertigo, nausea, vomiting). A history of difficulty clearing on descent may be endorsed, although IEBT can also become apparent during ascent due to gas expansion. On exam, signs of MEB may be appreciated, as well as ataxia and positional nystagmus.

There are a number of investigative techniques that may aid in diagnosis of IEBT if a definitive diagnosis remains uncertain after a thorough history and physical examination. These include audiometry, fistula test, high resolution CT scan (if there is concern for an anatomic predilection), electronystagmography, and surgical exploration.[24]

If a diagnosis of IEBT is suspected, the initial management is usually conservative allowing for self-healing. Tympanotomy should be pursued if vestibular symptoms or hearing loss are severe or deteriorating. Tympanotomy may also be considered if there is no improvement after a trial of conservative management. Corticosteroids are commonly used but without significant supporting evidence.[24]

Of note, IEBT should be distinguished from inner-ear decompression sickness (IEDCS), as the two may have a very similar symptom complex, although a thorough patient and dive profile history is typically sufficient to distinguish the two. Evidence of MEB on exam also supports a diagnosis of IEBT as the underlying pathology is of similar origin. One study suggests that in IEDCS dizziness is the most common symptom, while in IEBT tinnitus and hearing loss are the most reported symptoms.[39] This symptomatic difference is likely due to the air embolism in DCS affecting the labyrinth artery, while the pressure-related changes of IEBT primarily affect the cochlea. If IEDCS is unable to be excluded, a trial of HBO_2 has not been proven to be detrimental even if the true diagnosis is IEBT.[24] While prophylactic paracentesis of the tympanic membranes is not generally recommended, it may be warranted in the case where IEBT is the underlying pathology due to IEBT potentially being worsened by difficult ear clearing during pressurization in a chamber.[39]

Sinus Barotrauma

The sinuses of the skull provide an ideal environment to meet the requirements for barotrauma to occur. When barotrauma occurs on descent, it is known as a "sinus squeeze." When it occurs on ascent, it is known as a "reverse sinus squeeze." The risk factors for sinus barotrauma include history of sinus surgery, sinusitis, seasonal allergies, and anatomic variations. The most common symptom is sinus pain. Many divers will also develop epistaxis secondary to the frailty of the sinus vasculature. Although rare, infraorbital nerve involvement may be seen and presents as paresthesia under the orbit. Divers with sinus barotrauma will have tenderness on palpation of the affected sinus. The treatment is determined by the underlying cause of the barotrauma.

Barodontalgia

Barodontalgia, tooth squeeze, is a form of barotrauma that can occur on descent or ascent (reverse tooth squeeze). Small pockets of gas may be present under cracked teeth or poorly fitting dentures due to decay, which if present and unable to properly vent, may cause divers to develop significant tooth pain or pain that is referred to the maxillary sinus. In extreme cases, they may develop an exploding or imploding tooth. Risk factors for barodontalgia are known dental disease or recent dental work. The treatment is to decrease one's depth in the water column. If significant symptoms develop, and the dive must be aborted, treatment is aimed at providing pain relief and urgent dental referral.

Mask Barotrauma

The space under the divers mask is a place that is rarely associated with barotrauma, but barotrauma could occur if the diver fails to equalize pressure in the mask on descent. If a diver is wearing goggles, then there is no mechanism for equalization of pressure, and mask squeeze will undoubtedly occur. The signs and symptoms can be quite astounding and include periorbital pain, petechiae, swelling, and subconjunctival hemorrhage. The treatment is observation.

Skin Barotrauma

Skin barotrauma is also possible when exposure suits (wet/dry) are being used. If air pockets are trapped between the suit and the skin, the volume of air decreases during descent causing a "suctioning" effect on the skin. These may cause bruising at the sight of offense. There is no specific treatment other than time.

Thoracic Barotrauma

Thoracic barotrauma is a potential complication seen primarily in breath-hold diving and is different from the pulmonary overinflation syndrome injuries associated with ascent in the water column. If the depth of the breath-hold dive is sufficient, negative pressure may develop leading to edema, hemorrhage, and transudation of lung tissue. The symptoms include dyspnea, hemoptysis, and cardiovascular collapse. The treatment is supportive and may require artificial airway, oxygen, and hemodynamic support.

Gastrointestinal Barotrauma

The air in the gastrointestinal tract is also subject to Boyle's law. Therefore, barotrauma may occur if air is not properly vented through the mouth or anus. As the air expands on ascent, it may cause abdominal discomfort and, although rare, rupture. The signs and symptoms associated with this barotrauma are abdominal pain and distension with possible pneumoperitoneum, peritonitis, and shock. If symptoms are mild, then descent in the water column and venting of the gastrointestinal tract will relieve the discomfort. If rupture has occurred, surgical intervention is the appropriate course of action.

PREGNANCY AND DIVING

Diving is a great sport that can be shared by men and women alike, but one large factor that has only recently been evaluated due to the increase in female recreational divers is pregnancy. Should women dive while pregnant? Multiple factors come into play when assessing the risk-to-benefit value of diving during pregnancy. It is very difficult to study though, as human studies are limited primarily to retrospective studies in evaluating the potential detriments that follow, e.g., birth defects, fetal-maternal DCS, and fetal death.

In a nonfetal human being, the lungs serve as a large, efficient filter that helps prevent and limit the likelihood of DCS or AGE. But, due to the nature of fetal circulation and the reliance on the patent foramen ovale and ductus arteriosus, the lungs are completely bypassed, and therefore any bubbles formed maternally are then passed to the fetus via the umbilical vein and will likely end up in the fetal brain or the coronary arteries. Because of this, any bubble formation in the fetus is rather ominous.

Sheep studies have shown that fetal sheep are affected by bubbles when pressed in the womb. The first signs noted were cardiac arrhythmias. After arrhythmias, fetal cardiac malformations or death followed when pregnant maternal sheep were pressed, regardless of if the mother was symptomatic or asymptomatic in regards to DCS.[26,57]

The fetal environment is naturally hypoxic, and, as a result, fetal hemoglobin naturally have a higher affinity for oxygen with the oxygen dissociation curve shifted left. Therefore, when a fetus experiences a "dive" as the mother descends and consumes compressed air, the baby is put at risk for fetal oxygen toxicity. This comes to term secondary to the large increase in partial pressure of oxygen in fetal circulation, which then overwhelms the fetal hemoglobin and puts the fetus at risk for oxygen toxicity. Also, any time a mother-to-be descends in the water column, she is at risk of a diving accident, which would then potentially require hyperbaric therapy. Chamber therapy for the mother in an oxygen-saturated state then places the baby in an increased oxygen environment, and, as previously discussed, due to the strong binding capacity of fetal hemoglobin, the fetus is placed at risk of oxygen toxicity.

In a retrospective survey performed by M.E. Bolton, 109 women dove before and during gestation.[4] Although no official statistical analysis was performed, the survey noted that 69 women dove prior to pregnancy but ceased diving once pregnancy was discovered. The survey also noted that the 50 women who continued to dive throughout pregnancy reported a higher rate of low birth weight, birth defects, neonatal respiratory difficulties, and other problems with pregnancy, delivery, and fetal outcomes. Of note from this small surveyed population, the fetal defects reported from the 50 women who continued diving included cases of hemivertebrae, absence of hand, ventricular septal defect, coarctation of the aorta, hypertrophic pyloric stenosis, and a cutaneous birthmark. In opposition, the 69 women who ceased diving upon pregnancy reported no birth defects.

It is known that vasoconstriction occurs in divers. This is likely a combination of response to water temperatures, increased exercise demand, pregnancy, and anxiety. Regardless of the cause, this vasoconstriction leads to a risk for limited uterine blood flow, putting the fetus at risk of hypoxia.

Pregnancy also leads to natural anatomical changes in women to better provide a hospitable environment for a fetus. Increased interstitial fluid and adipose tissue during pregnancy potentially increase the reservoir for nitrogen on-gassing, which in turn requires a longer time for off-gassing. Therefore, standard dive tables for repeat dives may not apply to pregnant woman as they do to a nonpregnant individual. Naturally, a woman retains more fluids, and as a result may have mucus membrane swelling, which may lead to difficulty clearing sinuses, as a result putting her at an increased risk for a sinus squeeze.

In the early stages of pregnancy, women also experience nausea, vomiting, and gastric esophageal reflux disease (GERD). Increased acid reflux increases discomfort, and when at pressure the symptoms may worsen, which may lead to a less enjoyable dive. More dangerous than increased discomfort from GERD, becoming nauseous and potentially vomiting while underwater greatly puts individuals at risk of aspiration or drowning.

So, although no clear risk can be assessed, and a statistical number cannot be placed on the likelihood of fetal deformities or demise, the risk-to-reward just does not seem worth the dives. Although there are plenty of cases where women continue to dive while pregnant, it appears that a break from diving is well worth the potential alternatives.

DIVING IN THE ELDERLY

The feeling of floating effortlessly through the water while exploring another world is one all divers never forget, and that is what keeps us coming back for years of exploration. Unfortunately, as we age our bodies change whether we like it or not, and the things we used to be able to do become more difficult or near impossible. Diving as we age is no different, and it is important for providers and divers alike to be aware of the risks that are to come with diving as we age.

A systems-based approach can begin with the heart, as the known cardiovascular changes with age include increases in blood pressure and peripheral vascular resistance and decreases in oxygen uptake, work capacity in the form of increased preload and decrease in the contractility of the myocardium, and maximal heart rate.[45]

DAN fatality surveillance data reveal that cardiac conditions are the number two cause of death, second only to drowning. Approximately 80% of fatalities were in people 40 years or older, and, for those whose medical history was available, hypertension and heart disease were the most common conditions reported.[20]

Prospective divers' physicians must consider their patients' cardiac risk factors in light of the unique stresses diving puts on the heart. Aside from increased myocardial oxygen demands from swimming, preload is also increased because of immersion-induced increase in central venous return, whereas afterload is increased from cold-induced peripheral vasoconstriction. The Recreational Scuba Training Council, Undersea and Hyperbaric Medical Society (UHMS), and DAN recommend that divers over the age of 40 undergo risk assessment for coronary artery disease. Exercise stress testing may be recommended for asymptomatic divers with multiple cardiac risk factors.[20,30,45]

Physicians must also be aware of a prospective diver's lung function prior to clearance for diving. The lungs continue to develop until approximately 25 years of age, and, after turning 30 years old, they begin to decrease in their functional capabilities. This functional decline can be broken down into three categories: anatomy, immunology, and physiology.[63]

As an individual ages, anatomically their thoracic cage structurally changes primarily secondary to osteoporosis. Over time the diaphragm can become fatigued and lose its ability to contract as efficiently as it had in earlier years. Additionally, the degeneration of the elastic fibers surrounding the alveolar ducts leads to decreased functionality, resulting in both decreased lung compliance and air trapping, which directly leads to overinflation. This is called senile hyperinflation or "senile emphysema."

The immunological effects, although thought to be very real, are just not adequately studied and have not been proven as absolute as of yet. But, through multiple studies, it has been determined that as we age an increase in neutrophils and a decrease in macrophages can lead to a persistent low-grade inflammation of the lower respiratory tract and as a result lead to the loss of alveolar membrane gas exchange capability.(47)

Physiologically speaking, as we age our lungs have an increase in bronchial reactivity, which not only causes our airways to react in a more drastic manner to either a toxin or an irritant, but also requires a much longer time frame of recovery from the incident. There is an increase in dead space within the lungs as we age resulting from multiple factors, e.g., air trapping as previously discussed, as well as a decrease in vital capacity (VC). This decrease in dead space in combination with decreased heart rate response, cardiac output, and muscle mass leads to an overall decrease in exercise capacity, which can affect an elderly diver in multiple ways. It has also been determined that with age the lungs have a decreased response to hypoxia and hypercapnia, which greatly puts elderly divers at risk of diving casualties.(63)

According to Bove and Davis, additional contributing factors to consider in elderly diving include an alteration in the metabolic state, as primary insulin deficiency may lead to glucose intolerance leading to hyperglycemia. Those with these conditions should not be allowed to dive due to increased risk of morbidity and mortality. Additionally, the elderly are known to have an increased likelihood of reduced hypoglycemic awareness, which in turn increases susceptibility to symptomatic hypoglycemia (e.g., shakiness, anxiety, tachycardia, blurred vision, fatigue, numbness/tingling, decreased coordination, unconsciousness), which puts a diver at increased risk of injury and may mask the signs and symptoms of DCS, which also can lead to increased diving casualties.(6)

Elderly divers are also more susceptible to hypothermia due to a myriad of possibilities, e.g., thyroid dysfunction, reduced sensation of cold, medications countering thermal regulation, chronic illness, and a reduction in subcutaneous fat. As noted previously in thoracic cage function, osteoporosis throughout the body can limit an elderly diver's ability to function underwater, putting themselves and their dive partners at risk. It also has been found that as we age our tympanic membranes weaken, increasing the risk of TM rupture.(35)

Although there is no set age limit for when an individual should hang up his or her fins, a detailed risk assessment should be performed on all individuals over the age of 40, noting acute and chronic illnesses, as well as the general overall fitness, to ensure a safe diving experience.

LONG-TERM PHYSIOLOGICAL EFFECTS

According to the U.S. Navy Medicine Department at Naval Diving and Salvage Training Center (NDSTC), with references to Bove and Davis' *Diving Medicine*(14) and Bennett-Elliott's *The Physiology and Medicine of Diving,*(23) it has been determined that there are two well-documented long-term health effects related to diving.

Those two are dysbaric osteonecrosis (DON) and decreased hearing acuity. Although DON and decreased hearing acuity are both common in commercial and career-based divers, DON has not been known to affect recreational divers with a lifetime's worth of dives.

DON is destruction of bone tissue in the long bones, hips, and shoulders associated primarily with commercial diving and compressed-air work.[55] Proposed mechanism of DON, according to NDSTC, is categorized into two forms with a combination of the two being most likely the etiology of this avascular necrosis. Asymptomatic bubbles and extreme pressure, which acts on the cellular and molecular mechanisms of the body, are the hypothesized culprits that can lead to DON. Asymptomatic bubbles are noted to have a summation effect on the body in the form of biochemical, mechanical, and physiological changes. Biochemical changes occur as a result of lipid emboli, deformed red blood cells, and denatured proteins in combination with gaseous emboli damaging capillaries. Damaged capillaries in turn create an avascular environment and over time lead to an increased risk of developing DON.

According to Emmanuel Gempp, MD, a senior consultant in the department of diving and hyperbaric medicine and dive medical officer for the French military, although gas bubble formation during decompression is the primary cause of DON, it alone may not be sufficient to cause ischemic bone necrosis (bone death from lack of circulation). Dive-related factors associated with DON include the number of lifetime dives, dive depths greater than 115 to 130 feet, and empirical decompression procedures. Diver-related factors include previous musculoskeletal DCS (Type 1), older age, excessive alcohol consumption, tobacco use, high cholesterol, and coagulation abnormalities. Some researchers suspect rapid rates of compression and increased partial pressure of oxygen contribute to necrosis.[55] Per NDSTC, saturation diving may also increase the risk of DON secondary to the long time periods at depths greater than 90 fsw.

Of note, individuals with DON will usually present with arthritis-like symptoms and should be put on NSAIDs for symptomatic relief and followed annually. Divers should be considered disqualified from diving duty if imaging notes definitive juxta-articular lesions or notable radiographic proof of lesion progression or any lesion is found in a saturation diver. Joint replacement surgery may be considered for final symptomatic relief.

The other known long-term health effect from diving is decreased hearing acuity, primarily seen in the form of high-frequency sensorineural hearing loss. Per NDSTC, the etiology of such hearing loss is suspected to be result of either repeat inner- and middle-ear barotrauma, inner-ear DCS, or a combination of the two. As a result, it is recommended that regular hearing checks be performed on individuals who dive on a regular basis. In addition, although uncommon, permanent hearing loss secondary to ear barotrauma (repetitive or from an isolated incident) and inner-ear decompression sickness (IEDCS) is possible. If unilateral hearing loss occurs due to some form of trauma, it is important for physicians during follow-up to counsel divers following such injuries that they are at an increased risk of further hearing loss in one or both ears and, as a result, to recommend against diving in the future. In fact, it is recommended that, for hearing conservation, diving be deterred by all who have hearing loss due to its increased probability for worsening hearing.

Anyone who has had surgery involving the ear, e.g., cochlear implants, ossicle surgery, or tympanic membrane repair (myringoplasty) should avoid diving. The changes in pressure and underwater hazards put divers with this surgical history at risk of damage to the surgical repair, which likely will lead to further hearing loss. If diving cannot be suspended, divers who have undergone such procedures or suffered permanent hearing loss from ear barotrauma should have close monitoring and follow up with an ear, nose, and throat (ENT) specialist prior to clearance.[22]

MEDICATIONS

More than likely, at some time in his or her life, a diver will be taking some sort of medication at the same time he or she would like to dive. As a result, it is important for the diver and his or her doctor to be on the same page in regards to the potential risks and adverse outcomes that may result when diving under the influence of medication. All medications, whether bought over the counter or given by a licensed provider, adjust the body's natural state and therefore should be considered when diving.

Medications that may increase the risks associated with diving include medications that potentially impair physical ability, mental capacity, and decision-making capabilities. It is accepted worldwide that one should not dive while under the influence of alcohol. The same is to be said about any medications that can cause sedation or altered mental state. This is especially true when diving at increased depths where one is at risk of nitrogen narcosis. The summation of the two can be lethal. It is also not recommended to dive while on medications that increase the likelihood of prolonging the Q-T interval, due to the increased risk of arrhythmias. Also, peripheral vasoconstriction is a natural response when diving to conserve the essential organs, the brain and heart. If an individual is mismanaged on antihypertensive medication, the outcome can put the diver's life in danger for a multitude of reasons, e.g., ischemia, infarction, stroke.

Because diving is a recreational sport, and people travel at great lengths to participate in the sport that they love, divers do not want a simple ailment to keep them from diving. That may be a common cold, motion sickness, or general aches and pains. As a result, over-the-counter (OTC) medications are a part of every diver's arsenal for getting him or her to depth. The four most prevalent categories of OTC medications are antihistamines, decongestants, anti-motion sickness, and analgesics/anti-inflammatory medications. Each will be discussed further to include potential need, risks, and contraindications.

Antihistamines

Antihistamines are most often used to provide symptomatic relief of allergies, colds, and motion sickness. The active ingredient most commonly used is diphenhydramine hydrochloride. This is antagonistic in nature to the actions of histamine. Histamine is a powerful stimulant of gastric secretion, a constrictor of bronchial smooth muscle, and a dilator of capillaries and arterioles. These actions counteract the symptoms of allergies, colds, and motion sickness. Unfortunately, with any medication, a pharmacological alteration risks side effects and may include dryness of the mouth, nose, and throat, blurred vision, drowsiness, undesired sedation, tachycardia, and Torsades de Pointes, which can lead to cardiac arrest and death if experienced while diving.[44,53]

Decongestants

The primary mechanism of action of decongestants is vasoconstriction. This occurs via direct stimulation of alpha-adrenergic receptors in respiratory mucosa. The common active ingredients are pseudoephedrine hydrochloride and phenylpropanolamine hydrochloride. These medications provide a temporary relief of congestion in the nasal airways which increases one's ability to effectively Valsalva upon descent.

Decongestants also directly stimulate beta-adrenergic receptors causing bronchial relaxation and increased heart rate and contractility. This receptor stimulation can cause a myriad of side effects including CNS stimulation, headache, nausea, hypertension, tachycardia, dizziness, seizures, agitation, hyperstimulus, and possible psychosis. Decongestants are contraindicated in divers with hypertension or coronary artery disease. This is because the vasoconstriction may affect the coronary vasculature, leading to ischemia and possible infarction.

Anti-Motion Sickness

Many dives begin with the boat ride to the ideal location, and with that boat ride comes the opportunity for motion sickness. This sickness is secondary to the discordance between vestibular, visual, and proprioceptive signals, which leads to nonvertiginous dizziness, nausea, and vomiting. As a result, people combat the undesired symptoms with medications, but recreational divers should use these medications with caution. As with some antihistamines, these medications may contain promethazine, scopolamine, meclizine hydrochloride, dimenhydrinate, diphenhydramine hydrochloride, or cyclizine. Common side effects are drowsiness, fatigue, and respiratory depression. This may cause impairment of a diver's ability to perform hazardous activities requiring mental alertness or physical coordination. At a minimum, these side effects will decrease the pleasure of a dive and may very well increase the morbidity and mortality associated with diving.[44,53]

Analgesics/Anti-Inflammatories

Anti-inflammatories and analgesics are generally taken for the temporary relief of aches and pains. While they may provide temporary relief, one must remember that the injury itself is still present. Underlying injuries may limit range of movement or cause swelling and pain. This can place a diver at risk of additional injury. In addition, medication for pain relief may mask mild pain due to decompression sickness, and the diver may subsequently delay seeking treatment.[44,53]

Nonsteroidal anti-inflammatories (NSAIDs) include naproxen sodium and ibuprofen, with notable side effects such as heartburn, nausea, abdominal pain, gastric ulcers, and rebound headache. Standard precautions discourage their use by those with medical disorders involving heartburn, gastric ulcers, bleeding problems, or asthma. A careful risk-and-benefit analysis should be undertaken by anyone on these medications prior to engaging in diving.

DIVING HAZARDS

There are a number of hazards associated with the underwater environment. Some of them are innate to the environment, while some are the result of human interference. These hazards must be taken into account before, during, and after a dive.

The diver must be acutely aware of his or her surroundings at all times. Surface boat traffic in the area increases the risk of falling equipment such as propellers or anchors that break loose and can cause life-threatening injury to a diver. This threat is minimized with the use of surface floats or buoys that signal that divers are in the water.

Environmental toxins and infectious agents may also be present in the water. These are most likely encountered in commercial and military diving and require special protective gear.

Indigenous plant and animal life in the area of operation are an ever-present danger for divers. Divers and medical practitioners should be aware of the marine life in the area and know the risks associated with each and the treatments of potential injuries sustained.

While unlikely to be encountered in recreational diving, underwater explosions are a very real danger for many military and commercial divers. Indeed, the navy's underwater explosive ordinance disposal technicians work directly with bombs in attempts to render them safe. Underwater welders are also at risk of encountering explosions due to the oxygen and hydrogen produced with electrolysis of water. These gases collect under structures and are at risk of igniting in the presence of a spark or flame. The water acts as a conduit through which explosive pressure waves travel in all directions. Once the waves encounter an air-water interface, the energy translation causes a shearing/shredding effect known as the spalling effect. The effects of this are intuitively understood by imagining the effects of an underwater explosion at the surface seen by an observer as a shower of foam and water droplets. What the medical practitioner must also consider is that these effects are also realized at any air filled structure of the body. This includes the lung, middle ear, sinuses, and bowel. This explosive effect may lead to an injury known as blast lung and may have associated pneumothorax or arterial gas embolism. Bowel blast injury may also occur and can be severe enough to require an exploratory laparotomy. A victim may also suffer from orbital and basilar skull fractures. The treatment of these injuries requires prompt application of advanced trauma life-support principles and transport to the nearest trauma facility.

Military and commercial divers often use equipment powered by electricity (e.g., power tools and communication equipment), and these are associated with risk of electric shock. The most commonly encountered injuries from electricity are burn injuries and cardiac arrhythmias. Treatment principles are the same as electric shock in other environments. Victims should have basic and advanced life support, as well as monitoring for complications of rhabdomyolysis as the electric shock may be associated with a muscle tetany response. Victims may be at risk of life-threatening injuries up to 24 hours after the initial injury occurred.

Divers may also encounter high-intensity, underwater sound energy that can damage the hearing structures and lead to permanent hearing loss. Military divers may also be exposed to ionizing radiation as they work near nuclear reactors on the hulls of nuclear-powered ships and submarines. The military employs a strict set of guidelines to minimize a diver's exposure to ionizing radiation.

Human Factors

Human risk factors are a key consideration in any activity, physical or mental. The diving environment brings with it a requirement for a high degree of physiologic reliability and stamina. Much has been written on "fitness to dive" and will not be discussed here. However, as human error is common in diving mishaps, a general idea of the potential causes for pathology due to the "human factor" is necessary for medical practitioners working with divers.

General physical fitness is crucial in diving. Due to the high energy demand placed on the body while diving, good diver fitness decreases the risk of injury for those looking to enjoy the subaquatic environment. Fitness must be continually assessed for all interested in continuing diving activity. In addition, divers must be trained on the equipment in use and on emergency procedures associated with the equipment.

The diving reflex is innate to human physiology and therefore serves as a factor that must be assessed when anticipating a dive. It is a complex physiologic response to immersion in water that stimulates both the sympathetic and parasympathetic autonomic nervous system.[62] The series of events include bradycardia, peripheral arteriolar vasoconstriction, decreased cardiac output, and an increase in mean arterial pressure.[68] Collectively, these responses promote preferential conservation of oxygen for use by the heart and brain.[68] The diving reflex has been implicated in drowning and cardiac arrhythmias, especially in patients with prolonged QT syndromes.[62] The vagal-mediated bradycardia with concurrent increased sympathetic tone is thought to trigger fatal arrhythmias.[62] It has also been implicated in ischemic stroke in divers and intracerebral hemorrhage secondary to cerebral hypertension triggered by the diving reflex.[46] This reflex, while beneficial for oxygen conservation, may be a nidus for disaster in those with pathology that predisposes them to injury.

Hypothermia is defined as a core body temperature less than 95°F (35°C). Due to the high thermal conductivity of water, without proper planning and protective equipment, hypothermia may be encountered while diving. Tropical waters provide a false sense of security, but these waters may lead to progressive heat loss as the temperatures are most often significantly less than ideal body temperatures. While hypothermia is an important consideration in all diving environments, this is of particular importance when diving with breathing mediums containing helium because helium gas has greater thermal conductivity than other gases used in diving. The primary goal of treatment of hypothermia is rewarming in a controlled environment and monitoring for signs and symptoms that may require basic and advanced life support.

Divers may also experience hyperthermia, especially if diving in water that is greater than 95°F. The high work effort required of divers increases this risk. Presentation may include heat edema, heat cramps, heat syncope, heat tetany, heat exhaustion, and heat stroke. Complications may include electrolyte abnormalities, rhabdomyolysis, and acute renal injury. Treatment is aimed at lowering the core body temperature and judiciously applying life-support principles.

Other human factors that may lead to injury while diving include lack of experience, panic, disorientation, insufficient training for the level of diving complexity, and equipment failure from improper use or maintenance.

ALTITUDE

Diving throughout history has primarily been centered on the ocean. Our equipment, dive tables, and research are created for the idea of diving in the sea. But there has been an increase in intrigue for diving fresh bodies of water, which more than likely are found at a distance above sea level. The increase in altitude changes how one should approach the dive, as there are multiple factors that must be accounted for when diving at altitude versus when diving at sea level.

The primary and most focused factor to be taken into account is the idea that as an individual climbs in altitude the atmospheric pressure decreases. As a result, diving at specific altitudes changes depth parameters compared to at sea level, which directly affects the time allowed at depth. For example, when an individual diving at sea level dives to 60 fsw, he or she is allowed approximately 60 minutes of bottom time without need for decompression stops. But when an individual dives to 60 feet at 5,000 feet above sea level, his or her adjusted depth is actually 72.1 fsw, which allows for a bottom time of only approximately 39 minutes.[67]

How is this calculated? Well, through the last half century, multiple equations have been developed on how to appropriately adjust for altitude, with the Haldane method and Cross Correction being the most recent and widely accepted. The Haldane method uses current dive tables and converts the maximum depth a diver is planning to reach into an equivalent sea dive depth. This method adjusts the bottom time, reducing time allowed by using the time limit from a deeper depth.(14,64) Modern-day technology and dive watches/computers when recalibrated are able to make the calculations and adjustments for the diver on the fly, but, in terms of old-school pen and paper calculations, the U.S. Navy uses the Cross Correction and is focused on the adjustment calculations needing to be made to cover the difference at altitude and diving fresh- versus saltwater. Cross Correction can be created by taking altitude depth (fsw) multiplied by the quotient of pressure at sea level and pressure at altitude. This gives the calculated "Equivalent Depth" (fsw).(67)

Example: A diver makes a dive to 60 fsw at an altitude of 5,000 feet. The atmospheric pressure measured at 5,000 feet is 843 millibars (0.832 ATA). Atmospheric pressure at sea level is assumed to be 1,013 millibars (1.000 ATA). Sea level equivalent is then 72.1 fsw.

Equivalent Depth (fsw) = 60 fsw x 1.000 ATA / 0.832 ATA = 72.1 fsw(67)

According to the U.S. Navy dive manual, a dive table has been created allowing for quick reference with the parameters/suggestions of the following:

Any dive < 300 feet above sea level does not require adjustment to the dive table

Dives from 300–1,000 feet above sea level should be adjusted if diving deeper than 145 fsw (actual depth, not calculated)

Dives at altitudes of 1,000–10,000 feet above sea level should be adjusted appropriately no matter the depth

Any dive > 10,000 feet above sea water must be appropriately discussed with U.S. Navy Supervisor of Salvage and Diving (NAVSEA 00C) for appropriate parameters and calculations.(67)

In addition to needing to calculate the difference in depth secondary to pressure changes, one must take into account calibration/equilibration and acclimation. Calibration is the amount of time required to off-gas the natural inert gases in the tissues as an individual climbs in altitude due to the difference in partial pressures. The times required for this to occur are variable, being based on change of altitude and whether or not the gas inspired with ascension contains inert gas (e.g., breathing oxygen while climbing altitude). Operationally speaking, the military and police/fire rescue services push these limits, as at times divers may be at a certain altitude and, when called to duty/emergency, may be required to fly to a greater altitude and splash in less than the recommended time. That recommended time for complete calibration and off-gassing is 12 hours. If that full 12 hours cannot be met, then a dive must be calculated, and a group designator must be used to determine appropriate bottom time allowed.(67)

Acclimation is the body's natural way of adapting to the higher altitude, which presents a lesser atmospheric pressure and oxygen concentration. Both create a homeostatic imbalance that must be overcome to prevent acute altitude illness (AAI), which can come in the form of acute mountain sickness (AMS), high-altitude cerebral edema (HACE), and high-altitude pulmonary edema (HAPE). AAI can begin to present when traveling to altitudes greater than 2,000 meters (6561 feet).(51) AAI can be prophylactically treated with acetazolamide, dexamethasone, nifedipine, sildenafil, and ondansetron, but the only true treatment for cure is descent in altitude.

AMS presents in a more nonspecific subjective manner with symptoms of headache, malaise, nausea, and difficulty sleeping and usually presents itself within 6–36 hours upon arrival to new altitude. Due to the subjectivity, a physical exam is usually unremarkable for AMS, and it is treated symptomatically and either with time for acclimation or descent.

HACE, on the other hand, can be noted with physical exam as upon arrival to altitude an individual begins to have AMS symptoms in combination with neurological deficits. These deficits can be found in the form of ataxia, hallucinations, confusion, general stupor, and eventually coma. Treatment mandates immediate oxygen supplementation and descent in altitude.

Finally, HAPE, which is the most deadly of the altitude illnesses, presents itself initially as a subtle nonproductive cough and mild shortness of breath within 2–4 days of arrival to altitudes usually greater than 3,000 meters (9,842 feet). The symptoms progressively worsen to include dyspnea at rest, productive cough of pink frothy sputum, tachycardia, tachypnea, bilateral crackles with auscultation, lethargy, and inevitably coma. Oxygen and descent is an absolute necessity for treatment.

FLYING AFTER DIVING

Not every diving enthusiast lives near the tropical underwater wonderlands he or she enjoys, and, as a result, many divers have to travel to get their fill of bottom time. Frequently with travel to such places, planes are a means of transportation, but with planes comes the scenario of elevation change, and with elevation change comes pressure change. This pressure change can be quite hazardous to one's health if the correct guidelines aren't followed after squeezing in that last-minute dive to one's favorite reef.

Unfortunately, there is no absolute and obvious answer in regards to when to fly after a dive. The answer varies among sources and varies individually. Factors that weigh in are overall health/comorbidities, general diving fitness, depth, time at depth, number of dives, history of DCS, etc. The U.S. Navy follows a multifactorial guideline relating the Repetitive Group Designator (RGD) and anticipated flying altitude to then develop the recommended surface interval prior to flying. When calculating, one must use the highest RGD in the previous 24 hours. Situations which require a short surface interval (for example, surfacing and then getting on a transport aircraft within a matter of minutes, which is possible in the military) require an RGD group A, B, or C. This also applies for those traveling on commercial airlines, secondary to the cabin pressure being approximately 8,000 feet altitude. The U.S. Navy intervals can be as short as a couple hours for clearance, but, in order to be clear of all RGDs, a 24-hour surface interval is recommended.

Previously, a study conducted by DAN at the F.G. Hall Hypo/Hyperbaric Center of Duke Medical Center was created to help answer the dive-to-flight interval question. The study consisted of a 60 fsw chamber dive for approximately 55 minutes. Upon surfacing, various surface intervals (SI) were tested (3, 6, 9, and 12 hours), which were followed by simulated chamber flights at 8,000 feet for four hours. Determining presence of DCS signs and symptoms was the objective, and, due to the subjective nature of diagnosing DCS, any and all signs and symptoms reported by the participants were recorded. The three categories of DCS were further evaluated and documented by the research staff.

The three categories were as follows: (1) "Not DCS" referring to signs or symptoms that are clearly unrelated to the experiment, such as the diver who injured him- or herself during the preflight surface interval; (2) "Ambiguous DCS," which is noted as signs and symptoms that lasted only a short time, were very mild, and/or were uncertain in the judgment of the hyperbaric physician, or may not have responded to recompression therapy; and (3) "Definite DCS" was defined as clear and certain signs and symptoms that improved or resolved completely with recompression. Within the category of Definite DCS there are two types: pain only and neurological. We generally worry more about neurological symptoms than joint pain. Neurological signs and symptoms that occurred included numbness, tingling, weakness, confusion, and visual disturbances, all of which resolved with recompression.[21]

Upon completion, it was noted that at a 3-hour SI there was an estimated 10% risk of Definite DCS and a 20% risk of Ambiguous DCS. The 6- and 9-hour intervals were statistically discredited, and, at the 12-hour SI, there was roughly a 1% risk of Definite DCS and 2% risk of Ambiguous DCS.

Of note in regards to the previous research, the testing was performed in a chamber under very controlled conditions, and therefore cannot be used as determination for an absolute when determining the dive-to-flight interval time. Actual "wet" diving with individuals who have not been carefully evaluated and selected may result in additional factors, and an appropriate dive-to-flight interval should be left to the educated individual diver's discretion.

According to the Undersea and Hyperbaric Medicine Society, it is recommended to wait 12 hours before ascent on commercial aircraft for no-decompression dives but, if participating in a decompression dive or multiple-day diving excursions, a waiting period of greater than 12 hours is recommended. This 12-hour period can be a soft recommendation in military operations and can still be safe if appropriate precautions are taken. For example, if needing to fly in a pressurized aircraft (commercial) and if placed on oxygen nonrebreather upon ascension, the likelihood of developing DCS is decreased. Another example for a nonpressurized aircraft (helicopter) is remaining at a flying altitude less than 1,000 feet, which also limits DCS manifestations.[51]

Of side note, when diving other rigs aside from SCUBA and surface-supplied, various other time constraints/mandates are followed. For example, when diving heliox, one must wait for 12 hours if on a no-decompression dive and 24 hours if on a decompression dive. Saturation dives must wait a minimum of 72 hours from surfacing to takeoff, and closed-circuit oxygen dives are allowed to fly immediately after surfacing secondary to the lack of nitrogen saturation.[51]

It's clear that there is an obvious risk-to-benefit ratio that must be weighed. If one wants no risk of DCS secondary to altitude, either don't dive or don't fly. But, because all divers want to dive, and none want to be held to the confines of their backyard pool, it is left to an individual's best judgment in determining when to fly as each individual diver knows better than any other his or her personal state of health. It is also a personal decision to the reasoning behind the decision to take that one last dive before getting on the plane. Therefore, all that can be done is advise divers on the decision of diving within that 24-hour window of takeoff.

SATURATION DIVING

Saturation diving is a prolonged dive where all tissues are considered to be saturated with inert gas. With all tissues saturated, the diver can remain at depth for as long as is necessary without incurring additional decompression obligation. Once a diver has been at depth for a sufficient amount of time for saturation to occur, it doesn't matter if the diver remains under pressure for three days or three months. Additional time at pressure incurs no additional decompression penalty. The first intentional saturation dive was carried out by Edgar End and Max Nohl in 1938. The experiment was performed to gain insight into how to care for animals that were used for hauling muck cars in compressed-air tunnels and were kept under pressure for an extended period of time. They remained in a hyperbaric chamber for 27 hours at 101 feet breathing air and successfully decompressed in around 5 hours with only Nohl experiencing decompression sickness. The process was developed from that point on, and saturation diving is commonplace today with military, commercial, and scientific applications.

A saturation dive can be thought of conveniently as existing in three phases: the compression phase, the time at storage depth, and the decompression phase. The compression phase is typically slower than for a routine nonsaturation dive due to the need to prevent high-pressure nervous syndrome (HPNS) as well as compression arthralgia. Once at storage depth, divers typically conduct their work from a personnel transfer capsule (PTC). The PTC allows the divers to move between a dry, hyperbaric environment at the pressure of the storage depth and the corresponding underwater working environment. The decompression phase is lengthy and usually takes several days to complete, depending on the maximum depth of the deepest diver. There are emergency abort procedures in place, but these only minimally reduce the number of days required for decompression.

The austerity of the saturation diving environment is unlike any other environment that humankind is exposed to. Decompression takes days, and, as such, emergency medical help is not quickly accessible. For example, if the maximum depth attained during a saturation dive is a minimal 400 fsw, then the surface (and emergency medical help) is over 4 days away. A saturation dive tests the limits of human physiology in several unique ways that medical practitioners and divers alike should be aware of.

Selection of saturation divers is the first step in preventing untoward medical problems. Due to the extreme isolation, only the most physically and mentally healthy divers should undertake a saturation dive.

HPNS, as discussed previously, is usually only encountered in saturation dives. It is prevented (and treated) with slow compression, stopping compression for a period of time to allow the body to adapt, and addition of nitrogen or hydrogen to the breathing mix to balance the effects of helium (see section on abnormal gases in diving). There is inter-diver variability in propensity to develop HPNS, so diver selection is also a key component of preventing HPNS.

There is also a phenomenon known as compression arthralgia. It is typically associated with pressures greater than 200 fsw. Most saturation divers will experience this in the form of pain or cracking in joints, causing restriction of movements. The shoulder, knee, wrist, and hip seem to be most often involved. This is reversible and seems to improve with increased time at depth.

Fungal and bacterial skin infections are common, as one might expect in a warm, humid, and sealed environment.[42] Infections that are mild on the surface can wreak severe havoc during a saturation dive. Seemingly minor superficial lacerations can quickly deteriorate into life-threatening scenarios that require aggressive treatment. The high humidity and temperature of the environment at saturation also favor the proliferation of gram-negative bacteria in the external auditory meatus.[36] This leads to the development of otitis externa. This is often combated with the prophylactic use of aluminum acetate drops in the ears.

Hypothermia must also be combated during saturation dives due to the high thermal conductivity of helium. This effect increases with depth and necessitates active heating of divers during dives, as well as the heating of chambers and the diver's gas supply to prevent life-threatening hypothermia.[42]

The breathing mediums must be closely monitored as the various gases in the mixture must be kept within a tight range. Small changes in gas mixtures lead to large partial pressure changes of gases at depth. These may lead to toxic situations.

DCS may present as a complication from a saturation dive as well. Type 1 seems to have a higher prevalence than Type 2. Lower-extremity pain is the most common symptom of DCS in saturation dives.[(65)] Treatment principles are the same as for DCS in other diving scenarios.

CONCLUSION

Diving, although enjoyable, has a multitude of risks. Some risks are directly associated with diving, and others are associated with the undersea environment. Therefore, it is very important for a diver and a diver's clinician to be aware of an individual's risk factors and the risks inherent in diving. A risk assessment of every dive should be undertaken, and any risks should be discussed and accounted for prior to splashing. When the appropriate steps and precautions are taken, diving is rather safe and enjoyable for all parties involved.

DISCLAIMER

This chapter represents the views of the authors and in no way represents the views of the U.S. Department of Defense, Department of the Navy, or Department of Veterans Affairs.

REFERENCES

1. American Heart Association [Internet]. American Heart Association. Cardiovascular disease statistics [cited 2008 Feb 10]. Available from: http://www.americanheart.org/presenter.jhtml?identifier4478.
2. Aquatic deaths and injuries: United States. MMWR. 1982;31:417-22.
3. Azizi MH. Ear disorders in SCUBA divers. Int J Occup Environ Med. 2011 Jan;2(1):20-6
4. Bolton ME: Scuba diving and fetal well-being: a survey of 208 women. Undersea Biomed Res. 1980;7:183-9.
5. Bove AA, Clark JM, Thom SR. Toxicity of oxygen, carbon dioxide, and carbon monoxide. In: Bove and Davis' diving medicine. 4th ed. 2004. p. 244.
6. Bove AA. Diving in the elderly and the young: metabolic changes. Bove and Davis' diving medicine. 4th ed. 2004. p. 414.
7. Bove AA. Diving Medicine. Am J Respir Crit Care Med. 2014 Jun 15;189(12):1479-86.
8. Bove AA, Ferrigno M. Clinical aspects of breath hold diving: cardiovascular problems. In: Bove and Davis' diving medicine. 4th ed. 2004. p. 85.
9. Bove AA, Ferrigno M. Physiology of breath hold diving: cardiovascular system. In: Bove and Davis' diving medicine. 4th ed. 2004. p. 79.
10. Bove AA, Flynn ET. Medical supervision of diving operations. In: Bove and Davis' diving medicine. 4th ed. 2004. p. 355.
11. Bove AA. Neuman T. Near drowning: pathophysiology. Bove and Davis' diving medicine. 4th ed. 2004. p. 278.
12. Bove AA, Neuman T. Near drowning. Bove and Davis' diving medicine. 4th ed. 2004. p. 275.
13. Bove AA, Neuman T. Near drowning. Bove and Davis' diving medicine. 4th ed. 2004. p. 281.
14. Bove AA, Walder DN, Elliot DH. Aseptic necrosis of bone: causes of dysbaric osteonecrosis. Bove and Davis' diving medicine. 4th ed. 2004. pg 422.
15. Buzzacott P. Altitude diving [Internet]. [updated 2011 Apr]. Available from: http://www.altitude.org/high_altitude_diving.php
16. Causey AL, Tilelli JA, Swanson ME. Predicting discharge in uncomplicated near-drowning. Am J Emerg Med. 2000;18:9-11.
17. Clark JE. Moving in extreme environments: inert gas narcosis and underwater activities. Extrem Physiol Med. 2015 Feb 24;4:1. doi: 10.1186/s13728-014-0020-7. eCollection 2015.
18. Demchenko IT, Welty-Wolf KE, Allen BW, Piantadosi CA. Similar but not the same: normobaric and hyperbaric pulmonary oxygen toxicity, the role of nitric oxide. Am J Physiol Lung Cell Mol Physiol. 2007 Jul;293(1):L229-38. Epub 2007 Apr 6.
19. Dietz PE, Baker SP. Drowning: epidemiology and prevention. AM J Public Health. 1974;64:303-12.
20. Divers Alert Network Annual Diving Report 2007. Durham (NC): Divers Alert Network; 2007.
21. Divers Alert Network [Internet]. Divers Alert Network. DAN medical research: DAN flying after diving; 1993-1999. Available from: https://www.diversalertnetwork.org/research/projects/fad/index.asp
22. Divers Alert Network. Hearing loss as long term effect of diving.
23. Elliott DH, Moon RE. Long term health effects of diving. In: The physiology and medicine of diving. 4th ed. 1993.

24. Elliott EJ, Smart DR. The assessment and management of inner ear barotrauma in divers and recommendations for returning to diving. Diving Hyperb Med. 2014 Dec;44(4):208-22.
25. Ferrigno M, Ferretti G, Ellis A, et al. Cardiovascular changes during deep breath hold dives in a pressure chamber, J Appl Physiol. 1997;83:1282-90.
26. Fife WP, Simmang C, Kitzman JV. Susceptibility of fetal sheep in acute decompression sickness. Undersea Biomed Res. 1978;5(3):287-92.
27. Fine NL, Myerson DA, Myerson PJ, Pagliaro JJ. Near drowning presenting as the adult respiratory distress syndrome. Chest. 1974;65:347-9.
28. Golding FC, Griffiths P, Hempleman HV, Paton WD, Walder DN. Decompression sickness during construction of the Dartford Tunnel. Br J Ind Med. 1960 Jul;17:167-80.
29. Greer HD, Massey EW. Neurologic injury from undersea diving. Neurol Clin. 1992 Nov;10(4):1031-45.
30. Harrison D, Lloyd-Smith R, Khazei A, Hunte G, Lepawsky M. Controversies in the medical clearance of recreational SCUBA divers: updates on asthma, diabetes mellitus, coronary artery disease and patent foramen ovale. Curr Sports Med Rep. 2005;4:275-81.
31. Hayward, JS, Eckerson JD. Physiological responses and survival time prediction for humans in ice water. Aviat Space Environ Med. 1984;55:206-12.
32. Hickey MJ, Zanetti CL. Delayed-onset cerebral arterial gas embolism in a commercial airline mechanic. Aviat Space Environ Med. 2003 Sep;74(9):977-80.
33. Hoff BH. Multisystem failure: a review with special reference to drowning. Crit Care Med. 1979;7:310-8.
34. Hunter TB, Whitehouse WM. Fresh-water near drowning: radiological aspects. Radiology. 1974;112:51-6.
35. Jensen JH, Bonding P. Experimental pressure induced rupture of the tympanic membrane in man. Acta Otolaryngol. 1993;113:62-7.
36. Jones DM, Davis P. Upper respiratory tract and aural flora of saturation divers. J Clin Pathol. 1978 Aug;31(8):721-3.
37. Kaukinen L. Clinical course and prognostic signs in near-drowned patients. Ann Chir Gynaecol. 1984;73:34-9.
38. Kizer KW. Resuscitation of submersion casualties. Emerg Med Clin North Am. 1983;1:643-52.
39. Klingmann C, Praetorius M, Baumann I, Plinkert PK. Barotrauma and decompression illness of the inner ear: 46 cases during treatment and follow up. Otol Neurotol. 2007 Jun;28(4):447-54.
40. Kot J. Extremely deep recreational dives: the risk of carbon dioxide (CO(2)) retention and high pressure neurological syndrome (HPNS). Int Marit Health. 2012;63(1):49-55.
41. Lanphier EK. Application of decompression tables to repeated breath-hold dives. In: Rahn H, Yokoyama T, editors. Physiology of breath-hold diving and the AMA of Japan. Publication 1341. Washington (DC): National Academy of Sciences, National Research Council; 1965. p. 227-36.
42. Leitch DR. Complications of saturation diving. J R Soc Med. 1985 Aug;78(8):634-7.
43. Leitch DR, Green RD. Pulmonary barotrauma in divers and the treatment of arterial gas embolism. Aviat Space Environ Med. 1986 Oct;57(10 Pt 1):931-8.
44. Levano B. Taking medications when you dive. Divers Alert Network. 1999 Jan-Feb.
45. Lynch JH, Bove A. Diving medicine: a review of current evidence. J Am Board Fam Med. 2009;22:399-407.

46. McKee K, Nelson S, Batra A, Klein JP, Henderson GV. Diving into the ice bucket challenge: intraparenchymal hemorrhage and the mammalian diving reflex. Neurohospitalist. 2015 Jul;5(3):182-4. doi: 10.1177/1941874415573024.
47. Meyer KC, Ershler W, Rosenthal NS, et al. Immune dysregulation in the aging human lung. Am J Respir Crit Care Med. 1996;153:1072-9.
48. Modell JH, Graces SA, Ketover A. Clinical course of 91 consecutive near-drowning victims. Chest. 1976;70:231-8.
49. Moloff AL. Delayed onset arterial gas embolism. Aviat Space Environ Med. 1993 Nov;64(11):1040-3.
50. Mor A, Kuttner YY, Levy S, Mor M, Hollmann M. Grossman Y. Pressure-selective modulation of NMDA receptor subtypes may reflect 3D structural differences. Front Cell Neurosci. 2012 Sep 11;6:37. doi: 10.3389/fncel.2012.00037. eCollection 2012.
51. Naval Diving and Salvage Training Center Dive Medical Officer lectures.
52. Neuman TS. Near drowning. In: Moser KM, Spragg RS, editors. Respiratory emergencies. 2nd ed. St. Louis: Mosby; 1982. p. 282-4.
53. Nord DA. Over the counter medications. Divers Alert Network. 1996 May-Jun.
54. Orlowski J. Prognostic factors in pediatric cases of drowning and near drowning. JACEP. 1979;8:176-9.
55. Petar Denoble. Dysbaric osteonecrosis in recreational diving. Alert Diver. 2012 Fall.
56. Peterson B. Morbidity of childhood near drowning. Pediatrics. 1970;59:364-70.
57. Powell MR, Smith MT. Fetal and maternal bubbles detected noninvasively in sheep and goats following hyperbaric decompression. Undersea Biomed Res. 1985;12(1):59-67.
58. Putman CE. Drowning: another plunge. Am J Roentg Radium Ther Nucl Med. 1975;125:543-9.
59. Rosenbaum HT, Thompson WL, Fuller RH. Radiographic pulmonary changes in near drowning. Radiology. 1964;83:306-12.
60. Rosinska J, Lukasik M, Kozubski W. Neurological complications of underwater diving. Neurol Neurochir Pol. 2015;49(1):45-51. doi: 10.1016/j.pjnns.2014.11.004. Epub 2014 Dec 1.
61. Schuman SH, Rowe JR, Glazer HM. Risk of drowning: an iceberg phenomenon. JACEP. 1977;6:139-72.
62. Shamsuzzaman A, Ackerman MJ, Kunihoshi FS, Accurso V, Davison D, Amin RS, Somers VK. Sympathetic nerve activity and simulated diving in healthy humans. Auton Neurosci. 2014 Apr;181:74-8. doi: 10.1016/j.autneu.2013.12.001.
63. Sharma G, Goodwin J: Effect of aging on respiratory system physiology and immunology. Clin Interv Aging. 2006;1(3):253-60.
64. Sierra Diving Center. Altitude diving calculations. 2012 Dec.
65. Sowden LM, Kindwall EP, Francis TJ. The distribution of limb pain in decompression sickness. Aviat Space Environ Med. 1996 Jan;67(1):74-80.
66. Thomson L, Paton J. Oxygen toxicity. Paediatr Respir Rev. 2014 Jun;15(2):120-3. doi: 10.1016/j.prrv.2014.03.003. Epub 2014 Mar 26.
67. U.S. Navy Diving Manual. Vol. 2. Chapter 9, Air decompression: 9-13 diving at altitude; p. 489-91.
68. Wittmers LE, Pozos RS, Fall G, Beck L. Cardiovascular responses to face immersion (the diving reflex) in human beings after alcohol consumption. Ann Emerg Med. 1987 Sep;16(9):1031-6.

CHAPTER 44 CHAPTER

Closed-Circuit Rebreathers (CCRs)

CHAPTER FORTY-FOUR OVERVIEW

Introduction **1087**

Closed-Circuit Rebreathers Versus Open-Circuit **1088**

Components **1089**

Different Types of Rebreathers: eCCR, mCCR, and hCCR **1091**

Work of Breathing and Static Lung Loading **1092**

Pulmonary Gas Exchange at Depth **1093**

Mechanical Causes of Hypercarbia: Scrubber Failure **1093**

UBA and Respiratory Loads **1093**

Inertance 1093

Elastic Loads 1093

Resistive Loads: External and Internal Rebreather Design – External Resistance 1094

Gas Density – Internal Resistance. 1094

Case Report 1095

Summary 1095

3 H'S: Hypoxia, Hyperoxia, and Hypercarbia **1096**

Hypoxia 1096

Hyperoxia 1097

Hypercarbia 1098

Absorbent Aspiration and Ingestion (Caustic Cocktail) **1099**

CCR Fatalities **1101**

References **1103**

Closed-Circuit Rebreathers (CCRs)

Derek B. Covington, Charlotte Sadler, Richard L. Sadler

INTRODUCTION

Rebreather technology can arguably be attributed to primitive submarine design of the seventeenth century.[47] Rebreathers became commercially viable in 1878 with a unit developed by Henry Fleuss.[47] Mass production then started with Drager of Germany in 1912. Subsequent variants in the interwar years were adopted for military use by the Italian and German navies. Parallel development was done by an American medical student, Christian J. Lambertsen, in 1939. An enthusiastic swimmer and diver, he built a primitive rebreathing circuit using 100% oxygen and demonstrated the ability to stay submerged for a prolonged time.[18] Testing the unit on himself, he realized the limitations incurred by the accumulation of CO_2. Inspired by the newest technological innovations in anesthesia, he then incorporated chemical CO_2 absorbent, or "scrubber." One-way valves were then added to improve this scrubber contact time. The resulting "recirculating loop" allowed a relatively small amount of gas volume (oxygen) to be carried by the diver, which allowed for extended dive times with no exhaled bubbles. Developed during World War II, the tactical advantages of this early rebreather were obvious. Patented in 1944, it was dubbed the Lambertsen Amphibious Respiratory Unit (LARU) and was adopted by the U.S. Navy (USN) for use by the early operational swimmer groups, which were the forerunners of today's UDT/SEAL teams. It was then renamed in 1952 to self-contained underwater breathing apparatus (SCUBA).

These early rebreather designs utilized 100% oxygen, which minimized the volume carried by the diver but limited operational depth to less than 30 feet of water. In order to maximize the inherent efficiency of a rebreather, the addition of a gas diluent was added, allowing a constant partial pressure of oxygen, based on depth. This system is inherently more efficient than open-circuit systems as it requires lower volumes of gas and less inert gas loading. However, precise control of the oxygen and carbon dioxide partial pressures is critical. Failure to control these variables has led to deaths from hyperoxia, hypoxia, and hypercarbia (known as the "3 Hs"). Various designs include semi-closed-circuit, with active addition (constant mass flow rate) or passive addition (respiratory minute volume keyed). Electronic control with oxygen sensors is by far the most precise, but implementation is technically challenging. The first operational unit was developed by Stark in 1968 (Electrolung). This was followed in 1969 by the Biomarine 1000. A spinoff from General Electric Corporation, it was notable for using galvanic oxygen sensors originally developed for the National Atmospheric and Space Administration (NASA). This design subsequently became the USN Mark 15 rebreather, which is still in use today. With an operational depth of greater than 1,500 feet (500 m), long scrubber duration, and low work of breathing, it remains the standard for high performance.[31]

During the 1900s, consumer units were offered by Drager (Dolphin and Atlantis), as semi-closed technology. By 1999, the modern era was arguably initiated with the first electronically controlled unit (eCCR) made for the consumer market by Ambient Pressure Diving (Inspiration Classic), which is currently the most common model worldwide.[31]

CLOSED-CIRCUIT REBREATHERS VERSUS OPEN-CIRCUIT

Although closed-circuit SCUBA was invented prior to open-circuit equipment, open-circuit (OC) configurations continue to dominate the current market. Nonetheless, closed-circuit rebreathers (CCR) are becoming exponentially more popular. Once relegated only to military, research, and technical diving applications, CCR has even begun to be embraced by the recreational diving community.

Open-circuit gear is robust, simple, and reliable. It is also much cheaper to purchase and to maintain compared to closed-circuit equipment. Furthermore, users of one type or manufacturer of OC equipment can usually utilize other types or manufacturers without the need for a new certification or acquired skill set. However, OC equipment is not efficient for breathing-gas utilization, especially for deeper diving. In addition, OC regulators vent exhaled gas bubbles into the water column, which may scare underwater life (and prove frustrating for underwater photographers) or disrupt fragile structure above the diver, such as in certain cave systems or wrecks. Finally, it delivers cold, dry, compressed air to the user, which may irritate airways and dehydrate the diver; this is especially apparent during extended dives or for users with reactive airway disease.

Closed-circuit rebreathers (CCR) are extremely efficient with gas utilization as they vent gas bubbles only rarely (on ascent, if the loop is over-pressurized, or during mask clearing). As a result, wildlife often will be more approachable for photographic pursuits, and the chance of decreased visibility due to falling debris (caves and wrecks) from vented gas is limited (Figure 1, Figure 2). In addition, CCR become increasingly efficient with regard to breathing-gas utilization at greater depths because the metabolic consumption of oxygen remains stable regardless of depth. However, for open-circuit divers, the deeper one ventures, the larger the volume of gas breathed in and eventually exhaled into the water column, which would deplete the gas supply more quickly. Rebreathers also allow for more physiologically correct tidal volumes of warm, humidified gas, providing a more comfortable experience for long-duration dives and for those with reactive airway disease. Finally, CCR also allow for a constant partial pressure of inert gases and oxygen, leading to extremely efficient decompression schedules by varying the fraction of inspired gases (and maintaining a constant partial pressure) throughout the dive. On the other hand, open-circuit SCUBA utilizes a constant fraction of inspired gases that changes with depth, resulting in variable partial pressures of gases.

Closed-circuit rebreathers (CCR) are devices that recycle one's breath or, more specifically, a portion of one's breath. These machines allow a user to breathe in a mixture of gas (air, enriched air nitrox, and/or helium-based gases) and then

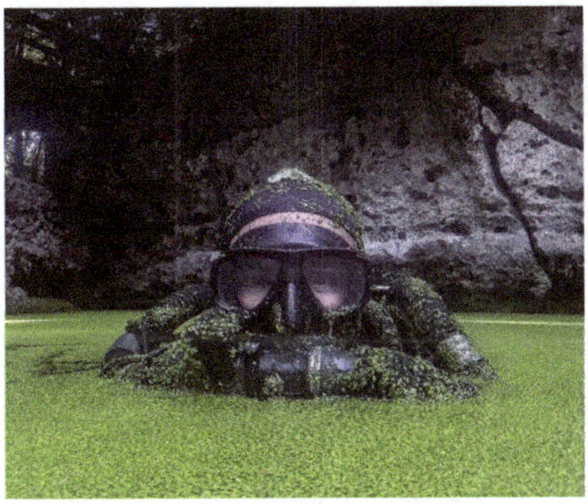

Figure 1. A closed-circuit rebreather diver surfaces in the duckweed covering Orange Grove Sink in Peacock Springs State Park (Luraville, FL). Photo courtesy of Laura de Armas.

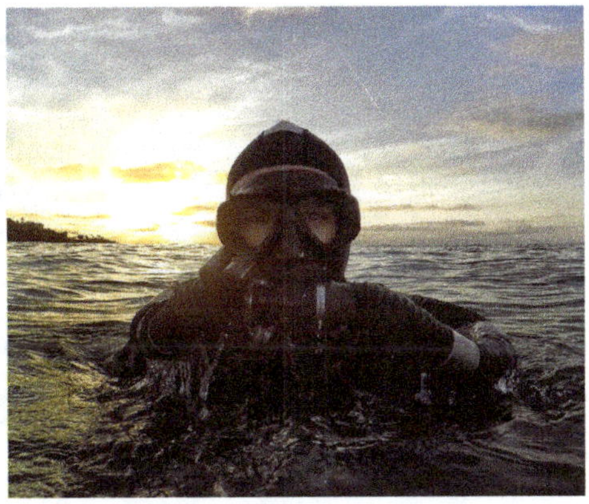

Figure 2. A closed-circuit rebreather diver emerges from a shore dive (La Jolla, CA). Photo courtesy of Laura de Armas.

breathe it out in a closed system. As the user draws a new breath, the previously exhaled breath is "pushed" along the remaining loop. Eventually the exhaled gas will encounter a carbon dioxide scrubber canister. The carbon dioxide scrubber contains soda lime or other material, which removes carbon dioxide from the exhaled breath through an exothermic reaction. The gas then encounters oxygen sensors that provide real-time partial-pressure-of-gas information to the user. Depending on the design of the rebreather, oxygen or other gas is added to the loop either by the user (manual, or mCCR) or directed by the computer (electronic, eCCR). There are also designs that allow the user and the computer to control the partial pressure of gases, commonly called "set points." In order to prevent mixture of exhaled and inhaled gases, there are a series of one-way valves throughout the loop that maintain gas flow in a single direction. The gas once again enters the mouthpiece and eventually the oropharynx and lungs of the user.

COMPONENTS

The loop constitutes all of the space the gas can occupy and allows the gas to flow in a circular direction. The loop is interrupted by the placement of a dive surface valve (DSV), which is a simple mechanism that allows the user to close the mouthpiece to the loop and prevents water from entering. Loop weights may be utilized to maintain the position of the loop and not impede diver vision or compromise streamlining of equipment. The counterlungs (CL) allow space for the exhaled and inhaled breath to travel along the loop. The CL may be placed in different locations (back mounted [BM], over the shoulder [OTS]) and have ramifications for work of breathing (WOB) in various trim positions in the water column depending on design and placement (see next section on work of breathing and static lung loading).

Cylinders containing both diluent and oxygen are also attached and plumbed into the system via low-pressure hoses. The diluent may be simply air, enriched air nitrox (EANx), or various mixes of heliox or trimix. Regardless of diluent choice, it must be able to "dilute" the oxygen in order to achieve a desired partial pressure of oxygen throughout the dive. It must also be nontoxic at the deepest part of the dive. Thus, a diver can perform what is known as a diluent flush ("dil flush") to verify function of oxygen cells, to lower the oxygen set point, or to take a sanity breath.

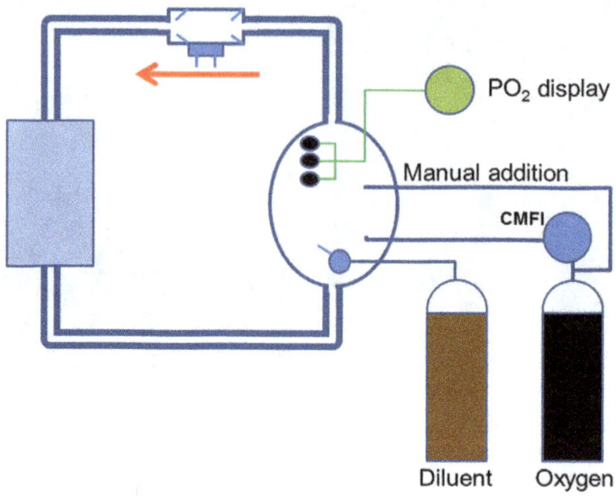

Figure 3. Simplified schematic of a manual closed-circuit rebreather, or mCCR. Note the direction of gas flow is indicated by the red arrow underneath the mouthpiece with one-way mushroom valves. The CO_2 scrubber is represented by the light-blue rectangle. Finally, the oxygen cells are depicted as being sited in the countering, but this is never the case. A manual injector for diluent has been omitted for simplicity. CMFI = constant mass flow injector.

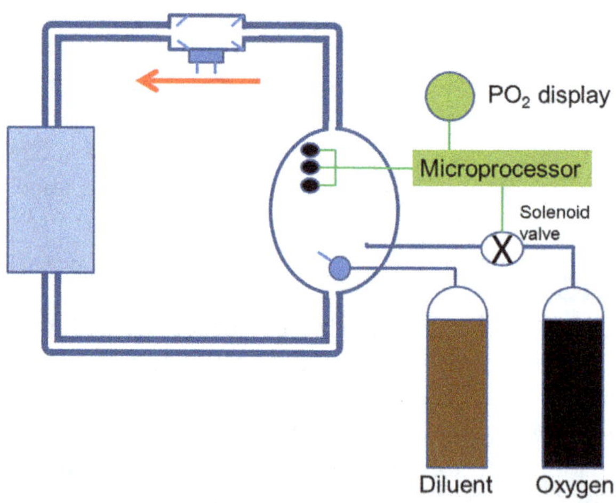

Figure 4. Simplified schematic of an electronic closed-circuit rebreather, or eCCR. Note that the manual injectors for both oxygen and the diluent gases have been omitted for simplicity.

The cylinders utilized for CCR are smaller in capacity in comparison to open-circuit gear secondary to the much-improved efficiency of the CCR. Cylinders constructed from aluminum, steel, and carbon fibers are all available and utilized by CCR divers.

Oxygen sensors are placed in the rebreather system and utilized to monitor real-time partial pressure of oxygen. These oxygen sensors are galvanic oxygen sensors, which convert oxygen partial pressures to electrical currents and display the information to the diver.[6,20] These sensors were designed for medical purposes, and manufacturers state these sensors may last 24–48 months. However, this is at normobaric pressure and room temperature. Sensors utilized in CCRs are exposed to humid and hyperbaric conditions and may fail in a variety of ways, such as current limitation, corrosion of contacts, and broken contacts.[39] Thus, it is prudent to monitor accuracy and longevity of these cells in this austere environment. Many CCR units utilize three or more sensors for safety and redundancy.

A diving computer then incorporates the partial pressure of loop gases and diving profiles and informs the user of no-decompression limits or of accrued decompression times and required stops. Current computers also tell the user water temperature, have compass functions, and allow the addition of gases in the event of a gas loss or gas addition from a team member. It is not uncommon for a CCR diver to utilize two or more computers for additional redundancy and verification of correct set points and decompression obligations.

Carbon dioxide scrubbers are crucial to prevent the buildup of carbon dioxide in the unit. Proper installation and adherence to strict usage durations prevent a common issue with rebreathers, which is hypercarbia. These carbon dioxide scrubbers are constructed in either a radial or axillary design depending on the flow of gas through the scrubber. More recently, scrubbers have been designed to accept scrubber cartridges, which are sheets of scrubber sprayed and then rolled. These are designed to prevent inaccurate filling leading to channeling through the canister. The media, or material which actually scrubs the CO_2, is usually composed of soda lime, which is a mixture of calcium hydroxide and sodium hydroxide. These compounds absorb the exhaled CO_2 and form calcium carbonate and water via an exothermic reaction.

The entire CCR unit is usually mounted on a backplate composed of metal (aluminum, stainless steel) or plastic. This allows the connection of a harness and a wing, which functions as a buoyancy compensator device. However, the use of CCR in a sidemount, or SM, configuration is gaining popularity, especially for divers desiring a smaller anterior-posterior profile that allows access to small areas, such as those found in wrecks or caves (Figure 5). Finally, the other crucial part of equipment is an open-circuit cylinder with a regulator in order to allow for "bail out" in case of CCR failure or diver discomfort. These bail-out cylinders are carried along the side of the diver to allow for quick access and to maintain streamlining. Technical divers pursuing extremely deep profiles have also begun to use a second CCR as a source of bail out. This bail-out CCR is usually side-mounted and carried like a decompression or OC bail-out cylinder.

DIFFERENT TYPES OF REBREATHERS: ECCR, MCCR, AND HCCR

Semi-closed rebreathers, or SCRs, function as "gas extenders." These units utilize EANx cylinders that constantly add this breathing gas to the loop. The diver then breathes on the loop for 2–3 breaths (and decreases the FiO_2 secondary to oxygen consumption) and then vents the gas. Additional fresh gas is then added to the loop. Some SCR units vent part of each exhalation and then add fresh gas to replace the lost volume.

In contrast to SCR designs, CCR machines recirculate entire breaths and remove the exhaled CO_2 via a CO_2 scrubber. Within the designation of CCR, there are various subtypes distinguished by the mechanisms of how the oxygen is added

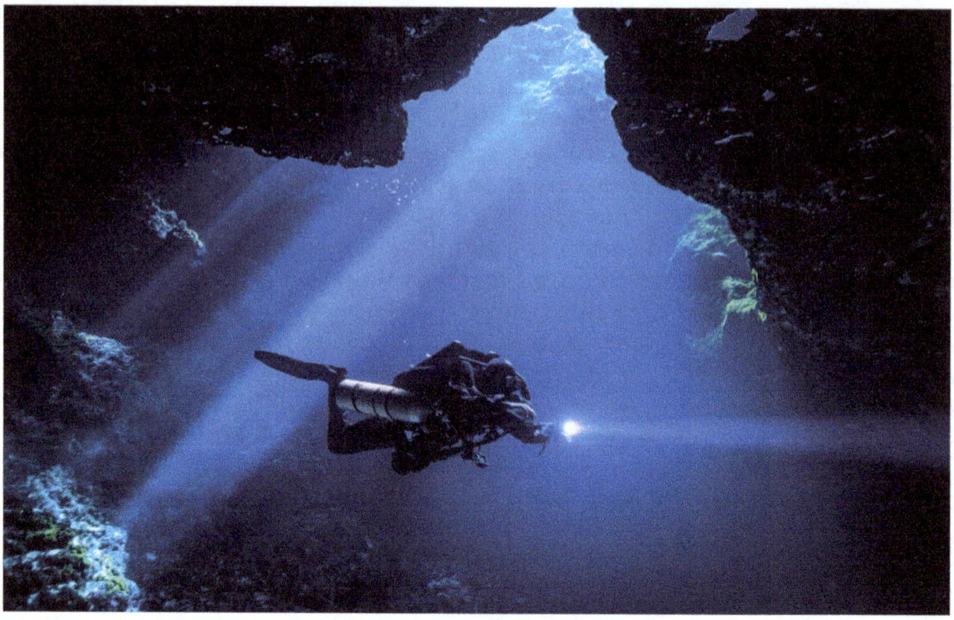

Figure 5. A closed-circuit rebreather diver explores the Blue Hole Spring Cavern at Ichetucknee Springs State Park (Fort White, FL). Photo courtesy of Laura de Armas.

to the loop. When a computer controls the set point of oxygen partial pressure, it's referred to as an electronically controlled CCR, or eCCR. When the user controls the set point via the addition of oxygen or diluent, it is referred to as a manual, or mCCR. These mCCR units also utilize a design known as a constant mass flow, or CMF, system which provides an ongoing input of oxygen into the loop. The rate of oxygen influx should be sufficient to maintain a minimum oxygen partial pressure consistent for life, but not lead to hyperoxia. A desired set point is then maintained by manual addition of oxygen via the diver. If a unit has both a computer-controlled and manual options, it is referred to as a hybrid, or hCCR. Users may then elect to have the computer maintain at least a minimum partial pressure of oxygen in the event that they are distracted or unable to, but then use the oxygen manual addition to supplement and maintain a higher partial pressure of gas. Finally, there is a specific type of CCR known as the oxygen rebreather. This CCR design utilizes one bottle of oxygen and allows addition of only oxygen to the loop. As a result, there is no diluent, and maximum operating depths must be closely adhered to in order to prevent oxygen toxicity. These units are typically utilized by military personnel.

WORK OF BREATHING AND STATIC LUNG LOADING

The inherent efficiency of rebreathers allows for deeper dive profiles, extended bottom times, and accelerated decompression profiles. This in turn has led to an increased utilization of this underwater breathing apparatus (UBA). The use of rebreathers has the same potential complications as conventional or open-circuit (OC) SCUBA, with a shift in relative risk. The performance advantages depend upon the recirculation of the breathing gas. This recirculating design has two unique requirements. First, the energy supplied to move gas around the breathing circuit, or loop, is supplied by the diver; thus the work of breathing (WOB) must be considered. Second, the recirculated gas contains CO_2, unlike gas from an open circuit. Therefore, the potential for hypercapnia is significant. Elevated partial pressures of CO_2 (pCO_2) levels may produce headache and dyspnea, but can also create debilitating shortness of breath, confusion, anxiety, impaired cognition, and ultimately death. WOB, static lung load (SLL), and hypercapnia are inextricably linked. An understanding of WOB and SLL (Transpulmonary Pressure – P_{TR}) is crucial for understanding the clinical picture of the rebreather diver.

PULMONARY GAS EXCHANGE AT DEPTH

Oxygen represents approximately 14% of alveolar gas. This is exchanged for CO_2 in the alveolus. The inspired gas, air at 1 ATA, is efficiently transported to the alveolus through the tracheobronchial tree. The gas density is approximately 1 gm/L.[32] The hyperbaric environment, with the linear increase in gas density and hemodynamic changes from immersion, degrades this efficiency. At a certain point, this failure to ventilate will lead to CO_2 retention (hypercarbia), with potentially fatal consequences. Critical to this concept is understanding gas exchange, which occurs by convective mixing in the larger airways and gaseous diffusion in the alveoli. Increasing gas density will reduce this diffusivity and loss of exchange efficiency.[46]

Effective diffusive gas exchange is crucial. A detailed explanation of the relationship between diffusion and concentration gradients is beyond the scope of this chapter. A detailed explanation is provided in Moon,[32] Sapoval,[38] and Weibel.[56]

MECHANICAL CAUSES OF HYPERCARBIA: SCRUBBER FAILURE

Rebreather design requires a mechanism for the removal of expired CO_2. In modern rebreathers, this is accomplished with the use of soda lime. Loss of effective chemical reaction due to shortened dwell time, inactive soda lime, or excess CO_2 production will inevitably lead to hypercarbia. These design issues are discussed elsewhere.

UBA AND RESPIRATORY LOADS

All rebreathers require some degree of breathing effort or respiratory loading. Respiratory loading has subcomponents consisting of inertance, elasticity (compliance and transpleural pressure), resistive effort (external and internal), and dead space.

The effort produced by the diver is correctly called resistive work,[52] though more commonly known as work of breathing (WOB).[52] The unit measure is joules/liter (J/L).

It is not a direct measurement of caloric work, but reflects the work required to overcome the pressure differential imposed by the hydrostatic loads. 1 J/L is equivalent to 1 kPa, which is equivalent to 10 cm H_2O. The distance measurement is relevant to measuring the static lung load. They are discussed in order of ascending importance.

Inertance

In this context, inertia refers to the energy required for movement of gas and the chest wall. The effects are relevant only at very high respiratory rates. Divers normally have a much lower respiratory rate; thus inertance is not a significant component of work in most circumstances.[14,33,36]

Elastic Loads

Compliance and Transpleural Pressure (P_{TR}) – The major component of elastic work is contributed by the transpleural pressure (P_{TR}) or static lung load and pulmonary compliance. Immersion causes increased venous return of approximately 500–800 ml of blood to the pulmonary vasculature.[22] This reduced compliance reduces lung volumes by reducing expiratory residual volume (ERV) and vital capacity (VC). Divers automatically compensate at depth by increasing the ERV to increase airway diameters and decrease resistance. This comes at the cost of raising elastic load.[14,53]

Of greater importance is P_{TR} or static lung load (Figure 3).[32] P_{TR} is a major determinant of exercise performance in divers and, by implication, subsequent CO_2 production. WOB in this context is categorized as external work of breathing, since the resistance is from the external UBA.

The diver's lung and the counterlung are affected by hydrostatic pressure within the column of water. The distance between the counterlung and diver's lung is measured as the relative difference in the water column. A counterlung that is deeper than the diver's lung is subject to higher hydrostatic pressure and thus is said to have a positive value. Conversely, a counterlung at a shallower depth is negative in value.

The word "static" does not refer to the pressure, which changes with the diver's position within the water column. Instead, the number (e.g., 10 cm) is the fixed distance between the counterlung and the central part of the diver's lung, known as the centroid. The centroid is that point within the tracheobronchial tree where the respiratory muscles are relaxed (ERV) and the expiratory reserve volume is the same as at 1 ATA. "Static" thus refers to the unchanging distance relationship inherent to the given rebreather design.[52] Optimal lung loading should remain within a maximum of 10–12 cm H_2O, or 1.2 kPa. Accepting elevated pCO_2 levels of 60 mmHg, the WOB should not exceed 1.5–2.0 J/L.[55]

When evaluating the difference between the inspiratory and expiratory limbs of the circuit, Warkander found that excess work required for inspiration (i.e., negative load) was predictive of hypercarbia.[53] Positive loading of the inspiratory component decreased perceived dyspnea. The beneficial effects of positive loading might be from decreased airway resistance (see section on gas density - internal resistance below). Positive loading seems to be preferred within physiologic limits.[22] Negative lung loading is associated with unacceptable dyspnea.[43] Negative P_{TR} has further implications. It enhances the normal redistribution of blood into the thoracic cavity, further distending pulmonary vessels and decreasing lung compliance, thus decreasing ERV. The result of the decreased ERV is that the airways are narrower at the initiation of inspiration, thus increasing resistance to gas flow. Combined with the increasing gas density seen at depth, relative alveolar hypoventilation is problematic.[42]

Resistive Loads: External and Internal Rebreather Design – External Resistance

Practically, this is a function of the EWOB (external work of breathing), or the design of the rebreather or underwater breathing apparatus (UBA). This was discussed above under P_{TR} or static lung load: it is the resistance created by the gas flow through all components of the UBA, e.g., hoses, valves, scrubbers, and counterlungs.

Gas Density – Internal Resistance

The largest contributor to this is gas density. Gas density depends upon the combination of gas mixture and pressure (depth). The increased density enhances turbulent flow into the more distal airways.[32] Under pressure, reductions in the FEV_1 /FVC ratio, maximum voluntary ventilation (MVV), and peak expiratory flow are noted.[21,26,50] As an example, MVV at 4 ATA is 50% compared to the surface,[29] which is attributed to the increase in gas density. Dynamic airway collapse and effort-independent expiration are increased with depth[29] further compromising alveolar gas exchange (V_A).[29]

Increased gas density also reduces gas phase diffusion.[46] As discussed above, the combination of acinar diffusional screening and reduced diffusion will compromise gas exchange. Although manipulation of the breathing gas mixture with the addition of lower molecular weight gas (e.g., helium) can mitigate this to some degree, increasing density is inexorable with increasing depth.

With exercise, the single most important predictor of increased pCO_2 is gas density.[16,19,23,36-37] High gas density can also raise internal respiratory resistance such that flow limitation severely limits exercise capacity at depth. A case report is given below.[28,57] Mechanical breathing resistance has less effect in raising the pCO_2.[53-55] Dead space is the gas remaining after expiration. Anatomically, it does not change significantly with depth. However, dead-space gas contains the expired CO_2. An increased respiratory rate will potentially decrease tidal volume. This increases the relative percent volume of the dead space. Therefore, CO_2 exchange is diminished, resulting in hypercarbia. The major predictor of hypercarbia is the combination of increased gas density and dead space (V_d/V_T).[7]

Case Report

A 51-year-old, fit, male diver started a dive to 264 m (792 ffw) in a South African cave with the intent of recovering the body of a deceased diver. His support team located him motionless on the bottom and was unable to recover him until three days later. Forensic analysis of the rebreather noted that the soda lime scrubber was assembled in a manner outside of normal approved parameters. This suggested the possibility of CO_2 "breakthrough" as a contributing factor to the accident. Audio tape demonstrated that the diver was aware of the hypercarbia and initiated mitigation by flushing the circuit with fresh gas supply. The oxygen solenoid was heard to be functioning appropriately. The dive profile itself was also a major contributor to presumed hypercarbic respiratory failure. The extreme depth exacerbated effort-independent expiratory flow, probably by 50% or more. The extreme gas density could even create effort-independent inspiratory flow. The larynx and soft tissues could act as flow restrictors with high negative inspiratory pressures. The precise cause of death will never be conclusive. However, this case does demonstrate the issues discussed above. At extreme depths and pressure, even a high-performance rebreather may have excessive WOB. The high gas densities combined with the physiologic changes of diminished ventilation, effort-independent expiratory and possibly inspiratory flow, and inadequate scrubber performance were terminal. The diver would be in the downward spiral described by Mitchell, wherein the increased WOB produced even more CO_2, possibly leading to mental confusion and incapacitation, resulting in respiratory failure and death.[30,51]

Summary

Work of breathing, static lung loading, and resistive effort are significant concerns in rebreather design and use. The risks of decreased alveolar ventilation (V_A) and hypercarbia are potentially fatal complications of rebreather use. The major external component is the rebreather circuit design combined with static lung loading. This is a fixed value linked to individual rebreather design. Positive static loading is associated with increased expiratory reserve volume and increased airway diameter. The major internal component of work is increased gas density and dead space. Gas density can be modified with the use of low molecular weight gas (e.g., helium). However, gas density inexorably increases with depth. When combined with dynamic airway closure and effort-independent expiratory flow, elevated pCO_2 levels and hypercapnia are certain.

Having summarized above the unique equipment used and physiologic conditions that occur in CCR diving, we now describe how these conditions can potentially lead to pathology in CCR divers. It is imperative to take a thorough dive history, to determine when in the dive the event occurred (surface, descent, at depth, or ascent), and to assess the accompanying symptoms and these may provide critical clues to the etiology of the event.

3 H'S: HYPOXIA, HYPEROXIA, AND HYPERCARBIA

The human body operates within a relatively narrow threshold with respect to oxygen and carbon dioxide (CO_2) levels. When exposed to levels of either oxygen or CO_2 outside of this range, there are potentially catastrophic outcomes. CCR divers are at risk for both hypoxia and hyperoxia, as well as hypercarbia.

Hypoxia

It is generally accepted that the human body can successfully function with O_2 levels as low as 0.16 ATA, and anything below this is considered hypoxia. There are a few ways in which a CCR diver can become hypoxic, including procedural problems directly related to the equipment. In contrast to open-circuit (OC) diving, errors such as forgetting to turn on the gas or open a valve may not be immediately obvious at the beginning of a dive. For example, failing to open the valve to the O_2 tank may not become evident until the dive is already underway, because as the diver descends there is a certain amount of oxygen in the loop from the prebreathe. The diver will continue to slowly metabolize this oxygen, but because the pO_2 in the loop will increase with depth and pressure, the diver may not become hypoxic until he or she is at depth. Additionally, failing to calculate the amount of O_2 needed for the dive can also result in exhaustion of gas supply and subsequent hypoxia, though O_2 supply is generally not the limiting factor in CCR diving. There are multiple mechanical failures that can result in hypoxia, though these are addressed elsewhere in this chapter (see previous section on components). Of note, however, O_2 sensors do not generally fail high (i.e., they do not generally produce artificially high readings).

Another potential mechanism for hypoxia in the CCR diver is a rapid ascent or decrease in pressure. If a diver makes a rapid ascent, the pO_2 in the loop will decrease as the pressure decreases and will not increase until additional gas is added. If a slow ascent is made, depending on the unit, this will happen automatically, or the diver can add the gas manually. However, if the ascent is too rapid, there is not enough time for the unit to equilibrate and add gas quickly enough, and the diver may become hypoxic.[9,47]

The potential for hypoxia is also dependent on the gas mixes that the diver is using for the diluent and bail out. Without going into the complexities of all the different potential combinations of gas, it is important to understand that there are technical divers who use deep mixes that are hypoxic at the surface. For example, the mixture may contain only 10% oxygen. Assuming that the minimum pO_2 necessary to function is 0.16 ATA, this mixture should not be breathed above 1.6 ATA. Inadvertently using this mixture at shallower depths or on the surface will result in hypoxia.

The symptoms of hypoxia may range from subtle to extreme, depending on the degree of hypoxia as well as the diver. Symptoms include euphoria, dizziness, tunnel vision, tingling and parasthesias, perioral/lip numbness, dysarthria, subjective dyspnea, and unconsciousness. Although there is not an absolute correlation between pO_2 and symptoms, the following are rough correlations:

- pO_2 above 0.16 ATA – asymptomatic, except possible loss of night vision
- 0.12–0.14 ATA – tingling, lip numbness, tunnel vision, increase in resting minute volume (RMV)
- 0.09–0.11 – difficult speech, dizziness, imminent collapse, and death

Unfortunately, there may be a rapid progression of initial symptoms to unconsciousness, or loss of consciousness may be the first symptom.[13]

Hyperoxia

Conversely, in addition to the dangers of hypoxia, the CCR diver is also at risk for hyperoxia. The two organ systems primarily affected by oxygen toxicity, at least with respect to divers, are the pulmonary and CNS systems. The primary concern of CNS O_2 toxicity in divers is the development of seizures. Although there is not a value below which a diver is considered absolutely safe from oxygen toxicity, many divers dive with a maximum O_2 set point of 1.3 ATA during the dive and 1.6 ATA during safety stops/shallow decompression. It is important to note that oxygen toxicity can still occur below these values that are thought to be "safe." Pulmonary O_2 toxicity can also occur with prolonged use of CCR while breathing high partial pressures of O_2. The mechanism is the same as pulmonary O_2 toxicity that may occur during hyperbaric oxygen treatments and is discussed in detail in Chapter 3.

Hyperoxia has been reported at a wide range of depths, including as shallow as 3 m (though this is very rare), and risk continues to increase dramatically with increased depth. The incidence of oxygen toxicity is unknown. Although, it was found to be 12% in a large study of Israeli military divers.[3] Just as with hypoxia, there are multiple points in the rebreather in which mechanical problems can result in hyperoxia, which are addressed in the components section. It is worth noting that one of the common failures that occurs with the sensors (either with the sensors themselves or the batteries) is the inability to detect high O_2 readings, which leads to the diver having an artificially low O_2 reading on his or her computer.[6,40]

The symptoms of hyperoxia, just as those associated with hypoxia, may range from subtle to extreme, and it is commonly thought that a diver may not experience any warning signs before experiencing a seizure or loss of consciousness. The range of symptoms reported is extremely broad, though some of the most common are nausea, limb twitching, hearing and visual disturbances (including tinnitus and tunnel vision), dizziness, and convulsions.[3] This is by no means an exhaustive list, and there have been over 30 different signs of oxygen toxicity reported and described in the literature. The greatest concern is loss of consciousness or seizure in the water.

When this occurs in a dry hyperbaric chamber, it can generally be managed effectively without any lasting effects. When it occurs in the water, it often leads to aspiration, drowning, and death, which is why CCR divers must be vigilant about monitoring themselves and their buddies for any signs of oxygen toxicity.

Arieli et al. performed a retrospective review of symptoms that occurred in oxygen toxicity accidents in the Israeli navy, all at depths less than 7 meters. They found that the most common symptoms that occurred before termination of a dive were limb convulsions (tremor), hyperventilation, difficulty maintaining a steady depth, and headache. The most common symptoms that occurred after termination of a dive (after detaching from a mouthpiece) were headache, loss of consciousness, confusion, weakness, facial twitching, and limb convulsions. [(2)] In another study, the probabilities of a diver to lose consciousness varied widely among the following three conditions: 26 times more likely for a diver who has experienced disorientation, 42 times more likely in a diver with hearing disturbances and 700 times more likely in a diver with facial twitching. [(3)] They also evaluated the occurrence of high CO_2 in these divers, and it was noted that loss of consciousness occurred in 40% of the high CO_2 group, and there were no occurrences of loss of consciousness in the oxygen toxicity group that had low CO_2. These symptoms differ slightly from those reported in prior studies, which may have had confounding factors at play, such as nitrogen narcosis. Interestingly, there were no incidences of loss of consciousness without a preceding warning symptom, and the shortest period of time from initial symptom to termination of dive was five minutes.[(2)] These observations bring into question the commonly held belief that loss of consciousness or seizure may be the only presenting symptom of oxygen toxicity, but further work needs to be done on the subject.

The susceptibility to oxygen toxicity has obviously been a concern of both the military and the recreational CCR communities, and multiple attempts have been made to identify risk factors, with somewhat varying results. Many of these risk factors are not unique to divers, such as medications and coexisting medical conditions that are discussed elsewhere in this book. In animal studies, it has been shown that a cold-induced increase in metabolic rate, as well as darkness, increased susceptibility to oxygen toxicity, though this has not been shown definitively in humans.[(3)] There are currently ongoing investigations into the effects of the ketogenic diet in preventing CNS oxygen toxicity, given its history of effectiveness in treating epilepsy. It is theorized that the ketogenic diet may have a neuroprotective effect via antioxidant effects. A pilot study has been done showing the feasibility of rapidly achieving ketosis (within 48 hours) through diet without negatively affecting performance during diving, and larger investigations are currently underway.[(45)]

Hypercarbia

There is conflicting data regarding whether particular individuals without other known risk factors have an intrinsically increased susceptibility to oxygen toxicity, and some evidence has tied a higher possibility of CNS oxygen toxicity in individuals with decreased responsiveness to elevated CO_2 levels [(2)] In animal studies, increased levels of CO_2 significantly decreased the latency to appearance of oxygen toxicity in rats.[(1)] It has also been reported that individuals with CO_2 retention have seized at even "safe" levels of oxygen exposure.[(11)] Even independent of its association with increased susceptibility to oxygen toxicity, hypercarbia presents its own danger to the diver. The possible causes of hypercarbia during a dive are numerous, including scrubber failure (over- or underpacking, "tunneling," exhaustion, flooding, etc.), "overbreathing" the scrubber due to increased work during the dive, and mechanical respiratory failure.[1] Other contributing factors to hypercarbia include nitrogen narcosis depressing central drive[24] and hypercapnic ventilatory response.[25] At extreme depths, with increased air density and turbulent flow, expiratory flow rates significantly decrease, leading to CO_2 retention.[30,38] This is discussed further in work of breathing and static lung loading section.

The symptoms of hypercarbia include subjective dyspnea/air hunger, tachypnea, dizziness, and headache. This may proceed to impaired judgment, poor decision-making, total incapacitation, loss of consciousness, and death. There does appear to be some individual variability in ability to detect higher levels of inhaled CO_2, as well as individual variation in the tendency to retain CO_2 and the ventilation response to high CO_2 levels. There is also some evidence that the ability to detect increased levels of CO_2 may be improved with training.[11]

Unfortunately, hypercarbia has been implicated in a number of CCR deaths and fatalities. However, a study performed by Warkander[54] suggests otherwise. In this study, Warkander assessed the physiologic responses to increased breathing resistance during exercise at 6.8 ATA in six divers. The subjects were closely monitored for subjective symptoms of dyspnea, unusual behavior, and continuous end-tidal pCO_2 levels. Significant incapacitation rapidly leading to unconsciousness was observed in one of their divers. However, perhaps most concerning, the diver had no subjective complaints or feelings of dyspnea prior to incapacitation. It is also well documented that individuals respond very differently and have very different tolerances to the same levels of pCO_2. These variations are observed among different divers and even amongst the same divers in varying situations.[54]

In addition to disturbance of oxygen and CO_2 levels, CCR divers are at risk for a unique condition, commonly referred to as a "caustic cocktail."

ABSORBENT ASPIRATION AND INGESTION (CAUSTIC COCKTAIL)

All rebreathers require a system for carbon dioxide (CO_2) removal based on an exothermic chemical reaction where CO_2 dissolved in water reacts with a strong base, NaOH (Sofnolime 797) or LiOH (Micropore). The fundamental reaction is:

$Ca(OH)_2 + CO_2$ catalysed by NaOH $CaCO_3 + H_2O$.

Regardless of the specific mix, the strong alkali nature of the absorbents poses serious hazards and unique challenges for care. Although modern rebreather design attempts to isolate the scrubber from any contact with water, the breathing circuit will always have potential ingress points. Typically, these include accidental loss of the mouthpiece or a break in the loop integrity at connection point. The pre-dive checklist must always include a positive and negative pressure "loop check," since faulty assembly is a common hazard. Additionally, a leak in the counterlung can also provide an ingress point. Most scrubbers are of sufficient size that a small amount of fluid is absorbed without difficulty. However, large volumes of water will create a slurry of the granules.

The slurry will move from the scrubber into the inhalation side of the loop. The diver is creating a negative airway pressure with inspiration, facilitating aspiration into the airway and/or esophagus. Should this slurry come into contact with oropharyngeal or respiratory mucosa, severe chemical burns result, producing mucosal sloughing, edema, and spasm. Symptoms will include severe pain, laryngospasm, stridor, and dysphagia.

Acidic injury (pH < 3), causes a coagulation necrosis, with protein denaturation and vascular thrombosis. In effect, a shallow eschar is rapidly established, thus limiting the depth of injury. The very high pH (11.5–13.5) of these alkali solutions is vastly more treacherous. Rather than an eschar formation, the injury is one of liquefaction necrosis. The tissue destruction will continue into the tissues until effectively diluted. Thus, the depth of injury is potentially full thickness, resulting in perforation of the tracheobronchial system or the esophagus.

The extent of tissue destruction depends on three factors: the concentration and pH of the solution, the contact duration, and the amount aspirated. Sofnolime 797, a common absorbent, has a pH of 12 to 14 (3% NaOH).[41] Micropore lithium hydroxide at 1% has a pH > 13.[27]

Both of these common absorbents are extremely caustic. Contact duration will usually be minimized due to the resulting gag reflex. Immediate washing of the oropharynx with ambient water will be instinctive, aiding in dilution. However, granules of solution aspirated into the trachea cannot be effectively diluted. The reflexive expelling of the mouthpiece, however, may exacerbate the loop flood, thus making gas supply problematic.

Immediate steps should include access to an uncontaminated air source ("bail out") and immediate dive termination as soon as safely possible. On the surface, thorough washing of the oropharynx is indicated with water only. No attempt should be made to neutralize the base with a weak acid. The resulting exothermic reaction can only increase tissue damage. Judicious ingestion of freshwater is a reasonable adjunct, especially if medical care is not available. However, the induction of emesis is strongly discouraged, which would expose the esophagus to additional contact. Any ongoing distress or abdominal pain implies impending tissue destruction and thus is a medical emergency. Ultimately, esophageal resection and reconstruction may be needed.

Tracheobronchial necrosis (TBN) is perhaps the worst complication because of the rapid intolerance to any airway compromise. In one series, prompt emergent surgery within < 6 hours still had a 45% mortality rate. Late presentation of airway perforation had a mortality of > 80%.[4] Without immediate intensive surgical care, the mortality rate is essentially 100%.

The severity of esophageal injury cannot be overstated. There is at least one case report of the esophageal necrosis extending beyond the muscularis level and into the posterior (membranous) section of the trachea, resulting in extensive corrosive injuries of the upper airways and gastrointestinal tract.[15]

Initial management must focus on airway assessment and protection. Initial contact with mucous membranes will result in edema followed by tissue sloughing. This may progress into mechanical obstruction and airway compromise. Rapid cricothyrotomy or tracheostomy may be indicated.

In summary, common absorbent materials of NaOH or LiOH have pH values of 13 or more. These severely caustic materials create a liquefaction necrosis that can quickly lead to full-thickness injury of the trachea or esophagus. Principles of treatment depend on dilution and minimization of contact time with water irrigation. Supportive care with intravenous fluids, steroids, antibiotics, and pain medications are appropriate. Chemical neutralization with dilute acids is contraindicated, as is blind esophageal or tracheal intubation. Prognosis is dependent upon the tissue depth of injury, with organ perforation having greater than 80% mortality.

CCR FATALITIES

Although CCR diving has long been used in the military and is rapidly gaining popularity in the recreational, scientific, and technical diving communities, there have been concerns about its safety and potential association with increased rates of diving fatalities. As with all diving fatality statistics, the numbers are problematic and inexact at best, as no one knows the total number of individual divers, and there is no way to capture data on all fatalities and accidents. Additionally, when these incidents occur, the investigations often do not uncover a definitive cause of the accident.

In the Divers' Alert Network (DAN) annual diving report reviewing fatalities and accidents from 2010–2013, 8% of fatalities involved CCR, with 30% occurring in the United States.[5] Although it is difficult to know the total number of CCR and OC divers, this likely represents a disproportionately high number of fatalities in CCR when compared to OC. When compared to open-circuit fatalities, there were a higher proportion of "human factors" involved, including mistakes such as forgetting to open tank valves and accidentally breathing the wrong gases.[5] The rise in CCR fatalities was also addressed in the annual American Academy of Underwater Sciences (AAUS) symposium in 2007. Their review showed a significant rise in total number of CCR deaths, likely reflecting a rise in their popularity and overall prevalence of CCR diving. Similar to the DAN data, their data identified more equipment trouble and buoyancy problems implicated in the deaths when compared to open-circuit deaths. These appeared to be more related to procedural problems/human error than true equipment failure. In only 3 of 80 deaths did they identify true equipment failures. There was a significant number of equipment-related problems that were more related to procedural issues, such as poor preparation, inappropriate equipment operation (including turning on all sensors/tanks), and poor equipment maintenance.[48] Similar findings were discussed at the Rebreather Forum 3 in 2012, in which a group of individuals representing hyperbaric and dive medicine, scientific and commercial diving, and the CCR industry met with the specific goal of increasing rebreather safety.[34]

There are multiple published case reports illustrating various causes of injuries and fatalities in CCR, including oxygen toxicity, cerebral arterial gas embolism, decompression sickness, and respiratory failure secondary to hypercarbia.[8,12,17,30,44] Although almost any of these things can also occur in open-circuit diving, there are some conditions that are more frequently seen among CCR divers. Not surprisingly, oxygen toxicity was more commonly a cause of death in CCR than OC deaths, and, as mentioned above, there appear to be more procedural and equipment-related deaths in CCR fatalities.[34] Hypercarbia is essentially not an issue in OC diving, since there is no recirculation of exhaled breaths, and the CO_2 is lost to the environment. Additionally, CCR allows divers to explore certain environments previously virtually inaccessible on open-circuit, such as extreme depths, overhead environments, and prolonged bottom times. These extreme conditions may result in previously unencountered environmental hazards, as well as new physiologic challenges, such as hypercarbia, subsequent respiratory failure and death from extreme depths.[30]

Just as with open-circuit divers, it is important to note that medical problems may occur while diving. By far the most common problems that occur during diving are cardiac related, including arrhythmias and myocardial infarctions. These are likely underreported, as many of these deaths are classified as "drownings" by pathologists simply because they occurred in the water.[35] Research is ongoing into the effects of CCR diving on cardiac physiology.[10]

The CCR community is invested in promoting the safety of CCR diving, and there have been multiple symposiums and reviews dedicated specifically to this task. In addition to the necessity of ensuring adequate training for CCR diving, there have been multiple calls to develop pre-dive checklists in an effort to prevent procedural-related and equipment problems before entering the water or just after entry in to the water.[5,48] There have also been efforts to educate divers on resuscitation and rescue specifically of CCR divers.[49]

REFERENCES

1. Arieli R. The effect of over- or underfilling the soda lime canister on CO2 absorption in two closed-circuit oxygen rebreathers. Undersea Hyperb Med. 2008;35:213-8.
2. Arieli R, Arieli Y, Daskalovic Y, Eynan M, Abramovich A. CNS oxygen toxicity in closed-circuit diving: signs and symptoms before loss of consciousness. Aviat Space Environ Med. 2006;77:1153-7.
3. Arieli R, Shochat T, Adir Y. CNS toxicity in closed-circuit oxygen diving: symptoms reported from 2527 dives. Aviat Space Environ Med. 2006;77:526-32.
4. Benjamin B, Agueb R, Vuarnesson H, et al. Tracheobronchial necrosis after caustic ingestion. Ann Surg. 2016;263:808-13.
5. Buzzacott P, Trout B, Caruso J, Nelson C, Denoble P. DAN Annual Diving Report 2012-2015. Divers Alert Network; 2015.
6. Chang SC, Stetter JR, Cha CS. Amperometric gas sensors. Talanta. 1993;40(4):461-77.
7. Cherry AD, Forkner IF, Frederick HJ, Naatoli MJ, Schinazi EA, Longphre JP, Conard JL, White WD, Freiberger JJ, Stolp BW, Pollock NW, Doar PO, Boso AE, Alford EL, Walker AJ, Ma AC, Rhodes MA, Moon RE. Predictors of increased PaCO2 during immersed prone exercise at 4.7 ATA. J Appl Physiol. 2009;106(1):316-25.
8. Chong SJ, Tan TW. Cerebral arterial gas embolism in a diver using closed circuit rebreather diving apparatus. Diving Hyperb Med. 2008;38:46-7.
9. Clark M. CCR trimix simplified. Silent Scuba LLC; 2009.
10. Covington DB, Bielawski A, Scalzini A, et al. Cardiovascular changes of closed-circuit rebreather divers assessed via transthoracic 2-D Doppler echocardiography [poster abstract]. Undersea and Hyperbaric Medical Society; 2016.
11. Eynan M, Daskalovic YI, Arieli Y, Arieli R, Shupak A, Eilender E, Kerem DH. Training improves divers' ability to detect increased CO2. Aviat Space Environ Med. 2003 May;74(5):537-45.
12. Frånberg O, Ericsson M, Larsson A, Lindholm P. Investigation of a demand-controlled rebreather in connection with a diving accident. Undersea Hyperb Med. 2011;38:61-72.
13. Hamilton B. Rebreather physiology. ed. 27. 1997. p. 57-60.
14. Hesser CM, Lind F, Linnarsson D. Significance of airway resistance for the pattern of breathing and lung volumes in exercising humans. J Appli Physiol. 1990;68:1875-82.
15. Jaillard S, Nseir S, Métois D, et al. Extensive corrosive injuries of the upper airways and gastrointestinal tract. J Thorac Cardiovasc Surg. 2002;123:186-8.
16. Jarrett AS. Alveolar carbon dioxide tension at increased ambient pressures. J Appl Physiol. 1966;21:158-62.
17. Johns K. Scientific diver rebreather fatality: an incident review. Curacao AAUS/ESDP Joint International Symposium; 2013. p. 139-46.
18. Juergensen K. Juergensen Marine's MK 15 Manual [Internet]. 1998 [updated 2005 Sep 7 personal communication]. Available from: http://www.nwdesigns.com/rebreathers/mk15_manual.htm
19. Kerem D, Daskalovic YI, Arieli R, Shupak A. CO2 retention during hyperbaric exercise while breathing 40/60 nitrox. Undersea Hyperb Med. 1995;22:339-46.
20. Lamb JS. The practice of oxygen measurement for divers. Best Publishing Co.; 1999 Jan.

21. Lambertsen C, Gelfand R, Peterson R, et al. Human tolerance to breathing He, Ne, and N2 at respiratory gas densities equivalent to He-O2 breathing at depths to 1200, 2000, 3000, 4000, and 5000 feet of sea water (predictive studies III). Aviat Space Environ Med. 1977;48:843-55.

22. Lanphier EH. Immersion effects and apparatus design: a view from Wisconsin. In: Physiological and human engineering aspects of underwater breathing apparatus. Proceedings of the 40th Undersea and Hyperbaric Medical Society Workshop; 1989. p. 45-56.

23. Lanphier EH. Nitrogen-oxygen mixture physiology. U.S. Navy Experimental Dive Unit; 1958. Phase 4: carbon dioxide sensitivity as a potential means of personnel selection. Phase 6: carbon dioxide regulation under diving conditions; p. 7-58. Available from: http://www.navsea.navy.mil/Home/SUPSALV/NEDU/.

24. Linnarsson D, Hesser CM. Dissociated ventilatory and central respiratory responses to CO2 at raised N2 pressure. J Appl Physiol. 1978;45(5):756-61.

25. Lundgren CEG, Miller JN. Carbon dioxide retention. Identification of CO2 retainers. In: Lung biology in health and disease: the lung at depth. New York: Dekker; 1999. p. 229.

26. Maio DA, Farhi LE. Effect of gas density on mechanics of breathing. J Appl Physiol. 1967;23:687-93.

27. Micropore lithium safety data sheet MSDS0001. Version 5. 2008.

28. Miller RD, Fleischer LA. Airway resistance. In: Miller's anesthesia. Philadelphia: Elsevier; 2005.

29. Mitchell S. Physiology of rebreather diving. Rebreather Forum 3; 2012. p. 80-91.

30. Mitchell SJ, Cronjé FJ, Meintjes WA, Britz HC. Fatal respiratory failure during a "technical" rebreather dive at extreme pressure. Aviat Space Environ Med. 2007;78:81-6.

31. Mitchell SJ, Doolette DJ. Recreational technical diving part 1: an introduction to technical diving methods and activities. Diving Hyperb Med. 2013 Jun;43(2):86-93.

32. Moon RE, Cherry AD, Stolp BW, Camporesi EM. Pulmonary gas exchange in diving. J Appl Physiol. 2009;106:668-77.

33. Mummery HJ, Stolp BW, Dear GDL, Doar PO, Natoli MJ, Boso AE, Archibald JD, Hobbs GW, El-Moalem HE, Moon RE. Effects of age and exercise on physiological dead space during simulated dives at 2.8 ATA. J Appl Physiol. 2003;94:507-15.

34. Rebreather Forum 3 Proceedings. Rebreather Forum 3; 2012.

35. Sadler CN, Grover I, Witucki P, Neuman T. Dilemma of natural death while scuba diving. Academ Forensic Pathol. 2013;3:202-12.

36. Salzano JV, Camporesi EM. Physiological responses to exercise at 47 and 66 ATA. J Appl Physiol. 1984;57:1055-68.

37. Salzano J, Rausch DC, Saltzman HA. Cardiorespiratory responses to exercise at a simulated seawater depth of 1,000 feet. J Appl Physiol. 1970:1055-68.

38. Sapoval B, Filoche M, Weibel ER. Smaller is better – but not too small: a physical scale for the design of the mammalian pulmonary acinus. Proc Natl Acad Sci U S A. 2002;99:10411-6.

39. Sieber A. Oxygen sensor technology for rebreathers. Rebreather Forum 3. Durham (NC): AAUS/DAN/PADI; 2014. p. 185-92.

40. Sieber A, L'abbate A, Bedini R. Oxygen sensor signal validation for the safety of the rebreather diver. Diving Hyperb Med. 2009;39:38-45.

41. SofnolimeSafetyData. Material safety data sheet. Version 13. 2012.

42. Taylor NAS, Morrison JB. Lung centroid pressure and its influence on respiratory and physical work during immersion. In: Physiological and human engineering aspects of underwater breathing apparatus. Proceedings of the 40th Undersea and Hyperbaric Medical Society Workshop; 1989. p. 33-42.

43. Thalmann ED, Sponholtz DK, Lundgren CE. Effects of immersion and static lung loading on submerged exercise at depth. Undersea Biomed Res. 1979;6:259-90.

44. Trytko B, Mitchell S. Extreme survival: a serious technical diving accident. SPUMS J. 2005;25:23-7.

45. Valadao JM, Vigilante JA, DiGeorge NW, et al. Ketogenic diet for high partial pressure oxygen diving. Undersea Hyperb Med. 2014;41:331-5.

46. Van Liew HD, Thalmann ED, Sponholtz DK. Hindrance to diffusive gas mixing in the lung in hyperbaric environments. J Appl Physiol. 1981;51(2):243-7.

47. Vann R. Lambertsen and O2: beginnings of operational physiology. Undersea Hyperb Med. 2004;31(1):21-31.

48. Vann R, Pollock NW, Denoble P. Rebreather fatality investigation. American Academy of Underwater Sciences 26th Symposium; 2007. p. 101-10.

49. Verdier C, Lee DA, Scoff H. Unconscious recreational rebreather diver and rescue techniques. In: Verdier, editor. Nitrox rebreather diving. 2008

50. Vorosmarti JR, Bradley ME, Anthonisen NR. The effects of increased gas density on pulmonary mechanics. Undersea Biomed Res. 1975;2:1-10.

51. Warkander DE. CO2 Retention with minimal symptoms but severe dysfunction during we simulated dives to 6.8 atm abs [abstract]. Undersea and Hyperbaric Medical Society Annual Scientific Meeting; 1987.

52. Warkander DE. Comprehensive performance limits for divers' underwater breathing gear: consequences of adopting diver-focused limits [Internet]. Naval Sea Systems Command Navy Experimental Diving Unit (US); 2007 Jan. TA05-12 NEDU TR 07-02. Available from: http://studylib.net/doc/8928010/consequences-of-adopting-diver

53. Warkander DE, Nagasawa GK, Lundgren CE. Effects of inspiratory and expiratory resistance in divers' breathing apparatus. Undersea Hyperb Med. 2001;28:63-73.

54. Warkander DE, Norfleet WT, Nagasawa GK, Lundgren CE. CO2 Retention with minimal symptoms by severe dysfunction during wet simulated dives to 6.8 atm abs. Undersea Biomed Res. 1990;17:515-23.

55. Warkander DE, Norfleet WT, Nagasawa GK, Lundgren CE. Physiologically and subjectively acceptable breathing resistance in divers' breathing gear. Undersea Biomed Res. 1992;19:427-45.

56. Weibel ER, Sapoval B, Filoche M. Design of peripheral airways for efficient gas exchange. Respir Physiol Neurobiol. 2005;148:p3-21.

57. Wood LD, Bryan AC, Bau SK, Weng TR, Levison H. Effect of increased gas density on pulmonary gas exchange in man. J Appl Phy

CHAPTER 45 CHAPTER

Maladies Specific to Technical and Rebreather Divers

CHAPTER FORTY-FIVE OVERVIEW

Introduction 1109
Technical Diving Defined 1109
History of Rebreathers 1110
Description of Rebreathers 1110
Specific Maladies 1114
Fatigue/Lethargy 1114
Hyperoxic Myopia 1114
Off-Gassing in the Eyes 1115
Caustic Cocktail 1115
Hypercapnia 1118
Middle-Ear Oxygen Absorption 1120
Pulmonary Oxygen Toxicity 1120
Pulmonary Disease 1122
Hypoxia 1122
Deep Water Blackout 1123
Isobaric (Inert Gas) Counter Diffusion 1123
CNS Oxygen Toxicity 1126
High-Pressure Nervous Syndrome 1127
Back Pain 1127
Compression Arthralgia 1128
References 1130

Maladies Specific to Technical and Rebreather Divers

Carla Renaldo, Joseph Dituri, Brian P. O'Connell

INTRODUCTION

Divers using rebreathers and other technical diving gear are subject to the same medical issues as those who dive using recreational open-circuit diving equipment. These divers potentially face ailments beyond what the conventional diver faces, since they are capable of diving deeper with different breathing media and for longer durations. This chapter focuses on maladies specific to these rebreathers and technical divers only and does not discuss in great detail those maladies common to both conventional as well as rebreather and technical divers since they are previously discussed throughout this text.

TECHNICAL DIVING DEFINED

Although the concept and term "technical diving" are relatively recent advents to Self-Contained Underwater Breathing Apparatus (SCUBA) diving vernacular, divers have been engaging in what is now commonly referred to as technical diving for decades. For the past 30–40 years, technical divers have been trying to find a way around Henry's law and the obligated decompression. Technical divers have done just that by:

1. modifying the amount of oxygen in the breathing medium,
2. modifying the amount and type of inert gas in the breathing medium,
3. increasing the size and number of cylinders used for the medium, and
4. developing methods for decompression using nontraditional algorithms.

There are several methods for technical divers to understand their decompression limits for a given dive. Commercial decompression tables are available for purchase, offering varying depth/time schedules. These tables include decompression stops based on varying gases such as helium, oxygen, or air enriched with oxygen. A diver can also plan the dive on computer software and print out a personalized depth/time schedule for a dive. Finally, most dive computer manufacturers offer real-time decompression calculations based on the actual dive parameters and gas mixtures that can be used for technical dives.

For the purposes of this chapter, technical, "Tec," or "Tek" diving is defined as any form of SCUBA that exceeds conventional recreational SCUBA diving limits. As defined by the Occupational Safety and Health Administration (OSHA), technical diving is merely a form of extended recreational SCUBA diving with respect to depth, breathing media, bottom time, and nature of dive. Contrary to commercial diving, OSHA rules do not apply to recreational or technical diving.

Technical diving requires additional experience, training, and specialized equipment. Technical divers are trained to plan their dives so that they stay at depth considerably longer than when using recreational SCUBA diving time schedules. When longer dives are planned, these plans detail the required decompression stops. Technical divers who plan decompression have been trained to understand the ramifications of failing to properly complete or altogether omitting required stops.

HISTORY OF REBREATHERS

Rebreathers were first conceptualized in the late 1600s by Giovanni Borelli, an Italian mathematician and physicist. Although his design was flawed, probably even deadly, Borelli's idea of removing the impurities from the exhaled breath is the basis for modern rebreathers. For the next 200 years, advances in rebreather technology came about due to the mining industry's need for a mine rescue unit that had nothing to do with the dive industry. In 1878, the first patent for a diving rebreather was granted to Henry Fluess.[4] Later that same year, Henry Fluess sold his patent to a manufacturing company, and that company later began producing rebreathers. After this, other inventors began to experiment with myriad types of configurations.

Since the rebreather was conceived prior to open-circuit (OC), many ask why rebreathers are not more popular than OC. The authors suppose that the rise in popularity of television shows and the explorations filmed by Jacques Cousteau, coupled with the extra work required when using a rebreather to ensure safe diving, led to the springboard effect for OC. It is also rumored that Jacques Cousteau had many problems with rebreathers and vowed not to use them.

DESCRIPTION OF REBREATHERS

There are three types of SCUBA diving: OC, semi-closed-circuit rebreather (SCR), and closed-circuit rebreather (CCR). While using OC, a person takes a breath of compressed gas from a cylinder, and that gas is subsequently exhaled into the water. With SCR and CCR, the diver takes a breath of gas from a flexible gas storage space (counterlung), and, instead of exhaling it into the surrounding water, the exhaled gas stays in the breathing loop where it is then breathed again (rebreathed).

A rebreather is a piece of technical diving equipment, represented in Figure 1, which affords a diver a number of benefits over recreational OC SCUBA equipment. One benefit is the ability for a diver to carry less gas on a dive. That, coupled with decreased decompression obligation because of the fixed partial pressure of oxygen as well as breathing a warm and moist breathing media, make rebreathers popular with divers seeking to extend the reach beyond normal OC diving limits.

Over the past ~140 years there have been many advances in rebreather technology, and currently all rebreathers fall into three basic categories: oxygen rebreathers, SCR, and CCR. All rebreathers have a loop which consists of the following:

1. Hoses to carry the exhaled gas to a counterlung and back to the diver
2. Check valves ensuring one-way flow around the loop
3. At least one counterlung
4. Some method of scrubbing carbon dioxide from the exhaled breath
5. Some method of volumetric makeup to compensate for the increasing pressure and decreasing volume associated with Boyle's law
6. Some method for metabolic makeup to counteract oxygen metabolism and maintain a breathable mixture

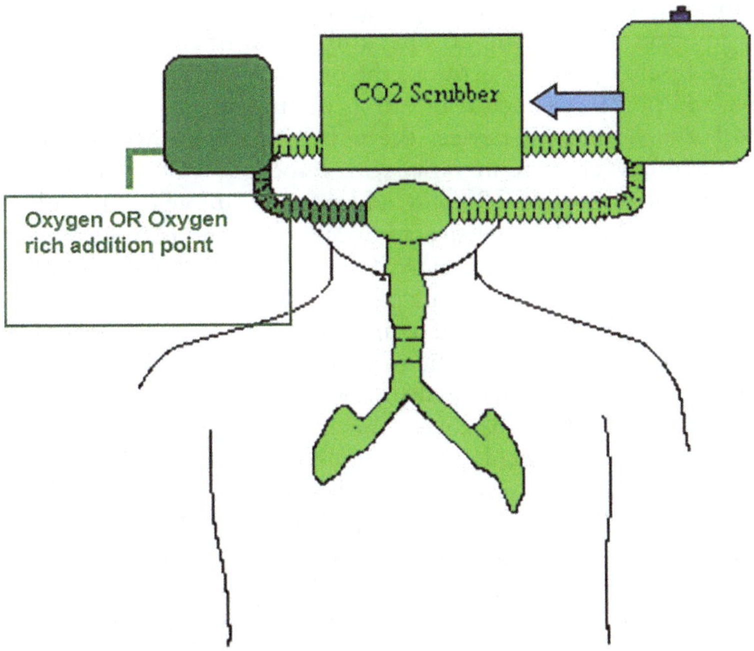

Figure 1. Simplified rebreather diagram.

The CO_2 scrubber canister is specifically designed for each rebreather with a specific kind of scrubbing material or soda lime which is predominantly calcium hydroxide ($Ca(OH)_2$). It is designed for use in water temperatures between 32°F–85°F (0°C–30°C). There are two sizes of mesh for the absorbent (mesh size 4–8 or 8–12). If the scrubber agent becomes wet, the canister duration is considerably less. If the dive plan details use of the rebreather in water temperatures below 50°F (10°C), divers should store the absorbent at room temperature for 12 hours prior to diving. The canister should be filled immediately before diving.

It is essential that correct handling procedures be observed when using absorbent. When filling, do so in a well-ventilated space, preferably outdoors, with any dust blowing away from all living creatures. As it is a chemical, care should be taken to avoid contact with children and pets. If it is ingested, call the poison control center for appropriate steps.

When packing the canister, ensure no gaps are allowed to form in the absorbent material. In order to do this, tap the sides of the canister briskly while filling. Do not forget to install the anti-channeling device (if equipped) when the canister is full. Tap the canister sides vigorously again to reduce gaps. Fill to the top, and level off the absorbent at the fill line.

Oxygen rebreathers are the least complex of the three types of rebreathers. Oxygen rebreathers only use pure oxygen within the breathing loop. These passive addition systems only add oxygen when the volume of the breathing loop decreases to a prescribed level. That is to say that oxygen is the gas used for volumetric and metabolic makeup. These devices generally have a maximum operating depth of approximately 20 feet because of the risk of central nervous system (CNS) oxygen toxicity.

SCRs use a single breathing mixture that is not pure oxygen. The oxygen required for metabolic makeup is "added" to the breathing loop with the other gases that make up the single breathing mixture. SCRs can either be active addition or passive addition. The maximum operating depth of this rebreather is derived using the maximum operating depth of the breathing mixture used for the dive.

Active-addition SCRs add the breathing mixture through a constantly flowing orifice or other such metering device. The added gas mixes with the rebreathed gas, and the inspired oxygen content varies with respect to VO_2, flow rate, and diver work rate. Passive-addition SCRs only add gas mixture when the volume of the entire loop is decreased. These passive-addition SCRs tend to have a lower inspired oxygen percentage than active-addition SCRs.

CCRs use two different breathing gases. One gas is always 100% oxygen, and the other is called a diluent which can be any combination of oxygen and other inert gases. The oxygen serves as metabolic makeup. The diluent dilutes the breathing mixture and serves as volumetric makeup. The oxygen is added to the breathing loop as it is metabolized by the diver. The "need to add" oxygen is determined by comparing the values calculated by the oxygen sensors. This comparison is calculated automatically by a computer (in the case of an electronically controlled or eCCR), mechanically by a constant flow orifice or metering device (in the case of a mechanically controlled or mCCR), or manually by the diver. Manual addition of oxygen can be accomplished at any time throughout the dive on most CCR because it is accomplished by the diver. Hybrids as well as home-built versions of the aforementioned types exist in some form but are beyond the scope of this chapter. The advantage of a CCR in general is the ability to allow the diver to maintain a constant partial pressure of oxygen (pO_2) throughout a dive regardless of depth, thereby reducing the decompression obligation.

Almost all oxygen sensors used for rebreathers are galvanic fuel cells, except for the cells produced for lifetime use in Poseidon rebreathers. Poseidon's sensor is based on unique luminescent dyes, which are excited with red light and show an oxygen-dependent luminescence in the range of near-infrared light. These "solid state" sensors appear to function well, but substantial testing is required to ensure lifetime accuracy.

Galvanic oxygen sensors are batteries that generate electrical current proportional to the number of oxygen molecules in the surrounding gas. Basic elements of these sensors are similar to those of a battery such as a lead anode, a noble-metal plated cathode, and a solution of potassium hydroxide as an electrolyte.

The cathode is a convex metal disc plated with gold or silver that has numerous perforations. The surface is designed to facilitate continuous wetting of the upper portion and contains a small amount of electrolyte between the membrane and the cathode. As oxygen diffuses into the sensor, the lead is oxidized into lead oxide. The chemical reaction produces a small current between the anode and cathode. An increase in the exposed pO_2 results in a proportional increase in the current generated by the sensor.

Continual accurate monitoring of the pO_2 within the loop of any rebreather is important to ensure the pO_2 of the breathing gas is not hypoxic or hyperoxic. Since CCR computers calculate decompression predicated upon inert gas content, and that content varies in a CCR with the pO_2, the knowledge of pO_2 is also important for determining decompression obligation. In order to ensure accurate monitoring, calibration is required. The calibration process is different for different rebreather models.

The current generated by an oxygen sensor is affected by temperature and humidity. Oxygen sensors have a normal operating range from 32°F–122°F (0°C–50°C) and may provide inaccurate readings outside those bounds. Build-up of humidity on the sensor membrane can also lead to inaccurate pO_2 being displayed. These oxygen sensors lose their ability to generate current over time just like any battery. It is characteristic to see a gradual decrease in millivolt output of the galvanic cell until near end of life. At near end of life, the cell often portrays uncharacteristically high millivoltage output which could be misinterpreted as a higher oxygen concentration and lead to potential hypoxia. To be safe, galvanic sensors should not be trusted if open for over one year or if they are starting to display seemingly abnormally high or low output.

The placement of the counterlung is important to the work of breathing resistance experienced by the rebreather diver. There are two main types of static lung load differential (SLLD) which are positive SLLD and negative SLLD. The higher the SLLD, the more work it takes for a diver to breathe. The centroid is the volumetric center of a compliant volume. In the case of a rebreather, the diver has two distinct breathing spaces. The first is the lungs, and the centroid of the lungs is illustrated in Figure 2 with a red X in the center of the diver's body. The second is the centroid of the counterlung which is pictured as an X inside the purple space. The change in pressure between these two spaces provides a representation of the SLLD. In the case of Figure 2a, there is a negative SLLD, making it more difficult for the diver to inhale from the counterlung but easier to exhale. Figure 2b is representative of a positive SLLD which makes it easier for the diver to inhale from the counterlung but more difficult to exhale. The over-the-shoulder counterlung is represented by Figure 2c, and in the case represented portrays an only slightly positive (almost neutral) SLLD, making inhaling and exhaling almost identically easy. Finally, Figure 2d represents a compensated bellows which has a weight that assists with compression of the bellows, thereby decreasing the SLLD no matter what position the diver takes. It is important to note that these positions are as represented and would change with the change in pressure represented by the diver's swim position (lung position) relative to the unit's position (counterlung position).

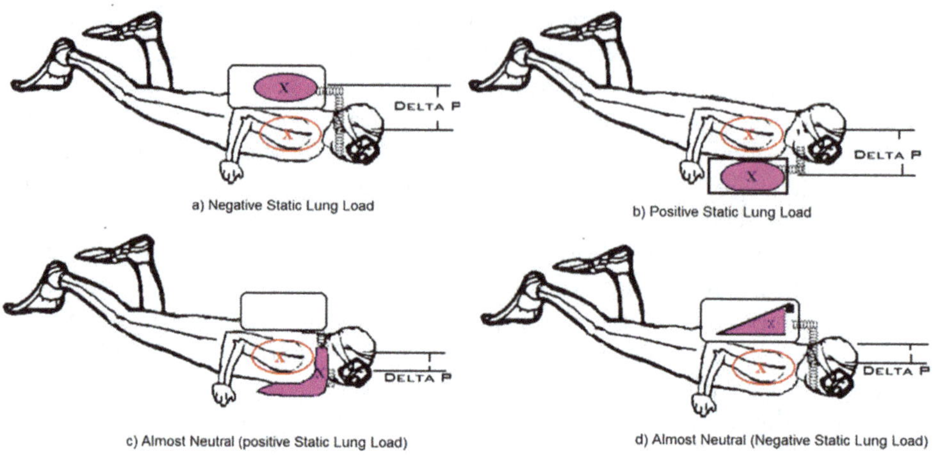

Figure 2. Pictorial representation of SLLD. [31]

SPECIFIC MALADIES

Fatigue/Lethargy

Fatigue can be the difficulty, inability, or a reduced capacity to perform and maintain activities and/or difficulties with concentration, memory, and emotional stability.[27] Post-dive fatigue is a common finding among technical or rebreather dives. Sometimes fatigue can be due to "normal" increased physical activity demands at depth for long durations, while other times it may signify oxidative stress from high pO_2 or decompressive stress which has been coined "subclinical" decompression sickness (DCS).[10] Additionally, the lethargy may be caused by the body's temperature maintenance requirement because water conducts heat away from the body 25 times faster than air.[25] Another contributing factor to fatigue is that removing the wet suit forces a decline in central blood volume and a corresponding drop in blood pressure following pressure immersion diuresis.[29]

It is important to differentiate appropriate fatigue from inappropriate fatigue. Any extraordinary fatigue may endanger the diver because it may impact the diver's decision-making process, thereby predisposing the diver to error. If the diver is feeling any unusual fatigue he or she should monitor him- or herself for more serious symptoms of DCS and consider the source of the fatigue. Hydration, rest, and oxygen may be indicated.

Hyperoxic Myopia

Hyperoxic myopia (HM), or "oxygen eye," is a reversible myopic shift in acuity and is potentially problematic with technical divers but more common in rebreather divers on long-duration, multi-day missions. Rebreathers allow the diver to set the oxygen partial pressure for the duration of a dive, and, in order to decrease decompression obligation, rebreather divers often increase oxygen to 1.3 pO_2 or more. It has been known for some time that that high a pO_2 can impair cellular function. The damage of hyperbaric oxygen is caused by the secondary generation of more reactive intermediaries and the products of lipid peroxidation versus the direct effects of the superoxide radical and hydrogen peroxide.[7]

It is postulated that, in HM, hyperoxygenation alters the shape or metabolism of the lens and increases the refractive power of the lens.

HM has been reported in a publicized case report in 1999 on a mixed-gas CCR diver whose dive profile was significant for prolonged dive times on multiple repetitive days.[7] The impact of HM is purportedly proportional to the pO_2 breathed and duration of exposure. While this process is reversible with exposure to normobaric air, it may take as long as 14 days for the impact to be reduced and up to 3 months to be completely reversed.

In dry chambers, this malady is a well-documented side effect of patients undergoing multiple HBO_2 therapy treatments, as well as the development of cataracts.[32] Reports from patients experiencing HM while receiving HBO_2 therapy indicate it may take as long as 6 to 12 months for the symptoms to resolve.[3] The difference in the resolution of the symptoms between the divers and the HBO_2 therapy is likely multifactorial including environment, exposure levels, as well as demographic.

There is at present no cure for HM; however, treatment includes exposure to normobaric air for long periods of time. The prolonged exposed to high pO_2 could exacerbate the issue, thus worsening the myopia until the diver is unsafe in his or her ability to perform dives. Divers experiencing HM should discontinue diving until symptoms resolve.

Off-Gassing in the Eyes

Technical and rebreather divers who wear contact lenses and have pushed the decompression envelope have reported blurred vision and decreased visible acuity with noted halos following deep and technical or decompression dives. One possible reason for this could be a gas buildup behind the contact lens and bubble collection. In a study by Simon and Bradley, these symptoms were reported in divers wearing hard contact lenses and notably absent in those divers wearing soft contact lenses.

The eye is purportedly one of the fastest tissues for off-gassing, so it may become saturated in the course of a technical dive. In Haldanian decompression, fast tissues absorb and release gas quickly even during ascent. A potential causality for this affliction is the escaping gas becoming trapped in the concave portion of the normally gas-permeable contact lenses, thereby distorting vision. Contact lenses are designed to be gas permeable on the convex side (greater surface area) moving toward the concave (lesser surface area). They are less effective at gas permeability on the concave side due to their curvature and the tighter structure.

It is a key point that the symptoms occurred in those divers who wore hard gas-permeable lenses and not in those divers wearing soft contact lenses. In the aforementioned study by Simon and Bradley, the bubbles were eliminated by removing the hard contact lenses. Alternatively, a 0.4-millimeter fenestration in the center of the contact lens allows the expanding gas carried by tears a path through which it can escape.[36]

Caustic Cocktail

A “caustic cocktail” (CC) is the “slurry” that results when water comes into contact with the chemical components of carbon dioxide (CO_2) absorbent, or soda lime. The main components of the most common soda lime are calcium hydroxide and sodium hydroxide; some manufacturers add potassium hydroxide.

Other manufacturers choose to make the main ingredient barium hydroxide or lithium hydroxide, but these are rarer. They are strong bases, each having a pH greater than 12, and, in the presence of water, an exothermic reaction ensues and a "cocktail" is created as the soda lime is liquefied; when ingested or inhaled by the diver, mild to severe chemical injury will result. Figure 3 below demonstrates the chemical bonds and reaction between the most common soda lime (calcium hydroxide) and CO_2. It is noteworthy to mention that, while the results of the lithium hydroxide reaction are largely similar to the other soda limes, it has a considerable exothermic property to its reaction and is vastly more efficient at CO_2 removal with greater duration for the same mass. Additionally, the causticity of lithium hydroxide is considerably more severe.

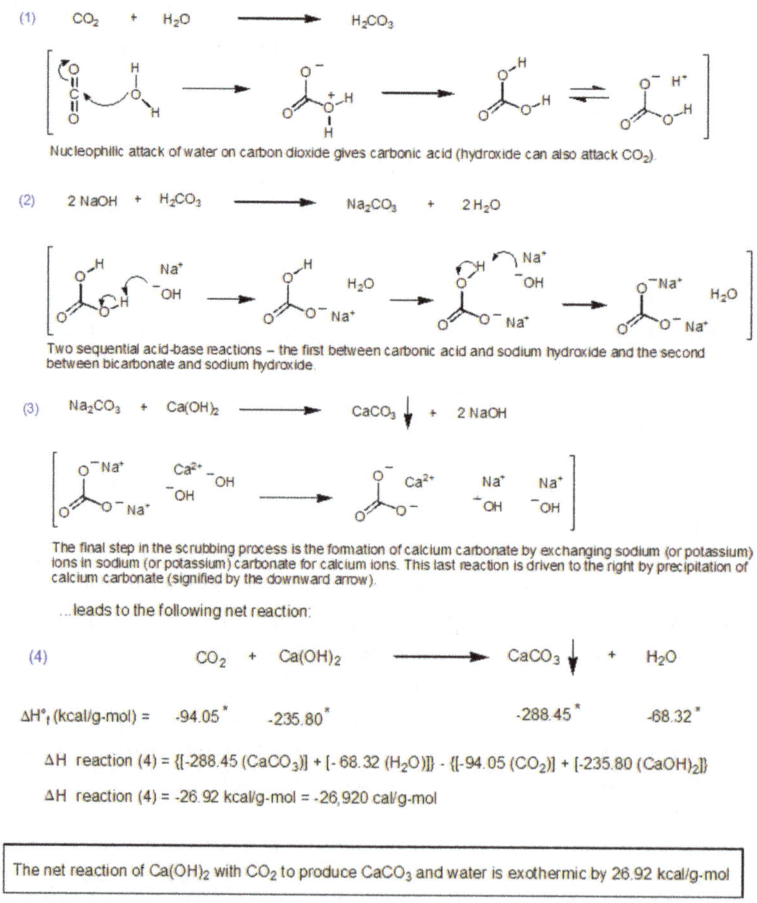

Figure 3. Chemical reaction in detail.

When a diver's body metabolizes oxygen, the byproduct is CO_2. The exhaled CO_2 reacts with the moisture in the exhaled breath to produce a weak carbonic acid (H_2CO_3). The presence of some moisture is necessary to catalyze the reaction needed to remove the diver's exhaled CO_2 as it passes through the scrubber bed. This acid can be neutralized with a base material such as the scrubber material (calcium hydroxide). As the carbonic acid passes through the base material, the CO_2 molecules bond to the granules and are removed from the exhaled gas.

Sodium hydroxide acts as a catalyst and contributes to a faster elimination of CO_2 than calcium hydroxide alone would. Reactions in aqueous state are generally faster than would occur in dry or solid state. Another key absorbent parameter is water content. Although water is needed to react with carbon dioxide to produce carbonic acid, some of the water in the absorbent is used to counteract the heat of the scrubber reaction by vaporization. If too much water is present, absorbent pores will fill and reduce the surface area available for reaction. Too little water and the absorbent dries out, shortening its life.(9)

NaOH and KOH are needed, along with the major scrubber component of $Ca(OH)_2$ in CO_2 absorbent, to promote fast and efficient reaction with carbon dioxide and carbonic acid in the scrubber. The reason is that NaOH and KOH are more reactive and more soluble than $Ca(OH)_2$.

Absorbent composed of $Ca(OH)_2$ alone is produced for medical applications under the trade name of Amsorb. The carbon dioxide absorption capacity of Amsorb has been reported as being as little as half that of soda lime.(23) This illustrates the importance of NaOH and KOH in small quantities along with $Ca(OH)_2$ in absorbents and the need to use only absorbents designed and approved for diving.

As stated previously, the symptoms of a CC which the diver will experience will range from mild to severe. The extent of injury depends on duration of contact, amount of chemical, and distribution. If ingested, the diver may experience sore throat, odynophagia, nausea with or without vomiting, and abdominal pain. He or she may complain of choking and gagging. Mucosal ulcerations can occur along the gastrointestinal tract including the oropharynx, hypopharynx, esophagus, and stomach. The injured diver may experience esophageal spasms. Long-term effects include strictures.

In the most severe cases, the diver sustains an inhalation injury which can result in swelling of the tissues in the oropharynx comprising the airway. The bronchial tree can be adversely affected, and consequences may not be seen for hours or days after the initial insult. Liquefactive necrosis is the type of tissue injury that occurs from strong bases and is the process of saponification of fats and the solubilization of proteins. This can lead to chemical pneumonitis and acute respiratory distress syndrome (ARDS), which can lead to placing the diver on mechanical ventilation.

The treatment of a CC includes (if the diver is in the water), assuming an upright position and making a controlled ascent to the surface. The diver's mouth should be rinsed with freshwater and forced swallowing. If only seawater is available, rinsing and spitting out is acceptable. One should not induce vomiting. It is not recommended to administer a weak acid solution such as vinegar or lemon juice.(37) If possible, administer intravenous (IV) or intramuscular (IM) steroids and benzocaine throat spray and monitor.

The source of the malfunction should be determined and repaired before the diver uses the rebreather to dive again. Pre-dive negative-pressure checks are important to help prevent such an occurrence. CCs are easily avoided by taking a few precautionary steps. The responsibility to reduce the possibility of this and any other potential problem is the divers'. Ensure the canister check is satisfactory prior to each dive. Also, avoid removing the mouthpiece from the mouth when the switch is in the "on" position. This should be practiced even when the diver is on the boat. If this habit is developed above water, it will be natural to never remove the mouthpiece unless the switch is in the "off" position below water.

Hypercapnia

Hypercapnia ($PaCO_2$ > 45 mmHg) or hypercarbia is the condition of abnormally high levels of carbon dioxide in the body's tissues. The early symptoms are often not recognized and can include headache, confusion, and lethargy. The symptomatology may progress to disorientation, panic, hyperventilation, convulsions, unconsciousness, and death in severe hypercapnia, which generally occurs at a $PaCO_2$ > 75 mmHg. Other signs and symptoms of hypercapnia include flushed skin, bounding pulse, tachypnea, dyspnea, premature contraction of the heart, other muscle twitches, asterixis, reduced neural activity, and hypertension.

Hypercapnia is commonly observed in rebreather divers and technical divers as well as skip-breathing divers.

For rebreather divers, the concerns stem from two separate but equally potentially devastating eventualities, the first being improper packing of the scrubber material into the canister. If the canister is improperly packed, insufficiently full, or has been overshaken allowing the settling of the scrubber material, a channeled path could allow CO_2 to take the path of least resistance through the scrubber material and circumvent the scrubbing process, allowing the CO_2 to be rebreathed. This is called channeling and is easily avoided by properly packing and regularly checking the scrubber material prior to diving. An antichannelling device contacts the side of the canister wall and makes it more difficult for gas to slip along the side of the smooth walls of the canister. Ensuring the mating surfaces of the canister and cover gasket are free from all dust and particles prior to closing the top will also help prevent failure. Applying pressure to the top while tightening the locking screw in a clockwise direction will compress the packing springs. This will make it easier to secure the top. Avoid overtightening the top of the canisters.

The second concern for rebreather divers is end of life or "breakthrough." When scrubber material is consumed, the binding sights around the external surfaces of each granular are activated. Once these sights are activated, they are essentially not usable again. The interaction between the exhaled breath of the diver and the scrubber material is a chemical reaction. All chemical reactions involve energy. Energy is used to break bonds in reactants, and energy (heat in this case) is released when new bonds form in products. In an exothermic reaction, it takes less energy to break bonds in the reactants than is released when new bonds form in the products. The reaction itself is exothermic in nature; heat is released and the binding sights become more efficient. Generally speaking, the center of the canister is considerably more efficient than the outside of the canister due to conductive heat loss on the outer surfaces. Therefore, the exhaled breath traveling through the scrubber canister would contain more CO_2 on the outside of the canister than in the center, allowing breakthrough nearer the outside of the canister.(31)

For rebreather divers, excess CO_2 in a closed breathing loop due to any of the failures mentioned above is problematic. CO_2 is removed from the body via alveolar mechanisms and is expelled into the breathing loop. Another supplemental mechanism for CO_2 removal exists that involves a nonalveolar process and suggests that excess CO_2 is eliminated via the digestive system. Gastric CO_2 can also be introduced into the rebreather loop, compounding hypercapnia due to the closed-loop nature of rebreathers.

The theory of gastric CO_2 ventilation or "pneumogastric ventilation" describes a previously unrecognized reflex mechanism controlled by neurons in the caudal solitary complex (cSC) for nonalveolar elimination of systemic CO_2 during respiratory acidosis.(11)

This cSC is also the site of cardiopulmonary receptor sensitivity for alveolar CO_2 elimination. The review article demonstrated a link between these two independent systems (respiratory and gastroesophageal) and how CO_2 is removed from the body. Illustrative of this point is the knowledge that U.S. Navy submariners who lived in higher concentrations of CO_2 (~25 x normal – .7%–1.5% CO_2 by concentration)[34] have reported gastrointestinal symptoms after being underway for several weeks.

A postprandial state, consumption of carbonated beverages, and systemic hypercapnic acidosis are all separate stimuli that induce gastric acid secretion and the production of HCO_3 – which react together to regenerate CO_2 in the gastric lumen. Dean describes a seven-step process for the conversion of cellular CO_2 into gastric CO_2 that is "exhaled" through the esophagus to be mixed with pulmonary gas in the oropharynx and exhaled primarily as alveolar CO_2 supplemented with gastric CO_2.[11] This extra CO_2 can be expelled into the closed breathing loop, compounding hypercapnia in the context of a failed scrubber which the authors have termed the "Dean effect." The excess CO_2, combined with an increase in depth, will have the multiplicative impact of increased partial pressure.

Possible mitigation techniques to decrease CO_2 production are not eating or drinking carbonated beverages before diving because it could over tax the CO_2 scrubber. There are a finite number of carbon dioxide binding sites in a scrubber canister, and an increase in CO_2 production would yield a corresponding decrease in scrubber duration. Additionally, in the event of a scrubber failure or the start of hypercapnia from any other failure, the diver should be removed from the rebreather loop as soon as possible because there is a greater chance of compounded production of CO_2 from the stomach. Since any stimulus that activates gastric acid secretion is expected to produce gastric CO_2, it may also be important to consider various stressful vocations and situations in the context of diving with a rebreather – for example, stress associated with first responders, sleep deprivation, and shift work, as well as emotional stress in general. Finally, consideration should be given to how preexisting gastrointestinal disorders contribute to the pneumogastric ventilation of CO_2.

CO_2 can be problematic in OC technical divers as well. Skip breathing, hypoventilation, or breath holding during dives increases CO_2. This is a common technique used to conserve gas, but it often acts contrarily, forcing respirations and actually increasing gas consumption over a given period of time. Additionally, rapid descents necessitate shallow or incomplete breathing, which leads to an increase in CO_2. Once a diver reaches the bottom and can fully ventilate, significant gas is used to ventilate the lungs of the built-up CO_2. Additionally, CO_2 exacerbates the symptoms of nitrogen narcosis and is known to be more narcotic than nitrogen due to the lipid solubility of CO_2.

Elevated metabolic activity, increasing equipment's dead space, increased work of breathing resistance,[37] and inadequate CO_2 elimination can lead to hypercapnia. Additionally, failure of the one-way valve, in the mouthpiece of a rebreather, would allow for CO_2 to flow back into the breathing loop, thereby increasing hypercapnia potential. Finally, large volumes of water or flooding of the rebreather will reduce the efficacy of the CO_2 scrubbing material, leading to CO_2 buildup.

Prevention is key; therefore, proper rebreather maintenance, including replacing the scrubber when recommended and pre-dive check for water leaks and proper one-way valve function, is best. The elevated levels of CO_2 trigger the respiratory drive, which increases the respiratory rate.[40] Divers experiencing hypercapnia and bailing out to OC can expect to have an insatiable thirst for OC gas. This situation is of great concern because it can rapidly become an out-of-air scenario.

Middle-Ear Oxygen Absorption

Middle-ear oxygen absorption, or "oxygen ear," refers to the negative pressure that may develop in the middle ear after a prolonged oxygen dive. Symptoms are usually mild and include a painless hearing loss with a sense of fullness in the ear, indicating acute serous otitis media. They most likely occur the morning after a dive upon awakening.

The proposed mechanism is that, following a high partial pressure oxygen dive, oxygen is slowly absorbed by the tissues of the middle ear and replaces the air-filled cavity. If the eustachian tubes do not open spontaneously, negative pressure builds because the absorbed gas is not replaced with air.

The treatment for oxygen ear is simple and straightforward: the diver is instructed to equalize the middle ear and repeat until the additional oxygen is absorbed.

It is important to take note of the onset of ear symptoms and their temporal relationship to the dive as well as associated symptoms. Although oxygen ear is unlikely to occur with the conventional OC SCUBA diver, the technical or rebreather diver will be susceptible to various maladies involving the ear. Therefore, it is critical to make the distinction between oxygen ear, ear barotrauma, and inner-ear DCS (IEDCS) in order to render appropriate treatment to the diver.

Pulmonary Oxygen Toxicity

Pulmonary oxygen toxicity is a form of oxygen toxicity that can result from prolonged exposure to elevated oxygen partial pressure. It is also termed the "Lorraine Smith effect" after the pathologist who, in the late nineteenth century, described deleterious pulmonary changes in experiments with mice after exposure to high partial pressures of oxygen for prolonged periods of time. It is less common that CNS oxygen toxicity and is more of a concern in extended dives, most notably with saturation diving, the high fraction of inspired oxygen (FiO_2) mixed gases with technical diving, and repeated chamber dives such as occurs with therapeutic recompression. Additionally, divers who set the pO_2 of their rebreather too high for long periods of time or technical divers who incorrectly plan or account for their oxygen exposure may experience pulmonary oxygen toxicity.

Early symptoms of pulmonary oxygen toxicity include mild tracheobronchitis and cough. These symptoms are worsened with deep inspiration and may progress to chest tightness and substernal discomfort. With prolonged exposure, the diver may experience dyspnea, which can be either exertional or nonexertional.

The degree to which a diver will experience pulmonary symptoms depends on a variety of factors, including the partial pressure of oxygen and the duration of the dive as well. Mild symptoms have been reported after 4 hours of oxygen breathing at 1.0 pO_2 and just after 1 hour of breathing oxygen at 3.0 pO_2. At higher partial pressures, similar symptoms reported after 4 hours at 1.0 pO_2 occur at 3 hours at 2.0 pO_2. More severe symptoms have been reported just after 3.5 hours at 3.0 pO_2.[38]

In addition to partial pressure of oxygen and dive duration, individual susceptibility can greatly influence the degree and the onset of symptoms of pulmonary oxygen toxicity.

Physical findings including rales, rhonchi, and fever have been reported. Chest X-ray changes reported by Hyde and Rawson revealed diffuse, bilateral pulmonary densities after prolonged oxygen therapy which cleared after the reduction in inspired pO_2.

Although clinical manifestations are more sensitive markers in tracking the progression of pulmonary oxygen toxicity, vital capacity (VC) is one method used to track the progression. A 2% decrease in VC is associated with mild pulmonary symptoms and is noted to be reversible whereby a 10% decrease in VC produces moderate symptoms and is reversible within a few days.[33] This decrease in VC is considered the allowable limit for most hyperbaric oxygen procedures. Other indices that have been studied to track the progression of pulmonary oxygen toxicity include inspiratory capacity, expiratory reserve volume, inspiratory flow rate, carbon monoxide diffusing capacity, and lung compliance. None have proven to be a single reliable marker for the onset, progression, or resolution of pulmonary oxygen toxicity.

Because the effects of hyperoxia on the lungs is dependent on both the inspired pO_2 and the duration of the exposure, it would make sense to track both to understand the point at which toxicity occurs in an effort to prevent it from occurring. The unit pulmonary toxic dose (UPTD) or oxygen tolerance unit (OTU) does just that. It is the equivalent of breathing 100% oxygen at 1 ATA. It is recommended that a maximum of 300 UPTD not be exceeded in a 24-hour period for multiple days of diving.

TABLE 1. OXYGEN TOLERANCE UNIT

UPTD Table

Time in Minutes (columns); Partial Pressue of Oxygen (rows)

	10	20	30	40	50	60	70	80	90	100	110	120	130	140	150	160	170	180	190	200	210	220	230	240	250	260	270	280	290	300
0.2	2	4	6	8	10	12	14	16	18	20	22	24	26	28	30	32	34	36	38	40	42	44	46	48	50	52	54	56	58	60
0.3	3	6	9	12	15	18	21	24	27	30	33	36	39	42	45	48	51	54	57	60	63	66	69	72	75	78	81	84	87	90
0.4	4	8	12	16	20	24	28	32	36	40	44	48	52	56	60	64	68	72	76	80	84	88	92	96	100	104	108	112	116	120
0.5	5	10	15	20	25	30	35	40	45	50	55	60	65	70	75	80	85	90	95	100	105	110	115	120	125	130	135	140	145	150
0.6	6	12	18	24	30	36	42	48	54	60	66	72	78	84	90	96	102	108	114	120	126	132	138	144	150	156	162	168	174	180
0.7	7	14	21	28	35	42	49	56	63	70	77	84	91	98	105	112	119	126	133	140	147	154	161	168	175	182	189	196	203	210
0.8	8	16	24	32	40	48	56	64	72	80	88	96	104	112	120	128	136	144	152	160	168	176	184	192	200	208	216	224	232	240
0.9	9	18	27	36	45	54	63	72	81	90	99	108	117	126	135	144	153	162	171	180	189	198	207	216	225	234	243	252	261	270
1	10	20	30	40	50	60	70	80	90	100	110	120	130	140	150	160	170	180	190	200	210	220	230	240	250	260	270	280	290	300
1.1	11	22	33	44	55	66	77	88	99	110	121	132	143	154	165	176	187	198	209	220	231	242	253	264	275	286	297	308	319	330
1.2	12	24	36	48	60	72	84	96	108	120	132	144	156	168	180	192	204	216	228	240	252	264	276	288	300	312	324	336	348	360
1.3	13	26	39	52	65	78	91	104	117	130	143	156	169	182	195	208	221	234	247	260	273	286	299	312	325	338	351	364	377	390
1.4	14	28	42	56	70	84	98	112	126	140	154	168	182	196	210	224	238	252	266	280	294	308	322	336	350	364	378	392	406	420
1.5	15	30	45	60	75	90	105	120	135	150	165	180	195	210	225	240	255	270	285	300	315	330	345	360	375	390	405	420	435	450
1.6	16	32	48	64	80	96	112	128	144	160	176	192	208	224	240	256	272	288	304	320	336	352	368	384	400	416	432	448	464	480
1.7	17	34	51	68	85	102	119	136	153	170	187	204	221	238	255	272	289	306	323	340	357	374	391	408	425	442	459	476	493	510
1.8	18	36	54	72	90	108	126	144	162	180	198	216	234	252	270	288	306	324	342	360	378	396	414	432	450	468	486	504	522	540
1.9	19	38	57	76	95	114	133	152	171	190	209	228	247	266	285	304	323	342	361	380	399	418	437	456	475	494	513	532	551	570
2	20	40	60	80	100	120	140	160	180	200	220	240	260	280	300	320	340	360	380	400	420	440	460	480	500	520	540	560	580	600
2.1	21	42	63	84	105	126	147	168	189	210	231	252	273	294	315	336	357	378	399	420	441	462	483	504	525	546	567	588	609	630
2.2	22	44	66	88	110	132	154	176	198	220	242	264	286	308	330	352	374	396	418	440	462	484	506	528	550	572	594	616	638	660
2.3	23	46	69	92	115	138	161	184	207	230	253	276	299	322	345	368	391	414	437	460	483	506	529	552	575	598	621	644	667	690
2.4	24	48	72	96	120	144	168	192	216	240	264	288	312	336	360	384	408	432	456	480	504	528	552	576	600	624	648	672	696	720
2.5	25	50	75	100	125	150	175	200	225	250	275	300	325	350	375	400	425	450	475	500	525	550	575	600	625	650	675	700	725	750
2.6	26	52	78	104	130	156	182	208	234	260	286	312	338	364	390	416	442	468	494	520	546	572	598	624	650	676	702	728	754	780
2.7	27	54	81	108	135	162	189	216	243	270	297	324	351	378	405	432	459	486	513	540	567	594	621	648	675	702	729	756	783	810
2.8	28	56	84	112	140	168	196	224	252	280	308	336	364	392	420	448	476	504	532	560	588	616	644	672	700	728	756	784	812	840
2.9	29	58	87	116	145	174	203	232	261	290	319	348	377	406	435	464	493	522	551	580	609	638	667	696	725	754	783	812	841	870
3	30	60	90	120	150	180	210	240	270	300	330	360	390	420	450	480	510	540	570	600	630	660	690	720	750	780	810	840	870	900

green line = Recreational Diving Limit; purple line = Hyperbaric Treatment Limit

yellow space = Exposure exceeds mutiple day diving UPTD; orange space = Exposure exceeds single day diving UPTD

Pulmonary Disease

The closed-loop system of a rebreather is a warm, dark, and moist environment ideal for growth of microorganisms. Many anecdotal reports exist from rebreather divers complaining of persistent or recurrent low-grade respiratory tract symptoms. It has been postulated that this is due to improper cleaning of breathing equipment and/or sharing of equipment. No standard exists regarding the proper cleaning solution or the frequency of cleaning equipment; however, one should refer to the manufacturer's recommendations when it comes to the care of the specific components of a breathing system.

A published study from 2002 checked validity of older cleaning agents and found Virkon S and TriGene II to be acceptable cleaning agents. Although they were not studied against a comprehensive list of cleaners, they were noted to meet the minimum criteria set forth, which included absence of components causing undue risk to human health, ability to kill full spectrum of virus bacteria and fungi, as well as compatibility with system components.[35]

In a more recent study conducted in 2012 by Jeffrey Bozanic, PhD, Steramine and Listerine provided slightly better results than the Betadine and Virkon. While all of the tested cleaners dramatically reduced bacterial growth when used with rinse or flood applications, only flood application of Steramine completely eliminated bacterial growth.[39]

Flood application is accomplished by rinsing thoroughly with freshwater and spraying entire area with a liberal coat of solution on and into the equipment. Let stand for 10 minutes, applying more solution if solution appears to be drying, keeping it wet for the full 10 minutes. After 10 minutes, rinse the entire assembly in a container of clean freshwater or rinse under running potable water.

There are limited studies touting the efficacy of one cleaning agent over another, and every manufacturer claims its product is superior. Regardless which cleaner is used, it is recommended to clean a rebreather after each dive versus after a multiday dive sequence or merely just storing it for a specified period of time. The following factors need to be considered when choosing a cleaning agent: potential health risks to the user once cleaned in the form of toxins left behind or vapor particle residue, disinfectant efficacy against bacteria, viruses, and fungi, and the potential destructive nature of the cleaner itself with respect to the degradation of equipment after use. Finally, it is clear that flood application is superior to other cleaning methods.

Hypoxia

Hypoxia is the condition in which the tissues do not receive sufficient oxygen to meet the metabolic needs of the body. In technical diving, it can occur due to a problem with the rebreather itself, a physiological problem, or breathing improper OC gas mixtures. Since hypoxia can be life threatening, it is best to avoid these issues.

Equipment problems that contribute to hypoxia include rebreather O_2 addition failure, electronics failure, inadequate purging of a hypoxic diluent, and inadequate gas flow for a given work rate. Physiological problems that can place a diver at risk for hypoxia include impaired oxygen exchange at the capillary-alveolar bed or alveolar hypoventilation due to increased density of gas at depth. A ventilation-perfusion mismatch has been noted in technical divers because the helium promotes lung cooling, and a decrease in temperature must have a corresponding decrease in volume which could lead to hypoxia.[17]

Myriad mistakes have been made concerning improperly labeled gas cylinders. OC divers using hypoxic surface mixtures (or back gas) to decrease the pO_2 at depth have accidentally breathed these hypoxic mixtures at the surface, causing hypoxic symptoms.

Keep in mind that CCR and SCR function best underwater because the pO_2 in the rebreather is increased due to Dalton's law at depth. The greatest risk of hypoxia on a rebreather is near the surface at the start or the end of a dive under high work rates.

Symptoms of hypoxia include incoordination, dizziness, inability to focus or concentrate, confusion, and convulsions.(20) Mild symptoms can start as early as 0.16 pO_2. Hypoxia occurs at 0.14 pO_2, and death can occur at 0.10 pO_2.

Treatment includes administration of oxygen, although preventative measures may be easiest, including pre-dive equipment checks, avoiding exertion at or near the surface on a rebreather, and gas analysis coupled with proper cylinder labeling. These are paramount in avoiding hypoxia.

Deep Water Blackout

Deep water blackout (DWB) is loss of consciousness due to extreme nitrogen narcosis. It is important to differentiate DWB caused by nitrogen narcosis from ascent syncope associated with hypoxia due to breath-hold diving. DWB occurs at deep diving depths in excess of 218 fsw, while ascent syncope occurs while a diver is on ascent from a free dive nearing shallow water.

DWB has more to do with rebreather and technical divers. Rebreather divers may be particularly susceptible to DWB if the scrubber canister has breakthrough or any failure leading to high loop CO_2 levels. The increased lipid solubility of CO_2 could exacerbate the narcosis felt in rebreather divers and decrease psychomotor performance(21) when combined with nitrogen narcosis, yielding a super narcosis of sorts.

Formerly, deep divers had no option save air on which to perform deeper dives. Because air contains only oxygen and nitrogen, these divers were truly taking their lives into their own hands when they performed dives deeper than 218 fsw. The partial pressure of oxygen in air at 218 fsw is 1.6 pO_2, which is above the recommended limit. At PPN_2s greater than 4.5, nitrogen narcosis is extreme. The option for using air deeper than 150 fsw has fallen out of favor with most training agencies(13) and technical divers in favor of mixes containing helium to combat nitrogen narcosis as well as decrease partial pressures of oxygen potentially leading to CNS oxygen toxicity.

The symptoms are consistent with those of nitrogen narcosis progressing to loss of consciousness.(18) Most importantly, this malady can be easily prevented with proper dive planning and depth maintenance as well as attention to scrubber canisters when rebreather diving.

Isobaric (Inert Gas) Counter Diffusion

Isobaric counter diffusion (ICD) is the theory of two inert gases moving in opposite directions in and out of tissues while under equal pressure. While ICD is not a malady, it is concerning because it potentially increases the likelihood of DCS. Technical and rebreather divers, because they are pushing to greater depths, need to consider ICD when planning dives.

The two types of ICD are "superficial" and "deep tissue."(22) It is important to first note the solubility and diffusion rate of the most commonly used inert gases to help illustrate each concept. The solubility of nitrogen is 0.067 and the solubility of helium is 0.015. Therefore, nitrogen is 4.46667 times more soluble than helium. Another important number is the speed of diffusivity or speed the gas goes into and out of solution. Helium diffuses 2.67 times faster than nitrogen. Additionally noteworthy is the molecular mass of the gas helium = 4 g/mol and the molecular mass of nitrogen = 14 g/mol.

Superficial ICD occurs when a diver's breathing gas has a slower diffusion rate than the gas surrounding the diver. For example, a diver in a dry suit breathing nitrogen as the prevalent inert gas who is using helium as the prevalent inert gas for dry suit inflation will create a theoretical supersaturated state, leading to the cutaneous manifestations of superficial ICD, including skin lesions and pruritus. This theoretically occurs because the rapidly diffusing helium coming from outside the body is creating inert gas tension as it is simultaneously absorbed into the tissues along with the nitrogen (slower diffusing) from inside the body. This was once a problem in early technical diving, but its practice has fallen out of favor for obvious reasons. Superficial ICD is easily avoided by ensuring dry suit media is of the highest solubility the diver is breathing on the dive.

Deep-tissue ICD occurs when gas switching from a slowly diffusing breathing medium to a rapidly diffusing breathing medium. The rapidly diffusing medium rushes into the tissues faster than the slower-diffusing medium has time to escape. The overall tissue gas supersaturation increases and can exceed the critical limit. Generally, this type of switch would be performed at very shallow depths (if at all) by technical and rebreather divers and it is not considered a problem.

Another historically problematic type of deep-tissue ICD theoretically occurs when gas switching from a rapidly diffusing breathing medium to a slower-diffusing breathing medium at great depths. This creates a situation of rapid off-gassing of the lighter gas versus the slower on-gassing of the heavier gas. There is apparently no mathematical reason for critical saturation of the tissue, but, nonetheless, technical and rebreather divers continue to suffer significant DCS when performing such a switch. A current theory of the authors is that the higher lipid solubility of nitrogen coupled with the increased pressure at depth causes a vacuum and subsequent critical saturation of the tissues following the inert gas shift to exceptionally high levels of nitrogen.

For example, a diver performs a dive with a mixture of helium, oxygen, and nitrogen (trimix) at 10 ATA that contains 40% helium, 45% nitrogen, and 15% oxygen; a switch to EAN32 would deliver a rapid spike of nitrogen (+23%) and a marked decrease in helium content (-40%). This type of deep-tissue ICD occurs every time a diver makes this kind of a significant switch from a helium-rich mixture to nitrogen-rich mixture or any time a diver has a marked increase in equivalent narcotic depth (END). Most often these switches will be asymptomatic, but the severity of the incident will likely correlate to the tissue that is controlling the ascent. If performed correctly, this example of deep-tissue ICD is uneventful because at this depth the limiting tissues are the slower ones. Slower tissues are less sensitive to a spike in END.

ICD can and does occur yielding asymptomatic results. The final gas switch from OC or rebreather to surface air is a change in END and may also cause ICD.

This, coupled with the effects of redistribution of fluids due to gravity, are very good reasons divers should not make haste to get out of the water following a deep dive. As a matter of exactness, every time a diver takes an air break from oxygen decompression, there is a significant change in END and therefore an ICD occurs.(12)

The mathematical inert gas uptake models are mostly predicated upon the absorption of inert gas from the blood. The ear is a slow tissue group that on-/off-gasses from both the blood as and the round window. There may be a time during the gas shift where there is a high partial pressure of helium in the middle ear. This indicates the helium partial pressure may not be able to fall because the helium is being replaced at the same time (and perhaps rate) as it diffuses out into the blood. Normal tissue compartment saturation rates are difficult to calculate, but the inner ear is especially difficult because of the multiple on-/off-gas methods in the ear.

Divers who get ICD often have issues with vestibulo-cochlear apparatus or IEDCS. The further technical divers expand the boundary of deep diving, the more we can expect to see this and other rare or previously undiscovered maladies. Currently, approximately 26% of patients suffering "serious" or "neurological" DCS exhibit evidence of inner-ear involvement. These numbers are confounding since residual deficits in balance and in hearing are common despite recompression treatment, and the window of opportunity for treatment is relatively short.(15) As seems evident, the differential diagnosis of ICD from an issue with a perforated eardrum or the most common form of barotraumas (middle ear) is required as well as a differential for IEDCS.

Most of the studies and trials observing ICD are conducted in dry chambers that simulate depth of seawater with increased pressure. Those body spaces that are exposed to dry environments as opposed to wet environments may on-gas at different rates given the different environments. Diffusion across the tympanic membrane accounts for most of the inert gas entering the middle ear from ambient and respiratory environments containing the inert gas.(16) Given this information, perhaps the literature involving testing for ICD in dry environments may be incorrect or in need of further work.

An accepted method for avoiding ICD is to ensure the decrease in helium content never exceeds the 4.46667 times increase in solubility from nitrogen to helium. The assumption herein is that the overall change in inert gas levels should be linked to the solubility of the gases. A 5:1 ratio is rounded for easy math and commonly used to avoid ICD DCS.(6) The 5:1 ratio indicates that a diver should not switch to a gas that has a helium drop of 5% (actual percent by volume) for every 1% (actual percent by volume) increase in nitrogen content. For instance, if the diver has completed a dive that has the first decompression ceiling at 150 fsw (45 msw) and decides to switch from trimix (helium 30%, nitrogen 50%, and oxygen 20%), the maximum EANx to which the diver should switch is 56%. A switch larger than this could lead to an ICD and DCS.

Another ICD avoidance technique is detailed in Sheck Exley's book *Caverns Measureless to Man.*(19) The main premise of this idea was to make the switch as "gradually as possible." The supposition is 1-2-2-1 for a "phase in." For example, take a single breath from a tank containing a mixture of nitrogen and oxygen (nitrox) and then back to trimix for two breaths and then switch back to nitrox for two breaths then back to trimix for one breath and finally back to nitrox for good. This gives your fast tissues an opportunity to phase-in the off-gassing. This is a complex maneuver, and, at this time in diving, significantly higher PPN_2s were more prevalent.

In Sheck's case, this also seemed to limit the amount of narcosis he experienced. The technical community no longer recommends switching to a nitrogen-based mixture deeper than 70 fsw.

As a growing trend, rebreather divers decompress on helium-rich mixtures all the way to the surface, instead of switching to nitrogen-based mixtures, making ICD less and less of a problem. OC technical divers may still experience these ICD issues due to the practicality of bringing too many tanks with varying inert gas mixes to avoid ICD. It is noteworthy that the same calculations could (and have been) be practiced using different inert gases if the diver intends on switching between, let's say, helium-rich and neon-rich mixes or neon-rich and nitrogen-rich mixture.

As a final thought, it is important to note the aforementioned avoidance methods are theory only, and there are no clinical trials to support these theories. To modify a quote from Dr. Bill Hamilton, "what works . . . works" . . . but may not for everyone. The above methods of avoidance show anecdotal evidence and appear to abate the symptoms associated with resultant DCS from ICD, but individual susceptibilities may vary.

CNS Oxygen Toxicity

CNS oxygen toxicity, aka the Paul Bert effect, is a serious consequence of hyperoxia. Rebreather divers who set the pO_2 of their system too high or technical divers who incorrectly switch to high fraction of oxygen gas mixes inadvertently may experience CNS oxygen toxicity. The symptoms may occur suddenly and are well known by the mnemonic CONVENTID:

- **Con**vulsions
- **V**isual changes
- **E**uphoria, Ear/Tinnitus
- **N**ausea
- **T**witching, Tingling
- **I**rritability
- **D**izziness

The most serious of these symptoms are convulsions which are often fatal as they ultimately end in drowning. Factors that will contribute to CNS oxygen toxicity include increased pO_2, prolonged immersion, strenuous physical exertion, CO_2 buildup, and shivering. Systemic illnesses that contribute to increased oxygen consumption can also increase the likelihood of CNS oxygen toxicity. These include thyroid or adrenal disorders as they tend to cause an increase in oxygen sensitivity.

While there is, generally speaking, no accepted methodology for the prediction of CNS oxygen toxicity, a 2012 paper[30] concluded that hyperoxic hyperpnea, a compound hyperoxic ventilatory response, is a predictor of an impending seizure while breathing poikilocapnic hyperoxic conditions at rest in unanesthetized rats. This could lead to future development of a correlation of increased breathing rate in mammals and the onset of CNS oxygen toxicity.

The following is the appropriate treatment if a seizure occurs in water: If the diver is wearing a full-face mask, or the regulator is retained in the mouth, a safety diver must make every attempt to hold the mask or regulator in place, and the diver should be kept at depth until the seizure is resolved.[28] The moment the seizure appears to abate, the diver should be brought directly to the surface and removed from the water as quickly as possible, and an ABC protocol instituted. If the regulator is lost from the mouth, and the airway is obviously unprotected, a safety diver should not attempt to replace the regulator. He or she should bring the diver to the surface immediately, even if the seizure appears to be continuing. Remove the diver from the water and initiate an ABC protocol.[28] Continue the administration of oxygen on the surface after ABCs are complete and the diver has been conscious for 15 minutes[14] or longer if required due to omitted decompression.

The following is the appropriate treatment if a nonseizure symptom of oxygen toxicity arises: The diver with symptoms should notify any accompanying diver of his or her symptoms immediately. The victim's breathing gas should be changed to air. Because the relationship of premonitory symptoms to the onset of a seizure is variable and unpredictable, as is the efficacy of lowering the inspired pO_2 in preventing progression to a seizure, the diver should exit the water as soon as possible over one to two minutes. Any diver must be ready to intervene immediately should a convulsion occur. The diver should be removed from the water and placed on surface oxygen if the diver had to omit decompression stops, and consider evacuation for recompression in a hyperbaric chamber.[14]

High-Pressure Nervous Syndrome

High-pressure nervous syndrome (HPNS) is also known as high-pressure neurological syndrome and refers to a constellation of signs and symptoms including electroencephalogram changes, muscle tremors, nausea, seizures, vomiting, and vertigo.[24] This malady is presumably outside the realm of technical and rebreather divers, but, as some divers expand the boundaries, symptoms of HPNS and issues attributed to HPNS have arisen. The exact mechanism is not well understood; however, it is generally accepted that many of the symptoms of HPNS are due to the compression effects on the lipid membrane of the cells.

Mild symptoms can occur at depths beyond 300 fsw using mixtures containing helium and oxygen (heliox) or high concentrations of helium within trimix. Another commonly reported symptom is "mind race" or "helium willies." That is to say, the diver has a lack of ability to concentrate on a task because his or her mind is racing through the task but not remembering what the task was or how it was accomplished. This experience is best represented by a diver looking at his or her watch to note bottom time and a few seconds later repeating the task of checking bottom time because of a failure to recall having completed the task.

If symptoms occur, the rate of descent should be reduced, or, if severe enough, the dive should be aborted. The combination of nitrogen in the breathing media retards the onset on HPNS.[1] This malady can be partially or possibly fully ameliorated if, when planning a dive, the diver could add enough nitrogen to offset the onset of high pressure issues.

Back Pain

Back pain is common in an aging population. Approximately 31 million Americans suffer from back pain in one form or another.[26] While this malady is not necessarily specific to technical or rebreather diving, the added weight of the equipment and its placement can be problematic for users and exacerbate chronic back pain.

As usual, warming up or stretching before exercising or physical activities is an important prophylactic measure to avoid acute and chronic back pain. Additionally, the maintenance of proper posture during both surface and diving activities can prevent acute pain. Simple recommendations for divers to lift with their knees, while keeping the equipment close to their body, and to avoid twisting when lifting can help avoid back pain.

Moreover, appropriate weighting while diving can not only help to avoid back pain but assist in reducing hydrodynamic drag in the water and make the experience of diving a more pleasant one. The importance of maintaining a healthy body weight and strong core muscles cannot be underscored.

The added weight of either double tanks or a rebreather could raise the center of gravity of the diver by necessarily placing weight high on the body. Properly fitting waist straps should bear 80% of the weight of the unit/tanks and drive the weight to the diver's hips and away from the shoulders. This can take some adjustment, especially if the divers are of smaller stature.[2] Finally, the proper placement of trim weights atop the shoulders will slightly raise the center of gravity but also serve to reduce the hydrodynamic position by trimming the diver in a horizontal position.

A great many divers have shifted the weight off their backs to a more distributed system such as side mount. This mounting system is generally construed as easier to fill and transport tanks as well as easier to carry to water since it divides the weight of the double tanks and distributes to single tanks on either side of the body.

Treatment of back pain in divers is as normally accomplished after a differential diagnosis ruling out decompression sickness. Equipment placement and fit along with proper lifting techniques are the important preventative measures that a technical diver can take to reduce acute back pain.

Compression Arthralgia

Deep divers sometimes experience a malady coined "Smithers" or compression arthralgia (CA). CA is characterized by a clicking or popping of the extremities at depth during use. CA is a syndrome of joint pain, popping, and cracking that generally occurs at depths greater than 200 fsw and most often on heliox dives.[20]

It was first described by Case and Haldane during compressed air dives at pressures of 10.7 ATA.[8] The report did not include complaints of pain. Studies on helium-oxygen performed by Bradley and Vorosmarti included dives ranging from 100 fsw to 850 fsw that included complaints of clicking, popping, and joint pain. It is theorized that the absence of pain noted on the compressed air dives could be attributed to the narcotic effect of the nitrogen masking any joint pain.

Symptoms have been described as deep, sharp, or achy joint pain in one or more joints with movement, aggravated by fast compression rates, although individual susceptibilities will vary. It should be noted that worsening of the symptoms can also occur with slower compression rates. Joints most commonly affected include the shoulders, knees, wrists, hips, and ankles. There is no associated soft-tissue swelling. The symptoms abate by return to shallower water or by longer bottom times.

There have been several theories as to why the symptoms of compression arthralgia occur, including increased hydrostatic pressure; another is that the dissolution of the inert gases cause fluid shifts in the articular cartilage leading to dehydration of the synovial cavity. The shift of fluid results from a pressure gradient that is generated by the higher pressure of inert gas in the blood that exceeds that of the poorly perfused articular cartilage. Loss of water from the joints interferes with lubrication of the joints, decreasing elasticity and increasing frictional resistance, which in turn are thought to stimulate pain receptors, thus causing the pain of CA. Generally speaking, the deeper the dive, the longer the pain persists.

Much of the literature supports that the symptoms disappear in reverse order on decompression; however, anecdotal reports from present technical and rebreather divers demonstrate a pain that starts from the CA at depth and remains long after surfacing. It is important to differentiate the resultant pain from CA, which may continue after the diver surfaces, with the pain from DCS. A key indication the pain has originated from CA is the pain does not respond to recompression. Experienced divers will report this symptom readily as they have likely experienced these symptoms before.

The symptoms are less likely with slow compression rates and abate with prolonged bottom times or by returning to shallower depths.[(5)] Since the symptoms can be exacerbated by rapid repetitive movement, divers should attempt to limit those motions causing the clicking while at depth.

REFERENCES

1. Bennett P, Coggin R, Roby J. Control of HPNS in humans during rapid compression with trimix to 650 m (2131 ft). Undersea Biomed Res. 1981 Jun;8(2).
2. Blum P. Equipment configuration for small divers. In: Tao of survival underwater. IANTD Press; 2008. p. 107-12.
3. Bove A. Toxicity of oxygen, carbon dioxide and carbon monoxide. In: Bove AA, Davis JC, editors. Diving medicine. 4th ed. Philadelphia: Saunders; 2004. p. 241-59.
4. Bozanic J. Mastering rebreathers. 2nd ed. West Palm Beach (FL): Best Publishing Co.; 2010. 704 p.
5. Bradley ME, Vorosmarti J. Hyperbaric arthralgia during helium-oxygen dives from 100 to 850 fsw. Undersea Biomed Res. 1974 Jun;1(2):151-67.
6. Burton S. ScubaEngineer.com; 2007 Feb 6. Available from: http://www.scubaengineer.com/isobaric_counter_diffusion.html
7. Butler, White, Twa, et al. Hyperoxic myopia in a closed-circuit mixed-gas scuba diver. UHM Journal. 1999.
8. Case E, Haldane J. Human physiology under high pressure. Effects of nitrogen, carbon dioxide and cold. J. Hyg. 41(3):225-49.
9. Collins V. Principles of anesthesiology. Philadelphia: Lea & Febiger; 1976.
10. Davis A. Subclinical DCS, decompression stress and post dive fatigue [Internet]. Scuba Tech Philippines; 2015 Dec 16. Available from: http://www.scubatechphilippines.com
11. Dean J. Theory of gastric CO2 ventilation and its control during respiratory acidosis: implications for central chemosensitivity, pH regulation, and diseases causing chronic CO2 retention. Respir Physiol Neurobiol. 2011 Feb 15;175(2):189-209. doi: 10.1016/j.resp.2010.12.001. Epub 2010 Dec 7.
12. Dituri J. Isobaric issues in diving. In: Tao of survival underwater. IANTD Press; 2008. p. 73-6.
13. Dituri J. Recompression chamber operations manual. International Board of Undersea Medicine Press. p. 1-45.
14. Dituri J, Sadler R, et al. Emergency management of stricken divers in remote areas. IANTD Press. p. 1-24.
15. Doolette D, Mitchell S. A biophysical basis for inner ear decompression sickness. J Appl Physiol. 2003:2. JAP-01090-2002-R1.
16. Dueker, Lambertsen, Rosowski, Sanders. Middle ear gas exchange in isobaric counter diffusion. J Appl Physiol. 1979;47(6):1239-44.
17. Edmonds C. Hypoxia, diving and sub aquatic medicine. 4th ed. p. 195-205.
18. Elliot D. Deep water blackout. SPUMS J. 1996 Sep;26(3).
19. Exley S. Caverns measureless to man. Cave Books; 1994 Jun. p. 176.
20. Flynn E. Medical supervision of diving operations. In: Bove A, Davis J, editors. Diving medicine. 4th ed. Philadelphia: Saunders; 2004. p. 343-79.
21. Fothergill D, Hedges D, Morrison J. Effects of CO2 and N2 partial pressures on cognitive and psychomotor performance. Undersea Biomed Res. 1991;18(1).
22. Hamilton R. Mixed gas diving. In: Bove AA, Davis JC, editors. Diving medicine. 4th ed. Philadelphia: Saunders; 2004. p. 95-126.
23. Higuchi H et al. International Anesthesia Research Society; 2001. 23. 221.
24. Hunter W, Bennet P. The causes, mechanisms and prevention of high pressure nervous syndrome. Undersea Biomed Res. 1974;1:1-28.

25. International Association of Nitrox and Technical Divers open water diver training manual. IANTD Press; 2016.

26. Jensen M, Brant-Zawadzki M, Obuchowski N, et al. Magnetic resonance imaging of the lumbar spine in people without back pain. N Engl J Med. 1994;331:69-116.

27. Markowitz A, Rabow M. Palliative management of fatigue at the close of life: "it feels like my body is just worn out." JAMA. 2007:298(2):217

28. Mitchell, Bennett, Bird, et al. Recommendations for rescue of a submerged unresponsive compressed-gas diver. Undersea Hyperb Med. 2012;39(6).

29. Nochetto M. Air, nitrox and fatigue. Alert Diver Online. 2014 Summer.

30. Pilla R, Landon C, Dean J. A potential early physiological marker for CNS oxygen toxicity: hyperoxic hyperpnea precedes seizure in unanesthetized rats breathing hyperbaric oxygen. J Appl Physiol (1985). 2013 Apr;114(8):1009-20. doi: 10.1152/japplphysiol.01326.2012. Epub 2013 Feb 21.

31. Rebreather FUNdamentals. Dituri, Pyle. Rebreather FUNdamentals [DVD]. Gallant Aquatic Ventures International; 2003.

32. Ross M, Yolton D, Yolton R, et al. Myopia associated with hyperbaric therapy. Optom Vis Sci. 1996 Aug;73(7):487-94.

33. Sawatzky D. Oxygen toxicity – signs and symptoms. Dive Rite [Internet]. 2016 Feb 11. 2017 Jan 21.

34. Schaefer K. Physiological stresses related to hypercapnia during patrols on submarines. Undersea Biomed Res. 1979;Submarine Suppl:S15-46.

35. Severs Y, Lamontagne M. A literature review of disinfectants: effects when used by CS divers in cleaning rebreather sets. Defense R&D Canada; 2002 Nov. DRDC Toronto TR 2002-209.

36. Simon D, Bradley M. Adverse effects of contact lens wear during decompression. JAMA. 1980;244:1213-4.

37. U.S. Navy Department. U.S. Navy diving manual. Revision 6. Diving medicine and recompression chamber operations. Washington (DC): Naval Sea Systems Command; 2008. NAVSEA 0910-LP-106–0957.

38. van Ooij, Hollmann, van Hulst, Sterk. Assessment of pulmonary oxygen toxicity: relevance to professional diving; a review. Respir Physiol Neurobiol. 189(1):117-28. P.J.A.M.

39. Vann R, Denoble P, Pollock N, editors. Rebreather Forum 3 proceedings. Durham (NC): AAUS/DAN/PADI; 2014. 324 p. ISBN: 978-0-9800423-9-9.

40. Warkander, Norfleet, Nagasawa, et al. CO2 retention with minimum symptoms but severe dysfunction during wet simulated dives to 6.8 ATA. Undersea Biomed Res. 1990;17:515-23.

CHAPTER 46 CHAPTER

Ocean Exploration: Living in the Deep Sea

CHAPTER FORTY-SIX OVERVIEW

Motivation 1135
Introduction 1135
Conshelf Series 1136
Sea Lab 1137
Cousteau's Project 1138
Poseidon Project 1139
Space "Spinoffs" and the Benefits to Humanity 1140
Oceans, the Breadbasket of the World 1141
With Technical Advance Comes Increased Access 1143
The Economy, Biotechnology, and Space Exploration 1143
Show Me the Money 1144
Intellectual Property 1144
Protecting the Future 1145
The Future of Undersea Housing 1147
Conclusion 1147
References 1148

Ocean Exploration: Living in the Deep Sea

Harry T. Whelan, Terrance L. Leighton III, Heather Annis, Joseph Dituri

MOTIVATION

After writing "Land to Sea,"[(73)] which investigated the growing number of pharmaceuticals and other bioderived products from the deep ocean, the authors were struck by the differences in spending between space and ocean research at the expense of bio-innovation and conservation and their direct contributions to improving and sustaining human existence on Earth.

INTRODUCTION

From the beginning of time, humanity has been limited, and therefore intrigued by, the sea. We are forever surrounded by it and have barely begun to explore and understand it. Centuries ago it was thought to be controlled by Poseidon, and still to this day humans are limited by the mighty ocean. We try to sail over it, cruise under it, and live in it, and yet she so many times gets the upper hand because humans still need what the sea can't provide . . . AIR.

Jules Vern continued with *Twenty Thousand Leagues Under the Sea* capturing humankind's continuous infatuation with living under the sea and as a result provided a blueprint for what was to come. Humans first started diving in what is documented approximately 300 BC, and, thanks to the development of technology, the progression of the diving process and length of time an individual is capable of being submersed has grown exponentially. We've gone from bags of air to primitive diving bells developed in the fifteen hundreds, from monster 300-pound dive suits to what we know today as wet/dry suit–based SCUBA and surface-supply diving (Figure 1). Simple submersibles originally drawn by Aristotle have developed into submarines that can dive to impressive depths and be underway for thousands of submersed miles. Once limited by diesel fuel and fumes, our now-clean-running nuclear underwater monsters can support a small community for as long as the food and water rations will allow.

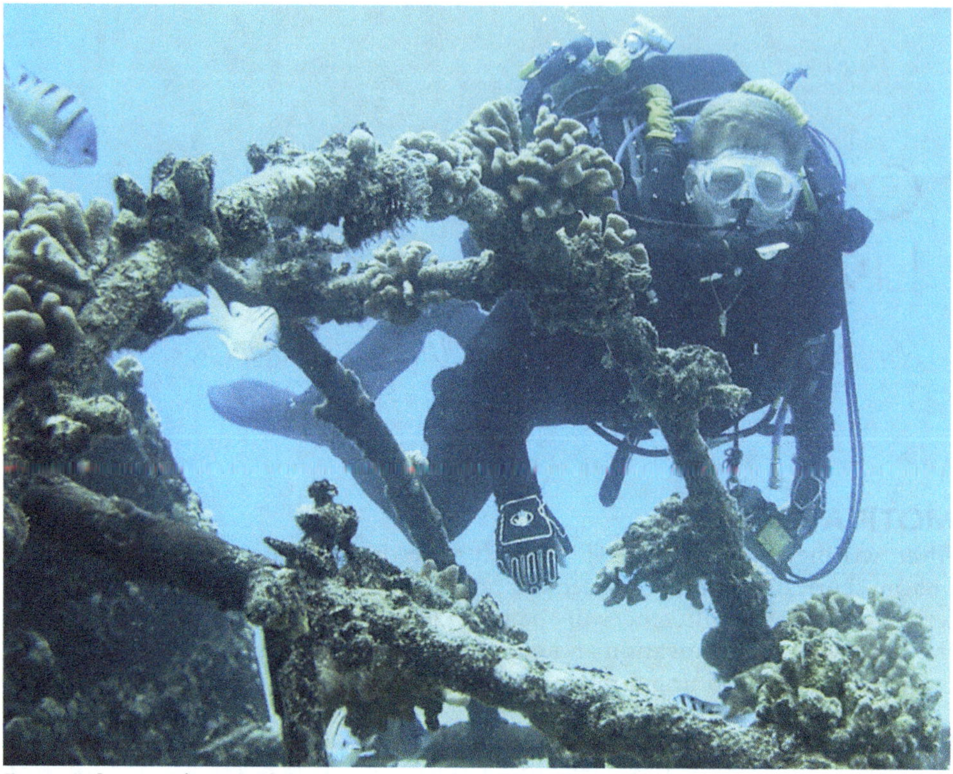

Figure 1. Commander Joseph Dituri doing a civilian wreck dive.

CONSHELF SERIES

In the 1960s, Jacques Cousteau and a French-based team developed and then inhabited a series of undersea habitats that served as research stations. They were called Continental Shelf Stations (ConShelf) with a goal to advance undersea technology and human physiology research and eventually increase awareness of oceanic preservation through public awareness.

ConShelf I was constructed in 1962 and was developed for a team of 2 to 33 fsw off the coast of Marseilles, France. This team lived here for seven days and obtained more than five hours a day of diving, undersea research. They were also subject to daily medical exams, which allowed for advancement in dive medicine and understanding how the human body reacts to and adapts to life undersea.

ConShelf II stepped up to the next level in 1963 with the development of 6 aquanauts in a submersed structure to 33 fsw in the Red Sea off the coast of Sudan for 30 days. In addition to the main habitat, a smaller habitat was stationed at 100 fsw and allowed for 2 divers to live for a week. It was during this time that the mixture of helium and oxygen (heliox) was used in efforts to ward off nitrogen narcosis. The experiment of breathing oxygen prior to and during ascent/decompression to decrease chances of the bends was also performed with a high success rate. It was also this deployment that Jacques Cousteau used to film the Academy Award–winning documentary, which again brought great intrigue to the ocean during a time when the world was so focused on space.

ConShelf III in 1965 was established at 336 fsw with 6 divers in the Mediterranean between Nice, France and Monaco for 3 weeks. This increased depth pushed the limits and allowed for further development of deep-sea diving tactics, as well as the studies and development of industrial protocols for drilling and building at depth.

SEA LAB

Underwater living was taken to the next level with the development of the SEA LAB projects created by the U.S. Navy, with a total of three projects: SEA LAB I off the coast of Aruba in 1964 and SEA LAB II and III being submerged off the coast of Southern California in the La Jolla Canyon. SEA LAB I was a first of its kind with its focus on saturation diving in the open ocean. The SEA LAB experiment, in addition to saturation diving, brought research data on habitat placement, air and communication umbilicals, and humidity, as well as helium speech descrambling.[48] SEA LAB I's crew consisted of 4 divers and was at a depth of 192 fsw. The expedition lasted for 11 days with the original goal of 21 days, but a tropical storm led to the abort of the mission (Figure 2).

Following the Caribbean attempt of SEA LAB I, its follow-up project, appropriately named SEA LAB II, gave it another go dropping a capsule to the ocean floor in the La Jolla Canyon to a depth of approximately 205 fsw. With multiple crews spending 15-day intervals at depth and under pressure, new research was able to emerge. New tools, salvage techniques, and dry suits were tested, while bottom time records were broken by astronaut/aquanaut Scott Carpenter, who stayed underway for 30 days.

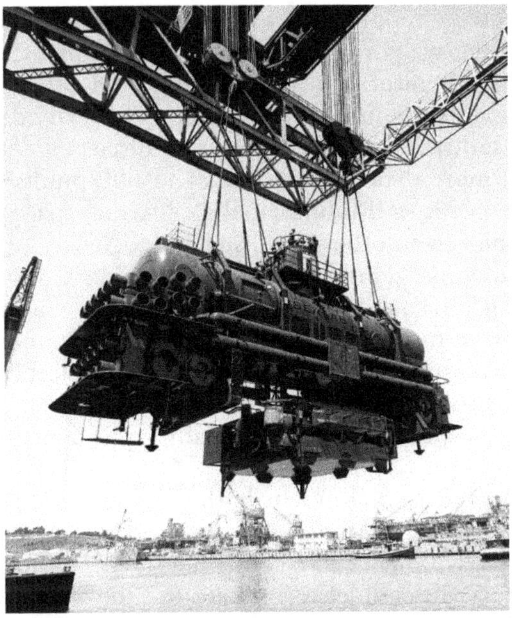

Figure 2. SEALAB III being hoisted in San Francisco. (U.S. Navy photo via Bill Gonyo)

In 1969, SEA LAB III, with a refurbished hull and updated technology, was deployed to 610 fsw off the coast of San Clemente Island near Southern California. Unfortunately, throughout multiple attempts, SEA LAB III just continued to be plagued with problems and technical difficulties. Leaks being the primary factor, multiple attempts were made to repair SEA LAB III underwater but were unsuccessful – one of which cost a diver his life. Berry L. Cannon died in an attempt to repair SEA LAB III while deployed due to carbon dioxide poisoning secondary to a failed scrubber in his diving apparatus.[17,64] After the catastrophic event, the SEA LAB program was terminated, and eventually SEA LAB III was scrapped. Fortunately, to this day, the original SEA LAB I vessel remains on display in Panama City Beach, Florida, mounted in front of the Museum of Man in the Sea.

COUSTEAU'S PROJECT

Learning from our previous SEA LAB experiments, combined with the continued calling to explore, we learn and have aspirations to one day live in the ocean. The most recent project has been built and currently resides in the Florida Keys. In just 19 meters (62 feet) of water is the world's only permanent undersea laboratory, Aquarius (Figure 3).[26,53] It was originally owned by the National Oceanic and Atmospheric Administration (NOAA) and operated by the University of North Carolina at Wilmington from its origin in 1986 until it was defunded of approximately $3 million of federal aid by NOAA in 2012, and now it survives under the stewardship of Florida International University and its use by the National Aeronautics and Space Administration (NASA), the U.S. Navy, and private research initiatives.[26] It was created and placed for the initial use of marine research, including coral studies and monitoring marine wild life. NASA has also borrowed Aquarius for its use in NEEMO (NASA Extreme Environment Mission Operations) to better prepare its astronauts for living onboard a spacecraft and working in hostile, weightless, and airless environments.[51] The U.S. Navy also utilizes Aquarius for saturation dive training and other underwater-related research, as its aquanauts are inhabitants at depth for extended periods of time, which leads to the saturation of the inert gases discussed elsewhere. From this single facility alone, more than 120 missions and 600 published research papers have been spawned.[51] It is in this one small facility that space and ocean research come together as equals in an otherwise disparate existence.

Picking up where his grandfather left off, Fabien Cousteau found himself living in Aquarius for a record 31 days in June of 2014. Summarizing Cousteau in his debrief interview: his mission was not to break his grandfather's record of 30 days but was to live underwater and experience the habitat without having to worry about on-/off-gassing. The amount of research that was able to be obtained in the 31 days of the expedition was potentially equivalent to 3 years' worth of surface dives.[47]

The research proved productive in both success stories and failures. Three individuals remained submerged for the full 31 days but entertained many visitors, both in person and via live video chat. Cousteau was able to regularly give live-feed interviews and interact with students from around the world. Creating this great connection hopefully instills a passion and curiosity in the minds of those that may help conserve our oceans and potentially open the doors for future sea exploration and hopefully habitation.

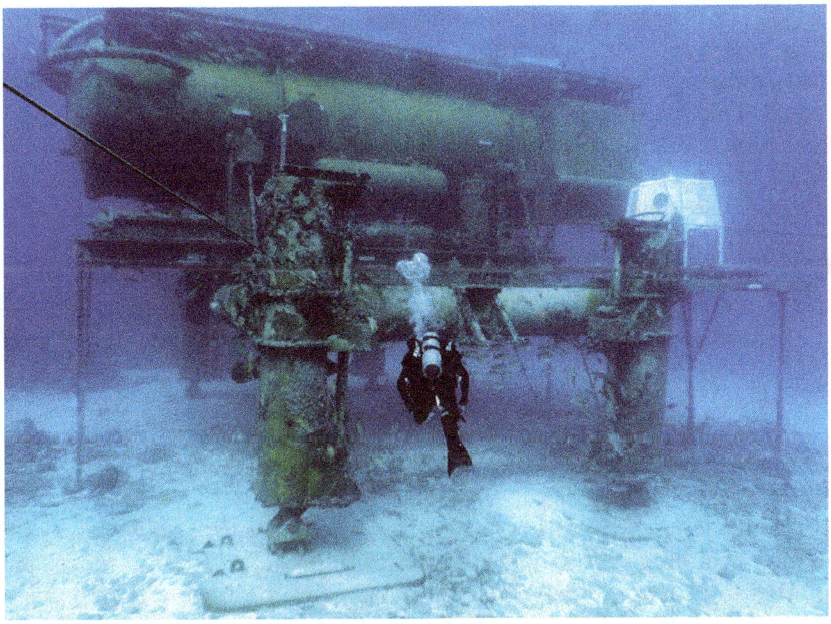

Figure 3. Aquarius Undersea Lab, located 63 feet below the surface in Florida Keys National Marine Sanctuary. Photo courtesy of the National Oceanic and Atmospheric Administration/ Department of Commerce.

Research was done and data collected on a wide spectrum during Cousteau's time and continues to be collected. An estimated 10 papers are to be published over time from the data collected. Examples of such research were the physiological and medical effects of long-term living in isolation and under approximately 3 atmospheres (Aquarius is located at 63 fsw). Cousteau noted increased hair growth rate and a highly dulled sense of taste over time.[(22,47)]

POSEIDON PROJECT

The Aquarius facility has far from lived out its final purpose and now has been adopted by NASA and the Sea Space Exploration & Research Society for Project Poseidon. Project Poseidon is a multidimensional planned endeavor that is slated to begin May 4, 2018, with marine research being just the beginning. For a record-breaking 100 straight days, many different doctors, divers, astronauts, aquanauts, and researchers will inhabit Aquarius. Few team members, including Nicole Stott, formerly of the NASA Extreme Environment Mission Operations NEEMO Mission 9 and a record-breaking female saturation diver,[(29)] will remain for the duration, with many more visiting the habitat for shorter, research-specific missions.

This Aquarius expedition will hopefully serve not only as a scientific research project, but also as a way to put undersea exploration in the public eye to increase the interest in such future research projects and hopefully the end goal of underwater living. Spotlighting the idea of long-term living under the sea can and hopefully will spark further innovation in utilizing such a vast, underutilized part of our world.

Project Poseidon will attempt to attack research in marine biology, human health and performance at depth for extended periods of time, human behavioral performance and group dynamics secondary to seclusion, engineering (e.g., aquatic, aerospace, etc.), telemedicine, space analog research, robotics, and human-machine interaction.

Project Poseidon is to consist of a multitude of professionals/subject-matter experts in a large scope of exploration, science, medicine, and engineering and is to be the ultimate collaboration of academia, government, and industry with the hopes to advance the understanding and utilization of the sea.[29]

NASA's key role in this project is to create a comparable scenario to that of Mars travel and exploration. Specific rovers are to be tested with the intention of learning how these new tools can and potentially will behave upon a Mars Mission.

SPACE "SPINOFFS" AND THE BENEFITS TO HUMANITY

The allure of interstellar travel and alien existence is as old as time itself. As such, modern humans, with the help of imaginative film and television, are firmly attached to the idea of space exploration and colonization as evidenced by the more than USD$575 billion spent by the North American Space Agency (NASA) between 1958 and 2014.[49-50,52] While this may seem an astronomic figure, it is dwarfed by the U.S. national debt of 17.9 trillion,[70] and the benefits to humanity are priceless.

Through the research efforts spawned by the race to space, we have satellites and satellite technology allowing us to monitor climate, weather, sea level, and the environment from space; to have instant global communication; to have television at the flick of a button from Antarctica to Zanzibar; to have protection of our shores through global monitoring of the skies; to have personal location devices, personal global positioning devices; and to have improved 2-D and 3-D imaging software for CT, MRI, and US thanks to computer chip technology developed for satellites.[6,24,28]

We have aerogel, a flexible, lightweight insulation now found in the insoles of mountain climbing boots and endurance running shoes, home insulation, construction, automobiles, and medical appliances;[18,23] we have lightweight heat- and flame-resistant textiles for firefighters and furniture;[10] and we have digital fly-by-wire technology replacing heavy hydraulics in aircraft.[69] Huge advances in robotics, especially in the medical field, allow for increasingly intricate neurosurgery and remote surgery.[3]

Then there is MELDOQ (Melanoma Recognition, Documentation and Quality Assurance System) which analyses magnified images of the skin to detect malignant melanoma;[42] endovascular brachytherapy that uses radiation to prevent arterial restenosis after balloon angioplasty;[46] miniature implantable dosimeters that can be used to monitor focal radiation therapy of tumors reducing risk of damage to surrounding tissue;[31,45] and shape-memory alloys used in staples that reapproximate and support healing bone fractures and are also used for orthodontic springs in dental braces.[21,54]

We also have Faint Object Camera technology, originally designed for the Hubble telescope, not only leapfrogging cell phone and video camera technology, but also that of photocopiers, and allowing scientists to "see" how chemicals, such as pesticides, interact with proteins in the brain.[1] We also have miniaturized high performance capillary electrophoresis (HPCE) allowing for the separation and identification of organic products such as blood and the identification of numerous diseases on a single chip.[32,34,66]

Thanks to spinoffs from space research, we have incredible advances in solar panels, implantable heart monitors, miniaturization technology, light-based anti-cancer treatments, tiny cell phone cameras, water purification systems, and hydrogen engines; methanol-to-hydrogen fuel converters making hydrogen technology safer for use in automobiles; electronic sniffer devices for detecting explosives, chemical warfare agents, cancer, and infection; also carbon brakes and inflatable airbags for the auto industry; anti-vibration technology used in cameras, construction, and engineering; wireless technology, freeze-dried food; and the development of 'intelligent' prosthetics.[40,59]

OCEANS, THE BREADBASKET OF THE WORLD

The ocean comprises 78.5%–97% of Earth's biosphere with only a tiny fraction explored.[9] While this statement is difficult to qualify, it may be more acceptable to claim that oceans comprise greater than 70% of the surface of the Earth, or 99% of the volume of the biosphere.[16] Home to 34 of 36 living animal phyla, there are an estimated 18,000 natural products and 4,900 patents associated with genetics of marine origin increasing at a rate of 12% per year.[4] The potential of maritime biodiversity is highlighted by the 600% increase in the use of marine products in 2007 compared to the period 1965–2005.[14] Areas previously inaccessible, such as the Marianas Trench, offer a variety of ocean habitats with organisms which have adapted to unique environments of extreme heat, cold, and pressure (Figure 4). As such, the abundance of novel and adapted organisms should yield many new genes that hold the key to their adaptive abilities. Aquatic species, having the luxury of more than a billion extra years of evolution and adaptation to these environments, could yield genes coding for the adaptive proteins potentially holding the key to commercially significant biomaterials for human use in extreme environments including space. Remarkable chemotherapy agents, antivirals, antifungals, antiprotozoans, antibiotics, and other bioproducts for use in medicine and surgery are being tested.[4,14,20,30,39,43,57,60,73] One major component of sea organisms, polyunsaturated fatty acids, has been utilized extensively in the development of novel delivery agents for medications, serving as a key part of various solutions (Table 1).[39]

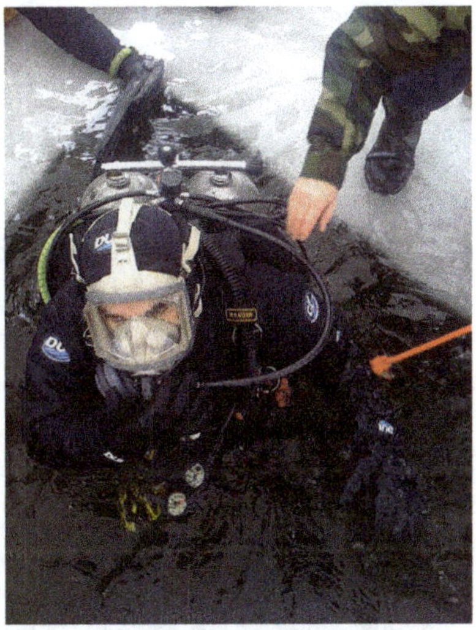

Figure 4. Capt. Whelan performing an Ice Dive with the U.S. Navy Experimental Diving Unit.

TABLE 1. NEW MARINE BIOLOGY NATURAL PRODUCTS

Use of sea urchin genetic code to better understand our own genome and how it relates to Alzheimer's Disease, Parkinson's disease and various types of cancers along with several different types of muscular dystrophy.
Microorganisms extracted from the ocean include a *Vibrio* species that produces an exopolysaccharide that is similar to heparin.
Cold can adversely affects nerve conduction but Antarctic fish continue to conduct at –50°C. Fish would freeze; however, this is countered by the production of special peptides and glycopeptides that act as a natural form of antifreeze.
Fish offer CAP or Cationic Antimicrobial Peptide augmentation of host immune function. CAPs have been shown to have broad antibacterial activity, as well as some propensity for activity against viruses, fungi, protozoa, and malignant cells. CAP's binding of exotoxin decreases in the likelihood of sepsis. Fish glide through the water with minimum friction due to either the mucous they produce or special macromolecules on their body surface. These hold promise for the medical world, where catheters, cardiac valves, and contact lenses could benefit. Of special relevance is the potential for intravascular use where these naturally derived products could prevent triggering the clotting cascade in intravascular implants.
The development of antifungal and anti-tuberculosis agents can give hope to immunocompromised patients.
Another antifungal, Ircinol A, is especially promising because of its low cytotoxicity and potential for side effects.
The Bryozoan, *Bugula neritina*, is the source Brostatin-1 which can protect bone marrow from lethal doses of radiation, stimulate production of progenitor cells, and also stimulate the immune system to respond to malignancy.
Antimicrobials are well represented among marine natural products. The ocean floor is home to a group of actinomycetes, bacteria Salinosporamide A that may have the ability to inhibit tumor growth such as breast, colon and non-small cell lung cancer.
Several medications have synthesized from natural products with anti-cancer properties (i.e., taxoids, vinca alkaloids and anthracyclines).
Trididemnum solidum, a Carribean Sea Squirt has been the source of several anti-tumor agents. Didemnim B inhibits protein synthesis by acting on Elongation Factor 1A and various ribosomes.
Didemnim B's in vitro properties generated great excitement, and several partial and complete responses were noted in non-Hodgkin's lymphoma.
Studies of acute lymphoblastic leukemia and acute myeloid leukemia demonstrate that Aplidine, a drug sourced from *Aplidium albicans* (another sea squirt), may have a role in both resistant forms of leukemia and leukemia's non-response to other drugs. Aplidine inhibits DNA synthesis and protein synthesis and it also starves the tumor of nutrients by inhibiting secretion of VEGF.
Sponges of the Tethva and Halichondria families have been utilized in the production of chemotherapy agents, antibiotics and antivirals.
Sea organisms' polyunsaturated fatty acids have been utilized extensively in the development of novel delivery agents for medications.
Pseudomonas species remove cadmium from solution by precipitating it on the cell wall. This could provide a means of heavy metal removal from the environment during toxic and hazardous spills.
Barnacles can bind tightly to a slippery surface; "Polyphenolic protein" allows a strong binding to metal, plastic, bone, and skin holding promise for the development of new forms of surgical adhesives.
Technological advances-NASA technology has been adapted for navy divers allowing for diving at high pressure, in extreme temperature zones, and areas exposed to chemical spills. A new suit under investigation is using a mechanism in which a diver would breathe a highly oxygenated perfluorocarbon mixture that would replace air in the lung, nose and ear cavities. The lungs would extract oxygen from the mixture and carbon dioxide would be "scrubbed" from the diver.

WITH TECHNICAL ADVANCE COMES INCREASED ACCESS

A new suit under investigation is using a mechanism in which a diver would breathe a highly oxygenated perfluorocarbon mixture that would replace air in the lung, nose, and ear cavities.[65] The lungs would extract oxygen from the mixture, and carbon dioxide would be "scrubbed" from the diver by a mechanical gill embedded in the diver's femoral vein (Figure 5).[19] New deep-sea research habitats are allowing divers to study and take part in research for extended periods of time.[19] Combine this with the use of vehicles adapted for deep-sea exploration, and it will not be long before industry has access to the deepest regions of our planet. The Deepsea Challenger that successfully took film director James Cameron deep in the Mariana Trench[68] was specifically designed for this purpose. Other autonomous underwater vehicles controlled by computers with artificial intelligence[19] are making deeper ocean travel more efficient and accessible. However, according to Dr. Sylvia Earle, China, France, India, and Russia are all creating manned subs capable of reaching 6,000 meters at a time when we are cutting funding to similar ventures.[63] This does not bode well for U.S. leadership in the field and certainly not for conservancy of resources.

THE ECONOMY, BIOTECHNOLOGY, AND SPACE EXPLORATION

The biotechnology sector of the American economy is impressive, with over 1.6 million employed in 2013,[7] and revenues already greater than USD$577 billion by 2008.[5] According to the 2012 BIO International Convention, during the recession, the industry has gained jobs in a climate of general job loss across the country, with industry growth of 6.4% against a general private sector loss of 2.9%.[8]

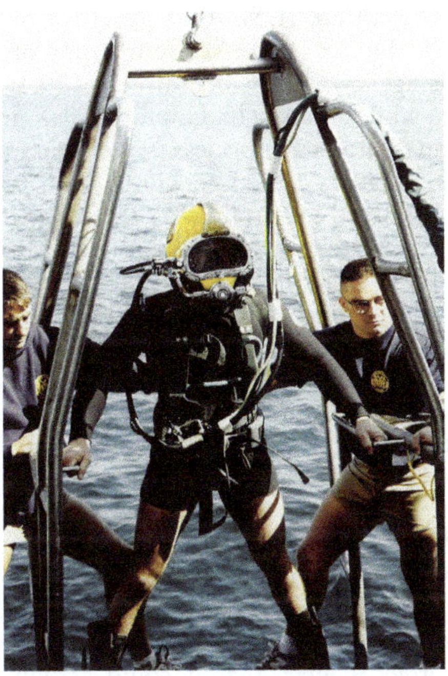

Figure 5. CDR Joseph Dituri wearing MK-21 on stage following a training dive.

Unfortunately, government investment has been less in the United States than in other nations. For example, China pledged over $308 billion to biotechnology research in 2011, while the U.S. government struggled not to cut the $32 billion in National Institutes of Health (NIH) funding for biotech research. Pharmaceutical companies like Novartis and Pfizer are spending billions collaborating with the Chinese in huge ventures[11] which would otherwise stimulate U.S. economic development if the tax and other incentives were available in the United States.

The space sector, on the other hand, employs 900,000 people worldwide in areas directly related to the space initiative such as space agencies, military initiatives, manufacturing of rocket satellites, construction of ground installations, and space industry component suppliers. This does not include university or private research and development, nor the industrial spinoffs discussed earlier. Worldwide, the direct space industry revenue amounted to over $250 billion from rocket components to satellite TV services.[62] Employment and revenue from spinoffs is very difficult to estimate, but the magnitude can be imagined when taking into account the more than 1,750 industries featured in NASA's *Spinoff* publication since 1976, where many of the innovations cataloged above as well as many others are highlighted.[38]

SHOW ME THE MONEY

Of the US$465.5 billion projected to be spent on research and development (R&D) in the United States in 2014, $123 billion comes from federal funding in the form of grants and appropriations.[76] This figure is slated to be $135.4 billion in 2015, with $64 billion to the Department of Defense, $30 billion to the NIH, $5.7 billion to the National Science Foundation (NSF) of which only $29 million is earmarked for biotech research, $11.6 billion to NASA (total NASA funding ~$18 billion, 0.476% of the federal budget),[27] $12.3 billion to the Department of Energy, $2.4 billion to the Department of Agriculture (USDA), a generous $688M to the National Oceanic and Atmospheric Agency (NOAA) (from a total of $5.5 billion in federal funding received by this agency,[55] of which a mere $29.1 million goes to ocean exploration and research, while almost a half billion dollars are allocated to fisheries research and $186 million to protected species research and management), while the Environmental Protection Agency (EPA) gets only $560 million. Comparatively, education and others are starved of funding.[76] The other major players in ocean research are the Woods Hole Oceanographic Institution with an operating revenue of $213.5 million including $58 million in research funding,[74] Scripps Institution of Oceanography with $165 million of its $190 million budget going to research,[61] and the Harbor Branch Oceanographic Institution with a budget according to the interim director of only $18–$20 million.[25] To put all this funding in perspective, Americans spend almost one trillion dollars on entertainment, alcohol, tobacco, gambling, toys, and pets. This is 63 times the space budget and about 5,000 times that spent on ocean research.[15]

INTELLECTUAL PROPERTY

The issue of intellectual property and patent protection is of serious concern to the authors. There is a hot debate over the effect of patent protection. Patent protection of genes could drive humanity to discover new genes and produce new marketable products. Others believe that it could actually stifle research.[2,35-36] Either way, there could be a rush to secure potential specimens for research, resulting in serious harm to the maritime environment. Furthermore, ethical concerns about the patenting of genes have resulted in a series of contradictory U.S. court decisions[13] which may eventually lead to cessation of gene patenting. How this would impact the rate or magnitude of bioprospecting is impossible to predict. Ultimately, corporate interest in new marine genes located on foreign soil or in international and foreign waters will raise issues of propriety and intellectual property.[41] It will open the floodgates of bioprospecting in place of biopiracy.[44] It is important that international law and the laws of developed countries reflect the importance of protecting the rights of those countries which do not have the means to utilize the bioproduct themselves. The Eli Lilly profit from the sale of two anticancer drugs obtained from Madagascar's Rosy Periwinkle plant with absolutely no financial gain by the nation of origin,[56] and the W.R. Grace–patented insecticide from the Indian Neem tree that caused riots in India,[44] led to the development of the Trade-Related Aspects of Intellectual Property Rights (TRIPS) agreement, the Biodiversity Treaty.[56] In 2003, the Convention on Biological Diversity (CBD) was ratified which attempts to ensure the "safe transfer, handling and use" of living modified organisms resulting from modern biotechnology that may have adverse effects on the conservation and sustainable use of biological diversity, taking also into account risks to human health, and specifically focusing on transboundary movements.[67] In 2010, the CBD, at the Nagoya Conference, established a protocol for improving access to genetic resources and the fair, equitable sharing of any advantages or profits gained from the use of these resources.[67] It would be convenient to believe that the United Nations Convention on the Law of the Sea (UNCLOS), which codifies modern international law regarding sovereignty of territorial water by defining the rights and responsibilities of nations in their use of the world's oceans and establishes guidelines for the management of marine natural resources, would ensure "ownership" of bioresources in territorial waters. However, we currently have numerous disputes between China and the various other nations surrounding the South China Sea over who actually "owns" the disputed territory. China, a full signatory of UNCLOS, states that it is not governed by the code because it has controlled the region for 2,000 years.[71] Despite these advances, profit drives "piracy," as we have seen with ivory, rhinoceros horn, and so many other "protected" species, and overfishing by foreign travelers in sovereign seas. Laws, codes, and treaties are only as good as the willingness of nations and individuals to uphold them and are almost impossible to enforce in international waters.

PROTECTING THE FUTURE

We are concerned these resources are not adequately protected from negative impact. One of the greatest threats to taking advantage of the sea's gene potential is loss of biodiversity through alteration and destruction. This is a legitimate concern because 30% to 50% of the world's species face extinction by mid-century, with extinctions occurring at dozens per day.[12] Threats such as overfishing, dumping of nuclear and other wastes, and destruction of coastal ecosystems imperils the biodiversity of the oceans and the utilization of potential resources. Global collapse of all commercially exploited fish populations is expected by 2048 at current rates of exploitation.[75] Despite tropical reefs sheltering as many as of all marine species,[58] between ⅓ and ⅔ of the coral reefs are damaged or dying, predicted to cause the extinction of as many as of reef species.[37]

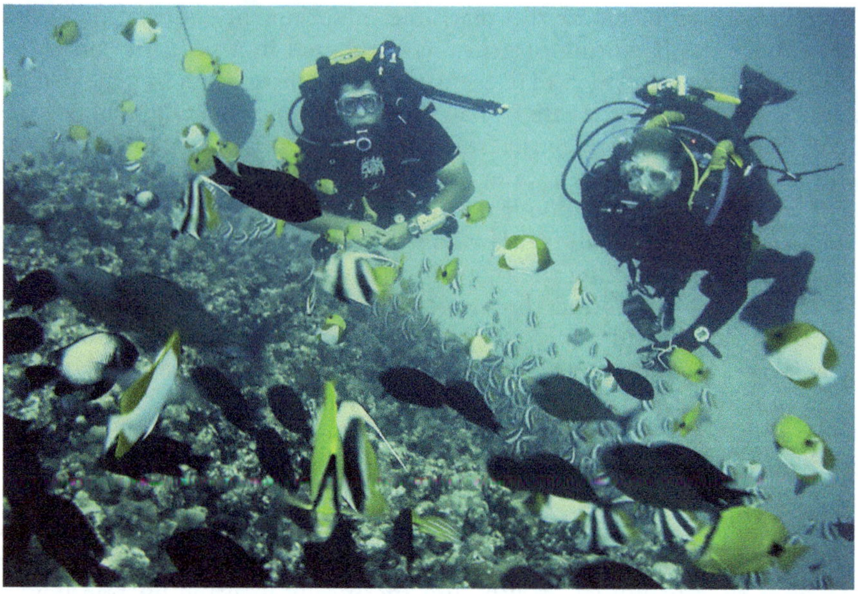

Figure 6. Ryan Wallace and CDR Joseph Dituri ascending from deep dive.

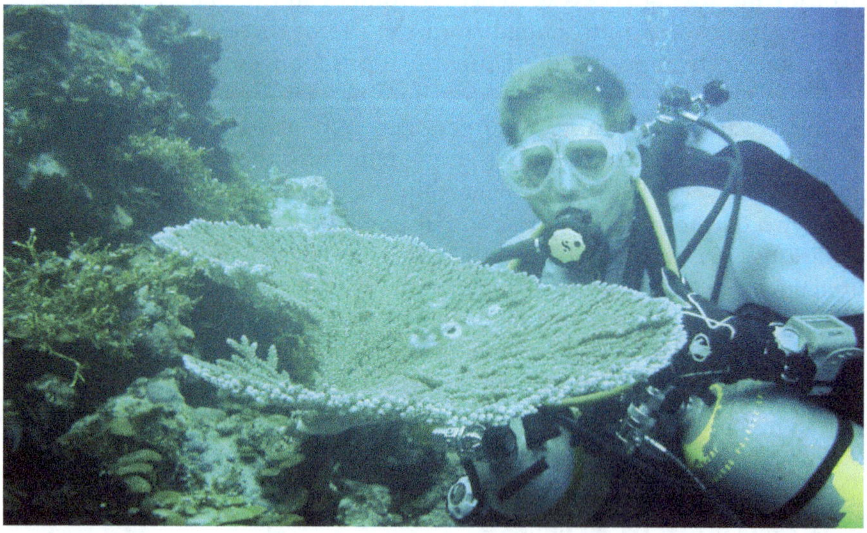

Figure 7. CDR Joseph Dituri ascending from a 100-meter deco dive using open-circuit.

It is vital that we act at the level of governmental and international policy to prevent irreparable damage to the last frontier even before we have the technology to benefit from the secrets of the deep (Figure 6, Figure 7). The authors suggest that research regulatory bodies such as the Institutional Review Board (IRB) implement approval processes for all bioderived product testing contingent upon sustainable harvesting and/or culture procedures and measures to protect the source environment and local interests. We must not neglect the local frontier in our efforts to colonize Mars because doing so would impede oceanic biotech innovations and allow current exploitation of the oceans to continue unchecked.

THE FUTURE OF UNDERSEA HOUSING

Imagine a life much like *The Jetsons*, but instead of an outer-space setting, it is 30 to 60 feet underwater – entire houses submersed with panoramic windows allowing for the opportunity to be entertained by a 360-degree aquarium.

Fortunately, private industry leaders in search of profits have taken what has been learned from previously discussed SEA LAB, Aquarius, and submarine design research and are now making the imagined future into the present. Currently there are multiple restaurants and resorts, in Fiji and Dubai primarily, that have submersed their businesses and brought what is only previously seen by divers and aquarium attendees to whoever is willing to pay.

U.S. Submarine Structures through H2OME currently is making to order 1250 and 3600 sq ft. underwater estates for USD$4 million and USD$12 million respectively, which does not include installation costs. The location is of the purchaser's choosing, pending U.S. Submarines' site evaluation and further detailed contract agreements.

A submersed hotel in Fiji, created by U.S. Submarine Structures, is currently under construction with the designs for the Poseidon Undersea Resort blueprints from 2009 with the lead contractors being U.S. Submarine Structures LLC. Their published overview article and blueprints provide insight on how an undersea dwelling is to be constructed, delivered, installed, and maintained. In general, the initial creation is built off of the inspiration of submarines, both of old and new generations.[33]

The viewports (floor-to-ceiling windows) are to be made of thick acrylic material, much like that of aquarium viewing stations. The rooms are constructed on land in individual pods and then delivered to their destination for installation at 30 feet below surface. The resort's main air supply, electricity, and communications are connected to land via umbilical, much like in surface-supplied diving. The rooms (pods) are connected to each other via a long, cylindrical, submerged structure that serves as a docking station and a hallway. Each pod can be attached and detached for maintenance purposes.[33]

The resort is accessed by the surface where its guests descend via elevator into a well-contained, -maintained, and safe underwater world with full service kitchen, dining rooms, and guest rooms.

The resort is minimally invasive to the environment with its only contact being the main pillars, which are the foundation in contact with the ocean floor. The goal for such is to over time allow coral growth and create in itself an underwater habitat and home to humans and marine life alike, which will then hopefully inspire many more to love and care for the future of the oceans.[33]

CONCLUSION

It is the opinion of the authors that, compared to space research, oceanic research has led to drugs and biomedical applications of value to humans at a far lower cost ratio. Five hundred people have been in space, 12 have stood on the moon, yet only 3 have been the depth of Everest below sea level, and 2 of those were in 1960 for a lengthy 20 minutes. While we would never consider calling for a decrease in space funding, oceanic funding needs to increase – if only to ensure the continuation of life as we know it here on Earth.

REFERENCES

1. Ahmed B et al. Advanced neuroscience technologies. In: Morris R, Tarasseno L, Kenword M, editors. Cognitive systems – information processing meets brain science. New York: Elsevier; 2006. p. 263-82.
2. Williamson AR. Gene patents: socially acceptable monopolies or an unnecessary hindrance to research? Trends Genet. 2001 Nov;17(11):670-3. ISSN: 0168-9525.
3. Andrade AO. Bridging the gap between robotic technology and health care. Biomed Signal Process Control. 2014;10:65-78.
4. Arrieta JM, Arnaud-Haond S, Duarte CM. What lies underneath: conserving the oceans' genetic resources. Proc Natl Acad Sci U S A. 2010;107:18318-24.
5. Battelle/Biotechnology Initiative Organization, State Bioscience Initiatives 2010 [Internet]. [cited 2014 Dec 6]. Available from: http://www3.bio.org/local/battelle2010/Battelle_Report_2010.pdf
6. Bille MA, Lishock ER. The first space race: launching the world's first satellites. Texas: Texas A&M University Press; 2004.
7. BIO Biotechnology Innovation Organization [Internet]. BIO Biotechnology Innovation Organization. BIO releases bioscience economic development report and guide [cited 2014 Jun 6]. Available from: http://www.bio.org/media/press-release/bio-releases-bioscience-economic-development-report-and-guide
8. Bioscience industry adds jobs over the last decade, despite economic setbacks for the nation. Battelle [Internet]. Battelle Memorial Institute. Bioscience industry adds jobs over the last decade, despite economic setbacks for the nation [cited 2014 Jun 6]. Available from: http://www.battelle.org/media/press-releases/bioscience-industry-adds-jobs-over-the-last-decade-despite-economic-setbacks-for-the-nation
9. Broad WJ. The universe below. New York: Simon and Schuster; 1997.
10. Ceylan O et al. Combustion characteristics of cellulosic loose fibers. Fire Mater. 2013;37(6):482-90.
11. China's 5-year biotech investment fires clear warning to US. GaBI Online Generics and Biosimilars Initiative [Internet]. Generics and Biosimilars Initiative (Gabl). China's 5-year biotech investment fires clear warning to US; 2011 [cited 2014 Jun 6]. Available from: http://www.gabionline.net/Biosimilars/News/China-s-5-year-biotech-investment-fires-clear-warning-to-US
12. Chivian E, Bernstein A, editors. Sustaining life: how human health depends on biodiversity. Center for Health and the Global Environment. New York: Oxford University Press; 2008.
13. Chojnacki B, White RF. The BRCA gene patents: arguments over patentability and social utility. World Med Health Policy. 2013;5:276–300.
14. Committee on Marine Biotechnology. Marine biotechnology in the twenty-first century: problems, promise, and products. Washington (DC): National Academies Press (U.S.); 2002.
15. Consumer expenditure survey [Internet]. Bureau of Labor Statistics [cited 2014 Dec 14]. Available from: http://www.bls.gov/cex/.
16. Costanza R. The ecological, economic, and social importance of the oceans. Ecol Econ. 1999 Nov;31(2):199-213. ISSN: 0921-8009.
17. Craven JP. The silent war: the Cold War battle beneath the sea. New York: Simon & Schuster; 2001.
18. Cuce E, Cuce PM, Wood CJ, Riffat SB. Toward aerogel based thermal superinsulation in buildings: a comprehensive review. Renew Sustain Energy Rev. 2014;34:273-99.

19. DeepSeaWaters.com [Internet]. DeepSeaWaters.com. Deep sea technology: tools for research; 2012 [cited 2014 Jun 6]. Available from: http://www.deepseawaters.com/deep_sea_technology.htm

20. Donia M, Hamann MT. Marine natural products and their potential applications as anti-infective agents. Lancet Infect Dis. 2003;3:338-48.

21. Espinar-Escalona E et al. Effect of temperature on the orthodontic clinical applications of niti closed-coil springs. Med Oral Patol Oral Cir Bucal. 2013;18(4):e721-4.

22. F. Cousteau. What I learned spending 31 days underwater. TED Talk. TED Global. 2014.

23. Fan Z, Gong F, Nguyen ST, Duong HM. Advanced multifunctional graphene aerogel – Poly (methyl methacrylate) composites: experiments and modeling. Carbon. 2015;81:396-404.

24. Finkl CW. Coastal hazards. New York: Springer; 2013.

25. Florida Atlantic University. FAU Harbor Branch at a glance [Internet]. Boca Raton (FL): Florida Atlantic University [updated 2013 Sep; cited 2017 Feb 2]. Available from: http://www.fau.edu/hboi/pdf/At-a-Glance%202013%20updated%209-2013.pdf

26. Florida International University Arts, Sciences & Education [Internet]. Miami (FL): Florida International University; 2013. Aquarius: School of Environment, Arts and Society: About [cited 2017 Feb 2]. Available from: http://aquarius.fiu.edu/about/.

27. FY 2015 president's budget request summary [Internet]. National Aeronautics and Space Administration. Available from: http://www.nasa.gov/news/budget/.

28. Gibson I. Advanced manufacturing technology for medical applications. Chichester: John Wiley & Sons; 2006.

29. Guined J. Project Poseidon 100-day undersea expedition names crew [Internet]. SeaSpace Exploration and Research Society; 2016 May 4. Available from: http://www.prweb.com/releases/2016/05/prweb13387063.htm

30. Haefner B. Drugs from the deep: marine natural products as drug candidates. Drug Discov Today. 2003;8:536-44.

31. Hardcastle, N. In vivo real-time rectal wall dosimetry for prostate radiotherapy. Phys Med Biol. 2010;55:3859-71.

32. He JB, Cui T, Zhang WW, Deng N. A chip-type thin-layer electrochemical cell coupled with capillary electrophoresis for online separation of electrode reaction products. Anal Chim Acta. 2013;786:159-65.

33. Jones LB. Technical considerations in the design, engineering, construction, and installation of the Poseidon Undersea Resort. U.S. Submarine Structures LLC; 2009 Mar.

34. Jung W, Han J, Choi JW, Ahn CH. Point-of-care testing (POCT) diagnostic systems using microfluidic lab-on-a-chip technologies. Microelectron Eng. 2015;132:46-57.

35. Klein RD. Gene patents and genetic testing in the United States. Nat Biotechnol. 2007;25:989-90.

36. Klein RD, Mahoney MJ. LabCorp v. Metabolite Laboratories: the Supreme Court listens, but declines to speak. J Law Med Ethics. 2008 Spring;36(1):141-9.

37. Knowlton N, Jackson JB. Shifting baselines, local impacts, and global change on coral reefs. PLoS Biol. 2008;6:e54.

38. Lam B. Searching for the ocean's secrets from the last undersea base [Internet]. Gizmodo.com; 2012 [cited 2014 Dec 6]. Available from: http://gizmodo.com/5925852/searching-for-the-oceans-secrets-from-the-last-undersea-base?tag=missionaquarius

39. Leal MC, Puga J, Serôdio J, Gomes NC, Calado R. Trends in the discovery of new marine natural products from invertebrates over the last two decade – where and what are we bioprospecting? PLoS One. 2012;7:30580.

40. Li Y, Zhang X, Huang Z, Hu Q. Design of wearable intelligent mind controlled prosthetic hand. In: International Conference on Mechatronics and Automation (ICMA); Chengdu. 2012. p. 2462-6.

41. Marine biotechnology: creating new value from the sea [Internet]. Available from: www.oceanpanel.nos.noaa.gov/backgroundpage/PDF_Background/Marine_Biotech.pdf This web site has since been retired and the article is imbedded within the archived site available from: http://oceanservice.noaa.gov/websites/retiredsites/oceanpanel.pdf Cited 2014 Mar 1.

42. Marsch A, High WA. Medicolegal issues with regard to melanoma and pigmented lesions in dermatopathology. Dermatol Clin. 2012;30(4):593-615.

43. McKie R. Marine treasure trove could bring revolution in medicine and industry. The Guardian [Internet]. 2012 Nov 10 [cited 2014 Dec 6]. Available from: http://www.guardian.co.uk/environment/2012/nov/10/marine-treasure-trove-medicine

44. Merson J. Bio-prospecting or bio-piracy: intellectual property rights and biodiversity in a colonial and postcolonial context. Osiris. 2000;15:282-96.

45. Metcalfe P et al. Review of four novel dosimeters developed for use in radiotherapy. J Phys Conf Ser. 2013;444:012008.

46. Mitchell D et al. Endovascular brachytherapy and restenosis following lower limb angioplasty: systematic review and meta-analysis of randomized clinical trials. Int J Surg. 2012;10:124-8.

47. Morton B. This man lived underwater for 31 days [Internet]. Red Bull; 2014 Jul 23. Available from: http://www.redbull.com/us/en/adventure/stories/1331665953342/how-fabien-cousteau-lived-underwater-for-31-days

48. Murray J. "Papa Topside," Captain George F. Bond, MC, USN. Faceplate. 2005;9(1):8-9.

49. Nasa budgets: US spending on space travel since 1958 UPDATED. The Guardian [Internet]. [cited 2017 Feb 2]. Available from: http://www.theguardian.com/news/datablog/2010/feb/01/nasa-budgets-us-spending-space-travel Compiled from data from the Federal Department of Management and Budget available at http://www.whitehouse.gov/omb/budget/Historicals/.

50. NASA historical databook .Van Nimmen J, Bruno LC, Rosholt RL. NASA historical databook, 1958-1968 [Internet]. Vol. I, NASA resources. Washington (DC): National Aeronautics and Space Administration, Scientific and Technical Information Office; 1976. p. 10 [cited 2014 Dec 6]. Available from: http://history.nasa.gov/SP-4012v1.pdf NASA SP-4012v1.

51. NASA [Internet]. Washington (DC): National Aeronautics and Space Administration. About NEEMO (NASA Extreme Environment Mission Operations) [updated 2015 Jul 30; cited 2017 Feb 2]. Available from: http://www.nasa.gov/mission_pages/NEEMO/about_neemo.html

52. NASA [Internet]. Washington (DC): National Aeronautics and Space Administration. Budget documents, strategic plans and performance reports [2016 Dec 1; cited 2017 Feb 2]. Available from: https://www.nasa.gov/news/budget/index.html

53. NASA [Internet]. Washington (DC): National Aeronautics and Space Administration. NEEMO [updated 2016 Aug 31; cited 2017 Feb 2]. Available from: http://www.nasa.gov/mission_pages/NEEMO/

54. Nespoli A et al. Design and thermo-mechanical analysis of a new NiTi shape memory alloy fixing clip. Mater Sci Eng C. 2014;37:171-6.

55. NOAA FY 2014 budget blue book [Internet]. National Oceanic and Atmospheric Administration [cited 2014 Dec 6]. Available from: http://www.corporateservices.noaa.gov/nbo/14bluebook_highlights.html

56. Oxley A. Developing effective approaches to access to genetic resources: a report published by the Australian APEC Study Centre, Monash University, Australia [Internet]. Australian APEC Study Centre, Monash University [cited 2014 Dec 6]. Available from: http://www.apec.org.au/docs/oxley2005.pdf

57. Patrzykat A, Douglas SE. Gone gene fishing: how to catch novel marine antimicrobials. Trends Biotechnol. 2003;21:362-9.

58. Plaisance L, Caley MJ, Brainard RE, Knowlton N. The diversity of coral reefs: what are we missing? PLoS One. 2011;6:e25026.

59. Santoni F et al. An orientable solar panel system for nanospacecraft. Acta Astronautica. 2014;101:120-8.

60. Schwartsmann G, Da Rocha AB, Mattei J, Lopes R. Marine-derived anticancer agents in clinical trials. Expert Opin Investig Drugs. 2003;12:1367-83.

61. Scripps Institution of Oceanography Annual Report 2012-2013 [Internet]. San Diego (CA): Scripps Institution of Oceanography; 2013 [cited 2017 Feb 2]. Available from: https://scripps.ucsd.edu/sites/scripps.ucsd.edu/files/node/21/edit/annual_report_2012-2013.pdf

62. Space economy at a glance [Internet]. Organisation for Economic Co-operation and Development; 2014 [cited 2014 Dec 6]. Available from: http://www.oecd.org/futures/oecdspaceforum.htm ISBN: 978-92-64-217294.

63. Spinoff 2011: a NASA publication [Internet]. National Aeronautics and Space Administration. Available from: http://spinoff.nasa.gov/back_issues_archives.html

64. Oceanography: death in the depths. Time. 1969 Feb 2 [cited 2011 Feb 18].

65. Taylor J. "Into the abyss: the diving suit that turns men into fish. The Independent [Internet]. 2010 Nov 20 [cited 2014 Dec 6]. Available from: http://www.independent.co.uk/news/science/into-the-abyss-the-diving-suit-that-turns-men-into-fish-2139167.html

66. Temiz Y, Lovchik RD, Kaigala GV, Delamarche E. Lab-on-a-chip devices: how to close and plug the lab? Microelectron Eng. 2015;132:156-75.

67. Text from Convention on Biological Diversity [Internet]. Cartagena Protocol on Biosafety, Nagoya Protocol on Access and Benefit Sharing [cited 2014 June 6]. Available from: http://bch.cbd.int/protocol/text/ and http://www.cbd.int/abs/.

68. Text from National Geographic [Internet]. National Geographic; 2013. James Cameron's Deepsea Challenge 3D the sub 2014 Mar 1]. Available from: http://deepseachallenge.com/the-sub/.

69. Tooley M. Aircraft digital electronic and computer systems. 2nd ed. New York: Routledge; 2011.

70. Treasury Direct [Internet]. U.S. Department of the Treasury, Bureau of the Fiscal Service [cited 2014 Dec 6]. Available from: http://www.treasurydirect.gov/NP/debt

71. UNCLOS cannot determine South China Sea dispute: China. Business Standard [Internet]. 2014 Jun 6 [cited 2014 Jun 6]. Available from: http://www.business-standard.com/article/pti-stories/unclos-cannot-determine-south-china-sea-dispute-china-114060201484_1.html

72. U.S. Submarine Structures LLC [Internet]. Rathdrum (ID): U.S. Submarine Structures LLC. Pricing; [cited 2017 Feb 2]. Available from: http://www.ussubstructures.com/pricing.html

73. Whelan HT, Annis H, Guajardo P. From land to sea; embracing a renewable future. J Biotechnol Biomater. 2013;4:163.

74. Woods Hole Oceanographic Institution [Internet]. Woods Hole (MA): Woods Hole Oceanographic Institution. Climate & oceans; [cited 2017 February 2]. Available from: http://www.whoi.edu/page.do?pid=8916#5

75. Worm B, Barbier EB, Beaumont N, Duffy JE, Folke C, et al. Impacts of biodiversity loss on ocean ecosystem services. Science. 2006;314:787-90.

76. 2014 global r&d funding forecast, a Battelle Memorial Institute publication [Internet]. Battelle Memorial Institute; 2013 Dec [cited 2014 Dec 6]. Available from: http://www.battelle.org/docs/tpp/2014_global_rd_funding_forecast.pdf

Index

A

ABG 72, 79-81, 90, 179, 183, 1061
ABI 566-569, 572, 595-596, 599, 612, 616
ability to heal 617
absolute contraindications 230, 973, 981, 1004
Doxorubicin (Adriamycin®) 132, 144, 157, 172-173, 182, 191-192, 196, 198, 230
mafenide acetate (Sulfamylon®) 131, 140, 174, 186, 196, 448, 458, 808
untreated pneumothorax 177, 230
acetazolamide 131, 140, 154, 157, 822, 824, 826, 1077
acidosis 304, 308, 312, 318, 420, 582, 793, 812, 886, 1061, 1118-1119, 1130
actinomyces spp. 469, 471, 478
acute
acute myocardial infarction 44, 47, 296, 816
acute renal failure 156, 323, 407, 422
acute respiratory distress syndrome 53, 183, 417, 1061, 1117
adipose 138, 372, 1003, 1009, 1013, 1070
adjunctive HBO 175, 189, 334, 465, 467, 472, 474, 481, 489, 497, 508, 568, 597-599, 601, 607, 610, 615, 652, 673, 711, 716, 801, 808-809, 886-887
advanced practice nurses 125
aerobic metabolism 381, 386-387, 439, 911, 934, 938, 943, 1054, 1155
air breaks 57-58, 82, 94, 140, 212, 216, 270, 419, 697, 931, 976-978, 980, 990
air embolism 63, 92, 142, 148-149, 152-153, 155, 157, 188, 198, 213, 226, 364, 369-377, 1067
Albert Behnke 41
albumin 249, 536, 571, 583-584, 586-587, 594, 702
alcohol 146-147, 151, 154, 213, 329, 448, 452, 770, 865, 1006, 1060, 1072-1073, 1084, 1144
alginates 580
alpha toxin 283, 410-411, 414
AMB 883-885, 888
ambient pressure oxygen 310
American College of Hyperbaric Medicine XVIII, 32
aminoglycosides 150, 284-285, 383-384, 394, 417, 492, 497
amphotericin B 149-150, 153, 385, 390-391, 401, 884-889, 891
amputation 92, 172, 240-241, 245-246, 271, 295, 409, 430, 448-449, 453, 488-489, 503-504, 506-508, 513-515, 518, 525, 531, 533, 543, 545, 550, 552-553, 557-558, 561, 565, 568-569, 572, 575-582, 584-585, 587, 593-596, 598-604, 606, 608, 610-613, 615-621, 632-634, 637-638, 643, 651-652, 674, 676, 678, 683, 687, 689, 715, 804
anaerobes 382, 389, 436, 438-439, 445-446, 450, 469, 471, 495, 506, 799
anaerobic VI, 41, 45, 47, 54, 113, 149, 252, 282-283, 285, 379, 382-385, 388-390, 392, 395, 397, 400-402, 404-405, 410, 415, 424-426, 428-431, 433, 435-436, 438-443, 445-447, 449, 455-456, 458-460, 469-474, 477-478, 481-483, 496-497, 514, 518-519, 545, 563, 695, 806, 920, 1059, 1153, 1170
anaerobic metabolism 252, 389, 402, 920, 1059
anaerobiosis 298, 379, 381, 384, 392, 398, 401, 404, 521
analgesics 73-74, 79, 86, 132, 143, 528, 697, 755, 769, 1044, 1050, 1073-1074
narcotic 528
anesthetic 147-148, 153, 165, 421, 444
angiogenesis 43, 176, 186, 192, 231, 247, 268, 276, 278-282, 296-297, 491, 497, 508, 512, 542-543, 545, 552, 621, 628-

630, 635, 668, 712, 716, 721, 725, 727, 729-730, 732-739, 751, 764, 774-775, 779, 786-787, 800, 804, 867, 877, 902, 941
angiogenesis response 738
ankle-brachial index (ABI) 566, 584, 621
anoxic brain injury 952
antibacterial 44, 379, 383-385, 389, 404, 593, 721, 890, 901
antibiotic 191, 231, 285, 291, 389, 394, 397, 400, 403-404, 407, 413-414, 417, 423, 426, 440, 446-447, 450, 453, 470, 472, 477, 481, 497, 499-500, 502, 505, 507-510, 513, 519, 563, 579, 595, 666, 704, 710, 718, 746, 798
antibiotic therapy 397, 407, 413-414, 417, 423, 453, 470, 497, 499, 505, 509-510, 513, 563, 579, 710, 718, 798
anticonvulsants 132, 140-141, 185, 950
antifungal 153, 379, 385, 390, 398, 883-885, 887-888, 890, 892
antimicrobial 42, 45, 47, 136, 140, 149, 186, 383-385, 391, 393-395, 398, 401-402, 404, 431, 451, 473, 518-519, 563, 806, 892
antioxidants 51-52, 146, 157, 198, 305, 313, 352, 382, 384, 391, 399, 402, 798, 884, 942, 999
antiparasitic 379, 385, 397
antivenin 899, 901
antiviral 330, 337, 343, 349, 359-360, 391, 402
anxiety 77, 125, 228-229, 253, 307, 312, 593, 888, 927, 929, 981, 998, 1006, 1011-1012, 1056, 1059, 1069, 1071, 1093
apoptosis 45, 47, 176, 305, 313, 316, 647, 654, 657, 804, 818, 830, 920, 931-933, 941, 943, 947-948, 950, 959
ARDS 53, 183, 187, 217, 407, 417-418, 420-421, 1061, 1117
arrhythmia 266, 307, 317, 417
arterial
arterial blood gas 179, 421, 1061
arterial carbon dioxide tension 72, 79
arterial gas embolism 55, 79, 87, 213, 215, 217, 231, 253, 255, 267, 270, 288, 363, 369-375, 413, 423, 683, 828, 982, 1049, 1059, 1062, 1064, 1075, 1083-1084, 1101, 1103
arterial oxygen tension 81, 94, 420, 472, 710
arteriography 595
arteriole thrombosis 647
aseptic necrosis 1082
aspergillosis 881, 883, 885, 888-893
aspirin 143, 250, 367, 538, 562, 826, 856, 859
asthma 179, 190, 230, 349, 363, 865, 1074, 1083
atelectasis 224, 311, 420
atmospheres absolute 70, 252, 271, 287, 293, 309, 367, 414, 494, 545, 630, 668, 674, 800, 839, 847, 888, 902, 997, 1002, 1034, 1052
atrial fibrillation 364
auditory (Eustachian) tube 161-163, 203-206, 226, 229-231, 1065-1066
Australia XVI, 468, 832, 839, 1151
autism 221, 231-232, 234-235, 273, 282, 843, 945, 952-954, 957
autoimmune 357, 360
autolytic debridement 580
automobile exhaust 303

B

bacteremia 413, 425
bacteria 41, 45, 48, 149, 154, 241, 280-285, 292, 379, 382, 384-386, 388-389, 392, 395, 397-398, 400, 403-404, 409-411, 437, 441, 446, 460-461, 469, 482-483, 491-492, 495-497, 514, 518, 534, 563, 666, 710, 799, 817, 966-968, 1080, 1122
aerobic bacteria 41, 379, 382, 385, 389, 496
anaerobic bacteria 45, 149, 385, 388, 395, 482-483, 514, 518, 563
bacterial
bacterial invasion 383, 439, 561, 793
bacterial synergy 436-437
bactericidal activity 384-385, 401, 403-404, 497, 519
bacteriostatic 39, 45, 282, 379, 382, 384-386, 388
bacteroides spp. 469-470
Bakker VI, XV, 127, 296, 435, 438, 456, 459, 461, 481, 521, 690, 787
bar 104, 138, 149-150, 156, 449, 478, 752, 841, 980, 989
barbiturates 132, 142, 950
Baromedical Nurses Association 32, 115-116, 120, 127
barosinusitis 161, 199, 207
barotitis 159, 161, 165-166, 202, 217
barotrauma 74, 89, 148, 163, 168, 171-173, 177-179, 191-192, 199, 201-211,

213, 215, 217-219, 225-226, 230, 253, 292, 311, 350, 363, 365, 367, 371, 373-374, 786, 809, 981-982, 1019, 1032, 1049-1050, 1052, 1060, 1063-1068, 1072-1073, 1083, 1120
Bartlett 427, 456, 458, 461, 686, 815, 891-892
basic fibroblast growth factor 44, 591, 734
beam collimation 727
Beckman 151-152, 859, 992
Behnke 41, 48, 59
Bennett VIII, XVI, 59, 92, 234-235, 316, 353, 356, 369-371, 429, 460, 618, 622, 640, 686, 719, 817-818, 839, 855-856, 858, 891, 893, 955, 992, 1130-1131
bends XI, 41, 148, 365, 1136
Bert 212, 217, 964, 997, 1059, 1126
bioburden 280, 282, 579, 662-663, 666
bladder 175-176, 193, 227, 376, 409, 415-416, 781, 953, 1004
bleomycin 132, 146, 151, 154, 156-157, 172-173, 183, 193-198, 224, 230
blood VII, 42-43, 45, 47, 52, 58-59, 70-72, 76, 78-80, 82, 84, 87, 92-95, 107, 124, 128, 134-136, 140, 143-147, 150-151, 154-155, 161, 163, 178-179, 185-186, 203-204, 206, 217, 224-225, 237-238, 240-243, 245, 247, 249-251, 253, 256-259, 261-262, 264-265, 267, 271-273, 275-276, 280, 285-287, 289, 294-297, 304-305, 308, 310, 313-314, 317, 320-322, 328, 330, 356, 359, 363-364, 366, 370-373, 381, 383-384, 388-389, 393-394, 399, 401, 403, 407, 410-413, 417-418, 420-421, 423, 440, 444, 469-470, 472, 491-493, 497, 505-506, 513, 534-536, 538-540, 552, 557, 559, 566-568, 571, 579, 581, 583-584, 593-596, 599-600, 612, 616, 621, 625-626, 629-630, 634-635, 639, 648, 651, 655, 662-663, 665-666, 668-670, 676-678, 682, 686-689, 691, 693-698, 700, 702-705, 710-713, 715, 717, 739, 759, 798, 801, 808, 814, 826, 844, 847, 849, 856-858, 863-866, 883, 885, 888, 892, 899, 901, 906, 911, 920, 927, 929-930, 934-935, 939-941, 947, 949, 951, 958-959, 975, 981-982, 984, 999-1000, 1002, 1004-1007, 1009, 1012-1013, 1022, 1041, 1056, 1058-1059, 1061, 1065, 1067, 1069-1070, 1072, 1094, 1114, 1125, 1128, 1140
    blood glucose 124, 128, 144-145, 151, 217, 420, 557, 583-584, 593, 595-596, 612, 616, 849, 1000, 1005
    blood loss *VII*, 80, 261, 418, 691, 693, 695-696, 702-703, 705
    blood oxygen 225, 237, 256-259
    blood pressure 71, 76, 78, 82, 87, 92-95, 144-146, 151, 304-305, 328, 356, 366, 566-568, 600, 621, 697-698, 717, 808, 849, 856, 982, 1059, 1070, 1114
    whole blood 418
board certification 31, 36
Boerema 42, 47, 113, 259, 295, 418, 425, 427, 430, 480, 686, 694, 703, 969
bone
    bone formation 47, 276, 281, 328, 505, 509, 625-626, 628-630, 632, 635, 739, 867, 878
    bone graft 517, 631, 634-635, 738-739, 741, 752, 767-768
    bone grafting 508, 630, 632-635, 637-638, 751, 764, 768
    bone morphogenetic protein 630, 637-638, 767
    bone necrosis *VIII*, 755, 861, 863, 1072
    bone scans 506
"boxcars" 365
Boyle's law 171, 214, 270-271, 287, 1049, 1052, 1062-1063, 1068, 1111
BP monitoring 78-79, 81, 86
brain
    brain abscess 396, 400-401, 428, 476, 480-483
    brain edema 857, 941-942, 958
    brain lesions 308, 940
bronchopulmonary dysplasia 221, 224-225
brown recluse spider VIII, 284-285, 296-297, 897-908
Brummelkamp 47, 295, 409, 418, 425, 427, 480, 686, 969
bubble size 42, 270-271
burn VII, 260, 264, 273, 276, 290, 296, 317, 409, 429, 461, 542, 584, 661-662, 682-683, 716, 720, 722, 789, 791-793, 798-801, 803-806, 808-818, 885, 1044, 1099
    burn shock 799
    burn wound 193, 715, 721, 793, 798-800, 804, 806, 808, 810, 812, 814-816, 891

C

caisson workers XI
Camporesi V, VIII, XVI, 41, 46-48, 92,

94, 155, 198, 217, 370, 374, 377, 398, 618, 863, 878, 880, 959, 1104
cancer XIII, XIV, 42, 144, 152-153, 157, 174-176, 186, 190-191, 193-194, 196-198, 231, 253, 397, 409, 429, 525, 558, 586, 709, 714, 725, 729, 739, 746, 755, 770-775, 779-781, 784-785, 787, 843, 888, 955, 968, 1141
  head and neck cancer 194, 729, 746, 773
capillary
  capillary basement membrane 246, 261-262, 492
  capillary perfusion 273, 275, 493, 664, 678, 680-681, 735
  capillary proliferation 712, 718
carbon dioxide (CO_2) 58, 72, 79, 95, 140, 243, 246, 252, 261, 295, 308, 370-371, 373-375, 396, 439, 492, 541, 554, 664, 937, 975, 988, 1053-1054, 1056, 1082-1083, 1087, 1089, 1091, 1096, 1099, 1103-1104, 1111, 1115, 1117-1119, 1130, 1138, 1143
carbon monoxide (CO) VI, XII, 41-42, 48, 87, 113, 116, 147, 163, 174-175, 179, 194-195, 197-198, 212-214, 218, 223-224, 226, 230-232, 234, 253, 261, 267, 271-272, 286-288, 291-292, 298, 301, 303-307, 309, 311, 313-314, 316-323, 381, 683, 800, 814, 817, 1049, 1055-1056, 1082, 1121, 1130
  carbon monoxide binding 304
  carbon monoxide poisoning 42, 44, 48, 87, 113, 116, 144, 163, 174-175, 195, 197-198, 212-214, 218, 226, 230-232, 234, 253, 267, 272, 288, 291, 301-314, 316-323, 657, 683, 800, 814, 817, 1049, 1055
carboxyhemoglobin (COHb) 287, 303-304, 306-309, 311-314, 316-318, 321-323, 1055
  carboxyhemoglobin (COHb) level 304, 308, 311-314
cardiac
  cardiac arrest 42, 60, 365, 370, 958, 981, 1061-1062, 1073
  cardiac depression 144
  cardiac failure 422
cardiogenic shock XII
cardiotoxic 307, 422
cardiovascular surgery 114
catalase 51, 364, 386, 388-389, 391, 397, 404, 414, 496, 884, 937
cataracts 55-56, 181, 191, 199, 211-212, 332, 352, 1057, 1115
causes of gas embolism 364
caustic cocktail 1085, 1099, 1107, 1115
cellular adhesion molecules 650
central venous pressure 419, 937
cerebral
  cerebral aerobic metabolism 911, 938, 943
  cerebral blood flow (CBF) 52, 140, 154, 224, 308, 310, 320, 322, 328, 356, 372, 472, 844, 847-849, 857-858, 911, 913, 917, 920, 925, 930-931, 934-935, 938-939, 941, 951, 958, 1006, 1009, 1013
  cerebral edema 93, 366, 375, 465, 472, 482-483, 849, 859, 921, 932, 941-943, 950, 958, 1077
  cerebral gas embolism 374
  cerebral metabolic rate of oxygen ($CMRO_2$) 913, 917, 920-921, 930-931, 934-935
  cerebral metabolism 155, 920, 934-936, 939-940, 942-943, 958
  cerebral palsy 221, 232, 234-235, 273, 291, 314, 843, 847, 856-858, 945, 951, 954-957
cerebrospinal fluid (CSF) 136, 154, 156, 162, 188-189, 193, 207, 340, 350, 399, 403, 470, 890, 913, 917, 920, 930-931, 934-935, 937-940, 956, 1001, 1011
cerumen 164, 202, 207, 1065
chamber material
  collapsible 161, 178, 364
  rigid 103, 161, 203, 478, 612, 634, 738-739, 763-764, 1063
chamber shapes
  combination 73, 144, 149-150, 182-183, 225, 228, 231, 266, 283, 330-332, 335-337, 340, 342-343, 353, 355, 359-360, 383, 414, 417, 431, 438, 440-442, 447, 451, 454, 472, 477, 481, 491, 497, 506, 521, 557, 561, 582, 592, 636, 644, 682-683, 775, 798, 804, 830, 902, 921, 950, 964, 968, 980, 1018, 1021, 1031, 1044, 1053, 1059-1060, 1067, 1069, 1071-1072, 1078, 1094-1095, 1112, 1127
cherry red lips 314
children 116, 125, 163, 165, 193, 221, 223-224, 226-232, 234-235, 303-304, 312, 314, 316-317, 319, 325, 342, 354, 422, 435, 444, 446, 456-457, 459, 480-482, 501, 630-631, 640, 808, 843,

857-858, 899-900, 912, 939, 941-942, 951-952, 954-955, 957-958, 1001-1002, 1004, 1011, 1111
Children's Hospital XVII, XIX, XX, XXI, 114
China 468, 631, 640, 833, 1143-1145, 1151
Christian J. Lambertsen 1087
chronic refractory osteomyelitis VII, 181, 191, 252, 485, 487-489, 491, 496, 498-499, 503, 508, 510, 512, 515-517, 521, 542, 550, 632, 637, 640
chronic wounds 260, 295, 349, 356, 492, 552, 584, 620, 622, 709, 804, 816, 997
Churchill-Davidson 42, 47
cigarette smoking 303, 323, 329
circulation 42, 134-135, 137, 155, 178, 234, 247-248, 265, 271, 294, 296, 321, 363-364, 366, 374, 376, 412, 416, 419, 425, 447, 492, 520, 619, 651, 654, 657, 686, 688, 690, 695, 709-714, 719, 722, 793, 798, 813, 821, 826, 832, 857, 865-866, 868, 878, 939, 982, 984, 988-989, 1057, 1064, 1069, 1072
cis-platinum 156
claudication 243, 567, 587
clindamycin 404, 417, 431, 447-448, 450, 455, 462, 478
clinical
  clinical nurse specialists 125
  clinical outcome 358, 460, 574, 800, 856, 911, 933-936, 938, 942
closed-circuit rebreather 1009, 1011, 1089-1090, 1103, 1110
closed-loop 1118, 1122
clostridial
  clostridial cellulitis 407, 413, 441-442, 449
  clostridial gas gangrene 70, 413, 423, 425-427, 431
  clostridial myonecrosis 252, 283, 285, 401, 407, 410-417, 420-421, 423, 427-428, 430, 446, 448, 455, 542
  clostridial organisms 282-284, 410-411, 414-416, 423
clostridium perfringens 283, 296, 385, 388, 397, 404, 410, 414, 424-428, 430-432, 470
CO
  CO binding 304
  CO poisoning 42, 44, 48, 87, 113, 116, 144, 163, 174-175, 195, 197-198, 212-214, 218, 226, 230-232, 234, 253, 267, 272, 288, 291, 301-314, 316-323, 657, 683, 800, 814, 817, 1049, 1055
collagen 43, 143, 278, 447, 496, 514, 518, 535, 542, 561, 563, 592, 626, 630, 668, 687, 709-710, 716, 718, 720, 727-728, 733-734, 751, 754, 779, 798
  collagen synthesis 143, 518, 563, 687, 709-710, 716, 720, 728, 733-734, 754, 779
colloid 419
coma 311, 696, 700, 914-916, 920, 930, 934, 942, 951, 957-958, 1078, 1159
compartment syndrome 230, 247, 273, 297, 521, 552, 648, 651-652, 657, 661-662, 664, 678, 680-682, 684, 686-689, 867
complications VI, XI, 62, 92, 118-119, 146, 153, 166, 174, 180, 185, 188-189, 192, 198-199, 201, 219, 224-227, 229, 301, 311-312, 319, 321, 332, 407, 414-416, 421-422, 451, 453, 483, 518, 520, 534, 552, 579, 582, 587, 618, 620, 635, 656, 670, 676, 678, 683, 686, 715, 717, 720, 738-739, 744, 756, 774, 781, 784-785, 792, 886, 888, 904, 937-938, 955, 985, 990, 998, 1060-1061, 1075-1076, 1083-1084, 1092, 1095, 1172
composite grafts 713-714, 718-719, 808
compression 41, 61, 70, 77-78, 82, 84, 87, 90, 101, 107, 133-134, 161-162, 178, 189, 203, 205-211, 218, 230, 248, 251, 367, 369, 372, 567, 614, 678, 781, 828, 864, 976, 987, 1058, 1062, 1072, 1080, 1107, 1113, 1127-1130
compromised
  compromised host 449, 455, 477, 485, 487-488, 503, 505-506, 508, 511-514, 517
  compromised tissue 416, 709
  compromised wounds 738
confinement anxiety 125, 593, 888
congenital spherocytosis 185, 230
contamination of wounds 411
contraindications VI, 80, 118, 133, 147, 169, 171-172, 177, 196, 206, 221, 230-231, 253, 351-352, 395, 567, 569, 937, 973, 981-982, 990, 1004, 1073
controversies 221, 223, 230, 482, 617, 1083
convulsions 52-53, 56-59, 141-143, 152, 155, 213, 987, 998, 1056-1058, 1097-1098, 1118, 1123, 1126
cost
  cost effectiveness 123, 605, 792, 805, 815
  cost factors 769

cost of care 525, 744, 791, 800-801, 805, 809-810, 813
cost savings 717, 770, 809
Cousteau 1110, 1136, 1138-1139, 1149
Cowley 369, 703
Cramer 61, 296, 314, 317, 374, 397, 481, 521, 690
critically ill patients V, 67, 69-74, 77-78, 82, 87, 90-94, 420, 478, 582, 937, 943
crush injury VII, 44, 217, 230, 272, 438, 493, 521, 651-652, 655, 659, 661-662, 672-675, 677-678, 682, 684-687, 689
crystalloid 84, 700
Cullen's ulcer 436, 441
Cunningham 219, 457, 964
cyanide 231, 286, 288, 298
antidote 148
poisoning 42, 44, 47-49, 51-53, 55, 60, 66, 87, 113, 116, 144, 163, 174-175, 195, 197-198, 212-214, 218, 226, 230-232, 234, 253, 260, 267, 272, 286, 288, 290-291, 298, 301, 303-314, 316-323, 657, 683, 800, 814, 817, 1049, 1055, 1138, 1165
toxicity V, VIII, XIV, 42, 49, 51-56, 58-62, 64, 66, 77, 82, 86-87, 89-90, 92, 131-132, 134, 139-144, 146-149, 151, 153-157, 171-173, 180, 183, 185-187, 193-198, 212-213, 215, 217-219, 223-226, 232, 235, 253, 261, 270-271, 292, 304, 317, 321, 386, 389, 396-397, 399, 402, 407, 412-414, 419-421, 430, 445-446, 449, 452, 455, 474, 631, 686, 697, 704, 729, 804, 808-809, 828, 856, 885, 889, 898, 902, 905, 907, 909, 934-938, 941-943, 973, 982, 984-985, 989-990, 995, 997-998, 1001, 1007, 1010-1011, 1013, 1049, 1054-1057, 1069, 1082, 1084, 1092, 1097-1098, 1101, 1103, 1107, 1112, 1120-1121, 1123, 1126-1127, 1130-1131, 1165, 1167, 1170
cytochrome oxidase 136, 304, 312, 940

D

Dalton's law 1049, 1052, 1123
dapsone 900-903, 905-908, 963, 967
Davis 60, 62, 93, 127-128, 153, 202, 217, 374, 398, 425, 427, 457-458, 460-461, 480, 482, 499, 502, 517-519, 583, 593, 618, 654, 686-687, 709, 719, 722, 774-775, 787, 814-815, 818, 892, 941, 969, 1012, 1059, 1071, 1083, 1130
debridement 231, 284, 388, 390, 407, 415-416, 419-421, 423, 440-441, 446-447, 450, 453-454, 456, 493, 499-501, 503, 505, 507-511, 513-514, 525, 531-533, 536, 543, 549-550, 553, 558, 568, 570, 579-581, 583-584, 592-594, 596, 599-600, 610-617, 631, 634, 673, 675, 677, 742, 745, 754, 757, 763, 770, 794, 806, 814, 883, 885-888, 890, 902, 1154, 1158, 1170
decompression XI, 41, 44, 55, 57-58, 64, 70, 87, 105-106, 114, 116, 118, 128, 133-134, 142, 147-149, 151, 153, 156-157, 172, 177-180, 185, 205-211, 213, 215-216, 227-228, 230-231, 253, 255, 261, 267, 270-271, 286-288, 364-377, 416, 419, 680-681, 683, 695, 700, 804, 865, 877-879, 937, 975-976, 979, 981, 984, 986, 988, 992, 997, 1007, 1015, 1019-1025, 1030, 1032-1035, 1037-1040, 1043-1046, 1049, 1052, 1062, 1064, 1067, 1072, 1074, 1076, 1079-1080, 1083-1084, 1088, 1091-1092, 1097, 1101, 1109-1110, 1112-1115, 1125, 1127-1131, 1136, 1165, 1171
decompression illness 153, 157, 366-369, 371, 373-377, 419, 992, 1007, 1035, 1040, 1045, 1083, 1165
decompression sickness (DCS) XI, 41, 44, 55, 64, 105, 116, 118, 128, 147-149, 151, 156, 172, 178, 230-231, 253, 255, 261, 267, 270-271, 287-288, 365-367, 369-373, 375, 377, 683, 804, 937, 975-977, 979-982, 984, 986-988, 990-992, 997, 1008, 1022-1024, 1044, 1049, 1052, 1055, 1062-1063, 1067, 1069, 1071-1072, 1074, 1078-1081, 1083-1084, 1101, 1114, 1120, 1123-1126, 1128-1130
recompression 41, 215, 217, 366-367, 370, 374, 632, 840, 976, 986-990, 992-993, 1018, 1020, 1022-1025, 1029, 1044-1048, 1062-1064, 1079, 1120, 1125, 1127, 1129-1131, 1169
type 1 ("*pain only*") 145, 191, 452, 558, 615, 999, 1062, 1072, 1081
type 2 ("*serious symptoms*") 157, 190, 452, 558, 579, 582, 587, 616, 1062, 1081
decongestants 159, 163, 206, 209, 1050, 1066, 1073-1074
deep vein thrombosis 250, 368, 407, 422

defibrillation 67, 71, 349
dehiscence 520, 614, 631, 640, 739, 742-745, 786
delayed neurologic sequelae 310, 317
demyelination 952
dental problems 173, 180
dextran 330, 336-338, 342-343, 346, 538, 682, 694, 698, 704, 717, 720, 900
diabetes 92, 116, 145, 151, 154, 157, 174, 180, 185, 190-191, 211, 294, 329, 353, 375, 409, 412, 415, 420, 424, 435, 440, 443, 445, 449, 451-452, 454, 459, 488, 492, 518, 520, 525, 534-535, 546, 549, 552-554, 557-558, 561-563, 568, 579, 581-587, 592, 598, 611, 618-622, 718-719, 780, 887, 893, 1083
diabetes mellitus 151, 154, 180, 190-191, 294, 329, 375, 412, 415, 420, 435, 440, 443, 445, 449, 451-452, 454, 459, 488, 492, 518, 525, 552, 554, 557-558, 561-563, 568, 579, 584, 586, 598, 611, 718, 780, 887, 1083
diabetic
diabetic foot infection 579
diabetic foot lesions 93, 622
diabetic foot ulcer *VII*, 192, 545, 552-553, 555, 557-559, 561, 564-565, 575, 577-580, 582-586, 591-592, 595, 597, 604, 615, 618, 620-621, 841
diabetic foot wound 245, 502, 553
diabetic peripheral neuropathy 584, 587
diabetic ulcer 561, 738, 899
Diazepam (Valium®) 58, 142-143, 155, 337, 1013
diffuse
diffuse sclerosing 485, 487, 503, 506, 509, 511-513
diffuse sclerosing osteomyelitis 485, 503, 506, 509
diffusion distance 246-247, 252, 260, 262-263, 271, 273, 382, 492, 663-664, 997
digitalis 132, 148, 151
digoxin 132, 148
disseminated intravascular coagulopathy 407, 421, 899, 908
Disulfiram (Antabuse®) 56, 60, 132, 146-147, 152-153, 174, 186, 191-192, 194, 230
diver medical technician 118
diving VIII, IX, XI, XII, XIII, XIV, XVI, XVII, XXI, XXIII, 32, 54, 59, 61, 63-64, 66, 92-93, 116-118, 128, 153, 157, 168, 172, 177-178, 188, 195, 198, 202-203, 205-206, 210, 214, 218-219, 235, 271, 286-287, 292, 297, 316, 359-360, 363-364, 370-377, 456, 518, 520, 700, 702, 812, 830, 855-856, 858, 865, 971, 976-978, 980-982, 984, 986, 988, 990, 992-993, 997-998, 1002, 1005, 1007, 1009-1011, 1014-1015, 1017-1018, 1020, 1023-1025, 1029, 1033, 1037, 1046, 1048-1060, 1062-1063, 1065-1066, 1068-1084, 1088, 1091, 1096, 1098, 1101-1105, 1107, 1109-1111, 1115, 1117-1125, 1127-1128, 1130-1131, 1135-1138, 1141, 1147, 1151, 1169
DNA 143, 146, 330, 384, 386-387, 391, 393, 397, 399-400, 404, 411, 547, 695
documenting 86, 119, 594, 810
Donald 60
doxorubicin 132, 144, 157, 172-173, 182, 191-192, 196, 198, 230
draining wounds 410
dressings 248, 411, 422, 504, 531, 533, 549, 558, 580, 583, 586, 742, 793, 799, 806, 1159-1160, 1173
ductus arteriosus 221, 224-225, 1069
Duke University XX, XXIII, 114, 194, 313, 482
Dutch Royal Navy 113
Dutka 155, 370-371, 858, 941, 957
dynamic cortical deformation 931
dysrhythmias 71, 73, 163, 422

E

ear squeeze 161
edema 53, 63, 93, 149, 161-162, 167, 204, 206-208, 231, 237, 243, 246-249, 253, 260, 262, 264, 267-268, 271, 273, 275-276, 284, 292, 297, 311, 323, 330, 333, 364-366, 370-371, 375, 377, 382, 411-412, 416, 421-422, 429, 432, 441, 444, 447, 465, 472, 477, 482-483, 492-493, 506, 512-513, 535, 538, 542, 550, 614, 648, 651, 656, 661-665, 669-670, 677-678, 680-682, 688-689, 710, 791-794, 796, 800, 802, 804-805, 813-814, 817, 832, 849, 857, 859, 864, 867, 921, 932, 941-943, 947-950, 958, 967, 1057, 1061, 1068, 1076-1077, 1100
edema fluid 249, 271, 273, 681
edema reduction 237, 243, 246-249, 253, 267-268, 273, 333, 535, 538, 550, 669-670, 682, 793-794
effective percentage 147

Efuni 154, 156
ejection fraction 184, 191, 1164
electrical stimulation 630, 637
electrolyte 330, 416, 419-420, 422, 808, 1076, 1112-1113, 1160
electrolyte status 419-420, 422
emergency medical technician 118
Edgar End XI, 1079
endarteritis 779
endothelial cells 43, 305, 322, 355, 432, 558, 644, 647, 650-651, 703, 728, 797, 892, 898, 1022
endothelial nitric oxide synthase 396, 591
endothelial proliferation 733
endothelium 44, 266, 285-286, 305, 363, 365, 645-649, 655, 663, 666, 671, 727, 793, 804, 1062, 1173
endotracheal tube (ET) 70, 73, 87, 102, 418
enterobacter 384, 448, 469-470
envenomation 297, 678, 897, 899, 901-908
enzymatic debridement 532, 806
enzyme-linked immunosorbent assay 899, 908
enzymes 45, 47, 51-52, 135-137, 139, 147, 153-154, 385-386, 389-390, 399, 402, 496, 531, 644, 701, 727, 898-899, 901, 1001
epidural empyemas 467
epilepsy 142, 193-194, 197, 951, 1000, 1002, 1004-1007, 1010-1013, 1098
epinephrine 73, 224, 412, 427, 431, 690
equipment XI, 31-32, 42, 69-71, 81, 91, 93, 99-100, 104-107, 113, 116-118, 124, 134, 147, 172, 215, 221, 228-230, 233, 244, 303, 309, 454, 531, 566, 598, 911, 938, 977, 982-984, 1021, 1031, 1033-1037, 1039, 1041, 1047, 1051, 1053-1054, 1063, 1074-1076, 1088-1089, 1091, 1096, 1101-1102, 1109-1110, 1122-1123, 1127-1128, 1130
erythema 204, 504, 793, 900, 903
eschar formation 900, 1100
etiology 180, 211, 307, 325, 327-329, 359, 369, 433, 435, 438-439, 453, 460, 462, 502, 525, 561-562, 577, 682, 775, 878, 999, 1055, 1063, 1072, 1096
evidence-based indication 515, 684
excision 436, 444, 449-450, 455, 763, 765, 792, 806, 809, 814, 816, 901-902, 908
exposed bone 504, 513, 533, 673, 756-759
exposure to hyperbaric oxygen 135, 139, 156, 224, 232, 448, 720, 939, 1057
external compression 678

F

fascia 437, 441-445, 449-450, 664
fasciotomy 455, 651, 680-681, 686, 690
faster healing 593, 801
fat embolism 407, 422-423
fatalities 305, 316, 1059, 1070, 1085, 1099, 1101
feces 290
Feldmeier 194, 719, 787
femoral head necrosis 46-47, 273, 276, 863, 868, 876, 878-880
fetus 116, 174, 313-314, 318, 320, 1069-1070
fibroblast 44, 143, 278-279, 297, 447, 492-493, 496, 513, 520, 543, 563, 591, 630, 677, 689, 709, 734
fibroblast growth factor 44, 591, 734, 1155
fibroplasia 56, 173, 182, 234, 725, 727, 729, 732, 734, 738-739, 751, 764, 1057
fire 32-34, 36, 71, 73, 78, 90, 93, 99-100, 103-106, 109, 124, 128, 134, 230, 307, 791, 1055, 1077, 1148
fire hazard 103
fire suppression 104
flap 167, 250-251, 510, 519, 533, 545, 597, 633, 648, 650-652, 655-657, 669, 682, 690, 710-723, 739, 742, 763-764, 766, 768, 775, 808
flesh eating bacteria 461
fluid 85, 136, 154, 156, 161-162, 188-189, 193, 204-211, 239, 241, 248-249, 252, 262-263, 271, 273, 275-276, 278, 280, 289, 330, 340, 399, 403, 419-422, 470, 492, 506, 662-666, 669-670, 677-678, 680-682, 701, 793-794, 797, 800-801, 803-805, 808, 812, 890, 920, 930, 934-935, 937, 939-941, 956, 982, 984, 1001, 1060-1061, 1070, 1099, 1128
fluid and electrolyte 419, 422, 808
fluorescein dye 712-713
Foam dressings 583
foot ulcers VII, 150, 272, 294, 526, 528-530, 542, 549, 552-554, 557, 568, 571, 577-580, 582-586, 589, 591, 599, 601, 603, 605, 610, 618-622, 640
Fournier's gangrene 149, 285, 435-437, 444-446, 452-453, 457-463, 542
fractionation 727

free radical scavenger 648
free radicals 45, 136, 141, 144, 146-147, 149, 330, 386-388, 390-392, 399, 401, 631, 641, 644-645, 654-656, 688, 815, 857-858, 937, 940, 1007, 1056
functional status 489, 504
fungi 382, 390, 395, 439, 445, 885, 891, 1122
fungicidal activity 883-884
fungus 283, 883, 888
Fusobacteria 469-471

G

Gagnon 584
"gangrenous spot of Chile" 897
gas
  gas abscess 413
  gas embolism *VI*, 55, 79, 87, 213, 215, 217, 219, 230-231, 253, 255, 267, 270-271, 288, 361, 363-366, 368-377, 413, 423, 427, 429, 683, 828, 982, 1049, 1059, 1062, 1064, 1075, 1083-1084, 1101, 1103, 1154, 1156, 1173
  gas gangrene *VI*, 42, 70, 82, 87, 113, 142, 144, 230-231, 267, 272, 296, 388, 399, 407, 409-415, 417-418, 420, 422-432, 435, 442, 445-446, 448-449, 455-456, 459, 467, 480, 683, 889, 1157
    gas gangrene protocol 455
  gas supply 74, 76, 1054-1055, 1080, 1088, 1095-1096, 1100
    compressed gas 33, 292, 364, 1110
Gasthuis 113
gauze 74, 133, 531, 536, 550, 580
gentamicin 136, 138, 150, 155-156, 401, 403-404
Glasgow
  Glasgow Coma Scale (GCS) 700, 912-916, 920, 922, 924, 926-927, 930, 933-935, 942, 951, 958
  Glasgow Outcome Scale (GOS) 913, 915, 920, 933-936, 942, 951, 958
glass vials 133-134
Gloucestershire 437, 458
glucose oxidation quotient 920
glutathione 51, 224, 305, 316, 322, 386-388, 1000, 1011
  glutathione peroxidase 51, 386
glycerol 47, 547, 822, 935, 938, 940-941
Gorman 318, 372, 374
gradient of injury 661, 664-665, 675, 681-682
grading 529-530, 533, 542, 549-550, 553, 572, 577, 587, 592-593, 596, 600, 605, 622, 665, 676, 900
grafts VII, 230, 247, 252, 260, 264, 266, 276, 282, 533, 542, 545, 550, 595, 661, 681-682, 707, 709-710, 713-715, 717-722, 739, 767, 808, 814, 1157, 1170
  graft survival 710
granulocytes 294, 442
Greenbaum 59, 61, 832

H

Haldane 1076, 1128, 1130
Hampson 62, 193, 195, 218, 318-319, 372, 480, 519, 719, 723, 787
Hansen's disease VIII, 961, 963-964, 966-969
  leprosy 901, 963-964, 967, 969
hard tissue 774-775
Hart 91, 93, 127, 149, 153, 194, 218, 234, 293, 295-297, 371-372, 404, 427, 458, 480, 516-518, 521, 553, 593, 620, 622, 640, 687, 689, 695, 703, 715, 719-720, 774-775, 801, 805, 814, 816, 831, 856-857, 859, 939, 966
health care XIX, XXII, 32-33, 36, 125, 128, 518, 552, 584, 621, 687, 769, 787, 1031-1032, 1148
Heimbach 60, 217, 427, 480, 774, 813-814
helium 287, 354, 700, 976, 1055, 1057-1058, 1076, 1080, 1095-1096, 1109, 1122-1125, 1127, 1136-1137
hematocrits 418
hemiparesis 188, 365, 475, 887, 949, 1062
hemoglobin 107, 141, 226, 256, 258-259, 261, 264, 289, 303-304, 308, 312-314, 323, 381, 389, 534, 571, 585, 587, 693, 696-697, 700, 704, 865, 899, 917, 975, 997, 1055-1056, 1069
hemolysis 185, 411, 413, 420, 693, 897-901, 903, 908
hemolytic
  hemolytic bacteria 441
  hemolytic streptococcal gangrene 436-437, 443-445
hemostasis 416, 878
hemotympanum 161, 230, 651
Henry's law 237, 256, 262, 1049, 1052, 1062, 1109
Henshaw 709
heparin 132, 148-149, 156-157, 330, 337, 343, 368, 417, 421-422, 426, 432, 538, 859, 901, 956

high pressure nervous syndrome 1130
high-volume 74
histamine 330, 719, 793, 1073
histopathology 360, 377, 884
history of spontaneous pneumothorax 173, 180
hospital gangrene 436, 444, 459-460
host factors 285, 292, 493, 496, 509, 514, 542-543, 545, 670, 674
host-function 670
Hunt 47, 60, 93, 128, 217, 239, 276, 279, 294, 399-400, 427, 460-461, 480, 482, 494, 518-519, 540, 553, 686-687, 703-704, 720-722, 734, 774-775, 787, 814-816, 818, 969
hydration 366, 562, 990, 1023-1024, 1114
Hydrogel dressings 583, 586
hydrogen peroxide 51, 364, 369-370, 372, 374-376, 379, 386-388, 399, 401, 644, 798, 1000, 1114
hydroxyl radical (OH) 51, 321, 387, 396, 431, 644, 772, 964, 1099, 1111, 1117
hyperbaric
- *hyperbaric chamber* V, 4, 33-34, 36, 42, 67, 69, 81, 84, 90, 92-95, 97, 99-107, 113, 116-118, 125, 127-128, 147, 168, 203, 209, 218-219, 228, 230, 234, 255, 292, 418, 423, 429, 542, 719, 729, 808-809, 942-943, 986, 989, 1024, 1039, 1041, 1051, 1062-1063, 1080, 1098, 1127
- *hyperbaric environment* 92, 106, 207, 210, 805, 997, 1040, 1080, 1093
- *hyperbaric facility accreditation* 31-32, 35-38
- *hyperbaric medicine procedures* 93, 831
- *hyperbaric nurse clinician* 115, 119
- *hyperbaric nursing* V, 31, 111, 113, 115-116, 118-119, 125, 127-128
- *hyperbaric oxygen (HBO_2)* V, VI, VII, VIII, XI, XII, 4-5, 32, 34-35, 38-39, 41-49, 51-52, 55-56, 61-63, 69-70, 79, 93-95, 99, 106, 113-115, 117, 120, 124, 127-129, 131-140, 143-158, 169, 171-172, 183, 187, 193-198, 201-202, 205, 211-214, 217-219, 224-226, 230-232, 234-235, 237-239, 242-244, 249-255, 259-260, 264-265, 268, 272-273, 279, 281-285, 289-290, 292, 294-298, 301, 309-313, 316-323, 326, 336, 344, 346, 352-360, 366, 368-375, 377, 379, 381, 383, 385-386, 388-392, 395-405, 407, 409, 414-415, 418, 420-432, 438, 440, 447-449, 451-463, 465, 467, 480-483, 485, 487-488, 493-495, 497-498, 502-503, 506, 508-521, 523, 525-526, 530, 538-539, 552-553, 558, 580, 582, 584-585, 589, 591-592, 604-605, 610, 618-623, 625, 629, 631-632, 634-635, 637-641, 643-644, 647-648, 651, 654-659, 661, 668-669, 671-672, 674-676, 680-691, 693, 702-705, 707, 709-723, 725, 727, 729, 731-739, 742-746, 748, 750, 752, 754, 756-760, 763-765, 768-775, 777, 779-780, 785-787, 789, 791-792, 794, 796, 798-800, 802-806, 808-818, 826-828, 830-833, 835, 837, 839-840, 843, 849-850, 855-859, 861, 863, 867, 876-881, 883-884, 886-888, 890-892, 895, 897, 900, 902-903, 905-909, 911, 920-921, 930, 933, 939-944, 947, 949, 951-953, 955-959, 961, 963-964, 969, 997, 1010-1011, 1013-1014, 1034, 1045, 1057, 1097, 1114, 1121, 1131
- *hyperbaric oxygen (HBO_2) therapy* VII, VIII, 5, 32, 34-35, 38, 41, 43, 45-49, 51-52, 56, 61-63, 69, 93-95, 99, 114-115, 117, 120, 127-129, 144, 151-152, 154-158, 171-172, 193, 195-198, 201-202, 205, 211, 214, 217-219, 224-225, 230, 234-235, 237, 239, 251, 253, 268, 290, 296-298, 309-310, 312, 316, 318-319, 321, 323, 326, 336, 344, 346, 352-360, 366, 368-370, 372-375, 377, 397, 400-401, 404, 421-432, 451, 453-454, 457, 459-462, 480-483, 510, 512, 516-521, 530, 538, 552-553, 580, 584, 589, 591-592, 604-605, 610, 618-622, 625, 631, 639-640, 654-655, 657, 684-690, 703-705, 709-711, 713-723, 774-775, 787, 789, 791-792, 794, 796, 798, 803-806, 808-813, 815-818, 827-828, 830-832, 837, 839, 843, 849, 855-859, 863, 878-880, 886, 891, 895, 897, 902-903, 906-908, 939-940, 942-943, 949, 951-952, 955-959, 964, 969, 1013-1014, 1034, 1045
- *hyperbaric oxygen therapy training* 117
- *hyperbaric unit* XIV, 67, 70-72, 129, 145, 227

hypercapnia 141, 174, 185, 213, 403, 856, 1049, 1054-1056, 1061, 1071, 1093, 1096, 1107, 1118-1119, 1131
hypercarbia 86-87, 1085, 1087, 1091, 1093-1096, 1098-1099, 1101, 1118

hyperemia 210, 241, 307, 802, 864
hyperfractionation 727
hyperopia 212
hyperoxia 41, 45, 51-52, 56, 60-61, 133, 135-138, 141, 143, 145-146, 152, 154-156, 174, 181-182, 185, 195-196, 231, 255, 283, 296, 311, 366, 379, 381-383, 385-394, 396-397, 399-404, 545, 619, 621-622, 640, 649, 654, 675, 709, 813, 849, 856, 859, 930, 932, 937, 940, 942-943, 956, 998, 1010, 1085, 1087, 1092, 1096-1097, 1121, 1126
hyperoxic 51, 55, 59-61, 133, 135-136, 139, 146, 148-149, 154-156, 182, 185, 197-198, 211, 213, 217, 224, 282, 389, 391, 396, 399, 403, 654, 833, 849, 959, 989, 1057, 1107, 1113-1114, 1126, 1130-1131
hyperoxygenation 55, 237-238, 242, 251-253, 255-256, 259-262, 266-268, 270-273, 280, 292-293, 333, 336, 637, 668-670, 677, 681, 683, 716, 1115
hypocellular 728-729, 744, 779
hypokalemia 420
hypotension 86-87, 214, 297, 304, 307, 309, 328, 358, 365, 681, 689, 703, 808, 950
hypothermia 139, 227-228, 291, 294, 298, 520, 686, 688, 950, 982, 992, 1018, 1031, 1044-1045, 1055, 1071, 1076, 1080
hypoxia 41, 44, 56, 137, 156, 175, 214, 239, 246-247, 249, 251, 255, 260, 278, 283, 285, 289, 292, 304, 306, 308, 312, 316, 319, 321, 330, 365-366, 379, 381, 383-385, 391-394, 397, 399-400, 402, 404, 412, 438, 455, 491-493, 506, 508, 518, 521, 535, 538, 550-551, 563, 582, 591, 595, 597-599, 610, 615-617, 629, 637, 640, 650, 654, 657, 661-663, 665-666, 674, 678, 681-682, 697, 709, 713, 721, 754, 812, 848-849, 883-884, 888, 891, 902, 931, 941, 947, 950, 987, 1011, 1049, 1054-1056, 1058-1060, 1069, 1071, 1085, 1087, 1096-1097, 1107, 1113, 1122-1123, 1130
hypoxic 42, 45-46, 176, 182, 197, 226, 231, 237, 239, 247, 256, 260-261, 272, 276, 278-282, 284-285, 304-305, 319, 325, 328, 382, 384, 388, 391-392, 399, 411-412, 416, 438, 472, 491-493, 495-497, 505, 513, 547, 550, 595, 629, 663, 666, 675, 709, 711, 716, 728-729, 738, 744, 774, 779, 794, 799, 883, 888, 1059, 1069, 1096-1097, 1113, 1122-1123

I

idling neurons 952
ileus
incomplete 173, 303, 343, 351, 439, 598, 608, 915, 1055, 1119
mechanical 4, 33, 53, 71-72, 79, 87, 89-92, 100, 133, 183, 219, 225, 230, 330, 421, 500, 559, 564, 598, 639, 791, 805, 857-858, 950, 976, 986, 1051, 1062-1063, 1072, 1085, 1093, 1095-1097, 1099-1100, 1117, 1143
paralytic 82
immune-compromised 435, 449
immunosuppressive 435
implanted pacemakers
in vitro 45, 137, 145, 149-150, 153, 155, 278, 297, 382, 384-386, 388-392, 398-400, 404-405, 414, 417, 427-428, 432, 516, 518, 520, 639, 649-650, 689, 703, 710, 814, 881, 884, 1007
increased intracranial pressure 205, 482, 941, 950, 1067
indications VIII, 5, 31, 51, 53, 55, 117, 159, 163, 174-175, 184, 217, 221, 223, 230, 235, 254, 267-268, 298, 344, 346, 357, 366, 429, 465, 477, 488, 510, 515-516, 518, 521, 551-552, 603, 618-622, 625, 637-639, 661, 680, 682, 684, 687-688, 691, 696, 779, 811, 827, 837, 839-843, 848, 855, 858-859, 905, 947-948, 980, 1014
industry 303, 307, 976, 979, 1101, 1110, 1140-1141, 1143-1144, 1147-1148, 1150
inert gases 224, 271, 287, 856, 976, 1055, 1057, 1077, 1088, 1112, 1123, 1126, 1128, 1138
infected wounds 563
infection 34, 54, 162, 167, 173, 183, 186, 193, 205, 209, 231, 234, 237, 239-243, 247, 249, 252-253, 261-262, 267, 276, 278, 280, 282, 294, 296, 329, 359, 379, 381-383, 390, 393-394, 397-398, 401-402, 404, 409-416, 421, 424-432, 436-437, 441, 443, 448-450, 452-462, 474, 481, 483, 487-488, 491-493, 495, 497-515, 517, 519-521, 526, 529-530, 534-535, 538-540, 549, 552-553, 560, 562-563, 571-572, 575-576, 578-581,

585-587, 591-592, 596-597, 599-601, 603, 607, 610-611, 613, 615-616, 633, 662-663, 666, 668, 670, 675-678, 682, 686-687, 690, 693, 704, 710, 715, 717-718, 739, 742, 744-745, 754, 757, 789, 792-794, 798-800, 804, 806, 809-810, 883-892, 899, 901, 937, 963, 1066, 1141

infectious diseases VI, XXIV, 387, 395, 427, 429, 456-457, 460, 472, 520, 553, 585, 620, 775, 887, 891, 893

inflammation 43, 45, 180, 204, 209-211, 249, 311, 330, 393, 396, 439-440, 495, 540, 562, 571, 583-584, 644, 751, 755-757, 760, 792, 799, 804, 810, 818, 901-902, 920, 941, 952, 1005, 1007, 1009, 1071

infusion pumps 71, 73, 84, 91-92, 94, 97, 107, 131, 134, 230

inhalation injury 789, 791-792, 803-805, 808-809, 816, 1117

inside-chamber attendants 116

Institutional Review Board 1146

insulin 73-74, 86, 132, 144-145, 155, 157-158, 186, 190, 294, 420, 593-596, 598-599, 601, 636, 999-1000, 1009, 1071
- *insulin deficiency* 1071

interface 491-493, 513, 648, 746, 1075

interleukin 920, 935

International Congress 193-196, 295-296, 320, 355-356, 369, 397, 426, 480-482, 517, 620, 719, 814-816, 830-832

intoxication XII, 54-55, 57, 147, 151, 154-155, 194, 223, 316-318, 320-322, 410, 1006, 1168

intracranial
- *intracranial abscess VI*, 230, 290-291, 400, 465, 467, 469, 472, 476-478, 480-483
- *intracranial pressure (ICP)* 81-82, 162, 189, 205, 207, 365-366, 376, 472, 482, 911, 913, 915-917, 920-21, 934-935, 937-939, 941-943, 950-951, 958, 1067

intrapulmonary shunts 363

intravenous fluid 419-420, 678, 982

Invasive Fungal Infections VIII, 881, 883, 889-890, 892

irradiation 195, 709, 715, 722, 892, 949, 956
- *postoperative irradiation* 709

irrigation 164, 364, 369, 376, 416, 500-501, 757, 1100

ischemia-reperfusion injury (I-R injury) 641, 643-645, 647-655, 658, 674, 714, 798-799, 818

ischemic 41, 43-45, 237, 239, 244, 250, 266-267, 271, 273, 278-280, 290-291, 296-297, 307, 310, 312, 316, 329, 333, 366, 375, 377, 383, 385, 388, 411, 493, 497, 574, 581, 595, 610-611, 618, 622, 644, 646, 648-651, 654, 656-657, 662, 666, 671, 678, 680-681, 687, 689-690, 695-696, 703, 710, 712, 714, 719, 722, 793, 799, 804, 810, 818, 826, 828, 830, 837, 844, 848-852, 854, 856-858, 866-867, 876, 879, 900, 902, 918, 932, 934, 942-943, 947-950, 954-955, 957-959, 1014, 1072, 1076

IV
- *IV line* 74, 82, 84-86, 309
- *IV solutions* 74, 83

J

Jacobson 115, 129, 154, 427, 482-483

James 704, 957, 1143, 1151

Japan 340, 359, 468, 814, 817, 1083

jaw 205, 488, 738-739, 744, 746, 751, 754, 761, 764, 774, 878

Journal of Hyperbaric Medicine 467

K

ketoacidosis 420, 885, 887, 999

kinins 793

L

lactate 44, 47, 308, 317, 629, 694, 696-697, 709, 734, 800, 815, 913, 917, 919-920, 931, 934-935, 940, 1003, 1009

Lanphier 376, 1083, 1104

laparotomy 1075

latency 140, 142-143, 154, 328, 542, 931, 1002-1003, 1005, 1007, 1010, 1098

learning disabilities 951

Lee XI, 59, 62, 151, 196-197, 217, 297, 317, 319, 354, 356-357, 373, 376, 656, 774, 787, 812-813, 815, 830, 879, 941, 957, 1014, 1105

left ventricular ejection fraction 184, 1164

lesions 43, 46, 93, 148, 191-192, 308, 319, 392, 412, 439, 461, 472, 561, 563, 572, 622, 863, 876, 889, 898, 900, 902-903, 916, 934, 940, 967, 1072, 1124

lethargy 188, 310, 1078, 1107, 1114, 1118

leukemia 350, 865, 887, 889, 893
leukocyte microbial killing 472, 687, 695
leukocytes 294, 305, 322, 365, 387, 399, 410, 438, 518, 644-646, 648-649, 654, 710, 793, 800, 814, 1022
lidocaine 73, 132, 138, 148, 152, 155, 157, 330, 367, 374, 377, 383, 822
lipid peroxidation 51-52, 59, 156, 305, 322, 387, 644, 649, 657, 666, 670, 690, 695, 704, 772, 798, 805, 849, 937-939, 957, 1114
liquid oxygen 72
logistical 169, 172, 223, 226-227, 973, 976, 979, 982-983, 986, 988, 1034, 1039, 1044
Lorazepam (Ativan®) 143
Lutheran General Hospital 114
lymphocytes 62, 393, 396, 400, 899

M

macrophage 155, 187, 281, 387-388, 392-393, 397, 402-404, 442, 513, 627, 703, 733-734, 774, 779, 792-793, 804, 883, 892-893, 937, 940, 1071
Mader 153-154, 193, 373, 396-399, 401, 404, 445, 447, 450-451, 460, 481, 488, 494-497, 501, 506, 511, 516-517, 519, 710, 721, 799, 815, 891-892, 939
mafenide acetate (Sulfamylon®) 131, 140, 174, 186, 196, 198, 230, 448, 458, 808
magnetic resonance imaging (MRI) 308, 317-318, 351, 440-441, 456, 458, 478, 493, 563, 569, 571, 579, 614-616, 848, 865-866, 877, 880, 890, 925, 930, 949-950, 953, 957, 1131, 1140
magnetic resonance study 506
malnutrition 445, 529, 535-536, 780
mandibular reconstruction 738, 774
mandibulotomy 755
Manson 655-656, 712, 721
Mazzone 157
mechanical breath 89
mediastinal emphysema 288, 365, 1049, 1063-1064
medical management 184, 240, 243, 249, 253, 523, 534-535, 538, 549, 552, 672, 683-684, 781, 866-867
Medicare 32, 35, 125, 252, 254, 276, 296, 510-511, 519, 545, 548-550, 553, 557, 585, 595, 621, 625, 684-685, 688
Meijne 47, 429, 686, 688, 969
Meleney
  Meleney's gangrene 436
  Meleney's ulcer 285, 436-437, 443-444
mental retardation 951
metabolic acidosis 308, 312, 793
metabolic conditions 387
methicillin resistant
  staphylococcus aureus (MRSA) 45, 149, 155, 392, 401-402, 436, 441, 445, 494-495, 497, 505, 514, 519-520
methylene blue 211, 964, 966, 968-969
metronidazole 385, 394-395, 401, 404, 417, 431, 447, 450, 478, 481
microaerophilic streptococci 469
microarterioles 647-648
microcirculation VII, 237, 247, 249-250, 262, 264-265, 273, 287, 290, 296, 491, 593, 641, 643-645, 647-648, 650-653, 656-657, 662, 664, 666, 668, 670, 677-678, 682-683, 690, 709, 793, 798, 800, 812, 818, 831, 864, 877
midazolam 74, 135, 143, 152
middle ear 161-163, 165, 168, 202-206, 217-218, 230, 786, 1060, 1065-1067, 1075, 1120, 1125, 1130
  middle-ear barotrauma 148, 163, 199, 202, 204-207, 226, 253, 982, 1049, 1065-1067, 1072
  middle-ear equalization 221, 229
minimal bactericidal concentrations (MBC) 45, 384
Minimal inhibitory concentrations (MIC) 45, 150, 384
mitochondria 51, 276, 304, 381, 387, 390, 404, 921, 932, 1010
  mitochondrial dysfunction 304-305, 920, 942
mobility 248, 514, 561, 612, 898, 1005
moist wound healing 193, 581
monocytes 45, 382, 402
monofilament 564-565, 584
monooxygenases 52, 60
monoplace chamber 55, 67, 69-72, 74, 77-84, 86-87, 89-94, 117, 216, 228-229, 367, 372, 428, 449, 454-455, 936-937, 940, 943
morbilliform rash 900
mortality 93, 141, 144, 146, 174, 194, 218, 290, 297, 303, 307, 310-312, 318, 320, 388-389, 391-392, 396, 404, 409, 414, 417, 425, 435-436, 445-446, 448-455, 458, 461, 465, 467-468, 475-476, 478, 480, 483, 500, 557, 577, 580-581, 583, 618, 695, 703, 715, 717, 791-792, 794, 799-802, 804-805, 809-810, 816, 848, 850, 852, 883, 886-888, 890-891,

904, 911, 915, 934-936, 938, 943, 950-951, 998, 1035, 1042, 1060, 1065, 1071, 1074, 1100-1101
mottling of the tongue 365
Mount Sinai Hospital 115
mucorales 390, 395, 885
mucormycosis 390, 397-398, 402, 881, 883, 885-887, 889-893, 1169
multibacillary 963, 968-969
multiplace chambers 99, 102, 117, 214-215, 227-228, 271, 937
multiplace hyperbaric facility 114, 118
multiple sclerosis 173, 180, 191, 196-197, 273, 276, 291, 350, 843, 856, 858, 945, 952, 954-959
mycobacterium (Leprae) 963-964, 966, 968-969
myelin 52, 1007
Myers 157, 198, 235, 298, 315, 320-321, 369, 401-402, 458, 462, 520, 656, 688, 719, 721-723, 892, 907
myocardial
myocardial infarct size 295, 690, 817
myocardial infarction 44, 47, 295-296, 307, 318, 322, 372, 375, 689, 816, 1063-1064, 1153
myocardial irritability 407, 417, 422
myocardium 304, 307-308, 383, 696, 799, 1070
myocutaneous flap 763, 775, 808
myoglobin 304
myopia 55, 59, 61, 181, 199, 211-212, 217, 219, 224, 1057, 1107, 1114-1115, 1130-1131
myringotomy VI, 159, 161, 163, 165-167, 183, 206, 230, 651, 915, 937

N

necrosis VIII, 46-47, 74, 209, 230, 273, 276, 278, 284, 297, 305, 308, 313, 330, 392, 402, 410-412, 416, 431, 437, 439, 441-446, 449-450, 635-636, 643-644, 647-648, 657, 662, 689, 711-714, 716-717, 719-722, 738, 746, 755, 765-766, 774, 777, 779-781, 784-787, 793-794, 800, 810, 821, 861, 863-864, 866-868, 876-880, 883, 887-889, 900-902, 905, 932, 941, 945, 949-950, 954, 956-959, 1061, 1072, 1082, 1100, 1103, 1117
necrotic wounds 786, 897
necrotizing
necrotizing enterocolitis 225
necrotizing fasciitis 72, 82, 87, 89, 144, 149, 227, 231, 234, 288, 433, 435-440, 443-446, 448, 450-452, 454, 456-463, 542, 545, 550, 841, 889
necrotizing infections 113, 226, 282, 457, 459, 716, 885
soft tissue infections 234, 456-463
negative pressure wound therapy (NWPT) 580
neonate 174, 369, 1010
neuroinflammation 231, 932, 938
neurologic
neurologic presentation 311
neurologic sequelae 213, 310, 317, 1158
neurological decompression illness 157, 369
neuronal shrinkage 948
neutrophil 43-44, 48, 231, 266, 280-282, 285-286, 294, 296, 298, 316, 375, 398, 442, 491, 495-496, 543, 564, 582, 644-651, 653-658, 690, 704, 798, 812, 817, 907, 955-956
neutrophil adhesion 644-645, 647, 650, 655-656, 798
neutrophil oxidative killing 280-282, 491, 496, 543
neutrophil-endothelial adhesion 645, 649, 658, 818
NFPA
NFPA code 134
NFPA guidelines 125
nicotinamide adenine dinucleotide 386
nitrogen 41-43, 105, 137, 142, 150, 224, 271, 287, 366, 419, 439, 535, 558, 563, 704, 846-847, 899, 976, 987-988, 999, 1006, 1021, 1049, 1055, 1057-1058, 1070, 1073, 1079-1080, 1098-1099, 1119, 1123-1125, 1127-1128, 1130, 1136
nitrogen narcosis 287, 1006, 1049, 1055, 1057, 1073, 1098-1099, 1119, 1123, 1136
Nohl 1079-1080
no-reflow phenomenon 149, 285
non-clostridial myonecrosis 455
non-healing wounds 775
non-traumatic osteonecrosis 879
normoxia 57, 145-146, 231, 381, 385-386, 389, 391, 393-394, 999
nurse 32, 34, 36, 70, 113-116, 118-120, 124-125, 127-128, 227
Nurse Practice Act 116
nurse practitioners 70, 125, 546-547
operating room nurse 113-114
registered nurse 114-115, 118

nursing
nursing diagnosis 120
nursing interventions 119-120
nutritional 86, 447, 571, 809, 849, 858, 995, 999, 1001-1003, 1005-1007, 1009

O

occlusion VII, 84, 178, 249, 264-265, 268, 328, 425, 593, 595, 678, 750, 793, 819, 821, 827, 830-833, 849, 856, 859, 864, 886, 947, 955, 959, 1065
oligodendroglia 321
omni-vent 90, 92-93
open-heart surgery 113, 294, 376, 688
operating-room nurses 113-114
optic neuritis 173, 180-181, 191-192, 194, 197, 826
osseointegration 746, 750-751
osteoblast 45, 47, 281, 493, 627, 630, 751, 878
osteoclast 45-47, 281-282, 493, 497, 509, 512-513, 629-630, 635, 866, 868, 876, 878
osteoclast activity 629, 866
osteoclast stimulation 512
osteointegrated prostheses 746
osteomyelitis VII, 54, 149, 155, 167, 181, 191, 230, 252, 280-282, 382, 384-385, 389, 392-393, 401-402, 465, 470-472, 481, 485, 487-489, 491-492, 494-506, 508-510, 512, 515-521, 528, 542, 545, 549-550, 563, 569-572, 579, 582-587, 600, 607, 610, 612-614, 616-617, 632, 635, 637, 640, 687, 710, 716, 721, 774, 815
osteoradionecrosis 191, 280, 517-519, 612, 621, 635, 715-718, 721, 723, 725, 738, 744, 746-748, 750-751, 754-756, 758-760, 764-765, 768-771, 773-775, 787
Stage I osteoradionecrosis 758
Stage III osteoradionecrosis 758-759
otic barotrauma 172, 191, 199, 201, 204-205, 207, 209, 226, 809
oxidative
oxidative burst 44, 382, 491
oxidative damage 56, 384, 391, 403, 892
oxidative stress 42, 44, 46, 48, 52, 62-63, 198, 305, 322, 389, 391, 397, 399, 403-404, 621, 650, 657, 800, 805, 813, 849, 937, 939, 999-1000, 1005, 1007, 1009-1010, 1012-1013, 1114
oxygen V, VI, VII, VIII, XI, XII, 4-5, 32, 34-35, 38-39, 41-49, 51-66, 69-70, 72, 79, 81, 90, 92-95, 99, 102-107, 113-115, 117-118, 120, 124, 127-129, 131-158, 169, 171-173, 175, 180-183, 185-187, 193-198, 201-202, 205, 211-219, 221, 223-226, 230-235, 237-244, 246-247, 249-273, 275-276, 278-285, 287, 289-292, 294-298, 301, 304-305, 309-314, 316-323, 326, 333, 336, 344, 346, 352-360, 364, 366-375, 377, 379-405, 407, 409-410, 414-416, 418-432, 438, 440, 447-463, 465, 467, 472, 474, 480-483, 485, 487-488, 491-498, 502-503, 506, 508-521, 523, 525-526, 530, 538-542, 550, 552-553, 558, 563-564, 568, 580, 582, 584-586, 589, 591-592, 594, 596, 598-601, 603-605, 610, 618-623, 625-632, 634-635, 637-641, 643-645, 647-648, 651, 654-659, 661-666, 668-677, 680-691, 693-697, 699, 701-705, 707, 709-723, 725, 727, 729-739, 742-746, 748, 750, 752, 754, 756-760, 763-765, 768-775, 777, 779-781, 785-787, 789, 791-794, 796, 798-800, 802-806, 808-818, 821, 826-833, 835, 837, 839-841, 843, 846-847, 849-850, 852-859, 861, 863-864, 867, 876-881, 883-884, 886-892, 895, 897, 900-903, 905-909, 911, 920-921, 930, 933-934, 936-944, 947-949, 951-953, 955-959, 961, 963-964, 966, 968-969, 973, 975-978, 980, 982-990, 992, 995, 997-1000, 1005-1014, 1019, 1021, 1023-1024, 1032, 1034, 1045-1046, 1049-1050, 1053-1062, 1064, 1066, 1068-1070, 1072, 1075-1079, 1082, 1084, 1087-1093, 1095-1099, 1101, 1103-1105, 1107, 1109-1114, 1116, 1120-1127, 1130-1131, 1136, 1143
as a drug 131, 133, 394, 840
oxygen exposure 51, 53, 56, 58-60, 64, 92-93, 137, 154, 183, 197, 224-225, 231, 253, 295, 393, 399, 517-518, 808, 1098, 1120
oxygen gradient 276, 382, 396, 591, 714, 721, 734-735, 738, 779
shallow 734-735, 779
steep 735, 738, 779
oxygen poisoning 49, 51-53, 55, 60, 66
oxygen tension 42, 58, 81, 94, 154, 225, 239, 262-264, 276, 280, 294, 379, 381, 391, 396, 398-400, 404, 420, 472, 492, 494-495, 497, 517-518,

552, 619, 630, 639-640, 694-695, 709-712, 716, 722-723, 734-735, 774, 794, 799, 814, 879, 892, 921, 964, 1011
oxygen tolerance 49, 56-57, 59-60, 62, 64, 66, 93, 181, 1121
oxygen toxicity *V, VIII*, 42, 49, 51-56, 59-62, 64, 66, 92, 131, 139-143, 146-147, 151, 153-157, 172-173, 180, 185-186, 193-194, 212-213, 215, 217-219, 223-226, 232, 235, 253, 261, 270-271, 292, 396-397, 419-421, 474, 631, 686, 697, 704, 804, 808, 828, 856, 889, 909, 936, 938, 941-943, 973, 982, 984-985, 989-990, 995, 997-998, 1007, 1010-1011, 1013, 1049, 1056-1057, 1069, 1082, 1084, 1092, 1097-1098, 1101, 1103, 1107, 1112, 1120-1121, 1123, 1126-1127, 1131
oxygen treatment *VI, VIII*, 47, 62, 144, 147, 153-154, 158, 169, 171, 197, 213, 215-216, 218, 234, 269, 295, 309, 311-312, 316, 318, 320, 360, 369, 374, 407, 418, 420-421, 425, 429-430, 463, 498, 510, 517-518, 521, 655, 674, 688, 714, 722-723, 733, 787, 796, 800, 803, 812, 814-815, 830-833, 858, 861, 863, 876, 902, 920, 930, 942-943, 957-959
oxygen-derived free radicals 401, 644, 688, 815
oxyhemoglobin 304, 313
oxyhemoglobin dissociation 304
oxyradicals 644
ozório de almeida 964

P

pain 82, 116, 143, 158, 161, 163-166, 181, 202-206, 208-211, 214, 218, 224, 228, 230-231, 243, 253, 333, 349, 369, 412, 414, 416, 429, 440, 444, 502, 508, 514, 518, 529, 542, 559, 564, 567, 603, 611, 631, 678, 680, 698, 781, 789, 792, 803, 810, 817, 848, 858-859, 865-867, 877, 897, 900-901, 907, 976, 985-986, 989, 1064-1066, 1068, 1074, 1079-1081, 1084, 1100, 1107, 1117, 1127-1129, 1131
parasites 389, 395, 397, 402, 446
partial pressures 41, 58, 64, 70, 136, 174, 225, 255, 267, 304, 312, 381, 420, 629, 657, 716, 884, 891, 978, 997, 1007, 1052, 1054-1055, 1066, 1077, 1087-1088, 1090, 1093, 1097, 1120, 1123, 1130
patent foramen ovale (PFO) 364, 376-377, 411, 987, 1069, 1083
pathologic fracture 757, 759
patient
patient care standards 120, 128
patient education 34, 123, 226, 351, 550
patient evaluation 209
patient's fluid status 419
patient's goals 253
pediatric VI, XX, XXI, 116, 125, 221, 223-224, 226-227, 229-235, 319, 327, 342, 359, 457, 473, 791, 950, 957, 999, 1084
pediatric advanced life support 116, 125, 229
pedicle flap 721
pelvic radiation 780, 787
penumbra 291, 849, 858, 932, 943, 947
peptostreptococci 437, 469
perfringolysin 411, 424
perfusion 135, 138-139, 231, 237, 239-245, 249-250, 252-253, 260, 264-265, 267, 273, 275, 278, 280, 285, 304, 307-308, 329, 382-383, 416, 421, 431, 491-494, 510, 523, 530-531, 535, 538-543, 549-551, 558, 562, 568-569, 572, 575, 582-583, 586, 600, 602, 605, 611, 614, 616, 625, 628, 635-637, 640, 643, 648, 656, 663-665, 670, 675, 677-678, 680-682, 710-714, 716-718, 728, 733-735, 821, 920, 937, 941, 947-949, 975, 982, 1061
perifocal
perifocal brain swelling 472
perifocal edema 472, 477
peripheral
peripheral arterial disease 557, 562-563, 565-566, 584, 586, 611, 670
peripheral vascular disease 409, 430, 435, 525, 689
periwound $TcPO_2$ 599
Perrins 498-499, 517, 520-521, 671, 688, 714, 722-723, 798, 816, 957
phagocytes 294, 389, 396, 495, 582, 883, 1022
phagocytosis 44-45, 294, 379, 382, 392, 403, 411, 794, 888, 891
Phenothiazines 132, 141, 149
Phenytoin (Dilantin®) 132, 136, 142, 151, 157

physical
  physical requirements 116
  physical therapy 532
physiology XV, XVI, XX, XXI, 5, 59, 61, 63, 70, 82, 91-92, 95, 118, 172, 176, 193-194, 196-197, 217, 219, 226, 237, 251, 256, 259, 262, 272, 275, 294-295, 371, 518, 552, 563, 623, 625, 690, 832, 856, 1070-1071, 1075, 1080, 1082-1084, 1102-1105, 1130, 1136
plasma 41, 107, 141, 145, 226, 252-253, 256-257, 259-260, 262-267, 271, 295, 335, 337, 365, 367, 369, 387, 418, 422, 637, 663-664, 668-669, 693-694, 697, 702, 704, 799, 804, 818, 997, 1062
platelets 264, 305, 410, 418, 421-422, 793, 899
plethysmography 179, 183
pmn 392, 650, 656, 898-899, 901
pneumonia 175, 214, 363, 370, 389, 391, 397, 400, 402, 404, 451, 791-792, 816, 941, 1061
pneumothorax 82, 171-173, 177, 180, 193, 195, 199, 213-219, 226, 230, 253, 367, 780, 981, 983, 1043, 1049, 1059, 1063-1064, 1075, 1153, 1161
  tension pneumothorax 171, 177, 213-219, 367, 1043, 1064
  untreated pneumothorax 177, 230, 1153
Pol 426, 428, 1084
polymicrobial sepsis 290, 297, 389, 404
polymorphonuclear
  polymorphonuclear cells 798
  polymorphonuclear leukocyte 371, 403, 495, 654, 794, 799
positive end expiration pressure (PEEP) 72, 79, 81, 87, 89-90, 107, 420-421, 423, 937, 1061
positron emission tomography (PET) 308, 317, 925, 930, 939-940, 949
potassium 148, 320, 328, 331, 420, 793, 950, 1002, 1004, 1112, 1115
prealbumin 536, 571, 582-583
pregnancy 116, 174-175, 194, 197, 225, 231, 253, 301, 308, 313-314, 318-319, 369, 372, 832, 901, 905, 1050, 1069-1070
pressure V, XI, 33, 36, 41-43, 45-48, 53, 55-56, 58-59, 61, 65, 70-72, 74, 76, 78-85, 87-90, 92-95, 99-109, 113-114, 127-129, 131, 133-134, 136-137, 139, 142-147, 149, 151-154, 156, 159, 161-164, 167, 171, 173, 176-178, 183-184, 188-189, 192-194, 196-198, 201, 203-213, 215-216, 218-219, 224-225, 229-230, 235, 247, 251-252, 255-257, 259, 262-263, 266-268, 270-271, 273, 275, 292, 295, 304-306, 309-310, 320-322, 328, 336, 340, 350, 356-357, 363-366, 369-370, 372, 374-376, 381, 385, 390-391, 398-401, 418-420, 422, 425, 428-429, 472, 474, 478, 480, 482, 493, 495, 501, 525, 528-529, 534, 548, 552-553, 559-561, 564, 566-570, 578, 582-583, 586-587, 592, 596, 600, 616, 621, 629, 648, 655, 662-665, 668, 670, 678, 680-681, 686-690, 694, 697-698, 703, 709-711, 717, 720, 729, 733, 781, 793-794, 796, 803, 808, 815, 828, 832, 846-847, 849, 856-857, 864-867, 877, 879, 884, 887-888, 911, 919-920, 930-931, 935, 937, 939-943, 948, 950, 952, 956, 958, 964, 966, 969, 975-976, 980, 982-983, 987, 997-998, 1006, 1009, 1014-1015, 1017-1019, 1021-1024, 1031-1032, 1035, 1046, 1051-1056, 1058-1070, 1072, 1075-1081, 1083, 1087-1096, 1099, 1104-1105, 1110-1114, 1118-1120, 1123-1125, 1127-1128, 1130, 1137, 1141
  pressure equalization tubes 159, 167, 206-207
  pressure ulcer 529, 553
preterm infants 224
progressive bacterial gangrene 433, 437-441, 443, 448-449, 454
propranolol 52, 61, 131, 141, 156-157
proteins 45, 51-52, 62, 136, 249, 264, 386-388, 898, 932, 943, 999, 1001, 1022, 1055, 1072, 1117, 1140-1141
proteus 392, 441, 448
protozoa 379, 382, 389
pulmonary
  pulmonary barotrauma 89, 179, 192, 199, 201, 213, 215, 363, 365, 367, 373-374, 1049, 1063-1065, 1083
  pulmonary edema 53, 63, 149, 271, 297, 311, 323, 364-366, 370-371, 377, 421, 1061, 1077
  pulmonary intoxication 54-55, 57
  pulmonary oxygen toxicity 49, 53-55, 59-61, 64, 66, 140-141, 146, 153, 156, 224-225, 253, 420-421, 697, 941, 943, 989-990, 997, 1057, 1082, 1107, 1120-1121, 1131
  pulmonary toxicity 49, 59, 64, 66, 146, 183, 186-187, 194-195, 197-198, 226, 389, 1056

purpura fulminans 231, 260, 542, 636, 899

Q

qualifications for hyperbaric nurses 116

R

radiated tissue 715, 725, 729, 731-736, 739, 741, 744, 746, 749, 757
radiation VII, XIV, 33, 42, 163, 175-176, 190-191, 194, 196, 205, 211, 230, 247, 252-253, 272, 280, 282, 542, 635, 709, 712, 714-717, 719-721, 725, 727-728, 734, 738-739, 744, 746, 751-752, 754-757, 765-766, 769-770, 773-775, 777, 779-781, 784-787, 865, 949, 956-959, 1044, 1047, 1075, 1140
radiation cystitis 190, 777, 781, 785-787
radiation damage 247, 746, 755
radiation dose 727, 734, 754-755, 1044
radiation injury *VII*, 175, 196, 230, 252, 272, 280, 282, 716, 725, 727, 734, 738, 755-756, 777, 780-781, 949
radiation necrosis 719, 765-766, 774, 777, 781, 786-787, 949, 956-959
radiation proctitis 777, 780, 785-787
radiation therapy 42, 175-176, 190-191, 194, 211, 253, 709, 714-715, 717, 721, 744, 751, 773, 779, 785, 958, 1140
radiation tissue injury 715-716, 719, 757, 786-787
radiation-induced necrosis 958
radionecrosis 54, 144, 167, 192, 716, 719, 727, 744, 774, 786, 956, 997
random flaps 713-714, 722
reactive oxygen species 43, 51-52, 61, 285, 305, 311, 388-389, 391, 400-402, 558, 670-671, 703, 710, 798, 1012, 1056
recompression 41, 215, 217, 366-367, 370, 374, 632, 840, 976, 986-990, 992-993, 1018, 1020, 1022-1025, 1029, 1044-1048, 1062-1064, 1079, 1120, 1125, 1127, 1129-1131
redox 47, 273, 297, 319, 382, 384-385, 395, 399, 621, 813, 921, 930, 935, 1001, 1006
reduced host defense 440
refractory osteomyelitis in a compromised host 506
registered nurses 114-115, 118
Reinisch 710, 722
reperfusion 44, 46-47, 238, 260-261, 264-268, 285-286, 290, 296, 298, 333, 531, 568, 643-651, 653-657, 666, 671, 677, 682-683, 686, 690, 695, 713, 793, 798-800, 817-818, 849, 948, 957
reperfusion injury 238, 260-261, 264-268, 285-286, 290, 298, 333, 643-644, 649, 651, 654-657, 666, 671, 677, 683, 690, 695, 798-800
research protocols 124, 604
respiratory
respiratory manifestations ("*chokes*") 364, 981
respiratory therapists 36, 70, 114-115
retinopathy of prematurity 173, 182, 195, 197, 221, 224-225, 234, 1057
retrolental fibroplasia 56, 173, 182, 234, 1057
revascularization 47, 237, 243-246, 249-252, 286, 295, 538, 550, 578, 587, 593, 595, 597, 603, 613, 629, 652, 674, 714, 721, 727, 733, 735, 814, 818, 864, 876
rhabdomyolysis 308, 687, 1061, 1075-1076
rhino-orbital-cerebral mucormycosis 885, 893
risks VI, 70, 79, 91, 93, 119, 133, 140, 146-147, 169, 171, 173-174, 178, 184, 187, 190-191, 221, 223, 226, 230, 251, 270, 292, 351, 545, 608, 774, 842, 846, 901, 949, 976, 980-981, 987, 990-991, 999, 1019, 1032, 1055, 1059, 1070, 1073, 1075, 1081, 1095, 1122, 1145
RNA 137, 386, 393, 695

S

saline 56, 62, 70, 74, 78-79, 94, 134, 418, 700, 950
saturation XVII, 55, 81, 107, 313, 542, 698, 700, 986, 1024, 1046, 1050, 1058, 1062, 1072, 1079-1081, 1083, 1120, 1124-1125, 1137-1139
saturation diving XVII, 986, 1050, 1072, 1079-1080, 1083, 1120, 1137
Saucerization 509
scar tissue 243, 249, 278, 492, 547, 668
scrotal gangrene 435, 444
scrubber 988, 1024, 1053, 1085, 1087-1091, 1093, 1095, 1099, 1111, 1116-1119, 1123, 1138
Sechrist 73-74, 76-78, 80-81, 86-88, 94, 943
sedation 82, 87, 89, 143, 221, 228-230, 234, 981, 1073

seizure 57-58, 62-63, 82, 116, 140-143, 149, 151, 174, 184-185, 188, 191, 194, 212-213, 218-219, 224, 253, 311-312, 321, 981, 983-985, 989, 998-1005, 1007, 1011, 1013-1014, 1097-1098, 1126-1127, 1131
seizure disorders 58, 185, 311, 1000-1001
selenium 51, 1004
sepsis 225, 273, 278, 282, 284-285, 289-290, 296-297, 330, 383, 389, 399, 404, 445, 456, 461, 494, 505, 545, 549, 663, 666, 687, 689, 792, 794, 799, 801, 812, 1168, 1173
sequestra 492, 495, 505
serotonin 149, 153, 647, 655, 1058
Severinghaus 147, 156
Sharp 42, 47, 165, 210-211, 322, 381, 435, 439, 531-532, 547, 550, 863, 877, 900, 1128
shunts 173, 184, 241, 363-364, 594, 710, 718, 1164
side effects VI, 46, 53, 55, 60, 62, 172, 182-183, 199, 201, 217, 219, 226, 253, 271, 292, 321, 332, 352, 422, 449, 474, 693, 786, 944, 963, 999, 1004, 1010, 1073-1074
single photon emission computed tomography (SPECT) 308, 310, 318, 320, 506, 844, 847-848, 857-858, 925, 930, 949, 952
sinus squeeze 208, 1068, 1070
skeletal
skeletal muscle 44, 47, 241, 285, 296-297, 410, 459, 644-645, 647-658, 678, 688-690, 798-799, 818
skeletal muscle-compartment syndrome 275, 493, 659, 664, 678, 684-685, 689
skin
skin flap 648, 652, 656-657, 669, 690, 710-711, 713-715, 717-719, 722-723
skin flap survival 648, 656-657, 669, 690, 711, 713, 715, 723
skin graft 502, 682, 714-715, 717
skin grafting 247, 549, 580, 710, 901-903
skin grafts and flaps *VII*, 533, 707, 709
skin lesions 902, 1124
skin substitute 580
skin-necrotizing factor 898
Smith 42, 47, 153, 157, 215-217, 295-296, 318-319, 322, 369, 373, 375, 397, 401-402, 428, 430, 436-437, 450, 461, 519, 552, 584, 686-687, 689, 723, 775, 787, 832, 858-859, 878, 892, 955, 1010, 1013, 1084, 1120
smoke inhalation 231, 273, 303, 306, 309, 804
smoking 162, 253, 303, 323, 329, 341, 535, 546, 597, 636, 714, 770, 877, 1047
soft tissue VI, 230, 234, 252, 413-414, 456-463, 501, 542, 570, 626, 636, 673, 675, 716-717, 722-723, 727, 739, 746, 759, 762-763, 787
soft tissue infections VI, 234, 456-463
aerobic soft tissue infections 460
anaerobic soft tissue infections VI, 459
mixed bacterial floras 435
somatosensory evoked potentials (SEP) 47-48, 94, 154-155, 168, 354-356, 358, 397-401, 403-404, 426, 481, 722, 775, 833, 957, 1048, 1083-1084, 1103, 1130, 1149
spasticity 951-952
St. Luke's Hospital XI, XII, 780, 785
staging 204, 311, 765, 773, 800, 1042
standard therapy 332, 392, 451, 476, 478
staphylococci 398, 403, 405, 438, 445, 448, 469
static lung loading (SLL) 1085, 1089, 1092-1093, 1095-1096, 1099, 1105
steroids 52, 140, 142, 178, 325, 330-332, 335, 337-343, 347, 349, 351-352, 354-356, 358-360, 477, 514, 535, 635, 698, 822, 866, 879, 901, 903, 942, 950, 953, 1100, 1117
stillborn 314
stoichiometric relationship 51
streptococcal infections 438-439, 446-447, 456-457, 460, 462
streptococci 397, 413, 436-437, 439, 441, 445-448, 450, 455, 458, 469-471, 473, 1165
anaerobic streptococci 446
microaerophilic streptococci 469, 1165
streptococcus gangrene 436, 460
stroke 291, 296, 329, 350, 357, 364-365, 370-372, 374-375, 557-558, 596, 612, 653, 655-656, 793, 817, 826, 828-829, 833, 837, 843-844, 846, 848-854, 856-859, 941, 945, 947-949, 951-952, 954-955, 957-958, 1007, 1014, 1063-1064, 1073, 1076
subcutaneous emphysema 365, 1049, 1063-1064
subdural empyema 469, 471, 480, 482
suction 71, 73-74, 76, 89, 91, 94, 435, 462, 500

suction apparatus 71, 94
superoxide
superoxide anion 305, 386-388, 396, 1000
superoxide dismutase (*SOD*) 51, 62, 137, 146, 153, 186, 386, 388-389, 391-392, 396, 400-401, 403-404, 496, 648-649, 655-656, 772, 884
supervoltage 727
suppurative fasciitis 444, 460
surface oxygen 311, 826, 978, 980, 982, 985-988, 990, 1064, 1127
surgery XV, XVI, XVII, XIX, XXI, XXII, XXIII, XXIV, 42, 47, 57, 93-94, 113-114, 147, 168, 173, 178, 180, 190-195, 214, 226, 231, 234, 242, 244-245, 249-250, 252-253, 265, 283, 291, 294, 296, 334, 339-340, 342, 350, 364, 370, 373-374, 376-377, 388, 398-399, 401, 409, 414, 416, 422, 425-430, 438-439, 448-451, 454-456, 460-462, 469, 472, 474, 477, 480, 488, 493, 498-500, 503, 507-508, 510, 512-515, 518, 520-521, 535-536, 538, 545, 548-549, 559, 565, 567, 576, 578-579, 582-585, 587, 595, 597-598, 600, 605, 607-608, 611-617, 620, 631, 634-636, 640, 654, 657, 673-674, 677-678, 680, 682, 684, 687-688, 690, 703-704, 709, 711, 713, 715, 717, 720-722, 725, 733, 738-739, 742, 744-746, 755, 757-759, 761-765, 769-770, 773-775, 786-787, 800-801, 805, 808, 810, 812-813, 815, 877-878, 885-890, 902, 904-905, 941, 1038, 1068, 1072, 1100, 1140-1141
surgical
surgical debridement 231, 388, 390, 416, 440, 447, 450, 454, 501, 505, 511, 513, 543, 570, 579-581, 584, 592, 594, 596, 610, 612, 615-617, 754, 763, 770, 883, 885-887, 890
surgical decompression 680-681
surgical trauma 756
surgical wounds 364, 423, 435, 604
survival function 884
syncope 188, 213, 998, 1076, 1123
synergistic
synergistic gangrene 436-437, 441, 448, 460
synergistic microorganisms 437
synergistic necrotizing cellulitis 435, 444-446, 454, 462

T

Taiwan 198, 335, 468
$TcPO_2$ 185, 568-569, 595-599, 601, 606-607, 610-613, 615-616, 1168
technetium scan 890
TEED scale 1066
teeth 208-210, 744, 746, 752, 754-755, 769-770, 982, 1068
therapeutic radiation 727
thermal
thermal injury 228, 682, 711, 791, 793-794, 798-799, 803, 805, 809-810, 812, 814, 816-817, 1018, 1031, 1034
thermal protection 221, 227, 983, 985
theta toxin 284, 411, 424
thoracic surgery 191
thrombolysis 295, 689, 816, 832, 848-849
thrombosis 247, 250, 264-265, 341, 358, 368, 382, 407, 410, 422, 440, 444, 567, 647, 651, 662, 728, 832, 858, 888, 1100
thyroid 131, 139-140, 224, 338, 343, 1071, 1126
tidal volume 73, 88-89, 108, 224, 1095
tissue VI, VII, 39, 42-45, 47, 52, 62, 80-81, 93, 134-136, 138, 143-144, 150, 154, 166, 178, 183, 191, 196, 203, 209, 214, 226, 230, 234, 238-239, 241, 243, 246-247, 249, 252-256, 260-268, 271-273, 275-276, 278-281, 283-288, 292, 294-295, 297, 304, 306-308, 312-313, 328, 330, 333, 366, 372, 381-383, 385, 388, 390-395, 400-401, 405, 410-416, 419-421, 425, 431, 437-445, 447-450, 454-463, 472-473, 480, 488, 491-492, 494-496, 501, 504, 506, 508, 513, 519, 525, 529, 532-533, 540-542, 545, 547, 562-563, 568, 570-572, 575, 579-581, 591-595, 597, 611-612, 614-615, 617, 621, 625-627, 629, 633-634, 636-637, 639, 643, 645, 648, 651, 656, 661-664, 666, 668, 670, 673-675, 678, 681-682, 688, 690, 694-695, 704, 709-719, 721-723, 725, 727-736, 738-739, 741-744, 746, 749, 751, 754-757, 759-763, 770, 774-775, 779-780, 786-787, 792-794, 798-799, 810, 815-817, 848, 867, 876-877, 883, 888-889, 892, 898, 902, 908, 920-921, 930, 932, 934-938, 942, 947-948, 950, 956, 964, 967, 987, 999-1000, 1003, 1007-1009, 1011, 1013, 1022, 1052, 1055-1057, 1062, 1064, 1066, 1068, 1070, 1072, 1100-1101, 1117, 1123-1125, 1140
tissue biopsies 415, 437, 440-441, 448

tissue damage 144, 183, 266, 268, 285, 449, 636, 661-662, 664, 755-756, 793, 956, 1100
tissue flaps 716
tissue fluids 246, 253, 256, 260-263, 268, 273, 275-276, 284, 491-492, 637, 663-664, 668
tissue hypoxia 255, 260, 304, 306, 308, 312, 330, 412, 438, 563, 615, 661-663, 678, 713, 902, 987
tissue injury 401, 405, 431, 562, 656, 666, 688, 715-716, 719, 727, 734, 756-757, 786-787, 815, 1117, 1169
tissue ischemia 306, 643, 709
tissue necrosis 284, 410, 431, 439, 442, 449, 643, 716, 888, 902
tissue perfusion 135, 307, 383, 416, 421, 562, 710, 713, 716, 718
tissue oxygen tensions 254, 271, 276, 279, 281, 381, 388, 390, 392-393, 496, 666, 718, 734

toe pressures 568-569
tongue function 746
tonometry 79
tooth
tooth extraction 478, 715, 755
tooth removal 725, 738, 744, 746-747, 755
tooth squeeze 1068

topical oxygen therapy 269, 295
total body surface area 791-792, 805, 809
total contact casting 552
toxicity V, VIII, XIV, 42, 49, 51-56, 58-62, 64, 66, 77, 82, 86-87, 89-90, 92, 131-132, 134, 139-144, 146-149, 151, 153-157, 171-173, 180, 183, 185-187, 193-198, 212-213, 215, 217-219, 223-226, 232, 235, 253, 261, 270-271, 292, 304, 317, 321, 386, 389, 396-397, 399, 402, 407, 412-414, 419-421, 430, 445-446, 449, 452, 455, 474, 631, 686, 697, 704, 729, 804, 808-809, 828, 856, 885, 889, 898, 902, 905, 907, 909, 934-938, 941-943, 973, 982, 984-985, 989-990, 995, 997-998, 1001, 1007, 1010-1011, 1013, 1049, 1054-1057, 1069, 1082, 1084, 1092, 1097-1098, 1101, 1103, 1107, 1112, 1120-1121, 1123, 1126-1127, 1130-1131
Toynbee maneuver 162, 205
transcutaneous
transcutaneous oximetry 619, 621, 640
transcutaneous oxygen 81, 93, 95, 118, 243, 249-254, 268, 294-295, 508, 521, 526, 540-541, 550, 552-553, 568, 585, 619, 621-622, 631, 637, 640, 673, 729, 756
transcutaneous oxygen measurements 249-251, 253-254, 295, 508, 521, 526, 540-541, 550, 553, 585, 621-622, 637, 640, 673, 729, 756
transcutaneous oxygen monitor 729

transport 41, 67, 70, 72-73, 92-93, 136, 155, 172, 227, 264, 267, 284, 290, 304, 309, 312-313, 316, 376, 384, 386-387, 391, 418, 492, 558, 693, 700, 988, 990, 1000, 1010-1011, 1017-1018, 1022, 1035, 1037, 1039-1040, 1046, 1054, 1056, 1075, 1078, 1128
trauma 53, 93, 147, 173, 180, 188-189, 196, 198, 204-207, 209, 213-214, 216, 219, 247, 261, 275-276, 283, 296, 309, 328, 334, 350, 355, 357, 363, 401, 409-412, 417, 421, 425, 427-429, 435, 439, 445, 450, 457-459, 461, 476, 481-482, 506, 513, 517-518, 525, 552, 560-562, 564, 635, 639-640, 643, 661-663, 674, 676, 678, 682-683, 686-689, 697, 702-703, 705, 714, 717, 722, 751, 755-756, 792, 813-814, 843, 856, 864, 879, 883, 885, 887, 891-892, 899, 939-943, 950, 955, 1018, 1031, 1065-1066, 1072, 1075
traumatic
traumatic brain injury *VIII*, 93, 188, 196, 221, 232, 235, 273, 298, 844, 856, 858-859, 909, 911, 920, 930, 939-945, 950-951, 954-955, 1007-1008
traumatic ischemias *VII*, 230, 260, 493, 644, 648, 659, 661-662, 664-666, 668, 670-672, 674-675, 681-685
traumatic wound 415

treatment 42-43, 46, 53, 55, 63-64, 113, 118-120, 124-125, 128, 145, 167, 171, 186, 202, 205-206, 209, 211-213, 215, 219, 224, 227-228, 230, 244, 250-254, 262, 265-268, 272, 276, 280, 282, 307, 310-311, 325, 331, 335, 338, 342-343, 349-350, 353, 366-367, 390-391, 407, 414-415, 418-421, 449, 453-454, 474-475, 478, 494, 499-500, 502, 508-514, 541, 543, 545, 549-551, 593-601, 603, 612, 625, 631-635, 637, 651, 670-675, 677-678, 680-684, 697-698, 700, 702, 710, 712-713, 715-716, 733, 756, 781, 798, 804, 808, 827-828, 839, 844-846, 850-851, 854, 865-867, 877, 884, 886,

888-889, 897, 902-904, 912, 914-916, 918, 922, 924, 926-928, 930-931, 933-938, 947-954, 988, 997, 1012, 1039, 1057, 1075, 1097, 1115, 1140
treatment protocol 53, 58, 146, 287, 349-350, 449, 454-455, 508, 691, 697, 702, 725, 738, 756, 867, 968
Trendelenburg position 370
Tucker 704
tumor 175-176, 182, 188, 197, 241, 273, 330, 440, 492, 540, 727, 734, 754-755, 770-772, 774-775, 794, 918, 920, 949-950
tympanic membrane 148, 153, 161-167, 202-204, 206-207, 253, 333, 1065-1066, 1072, 1083, 1125
tympanum 161, 166-167

U

U.S. Navy XI, XII, XIII, 4, 41, 54, 61, 63, 66, 105-106, 114, 140, 203, 219, 374, 419, 632, 695, 978, 988, 993, 1017-1020, 1024-1025, 1031, 1035, 1063, 1066, 1071, 1077-1078, 1084, 1087, 1104, 1119, 1131, 1137-1138, 1141
U.S. Navy Treatment Table 5 632
ulcer VII, 190-192, 247, 249, 285, 332, 436-437, 441, 443-444, 457, 525, 528-529, 545, 549, 552-553, 555, 557-562, 564-565, 567, 569-572, 575, 577-586, 591-593, 595-597, 599, 601, 604, 607, 610, 614-616, 618, 620-621, 700, 738, 841, 899, 904
ulcerations 529, 547, 562, 564, 593, 898, 1117
Undersea and Hyperbaric Medical Society (UHMS) 4-5, 31, 59, 61, 94, 116, 118, 153, 217-219, 230, 235, 290, 350, 367, 370, 373, 377, 467, 480, 510, 512, 516, 519, 605, 625, 639, 684, 687, 830, 832, 839, 844, 992, 997, 1014, 1059, 1070, 1103-1105
UHMS Annual Scientific Meeting 217-218
unit pulmonary toxic dose 55, 1121
United States Air Force XVIII
upper respiratory infections 327, 1065
urology 194, 457, 459, 787
USS Squalus 1022, 1048

V

vacuum regulator 89
valsalva maneuver 161-162, 205, 1065
vascular XXI, 44, 52, 86, 138, 146, 154, 176, 198, 203, 225, 227, 241, 244-245, 247, 250, 256, 273, 279-280, 295, 304-305, 307, 312-313, 322, 328-330, 333, 341, 353, 358, 366, 382, 409-411, 425-426, 430, 435, 440, 442, 472, 493, 514, 525-526, 535, 542, 546, 555, 557-558, 561, 564-569, 571-572, 576, 578-579, 581, 583-585, 587, 591-592, 594, 596, 598-600, 603, 605, 607, 611-617, 620, 622, 629, 631, 635-636, 639-640, 647, 650-651, 654, 656, 662-663, 673, 686, 688-689, 703-704, 713-715, 722, 728, 730-731, 733-735, 738-739, 754-756, 761-763, 766, 793, 798, 804, 813, 830-832, 848, 858, 864-865, 876, 879, 889, 920, 941, 947, 1044, 1047, 1065, 1070, 1100
vascular endothelial growth factor (VEGF) 176, 279, 295, 297, 591, 622, 651, 654, 734, 804, 879
vascular endothelium 44, 305
vascular intervention 578, 599
vascularization 182, 721
vasculitis 542, 666, 865, 899
vasoconstriction 41, 52, 134-135, 138, 146, 163, 182, 186, 238, 273, 275-276, 285, 292, 311, 381, 394, 419, 472, 563, 565, 635, 647-649, 653, 656, 658, 662, 666, 669-670, 675, 867, 959, 1059, 1069-1070, 1073-1074, 1076
vasodilation 58, 140, 143, 186, 250, 304-305, 338, 411, 647, 689
veillonella 469-470
venom 895, 897-900, 902, 904-907
venous gas embolism 363-364, 375
ventilation 34, 67, 71-73, 79, 81, 87, 89-92, 106-108, 143, 147, 166, 179-180, 183, 190, 192, 225, 227, 230, 233, 253, 303-304, 314, 363, 366, 369, 421, 474, 500, 694, 791, 805, 809, 833, 937, 1054, 1061, 1095, 1099, 1117-1119, 1130
ventilator 70-74, 76, 79-81, 87-90, 92-94, 99, 107, 234, 808, 943, 1061
ventilator pass-through 89
ventricular fibrillation 148, 307, 317, 422
vertiginous 343
Vickers chamber 114
viral infections 328, 379, 391-392
viruses 391, 446, 1122
vision 56, 61, 84, 92, 101-102, 165, 180-182, 191-192, 196, 211-212, 253, 821, 826-831, 876, 1056-1057, 1071, 1073, 1089, 1097, 1115

vitamins
vitamin C 51, 341
vitamin E (*alpha tocopherol*) 51, 131, 141, 154-156, 343, 387
volume 42, 59, 73, 80, 84-85, 87-89, 107-108, 138, 171, 177, 188-189, 210, 219, 224, 241, 259, 267, 270-271, 287, 297, 330, 340, 363, 384, 411, 419, 472, 493, 539, 663, 677, 682, 686, 694-695, 697-698, 714, 781, 793, 808, 850-851, 932, 948, 958, 982, 984, 988, 1021-1022, 1032, 1052-1053, 1063, 1068, 1087-1088, 1091, 1094-1097, 1111-1114, 1121-1122, 1125, 1141, 1172
volumetric pump 84

W

Waite 148, 157
Weaver V, XXIII, 48, 63, 69, 92-95, 157, 195, 217, 298, 310, 318-319, 323, 377, 518, 585, 618, 622, 639, 687, 811, 827, 844, 856, 858-859, 937, 939, 941, 943, 1014
Western Infirmary 113
whole blood 418
work of breathing (WOB) 107, 1085, 1088-1089, 1092-1095, 1099, 1113, 1119
Workman V, XXIV, 31, 38, 109, 148, 156, 723
World Health Organization (WHO) 352, 354-355, 360, 584, 605, 963, 969
wound XVIII, XX, XXII, 5, 41, 43-47, 62, 69, 74, 118, 124-125, 128, 143-144, 150, 154, 156, 186, 190-193, 197, 221, 231, 237, 239-254, 261-262, 267-268, 276, 278-282, 294-297, 369, 383, 388, 400, 410-413, 415-416, 421, 430, 432, 437, 444, 447-451, 461, 497, 502-510, 512, 517-518, 520-521, 523, 525-526, 528-536, 538-543, 545, 547, 549-550, 552-555, 558, 561, 563-565, 568-572, 576-582, 584-587, 591-600, 602-603, 605, 610, 612-619, 621-622, 626, 628, 631-632, 636, 640, 663, 666, 668, 670, 674-677, 680-683, 687, 689, 698, 704-705, 710-713, 715-717, 719-721, 723, 727, 733-736, 738-739, 742-746, 754, 756-757, 763, 774-775, 787, 792-793, 796, 798-802, 804, 806, 808, 810, 812-818, 891, 897, 900-904, 908, 920
wound area 605
wound care *XVIII*, *XX*, *XXII*, 69, 118, 125, 128, 186, 192, 246, 294-295, 297, 416, 448, 502-504, 521, 531, 534, 550, 552-553, 558, 563, 570, 577-580, 584, 586-587, 593-595, 602, 610, 612, 618, 622, 704-705, 742, 806, 816, 897, 901
wound care management 578
wound classification 529, 552, 586
wound cleansing 808
wound complications 739
wound contamination 410, 413
wound dehiscence 614, 631, 640, 739, 742-743, 745
wound dressings 549, 558, 580
wound healing 41, 43-45, 47, 62, 118, 124, 144, 156, 186, 193, 197, 221, 231, 237, 239-247, 253, 262, 267, 276, 278, 294-295, 416, 447-450, 497, 508, 518, 530, 533-535, 539-540, 542, 547, 553, 555, 558, 563, 568-569, 571-572, 576-577, 579-582, 584, 586-587, 591, 593-595, 597, 600, 603, 610, 614, 618-619, 621-622, 626, 631, 663, 666, 670, 675, 681, 683, 710, 712-713, 715-716, 719-721, 723, 733-734, 738-739, 744-746, 754, 756, 774-775, 787, 792, 800, 804, 810, 812-813, 815-816, 902
wound infection 294, 416, 432, 461, 517, 553, 600, 687, 739, 742, 744, 792, 799
wound irrigations 742
wound sepsis 801

XYZ

Zamboni VII, XXIV, 93, 266, 286, 296, 298, 405, 447, 451, 455, 461, 463, 596, 622, 643-644, 648, 654-658, 690, 723, 798, 815, 818
zygomycetes 150, 153

www.ingramcontent.com/pod-product-compliance
Lightning Source LLC
LaVergne TN
LVHW081330021026
849161LV00008BA/1828